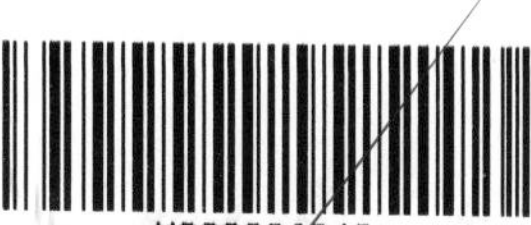

Hydroxyzine	Meperidine	Metoclopra	Midazola	Morphin	Nalbuphi	Pentazoc	Pentobar	Perphena	Prochlor	Promazi	Prometh	Ranitidi	Scopola	Secobar	Thiethylperazine
C	C	C	C	C	C	C	C	C	C	C	C	C	C	I	
C	C	C	C	C		C	I	C	C		C		C	I	C
C	C	C	C	C		C	I	C	C	C	C	C	C	I	
							I							I	
I	I	I		I	I	I	I	I	I	I	I		I	I	I
I	C	C	I	C		C	I	C	I	I	I	C	C	I	
C	C	C	C	C		C	I	C	C	C	C	C	C	I	
C	C	C		C	C	C	I	C	C	C	C		C	I	
C	C	C		C		C	I	C	C	C	C	C	C	I	
C	C			C		I	I		C	C	C	C	C	I	
	I			I		I					I				
	C	C		C	C	C	I		C	C	C	I	C	I	
C		C		I		C	I	C	C	C	C	C	C	I	
C	C			C		C		C	C	C	C	C	C	I	
C		C		C	C		I	I	I	C	C	I	C		C
C	I	C				C	I	C	C	C	C	C	C	I	
C							I		C		*	C	C	I	C
C	C	C		C			I	C	C	C	C	C	C	I	
I	I			I	I	I		I	I	I	I		C	I	
	C	C		C		C	I		C		C	C	C	I	I
C	C	C		C	C	C	I	C		C	C	C	C	I	
C	C	C		C		C	I		C		C		C	I	
C	C	C		C	C	C	I	C	C	C		C	C	I	
	C	C	I	C	C	C		C	C		C		C		C
C	C	C		C	C	C	C	C	C	C	C	C		I	
I	I	I		I	I	I	I	I	I	I	I		I		I
					C			I				C		I	

Parenteral compatibility occurs when two or more drugs are successfully mixed without liquefaction, deliquescence, or precipitation.

Consultants

Jean Krajicek Bartek, PhD, APRN
Nurse Practitioner
University of Nebraska Medical Center
College of Nursing
Courtesy Faculty
College of Medicine (Pharmacology)
Omaha, Nebraska

Doris M. Bates, RN
Oncology/OB Staff Nurse
Penobscot Valley Hospital
Lincoln, Maine

Rita Hanover Berdan, MS, RN, C
Nursing Faculty
St. Joseph's Hospital Health Center School of Nursing
Syracuse, New York

Barbara L. Cary, MSN, RN
Adjunct Faculty
University of Maine
Augusta, Maine

Tamara Conroy, RMA, CPT, SPN
Pittston, Pennsylvania

Linda M. DeLamar-Gallos, CRNA, MSN, MS
Capital Health Systems
Mercer Campus
Trenton, New Jersey

Jennifer L. DiGiacinto, Pharm D
Clinical Pharmacologist
Office of Clinical Pharmacology and Biopharmaceutics
US Food and Drug Administration
Rockville, Maryland

Henry B. Geiter, Jr, RN, C, CCRN
Vencor Hospital
St. Petersburg Junior College
St. Petersburg, Florida

F. James Grogan, PharmD
Executive Director
Grogan Communications
Swansea, Illinois

Jennifer L. Gudeman, PharmD
Product Surveillance Specialist
Corporate Product Monitoring
Mallinckrodt/Tyco Healthcare
St. Louis, Missouri

Scott Harrington, PharmD, RPh
Harrington Health Informatics
Tucson, Arizona

Phyllis Howard, RN, BSN
Associate Professor of Practical Nursing
Ashland Technical College
Ashland, Kentucky

Peter Huynh, PharmD
Pharmacotherapy Fellow
Washington State University
Spokane, Washington

Joan Ann Leach, RNC, MS, ME
Professor of Nursing
Capital Community College
Hartford, Connecticut

Mary Jo Mattocks, PhD, MN, BSN
Assistant Professor
Montana State University
Northern Great Falls Campus
Great Falls, Montana

Jennifer L. McQuade, PharmD
Medical Information Consultant
St. Louis, Missouri

Michelle M. Montpas, RN, MSN, OCN
CS Mott Community College
Flint, Michigan

Janet Rentfro, RN, ADN, ACLS
Medical Supervisor
Ascension Island
South Atlantic Ocean

Becky A. Ridenhour, PharmD
St. Louis College of Pharmacy
St. Louis, Missouri

Roberta J. Secrest, PhD, PharmD, RPh
Eli Lilly and Company
Indianapolis, Indiana

Patricia R. Teasley, APRN, BC
Professor
Nursing Department
Central Texas Collge
Killeen, Texas

Brenda L. Thompson, PharmD
Assistant Professor
Pharmacy Practice Division
St. Louis College of Pharmacy
St. Louis, Missouri

Joyce S. Willens, PhD, RN
Assistant Professor
College of Nursing
Villanova University
Villanova, Pennsylvania

Preface

Since the first publication of *Mosby's Nursing Drug Reference* in 1988, more than 100 U.S. and Canadian pharmacists and consultants have reviewed the book's content closely. Today, *Mosby's 2005 Nursing Drug Reference* is more up-to-date than ever—with features that make it easy to find critical information fast!

New facts

This edition features more than 2000 new drug facts, including:

- new drugs and new dosage information
- newly researched side effects and adverse reactions
- the latest precautions, interactions, and contraindications
- IV therapy updates
- revised nursing considerations
- updated patient/family teaching guidelines
- updates on key new drug research

New features

- "Tall Man" lettering required by the FDA helps distinguish 35 look-alike generic drug names
- Error-prone abbreviations (µg, IU, U, MgSO4, MS, MSO4) no longer used as recommended by JCAHO
- Cross-references throughout make it easier than ever to find information
- Appendix A, "Selected new drugs," provides detailed monographs for 17 drugs and brief monographs for 6 rarely used drugs recently approved by the FDA. (See Table of Contents for a complete list.) Included are monographs for:
  - fosamprenavir (Lexiva)—for treatment of HIV infection
  - memantine (Namenda)—for treatment of Alzheimer's disease
  - rosuvastatin (Crestor)—for treatment of hypercholesterolemia
  - vardenafil (Levitra)—for treatment of erectile dysfunction
- Appendix B, "Recent FDA drug approvals," lists generic/trade names and uses for 8 of the most recently approved drugs

Organization

This reference is organized into four main sections:

- Drug categories
- Individual drug monographs (in alphabetical order by generic name)
- Drug identification guide
- Appendixes (identified by the wide dark blue thumb tabs on the edge)

The guiding principle behind this book is to provide fast, easy access to drug information and nursing considerations. Every detail—from the paper, typeface, cover, binding, use of color, and appendixes—has been carefully chosen with the user in mind.

Individual Drug Monographs

This book includes monographs for more than 1300 generic and 4500 trade medications. Common trade names are given for all drugs regularly used in the United States and Canada, with drugs available only in Canada identified by an asterisk.

The following information is provided, whenever possible, for safe, effective administration of each drug:

High-alert status: Identifies high-alert drugs; labeled and screened light-blue for easy identification.

Pronunciation: Helps the nurse master complex generic names.

℞/OTC: Identifies prescription or over-the-counter drugs.

Functional and chemical classifications: Allows the nurse to see similarities and dissimilarities among drugs in the same functional but different chemical classes.

Controlled-substance schedule: Includes schedules for the United States (I, II, III, IV, V) and Canada (F, G).

Action: Describes pharmacologic properties concisely.

Uses: Lists the conditions the drug is used to treat.

Investigational uses: Describes drug uses that may be encountered in practice but are not yet FDA-approved.

Research notes: Describes key studies on new drug uses, doses, and interactions with specific references.

Dosages and routes: Lists all available and approved dosages and routes for adult, pediatric, and geriatric patients.

Available forms: Includes tablets, capsules, extended-release, injectables (IV, IM, SC), solutions, creams, ointments, lotions, gels, shampoos, elixirs, suspensions, suppositories, sprays, aerosols, and lozenges.

Side effects/adverse reactions: Groups these reactions by body system, with common side effects *italicized* and life-threatening reactions in ***bold italic type*** for emphasis.

Contraindications: Lists conditions under which the drug absolutely should not be given, including FDA pregnancy safety categories D or X.

Precautions: Lists conditions that require special consideration when the drug is prescribed, including FDA pregnancy safety categories A, B, and C.

Pharmacokinetics: Outlines metabolism, distribution, and elimination.

Interactions: Includes confirmed drug and food interactions, followed by the drug or nutrient causing that interaction, when applicable.

"Herb-Drug Interaction" icon (🍃): Highlights more than 400 potential interactions between herbal products and prescription or OTC drugs.

Do not confuse: Presents drug names that might easily be confused, within each appropriate monograph.

Lab test interferences: Identifies how the drug may affect lab test results.

Nursing considerations: Identifies key nursing considerations for each step of the nursing process: Assess, Administer, Perform/provide, Evaluate, and Teach patient/family. Instructions for giving drugs by various routes (e.g., IV, IM, PO) are included, with route subheadings in bold.

Compatibilities: Lists syringe, Y-site, and additive compatibilities and incompatibilities. If no compatibilities are listed for a drug, the necessary compatibility testing has not been done and that compatibility information is unknown. To ensure safety, assume that the drug may not be mixed with other drugs unless specifically stated.

"Nursing Alert" icon (◆): Highlights a critical consideration.

"Do Not Crush" icon (⊘): Denotes drugs that may not be administered in crushed form.

Treatment of overdose: Provides drugs and treatment for overdoses where appropriate.

Appendixes

Selected new drugs: Includes comprehensive information on 23 key drugs approved by the FDA during the last 12 months.

Recent FDA drug approvals: Summarizes basic information, such as generic name, trade name and uses, for drugs so recently approved by the FDA that complete information was not yet available when this book went to press.

Ophthalmic, otic, nasal, and topical products: Provides monographs for more than 140 ophthalmic, otic, nasal, and topical products commonly used today, grouped by chemical drug class.

Commonly used antiinfectives in adults and children: Presents at-a-glance adult and pediatric dosage information for common antiinfectives.

Vaccines and toxoids: Features an easy-to-use table with generic and trade names, uses, dosages and routes, and contraindications for 32 key vaccines and toxoids.

Antitoxins and antivenins: Provides dosages and contraindications.

Combination products: Provides details on the forms and uses of more than 700 combination products.

Less frequently used antihistamines: Includes names, uses, doses, forms, interactions and contraindications.

High-alert drugs: Lists the 118 drugs in *Mosby's Nursing Drug Reference* that are considered high-alert because of their potential to cause significant harm to patients.

Look-alike/sound-alike drug names: Includes 200 pairs of generic and trade drug names that are easily confused.

Herbal products: Features basic usage information on more than 70 common herbs and natural supplements.

FDA pregnancy categories: Explains the 5 FDA pregnancy categories.

Controlled substance chart: Covers both United States and Canadian drug schedules, with examples.

Abbreviations: Lists abbreviations alphabetically with their meanings.

Weights and equivalents: Provides the conversion for weight and volume among the metric, apothecary, and avoirdupois systems.

Formulas for drug calculations: Lists some of the most common and useful drug calculation formulas.

Nomogram for calculation of body surface area: Provides a quick, handy chart for calculating body surface area for patient drug calculations.

Bibliography: Lists key resources used in creating and updating *Mosby's 2005 Nursing Drug Reference*.

I am indebted to the nursing and pharmacology consultants who reviewed the manuscript and galley pages and thank them for their criticism and encouragement. I would also like to thank Darlene Como, Laura Selkirk, and Brian Dennison, my editors, whose active encouragement and enthusiasm have made this book better than it might otherwise have been. I am likewise grateful to Melissa Lastarria and Graphic World, Inc., for the coordination of the production process and assistance with the development of the new edition.

Linda Skidmore-Roth

Contents

Drug categories, 1

Drug Monographs New to This Edition (Appendix A)

agalsidase beta
alefacept
alfuzosin
aprepitant
atazanavir
bortezomib
daptomycin
desirudin
efalizumab
emtricitabine
enfuvirtide
fosamprenavir
gefitinib
gemifloxacin
laronidase
memantine
miglustat
omalizumab
palonosetron
pegvisomant
rosavastatin
tadalafil
vardenafil

ALPHA-ADRENERGIC BLOCKERS

Action: Acts by binding to α-adrenergic receptors, causing dilation of peripheral blood vessels. Lowers peripheral resistance, resulting in decreased blood pressure.
Uses: Used for pheochromocytoma, prevention of tissue necrosis and sloughing associated with extravasation of IV vasopressors.
Side effects/adverse reactions: The most common side effects are hypotension, tachycardia, nasal stuffiness, nausea, vomiting, and diarrhea.
Contraindications: Hypersensitive reactions may occur, and allergies should be identified before these products are given. Patients with myocardial infarction, coronary insufficiency, angina, or other evidence of coronary artery disease should not use these products.
Pharmacokinetics: Onset, peak, and duration vary among products.
Interactions: Vasoconstrictive and hypertensive effects of epINEPHrine are antagonized by α-adrenergic blockers.
Possible nursing diagnoses:
- Altered tissue perfusion *[uses]*
- Risk for injury *[adverse reactions]*
- Sleep pattern disturbance *[adverse reactions]*

NURSING CONSIDERATIONS

Assess:
- Electrolytes: K, Na, Cl, CO_2
- Weight daily, I&O
- B/P lying, standing before starting treatment, q4h thereafter
- Nausea, vomiting, diarrhea
- Skin turgor, dryness of mucous membranes for hydration status

Administer:
- Starting with low dose, gradually increasing to prevent side effects
- With food or milk for GI symptoms

Evaluate:
- Therapeutic response: decreased B/P, increased peripheral pulses

Teach patient/family:
- To avoid alcoholic beverages
- To report dizziness, palpitations, fainting
- To change position slowly or fainting may occur
- To take drug exactly as prescribed
- To avoid all OTC products (cough, cold, allergy) unless directed by prescriber

Selected generic names

phentolamine

ANESTHETICS—GENERAL/LOCAL

Action: Anesthetics (general) act on the CNS to produce tranquilization and sleep before invasive procedures. Anesthetics (local) inhibit conduction of nerve impulses from sensory nerves.

Uses: General anesthetics are used to premedicate for surgery, induction and maintenance in general anesthesia. For local anesthetics, refer to individual product listing for indications.

Side effects/adverse reactions: The most common side effects are dystonia, akathisia, flexion of arms, fine tremors, drowsiness, restlessness, and hypotension. Also common are chills, respiratory depression, and laryngospasm.

Contraindications: Persons with CVA, increased intracranial pressure, severe hypertension, cardiac decompensation should not use these products, since severe adverse reactions can occur.

Precautions: Anesthetics (general) should be used with caution in the elderly, cardiovascular disease (hypotension, bradydysrhythmias), renal disease, liver disease, Parkinson's disease, children <2 yr. The precaution for anesthetics (local) is pregnancy.

Pharmacokinetics: Onset, peak, and duration vary widely among products. Most products are metabolized in the liver and excreted in urine.

Interactions: MAOIs, tricyclics, phenothiazines may cause severe hypotension or hypertension when used with local anesthetics. CNS depressants will potentiate general and local anesthetics.

Possible nursing diagnoses:

General:

- Risk for injury *[adverse reactions]*
- Knowledge deficit *[teaching]*

Local:

- Pain *[uses]*
- Knowledge deficit *[teaching]*

NURSING CONSIDERATIONS

Assess:

- VS q10min during IV administration, q30min after IM dose

Administer:

- Anticholinergic preoperatively to decrease secretions
- Only with crash cart, resuscitative equipment nearby

Perform/provide:

- Quiet environment for recovery to decrease psychotic symptoms

Evaluate:

- Therapeutic response: maintenance of anesthesia, decreased pain

Selected generic names (Injectables only)

General anesthetics
droperidol
etomidate
fentanyl
fentanyl/droperidol
fentanyl transdermal
ketamine
methohexital
midazolam
propofol
thiopental

Local anesthetics
lidocaine
procaine
ropivacaine
tetracaine

ANTACIDS

Action: Antacids are basic compounds that neutralize gastric acidity and decrease the rate of gastric emptying. Products are divided into those containing aluminum, magnesium, calcium, or a combination of these.
Uses: Hyperacidity is decreased by antacids in conditions such as peptic ulcer disease, reflux esophagitis, gastritis, and hiatal hernia.
Side effects/adverse reactions: The most common side effect caused by aluminum-containing antacids is constipation, which may lead to fecal impaction and bowel obstruction. Diarrhea occurs often when magnesium products are given. Alkalosis may occur when systemic products are used. Constipation occurs more frequently than laxation with calcium carbonate. The release of CO_2 from carbonate-containing antacids causes belching, abdominal distention, and flatulence. Sodium bicarbonate may act as a systemic antacid and produce systemic electrolyte disturbances and alkalosis. Calcium carbonate and sodium bicarbonate may cause rebound hyperacidity and milk-alkali syndrome. Alkaluria may occur when products are used on a long-term basis, particularly in persons with abnormal renal function.
Contraindications: Sensitivity to aluminum or magnesium products may cause hypersensitive reactions. Aluminum products should not be used by persons sensitive to aluminum; magnesium products should not be used by persons sensitive to magnesium. Check for sensitivity before administering.
Precautions: Magnesium products should be given cautiously to patients with renal insufficiency and during pregnancy and lactation. Sodium content of antacids may be significant; use with caution for patients with hypertension, CHF, or those on a low-sodium diet.
Pharmacokinetics: Duration is 20-40 min. If ingested 1 hr after meals, acidity is reduced for at least 3 hr.

Interactions: Drugs whose effects may be increased by some antacids: quinidine, amphetamines, pseudoephedrine, levodopa, valproic acid, dicumarol. Drugs whose effects may be decreased by some antacids: cimetadine, corticosteroids, ranitidine, iron salts, phenothiazines, phenytoin, digoxin, tetracyclines, ketoconazole, salicylates, isoniazid.

Possible nursing diagnoses:

- Pain *[uses]*
- Constipation *[adverse reactions]*
- Diarrhea *[adverse reactions]*

NURSING CONSIDERATIONS

Assess:

- Aggravating and alleviating factors of epigastric pain or hyperacidity; identify the location, duration, and characteristics of epigastric pain
- GI symptoms, including constipation, diarrhea, abdominal pain; if severe abdominal pain with fever occurs, these drugs should not be given
- Renal symptoms, including increasing urinary pH, electrolytes

Administer:

- All products with an 8-oz glass of water to ensure absorption in the stomach
- Another antacid if constipation occurs with aluminum products

Evaluate:

- The therapeutic effectiveness of the drug; absence of epigastric pain and decreased acidity should occur

Teach patient/family:

- Not to take other drugs within 1-2 hr of antacid administration, since antacids may impair absorption of other drugs

---

Selected generic names

aluminum hydroxide
bismuth subsalicylate
calcium carbonate
dihydroxyaluminum sodium carbonate
magaldrate
magnesium oxide
sodium bicarbonate

ANTIANGINALS

Action: The antianginals are divided into the nitrates, calcium channel blockers, and β-adrenergic blockers. The nitrates dilate coronary arteries, causing decreased preload, and dilate systemic arteries, causing decreased afterload. Calcium channel blockers dilate coronary arteries, decrease SA/AV node conduction. β-Adrenergic blockers decrease heart rate so that myocardial O_2 use is decreased. Dipyridamole selectively dilates coronary arteries to increase coronary blood flow.

Uses: Antianginals are used in chronic stable angina pectoris, unstable angina, vasospastic angina. Some (i.e., calcium channel blockers and β-blockers) may be used for dysrhythmias and in hypertension.

Side effects/adverse reactions: The most common side effects are postural hypotension, headache, flushing, dizziness, nausea, edema, and drowsiness. Also common are rash, dysrhythmias, and fatigue.

Contraindications: Persons with known hypersensitivity, increased intracranial pressure, or cerebral hemorrhage should not use some of these products.

Precautions: Antianginals should be used with caution in postural hypotension, pregnancy, lactation, children, renal disease, and hepatic injury.

Pharmacokinetics: Onset, peak, and duration vary widely among coronary products. Most products are metabolized in the liver and excreted in urine.

Interactions: Please check individual monographs since interactions vary widely among products.

Possible nursing diagnoses:

- Altered tissue perfusion: cardiopulmonary *[uses]*
- Pain *[uses]*
- Risk for injury *[uses]*
- Knowledge deficit *[teaching]*
- Decreased cardiac output *[adverse reactions]*

NURSING CONSIDERATIONS

Assess:

- Orthostatic B/P, pulse
- Pain: duration, time started, activity being performed, character
- Tolerance if taken over long period
- Headache, light-headedness, decreased B/P; may indicate a need for decreased dosage

Perform/provide:

- Storage protected from light, moisture; place in cool environment

Evaluate:

- Therapeutic response: decrease, prevention of anginal pain

Teach patient/family:

- To keep tabs in original container
- Not to use OTC products unless directed by prescriber
- To report bradycardia, dizziness, confusion, depression, fever
- To take pulse at home, advise when to notify prescriber
- To avoid alcohol, smoking, sodium intake
- To comply with weight control, dietary adjustments, modified exercise program
- To carry emergency ID to identify drug that you are taking, allergies
- To make position changes slowly to prevent fainting

Selected generic names

Nitrates
amyl nitrite
isosorbide
nitroglycerin

β-*Adrenergic blockers*
atenolol
dipyridamole
metoprolol
nadolol
propranolol

Calcium channel blockers
amlodipine
bepridil
diltiazem
niCARdipine
NIFEdipine
verapamil

ANTICHOLINERGICS

Action: Anticholinergics inhibit the muscarinic actions of acetylcholine at receptor sites in the autonomic nervous system; anticholinergics are also known as antimuscarinic drugs.

Uses: Anticholinergics are used for a variety of conditions: gastrointestinal anticholinergics are used to decrease motility (smooth muscle tone) in the GI, biliary, and urinary tracts and for their ability to decrease gastric secretions (propantheline, glycopyrrolate); decreasing involuntary movements in parkinsonism (benztropine, trihexyphenidyl); bradydysrhythmias (atropine); nausea and vomiting (scopolamine); and as cycloplegic mydriatics (atropine, hematropine, scopolamine, cyclopentolate, tropicamide).

Side effects/adverse reactions: The most common side effects are dry mouth, constipation, urinary retention, urinary hesitancy, headache, and dizziness. Also common is paralytic ileus.

Contraindications: Persons with narrow-angle glaucoma, myasthenia gravis, or GI/GU obstruction should not use some of these products.

Precautions: Anticholinergics should be used with caution in patients who are elderly, pregnant, or lactating or in those with prostatic hypertrophy, CHF, or hypertension; use with caution in presence of high environmental temp.

Pharmacokinetics: Onset, peak, and duration vary widely among products. Most products are metabolized in the liver and excreted in urine.

Interactions: Increased anticholinergic effects may occur when used with MAOIs and tricyclic antidepressants and amantadine. Anticholinergics may cause a decreased effect of phenothiazines and levodopa.

Possible nursing diagnoses:

- Decreased cardiac output *[uses]*
- Constipation *[adverse reactions]*
- Knowledge deficit *[teaching]*

NURSING CONSIDERATIONS

Assess:

- I&O ratio; retention commonly causes decreased urinary output
- Urinary hesitancy, retention; palpate bladder if retention occurs
- Constipation; increase fluids, bulk, exercise if this occurs
- For tolerance over long-term therapy, dose may need to be increased or changed
- Mental status: affect, mood, CNS depression, worsening of mental symptoms during early therapy

Administer:

- Parenteral dose with patient recumbent to prevent postural hypotension
- With or after meals to prevent GI upset; may give with fluids other than water
- Parenteral dose slowly; keep in bed for at least 1 hr after dose; monitor vital signs
- After checking dose carefully; even slight overdose can lead to toxicity

Perform/provide:

- Storage at room temp
- Hard candy, frequent drinks, sugarless gum to relieve dry mouth

Evaluate:

- Therapeutic response: decreased secretions, absence of nausea and vomiting

Teach patient/family:

- To avoid driving or other hazardous activities; drowsiness may occur

• To avoid OTC medication: cough, cold preparations with alcohol, antihistamines unless directed by prescriber

Selected generic names

atropine
benztropine
biperiden
dicyclomine
glycopyrrolate
hyoscyamine
propantheline
scopolamine (transdermal)
trihexyphenidyl

ANTICOAGULANTS

Action: Anticoagulants interfere with blood clotting by preventing clot formation.

Uses: Anticoagulants are used for deep vein thrombosis, pulmonary emboli, myocardial infarction, open-heart surgery, disseminated intravascular clotting syndrome, atrial fibrillation with embolization, transfusion, and dialysis.

Side effects/adverse reactions: The most serious adverse reactions are hemorrhage, agranulocytosis, leukopenia, eosinophilia, and thrombocytopenia, depending on the specific product. The most common side effects are diarrhea, rash, and fever.

Contraindications: Persons with hemophilia and related disorders, leukemia with bleeding, peptic ulcer disease, thrombocytopenic purpura, blood dyscrasias, acute nephritis, and subacute bacterial endocarditis should not use these products.

Precautions: Anticoagulants should be used with caution in alcoholism, elderly, and pregnancy.

Pharmacokinetics: Onset, peak, and duration vary widely among products. Most products are metabolized in the liver and excreted in urine.

Interactions: Salicylates, steroids, and nonsteroidal antiinflammatories will potentiate the action of anticoagulants. Anticoagulants may cause serious effects; please check individual monographs.

Possible nursing diagnoses:

- Altered tissue perfusion *[uses]*
- Risk for injury *[side effects]*
- Knowledge deficit *[teaching]*

NURSING CONSIDERATIONS

Assess:

- Blood studies (Hct, platelets, occult blood in stools) q3mo
- Partial prothrombin time, which should be 1½-2 × control PPT qd, also APTT, ACT
- B/P, watch for increasing signs of hypertension
- Bleeding gums, petechiae, ecchymosis; black, tarry stools; hematuria
- Fever, skin rash, urticaria
- Needed dosage change q1-2wk

Administer:

- At same time each day to maintain steady blood levels
- Do not massage area or aspirate when giving SC injection; give in abdomen between pelvic bone, rotate sites; do not pull back on plunger; leave in for 10 sec; apply gentle pressure for 1 min
- Without changing needles
- Avoiding all IM injections that may cause bleeding

Perform/provide:

- Storage in tight container

Evaluate:

- Therapeutic response: decrease of deep vein thrombosis

Teach patient/family:

- To avoid OTC preparations that may cause serious drug interactions unless directed by prescriber
- That drug may be held during active bleeding (menstruation), depending on condition
- To use soft-bristle toothbrush to avoid bleeding gums, avoid contact sports, use electric razor
- To carry emergency ID identifying drug taken
- To report any signs of bleeding: gums, under skin, urine, stools

---

Selected generic names

ardeparin
argatroban
dalteparin
danaparoid
desirudin (Appx A)
enoxaparin
fondaparinux
heparin
lepirudin
tinzaparin
warfarin

ANTICONVULSANTS

Action: Anticonvulsants are divided into the barbiturates (p. 35), benzodiazepines (p. 37), hydantoins, succinimides, and miscellaneous products. Barbiturates and benzodiazepines are discussed in separate sections. Hydantoins act by inhibiting the spread of seizure activity in the motor cortex. Succinimides act by inhibiting spike and wave formation; they also decrease amplitude, frequency, duration, and spread of discharge in seizures.

Uses: Hydantoins are used in generalized tonic-clonic seizures, status epilepticus, and psychomotor seizures. Succinimides are used for absence (petit mal) seizures. Barbiturates are used in generalized tonic-clonic and cortical focal seizures.

Side effects/adverse reactions: Bone marrow depression is the most life-threatening adverse reaction associated with hydantoins or succinimides. The most common side effects are GI symptoms. Other common side effects for hydantoins are gingival hyperplasia and CNS effects such as nystagmus, ataxia, slurred speech, and mental confusion.

Contraindications: Hypersensitive reactions may occur, and allergies should be identified before these products are given.

Precautions: Persons with renal or hepatic disease should be watched closely.

Pharmacokinetics: Onset, peak, and duration vary widely among products. Most products are metabolized in the liver and excreted in urine, bile, and feces.

Interactions: Decreased effects of estrogens, oral contraceptives (hydantoins).

Possible nursing diagnoses:

- Risk for injury *[uses]*
- Noncompliance *[teaching]*
- Sleep pattern disturbance *[adverse reactions]*

NURSING CONSIDERATIONS

Assess:

- Renal studies, including BUN, creatinine, serum uric acid, urine creatinine clearance before and during therapy
- Blood studies: RBC, Hct, Hgb, reticulocyte counts qwk for 4 wk then qmo
- Hepatic studies: AST, ALT, bilirubin, creatinine
- Mental status, including mood, sensorium, affect, behavorial changes; if mental status changes, notify prescriber
- Eye problems, including need for ophthalmic exam before, during, and after treatment (slit lamp, fundoscopy, tonometry)

• Allergic reactions, including red, raised rash; if this occurs, drug should be discontinued
• Blood dyscrasia, including fever, sore throat, bruising, rash, jaundice
• Toxicity, including bone marrow depression, nausea, vomiting, ataxia, diplopia, cardiovascular collapse, Stevens-Johnson syndrome

Administer:

• With food, milk to decrease GI symptoms

Perform/provide:

• Good oral hygiene is important for hydantoins

Evaluate:

• Therapeutic response, including decreased seizure activity; document on patient's chart

Teach patient/family:

• To carry emergency ID stating drugs taken, condition, prescriber's name, phone number
• To avoid driving, other activities that require alertness

Selected generic names

Hydantoins
fosphenytoin
phenytoin

Succinimides
ethosuximide
methsuximide

Miscellaneous
acetaZOLAMIDE
carbamazepine
clonazepam
diazepam
felbamate
gabapentin
lamotrigine
magnesium sulfate
paraldehyde
paramethadione
phenacemide
phenobarbital
primidone
tiagabine
topiramate
valproate/valproic acid, divalproex sodium
zonisamide

ANTIDEPRESSANTS

Action: Antidepressants are divided into the tricyclics, MAOIs, and miscellaneous antidepressants (SSRIs). The tricyclics work by blocking reuptake of norepinephrine and serotonin into nerve endings and increasing action of norepinephrine and serotonin in nerve cells. MAOIs act by increasing concentrations of endogenous epINEPHrine, norepinephrine, serotonin, DOPamine in storage sites in CNS by inhibition of MAO; increased concentration reduces depression.

Uses: Antidepressants are used for depression and, in some cases, enuresis in children.

Side effects/adverse reactions: The most serious adverse reactions are paralytic ileus, acute renal failure, hypertension, and hypertensive crisis, depending on the specific product. Common side effects are dizziness, drowsiness, diarrhea, dry mouth, urinary retention, and orthostatic hypotension.

Contraindications: The contraindications to antidepressants are convulsive disorders, prostatic hypertrophy, severe renal, hepatic, cardiac disease depending on the type of medication.

Precautions: Antidepressants should be used cautiously in suicidal patients, severe depression, schizophrenia, hyperactivity, diabetes mellitus, pregnancy, and the elderly.

Pharmacokinetics: Onset, peak, and duration vary widely among products. Most products are metabolized in the liver and excreted in urine.

Interactions: Please check individual monographs since interactions vary widely among products.

Possible nursing diagnoses:

- Ineffective individual coping *[uses]*
- Risk for injury *[uses/adverse reactions]*
- Knowledge deficit *[teaching]*

NURSING CONSIDERATIONS

Assess:

- B/P (lying, standing), pulse q4h; if systolic B/P drops 20 mm Hg, hold drug, notify prescriber; take vital signs q4h in patients with cardiovascular disease
- Blood studies: CBC, leukocytes, differential, cardiac enzymes if patient is receiving long-term therapy
- Hepatic studies: AST, ALT, bilirubin, creatinine
- Weight qwk; appetite may increase with drug
- EPS, primarily in elderly: rigidity, dystonia, akathisia
- Mental status: mood, sensorium, affect, suicidal tendencies, increase in psychiatric symptoms: depression, panic
- Urinary retention, constipation; constipation is more likely to occur in children, elderly
- Withdrawal symptoms: headache, nausea, vomiting, muscle pain, weakness; do not usually occur unless drug was discontinued abruptly
- Alcohol consumption; if alcohol is consumed, hold dose until morning

Administer:

- Increased fluids if urinary retention occurs, bulk in diet, if constipation occurs
- With food or milk for GI symptoms
- Gum, hard candy, or frequent sips of water for dry mouth

Perform/provide:

- Storage in tight container at room temp; do not freeze
- Assistance with ambulation during beginning therapy, since drowsiness, dizziness occur
- Safety measures including side rails primarily in elderly
- Checking to see PO medication swallowed

Evaluate:

- Therapeutic response: decreased depression

Teach patient/family:

- That therapeutic effects may take 2-3 wk
- To use caution in driving, other activities requiring alertness because of drowsiness, dizziness, blurred vision
- To avoid alcohol ingestion, other CNS depressants
- Not to discontinue medication quickly after long-term use; may cause nausea, headache, malaise
- To wear sunscreen or wide-brimmed hat, since photosensitivity may occur

---

Selected generic names

Tetracyclics
mirtazapine

Tricyclics
amitriptyline
amoxapine
clomipramine
desipramine
doxepin
imipramine
nortriptyline
trimipramine

Miscellaneous
buPROPion
nefazodone
trazodone
venlafaxine

MAOIs
phenelzine
tranylcypromine

SSRIs
citalopram
escitalopram
fluoxetine
fluvoxamine
paroxetine
sertraline

ANTIDIABETICS

Action: Antidiabetics are divided into the insulins that decrease blood glucose, phosphate, and potassium and increase blood pyruvate and lactate; and oral antidiabetics that cause functioning β-cells in the pancreas to release insulin, improve the effect of endogenous and exogenous insulin.
Uses: Insulins are used for ketoacidosis and diabetes mellitus types 1 and 2; oral antidiabetics are used for stable adult-onset diabetes mellitus type 2.

Side effects/adverse reactions: The most common side effect of insulin and oral antidiabetics is hypoglycemia. Other adverse reactions to oral antidiabetics include blood dyscrasias, hepatotoxicity, and rarely, cholestatic jaundice. Adverse reactions to insulin products include allergic responses and more rarely, anaphylaxis.

Contraindications: Hypersensitive reactions may occur, and allergies should be identified before these products are given. Oral antidiabetics should not be used in juvenile or brittle diabetes, diabetic ketoacidosis, severe renal disease, or severe hepatic disease.

Precautions: Oral antidiabetics should be used with caution in the elderly, in cardiac disease, pregnancy, lactation, and in the presence of alcohol.

Pharmacokinetics: Onset, peak, and duration vary widely among products. Oral antidiabetics are metabolized in the liver, with metabolites excreted in urine, bile, and feces.

Interactions: Interactions vary widely among products. Check individual monographs for specific information.

Possible nursing diagnoses:

• Altered nutrition: more than body requirements *[uses]*

NURSING CONSIDERATIONS

Assess:

• Blood, urine glucose levels during treatment to determine diabetes control (oral products)

• Fasting blood glucose, 2 hr PP (60-100 mg/dl normal fasting level) (70-130 mg/dl normal 2-hr level)

• Hypoglycemic reaction that can occur during peak time

Administer:

• Insulin after warming to room temp by rotating in palms to prevent lipodystrophy from injecting cold insulin

• Human insulin to those allergic to beef or pork

• Oral antidiabetic 30 min before meals

Perform/provide:

• Rotation of injection sites when giving insulin; use abdomen, upper back, thighs, upper arm, buttocks; rotate sites within one of these regions; keep a record of sites

Evaluate:

• Therapeutic response, including decrease in polyuria, polydipsia, polyphagia, clear sensorium, absence of dizziness, stable gait

Teach patient/family:

• To avoid alcohol and salicylates except on advice of prescriber

• Symptoms of ketoacidosis: nausea, thirst, polyuria, dry mouth, decreased B/P; dry, flushed skin; acetone breath, drowsiness, Kussmaul respiration

- Symptoms of hypoglycemia: headache, tremors, fatigue, weakness; and that candy or sugar should be carried to treat hypoglycemia
- To test urine for glucose/ketones tid if this drug is replacing insulin
- To continue weight control, dietary restrictions, exercise, hygiene
- Obtain yearly eye exams

Selected generic names

chlorproPAMIDE
glipiZIDE
glyBURIDE
insulin aspart
insulin glargine
insulin lispro
insulin, regular
insulin, regular concentrated
insulin, zinc suspension (Lente)
insulin, zinc suspension extended (Ultralente)
insulin, zinc suspension, prompt (Semilente)
metformin
miglitol
pioglitazone
repaglinide
rosiglitazone
TOLBUTamide

ANTIDIARRHEALS

Action: Antidiarrheals work by various actions, including direct action on intestinal muscles to decrease GI peristalsis; by inhibiting prostaglandin synthesis responsible for GI hypermotility; by acting on mucosal receptors responsible for peristalsis; or by decreasing water content of stools.

Uses: Antidiarrheals are used for diarrhea of undetermined causes.

Side effects/adverse reactions: The most serious adverse reactions of some products are paralytic ileus, toxic megacolon, and angioneurotic edema. The most common side effects are constipation, nausea, dry mouth, and abdominal pain.

Contraindications: Persons with severe ulcerative colitis, pseudomembranous colitis with some products.

Precautions: Antidiarrheals should be used with caution in the elderly, pregnancy, lactation, children, dehydration.

Pharmacokinetics: Onset, peak, and duration vary widely among products. Most products are metabolized in the liver and excreted in urine.

Interactions: Please check individual monographs, since interactions vary widely among products.

Possible nursing diagnoses:

- Diarrhea *[uses]*
- Constipation *[adverse reactions]*
- Fluid volume deficit *[adverse reactions]*
- Knowledge deficit *[teaching]*

NURSING CONSIDERATIONS

Assess:

- Electrolytes (K, Na, Cl) if on long-term therapy
- Bowel pattern before; for rebound constipation after termination of medication
- Response after 48 hr; if no response, drug should be discontinued
- Dehydration in children

Administer:

- For 48 hr only

Evaluate:

- Therapeutic response: decreased diarrhea

Teach patient/family:

- To avoid OTC products
- Not to exceed recommended dose

Selected generic names

bismuth subsalicylate
difenoxin
kaolin/pectin
loperamide
opium tincture

ANTIDYSRHYTHMICS

Action: Antidysrhythmics are divided into four classes and miscellaneous antidysrhythmics:

- Class I increases the duration of action potential and effective refractory period and reduces disparity in the refractory period between a normal and infarcted myocardium; further subclasses include Ia, Ib, Ic
- Class II decreases the rate of SA node discharge, increases recovery time, slows conduction through the AV node, and decreases heart rate, which decreases O_2 consumption in the myocardium
- Class III increases the duration of action potential and the effective refractory period
- Class IV inhibits calcium ion influx across the cell membrane during cardiac depolarization; decreases SA node discharge, decreases conduction velocity through the AV node
- Miscellaneous antidysrhythmics include those such as adenosine, which slows conduction through the AV node, and digoxin, which decreases conduction velocity and prolongs the effective refractory period in the AV node

Uses: These products are used for PVCs, tachycardia, hypertension, atrial fibrillation, angina pectoris.

Side effects/adverse reactions: Side effects and adverse reactions vary widely among products.
Contraindications: Contraindications vary widely among products.
Precautions: Precautions vary widely among products.
Pharmacokinetics: Onset, peak, and duration vary widely among products.
Interactions: Interactions vary widely among products; check individual monographs for specific information.
Possible nursing diagnoses:
- Decreased cardiac output *[uses]*
- Altered tissue perfusion: cardiopulmonary *[uses]*
- Diarrhea *[adverse reactions]*
- Impaired gas exchange *[adverse reactions]*

NURSING CONSIDERATIONS

Assess:
- ECG continuously to determine drug effectiveness, PVCs, or other dysrhythmias
- IV infusion rate to avoid causing nausea, vomiting
- For dehydration or hypovolemia
- B/P continuously for hypotension, hypertension
- I&O ratio
- Serum potassium
- Edema in feet and legs daily

Evaluate:
- Therapeutic response, including decrease in B/P in hypertension; decreased B/P, edema, moist rales in CHF

Teach patient/family:
- To comply with dosage schedule, even if patient is feeling better
- To report bradycardia, dizziness, confusion, depression, fever

Selected generic names

Class I
moricizine

Class Ia
disopyramide
procainamide
quinidine

Class Ib
lidocaine
mexiletine
phenytoin
tocainide

Class Ic
flecainide
indecainide
propafenone

Class II
acebutolol
esmolol
propranolol
sotalol

Class III
amiodarone
bretylium
ibutilide

Class IV
verapamil

Miscellaneous
adenosine
atropine
digoxin

ANTIFUNGALS (SYSTEMIC)

Action: Antifungals act by increasing cell membrane permeability in susceptible organisms by binding sterols and decreasing potassium, sodium, and nutrients in the cell.

Uses: Antifungals are used for infections of histoplasmosis, blastomycosis, coccidiomycosis, cryptococcosis, aspergillosis, phycomycosis, candidiasis, sporotrichosis causing severe meningitis, septicemia, and skin infections.

Side effects/adverse reactions: The most serious adverse reactions include renal tubular acidosis, permanent renal impairment, anuria, oliguria, hemorrhagic gastroenteritis, acute liver failure, and blood dyscrasias. Some common side effects include hypokalemia, nausea, vomiting, anorexia, headache, fever, and chills.

Contraindications: Persons with severe bone depression or hypersensitivity should not use these products.

Precautions: Antifungals should be used with caution in renal disease, pregnancy, and hepatic disease.

Pharmacokinetics: Onset, peak, and duration vary widely among products. Most products are metabolized in the liver and excreted in urine.

Interactions: Please check individual monographs since interactions vary widely among products.

Possible nursing diagnoses:
- Risk for infection *[uses]*
- Risk for injury *[adverse reactions]*
- Knowledge deficit *[teaching]*

NURSING CONSIDERATIONS

Assess:
- VS q15-30min during first infusion; note changes in pulse, B/P
- I&O ratio; watch for decreasing urinary output, change in specific gravity; discontinue drug to prevent permanent damage to renal tubules
- Blood studies: CBC, K, Na, Ca, Mg q2wk
- Weight weekly; if weight increases over 2 lb/wk, edema is present; renal damage should be considered
- For renal toxicity: increasing BUN, if >40 mg/dl or if serum creatinine >3 mg/dl; drug may be discontinued or dosage reduced
- For hepatotoxicity: increasing AST, ALT, alk phosphatase, bilirubin
- For allergic reaction: dermatitis, rash; drug should be discontinued, antihistamines (mild reaction) or epINEPHrine (severe reaction) administered
- For hypokalemia: anorexia, drowsiness, weakness, decreased reflexes, dizziness, increased urinary output, increased thirst, paresthesias
- For ototoxicity: tinnitus (ringing, roaring in ears), vertigo, loss of hearing (rare)

Administer:
- IV using in-line filter (mean pore diameter >1 μm) using distal veins; check for extravasation, necrosis q8h
- Drug only after C&S confirms organism, drug needed to treat condition; make sure drug is used in life-threatening infections

Perform/provide:
- Protection from light during infusion, cover with foil
- Symptomatic treatment as ordered for adverse reactions: aspirin, antihistamines, antiemetics, antispasmodics
- Storage protected from moisture and light; diluted sol is stable for 24 hr

Evaluate:
- Therapeutic response: decreased fever, malaise, rash, negative C&S for infecting organism

Teach patient/family:
- That long-term therapy may be needed to clear infection (2 wk-3 mo depending on type of infection)

Selected generic names

amphotericin B
fluconazole
griseofulvin
itraconazole
ketoconazole
nystatin
voriconazole

ANTIHISTAMINES

Action: Antihistamines compete with histamines for H_1-receptor sites. They antagonize in varying degrees most of the pharmacologic effects of histamines.

Uses: Products are used to control the symptoms of allergies, rhinitis, and pruritus.

Side effects/adverse reactions: Most products cause drowsiness; however, fexofenadine and loratadine produce little, if any, drowsiness. Other common side effects are headache and thickening of bronchial secretions. Serious blood dyscrasias may occur, but are rare. Urinary retention, GI effects occur with many of these products.

Contraindications: Hypersensitivity to H_1-receptor antagonists occurs rarely. Patients with acute asthma and lower respiratory tract disease should not use these products since thick secretions may result. Other contraindications include narrow-angle glaucoma, bladder neck obstruction, stenosing peptic ulcer, symptomatic prostatic hypertrophy, newborn, lactation.

Precautions: These products must be used cautiously in conjunction with intraocular pressure since they increase intraocular pressure. Caution should also be used in patients with renal and cardiac disease, hypertension, seizure disorders, pregnancy, lactation, and in the elderly.

Pharmacokinetics: Onset varies from 20-60 min, with duration lasting 4-24 hr. In general, pharmacokinetics vary widely among products.

Interactions: Barbiturates, opioids, hypnotics, tricyclic antidepressants, or alcohol can increase CNS depression when taken with antihistamines.

Possible nursing diagnoses:

• Ineffective airway clearance *[uses]*

NURSING CONSIDERATIONS

Assess:

• I&O ratio; be alert for urinary retention, frequency, dysuria; drug should be discontinued if these occur

• CBC during long-term therapy, since hemolytic anemia, although rare, may occur

• Blood dyscrasias: thrombocytopenia, agranulocytosis (rare)
• Respiratory status, including rate, rhythm, increase in bronchial secretions, wheezing, chest tightness
• Cardiac status, including palpitations, increased pulse, hypotension

Administer:
• With food or milk to decrease GI symptoms; absorption may be decreased slightly
• Whole (sustained release tabs)

Perform/provide:
• Hard candy, gum, frequent rinsing of mouth for dryness

Evaluate:
• Therapeutic response, including absence of allergy symptoms, itching

Teach patient/family:
• To notify prescriber if confusion, sedation, hypotension occur
• To avoid driving, other hazardous activity if drowsiness occurs
• To avoid concurrent use of alcohol, other CNS depressants
• To discontinue a few days before skin testing

Selected generic names

brompheniramine
budesonide
cetirizine
chlorpheniramine
cyproheptadine
desloratadine
diphenhydrAMINE
fexofenadine
loratadine
promethazine
triprolidine

ANTIHYPERTENSIVES

Action: Antihypertensives are divided into angiotensin-converting enzyme (ACE) inhibitors, β-adrenergic blockers, calcium channel blockers, centrally acting adrenergics, diuretics, peripherally acting antiadrenergics, and vasodilators. β-Blockers, calcium channel blockers, and diuretics are discussed in separate sections. Angiotensin-converting enzyme inhibitors act by selectively suppressing renin-angiotensin I to angiotensin II; dilation of arterial and venous vessels occurs. Centrally acting adrenergics act by inhibiting the sympathetic vasomotor center in the CNS that reduces impulses in the sympathetic nervous system; blood pressure, pulse rate, and cardiac output decrease. Peripherally acting antiadrenergics inhibit sympathetic vasoconstriction by inhibiting release of norepinephrine and/or depleting norepinephrine stores in adrenergic nerve endings. Vasodilators act on arteriolar smooth muscle by producing direct relaxation or vasodilation; a reduction in blood pressure, with concomitant increases in heart rate and cardiac output, occurs.

Uses: Used for hypertension and some products are used for heart failure not responsive to conventional therapy. Some products are used in hypertensive crisis, angina, and for some cardiac dysrhythmias.

Side effects/adverse reactions: The most common side effects are hypotension, bradycardia, tachycardia, headache, nausea, and vomiting. Side effects and adverse reactions may vary widely between classes and specific products.

Contraindications: Hypersensitive reactions may occur, and allergies should be identified before these products are given. Antihypertensives should not be used in patients with heart block or in children.

Precautions: Antihypertensives should be used with caution in the elderly, in dialysis patients, and in the presence of hypovolemia, leukemia, and electrolyte imbalances.

Pharmacokinetics: Onset, peak, and duration vary widely among products. Most products are metabolized in the liver, with metabolites excreted in urine, bile, and feces.

Interactions: Interactions vary widely among products; check individual monographs for specific information.

Possible nursing diagnoses:

- Altered tissue perfusion *[uses]*
- Decreased cardiac output *[uses]*
- Diarrhea *[adverse reactions]*
- Impaired gas exchange *[adverse reactions]*

NURSING CONSIDERATIONS

Assess:

- Blood studies: neutrophil; decreased platelets occur with many of the products
- Renal studies: protein, BUN, creatinine; watch for increased levels that may indicate nephrotic syndrome; obtain baselines in renal and liver function studies before beginning treatment
- Edema in feet and legs daily
- Allergic reaction, including rash, fever, pruritus, urticaria: drug should be discontinued if antihistamines fail to help
- Symptoms of CHF: edema, dyspnea, wet rales, B/P
- Renal symptoms: polyuria, oliguria, frequency

Perform/provide:

- Supine or Trendelenburg position for severe hypotension

Evaluate:

• Therapeutic response, including decrease in B/P in hypotension; decreased B/P, edema, moist rales in CHF

Teach patient/family:

• To comply with dosage schedule, even if feeling better

• To rise slowly to sitting or standing position to minimize orthostatic hypotension

---

Selected generic names

Aldosterone receptor antagonist
eplerenone

Angiotensin-converting enzyme inhibitors
benazepril
enalapril
fosinopril
quinapril
ramipril
trandolapril

Angiotensin II receptor blockers
candesartan
eprosartan
irbesartan
losartan
olmesartan
telmisartan
valsartan

Centrally acting adrenergics
clonidine
guanfacine
methyldopa

Peripherally acting antiadrenergics
prazosin
reserpine
terazosin

Vasodilators
diazoxide
fenoldopam
hydralazine
minoxidil
nitroprusside

Antiadrenergic combined α-/β-blocker
labetalol

ANTIINFECTIVES

Action: Antiinfectives are divided into several groups, which include but are not limited to penicillins, cephalosporins, aminoglycosides, sulfonamides, tetracyclines, monobactam, erythromycins, and quinolones. These drugs act by inhibiting the growth and replication of susceptible bacterial organisms.

Uses: Used for infections of susceptible organisms. These products are effective against bacterial, rickettsial, and spirochete infections.

Side effects/adverse reactions: The most common side effects are nausea, vomiting, and diarrhea. Adverse reactions include bone marrow depression and anaphylaxis.

Contraindications: Hypersensitivity reactions may occur, and allergies should be identified before these products are given. Cross-sensitivity can occur between products of different classes (penicillins and cephalosporins). Many persons allergic to penicillins are also allergic to cephalosporins.

Precautions: Antiinfectives should be used with caution in persons with renal and liver disease.

Pharmacokinetics: Onset, peak, and duration vary widely among products. Most products are metabolized in the liver, and metabolites are excreted in urine, bile, and feces.

Interactions: Interactions vary widely among products; check individual monographs for specific information.

Possible nursing diagnoses:

- Risk for infection *[uses]*
- Diarrhea *[adverse reactions]*

NURSING CONSIDERATIONS

Assess:

- Nephrotoxicity, including increased BUN, creatinine
- Blood studies: AST, ALT, CBC, Hct, bilirubin; test monthly if patient is on long-term therapy
- Bowel pattern qd; if severe diarrhea occurs, drug should be discontinued
- Urine output; if decreasing, notify prescriber; may indicate nephrotoxicity
- Allergic reaction, including rash, fever, pruritus, urticaria; drug should be discontinued
- Bleeding: ecchymosis, bleeding gums, hematuria, stool guaiac daily
- Overgrowth of infection: perineal itching, fever, malaise, redness, pain, swelling, drainage, rash, diarrhea, change in cough, sputum

Administer:

- For 10-14 days to ensure organism death, prevention of superinfection
- Drug after C&S completed; drug may be taken as soon as C&S is drawn

Evaluate:

- Therapeutic response, including absence of fever, fatigue, malaise, draining wounds

Teach patient/family:

- To comply with dosage schedule, even if feeling better
- To report sore throat, bruising, bleeding, joint pain; may indicate blood dyscrasias (rare)

Selected generic names

Aminoglycosides
amikacin
azithromycin
clarithromycin
gentamicin
kanamycin
neomycin
streptomycin
tobramycin

Cephalosporins
cefaclor
cefadroxil
cefamandole
cefazolin
cefdinir
cefditoren
cefepime
cefixime
cefmetazole
cefonicid
cefoperazone
ceforanide
cefotaxime
cefprozil
ceftibuten
cefuroxime
cephalexin
cephalothin
cephapirin
cephradine
moxalactam

Fluoroquinolones
alatrofloxacin/trovafloxacin
ciprofloxacin
enoxacin
gemifloxacin (Appx A)
levofloxacin
lomefloxacin
nalidixic acid
norfloxacin
ofloxacin
sparfloxacin

Miscellaneous
adefovir dipivoxil
daptomycin (Appx A)
ertapenem
meropenem
peginterferon alfa-2a

Penicillins
amoxicillin/clavulanate
ampicillin/sulbactam
cloxacillin
dicloxacillin
imipenem/cilastatin
mezlocillin
nafcillin
oxacillin
penicillin G benzathine
penicillin G potassium
penicillin G procaine
penicillin G sodium
penicillin V potassium
piperacillin
ticarcillin
ticarcillin/clavulanate

Sulfonamides
sulfasalazine
sulfiSOXAZOLE

Tetracyclines
demeclocycline
doxycycline
minocycline
tetracycline

ANTINEOPLASTICS

Action: Antineoplastics are divided into alkylating agents, antimetabolites, antibiotic agents, hormonal agents, and miscellaneous agents. Alkylating agents act by cross-linking strands of DNA. Antimetabolites act by inhibiting DNA synthesis. Antibiotic agents act by inhibiting RNA synthesis and by delaying or inhibiting mitosis. Hormones alter the effects of androgens, luteinizing hormone, follicle-stimulating hormone, and estrogen by changing the hormonal environment.

Uses: Uses vary widely among products and classes of drugs. They are used to treat leukemia, Hodgkin's disease, lymphomas, and other tumors throughout the body.

Side effects/adverse reactions: Most products cause thrombocytopenia, leukopenia, and anemia, and if these reactions occur, the drug may have to be stopped until the problem is corrected. Other side effects include nausea, vomiting, glossitis, and hair loss. Some products also cause hepatotoxicity, nephrotoxicity, and cardiotoxicity.

Contraindications: Hypersensitive reactions may occur, and allergies should be identified before these products are given. Also, persons with severe liver and kidney disease should not use these products unless the benefits outweigh the risks.

Precautions: Persons with bleeding, severe bone marrow depression, or renal or hepatic disease should be watched closely.

Pharmacokinetics: Onset, peak, and duration vary widely among products. Most products cross the placenta and are excreted in breast milk and in urine.

Interactions: Toxicity may occur when used with other antineoplastics or radiation.

Possible nursing diagnoses:

- Risk for infection *[adverse reactions]*
- Altered nutrition: less than body requirements *[adverse reactions]*
- Altered oral mucous membrane *[adverse reactions]*

NURSING CONSIDERATIONS

Assess:

- CBC, differential, platelet count weekly; withhold drug if WBC is $<4000/\text{mm}^3$ or platelet count is $<75{,}000/\text{mm}^3$; notify prescriber of results
- Renal function studies, including BUN, creatinine, serum uric acid, and urine creatinine clearance before and during therapy
- I&O ratio; report fall in urine output of 30 ml/hr
- Monitor temp q4h (may indicate beginning infection)
- Liver function tests before and during therapy (bilirubin, AST, ALT, LDH) as needed or monthly
- Bleeding, including hematuria, guaiac, bruising or petechiae, mucosa, or orifices q8h; obtain prescription for viscous Xylocaine (lidocaine)
- Yellowing of skin, sclera, dark urine, clay-colored stools, itchy skin, abdominal pain, fever, diarrhea
- Edema in feet, joint pain, stomach pain, shaking
- Inflammation of mucosa, breaks in skin

Administer:

- Checking IV site for irritation; phlebitis
- EpINEPHrine for hypersensitivity reaction
- Antibiotics for prophylaxis of infection

Perform/provide:

- Strict asepsis, protective isolation if WBC levels are low
- Comprehensive oral hygiene, using careful technique and soft-bristle brush

Evaluate:

- Therapeutic response, including decreased tumor size

Teach patient/family:

- To report signs of infection, including increased temp, sore throat, malaise
- To report signs of anemia, including fatigue, headache, faintness, shortness of breath, irritability
- To report bleeding and avoid use of razors or commercial mouthwash

---

Selected generic names

Alkylating agents
busulfan
carboplatin
carmustine
chlorambucil
cisplatin
cyclophosphamide
dacarbazine
lomustine
mechlorethamine
melphalan
oxaliplatin
thiotepa

Antimetabolites
capecitabine
cytarabine
etoposide
fludarabine
fluorouracil
mercaptopurine
thioguanine (6-TG)

Antibiotic agents
bleomycin
dactinomycin
DAUNOrubicin
DOXOrubicin
epirubicin
methotrexate
mitomycin
mitoxantrone
plicamycin

Hormonal agents
aminoglutethimide
estramustine
flutamide
fulvestrant
goserelin
irinotecan
leuprolide
megestrol
mitotane
nilutamide
tamoxifen
testolactone
topotecan

Miscellaneous
altretamine
anastrozole
arsenic trioxide
asparaginase
bortezomib (Appx A)
cladribine
gefitinib (Appx A)
gemcitabine
ibritumomab
interferon alfa-2A
interferon alfa-2B
irinotecan
pentostatin
porfimer
procarbazine
rituximab
vinBLAStine
vinCRIStine
vinorelbine

ANTIPARKINSON AGENTS

Action: Antiparkinson agents are divided into cholinergics and dopamine agonists. Cholinergics work by blocking or competing at central acetylcholine receptors; dopamine agonists work by decarboxylation to dopamine or by activation of dopamine receptors; monoamine oxidase type B inhibitors work by increasing dopamine activity by inhibiting MAO type B activity.

Uses: Antiparkinson agents are used alone or in combination for patients with Parkinson's disease.

Side effects/adverse reactions: Side effects and adverse reactions vary widely among products. The most common side effects include involuntary movements, headache, numbness, insomnia, nightmares, nausea, vomiting, dry mouth, and orthostatic hypotension.

Contraindications: Persons with hypersensitivity, narrow-angle glaucoma, and undiagnosed skin lesions should not use these products.

Precautions: Antiparkinson agents should be used with caution in pregnancy, lactation, children, renal, cardiac, hepatic disease, and affective disorder.

Pharmacokinetics: Onset, peak, and duration vary widely among products. Most products are metabolized in the liver and excreted in urine.

Interactions: Please check individual monographs since interactions vary widely among products.

Possible nursing diagnoses:

- Risk for injury *[uses]*
- Risk for impaired physical mobility *[uses]*
- Knowledge deficit *[teaching]*

NURSING CONSIDERATIONS

Assess:

- B/P, respiration
- Mental status: affect, mood, behavioral changes, depression, complete suicide assessment

Administer:

- Drug up until NPO before surgery
- Adjust dosage depending on patient response
- With meals; limit protein taken with drug
- Only after MAOIs have been discontinued for 2 wk

Perform/provide:

- Assistance with ambulation, during beginning therapy
- Testing for diabetes mellitus, acromegaly if on long-term therapy

Evaluate:

- Therapeutic response: decrease in akathisia, increased mood

Teach patient/family:

- To change positions slowly to prevent orthostatic hypotension
- To report side effects: twitching, eye spasm; indicate overdose
- To use drug exactly as prescribed; if drug is discontinued abruptly, parkinsonian crisis may occur

Selected generic names

amantadine
benztropine
biperiden
bromocriptine
cabergoline
carbidopa-levodopa
levodopa
pramipexole
selegiline
tolcapone
trihexyphenidyl

ANTIPSYCHOTICS

Action: Antipsychotics/neuroleptics are divided into several subgroups: phenothiazines, thioxanthenes, butyrophenones, dibenzoxazepines, dibenzodiazepines, and indolones and other heterocyclic compounds. Although chemically different, these subgroups share many pharmacologic and clinical properties. All antipsychotics work to block postsynaptic dopamine receptors in the brain that are responsible for psychotic behavior, including hallucinations, delusions, and paranoia.

Uses: Antipsychotic behavior is decreased in conditions such as schizophrenia, paranoia, and mania. These agents are also effective for severe anxiety, intractable hiccups, nausea, vomiting, behavioral problems in children, and for relaxation before surgery.

Side effects/adverse reactions: The most common side effects include EPS such as pseudoparkinsonism, akathisia, dystonia, and tardive dyskinesia, which may be controlled by use of antiparkinsonian agents. Serious adverse reactions such as hypotension, agranulocytosis, cardiac arrest, and laryngospasm have occurred. Other common side effects include dry mouth and photosensitivity.

Contraindications: Persons with liver damage, severe hypertension or coronary disease, cerebral arteriosclerosis, blood dyscrasias, bone marrow depression, parkinsonism, severe depression, narrow-angle glaucoma, children <12 yr, or persons withdrawing from alcohol or barbiturates should not use antipsychotics until these conditions are corrected.

Precautions: Caution must be used when antipsychotics are given to the elderly since metabolism is slowed and adverse reactions can occur rapidly. Hepatic and renal disease may cause poor metabolism and excretion of the drug. Seizure threshold is decreased with these products; increases in the dose of anticonvulsants may be required. Persons with diabetes mellitus, prostatic hypertrophy, chronic respiratory disease, and peptic ulcer disease should be monitored closely.

Pharmacokinetics: Onset, peak, and duration vary widely with different products and routes. Products are metabolized by the liver, are excreted in urine as metabolites, are highly bound to plasma proteins, cross the placenta, and enter breast milk. Half-life can be extended over 3 days.

Interactions: Because other CNS depressants can cause oversedation, these combinations should be used carefully. Anticholinergics may decrease the therapeutic actions of phenothiazines and also cause increased anticholinergic effects.

Possible nursing diagnoses:

- Altered thought processes *[uses]*
- Sensory/perceptual alterations *[uses]*

NURSING CONSIDERATIONS

Assess:

- Bilirubin, CBC, hepatic studies qmo, since these drugs are metabolized in the liver and excreted in urine
- I&O ratio: palpate bladder if low urinary output occurs, since urinary retention occurs with many of these products
- Affect, orientation, LOC, reflexes, gait, coordination, sleep pattern disturbances
- Dizziness, faintness, palpitations, tachycardia on rising
- B/P lying and standing; wide fluctuations between lying and standing B/P may require dosage or product change, since orthostatic hypotension is occurring
- EPS, including akathisia, tardive dyskinesia, pseudoparkinsonism

Administer:

- Antiparkinsonian agent if EPS occur
- Liquid concentrates mixed in glass of juice or cola, since taste is unpleasant; avoid contact with skin when preparing liquid concentrate or parenteral medications

Perform/provide:

- Supervised ambulation until stabilized on medication; do not involve in strenuous exercise program because fainting is possible; patient should not stand still for long periods
- Increased fluids to prevent constipation
- Sips of water, candy, gum for dry mouth

Evaluate:

• Therapeutic response: decrease in excitement, hallucinations, delusions, paranoia, reorganization of thought patterns, speech

Teach patient/family:

• To rise from sitting or lying position gradually, since fainting may occur
• To remain lying down for at least 30 min after IM injections
• To avoid hot tubs, hot showers, or tub baths, since hypotension may occur
• To wear a sunscreen or protective clothing to prevent burns
• To take extra precautions during hot weather to stay cool; heat stroke can occur
• To avoid driving, other activities requiring alertness until response to medication is known
• That drowsiness or impaired mental/motor activity is evident the first 2 wk, but tends to decrease over time

---

Selected generic names

Phenothiazines
chlorproMAZINE
fluphenazine
mesoridazine
perphenazine
prochlorperazine
thioridazine
thiothixene
trifluoperazine

Butyrophenone
haloperidol

Miscellaneous
aripiprazole
loxapine
molindone
olanzapine
quetiapine
risperidone
ziprasidone

ANTITUBERCULARS

Action: Antituberculars act by inhibiting RNA or DNA, or interfering with lipid and protein synthesis, thereby decreasing tubercle bacilli replication.

Uses: Antituberculars are used for pulmonary tuberculosis.

Side effects/adverse reactions: They vary widely among products. Most products can cause nausea, vomiting, anorexia, and rash. Serious adverse reactions include renal failure, nephrotoxicity, ototoxicity, and hepatic necrosis.

Contraindications: Persons with severe renal disease or hypersensitivity should not use these products.

Precautions: Antituberculars should be used with caution with pregnancy, lactation, and hepatic disease.

Pharmacokinetics: Onset, peak, and duration vary widely among products. Most products are metabolized in the liver and excreted in urine.
Interactions: Please check individual monographs since interactions vary widely among products.
Possible nursing diagnoses:
- Risk for infection *[uses]*
- Risk for injury *[adverse reactions]*
- Knowledge deficit *[teaching]*
- Noncompliance *[teaching]*

NURSING CONSIDERATIONS

Assess:
- Signs of anemia: Hct, Hgb, fatigue
- Hepatic studies qwk: ALT, AST, bilirubin
- Renal status before, qmo: BUN, creatinine, output, specific gravity, urinalysis
- Hepatic status: decreased appetite, jaundice, dark urine, fatigue

Administer:
- For some of these agents on empty stomach, 1 hr ac (only for isoniazid and rifampin) or 2 hr pc
- Antiemetic if vomiting occurs
- After C&S is completed; qmo to detect resistance

Evaluate:
- Therapeutic response: decreased symptoms of TB, culture negative

Teach patient/family:
- That compliance with dosage schedule, duration is necessary
- That scheduled appointments must be kept; relapse may occur
- To avoid alcohol while taking drug
- To report flulike symptoms: excessive fatigue, anorexia, vomiting, sore throat; unusual bleeding, yellowish discoloration of skin/eyes

Selected generic names

ethambutol
isoniazid
pyrazinamide
rifabutin
rifampin
streptomycin

ANTITUSSIVES/EXPECTORANTS

Action: Antitussives act by suppressing the cough reflex by direct action on the cough center in the medulla. Expectorants act by liquefying and reducing the viscosity of thick, tenacious secretions.

Uses: Antitussives/expectorants are used to treat cough occurring in pneumonia, bronchitis, TB, cystic fibrosis, and emphysema; as an adjunct in atelectasis (expectorants); and nonproductive cough (antitussives).
Side effects/adverse reactions: The most common side effects are drowsiness, dizziness, and nausea.
Contraindications: Some products are contraindicated in hypothyroidism, pregnancy, and lactation.
Precautions: Some products should be used cautiously in asthmatic, elderly, and debilitated patients.
Pharmacokinetics: Onset, peak, and duration vary widely among products. Some products are metabolized in the liver and excreted in urine.
Interactions: Please check individual monographs since interactions vary widely among products.
Possible nursing diagnoses:
- Ineffective breathing pattern *[uses]*
- Ineffective airway clearance *[uses]*
- Knowledge deficit *[teaching]*

NURSING CONSIDERATIONS

Assess:
- Cough: type, frequency, character (including sputum)

Administer:
- Decreased dose to elderly patients; their metabolism may be slowed

Perform/provide:
- Increased fluids to liquefy secretions
- Humidification of patient's room

Evaluate:
- Therapeutic response: absence of cough

Teach patient/family:
- To avoid driving, other hazardous activities until patient is stabilized on this medication
- To avoid smoking, smoke-filled rooms, perfumes, dust, environmental pollutants, cleaners that increase cough

---

Selected generic names

acetylcysteine
ammonium chloride
benzonatate
codeine
dextromethorphan
guaifenesin
hydrocodone

ANTIVIRALS/ANTIRETROVIRALS

Action: Antivirals act by interfering with DNA synthesis that is needed for viral replication.

Uses: Antivirals are used for mucocutaneous herpes simplex virus, herpes genitalis (HSV_1, HSV_2), advanced HIV infections, herpes simplex virus encephalitis, varicella-zoster encephalomyelitis.

Side effects/adverse reactions: Serious adverse reactions are fatal metabolic encephalopathy, blood dyscrasias, and acute renal failure. Common side effects are nausea, vomiting, anorexia, diarrhea, headache, vaginitis, and moniliasis.

Contraindications: Persons with hypersensitivity, or immunosuppressed individuals with herpes zoster should not use these products.

Precautions: Antivirals should be used with caution in renal disease, hepatic disease, lactation, pregnancy, and dehydration.

Pharmacokinetics: Onset, peak, and duration vary widely among products. Most products are metabolized in the liver and excreted in urine.

Interactions: Please check individual monographs since interactions vary widely among products.

Possible nursing diagnoses:

- Risk for infection *[uses]*
- Risk for injury *[adverse reactions]*
- Knowledge deficit *[teaching]*

NURSING CONSIDERATIONS

Assess:

- Signs of infection, anemia
- I&O ratio; report hematuria, oliguria, fatigue, weakness; may indicate nephrotoxicity; check for protein in urine during treatment
- Any patient with compromised renal system, since drug is excreted slowly in poor renal system function; toxicity may occur rapidly
- Hepatic studies: AST, ALT
- Blood studies: WBC, RBC, Hct, Hgb, bleeding time; blood dyscrasias may occur; drug should be discontinued
- Renal studies: urinalysis, protein, BUN, creatinine, CCr
- C&S before drug therapy; drug may be taken as soon as culture is taken; repeat C&S after treatment
- Bowel pattern before, during treatment; if severe abdominal pain with bleeding occurs, drug should be discontinued
- Skin eruptions: rash, urticaria, itching
- Allergies before treatment, reaction of each medication; record allergies on chart in bright red letters

Administer:

• Increased fluids to 3 L/day to decrease crystalluria when given IV

Perform/provide:

• Storage at room temp for up to 12 hr after reconstitution

• Adequate intake of fluids (2 L) to prevent deposit in kidneys

Evaluate:

• Therapeutic response: absence or control of infection

Teach patient/family:

• That drug does not cure infection, just controls symptoms

• To report sore throat, fever, fatigue; could indicate superinfection

• That drug must be taken in equal intervals around the clock to maintain blood levels for duration of therapy

• To notify prescriber of side effects of bruising, bleeding, fatigue, malaise; may indicate blood dyscrasias

---

Selected generic names

abacavir
acyclovir
amantadine
atazanavir (Appx A)
cidofovir
delavirdine
didanosine
emtricitabine (Appx A)
enfuvirtide (Appx A)
famciclovir
fosamprenavir (Appx A)
foscarnet
ganciclovir
indinavir
nelfinavir
nevirapine
rimantadine
ritonavir
saquinavir
stavudine
tenofovir
valganciclovir
zalcitabine
zidovudine

BARBITURATES

Action: Barbiturates act by decreasing impulse transmission to the cerebral cortex.

Uses: All forms of epilepsy can be controlled, since the seizure threshold is increased. Uses also include febrile seizures in children, sedation, insomnia, hyperbilirubinemia, chronic cholestasis with some of these products. Ultra-short-acting barbiturates are used as anesthetics.

Side effects/adverse reactions: The most common side effects are drowsiness and nausea. Serious adverse reactions such as Stevens-Johnson syndrome and blood dyscrasias may occur with high doses and long-term treatment.

Contraindications: Hypersensitivity may occur, and allergies should be identified before administering. Barbiturates are identified as pregnancy category D and should not be used in pregnancy. Other contraindications include porphyria and marked impairment of liver function.

Precautions: Caution must be used when these products are given to the elderly or debilitated; usually smaller doses are needed since metabolism is slowed. Persons with renal and hepatic disease may show delayed excretion. Barbiturates may produce excitability in children.

Pharmacokinetics: Onset of action can be slow, up to 1 hr, with a peak of 8 hr and a duration of 3-10 hr. These drugs are metabolized by the liver, excreted by the kidneys, cross the placenta, and enter breast milk.

Interactions: Increased CNS depressant effect may occur with alcohol, MAOIs, sedatives, or opioids. These products should be used together cautiously. Oral anticoagulants, corticosteroids, griseofulvin, quinidine, oral contraceptives, and theophylline may show a decreased effect when used with barbiturates.

Possible nursing diagnoses:

- Sleep pattern disturbance *[uses]*
- Risk for injury *[adverse reactions]*

NURSING CONSIDERATIONS

Assess:

- Hepatic and renal studies: AST, ALT, bilirubin, creatinine, LDH, phosphatase, BUN if patient is on long-term therapy, since these products are metabolized and excreted by the liver and kidneys
- Blood studies: CBC, hematocrit, hemoglobin, and prothrombin time if patient is on long-term therapy, since these products increase the possibility of bleeding and blood dyscrasias
- Barbiturate toxicity: hypotension, pulmonary constriction; cold, clammy skin; cyanosis of lips, insomnia, nausea, vomiting, hallucinations, delirium, weakness

Evaluate:

- Therapeutic response, including appropriate sedation or seizure control

Teach patient/family:

- That physical dependency may result when used for extended periods (45-90 days, depending on dose)
- To avoid driving, activities that require alertness since drowsiness and dizziness may occur
- To abstain from alcohol or other psychotropic medications unless directed by prescriber
- Not to discontinue medication abruptly after long-term use; withdrawal symptoms will occur

Selected generic names

pentobarbital
phenobarbital
secobarbital
thiopental

BENZODIAZEPINES

Action: Benzodiazepines potentiate the effects of γ-aminobutyric acid (GABA), including any other inhibitory transmitters in the CNS, resulting in decreased anxiety.

Uses: Anxiety is relieved in conditions such as phobic disorders. Benzodiazepines are also used for acute alcohol withdrawal to relieve the possibility of delirium tremens, and some products are used for relaxation before surgery.

Side effects/adverse reactions: The most common side effects are dizziness, drowsiness, blurred vision, and orthostatic hypotension. Most adverse effects are mediated through the CNS. There is a risk of physical dependence and abuse.

Contraindications: Hypersensitivity, acute narrow-angle glaucoma, children <6 mo, liver disease (clonazepam), lactation (diazepam).

Precautions: Caution must be used when these products are given to the elderly or debilitated; usually smaller doses are needed, since metabolism is slowed. Persons with renal and hepatic disease may show delayed excretion. Clonazepam may increase incidence of seizures.

Pharmacokinetics: Onset of action is ½-1 hr, with a peak of 1-2 hr and a duration of 4-6 hr. These drugs are metabolized by the liver, excreted by the kidneys, cross the placenta, and enter breast milk.

Interactions: Increased CNS depressant effect may occur with other CNS depressants. These products should be used together cautiously. Alcohol should not be used; fatal reactions can occur. The serum concentration and toxicity of digoxin may be increased.

Possible nursing diagnoses:

- Anxiety *[uses]*
- Risk for injury *[adverse reactions]*

NURSING CONSIDERATIONS

Assess:

- B/P (lying, standing), pulse; if systolic B/P drops 20 mm Hg, hold drug, notify prescriber; orthostatic hypotension is severe
- Hepatic and renal studies: AST, ALT, bilirubin, creatinine, LDH, alk phosphatase

• Physical dependency, withdrawal symptoms, including headache, nausea, vomiting, muscle pain, weakness after long-term use

Administer:

• With food or milk for GI symptoms; may give crushed if patient is unable to swallow medication whole

Evaluate:

• Therapeutic response, including relaxation or decreased anxiety

Teach patient/family:

• That drug should not be used for everyday stress or long-term; not to take more than prescribed amount since drug is habit-forming

• To avoid driving and activities that require alertness since drowsiness and dizziness occur

• To abstain from alcohol, other psychotropic medications unless directed by prescriber

• Not to discontinue medication abruptly after long-term use; withdrawal symptoms will occur

Selected generic names

alprazolam
chlordiazepoxide
clonazepam
diazepam
flurazepam
lorazepam
midazolam
oxazepam
temazepam
triazolam

BETA-ADRENERGIC BLOCKERS

Action: β-Blockers are divided into selective and nonselective blockers. Nonselective blockers produce a fall in blood pressure without reflex tachycardia or reduction in heart rate through a mixture of β-blocking effects; elevated plasma renins are reduced. Selective β-blockers competitively block stimulation of β_1-receptors in cardiac smooth muscle; these drugs produce chronotropic and inotropic effects.

Uses: β-Blockers are used for hypertension, ventricular dysrhythmias, and prophylaxis of angina pectoris.

Side effects/adverse reactions: The most common side effects are orthostatic hypotension, bradycardia, diarrhea, nausea, vomiting. Serious adverse reactions include blood dyscrasias, bronchospasm, and CHF.

Contraindications: Hypersensitive reactions may occur, and allergies should be identified before these products are given. β-Adrenergic blockers should not be used in heart block, CHF, or cardiogenic shock.

Precautions: β-Blockers should be used with caution in the elderly or in renal and thyroid disease, COPD, CAD, diabetes mellitus, pregnancy, or asthma.

Pharmacokinetics: Onset, peak, and duration vary widely among products. Most products are metabolized in the liver, with metabolites excreted in urine, bile, and feces.

Interactions: Interactions vary widely among products; check individual monographs for specific information.

Possible nursing diagnoses:

- Altered tissue perfusion *[uses]*
- Decreased cardiac output *[uses]*
- Diarrhea *[adverse reactions]*
- Impaired gas exchange *[adverse reactions]*

NURSING CONSIDERATIONS

Assess:

- Renal studies, including protein, BUN, creatinine; watch for increased levels that may indicate nephrotic syndrome; obtain baselines in renal and liver function studies before beginning treatment
- I&O, weight daily
- B/P during beginning treatment and periodically thereafter; pulse q4h, note rate, rhythm, quality
- Apical/radial pulse before administration; notify prescriber of significant changes
- Edema in feet and legs daily

Administer:

- PO ac, hs; tablets may be crushed or swallowed whole
- Reduced dosage in renal dysfunction

Evaluate:

- Therapeutic response, including decrease in B/P in hypertension, decreased B/P, edema, moist rales in CHF

Teach patient/family:

- To comply with dosage schedule, even if feeling better
- To rise slowly to sitting or standing position to minimize orthostatic hypotension
- To report bradycardia, dizziness, confusion, depression, fever
- To take pulse at home; advise when to notify prescriber
- To comply with weight control, dietary adjustment, modified exercise program
- To wear support hose to minimize effects of orthostatic hypotension
- Not to discontinue drug abruptly; taper over 2 wk; may precipitate angina

Selected generic names

Selective β_1-receptor blockers
acebutolol
atenolol
esmolol
metoprolol

Combined α_1-, β_1-, and β_2-receptor blocker
labetalol

Nonselective β_1- and β_2-blockers
carteolol
nadolol
pindolol
propranolol
timolol

BRONCHODILATORS

Action: Bronchodilators are divided into anticholinergics, α/β-adrenergic agonists, β-adrenergic agonists, and phosphodiesterase inhibitors. Anticholinergics act by inhibiting interaction of acetylcholine at receptor sites on bronchial smooth muscle; α/β-adrenergic agonists by relaxing bronchial smooth muscle and increasing diameter of nasal passages; β-adrenergic agonists by action on β_2-receptors, which relaxes bronchial smooth muscle; phosphodiesterase inhibitors by blocking phosphodiesterase and increasing cAMP, which mediates smooth muscle relaxation in the respiratory system.

Uses: Bronchodilators are used for bronchial asthma, bronchospasm associated with bronchitis, emphysema, or other obstructive pulmonary diseases, Cheyne-Stokes respirations, prevention of exercise-induced asthma.

Side effects/adverse reactions: The most common side effects are tremors, anxiety, nausea, vomiting, and irritation in throat. The most serious adverse reactions include bronchospasm and dyspnea.

Contraindications: Persons with hypersensitivity, narrow-angle glaucoma, tachydysrhythmias, and severe cardiac disease should not use some of these products.

Precautions: Bronchodilators should be used with caution in lactation, pregnancy, hyperthyroidism, hypertension, prostatic hypertrophy, and seizure disorders.

Pharmacokinetics: Onset, peak, and duration vary widely among products. Most products are metabolized in the liver and excreted in urine.

Interactions: Please check individual monographs since interactions vary widely among products.

Possible nursing diagnoses:

- Ineffective airway clearance *[uses]*
- Activity intolerance *[uses]*

- Risk for injury *[adverse reactions]*
- Knowledge deficit *[teaching]*

NURSING CONSIDERATIONS

Assess:

- Respiratory function: vital capacity, forced expiratory volume, ABGs, lung sounds, heart rate and rhythm

Administer:

- After shaking, exhale, place mouthpiece in mouth, inhale slowly, hold breath, remove, exhale slowly
- Gum, sips of water for dry mouth
- PO with meals to decrease gastric irritation

Perform/provide:

- Storage in light-resistant container, do not expose to temps over 86° F (30° C)

Evaluate:

- Therapeutic response: absence of dyspnea, wheezing

Teach patient/family:

- Not to use OTC medications; extra stimulation may occur
- Use of inhaler; review package insert with patient
- To avoid getting aerosol in eyes
- To wash inhaler in warm water qd and dry
- To avoid smoking, smoke-filled rooms, persons with respiratory infections

Selected generic names

albuterol
aminophylline
atropine
bitolterol
dyphylline
epHEDrine
epINEPHrine
formoterol
ipratropium
isoproterenol
levalbuterol
metaproterenol
oxtriphylline
pirbuterol
terbutaline
theophylline

CALCIUM CHANNEL BLOCKERS

Action: These products act by inhibiting calcium ion influx across the cell membrane in cardiac and vascular smooth muscle. This action produces relaxation of coronary vascular smooth muscle, dilates coronary arteries, slows SA/AV node conduction, and dilates peripheral arteries.

Uses: These products are used for chronic stable angina pectoris, vasospastic angina, dysrhythmias, hypertension, and unstable angina.

Side effects/adverse reactions: The most common side effects are dysrhythmias and edema. Also common are headache, fatigue, drowsiness, and flushing.

Contraindications: Persons with 2nd- or 3rd-degree heart block, sick sinus syndrome, hypotension of <90 mm Hg systolic, Wolff-Parkinson-White syndrome, or cardiogenic shock should not use these products since worsening of those conditions may occur.

Precautions: CHF may worsen since edema may be increased. Hypotension may worsen since B/P is decreased. Patients with renal and hepatic disease should use these products cautiously since they are metabolized in the liver and excreted by the kidneys.

Pharmacokinetics: Onset, peak, and duration vary widely with route of administration. Drugs are metabolized by the liver and excreted in the urine primarily as metabolites.

Interactions: Increased levels of digoxin and theophylline may occur when used with these products. Increased effects of β-blockers and antihypertensives may occur with calcium channel blockers.

Possible nursing diagnoses:

- Altered tissue perfusion: cardiopulmonary *[uses]*
- Decreased cardiac output *[adverse reactions]*

NURSING CONSIDERATIONS

Assess:

- Cardiac system, including B/P, pulse, respirations, ECG intervals (PR, QRS, QT)

Administer:

- PO before meals and hs

Evaluate:

- Therapeutic response, including decreased anginal pain, decreased B/P, dysrhythmias

Teach patient/family:

- How to take pulse before taking drug; patient should record or graph pulses to identify changes
- To avoid hazardous activities until stabilized on this drug, since dizziness commonly occurs
- Need for compliance in all areas of medical regimen, including diet, exercise, stress reduction, drug therapy

Selected generic names

diltiazem
felodipine
niCARdipine
NIFEdipine
verapamil

CARDIAC GLYCOSIDES

Action: Products act by inhibiting sodium and potassium ATPase and then making more calcium available to activate contracted proteins. Cardiac contractility and cardiac output are increased.

Uses: These products are used for CHF, atrial fibrillation, atrial flutter, atrial tachycardia, and rapid digitalization in these disorders.

Side effects/adverse reactions: The most common side effects are cardiac disturbances, headache, hypotension, GI symptoms. Also common are blurred vision and yellow-green halos.

Contraindications: Hypersensitive reactions may occur, and allergies should be identified before these products are given. Also, persons with ventricular tachycardia, ventricular fibrillation, and carotid sinus syndrome should not use these products.

Precautions: Persons with acute MI and those who have or may develop serum potassium, calcium, or magnesium imbalances should use these products cautiously. Also, persons with AV block, severe respiratory disease, hypothyroidism, renal and hepatic disease, and the elderly should exercise caution when these drugs are prescribed.

Pharmacokinetics: Onset, peak, and duration vary widely with the route of administration. Digitoxin is inactivated by the liver, and inactive metabolites are excreted in urine. Digoxin is excreted in urine mainly as the parent drug and metabolites.

Interactions: Toxicity may occur when used with diuretics, succinylcholine, quinidine, and thioamines. Increased blood levels may occur with propantheline bromide, spironolactone, quinidine, verapamil, aminoglycosides (PO), amiodarone, anticholinergics, and quinine. Diuretics may increase toxicity.

Possible nursing diagnoses:

- Altered tissue perfusion: cardiopulmonary *[uses]*
- Decreased cardiac output *[adverse reactions]*

NURSING CONSIDERATIONS

Assess:

- Cardiac system, including B/P, pulse, respirations, and increased urine output

• Apical pulse for 1 min before giving drug; if pulse <60 bpm, take again in 1 hr; if still <60 bpm, notify prescriber
• Electrolytes, including K, Na, Cl, Mg; renal function studies, including BUN and creatinine; and blood studies, including AST, ALT, bilirubin
• I&O ratio, daily weights
• Monitor therapeutic drug levels

Administer:
• K supplements if ordered for K levels <3 mg/dl

Evaluate:
• Therapeutic response, including decreased weight, edema, pulse, respiration, and increased urine output

Teach patient/family:
• How to take pulse before taking drug; patient should record or graph pulse to identify changes
• To avoid hazardous activities until stabilized on this drug, since dizziness commonly occurs
• Need for compliance in all areas of medical regimen, including diet, exercise, stress reduction, drug therapy

---

Selected generic name

digoxin

CHOLINERGICS

Action: Cholinergics act by preventing destruction of acetylcholine, which increases concentration at sites where acetylcholine is released; this exaggerates the effects of acetylcholine and facilitates transmission of impulses across the myoneural junction. Cholinergics may also act by stimulating receptors for acetylcholine.

Uses: Cholinergics are used for myasthenia gravis, as antagonists of nondepolarizing neuromuscular blockade, postoperative bladder distention and urinary distention, and postoperative ileus.

Side effects/adverse reactions: The most serious adverse reactions are respiratory depression, bronchospasm, constriction, laryngospasm, respiratory arrest, convulsions, and paralysis. The most common side effects are nausea, diarrhea, and vomiting.

Contraindications: Persons with obstruction of the intestine or renal system should not use these products.

Precautions: Caution should be used in patients with bradycardia, hypotension, seizure disorders, bronchial asthma, coronary occlusion, hyperthyroidism, lactation, and in children.

Pharmacokinetics: Onset, peak, and duration vary widely among products. Most products are metabolized in the liver and excreted in urine.

Interactions: Please check individual monographs since interactions vary widely among products.

Possible nursing diagnoses:

- Altered urinary elimination *[uses]*
- Ineffective breathing pattern *[uses]*
- Knowledge deficit *[teaching]*
- Noncompliance *[teaching]*

NURSING CONSIDERATIONS

Assess:

- VS, respiration q8h
- I&O ratio; check for urinary retention or incontinence
- Bradycardia, hypotension, bronchospasm, headache, dizziness, convulsions, respiratory depression; drug should be discontinued if toxicity occurs

Administer:

- Only with atropine sulfate available for cholinergic crisis
- Only after all other cholinergics have been discontinued
- Increased doses if tolerance occurs
- Larger doses after exercise or fatigue
- On empty stomach for better absorption

Perform/provide:

- Storage at room temp

Evaluate:

- Therapeutic response: increased muscle strength, hand grasp, improved muscle gait, absence of labored breathing (if severe)

Teach patient/family:

- That drug is not a cure; it only relieves symptoms (myasthenia gravis)
- To carry emergency ID specifying myasthenia gravis, drugs taken

---

Selected generic names

bethanechol
edrophonium
neostigmine
physostigmine
pyridostigmine

CHOLINERGIC BLOCKERS

Action: Cholinergic blockers inhibit or block acetylcholine at receptor sites in the autonomic nervous system.

Uses: Many products are used to decrease secretions before surgery, to reverse neuromuscular blockade, and to decrease motility of GI, biliary, urinary tracts. Other products are used for parkinsonian symptoms, including dystonia associated with neuroleptic drugs.

Side effects/adverse reactions: The most common side effects are dryness of the mouth and constipation, which can be prevented by frequent rinsing of the mouth and by increasing water and bulk in the diet.

Contraindications: Hypersensitivity can occur, and allergies should be identified before administering these products. Persons with GI and GU obstruction should not use these products since constipation and urinary retention may occur. They are also contraindicated in angle-closure glaucoma and myasthenia gravis.

Precautions: Caution must be used when these products are given to the elderly, since metabolism is slowed. Also, persons with tachycardia or prostatic hypertrophy should use these products with caution.

Pharmacokinetics: Onset, peak, and duration vary with route.

Interactions: Increase in anticholinergic effect occurs when used with opioids, barbiturates, antihistamines, MAOIs, phenothiazines, and amantadine.

Possible nursing diagnoses:

- Impaired physical mobility *[uses]*
- Pain *[uses]*

NURSING CONSIDERATIONS

Assess:

- I&O ratio; be alert for urinary retention, frequency, dysuria; drug should be discontinued if these occur
- Urinary hesitancy, retention; palpate bladder if retention occurs
- Constipation; increase fluids, bulk, exercise
- For tolerance over long-term therapy, dose may have to be increased or changed
- Mental status: affect, mood, CNS depression, worsening of mental symptoms during early therapy

Administer:

- With food or milk to decrease GI symptoms
- Parenteral dose with patient recumbent to prevent postural hypotension; give parenteral dose slowly, monitoring vital signs

Perform/provide:

• Hard candy, gum, frequent rinsing of mouth for dryness

Evaluate:

• Therapeutic response, including absence of cramps and EPS

Teach patient/family:

• To avoid driving, other hazardous activity if drowsiness occurs

• To avoid concurrent use of cough, cold preparations with alcohol, antihistamines unless directed by prescriber

• To use with caution in hot weather since medication may increase susceptibility to heat stroke

Selected generic names

atropine
benztropine
biperiden
glycopyrrolate
scopolamine
trihexyphenidyl

CORTICOSTEROIDS

Action: Corticosteroids are divided into glucocorticoids and mineralocorticoids. Glucocorticoids decrease inflammation by the suppression of migration of polymorphonuclear leukocytes, fibroblasts, increased capillary permeability, and lysosomal stabilization. They also have varied metabolic effects and modify the body's immune responses to many stimuli. Mineralocorticoids act by increasing resorption of sodium by increasing hydrogen and potassium excretion in the distal tubule.

Uses: Glucocorticoids are used to decrease inflammation and for immunosuppression. In addition, some products may be given for allergy, adrenal insufficiency, or cerebral edema. Mineralocorticoids are given for adrenal insufficiency or adrenogenital syndrome.

Side effects/adverse reactions: The most common side effects include change in behavior, including insomnia and euphoria; GI irritation, including peptic ulcer; metabolic reactions, including hypokalemia, hyperglycemia, and carbohydrate intolerance; and sodium and fluid retention. Most adverse reactions are dose dependent.

Contraindications: Hypersensitivity may occur and should be identified before administering. Since these products mask infection, they should not be used in systemic fungal infections or amebiasis. Mothers taking pharmacologic doses of corticosteroids should not nurse.

Precautions: Caution must be used when these products are prescribed for diabetic patients since hyperglycemia may occur. Also, patients with glaucoma, seizure disorders, peptic ulcer, impaired renal function, CHF, hypertension, ulcerative colitis, or myasthenia gravis should be monitored closely if corticosteroids are given. Use with caution in children and the elderly and during pregnancy.

Pharmacokinetics: For oral preparations, the onset of action occurs between 1 and 2 hr, and duration can be up to 2 days, with a half-life of 2-4 days. Pharmacokinetics vary widely among products. These products cross the placenta and appear in breast milk.

Interactions: Decreased corticosteroid effect may occur with barbiturates, rifampin, phenytoin; corticosteroid dose may have to be increased. There is a possibility of GI bleeding when used with salicylates, indomethacin. Steroids may reduce salicylate levels. When using with digitalis glycosides, potassium-depleting diuretics, and amphotericin, serum potassium levels should be monitored.

Possible nursing diagnoses:

- Risk for infection *[adverse reactions]*
- Body image disturbance *[adverse reactions]*
- Risk for violence: self-directed (suicide) *[adverse reactions]*

NURSING CONSIDERATIONS

Assess:

- Potassium, blood glucose, urine glucose while on long-term therapy; hypokalemia and hyperglycemia are common
- Weight daily; notify prescriber of weekly gain >5 lb, since these products alter fluid and electrolyte balance
- I&O ratio; be alert for decreasing urinary output and increasing edema
- Plasma cortisol levels during long-term therapy (normal level is 138-635 nmol/L SI units when drawn at 8 AM)
- Infection, including increased temp, WBC, even after withdrawal of medication; drug masks symptoms of infection
- Adrenal insufficiency: nausea, anorexia, fatigue, dizziness, dyspnea, weakness, joint pain
- Potassium depletion, including paresthesias, fatigue, nausea, vomiting, depression, polyuria, dysrhythmias, weakness
- Mental status, including affect, mood, behavioral changes, aggression; if severe personality changes occur, including depression, drug may have to be tapered and then discontinued

Administer:

- With food or milk to decrease GI symptoms

Evaluate:

- Therapeutic response, including decreased inflammation

Teach patient/family:

- That emergency ID as steroid user should be carried
- Not to discontinue this medication abruptly, or adrenal crisis can result
- Teach patient all aspects of drug use, including cushingoid symptoms
- That single daily or alternate-day doses should be taken in the morning before 9 AM (for replacement therapy)
- To take with meals or a snack
- If taking immunosuppressives, avoid exposure to chickenpox or measles

Selected generic names

Glucocorticoids
beclomethasone
betamethasone
cortisone
dexamethasone
hydrocortisone
hydrocortisone sodium phosphate
methylPREDNISolone
prednisoLONE
predniSONE
triamcinolone

Mineralocorticoid
fludrocortisone

DIURETICS

Action: Diuretics are divided into subgroups: thiazides and thiazide-like diuretics, loop diuretics, carbonic anhydrase inhibitors, osmotic diuretics, and potassium-sparing diuretics. Each one of these subgroups has its own mechanism of action. Thiazides and thiazide-like diuretics increase excretion of water and sodium by inhibiting resorption in the early distal tubule. Loop diuretics inhibit resorption of sodium and chloride in the thick ascending limb of the loop of Henle. Carbonic anhydrase inhibitors increase sodium excretion by decreasing sodium-hydrogen ion exchange throughout the renal tubule. Carbonic anhydrase inhibitors also decrease secretion of aqueous humor in the eye and thus decrease intraocular pressure. Osmotic diuretics increase the osmotic pressure of glomerular filtrate, thus decreasing net absorption of sodium. The potassium-sparing diuretics interfere with sodium resorption at the distal tubule, thus decreasing potassium excretion.

Uses: B/P is reduced in hypertension; edema is reduced in CHF; intraocular pressure is decreased in glaucoma.

Side effects/adverse reactions: Hypokalemia, hyperuricemia, and hyperglycemia occur most frequently with thiazide diuretics. Aplastic anemia, blood dyscrasias, volume depletion, and dehydration may occur when thiazide-like diuretics, loop diuretics, or carbonic anhydrase inhibitors are given. Side effects and adverse reactions vary widely for the miscellaneous products.

Contraindications: Persons with electrolyte imbalances (Na, Cl, K), dehydration, or anuria should not be given these products until the problem is corrected.

Precautions: Caution must be used when diuretics are given to the elderly, since electrolyte disturbances and dehydration can occur rapidly. Hepatic and renal disease may cause poor metabolism and excretion of the drug.

Pharmacokinetics: Onset, peak, and duration vary widely among the different subgroups of these drugs.

Interactions: Cholestyramine and colestipol will decrease the absorption of thiazide diuretics. Concurrent use of thiazides with diazoxide may increase hyperuricemia, hyperglycemia, and antihypertensive effects of thiazides. Ototoxicity may occur when loop diuretics are used with aminoglycosides. Thiazide and loop diuretics may increase therapeutic and toxic effects of lithium.

Possible nursing diagnoses:

- Fluid volume excess *[uses]*
- Decreased cardiac output *[adverse reactions]*

NURSING CONSIDERATIONS

Assess:

- Weight, I&O daily to determine fluid loss; check skin turgor for dehydration
- Electrolytes: K, Na, Cl; include BUN, blood glucose, CBC, serum creatinine, blood pH, ABGs, uric acid, Ca; electrolyte imbalances may occur quickly
- B/P lying, standing; postural hypotension may occur since fluid loss occurs first from intravascular spaces
- Signs of metabolic alkalosis, including drowsiness and restlessness
- Signs of hypokalemia with some products, including postural hypotension, malaise, fatigue, tachycardia, leg cramps, weakness

Administer:

- In AM to avoid interference with sleep if using drug as a diuretic
- K replacement if K is less than 3 mg/dl

Evaluate:

- Therapeutic response: improvement in edema of feet, legs, sacral area daily if medication is being used in CHF; improvement in B/P if medication is being used as a diuretic; improvement in intraocular pressure if medication is being used to decrease aqueous humor in the eye

Teach patient/family:

- To take drug early in the day (diuretic) to prevent nocturia

Selected generic names

Thiazides
chlorothiazide
hydrochlorothiazide

Thiazide-like
chlorthalidone
indapamide
metolazone

Loop
bumetanide
furosemide
torsemide

Carbonic anhydrase inhibitor
acetaZOLAMIDE

Potassium-sparing
amiloride
spironolactone
triamterene

Osmotics
mannitol
urea

HISTAMINE H_2 ANTAGONISTS

Action: Histamine H_2 antagonists act by inhibiting histamine at the H_2-receptor site in parietal cells, which inhibits gastric acid secretion.

Uses: Histamine H_2 antagonists are used for short-term treatment of duodenal and gastric ulcers and maintenance therapy for duodenal ulcer; gastroesophageal reflux disease.

Side effects/adverse reactions: The most serious adverse reactions are agranulocytosis, thrombocytopenia, neutropenia, aplastic anemia, exfoliative dermatitis. The most common side effects are confusion (not with ranitidine), headache, and diarrhea.

Contraindications: Persons with hypersensitivity should not use these products.

Precautions: Caution should be used in pregnancy, lactation, child <16 yr, organic brain syndrome, hepatic disease, renal disease.

Pharmacokinetics: Onset, peak, and duration vary widely among products. Most products are metabolized in the liver and excreted in urine.

Interactions: Antacids interfere with absorption of histamine H_2 antagonists. Check individual monographs for other interactions.

Possible nursing diagnoses:

- Pain *[uses]*
- Risk for injury *[bleeding]*
- Knowledge deficit *[teaching]*

NURSING CONSIDERATIONS

Assess:

- Gastric pH (>5 should be maintained)
- I&O ratio, BUN, creatinine

Administer:

- With meals for prolonged drug effect
- Antacids 1 hr before or 1 hr after cimetidine
- IV slowly; bradycardia may occur; give over 30 min

Perform/provide:

- Storage of diluted sol at room temp for up to 48 hr

Evaluate:

- Therapeutic response: decreased pain in abdomen

Teach patient/family:

- That gynecomastia, impotence may occur, but are reversible
- To avoid driving, other hazardous activities until patient is stabilized on this medication
- To avoid black pepper, caffeine, alcohol, harsh spices, extremes in temp of food
- To avoid OTC preparations: aspirin, cough, cold preparations
- That drug must be continued for prescribed time to be effective
- To report bruising, fatigue, malaise; blood dyscrasias may occur

Selected generic names

cimetidine
famotidine
ranitidine

IMMUNOSUPPRESSANTS

Action: Immunosuppressants act by inhibiting lymphocytes (T).

Uses: Most products are used for organ transplants to prevent rejection.

Side effects/adverse reactions: The most serious adverse reactions are albuminuria, hematuria, proteinuria, renal failure, and hepatotoxicity. The most common side effects are overgrowth of oral *Candida,* gum hyperplasia, tremors, and headache. The most serious adverse reactions for azathioprine are hematologic (leukopenia and thrombocytopenia) and GI (nausea and vomiting). There is a risk of secondary infection.

Contraindications: Products are contraindicated in hypersensitivity.

Precautions: Caution should be used in severe renal disease, severe hepatic disease, and pregnancy.

Pharmacokinetics: Onset, peak, and duration vary widely among products. Most products are metabolized in the liver and excreted in urine.

Interactions: Please check individual monographs since interactions vary widely among products.

Possible nursing diagnoses:

- Risk for infection *[adverse reactions]*
- Risk for injury *[uses]*
- Knowledge deficit *[teaching]*

NURSING CONSIDERATIONS

Assess:

- Renal studies: BUN, creatinine at least qmo during treatment, 3 mo after treatment
- Hepatic studies: alk phosphatase, AST (SGOT), ALT (SGPT), bilirubin
- Drug blood levels during treatment
- Hepatotoxicity: dark urine, jaundice, itching, light-colored stools; drug should be discontinued

Administer:

- For several days before transplant surgery
- With meals for GI upset or drug mixed with chocolate milk
- With oral antifungal for *Candida* infections

Evaluate:

- Therapeutic response: absence of rejection

Teach patient/family:

- To report fever, chills, sore throat, fatigue, since serious infections may occur
- To use contraceptive measures during treatment, for 12 wk after ending therapy

---

Selected generic names

azathioprine
basiliximab
cycloSPORINE
muromonab-CD3
sirolimus
tacrolimus

LAXATIVES

Action: Laxatives are divided into bulk products, lubricants, osmotics, saline laxative stimulants, and stool softeners. Bulk laxatives work by absorbing water and expanding to increase moisture content and bulk in the stool. Lubricants increase water retention in the stool, causing reabsorption of water in the bowel. Stimulants act by increasing peristalsis by direct effect on the intestine. Saline draws water into the intestinal lumen.

Osmotics increase distention and promote peristalsis. Stool softeners reduce surface tension of liquids of the bowel.

Uses: Laxatives are used as a preparation for bowel and rectal exam, constipation, and stool softener.

Side effects/adverse reactions: The most common side effects are nausea, abdominal cramps, and diarrhea.

Contraindications: Persons with GI obstruction, perforation, gastric retention, toxic colitis, megacolon, abdominal pain, nausea, vomiting, or fecal impaction should not use these products.

Precautions: Caution should be used in rectal bleeding, large hemorrhoids, and anal excoriation.

Pharmacokinetics: Onset, peak, and duration vary among products.

Interactions: Please check individual monographs since interactions vary widely among products.

Possible nursing diagnoses:

- Constipation *[uses]*
- Diarrhea *[adverse reactions]*
- Knowledge deficit *[teaching]*

NURSING CONSIDERATIONS

Assess:

- Blood, urine electrolytes if drug is used often by patient
- I&O ratio: to identify fluid loss
- Cause of constipation; identify whether fluids, bulk, or exercise is missing from lifestyle
- Cramping, rectal bleeding, nausea, vomiting; if these symptoms occur, drug should be discontinued

Administer:

- Alone only with water for better absorption; do not take within 1 hr of antacids, milk, or cimetidine

Evaluate:

- Therapeutic response: decrease in constipation

Teach patient/family:

- To swallow tabs whole; not to chew
- Not to use laxatives for long-term therapy; bowel tone will be lost
- That normal bowel movements do not always occur daily
- Not to use in presence of abdominal pain, nausea, vomiting
- To notify prescriber of abdominal pain, nausea, vomiting
- To notify prescriber if constipation is unrelieved or if symptoms of electrolyte imbalance: muscle cramps, pain, weakness, dizziness

Selected generic names

Bulk laxatives
calcium polycarbophil
methylcellulose
psyllium

Lubricant
mineral oil

Osmotic agents
glycerin
lactulose

Saline laxatives
magnesium salts
sodium biphosphate/phosphate

Stimulants
bisacodyl
cascara sagrada
senna

Stool softener
docusate

NEUROMUSCULAR BLOCKING AGENTS

Action: Neuromuscular blocking agents are divided into depolarizing and nondepolarizing blockers. They act by inhibiting transmission of nerve impulses by binding with cholinergic receptor sites.

Uses: Neuromuscular blocking agents are used to facilitate endotracheal intubation and skeletal muscle relaxation during mechanical ventilation, surgery, or general anesthesia.

Side effects/adverse reactions: The most serious adverse reactions are prolonged apnea, bronchospasm, cyanosis, respiratory depression, and malignant hyperthermia. The most common side effects are bradycardia and decreased motility.

Contraindications: Persons who are hypersensitive should not be given this product.

Precautions: Caution should be used in pregnancy, thyroid disease, collagen disease, cardiac disease, lactation, children <2 yr, electrolyte imbalances, dehydration, neuromuscular disease (myasthenia gravis), and respiratory disease.

Pharmacokinetics: Onset, peak, and duration vary widely among products. Most products are metabolized in the liver and excreted in urine.

Interactions: Aminoglycosides potentiate neuromuscular blockade. See individual monographs.

Possible nursing diagnoses:

- Ineffective breathing pattern *[uses]*
- Risk for injury *[adverse reactions]*
- Knowledge deficit *[teaching]*

NURSING CONSIDERATIONS

Assess:

- For electrolyte imbalances (K, Mg); may lead to increased action of this drug
- Vital signs (B/P, pulse, respirations, airway) q15min until fully recovered; rate, depth, pattern of respirations, strength of hand grip
- I&O ratio; check for urinary retention, frequency, hesitancy
- Recovery: decreased paralysis of face, diaphragm, leg, arm, rest of body
- Allergic reactions: rash, fever, respiratory distress, pruritus; drug should be discontinued

Administer:

- Using nerve stimulator by anesthesia provider to determine neuromuscular blockade
- Anticholinesterase to reverse neuromuscular blockade
- IV undiluted over 1-2 min (only by qualified person, usually an anesthesiologist)

Perform/provide:

- Storage in light-resistant container, cool area
- Reassurance if communication is difficult during recovery from neuromuscular blockade

Evaluate:

- Therapeutic response: paralysis of jaw, eyelid, head, neck, rest of body

Selected generic names

atracurium
cisatracurium
doxacurium
gallamine
mivacurium
pancuronium
pipecuronium
rocuronium
succinylcholine
tubocurarine
vecuronium

NONSTEROIDAL ANTIINFLAMMATORIES

Action: Nonsteroidals decrease prostaglandin synthesis by inhibiting an enzyme needed for biosynthesis.

Uses: Nonsteroidal antiinflammatories are used to treat mild to moderate pain, osteoarthritis, rheumatoid arthritis, and dysmenorrhea.

Side effects/adverse reactions: The most serious adverse reactions are nephrotoxicity (dysuria, hematuria, oliguria, azotemia), blood dyscrasias, and cholestatic hepatitis. The most common side effects are nausea, abdominal pain, anorexia, dizziness, and drowsiness.

Contraindications: Persons with hypersensitivity, asthma, severe renal disease, and severe hepatic disease should not use these products.
Precautions: Caution should be used in pregnancy, lactation, children, bleeding disorders, GI disorders, cardiac disorders, hypersensitivity to other antiinflammatory agents, and the elderly.
Pharmacokinetics: Onset, peak, and duration vary widely among products. Most products are metabolized in the liver and excreted in urine.
Interactions: Please check individual monographs since interactions vary widely among products.
Possible nursing diagnoses:

- Chronic pain *[uses]*
- Impaired physical mobility *[uses]*
- Knowledge deficit *[teaching]*
- Noncompliance *[teaching]*

NURSING CONSIDERATIONS

Assess:

- Renal, hepatic, blood studies: BUN, creatinine, AST, ALT, Hgb, before treatment, periodically thereafter
- Audiometric, ophthalmic examination before, during, and after treatment
- For eye, ear problems: blurred vision, tinnitus; may indicate toxicity

Administer:

- With food to decrease GI symptoms; however, best to take on empty stomach to facilitate absorption

Perform/provide:

- Storage at room temp

Evaluate:

- Therapeutic response: decreased pain, stiffness in joints, decreased swelling in joints, ability to move more easily

Teach patient/family:

- To report blurred vision, ringing, roaring in ears; may indicate toxicity
- To avoid driving, other hazardous activities if dizziness, drowsiness occur, especially elderly
- To report change in urine pattern, increased weight, edema, increased pain in joints, fever, blood in urine; indicate nephrotoxicity
- That therapeutic effects may take up to 1 mo

Selected generic names

celecoxib
diclofenac
etodolac
fenoprofen
ibuprofen
indomethacin
ketoprofen
ketorolac
nabumetone
naproxen
piroxicam
sulindac
valdecoxib

OPIOID ANALGESICS

Action: Opioid analgesics act by depressing pain impulse transmission at the spinal cord level by interacting with opioid receptors. Products are divided into opiates and nonopiates.

Uses: Most products are used to control moderate to severe pain and are used before and after surgery.

Side effects/adverse reactions: GI symptoms, including nausea, vomiting, anorexia, constipation, and cramps are the most common side effects. Other common side effects include light-headedness, dizziness, sedation. Serious adverse reactions such as respiratory depression, respiratory arrest, circulatory depression, and increased intracranial pressure may result but are less common and usually dose dependent.

Contraindications: Hypersensitive reactions occur frequently. Check for sensitivity before administering. These drugs should be used cautiously if narcotic addiction is suspected.

Precautions: Caution must be used when these products are given to a person with an addictive personality since the possibility of addiction is so great. Also, they may worsen intracranial pressure. Persons with severe heart disease, hepatic or renal disease, respiratory conditions, or seizure disorders should be monitored closely for worsening condition.

Pharmacokinetics: Onset of action is immediate by IV route and rapid by IM and PO routes. Peak occurs from 1-2 hr, depending on route, with a duration of 2-8 hr. These agents cross the placenta and appear in breast milk.

Interactions: Barbiturates, other opioids, hypnotics, antipsychotics, or alcohol can increase CNS depression when taken with opioids.

Possible nursing diagnoses:

- Pain *[uses]*
- Impaired gas exchange *[adverse reactions]*

NURSING CONSIDERATIONS

Assess:

- I&O ratio; be alert for urinary retention, frequency, dysuria; drug should be discontinued if these occur
- Respiratory dysfunction, including respiratory depression, rate, rhythm, character; notify prescriber if respirations are <12/min
- CNS changes: dizziness, drowsiness, hallucinations, euphoria, LOC, pupil reaction
- Allergic reactions: rash, urticaria
- Need for pain medication; use pain scoring

Administer:

- With antiemetic if nausea or vomiting occurs
- When pain is beginning to return; determine dosage interval by response

Perform/provide:

- Assistance with ambulation; patient should not be ambulating during drug peak

Evaluate:

- Therapeutic response, including decrease in pain

Teach patient/family:

- To report any symptoms of CNS changes, allergic reactions, or shortness of breath
- That physical dependency may result when used for extended periods
- That withdrawal symptoms may occur, including nausea, vomiting, cramps, fever, faintness, anorexia
- To avoid alcohol and other CNS depressants

Selected generic names

alfentanil
buprenorphine
butorphanol
codeine
dezocine
fentanyl
fentanyl transdermal
hydromorphone
levorphanol
meperidine
methadone
morphine
nalbuphine
oxycodone
oxymorphone
pentazocine
propoxyphene
remifentanil

SALICYLATES

Action: Salicylates have analgesic, antipyretic, and antiinflammatory effects. The antiinflammatory and analgesic activities may be mediated through the inhibition of prostaglandin synthesis. Antipyretic action results from inhibition of the hypothalamic heat-regulating center.

Uses: The primary uses of salicylates are relief of mild to moderate pain and fever and in inflammatory conditions such as arthritis, thromboembolic disorders, and rheumatic fever.

Side effects/adverse reactions: The most common side effects are GI symptoms and rash. Serious blood dyscrasias and hepatotoxicity may result when used for long periods at high doses. Tinnitus or impaired hearing may indicate that blood salicylate levels are reaching or exceeding the upper limit of the therapeutic range.

Contraindications: Hypersensitivity to salicylates is common. Check for sensitivity before administering. Persons with bleeding disorders, GI bleeding, and vit K deficiency should not use these products since salicylates increase prothrombin time. Children should not use these products since salicylates have been associated with Reye's syndrome.

Precautions: Caution is needed when salicylates are given to patients with anemia, hepatic or renal disease, or Hodgkin's disease. Caution should also be exercised in pregnancy and lactation.

Pharmacokinetics: Onset of action occurs in 15-30 min, with a peak of 1-2 hr and a duration up to 6 hr. These drugs are metabolized by the liver and excreted by the kidneys.

Interactions: Increased effects of anticoagulants, insulin, methotrexate, heparin, valproic acid, and oral sulfonylureas may occur when used with salicylates. Aspirin may decrease serum concentrations of nonsteroidal antiinflammatory agents.

Possible nursing diagnoses:

- Pain *[uses]*
- Impaired physical mobility *[uses]*
- Activity intolerance *[uses]*
- Sensory/perceptual alterations: auditory *[adverse reactions]*
- Ineffective thermoregulation *[uses]*

NURSING CONSIDERATIONS

Assess:

- Hepatic and renal studies: AST, ALT, bilirubin, creatinine, LDH, alk phosphatase, BUN if patient is on long-term therapy, since these products are metabolized and excreted by the liver and kidney
- Blood studies: CBC, hematocrit, hemoglobin, and prothrombin time if

patient is on long-term therapy, since these products increase the possibility of bleeding and blood dyscrasias

• Hepatotoxicity: dark urine, clay-colored stools; yellowing of skin, sclera; itching, abdominal pain, fever, diarrhea, which may occur with long-term use

• Ototoxicity: tinnitus; ringing, roaring in ears; audiometric testing is needed before and after long-term therapy

Administer:

• With food or milk to decrease gastric irritation; give 30 min before or 1 hr after meals with a full glass of water

Evaluate:

• Therapeutic response, including decreased pain, fever

Teach patient/family:

• That blood glucose levels should be monitored closely if patient is diabetic

• Not to exceed recommended dosage; acute poisoning may result

• That therapeutic response takes 2 wk in arthritis

• To avoid use of alcohol, since GI bleeding may result

• To notify prescriber of ringing in the ears or persistent GI pain

• To take with full glass of water to reduce risk of lodging in esophagus

---

Selected generic names

aspirin
choline salicylate
magnesium salicylate
salsalate

THROMBOLYTICS

Action: Thrombolytics act by activating conversion of plasminogen to plasmin (fibrinolysin): plasmin is able to break down clots (fibrin).

Uses: Thrombolytics are used to treat deep vein thrombosis, pulmonary embolism, arterial thrombosis, arterial embolism, arteriovenous cannula occlusion, lysis of coronary artery thrombi after MI, and acute, evolving transmural MI.

Side effects/adverse reactions: Serious adverse reactions include GI, GU, intracranial retroperitoneal bleeding, and anaphylaxis. The most common side effects are decreased Hct, urticaria, headache, and nausea.

Contraindications: Persons with hypersensitivity, active bleeding, intraspinal surgery, neoplasms of the CNS, ulcerative colitis/enteritis, severe hypertension, renal disease, hepatic disease, hypocoagulation, COPD, subacute bacterial endocarditis, rheumatic valvular disease, cerebral embolism/thrombosis/hemorrhage, recent intraarterial diagnostic procedure or surgery (10 days), and recent major surgery should not use these products.

Precautions: Caution should be used in arterial emboli from left side of heart and pregnancy.

Pharmacokinetics: Onset, peak, and duration vary widely among products. Most products are metabolized in the liver and excreted in urine.

Interactions: Please check individual monographs since interactions vary widely among products.

Possible nursing diagnoses:

- Risk for injury *[uses]*

NURSING CONSIDERATIONS

Assess:

- VS, B/P, pulse, resp, neuro signs, temp at least q4h; temp >104° F (40° C) indicator of internal bleeding; cardiac rhythm following intracoronary administration; systolic pressure increase of >25 mm Hg should be reported to prescriber
- For neurologic changes that may indicate intracranial bleeding
- Retroperitoneal bleeding: back pain, leg weakness, diminished pulses
- Allergy: fever, rash, itching, chill; mild reaction may be treated with antihistamines
- For bleeding during 1st hr of treatment: hematuria, hematemesis, bleeding from mucous membranes, epistaxis, ecchymosis
- Blood studies (Hct, platelets, PTT, PT, TT, APTT) before starting therapy; PT or APTT must be less than ×2 control before starting therapy; TT or PT q3-4h during treatment

Administer:

- As soon as thrombi identified; not useful for thrombi over 1 wk old
- Cryoprecipitate or fresh, frozen plasma if bleeding occurs
- Loading dose at beginning of therapy; may require increased loading doses
- Heparin after fibrinogen level is over 100 mg/dl; heparin infusion to increase PTT to 1.5-2 × baseline for 3-7 days
- About 10% of patients have high streptococcal antibody titers requiring increased loading doses
- IV therapy using 0.8 μm filter

Perform/provide:

- Storage of reconstituted drug in refrigerator; discard after 24 hr
- Bed rest during entire course of treatment
- Avoidance of venous or arterial puncture, inj, rectal temp
- Treatment of fever with acetaminophen or aspirin
- Pressure for 30 sec to minor bleeding sites; inform prescriber if this does not attain hemostasis; apply pressure dressing

Evaluate:

- Therapeutic response: resolution of thrombosis, embolism

Selected generic names

alteplase
anistreplase
drotrecogin alfa
streptokinase
tenecteplase
urokinase

THYROID HORMONES

Action: Acts by increasing metabolic rates, resulting in increased cardiac output, O_2 consumption, body temp, blood volume, growth, development at cellular level, respiratory rate, enzyme system activity.
Uses: Products are used for thyroid replacement.
Side effects/adverse reactions: The most common side effects include insomnia, tremors, tachycardia, palpitations, angina, dysrhythmias, weight loss, and changes in appetite. Serious adverse reactions include thyroid storm.
Contraindications: Persons with adrenal insufficiency, myocardial infarction, or thyrotoxicosis should not use these products.
Precautions: The elderly and patients with angina pectoris, hypertension, ischemia, cardiac disease, or diabetes mellitus or insipidus should be watched closely when using these products. Caution should be used in pregnancy (A) and lactation.
Pharmacokinetics: Pharmacokinetics vary widely among products; check specific monographs.
Interactions:
- Impaired absorption of thyroid products may occur when administered with cholestyramine, iron products (separate by 4-5 hr)
- Increased effects of anticoagulants, sympathomimetics, tricyclic antidepressants, catecholamines may occur
- Decreased effects of digitalis, glycosides, insulin, hypoglycemics may occur
- Decreased effects of thyroid products may occur with estrogens

Possible nursing diagnoses:
- Knowledge deficit *[teaching]*
- Noncompliance *[teaching]*
- Body image disturbance *[adverse reactions]*

NURSING CONSIDERATIONS

Assess:
- B/P, pulse before each dose
- I&O ratio
- Weight qd in same clothing, using same scale, at same time of day
- PT should be closely monitored and dosage of anticoagulant therapy may need adjustment

• Height, growth rate if given to a child
• T_3, T_4, which are decreased; radioimmunoassay of TSH, which is increased; ratio uptake, which is decreased if patient is on too low a dosage of medication
• Increased nervousness, excitability, irritability; may indicate overdosage, usually after 1-3 wk of treatment
• Cardiac status: angina, palpitation, chest pain, change in VS

Administer:
• At same time each day to maintain drug level
• Only for hormone imbalances, not to be used for obesity, male infertility, menstrual conditions, lethargy

Perform/provide:
• Removal of medication 4 wk before RAIU test

Evaluate:
• Therapeutic response: absence of depression; increased weight loss; diuresis; pulse; appetite; absence of constipation; peripheral edema; cold intolerance; pale, cool, dry skin; brittle nails; alopecia; coarse hair; menorrhagia; night blindness; paresthesias; syncope; stupor; coma; rosy cheeks

Teach patient/family:
• That hair loss will occur in child and is temporary
• To report excitability, irritability, anxiety, chest pain, palpitations, increased pulse, excessive sweating, heat intolerance; indicates overdose
• Not to switch brands unless directed by prescriber
• That hypothyroid child will show almost immediate behavior/personality change
• That treatment drug is not to be taken to reduce weight
• To avoid OTC preparations with iodine; read labels
• To avoid iodine in food, iodinized salt, soybeans, tofu, turnips, some seafood, some bread

Selected generic names

levothyroxine (T_4)
liothyronine (T_3)
liotrix
thyroid USP

VASODILATORS

Action: Vasodilators have various modes of action. Please check individual monographs for specific action.

Uses: Vasodilators are used to treat intermittent claudication, arteriosclerosis obliterans, vasospasm and muscular ischemia, ischemic cerebral vascular disease, hypertension, and angina.

Side effects/adverse reactions: The most common side effects are headache, nausea, hypotension or hypertension, and ECG changes.

Contraindications: Some drugs are contraindicated in acute MI, paroxysmal tachycardia, and thyrotoxicosis.

Precautions: Caution should be used in uncompensated heart disease or peptic ulcer disease.

Pharmacokinetics: Onset, peak, and duration vary widely among products. Most products are metabolized in the liver and excreted in urine.

Interactions: Please check individual monographs since interactions vary widely among products.

Possible nursing diagnoses:

- Decreased cardiac output *[uses]*
- Altered tissue perfusion: cardiopulmonary *[uses]*
- Knowledge deficit *[teaching]*

NURSING CONSIDERATIONS

Assess:

- Bleeding time in individuals with bleeding disorders
- Cardiac status: B/P, pulse, rate, rhythm, character; watch for increasing pulse

Administer:

- With meals to reduce GI symptoms

Perform/provide:

- Storage in tight container at room temp

Evaluate:

- Therapeutic response: ability to walk without pain, increased temp in extremities, increased pulse volume

Teach patient/family:

- That medication is not cure; may need to be taken continuously
- That it is necessary to quit smoking to prevent excessive vasoconstriction
- That improvement may be sudden, but usually occurs gradually over several wk
- To report headache, weakness, increased pulse, as drug may have to be decreased or discontinued
- To avoid hazardous activities until stabilized on medication; dizziness may occur

---

Selected generic names

amyl nitrite
bosentan
dipyridamole
hydralazine
isoxsuprine
midodrine
minoxidil
nesiritide
papaverine

VITAMINS

Action: Action varies widely among products and classes; check specific monographs.

Uses: Vitamins are used to correct and prevent vitamin deficiencies.

Side effects/adverse reactions: There are no side effects or adverse reactions with the water-soluble vitamins (C, B). However, fat-soluble vitamins (A, D, E, K) may accumulate in the body and cause adverse reactions (see specific monographs).

Contraindications: Hypersensitive reactions may occur, and allergies should be identified before these products are given.

Pharmacokinetics: Onset, peak, and duration vary widely among products; check individual monographs for specific information.

Possible nursing diagnoses:

- Altered nutrition: less than body requirements *[uses]*

NURSING CONSIDERATIONS

Administer:

- PO with food for better absorption

Perform/provide:

- Storage in tight, light-resistant container

Evaluate:

- Therapeutic response: no vitamin deficiency

Teach patient/family:

- Not to take more than prescribed amount

Selected generic names

Fat-soluble
phytonadione (vitamin K_1)
vitamin A
vitamin D
vitamin E

Water-soluble
ascorbic acid (C)
cyanocobalamin B_{12}/hydroxocobalamin ($B_{12}a$)
pyridoxine (B_6)
riboflavin (B_2)
thiamine (B_1)

Miscellaneous
multivitamins

abacavir (℞)

(ah-bak'ah-veer)
Ziagen
Func. class.: Antiretroviral
Chem. class.: Nucleoside reverse transcriptase inhibitor (NRTI)

Action: A synthetic nucleoside analog with inhibitory action against HIV. Inhibits replication of the virus by incorporating into cellular DNA by viral reverse transcriptase, thereby terminating the cellular DNA chain
Uses: In combination with other antiretroviral agents for HIV-1 infection
Research note: One study has reported a reduced viral load in adults and children with HIV when abacavir[1] is combined with lamivudine, zidovudine
Dosage and routes:
- *Adult:* **PO** 300 mg bid with other antiretrovirals
- *Adolescents and child ≥3 mo:* 8 mg/kg bid, max 300 mg bid with other antiretrovirals

Available forms: Tabs 300 mg; oral sol 20 mg/ml
Side effects/adverse reactions:
HEMA: ***Granulocytopenia, anemia, lymphopenia***
CNS: Fever, headache, malaise, insomnia, paresthesia
GI: Nausea, vomiting, diarrhea, anorexia, cramps, abdominal pain, increased AST, ALT
RESP: Dyspnea
INTEG: Rash, ***fatal hypersensitivity reactions,*** urticaria
META: ***Lactic acidosis***
OTHER: Increased CPK
Contraindications: Hypersensitivity
Precautions: Granulocyte count <1000/mm^3 or Hgb <9.5 g/dl, pregnancy (C), lactation, children, severe renal disease, impaired hepatic function
Pharmacokinetics: 50% plasma protein binding, metabolized to inactive metabolites, half-life 1½-2 hr
Interactions:
- ↑ abacavir levels: alcohol
- Possible lactic acidosis: ribavirin
- Do not drink alcohol while taking this drug

NURSING CONSIDERATIONS
Assess:
- For lactic acidosis (elevated lactate levels, increased LFTs, severe hepatomegaly) with steatosis, discontinue treatment
- For fatal hypersensitivity reactions: fever, rash, nausea, vomiting, fatigue, cough, dyspnea, diarrhea, abdominal discomfort; treatment should be discontinued and not restarted
- For blood dyscrasias (anemia, granulocytopenia): bruising, fatigue, bleeding, poor healing
- For increased temp, may indicate beginning infection
- Renal studies: BUN, serum uric acid, CCr before, during therapy; these may be elevated throughout treatment
- Hepatic studies before and during therapy: bilirubin, AST, ALT, amylase, alk phosphatase q mo
- Blood counts q2wk; monitor viral load and CD4 counts during treatment; watch for decreasing granulocytes, Hgb; if low, therapy may have to be discontinued and restarted after hematologic recovery; blood transfusions may be required

Administer:
- Give in combination with other antiretrovirals with or without food

Perform/provide:
- Storage in cool environment; protect from light; do not freeze

Teach patient/family:

- That drug is not cure for AIDS but will control symptoms
- To notify prescriber of sore throat, swollen lymph nodes, malaise, fever; other infections may occur; to stop drug if skin rash, fever, cough, shortness of breath, GI symptoms, notify prescriber immediately; advise all health care providers that allergic reaction has occurred with abacavir
- That patient is still infective, may pass AIDS virus on to others
- That follow-up visits must be continued since serious toxicity may occur; blood counts must be done
- To use contraception during treatment
- Give patient Medication Guide and Warning Card, discuss points on guide
- That other drugs may be necessary to prevent other infections

RARELY USED/HIGH ALERT

abciximab (℞)

(ab-six′i-mab)

ReoPro

Func. class.: Platelet aggregation inhibitor

Uses: Used with heparin and aspirin to prevent acute cardiac ischemia following percutaneous transluminal angioplasty (PTCA) in patients at high risk for reclosure of affected arteries

Dosage and routes:

- *Adult:* **IV** 250 mcg (0.25 mg)/kg bolus 10-60 min prior to PTCA, followed by 125 mcg/kg/min **CONT INF** for 12 hr

Contraindications: Hypersensitivity to this drug or murine protein; GI, GU bleeding; CVA within 2 yr, bleeding disorders, intracranial neoplasm, intracranial arteriovenous malformations, intracranial aneurysm, platelet count <100,000/mm^3, recent surgery, aneurysm, uncontrolled severe hypertension, vasculitis

acarbose (℞)

(ay-car′bose)

Prandese✱, Precose

Func. class.: Oral antidiabetic

Chem. class.: α-Glucosidase inhibitor

Action: Delays digestion of ingested carbohydrates, results in smaller rise in blood glucose after meals; does not increase insulin production

Uses: Non–insulin-dependent diabetes mellitus (NIDDM) type 2, alone or in combination with a sulfonylurea

Dosage and routes:

- *Adult:* **PO** 25 mg tid initially, with first bite of meal; maintenance dose may be increased to 50-100 mg tid; dosage adjustment at 4-8 wk intervals
- *Adult <60 kg:* Not to exceed 100 mg PO tid
- ***Available forms:*** Tabs 25, 50, 100 mg

Side effects/adverse reactions:

GI: Abdominal pain, diarrhea, flatulence, increased serum transaminase level

Contraindications: Hypersensitivity, diabetic ketoacidosis, cirrhosis, inflammatory bowel disease, colonic ulceration, partial intestinal obstruction, chronic intestinal disease, serum creatinine >2 mg/dl

Precautions: Pregnancy (B), renal disease, lactation, children, hepatic disease

Do not confuse:

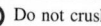

Precose/PreCare

Pharmacokinetics: Peak 1 hr, metabolized in GI tract, excreted as intact drug in urine, half-life 2 hr

Interactions:

• ↓ effect, ↑ hyperglycemia: digestive enzymes, intestinal absorbents, thiazide diuretics, loop diuretics, corticosteroids, estrogen, progestins, oral contraceptives, sympathomimetics, calcium channel blockers, isoniazid, phenothiazines, digoxin

• ↑ hypoglycemia: sulfonylureas, insulin

↑ hypoglycemia: alfalfa, aloe, basil, bay, bilberry, bitter melon, black cohosh, buchu, burdock, chromium, coenzyme Q-10, coriander, eyebright (PO), fenugreek, garlic, ginseng *(Panax),* glucomannan, glucosamine, goat's rue, gymnema, horehound, horse chestnut, jambul, myrrh, myrtle, raspberry, Siberian ginseng

↓ hypoglycemia: bee pollen, blue cohosh, broom chromium, elecampane, eucalyptus, gotu kola, senega

Lab test interferences:

Decrease: Calcium, vit B_6

Increase: AST, bilirubin

NURSING CONSIDERATIONS

Assess:

• Hypoglycemia (weakness, hunger, dizziness, tremors, anxiety, tachycardia, sweating), hyperglycemia; even though drug does not cause hypoglycemia, if patient is on sulfonylureas or insulin, hypoglycemia may be additive; if hypoglycemia occurs, treat with dextrose, or if severe, IV glucose or glucagon.

• 1 hr postprandial for establishing effectiveness, then glycosylated Hgb q3mo

• Monitor AST, ALT q3mo × 1 yr and periodically thereafter; if elevated, dose may need to be reduced or discontinued; obtain glycosylated Hgb periodically

Administer:

PO route

• Tid with first bite of each meal

Perform/provide:

• Storage in tight container in cool environment

Evaluate:

• Therapeutic response: improved signs/symptoms of diabetes mellitus (decreased polyuria, polydipsia, polyphagia; clear sensorium, absence of dizziness, stable gait)

Teach patient/family:

• The symptoms of hypo/hyperglycemia, what to do about each

• That medication must be taken as prescribed; explain consequences of discontinuing medication abruptly; that insulin may need to be used for stress, including trauma, surgery, fever

• To avoid OTC medications, herbal supplements unless approved by health-care provider

• That diabetes is lifelong illness; that this drug is not a cure

• To carry emergency ID for emergency purposes

• That diet and exercise regimen must be followed

acebutolol (℞)

(a-se-byoo′toe-lole)

Monitan✤, Sectral

Func. class.: Antihypertensive, β_1-blocker, antidysrhythmic (II)

Action: Competitively blocks stimulation of β-adrenergic receptors within vascular smooth muscle; decreases rate of SA node discharge, increases recovery time, slows conduction of AV node resulting in decreased heart rate (negative chronotropic effect), which decreases O_2 consumption in myocardium due to β_1-receptor antagonism; also decreases renin-aldosterone-angiotensin system at high doses, inhibits β_2-receptors in bronchial system (high doses)

Uses: Mild to moderate hypertension, sinus tachycardia, persistent atrial extrasystoles, tachydysrhythmias, management of PVCs

Investigational uses: Prophylaxis of MI, treatment of angina pectoris, tremor, mitral valve prolapse, thyrotoxicosis, idiopathic hypertrophic subaortic stenosis

Dosage and routes:

Hypertension

• *Adult:* **PO** 400 mg qd or in 2 divided doses; may be increased to desired response; maintenance 200-1200 mg/qd in 2 divided doses

Ventricular dysrhythmia

• *Adult:* **PO** 200 mg bid, may increase gradually, usual range 600-1200 mg daily; should be tapered over 2 wk before discontinuing

• *Geriatric:* not to exceed 800 mg qd

Renal dose

• *Adult:* **PO** CCr 25-50 ml/min, reduce dose by 50%; if <25 ml/min reduce dose by 75%

Available forms: Caps 200, 400 mg; tabs 100, 200; 400 mg

Side effects/adverse reactions:

CV: ***Profound hypotension, bradycardia, CHF,*** *cold extremities, postural hypotension,* ***2nd- or 3rd-degree heart block***

CNS: Insomnia, fatigue, dizziness, mental changes, memory loss, hallucinations, depression, lethargy, drowsiness, strange dreams, catatonia

GI: Nausea, diarrhea, vomiting, ***mesenteric arterial thrombosis, ischemic colitis, flatulence***

INTEG: Rash, flushing, pruritus, sweating, alopecia, dry skin

HEMA: ***Agranulocytosis, thrombocytopenia, purpura***

EENT: Sore throat; dry, burning eyes

GU: Impotence, decreased libido, dysuria, nocturia

ENDO: Increased hypoglycemic response to insulin

RESP: ***Bronchospasm,*** dyspnea, wheezing, cough

MS: Joint pain, cramping

MISC: Facial swelling, weight gain, decreased exercise tolerance

Contraindications: Hypersensitivity to β-blockers, cardiogenic shock, heart block (2nd, 3rd degree), sinus bradycardia, CHF, cardiac failure

Precautions: Major surgery, pregnancy (B), lactation, peripheral vascular disease, children, diabetes mellitus, renal disease, thyroid disease, COPD, asthma, well-compensated heart failure, hepatic disease

Pharmacokinetics:

PO: Onset 1-1½ hr, peak 2-4 hr, duration 10-12 hr, half-life 3-4 hr, metabolized in liver, 30%-40% excreted in urine, protein binding 26%

Interactions:

• ↑ hypotension, bradycardia: reserpine, hydralazine, methyldopa, prazosin, anticholinergics, cardiac glycosides, diltiazem, verapamil, diuretics, other antihypertensives, calcium channel blockers, cimetidine

• Attenuated effects: oral sulfonylureas

• ↓ antihypertensive effects: NSAIDs, calcium, cholestyramine, colestipol

• ↑ hypoglycemic effect: insulin

• ↓ bronchodilation: theophyllines, β_2-agonists

• Peripheral ischemia: ergots

May ↑ acebutolol effect: aloe, buckthorn bark/berry, betel palm, butterbur, cola tree, figwort, fumitory, guarana, hawthorn, lily of the valley, motherwort, plantain, rhubarb root, senna leaf/fruits, cascara sagrada bark

↓ antihypertensive effect: coenzyme Q10, yohimbe

Toxicity/death: aconite

Lab test interferences:

Positive: ANA titer

Increase: Serum lipoprotein levels, BUN, potassium, triglyceride, uric acid, LDH, AST, ALT, blood glucose, alk phosphatase

NURSING CONSIDERATIONS

Assess:

- B/P during beginning treatment, periodically thereafter; pulse q4h; note rate, rhythm, quality
- Apical/radial pulse before administration; notify prescriber of any significant changes (pulse <50 bpm); signs of CHF (dyspnea, crackles, weight gain, jugular vein distention)
- Baselines in renal, hepatic studies before therapy begins
- Edema in feet, legs daily: monitor I&O
- Skin turgor, dryness of mucous membranes for hydration status, especially elderly

Administer:

PO route

- Drug ac, hs, tablet may be crushed or swallowed whole; give with food to prevent GI upset

Perform/provide:

- Storage protected from light, moisture; place in cool environment

Evaluate:

- Therapeutic response: decreased B/P after 1-2 wk; decreased dysrhythmias

Teach patient/family:

- Not to discontinue drug abruptly, severe cardiac reactions may occur, taper over 2 wk; do not double dose; if a dose is missed, take as soon as remembered up to 4 hr before next dose
- Drug may mask signs of hypoglycemia or alter blood glucose levels
- Not to use OTC products containing α-adrenergic stimulants (such as nasal decongestants, OTC cold preparations) unless directed by prescriber
- To report low pulse, dizziness, confusion, depression, fever
- To take pulse, B/P at home, advise when to notify prescriber
- To comply with weight control, dietary adjustments, modified exercise program
- To carry emergency ID to identify drug, allergies
- To avoid hazardous activities if dizziness, drowsiness is present
- To report symptoms of CHF: difficult breathing, especially on exertion or when lying down, night cough, swelling of extremities
- To continue with required lifestyle changes (exercise, diet, weight loss, stress reduction)

Treatment of overdose: Lavage, IV atropine for bradycardia, IV theophylline for bronchospasm, digitalis, O_2, diuretic for cardiac failure, IV glucose for hypoglycemia, IV diazepam (or phenytoin) for seizures

acetaminophen (OTC)

(a-seat-a-mee'noe-fen)

Abenol♣, Acephen, Aceta, Actimol, Aminofen, Apacet, APAP, Apo-Acetaminophen♣, Arthritis Foundation Pain Reliever Aspirin-Free, Aspirin Free Anacin, Aspirin Free Pain Relief, Atasol♣, Banesin, Children's Feverall, Dapa, Dapacin, Datril, Exdol♣, FemEtts, Genapap, Genebs, Halenol, Liquiprin, Mapap, Maranox, Meda, Neopap, Oraphen-PD, Panadol, Redutemp, Robigesic♣, Rounax♣, Silapap, Tapanol, Tempra, Tylenol

Func. class.: Nonopioid analgesic, antipyretic

Chem. class.: Nonsalicylate, paraaminophenol derivative

Action: May block pain impulses peripherally that occur in response to inhibition of prostaglandin synthesis; does not possess antiinflammatory properties; antipyretic action results from inhibition of prostaglandins in the CNS (hypothalamic heat-regulating center)

Uses: Mild pain or fever

Dosage and routes:

• *Adult and child >12 yr:* **PO/RECT** 325-650 mg q4h prn, max 4 g/day

• *Child:* **PO** 10-15 mg/kg q4h

• *Child 6-12 yr:* **RECT** 325 mg q4-6h, max 2.6 g/day

• *Child 3-6 yr:* **RECT** 125 mg q4-6h, max 720 mg/day

• *Child 1-3 yr:* **RECT** 80 mg q4h

• *Child 3-11 mo:* **RECT** 80 mg q6h

Available forms: Rect supp 80, 120, 125, 325, 600, 650 mg; soft chew tabs 80, 160 mg; caps 500 mg; elix 120, 160, 325 mg/5 ml; liq 160 mg/5 ml, 500 mg/15 ml; sol 100 mg/1 ml, 120 mg/2.5 ml; granules 80 mg/packet, 80 mg/cap; tabs 160, 325, 500, 650 mg

Side effects/adverse reactions:

SYST: Hypersensitivity

HEMA: ***Leukopenia, neutropenia, hemolytic anemia (long-term use), thrombocytopenia, pancytopenia***

CNS: Stimulation, drowsiness

GI: Nausea, vomiting, abdominal pain; ***hepatotoxicity, hepatic seizure (overdose)***

INTEG: Rash, urticaria

TOXICITY: ***Cyanosis, anemia, neutropenia, jaundice, pancytopenia, CNS stimulation, delirium followed by vascular collapse, convulsions, coma, death***

GU: ***Renal failure (high, prolonged doses)***

Contraindications: Hypersensitivity, intolerance to tartrazine (yellow dye #5), alcohol, table sugar, saccharin, depending on product

Precautions: Anemia, hepatic disease, renal disease, chronic alcoholism, pregnancy (B), elderly, lactation

Pharmacokinetics: Well absorbed PO, rectal absorption varies; 85%-90% metabolized by liver, excreted by kidneys; metabolites may be toxic if overdose occurs; widely distributed, crosses placenta in low concentrations, excreted in breast milk, half-life 1-4 hr

PO: Onset 10-30 min, peak ½-2 hr, duration 3-4 hr

RECT: Onset slow, peak 1-2 hr, duration 3-4 hr

Interactions:

• ↓ effect; ↑ hepatotoxicity: barbiturates, alcohol, carbamazepine, hydantoins, rifampin, rifabutin, isoniazid, diflunisal, sulfinpyrazone

• Hypoprothrombinemia: warfarin, long-term use, high doses of acetaminophen
• Bone marrow suppression: zidovudine
• ↓ absorption: colestipol, cholestyramine
• Renal adverse reactions: NSAIDs, salicylates

Lab test interferences:
Interference: Chemstrip G, Dextrostix, Visidex II, 5-HIAA

NURSING CONSIDERATIONS

Assess:
• Hepatic studies: AST, ALT, bilirubin, creatinine prior to therapy if long-term therapy is anticipated; may cause hepatic toxicity at doses >4 g/day with chronic use
• Renal studies: BUN, urine creatinine, occult blood, albumin, if patient is on long-term therapy; presence of blood or albumin indicates nephritis
• Blood studies: CBC, PT if patient is on long-term therapy
• I&O ratio; decreasing output may indicate renal failure (long-term therapy)
• For fever and pain: type of pain, location, intensity, duration
• For chronic poisoning: rapid, weak pulse; dyspnea; cold, clammy extremities; report immediately to prescriber
• Hepatotoxicity: dark urine; clay-colored stools; yellowing of skin, sclera; itching, abdominal pain; fever; diarrhea if patient is on long-term therapy
• Allergic reactions: rash, urticaria; if these occur, drug may have to be discontinued

Administer:

PO route
• Crushed or whole; chewable tablets may be chewed; give with full glass of water
• With food or milk to decrease gastric symptoms if needed

Perform/provide:
• Storage of suppositories <80° F (27° C)

Evaluate:
• Therapeutic response: absence of pain, fever

Teach patient/family:
⬘ Not to exceed recommended dosage; acute poisoning with liver damage may result
⬘ That acute toxicity includes symptoms of nausea, vomiting, abdominal pain; prescriber should be notified immediately
• To read label on other OTC drugs; many contain acetaminophen and may cause toxicity if taken concurrently
• To recognize signs of chronic overdose: bleeding, bruising, malaise, fever, sore throat
• To notify prescriber of pain or fever lasting over 3 days

Treatment of overdose: Drug level, gastric lavage, activated charcoal; administer oral acetylcysteine to prevent hepatic damage *(see acetylcysteine monograph),* monitor for bleeding

*acetaZOLAMIDE (℞)

(a-set-a-zole′a-mide)
acetaZOLAMIDE, Apo-Acetazolamide ✤, Dazamide, Diamox, Diamox Sequels

Func. class.: Diuretic, carbonic anhydrase inhibitor, antiglaucoma agent, antiepileptic

Chem. class.: Sulfonamide derivative

Action: Inhibits carbonic anhydrase activity in proximal renal tubules to decrease reabsorption of water, sodium, potassium, bicarbonate; decreases carbonic anhydrase in CNS,

increasing seizure threshold; able to decrease aqueous humor in eye, which lowers intraocular pressure
Uses: Open-angle glaucoma, narrow-angle glaucoma (preoperatively, if surgery delayed), epilepsy (petit mal, grand mal, mixed), edema in CHF, drug-induced edema, acute mountain sickness
Investigational uses: Prevention of uric acid/cystine renal stones, decrease CSF production in infants with hydrocephalus
Dosage and routes:
Closed-angle glaucoma
• *Adult:* **PO/IM/IV** 250 mg q4h or 250 mg bid, to be used for short-term therapy
Open-angle glaucoma
• *Adult:* **PO/IM/IV** 250 mg-1 g/day in divided doses for amounts over 250 mg or 500 mg SR bid
Edema in CHF
• *Adult:* **IM/IV** 250-375 mg/day in AM
• *Child:* **IM/IV** 5 mg/kg/day in AM
Seizures
• *Adult:* **PO/IM/IV** 4-30 mg/kg/day, in 1-4 divided doses usual range 375-1000 mg/day
• *Child:* **PO/IM/IV** 8-30 mg/kg/day in divided doses tid or qid, or 300-900 mg/m^2/day, not to exceed 1 g/day
Mountain sickness
• *Adult:* **PO** 250 mg q8-12h
Renal stones
• *Adult:* **PO** 250 mg hs
Infants with hydrocephalus
• *Infant:* **IV** 5 mg/kg/dose q6h, may be increased up to 100 mg/kg/day if tolerated
Available forms: Tabs 125, 250 mg; caps sust rel 500 mg; inj 500 mg
Side effects/adverse reactions:
GU: Frequency, polyuria, ***uremia,*** glucosuria, hematuria, dysuria, crystalluria, renal calculi
CNS: Drowsiness, paresthesia, anxiety, depression, headache, dizziness, confusion, stimulation, fatigue, ***convulsions,*** sedation, nervousness
GI: Nausea, vomiting, anorexia, constipation, diarrhea, melena, weight loss, ***hepatic insufficiency,*** taste alterations
EENT: Myopia, tinnitus
INTEG: Rash, pruritus, urticaria, fever, ***Stevens-Johnson syndrome,*** photosensitivity
ENDO: Hyperglycemia
HEMA: ***Aplastic anemia, hemolytic anemia, leukopenia, agranulocytosis, thrombocytopenia, purpura, pancytopenia***
META: Hypokalemia, hyperchloremic acidosis
Contraindications: Hypersensitivity to sulfonamides, severe renal disease, severe hepatic disease, electrolyte imbalances (hyponatremia, hypokalemia), hyperchloremic acidosis, Addison's disease, long-term use in narrow-angle glaucoma, COPD
Precautions: Hypercalciuria, pregnancy (C), lactation
Do not confuse:
acetaZOLAMIDE/acetoHEXAMIDE
Diamox/Trimox
Diamox/Dobutrex
Pharmacokinetics:
PO: Onset 1-1½ hr, peak 2-4 hr, duration 8-12 hr
PO-SUS REL: Onset 2 hr, peak 3-6 hr, duration 18-24 hr
IV: Onset 2 min, peak 15 min, duration 4-5 hr, 65% absorbed if fasting (oral), 75% absorbed if given with food; half-life 2½-5½ hr; excreted unchanged by kidneys (80% within 24 hr), crosses placenta
Interactions:
• ↑ action of amphetamines, procainamide, quinidine, anticholinergics
• ↑ excretion of lithium

• ↑ toxicity: salicylates
• Toxicity: cycloSPORINE
• ↓ acetaZOLAMIDE effect: methenamine
• ↑ side effects: diflunisal
• ↓ primidone levels

Lab test interferences:
False positive: Urinary protein, 17 hydroxysteroid
Decrease: Thyroid iodine uptake

NURSING CONSIDERATIONS

Assess:
• Weight daily, I&O daily to determine fluid loss; effect of drug may be decreased if used qd; monitor the elderly for dehydration
• For cross-sensitivity between other sulfonamides and this drug
• B/P lying, standing; postural hypotension may occur
• Electrolytes: K, Na, Cl; also BUN, blood sugar, CBC, serum creatinine, blood pH, ABGs, LFTs; I&O, glucose, patient may need to be on a high-potassium diet

Administer:
• In AM to avoid interference with sleep if using drug as diuretic
• Potassium replacement if potassium level is less than 3.0 mg/dl

PO route
• With food if nausea occurs; absorption may be decreased slightly
⊘ Do not break, crush, or chew sus rel caps

IV route
• After diluting 500 mg in >5 ml sterile H_2O for injection; direct IV—give at 100-500 mg/min; may be diluted further in LR, D_5W, $D_{10}W$, 0.45% NaCl, 0.9% NaCl, or Ringer's sol and infused over 4-8 hr; use within 24 hr of dilution

Additive compatibilities: Cimetidine, ranitidine

Perform/provide:
• Storage in dark, cool area; use reconstituted solution within 24 hr

Evaluate:
• Therapeutic response: improvement in edema of feet, legs, sacral area daily if medication is being used in CHF; or decrease in aqueous humor if medication is being used in glaucoma

Teach patient/family:
• To take exactly as prescribed; if dose is missed, take as soon as remembered; do not double dose
• To notify prescriber if sore throat, unusual bleeding, bruising, paresthesias, tremors, flank pain, or skin rash occurs
• To use sunscreen to prevent photosensitivity; to monitor blood glucose and urine for sugar
• To avoid hazardous activities if drowsiness occurs
• Increase fluids to 2-3 L/day if not contraindicated
• Report nausea, vertigo, rapid weight gain, change in stools

Treatment of overdose: Lavage if taken orally; monitor electrolytes; administer dextrose in saline; monitor hydration, CV, renal status

acetylcysteine (℞)

(a-se-teel-sis'tay-een)
Mucomyst✤, Mucosil, Parvolex✤

Func. class.: Mucolytic; antidote—acetaminophen
Chem. class.: Amino acid L-cysteine

Action: Decreases viscosity of secretions by breaking disulfide links of mucoproteins; increases hepatic glutathione, which is necessary to inactivate toxic metabolites in acetaminophen overdose

Uses: Acetaminophen toxicity; bronchitis; pneumonia; cystic fibrosis; emphysema; atelectasis; tuberculosis; complications of thoracic, cardiovascular surgery; diagnosis in bronchial lab tests

Investigational uses: Prevention of contrast medium nephrotoxicity

Dosage and routes:

Mucolytic

• *Adult and child:* **INSTILL** 1-2 ml (10%-20% sol) q1-4h prn or 3-5 ml (20% sol) or 6-10 ml (10% sol) tid or qid

Acetaminophen toxicity

• *Adult and child:* **PO** 140 mg/kg, then 70 mg/kg q4h × 17 doses to total of 1330 mg/kg

Available forms: Sol 10%, 20%

Side effects/adverse reactions:

CNS: Dizziness, drowsiness, headache, fever, chills

GI: Nausea, stomatitis, constipation, vomiting, anorexia, ***hepatotoxicity***

EENT: Rhinorrhea, tooth damage

CV: Hypotension

INTEG: Urticaria, rash, fever, clamminess

RESP: ***Bronchospasm,*** burning, ***hemoptysis,*** chest tightness

Contraindications: Hypersensitivity, increased intracranial pressure, status asthmaticus

Precautions: Hypothyroidism, Addison's disease, CNS depression, brain tumor, asthma, hepatic disease, renal disease, COPD, psychosis, alcoholism, convulsive disorders, lactation, pregnancy (B)

Pharmacokinetics:

INH/INSTILL: Onset 1 min, duration 5-10 min, metabolized by liver, excreted in urine

Interactions:

• Do not use with iron, copper, rubber

• Do not mix with antibiotics: tetracycline, chlortetracycline, oxytetracycline, erythromycin lactobionate, amphotericin B, sodium ampicillin; iodized oil, chymotrypsin, trypsin, hydrogen peroxide

NURSING CONSIDERATIONS

Assess:

• Cough: type, frequency, character, including sputum

• Rate, rhythm of respirations, increased dyspnea; sputum; discontinue if bronchospasm occurs

• VS, cardiac status including checking for dysrhythmias, increased rate, palpitations

• ABGs for increased CO_2 retention in asthma patients

• Antidotal use: LFTs, PT, BUN, glucose, electrolytes, acetaminophen levels; inform prescriber if dose is vomited or vomiting is persistent

• Nausea, vomiting, rash; notify prescriber if these occur

Administer:

PO route

• Antidotal use: give within 24 hr; give with cola or soft drink to disguise taste; can be given with H_2O through tubes; use within 1 hr

INSTILL route

• By syringe 2-3 doses of 1-2 ml of 20% or 2-4 ml of 10% solution

• Decreased dose to elderly patients; their metabolisms may be slowed

• Only if suction machine is available

• Before meals ½-1 hr for better absorption, to decrease nausea

• 20% solutions diluted with NS or water for injection; may give 10% solution undiluted

• Only after patient clears airway by deep breathing, coughing

Perform/provide:

• Storage in refrigerator; use within 96 hr of opening

• Assistance with inhaled dose: bronchodilator if bronchospasm occurs

• Mechanical suction if cough insufficient to remove excess bronchial secretions

• Gum, hard candy, frequent rinsing of mouth for dryness of oral cavity

Evaluate:

• Therapeutic response: absence of purulent secretions when coughing; absence of hepatic damage in acetaminophen toxicity

Teach patient/family:

• About mucolytic use
• That unpleasant odor will decrease after repeated use
• That discoloration of solution after bottle is opened does not impair its effectiveness

activated charcoal (OTC)

Actidose-Aqua, CharcoAid, CharcoAid 2000, Liqui-Char

Func. class.: Antiflatulent; antidote

Action: Binds poisons, toxins, irritants; increases adsorption in GI tract; inactivates toxins and binds until excreted

Uses: Poisoning

Dosage and routes:

• Children should not get more than 1 dose of products with sorbitol

Poisoning

• *Adult and child:* **PO** 30-100 g or 1 g/kg, minimum dose 30 g/250 ml of water, may give 20-40 g q6h for 1-2 days in severe poisoning

Available forms: Powder 15, 25✤, 30, 40, 120, 125, 240 g/container; oral susp 12.5 g/60 ml, 15 g/72 ml, 15 g/120 ml, 25 g/120 ml, 30 g/120 ml, 50 g/240 ml; Canada 15 g/120 ml, 25 g/125 ml, 50 g/225 ml, 50 g/250 ml

Side effects/adverse reactions:

GI: Nausea, black stools, vomiting, constipation, diarrhea

Contraindications: Hypersensitivity to this drug, unconsciousness, semiconsciousness, poisoning of cyanide, mineral acids, alkalis

Pharmacokinetics:

PO: Excreted in feces

Interactions:

• Inactivation of: ipecac, acetylcysteine

NURSING CONSIDERATIONS

Assess:

• Respiration, pulse, B/P to determine charcoal effectiveness if taken for barbiturate/opiate poisoning

Administer:

PO route

• After inducing vomiting unless vomiting contraindicated (i.e., cyanide or alkalis)
• After mixing with water or fruit juice to form thick syrup; do not use dairy products to mix charcoal
• Repeat dose if vomiting occurs soon after dose; give with a laxative to promote elimination; alone, do not administer with ipecac
• After spacing at least 1 hr before or after other drugs, or absorption will be decreased

Perform/provide:

• Container closed tightly to prevent absorption of gases

NG

• Through a nasogastric tube if patient unable to swallow

Evaluate:

• Therapeutic response: LOC alert (poisoning)

Teach patient/family:

• That stools will be black
• How to prevent further poisonings

acyclovir (℞)

(ay-sye'kloe-ver)

Avirax🍁, Zovirax

Func. class.: Antiviral

Chem. class.: Acyclic purine nucleoside analog

See Topical Appendix for Topical Product

Action: Interferes with DNA synthesis by conversion to acyclovir triphosphate, causing decreased viral replication, time of lesional healing

Uses: Mucocutaneous herpes simplex virus, herpes genitalis (HSV-1, HSV-2), varicella infections, herpes zoster, herpes simplex encephalitis

Investigational uses: Cytomegalovirus, HSV after transplant, mononucleosis, herpes simplex

Dosage and routes:

Renal dose

• *Adult and child:* **PO/IV** CCr >50 ml/min dose q8h, CCr 25-50 ml/min dose q12h, CCr 10-25 ml/min dose q24h, CCr 0-10 ml/min 50% of dose q24h

Herpes simplex

• *Adult and child >12 yr:* **IV INF** 5 mg/kg over 1 hr q8h × 5 days

• *Child <12 yr:* **IV INF** 250 mg/m^2 or 30 mg/kg/day divided q8h over 1 hr × 5 days

Genital herpes

• *Adult:* **PO** 200 mg q4h (5×/day while awake) for 5 days to 6 mo depending on whether initial, recurrent, or chronic

Herpes simplex encephalitis

• *Adult:* **IV** 10 mg/kg over 1 hr q8h × 10 days

• *Child 3 mo-12 yr:* **IV** 20 mg/kg q8h × 10 days

• *Child birth-3 mo:* **IV** 10 mg/kg q8h × 10 days

Herpes zoster

• *Adult:* **PO** 800 mg q4h while awake × 7-10 days; **IV** 5 mg/kg q8h

Varicella-zoster

• *Adult:* **PO** 1000 mg q6h × 5 days or 600-800 mg q4h (5×/day while awake); **IV** 500 mg/m^2 q8h or 10 mg/kg q8h × 7 days

• *Child:* **PO** 10-20 mg/kg (max 800 mg) qid × 5 days; **IV** 500 mg/m^2 q8h or 10 mg/kg q8h × 7 days

Chickenpox

• *Adult and child:* **PO** 20 mg/kg qid × 5 days, max 800 mg/dose

Available forms: Caps 200 mg; inj 500 mg, oral susp, tabs 400, 800 mg

Side effects/adverse reactions:

CNS: Tremors, confusion, lethargy, hallucinations, ***seizures,*** dizziness, *headache,* encephalopathic changes

GI: Nausea, vomiting, diarrhea, increased ALT, AST, abdominal pain, glossitis, colitis

GU: ***Oliguria, proteinuria, hematuria,*** vaginitis, moniliasis, ***glomerulonephritis, acute renal failure,*** changes in menses, polydipsia

EENT: Gingival hyperplasia

INTEG: Rash, urticaria, pruritus, pain or phlebitis at IV site, unusual sweating, alopecia

MS: Joint pain, leg pain, muscle cramps

HEMA: ***Thrombotic thrombocytopenia purpura, hemolytic uremic syndrome*** (immunocompromised patients)

Contraindications: Hypersensitivity

Precautions: Lactation, hepatic disease, renal disease, electrolyte imbalance, dehydration, pregnancy (B)

Pharmacokinetics:

Distributed widely; crosses placenta, CSF concentrations are 50% plasma

IV: Onset immediate, peak immediate, duration unknown, half-life 20 min-3 hr (terminal); metabolized by liver, excreted by kidneys as unchanged drug (95%)

PO: Absorbed minimally; onset unknown, peak 1½-2 hr, terminal half-life 3½ hr

Interactions:

- ↑ levels, toxicity: probenecid
- Synergistic effect: interferon
- CNS side effects: zidovudine

NURSING CONSIDERATIONS

Assess:

- Signs of infection, anemia
- Any patient with compromised renal system, since drug is excreted slowly in poor renal system function; toxicity may occur rapidly
- Hepatic studies: AST, ALT
- Blood studies: WBC, RBC, Hct, Hgb, bleeding time; blood dyscrasias may occur; drug should be discontinued
- Renal studies: urinalysis, protein, BUN, creatinine, CCr, watch for increasing BUN and serum creatinine or decreased CCr, may indicate nephrotoxicity; I&O ratio; report hematuria, oliguria, fatigue, weakness; may indicate nephrotoxicity; check for protein in urine during treatment
- C&S before drug therapy; drug may be taken as soon as culture is taken; repeat C&S after treatment; determine the presence of other sexually transmitted diseases
- Bowel pattern before, during treatment; if severe abdominal pain with bleeding occurs, drug should be discontinued
- Skin eruptions: rash, urticaria, itching
- Allergies before treatment, reaction of each medication; place allergies on chart in bright red letters

Administer:

PO route

- Do not break, crush, or chew caps
- May give without regard to meals, with 8 oz of water
- Shake suspension before use
- Lower dose in acute or chronic renal failure

IV route

- Increased fluids to 3 L/day to decrease crystalluria
- After reconstituting with 10 ml compatible sol/500 mg of drug, concentration of 50 mg/ml, shake, further dilute in 50-100 ml compatible sol; use within 12 hr; give over at least 1 hr (constant rate) by infusion pump to prevent nephrotoxicity; do not reconstitute with sol containing benzyl alcohol in neonates

Additive compatibilities: Fluconazole

Solution compatibilities: D_5W, LR, or NaCl (D_5 0.9% NaCl, 0.9% NaCl) solutions

Y-site compatibilities: Allopurinol, amikacin, ampicillin, amphotericin B, cefamandole, cefazolin, cefonicid, cefoperazone, cefotaxime, cefoxitin, ceftazidime, ceftizoxime, ceftriaxone, cefuroxime, cephapirin, chloramphenicol, cholesteryl sulfate complex, cimetidine, clindamycin, dexamethasone sodium phosphate, dimenhyDRINATE, diphenhydrAMINE, DOXOrubicin, doxycycline, erythromycin, famotidine, filgrastim, fluconazole, gallium, gentamicin, granisetron, heparin, hydrocortisone sodium succinate, hydromorphone, imipenem/cilastatin, lorazepam, magnesium sulfate, melphalan, methylPREDNISolone sodium succinate, metoclopramide, metronidazole, multivitamin, nafcillin, oxacillin, paclitaxel, penicillin G potassium, pentobarbital, perphenazine, piperacillin, potassium chloride, propofol, ranitidine, remifentanil, sodium bicarbonate, tacrolimus, teniposide, theophylline, thiotepa, ticarcillin, tobramycin, trimethoprim-sulfamethoxazole, vancomycin, zidovudine

Perform/provide:

• Storage at room temperature for up to 12 hr after reconstitution; if refrigerated, sol may show a precipitate that clears at room temperature, yellow discoloration does not affect potency

• Adequate intake of fluids (2 L) to prevent deposit in kidneys

Evaluate:

• Therapeutic response: absence of itching, painful lesions; crusting and healed lesions; decreased symptoms of chickenpox

Teach patient/family:

• To take as prescribed; if dose is missed, take as soon as remembered up to 1 hr before next dose; do not double dose; that drug does not cure the condition

• That drug may be taken orally before infection occurs; drug should be taken when itching or pain occurs, usually before eruptions

• That sexual partners need to be told that patient has herpes; they can become infected; condoms must be worn to prevent reinfections

• Not to touch lesions to avoid spreading infection to new sites

• That drug does not cure infection, just controls symptoms and does not prevent infecting others

• To report sore throat, fever, fatigue (may indicate superinfection)

• That drug must be taken in equal intervals around the clock to maintain blood levels for duration of therapy

• To notify prescriber of side effects of bruising, bleeding, fatigue, malaise; may indicate blood dyscrasias

• To seek dental care during treatment to prevent gingival hyperplasia

• That women with genital herpes are more likely to develop cervical cancer; to keep all gynecologic appointments

Treatment of overdose: Discontinue drug, hemodialysis, resuscitate if needed

adalimumab (℞)

(add-a-lim'yu-mab)

Humira

Func. class.: Antirheumatic agent (disease modifying), immunomodulator

Chem. class.: Recombinant human IgG1 monoclonal antibody

Action: A form of human IgG1 monoclonal antibody specific for human tumor necrosis factor (TNF). Elevated levels of TNF are found in patients with rheumatoid arthritis.

Uses: Reduction in signs and symptoms and inhibiting progression of structural damage in patients with moderate to severe active rheumatoid arthritis in patients ≥18 years of age who have not responded to other disease-modifying agents

Dosage and routes:

• *Adult:* **SC** 40 mg ever other wk

Available form: Inj 40 mg/0.8 ml

Side effects/adverse reactions:

CNS: Headache

EENT: Sinusitis

GI: Abdominal pain, nausea

INTEG: Rash, *inj site reaction*

MISC: Flulike symptoms, UTI, hypertension, back pain, lupuslike syndrome

RESP: URI

Contraindications: Hypersensitivity

Precautions: Pregnancy (B), lactation, children, elderly, CNS demyelinating disease, lymphoma, latent TB

Pharmacokinetics: Terminal half-life 2 wk

Interactions:

• Do not give concurrently with vaccines; immunizations should be brought up to date before treatment

NURSING CONSIDERATIONS

Assess:

• Pain, stiffness, ROM, swelling of joints during treatment

• For inj site pain, swelling; usually occur after 2 inj (4-5 days)

⇔ For infections, stop treatment if present, some serious infections including sepsis may occur; patients with active infections should not be started on this drug

Administer:

• Do not admix with other sol or medications, do not use filter, protect from light

Evaluate:

• Therapeutic response: decreased inflammation, pain in joints

Teach patient/family:

• About self-administration if appropriate: inj should be made in thigh, abdomen, upper arm; rotate sites at least 1 inch from old site, do not inject in areas that are bruised, red, hard

• That if medication is not taken when due, inject next dose as soon as remembered and inject next dose as scheduled

adefovir dipivoxil (℞)

(add-ee-foh'veer)

Hepsera

Func. class.: Antiviral

Chem. class.: Adenosine monophosphate analog

Action: Inhibits hepatitis B virus DNA polymerase by competing with natural substrates and by causing DNA termination after its incorporation into viral DNA; causes viral DNA death

Uses: Chronic hepatitis B

Dosage and routes:

• *Adult:* **PO** 10 mg qd, optimal duration unknown

Renal dose

• *Adult:* **PO** CCr ≥50 ml/min 10 mg q24h; CCr 20-49 ml/min 10 mg q48h; CCr 10-19 ml/min 10 mg q72h; hemodialysis 10 mg q7 days following dialysis

Available forms: Tabs 10 mg

Side effects/adverse reactions:

CNS: Headache

GI: Dyspepsia, abdominal pain

Contraindications: Hypersensitivity

Precautions: Pregnancy (C), lactation, child, severe renal disease, impaired hepatic disease, elderly

Pharmacokinetics:

PO: Rapidly absorbed from GI tract, peak 1¾ hr, excreted by kidneys 45%; terminal half-life 7.48 hr

Interactions:

• ↑ serum concentration and possible toxicity: amphotericin B, dapsone, flucytosine, adriamycin, interferon, vinCRIStine, vinBLAStine, pentamidine, probenecid, experimental nucleoside analogs, benzodiazepines, cimetidine, morphine, sulfonamides, acyclovir, ganciclovir, DOXOrubicin, acetaminophen, indomethacin, fluconazole, phenytoin, trimethoprim

• Granulocytopenia: acetaminophen, aspirin, indomethacin

NURSING CONSIDERATIONS

Assess:

• For nephrotoxicity: increasing CCr, BUN

• For HIV before beginning treatment, because HIV resistance may occur in chronic hepatitis B patients

• For lactic acidosis, severe hepatomegaly with stenosis

• Elderly patients more carefully; may develop renal, cardiac symptoms more rapidly
• For exacerbations of hepatitis after discontinuing treatment, monitor LFTs

Administer:
• By mouth without regard to food

Perform/provide:
• Storage in cool environment; protect from light

Evaluate:
• Therapeutic response: decreased symptoms of chronic hepatitis B, improving LFTs

Teach patient/family:
• That optimal duration of treatment is unknown
• To avoid use with other medications unless approved by prescriber
• To notify prescriber of decreased urinary output

HIGH ALERT

adenosine (℞)

(a-den′oh-seen)
Adenocard, Adenoscan
Func. class.: Antidysrhythmic
Chem. class.: Endogenous nucleoside

Action: Slows conduction through AV node, can interrupt reentry pathways through AV node, and can restore normal sinus rhythm in patients with supraventricular tachycardia (SVT)

Uses: SVT, as a diagnostic aid to assess myocardial perfusion defects in CAD

Dosage and routes:
Antidysrhythmic
• *Adult:* **IV BOL** 6 mg; if conversion to normal sinus rhythm does not occur within 1-2 min, give 12 mg by rapid **IV BOL;** may repeat 12 mg dose again in 1-2 min
• *Infants and children:* 0.05 mg/kg, if not effective, increase dose by 0.05 mg/kg q2min to a max of 0.25 mg/kg or 12 mg

Diagnostic use
• *Adult:* 140 mcg/kg/min × 6 min

Available forms: Inj 3 mg/ml vial, 6 mg/2 ml vial

Side effects/adverse reactions:
GI: Nausea, metallic taste, throat tightness, groin pressure
RESP: Dyspnea, chest pressure, hyperventilation
CNS: Lightheadedness, dizziness, arm tingling, numbness, apprehension, blurred vision, headache
CV: Chest pain, pressure, ***atrial tachydysrhythmias,*** sweating, palpitations, hypotension, *facial flushing*

Contraindications: Hypersensitivity, 2nd- or 3rd-degree heart block, AV block, sick sinus syndrome, atrial flutter, atrial fibrillation

Precautions: Pregnancy (C), lactation, children, asthma, elderly

Do not confuse:
Adenocard/adenosine phosphate

Pharmacokinetics: Cleared from plasma in <30 sec, half-life 10 sec

Interactions:
• ↑ effects of adenosine: dipyridamole
• ↓ activity of adenosine: theophylline or other methylxanthines (caffeine)
• Higher degree of heart block: carbamazepine
• Possible ventricular fibrillation: digoxin
• Smoking: ↑ tachycardia
↑ Toxicity/death: aconite
↑ adenosine effect: aloe, broom, buckthorn, cascara sagrada, figwort, fumitory, goldenseal, kudzu, licorice, rhubarb, senna

↓ adenosine effect: coltsfoot, guarana

↑ serotonin effect: horehound

NURSING CONSIDERATIONS

Assess:

- I&O ratio, electrolytes (K, Na, Cl)
- Cardiopulmonary status: B/P, pulse, respiration, ECG intervals (PR, QRS, QT); check for transient dysrhythmias (PVCs, PACs, sinus tachycardia, AV block)
- Respiratory status: rate, rhythm, lung fields for rales, watch for respiratory depression; bilateral rales may occur in CHF patient; increased respiration, increased pulse, drug should be discontinued
- CNS effects: dizziness, confusion, psychosis, paresthesias, convulsions; drug should be discontinued

Administer:

IV BOLUS route

- Undiluted; give 6 mg or less by rapid inj; if using an IV line, use port near insertion site, flush with normal saline (50 ml)

CONT INF route

- Give 30 ml vial, undiluted, by peripheral vein

Solution compatibilities: D_5LR, D_5W, LR, 0.9% NaCl

Perform/provide:

- Storage at room temperature; sol should be clear; discard unused drug

Evaluate:

- Therapeutic response: normal sinus rhythm or diagnosis of perfusion defect

Teach patient/family:

- To report facial flushing, dizziness, sweating, palpitations, chest pain
- To rise from sitting or standing slowly to prevent orthostatic hypotension

Treatment of overdose: Defibrillation, vasopressor for hypotension

A

alatrofloxacin (℞)

(ah-lat-troh-floks'ah-sin)

Trovan IV

trovafloxacin (℞)

(tro-vah-floks'ah-sin)

Trovan (oral)

Func. class.: Antiinfective

Chem. class.: Fluoroquinolone

Action: Interferes with conversion of intermediate DNA fragments into high-molecular-weight DNA in bacteria; DNA gyrase inhibitor

Uses: Nosocomial pneumonia; *Escherichia coli, Proteus aeruginosa, Haemophilus influenzae, Staphylococcus aureus*; community-acquired pneumonia: *Streptococcus pneumoniae, H. influenzae, S. aureus, Klebsiella pneumoniae, Mycoplasma pneumoniae, Moraxella catarrhalis, Legionella pneumophila, Chlamydia pneumoniae*; chronic bronchitis, acute sinusitis, complicated intraabdominal infections, gynecologic/pelvic infections, skin/skin structure infections, UTIs, chronic bacterial prostatitis, urethral gonorrhea in males, PID, cervicitis caused by susceptible organisms

Dosage and routes:

Alatrofloxacin—serious infections

- *Adult:* **IV** 300 mg q24h

Other infections

- *Adult:* **IV** 200 mg q24h

Perioperative prophylaxis

- *Adult:* **IV** 200 mg ½-4 hr prior to surgery

Trovafloxacin—gonorrhea

- *Adult:* **PO** 100 mg as a single dose

Other infections

- *Adult:* **PO** 100-200 mg q24h

Perioperative prophylaxis

- *Adult:* **PO** 200 mg ½-4 hr prior to surgery

Available forms: Conc sol for inj 5 mg/ml (200 mg/40 ml, 300 mg/60 ml) (alatrofloxacin); tabs 100, 200 mg (trovafloxacin)

Side effects/adverse reactions:

CNS: Headache, *dizziness,* insomnia, anxiety, psychosis, ***seizures***

HEMA: Anemia, ***thrombocytopenia, leukopenia,*** decreased Hgb; Hct, increased platelets

GI: Nausea, flatulence, vomiting, diarrhea, abdominal pain, ***pseudomembranous colitis, hepatotoxicity, fatal hepatitis***

MS: Arthralgia, myalgia

GU: Vaginitis, crystalluria, increased BUN, creatinine

INTEG: Rash, pruritus, photosensitivity

SYST: ***Anaphylaxis, Stevens-Johnson syndrome***

Contraindications: Hypersensitivity to quinolones, seizure disorders, cerebral atherosclerosis, photosensitivity

Precautions: Pregnancy (C), lactation, children

Do not confuse:

Trovan/Tenormin

Pharmacokinetics: Metabolized in liver, excreted in urine unchanged

Interactions:

- May ↑ theophylline level, lead to toxicity
- May ↑ warfarin level
- Nephrotoxicity may occur with cycloSPORINE
- ↓ absorption of trovafloxacin: IV morphine
- ↓ absorption: antacids with aluminum, magnesium, citric acid buffered with sodium citrate, sucralfate, iron products, IV morphine

Do not use acidophilus concurrently with antiinfectives

↑ antiinfective effect: cola tree

NURSING CONSIDERATIONS

Assess:

- For hepatic toxicity, use only for serious or life-threatening infections
- For previous sensitivity reaction to fluoroquinolones
- For signs and symptoms of infection: characteristics of sputum, WBC >10,000, fever; obtain baseline information before and during treatment
- For CNS disorders, since other quinolones can cause CNS stimulation, seizures
- C&S before beginning drug therapy to identify if correct treatment has been initiated
- For allergic reactions and anaphylaxis: rash, urticaria, pruritus, chills, fever, joint pain; may occur a few days after therapy begins; epinephrine and resuscitation equipment should be available for anaphylactic reaction
- Bowel pattern qd; if severe diarrhea occurs, drug should be discontinued
- For overgrowth of infection, perineal itching, fever, malaise, redness, pain, swelling, drainage, rash, diarrhea, change in cough, sputum

Hepatic studies: AST; ALT, alk phosphatase, bilirubin; identify hepatotoxicity, fatal hepatitis

Administer:

Solution compatibilities: D_5, ½NaCl, D_5 ½NaCl, D_5/0.2% NaCl

Intermittent INF route

- Dilute with compatible solution to a concentration of 1-2 mg/ml, run over 1 hr

Y-site compatibilities: Amikacin, cycloSPORINE, DOPamine, droperidol, fentanyl, gentamicin, ketorolac, lorazepam, midazolam, nitroglycerin, ondansetron, tobramycin, vancomycin

(Rotahaler inhalation) 200 mcg cap inhaled q4-6h; may use 15 min before exercise

Available forms: Aerosol 90 mcg/actuation; oral sol 2 mg/5 ml; tabs 2, 4 mg; ext rel 4, 8 mg; INH sol 0.83, 0.5, 1, 2, 5 mg/ml; powder for INH (RotaCaps) 200, 400 mcg; powder for INH (Ventodisk) 200, 400 mcg; INH cap 200 mcg; 100 mcg/spray, 80 INH/canister, 200 INH/canister

Side effects/adverse reactions:

CNS: *Tremors, anxiety,* insomnia, headache, dizziness, stimulation, *restlessness,* hallucinations, flushing, irritability

CV: Palpitations, tachycardia, hypertension, angina, hypotension, dysrhythmias

EENT: Dry nose, irritation of nose and throat

GI: Heartburn, nausea, vomiting

MISC: Flushing, sweating, anorexia, bad taste/smell changes

MS: Muscle cramps

RESP: Cough, wheezing, dyspnea, ***bronchospasm,*** dry throat

Contraindications: Hypersensitivity to sympathomimetics, tachydysrhythmias, severe cardiac disease, heart block

Precautions: Lactation, pregnancy (C), cardiac disorders, hyperthyroidism, diabetes mellitus, hypertension, prostatic hypertrophy, narrow-angle glaucoma, seizures, exercise-induced bronchospasm (aerosol) in children <12 years

Do not confuse:

albuterol/atenolol
Ventolin/Vantin
Volmax/Flomax
Proventil/Prinivil
Salbutamol/salmeterol

Pharmacokinetics: Well absorbed PO, extensively metabolized in the liver and tissues, crosses placenta, breast milk, blood-brain barrier

PO: Onset ½ hr, peak 2½ hr, duration 4-6 hr, half-life 2½ hr

PO-ER: Onset ½ hour; peak 2-3 hr; duration 12 hr

INH: Onset 5 min, peak 1-1½ hr, duration 4-6 hr, half-life 4 hr

Interactions:

- ↑ action of aerosol bronchodilators
- ↑ action of albuterol: tricyclic antidepressants, MAOIs, other adrenergics; do not use together
- May inhibit action of albuterol: other β-blockers
- Severe hypotension: oxytocics
- Toxicity: theophylline
- ECG changes/hypokalemia: potassium-losing diuretics

↑ stimulation: caffeine (cola nut, green/black tea, guarana, mate, coffee, chocolate)

NURSING CONSIDERATIONS

Assess:

- Respiratory function: vital capacity, forced expiratory volume, ABGs; lung sounds, heart rate and rhythm, B/P, sputum (baseline and peak)
- That patient has not received theophylline therapy before giving dose
- Patient's ability to self-medicate
- For evidence of allergic reactions
- Paradoxical bronchospasm, hold medication, notify prescriber if bronchospasm occurs

Administer:

Inhalation route

- In geriatric patients, a spacing device is advised
- After shaking metered dose inhaler, exhale, place mouthpiece in mouth, inhale slowly, while depressing inhaler, hold breath, remove, exhale slowly; give INH at least 1 min apart
- NEB/IPPB diluting 5 mg/ml sol/2.5 ml 0.9% NaCl for INH; other sol do not require dilution; for neb O_2 flow or compressed air 6-10 L/min
- Gum, sips of water for dry mouth

PO route

• With meals to decrease gastric irritation

• Oral solution to children (no alcohol, sugar)

Do not crush, break, or chew ext rel tabs

Perform/provide:

• Storage in light-resistant container, do not expose to temperatures over 86° F (30° C)

Evaluate:

• Therapeutic response: absence of dyspnea, wheezing after 1 hr, improved airway exchange, improved ABGs

Teach patient/family:

• To use exactly as prescribed; take missed dose when remembered, alter dosing schedule

• Not to use OTC medications; excess stimulation may occur

• Use of inhaler; review package insert with patient; use demonstration, return demonstration

• To avoid getting aerosol in eyes; blurring of vision may result

• To wash inhaler in warm water qd and dry

• To avoid smoking, smoke-filled rooms, persons with respiratory infections

That paradoxic bronchospasm may occur and to stop drug immediately, call prescriber

• To limit caffeine products such as chocolate, coffee, tea, and colas

Treatment of overdose: Administer a β_1-adrenergic blocker

alclometasone topical

See appendix c

HIGH ALERT

aldesleukin (℞)

(al-dess-loo'ken)

Interleukin-2, IL-2, Proleukin

Func. class.: Miscellaneous antineoplastic

Chem. class.: Interleukin-2, human recombinant (cytokine)

Action: Enhancement of lymphocyte mitogenesis and stimulation of IL-2–dependent cell lines; enhancement of lymphocyte cytotoxicity; induction of killer cell activity; induction of interferon-γ production; results in activation of cellular immunity, cytokines, and inhibition of tumor growth

Uses: Metastatic renal cell carcinoma in adults, phase II for HIV in combination with zidovudine, melanoma

Investigational uses: Kaposi's sarcoma given with zidovudine, metastatic melanoma given with cyclophosphamide, non-Hodgkin's lymphoma given with lymphokine-activated killer cells, AIDS (phase I) given with zidovudine

Dosage and routes:

• *Adult:* **IV INF** 600,000 international units/kg (0.037 mg/kg) over 15 min q8h × 14 doses; off 9 days, repeat schedule for another 14 doses, for a max of 28 doses/course

Available forms: Powder for inj 22 million international units/vial

Side effects/adverse reactions:

CV: Hypotension, sinus tachycardia, dysrhythmias, bradycardia, PVCs, PACs, myocardial ischemia, ***myocardial infarction, cardiac arrest, capillary leak syndrome, CVA***

RESP: Pulmonary congestion, dyspnea, ***pulmonary edema, respira-***

tory failure, apnea, tachypnea, pleural effusion, wheezing
GI: Nausea, vomiting, *diarrhea,* stomatitis, anorexia, GI bleeding, dyspepsia, constipation, ***intestinal perforation***/ileus, jaundice, ascites
HEMA: Anemia, ***thrombocytopenia, leukopenia, coagulation disorders, leukocytosis, eosinophilia***
CNS: Mental status changes, dizziness, sensory dysfunction, syncope, motor dysfunction, fever, chills, headache, impaired memory, depression, sleep disturbances, hallucinations, rigors
GU: ***Oliguria/anuria, proteinuria, hematuria,*** dysuria, ***renal failure***
INTEG: Pruritus, *erythema, rash,* dry skin, ***exfoliative dermatitis,*** purpura, petechiae, urticaria
MS: Arthralgia, myalgia
SYST: Infection
EENT: Reversible visual changes

Contraindications: Hypersensitivity, abnormal thallium stress test or pulmonary function tests, organ allografts

Precautions: CNS metastases, bacterial infections, renal/hepatic/cardiac/pulmonary disease, pregnancy (C), lactation, children, anemia, thrombocytopenia

Do not confuse:
aldesleukin/oprelvekin
Proleukin/oprelvekin
Proleukin/Prokine

Pharmacokinetics: Renal elimination half-life 85 min; onset 4 wk, duration ≤12 mo

Interactions:
- Potentiate hypotension: antihypertensives
- Reduced antitumor effectiveness: glucocorticoids
- ↑ toxicity: aminoglycosides, indomethacin, cytotoxic chemotherapy, methotrexate, asparaginase, DOXOrubicin
- Unpredictable reactions: psychotropics

Lab test interferences:
Increase: Bilirubin, BUN, serum creatinine, transaminase, alk phosphatase; hypomagnesemia, acidosis hypocalcemia, hypophosphatemia, hypokalemia, hyperuricemia, hypoalbuminemia, hypoproteinemia, hyponatremia, hyperkalemia, alkalosis (toxic effect of drug)

NURSING CONSIDERATIONS

Assess:
- CBC, differential, platelet count weekly; withhold drug if WBC is <2000/mm^3 or platelet count is <75,000/mm^3; notify prescriber of these results
- ⬄ Capillary leak syndrome including a drop in mean arterial pressure (2-12 hr after initiating therapy); hypotension and hypoperfusion will occur; if B/P <90 mm Hg, use CVP, ECG, VS
- Renal studies: BUN, serum uric acid, urine CCr, electrolytes before, during therapy; I&O ratio; report fall in urine output to <30 ml/hr
- Monitor temp q4h; fever may indicate beginning infection
- Hepatic studies before, during therapy: bilirubin, AST, ALT, alk phosphatase, LDH as needed or monthly
- ECG; ST-T wave changes, low QRS and T, possible dysrhythmias (sinus tachycardia, PVCs)
- ⬄ Baselines in pulmonary function; document FEV >2 L or ≥75% prior to therapy; check daily VS, pulse oximetry, dyspnea, rales, ABGs; watch for respiratory failure, intubate if necessary
- Stress thallium study prior to therapy; document normal ejection fraction, unimpaired wall motion
- Bleeding: hematuria, guaiac, bruising petechiae, mucosa or orifices q8h
- Buccal cavity q8h for dryness,

sores, ulceration, white patches, oral pain, bleeding, dysphagia
• Local irritation, pain, burning at inj site
• GI symptoms: frequency of stools, cramping; acidosis, signs of dehydration: rapid respirations, poor skin turgor, decreased urine output, dry skin, restlessness, weakness

Administer:

IV, Intermittent INF routes

• Hydrocortisone, dexamethasone or sodium bicarbonate (1 mEq/1 ml) for extravasation, apply ice compresses
• Antiemetic 30-60 min before giving drug to prevent vomiting
• IV after diluting 22 million international units (1.3 mg)/1.2 ml sterile H_2O for inj at site of vial and swirl, do not shake; dilute dose with 50 ml D_5W and give over 15 min; use plastic bag; do not use an in-line filter, give through Y-tube or 3-way stopcock
• Dopamine 1-5 kg/min before onset of hypotension; decreased dose preserves kidney output

Y-site compatibilities: Amikacin, amphotericin B, calcium gluconate, diphenhydramine, DOPamine, fluconazole, foscarnet, gentamicin, heparin, IV fat emulsion, magnesium sulfate, metoclopramide, morphine, ondansetron, piperacillin, potassium chloride, ranitidine, ticarcillin, tobramycin, TPN #145, trimethoprim-sulfamethoxazole

Perform/provide:

• Liquid diet: carbonated beverage, gelatin (Jell-O) may be added if patient is not nauseated or vomiting
• Rinsing of mouth tid-qid with water, club soda; brushing of teeth bid-tid with soft brush or cotton-tipped applicators for stomatitis; use unwaxed dental floss
• Storage in refrigerator of diluted drug; do not freeze; administer within 48 hr; bring to room temperature before infusing; discard unused portion

Evaluate:

• Therapeutic response: decreased tumor size, spread of malignancy

Teach patient/family:

• To use a nonhormonal contraceptive method during therapy
• To report any complaints, side effects to nurse or prescriber
• To avoid foods with citric acid, hot or rough texture
• To avoid alcohol, NSAIDs, salicylates; GI bleeding may occur
• To report any bleeding, white spots, ulcerations in mouth to prescriber; tell patient to examine mouth qd
• To avoid crowds and persons with infections when granulocyte count is low
• Visual problems may occur, but are reversible

alefacept

See appendix a—selected new drugs

alemtuzumab (℞)

(al-em-tuz′uh-mab)

Campath

Func. class.: Misc. antineoplastic

Chem. class.: Monoclonal antibody

Action: Composed of recombinant DNA-derived humanized monoclonal antibody (campath-1H), binds to CD52 antigen that is present on surface of B and T lymphocytes, causes lysis of leukemic cells

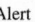

Uses: B-cell chronic lymphocytic leukemia that has been treated with alkylating agents

Dosage and routes:

• *Adult:* **IV** 3 mg over 2 hr daily; when tolerated, increase to 10 mg; when 10 mg tolerated increase to 30 mg qd, maintenance is 30 mg/day 3×/wk on alternate days

Available forms: Sol for inj 30 mg/ 3 ml

Side effects/adverse reactions:

CNS: Dizziness, insomnia, depression, headache, tremor, somnolence, fatigue

CV: Hypotension, tachycardia, hypertension, edema, chest pain, supraventricular tachycardia

GI: Anorexia, diarrhea, constipation, *nausea, stomatitis, vomiting, abdominal pain, dyspepsia*

HEMA: ***Anemia, neutropenia, thrombocytopenia, pancytopenia,*** purpura, epistaxis

INTEG: Rash, local reaction, pruritus

META: Hypokalemia, hypomagnesemia

MISC: Rigors, fever

RESP: Cough, pneumonia, rhinitis, ***bronchospasm***, dyspnea, pharyngitis

Contraindications: Hypersensitivity, active systemic infection, immunodeficiency

Precautions: Pregnancy (C), lactation, children

Pharmacokinetics: Steady state 6 wk

Interactions:

• Do not give live virus vaccines

Lab test interferences:

• *Interference:* Diagnostic tests using antibodies

NURSING CONSIDERATIONS

Assess:

• CBC, platelets qwk or more often if myelosuppression occurs; $CD4^+$ after therapy until recovery of >200 cells/μl

• For symptoms of infection; chills, fever, headache, may be masked by drug fever; do not administer drug if infection is present

• CNS reaction: LOC, mental status, dizziness, confusion

• Cardiac status: lung sounds; ECG before and during treatment, especially in those with cardiac disease

• Bone marrow depression: bruising, bleeding, blood in stools, urine, sputum, emesis

Administer:

IV route

• Do not give IV push or bolus

• Withdraw amount needed, use 5 μm filter before dilution, check for particulate matter and discoloration; inject into 100 ml sterile 0.9% NaCl or D_5W, invert to mix; do not add other drugs or infuse in same IV tubing

• Do not shake ampule

Perform/provide:

• Storage of reconstituted sol for ≤8 hr at room temperature, do not freeze; protect from light

Evaluate:

• Therapeutic response: decrease in production of malignant lymphocytes

Teach patient/family:

• To take acetaminophen for fever

• To avoid hazardous tasks, because confusion, dizziness may occur

• To report signs of infection: sore throat, fever, diarrhea, vomiting

• To avoid breastfeeding, effects are unknown, do not resume for ≥3 mo after last dose

alendronate (℞)

(al-en-drone′ate)

Fosamax

Func. class.: Bone-resorption inhibitor

Chem. class.: Biphosphonate

Action: Absorbs calcium phosphate crystal in bone and may directly block dissolution of hydroxyapatite crystals of bone; inhibits normal and abnormal bone resorption, mineralization

Uses: Treatment and prevention of osteoporosis in postmenopausal women, treatment of osteoporosis in men, Paget's disease, treatment of corticosteroid-induced osteoporosis in postmenopausal women not receiving estrogen and men who are on continuing corticosteroid treatment with low bone mass

Dosage and routes:

Osteoporosis in postmenopausal women

• *Adult and elderly:* **PO** 10 mg qd or 70 mg qwk

Paget's disease

• *Adult and elderly:* **PO** 40 mg qd × 6 mo, consider retreatment for relapse

Prevention of osteoporosis

• *Adult:* **PO** 5 mg qd or 35 mg qwk

Corticosteroid-induced osteoporosis in postmenopausal women (not receiving estrogen)

• *Adult:* **PO** 10 mg qd

Corticosteroid-induced osteoporosis in men or premenopausal women

• *Adult:* **PO** 5 mg qd

Available forms: Tabs 5, 10, 35, 40, 70 mg

Side effects/adverse reactions:

CNS: Headache

META: Anemia, hypokalemia, hypomagnesemia, hypophosphatemia

GI: Abdominal pain, anorexia, constipation, nausea, vomiting, esophageal ulceration

MS: Bone pain

Contraindications: Hypersensitivity to biphosphonates, delayed esophageal emptying, inability to sit or stand for 30 min

Precautions: Children, lactation, pregnancy (C), CCr <35 ml/min, esophageal disease, ulcers, gastritis

Do not confuse:

Fosamax/Flomax

Pharmacokinetics: Rapidly cleared from circulation, taken up mainly by bones, eliminated primarily through kidneys

Interactions:

• ↓ absorption: antacids, calcium supplements

• Possible GI reactions: NSAIDs, salicylates

• ↑ alendronate effect: ranitidine

• Drug/food: ↓ absorption when used with caffeine, orange juice

NURSING CONSIDERATIONS

Assess:

• For osteoporosis: bone density test

• For Paget's disease: increased skull size, bone pain, headache

• Electrolytes; renal function studies; Ca, P, Mg, K

• For hypercalcemia: paresthesia, twitching, laryngospasm, Chvostek's, Trousseau's signs

• Alk phosphatase levels, baseline and periodically, 2 × upper limit of normal are indicative of Paget's disease

Administer:

PO route

• For 6 months to be effective in Paget's disease; take with 8 oz of water 30 min before 1st food, beverage, or medication of the day

Perform/provide:

• Storage in cool environment, out of direct sunlight

A

Evaluate:
• Therapeutic response: increased bone mass, absence of fractures

Teach patient/family:
• To remain upright for 30 min after dose to prevent esophageal irritation, if dose is missed, skip dose, do not double doses or take later in day
• To take in AM before food, other meds, take with 6-8 oz of water only (no mineral water)
• To take calcium, vit D if instructed by health care provider
• To use weight-bearing exercise to increase bone density
• To let health care provider know if pregnant or if pregnancy is planned or if nursing

RARELY USED

alfentanil (℞)

(al-fen'ta-nil)
Alfenta, Rapifen✤
Func. class.: Opioid analgesic

Controlled Substance Schedule II
Uses: In combination with other drugs in general anesthesia, as a primary anesthetic in general surgery, monitored anesthesia care (MAC)
Dosage and routes:
Anesthesia <30 min
Combination
• *Adult:* **IV** 8-50 mcg/kg, may increase by 3-15 mcg/kg
Anesthetic induction
• *Adult:* **IV** 3-5 mcg/kg, then 0.5-1.5 mcg/kg/min; total dose is 8-40 mcg/kg
Anesthesia 30-60 min
Induction
• *Adult:* **IV** 20-50 mcg/kg
Maintenance
• *Adult:* **IV** 5-15 mcg/kg; may give up to 75 mcg/kg total dose
Continuous anesthesia >45 min
Induction
• *Adult:* **IV** 50-75 mcg/kg
Maintenance
• *Adult:* **IV** 0.5-3.0 mcg/kg/min; rate should be decreased by 30%-50% after 1 hr maintenance **INF;** may be increased to 4 mcg/kg/min or **BOL** doses of 7 mcg/kg
Induction of anesthesia >45 min
• *Adult:* **IV** 130-245 mcg/kg, then 0.5-1.5 mcg/kg/min
MAC
Induction
• *Adult:* **IV** duration ≤½ hr 3-8 mcg/kg
Maintenance
• *Adult:* 3-5 mcg/kg q5-20 min to 1 mcg/kg/min, total dose 3-40 mcg/kg
Contraindications: Child <12 yr, hypersensitivity

alitretinoin (℞)

(a-li-tret'i-noyn)
Panretin
Func. class.: Retinoid, 2nd generation

Action: Controls cellular differentiation and proliferation of neoplastic and healthy cells by binding to retinoid receptors
Uses: Kaposi's sarcoma cutaneous lesions
Dosage and routes:
• *Adult:* **TOP** Apply enough gel to cover lesions with a generous coating, allow to dry for 3-5 min, before covering with clothing, do not apply near mucosal areas, apply as long as benefit occurs
Available forms: Gel 0.1%
Side effects/adverse reactions:
INTEG: Rash, stinging, warmth, redness, erythema, blistering, crusting, peeling, contact dermatitis, *pain*
Contraindications: Hypersensitivity to retinoids, pregnancy (D)

Precautions: Lactation, eczema, sunburn, elderly, cutaneous T-cell lymphoma

Pharmacokinetics:

TOP: Poor systemic absorption

Interactions:

• Do not use around DEET (an insect repellant agent)

NURSING CONSIDERATIONS

Assess:

• Area of body involved, what helps or aggravates condition; cysts, dryness, itching; lesions may worsen at beginning of treatment

• Dermal toxicity that may start as erythema, then edema, may need to be discontinued and restarted

Administer:

• Bid initially to lesions, can be increased to tid-qid according to tolerance

Perform/provide:

• Storage at room temperature

• Hand washing after application

Evaluate:

• Therapeutic response: decrease in size and number of lesions

Teach patient/family:

• To avoid application on normal skin, getting cream in eyes, nose, other mucous membranes

• To avoid sunlight, sunlamps, or use protective clothing, sunscreen

• That treatment may cause warmth, stinging, dryness, peeling will occur

• That drug does not cure condition; only relieves symptoms

• That therapeutic results may be seen in 2-3 wk but may not be optimal until after 6 wk

allopurinol (℞)

(al-oh-pure'i-nole)

Alloprim, allopurinol, Apo-Allopurinol✱, Lopurin✱, Purimol✱, Zyloprim

Func. class.: Antigout drug

Chem. class.: Xanthene oxidase inhibitor

Action: Inhibits the enzyme xanthine oxidase, reducing uric acid synthesis

Uses: Chronic gout, hyperuricemia associated with malignancies, recurrent calcium oxalate calculi, Chagas' disease, cutaneous/visceral leishmaniasis

Investigational uses: Stomatitis (mouthwash)

Dosage and routes:

Increased uric acid levels in malignancies

• *Adult:* **IV INF** 200-400 mg/m^2/day, max 600 mg/day

• *Child:* **IV INF** 200 mg/m^2/day, initially

Gout/hyperuricemia

• *Adult:* **PO** 200-600 mg qd depending on severity, not to exceed 800 mg/day

• *Child 6-10 yr:* 300 mg qd

• *Child <6 yr:* 150 mg qd

Impaired renal function

• *Adult:* **PO** 200 mg qd (CCr is 20 to 30 ml/min); 100 mg qd (CCr <20 ml/min); **IV** CCr 10-20 ml/min 200 mg/day; CCr 3-10 ml/min 100 mg/day; CCr <3 ml/min 100 mg/day at intervals

Recurrent calculi

• *Adult:* **PO** 200-300 mg qd

Uric acid nephropathy prevention

• *Adult and child >10 yr:* **PO** 600-800 mg qd × 2-3 days

Stomatitis

• *Adult:* Mouthwash dose varies, do not swallow

Available forms: Tabs, scored 100, 300 mg; inj 500 mg/vial

Side effects/adverse reactions:

HEMA: ***Agranulocytosis, thrombocytopenia, aplastic anemia, pancytopenia, leukopenia, bone marrow suppression, eosinophilia***

CNS: Headache, drowsiness, neuritis, paresthesia

GI: Nausea, vomiting, anorexia, malaise, metallic taste, cramps, peptic ulcer, diarrhea, stomatitis

MISC: Myopathy, arthralgia, hepatomegaly, ***cholestatic jaundice, renal failure, exfoliative dermatitis***

EENT: Retinopathy, cataracts, epistaxis

INTEG: Fever, chills, dermatitis, pruritus, purpura, erythema, ecchymosis, alopecia

Contraindications: Hypersensitivity

Precautions: Pregnancy (C), lactation, renal disease, hepatic disease, children

Do not confuse:

allopurinol/apresoline

Lopurin/Lupron

Pharmacokinetics:

PO: Peak 2-4 hr; excreted in feces, urine; half-life 2-3 hr, terminal half-life 18-30 hr

IV: Half-life 1 hr

Interactions:

- ↑ action of oral anticoagulants, chlorpropamide, cyclophosphamide, hydantoin, theophylline, vidarabine, ACE inhibitors, mercaptopurine azathioprine
- Possible kidney stone formation: ammonium chloride, vit C, potassium/sodium phosphate
- ↓ effects of probenecid
- Rash: ampicillin, amoxicillin, bacampicillin
- ↑ allopurinol toxicity: thiazide diuretics
- ↓ effects of allopurinol: aluminum salts
- ↑ bone marrow depression: antineoplastics

NURSING CONSIDERATIONS

Assess:

- Uric acid levels q2wk; uric acid levels should be 6 mg/dl or less
- CBC, AST, BUN, creatinine before starting treatment, monthly
- I&O ratio; increase fluids to 2 L/day to prevent stone formation
- Nutritional status: discourage organ meat, sardines, salmon, legumes, gravies (high-purine foods), alcohol

Administer:

PO route

- With meals, to prevent GI symptoms
- A few days before antineoplastic therapy

IV INF route

- Reconstitute of 30 ml vial with 25 ml of sterile water for inj; dilute to desired conc with 0.9% NaCl for inj or D_5 for inj, begin inf within 10 hr

Solution incompatibilities: Amikacin, amphotericin B, carmustine, cefotaxime, chlorproMAZINE, cimetidine, clindamycin, cytarabine, dacarbazine, DAUNOrubicin, diphenhydrAMINE, DOXOrubicin, doxycycline, droperidol, floxuridine, gentamicin, haloperidol, hydrOXYzine, idarubicin, imipenem, cilastatin, mechlorethamine, meperidine, metoclopramide, methylPREDNISolone, minocycline, nalbuphine, netilmicin, ondansetron, prochlorperazine, promethazine, sodium bicarbonate, streptozocin, tobramycin, vinorelbine

Evaluate:

- Therapeutic response: decreased pain in joints, decreased stone formation in kidneys

Teach patient/family:

- That tabs may be crushed
- To take as prescribed; if dose is

missed, take as soon as remembered; do not double dose
• To increase fluid intake to 2 L/day
• To report skin rash, stomatitis, malaise, fever, aching; drug should be discontinued
• To avoid hazardous activities if drowsiness or dizziness occurs
• To avoid alcohol, caffeine; will increase uric acid levels
• To avoid large doses of vit C; kidney stone formation may occur
• To maintain a diet enhancing urine alkalinity (e.g., dairy products)
• To reduce dairy products, refined sugars, sodium, meat if taking for calcium oxalate stones

almotriptan (℞)

(al-moh-trip'tan)
Axert
Func. class.: Antimigraine agent
Chem. class.: 5-HT_1-Receptor agonist

Action: Binds selectively to the vascular 5-HT_1-receptor subtype, exerts antimigraine effect; causes vasoconstriction in cranial arteries
Uses: Acute treatment of migraine with or without aura
Dosage and routes:
• *Adult:* **PO** may use the 6.25-mg dose initially, but 12.5 mg is more effective; may repeat dose after 2 hr; do not give more than 2 doses/ 24 hr
Hepatic/renal dose
• *Adult:* **PO** 6.25 mg initially, max 12.5 mg
Available forms: Tabs 6.25, 12.5 mg
Side effects/adverse reactions:
CV: Flushing, palpitations, tachycardia, ***coronary artery vasospasm, MI, ventricular fibrillation, ventricular tachycardia***
EENT: Throat, mouth, nasal discomfort; vision changes
GI: Abdominal discomfort
INTEG: Sweating
MS: Weakness, neck stiffness, myalgia
NEURO: Tingling, hot sensation, burning, feeling of pressure, tightness, numbness, dizziness, sedation, headache, anxiety, fatigue, cold sensation
RESP: Chest tightness, pressure
Contraindications: Concurrent use of ergotamine-containing preparations, uncontrolled hypertension, hypersensitivity, basilar or hemiplegic migraine; concurrent MAO inhibitor therapy or within 2 wk
Precautions: Postmenopausal women, men >40 yr, risk factors for CAD, hypercholesterolemia, obesity, diabetes, impaired hepatic or renal function, pregnancy (C), lactation, children, elderly
Pharmacokinetics: Onset of pain relief 2 hr, peak 1-3 hr, duration 3-4 hr; metabolized in the liver (metabolite), metabolized by MAO-A, CYP2D6, CYP3A4; excreted in urine, feces, half-life 3-4 hr
Interactions:
• Extended vasospastic effects: ergot, ergot derivatives, other 5-HT_1 agonists
• ↑ almotriptan effect: MAOIs, CYP2D6 inhibitors
• ↑ plasma concentration of almotriptan: ketoconazole
↑ almotriptan effect: butterbur

NURSING CONSIDERATIONS
Assess:
• B/P; signs/symptoms of coronary vasospasms
• Tingling, hot sensation, burning, feeling of pressure, numbness, flushing
• For stress level, activity, recreation, coping mechanisms
• Neurologic status: LOC, blurring

vision, nausea, vomiting, tingling in extremities preceding headache
• Ingestion of tyramine foods (pickled products, beer, wine, aged cheese), food additives, preservatives, colorings, artificial sweeteners, chocolate, caffeine, which may precipitate these types of headaches

Administer:

⊘ PO, swallow whole

Perform/provide:

• Quiet, calm environment with decreased stimulation from noise, bright light, excessive talking

Evaluate:

• Therapeutic response: decrease in severity of migraine

Teach patient/family:

• To report chest pain, drowsiness, dizziness, tingling, flushing, pressure
• To use contraception while taking drug, notify prescriber if pregnancy is planned or suspected, avoid breastfeeding
• To provide dark, quiet environment
• That drug does not prevent or reduce number of migraine attacks

alprazolam (℞)

(al-pray′zoe-lam)

Apo-Alpraz✤, Novo-Alprazol✤, Nu-Alpraz✤, Xanax

Func. class.: Antianxiety

Chem. class.: Benzodiazepine

Controlled Substance Schedule IV

Action: Depresses subcortical levels of CNS, including limbic system, reticular formation

Uses: Anxiety, panic disorders, anxiety with depressive symptoms

Investigational uses: Depression, social phobia, premenstrual dysphoric disorders

Dosage and routes:

Anxiety disorder

• *Adult:* **PO** 0.25-0.5 mg tid, not to exceed 4 mg/day in divided doses
• *Elderly:* **PO** 0.125-0.25 mg bid; increase by 0.125 as needed

Panic disorder

• *Adult:* **PO** 0.5 mg tid may increase, max 10 mg/day

Premenstrual dysphoric disorders

• *Adult:* **PO** 0.25 mg bid-qid, starting on day 16-18 of menses, taper over 2-3 days when menses occurs

Social phobia

• *Adult:* **PO** 2-8 mg/day

Hepatic dose

Reduce dose by 50%

Available forms: Tabs 0.25, 0.5, 1, 2 mg; oral sol 0.1, 1 mg/ml

Side effects/adverse reactions:

CNS: Dizziness, drowsiness, confusion, headache, anxiety, tremors, stimulation, fatigue, depression, insomnia, hallucinations

GI: Constipation, dry mouth, nausea, vomiting, anorexia, diarrhea

INTEG: Rash, dermatitis, itching

CV: Orthostatic hypotension, ***ECG changes, tachycardia,*** hypotension

EENT: Blurred vision, tinnitus, mydriasis

Contraindications: Hypersensitivity to benzodiazepines, narrow-angle glaucoma, psychosis, pregnancy (D), lactation, addiction

Precautions: Elderly, debilitated, hepatic disease

Do not confuse:

alprazolam/lorazepam
Xanax/Lanoxin
Xanax/Tylox
Xanax/Zantac

Pharmacokinetics:

PO: Onset 30 min, peak 1-2 hr, duration 4-6 hr, therapeutic response 2-3 days; metabolized by liver, excreted by kidneys; crosses placenta, breast milk; half-life 12-15 hr

Interactions:

- ↓ sedation: xanthines
- ↓ alprazolam action: barbiturates, rifampin
- A substrate of CYP 3A4
- ↑ alprazolam action: cimetidine, disulfiram, erythromycin, fluoxetine, isoniazid, ketoconazole, metoprolol, propoxyphene, propanolol, valproic acid
- ↑ CNS depression: anticonvulsants, alcohol, antihistamines, sedative/hypnotics
- ↓ action of levodopa
- Drug/food: ↑ drug level; grapefruit juice

↑ CNS depression: cat's claw, chamomile, cowslip, echinacea, goldenseal, hops, kava, licorice, Queen Anne's lace, skullcap, St. John's wort, valerian, wild cherry

Lab test interferences:

Increase: AST/ALT, alk phosphatase

NURSING CONSIDERATIONS

Assess:

- Mental status: anxiety, mood, sensorium, affect, sleeping pattern, drowsiness, dizziness, especially in elderly
- B/P lying, standing; pulse; if systolic B/P drops 20 mm Hg, hold drug, notify prescriber
- Hepatic, blood studies: AST, ALT, bilirubin, creatinine, LDH, alk phosphatase, CBC; may cause neutropenia, decreased Hct, increased LFTs
- For indications of increasing tolerance and abuse

Physical dependency, withdrawal symptoms: anxiety, panic attacks, agitation, convulsions, headache, nausea, vomiting, muscle pain, weakness; withdrawal seizures may occur after rapid decrease in dose or abrupt discontinuation; since duration of action is short, considered to be the drug of choice in the elderly

Administer:

PO route

- With food or milk for GI symptoms
- Crushed, mixed with food or fluids if patient is unable to swallow medication whole
- May divide total daily doses into more times/day, if anxiety occurs between doses

Evaluate:

- Therapeutic response: decreased anxiety, restlessness, sleeplessness

Teach patient/family:

- Not to double doses; take exactly as prescribed; if dose is missed, take within 1 hr as scheduled
- That drug may be taken with food
- Not to use for everyday stress or longer than 4 mo unless directed by prescriber; not to take more than prescribed amount; may be habit forming; memory impairment is a sign of long-term use
- To avoid OTC preparations unless approved by prescriber
- To avoid driving, activities that require alertness, since drowsiness may occur
- To avoid alcohol ingestion or other psychotropic medications unless directed by prescriber
- Not to discontinue medication abruptly after long-term use
- To rise slowly or fainting may occur, especially elderly
- That drowsiness may worsen at beginning of treatment

Treatment of overdose: Lavage, VS, supportive care, flumazenil

A

RARELY USED

alprostadil (℞)

(al-pros'ta-dil)

Caverject, Edex, Muse, PGEI, prostaglandin E_1, Prostin VR♣, Prostin VR Pediatric

Func. class.: Hormone

Uses: To maintain patent ductus arteriosus (temporary treatment), erectile dysfunction

Dosage and routes:

Patent ductus arteriosus

• *Infants:* **IV INF** 0.1 mcg/kg/min, until desired response, then reduce to lowest effective amount, 0.4 mcg/kg/min not likely to produce greater beneficial effects

Erectile dysfunction of vasculogenic or mixed etiology, psychogenic

• *Men:* **INTRACAVERNOSAL** 2.5 mcg may increase by 2.5 mcg; may then increase by 5-10 mcg until adequate response occurs; **INTRAURETHRAL:** administer as needed to achieve erection

Contraindications: Hypersensitivity, respiratory distress syndrome (RDS)

HIGH ALERT

alteplase (℞)

(al-ti-plaze')

Activase, Activase rt-PA♣, Cathflo, Lysatec-rt-PA♣, tissue plasminogen activator, t-PA

Func. class.: Thrombolytic enzyme

Chem. class.: Tissue plasminogen activator (TPA)

Action: Produces fibrin conversion of plasminogen to plasmin; able to bind to fibrin, convert plasminogen in thrombus to plasmin, which leads to local fibrinolysis, limited systemic proteolysis

Uses: Lysis of obstructing thrombi associated with acute MI, ischemic conditions requiring thrombolysis (i.e., PE, DVT, unclotting arteriovenous shunts, acute ischemic CVA)

Investigational uses: Unstable angina, occluded central venous catheters

Dosage and routes:

Myocardial Infarction (Standard INF)

• *Adult >65 kg:* **IV** a total of 100 mg; 6-10 mg given **IV BOL** over 1-2 min, 60 mg given over 1st hr, 20 mg given over 2nd hr, 20 mg given over 3rd hr; or 1.25 mg/kg given over 3 hr for patients <65 kg

• *Adult <65 kg:* **IV** 0.75 mg over 1st hr, 0.075-0.125 mg/kg given **IV BOL** over 1st 1-2 min; 0.25 mg/kg over 2nd hr, 0.25 mg/kg over 3rd hr to a total dose of 1.25 mg/kg, max 100 mg total

Myocardial Infarction (Accelerated INF)

• *Adult:* **IV BOL** 15 mg; then 0.75 mg/kg over ½ hr; then 0.5 mg/kg over 1 hr, usually given with heparin

Pulmonary embolism

• *Adult:* **IV** 100 mg over 2 hr, then heparin

Acute ischemic stroke

• *Adult:* **IV** 0.9 mg/kg, max 90 mg; give as **INF** over 1 hr, give 10% of dose **IV BOL** over 1st min

Occluded central venous catheters

• *Adult:* 2 mg/2 ml infused in each port of dual-lumen catheter, dwell time varies widely

Available forms: Powder for inj 50 mg (29 million international units/vial), 100 mg (58 million international units/vial)

Side effects/adverse reactions:
SYST: ***GI, GU, intracranial, retroperitoneal bleeding,*** *surface bleeding,* ***anaphylaxis***
CV: ***Sinus bradycardia, ventricular tachycardia, accelerated idioventricular rhythm, bradycardia***
INTEG: Urticaria, rash

Contraindications: Hypersensitivity, active internal bleeding, recent CVA, severe uncontrolled hypertension, intracranial/intraspinal surgery/trauma, aneurysm

Precautions: Pregnancy (C), lactation, children, elderly, neurological deficits

Do not confuse:
alteplace/Altace

Pharmacokinetics: Cleared by liver, 80% cleared within 10 min of drug termination, onset immediate, peak 45 min, duration 4 hr, half-life 35 min

Interactions:
- ↑ bleeding: anticoagulants, salicylates, dipyridamole, other NSAIDs, abciximab, eptifibatide, tirofiban, clopidogrel, ticlopidine, some cephalosporins, plicamycin, valproic acid

Herb: ↑ risk of bleeding: agrimony, alfalfa, angelica, anise, basil, bay, bilberry, black haw, bogbean, bromelain, buchu, chondroitin, cinchona bark, dong quai, fenugreek, feverfew, garlic, ginger, ginkgo, ginseng, horse chestnut, Irish moss, kelp, kelpware, khella, lovage, lungwort, meadowsweet, mother wort, mugwort, nettle, papaya, parsley (large amts), Pau D'arco, pineapple, poplar, prickly ash, safflower, saw palmetto, tonka bean, tumeric, wintergreen, yarrow

Herb: ↓ anticoagulant effect: chamomile, coenzyme Q10, flax, glucomannan, goldenseal, guar gum

Lab test interferences:
Increase: PT, APTT, TT

NURSING CONSIDERATIONS

Assess:
- VS, B/P, pulse, respirations, neurologic signs, temperature at least q4h; temp >104° F (40° C) indicates internal bleeding; monitor rhythm closely; ventricular dysrhythmias may occur with hyperfusion; monitor heart, breath sounds, neurologic status, peripheral pulses; assess neurologic status, neurologic change may indicate intracranial bleeding

Alert: For bleeding during first hour of treatment and 24 hr after procedure: hematuria, hematemesis, bleeding from mucous membranes, epistaxis, ecchymosis; guaiac all body fluids, stools. Do not use 150 mg or more total dose; intracranial bleeding may occur

Alert: Hypersensitivity: fever, rash, itching, chills, facial swelling, dyspnea, notify prescriber immediately; stop drug, keep resusciatative equipment nearby; mild reaction may be treated with antihistamines

- Blood studies (Hct, platelets, PTT, PT, TT, APTT) before starting therapy; PT or APTT must be less than 2 × control before starting therapy TT or PT q3-4h during treatment
- ECG continuously, cardiac enzymes, radionuclide myocardial scanning/coronary angiography

Administer:

Intermittent IV INF route
- After reconstituting with provided diluent, add appropriate amount of sterile water for inj (no preservatives) 20 mg vial/20 ml or 50 mg vial/50 ml to make 1 mg/ml, mix by slow inversion or dilute with NaCl, D_5W to a concentration of 0.5 mg/ml; 1.5 to <0.5 mg/ml may result in precipitation of drug; use 18 G needle; flush line with NaCl after administration, give over 3 hr for MI, 2 hr for pulmonary embolism

• Heparin therapy after thrombolytic therapy is discontinued, TT, ACT, or APTT less than 2 × control (about 3-4 hr)
• Reconstituted IV solution within 8 hr or discard
• Within 6 hr of coronary occlusion for best results

Additive compatibilities: Lidocaine, morphine, nitroglycerin

Y-site compatibilities: Lidocaine, metoprolol, propranolol

Perform/provide:
• Avoidance of invasive procedures, injection, rectal temp
• Pressure for 30 sec to minor bleeding sites; 30 min to sites of atrial puncture, followed by pressure dressing; inform prescriber if this does not attain hemostasis; apply pressure dressing
• Storage of powder at room temperature or refrigerate; protect from excessive light

Evaluate:
• Therapeutic response: lysis of thrombi

Teach patient/family:
• The purpose and expected results of the treatment; to report adverse reactions

RARELY USED

altretamine (℞)

(al-tret′a-meen)

Hexalen, hexamethylmelamine, Hexastat✤

Func. class.: Misc. antineoplastic

Uses: Palliative treatment of recurrent, persistent ovarian cancer following first-line treatment with cisplatin or alkylating agent–based combination

Dosage and routes:
• *Adult:* **PO** 260 mg/m²/day for 14 or 21 days in a 28-day cycle; give in 4 divided doses after meals and at hs

Contraindications: Hypersensitivity, severe bone marrow depression, severe neurologic toxicity, pregnancy (D)

aluminum hydroxide (OTC)

AlternaGEL, Alu-Cap, Alugel✤, Aluminet, aluminum hydroxide, Alu-Tab, Amphojel, Basal gel, Dialume

Func. class.: Antacid, hypophosphatemic, antiulcer

Chem. class.: Aluminum product, phosphate binder

Action: Neutralizes gastric acidity, binds phosphates in GI tract; these phosphates are excreted

Uses: Antacid, hyperphosphatemia in chronic renal failure; adjunct in gastric, peptic, duodenal ulcers; hyperacidity, reflux esophagitis, heartburn, stress ulcer prevention in critically ill, GERD

Investigational uses: GI bleeding

Dosage and routes:

Antacid
• *Adult:* **SUSP** 5-10 ml 1 hr pc, hs; **PO** 600 mg 1 hr pc, hs, chewed with milk or water

Hyperphosphatemia in renal failure
• *Adult:* **SUSP** 500 mg-2 g bid-qid

GI bleeding
• *Infant:* 2-5 ml/dose q1-2h
• *Child:* **PO** 5-15 ml/dose q1-2h

Available forms: Caps 475, 500 mg; tabs 300, 500, 600 mg; susp 320 mg/5 ml, 450 mg/5 ml, 600 mg/5 ml, 675 mg/5 ml

Side effects/adverse reactions:
GI: Constipation, anorexia, ***obstruction,*** fecal impaction
META: Hypophosphatemia, hypercalciuria

Contraindications: Hypersensitivity to this drug or aluminum products

Precautions: Elderly, fluid restriction, decreased GI motility, GI obstruction, dehydration, renal disease, sodium-restricted diets, pregnancy (C), lactation

Pharmacokinetics:
PO: Onset 20-40 min, duration 1-3 hr, excreted in feces

Interactions:
• ↓ effectiveness of allopurinol, amprenavir, cephalosporins, ciprofloxacin, corticosteroids, delavirdine, diflunisal, digitalis, gabapentin, gatifloxacin, H_2-antagonists, iron salts, isoniazid, ketoconazole, penicillamine, phenothiazines, phenytoin, quinidine, tetracyclines, thyroid hormones, ticlopidine anticholinergics, warfarin; separate by at least 2 hr
↓ action of buckthorn, cascara sagrada, castor, Chinese rhubarb

NURSING CONSIDERATIONS
Assess:
• Pain: location, intensity, duration, character
• Phosphate levels, since drug is bound in GI system
• Hypophosphatemia: anorexia, weakness, fatigue, bone pain, hyporeflexia
• Constipation; increase bulk in diet if needed
• Urinary pH, Ca^{++}, electrolytes

Administer:
• 2 tsp (10 ml) will neutralize 20 mEq of acid; 2 tabs will neutralize 16 mEq of acid

PO route
• Give with 8 oz water for hyperphosphatemia, unless contraindicated
• Tablets must be chewed well, then give 8 oz water
• Laxatives or stool softeners if constipation occurs, especially elderly
• After shaking liquid
• With small amount of water or milk

NG route
• By nasogastric tube if patient unable to swallow

Evaluate:
• Therapeutic response: absence of pain, decreased acidity, healed ulcers

Teach patient/family:
• To increase fluids to 2 L/day unless contraindicated; measures to prevent constipation
• To avoid phosphate foods (most dairy products, eggs, fruits, carbonated beverages) during drug therapy for hyperphosphatemia
• Not to use for prolonged periods in patients with low serum phosphate or if on a low-sodium diet
• To add cheese, corn, pasta, plums, prunes, lentils after drug is discontinued
• That stools may appear white or speckled
• To check with prescriber after 2 wk of self-prescribed antacid use
• To separate other medications by 2 hr

amantadine (℞)

(a-man'ta-deen)
amantadine HCl, Symadine, Symmetrel
Func. class.: Antiviral, antiparkinsonian agent
Chem. class.: Tricyclic amine

Action: Prevents uncoating of nucleic acid in viral cell, preventing penetration of virus to host; causes release of dopamine from neurons

Uses: Prophylaxis or treatment of influenza type A, extrapyramidal reactions, parkinsonism, respiratory tract infections

Investigational uses: Neuroleptic malignant syndrome, cocaine dependency, enuresis

Dosage and routes:

Influenza type A

- *Adult and child >12 yr:* **PO** 200 mg/day in single dose or divided bid
- *Child 9-12 yr:* **PO** 100 mg bid
- *Child 1-9 yr:* **PO** 4.4-8.8 mg/kg/day divided bid-tid, not to exceed 200 mg/day

Extrapyramidal reaction/parkinsonism

- *Adult:* **PO** 100 mg bid, up to 400 mg/day in EPS; give for 1 wk, then 100 mg as needed up to 400 mg in parkinsonism; CCr 40-50 ml/min 100 mg/day; CCr 30 ml/min 200 mg 2×/wk; CCr 20 ml/min 100 mg 3×/wk; CCr <10 ml/min 100 mg alternating with 200 mg q7days

Available forms: Caps 100 mg; syr 50 mg/5 ml

Side effects/adverse reactions:

CNS: Headache, dizziness, drowsiness, fatigue, *anxiety,* psychosis, *depression, hallucinations,* tremors, ***convulsions***, confusion, *insomnia*

CV: Orthostatic hypotension, ***CHF***

INTEG: Photosensitivity, dermatitis

EENT: Blurred vision

HEMA: ***Leukopenia***

GI: Nausea, vomiting, constipation, dry mouth

GU: Frequency, retention

Contraindications: Hypersensitivity, lactation, child <1 yr, eczematic rash

Precautions: Epilepsy, CHF, orthostatic hypotension, psychiatric disorders, hepatic disease, renal disease, peripheral edema, elderly, pregnancy (C)

Do not confuse:

amantadine/ranitidine

amantadine/rimantidine

Symmetrel/Synthroid

Pharmacokinetics:

PO: Onset 48 hr, half-life 24 hr, not metabolized, excreted in urine (90%) unchanged, crosses placenta, excreted in breast milk

Interactions:

- ↑ anticholinergic response: atropine, other anticholinergics
- ↑ CNS stimulation: CNS stimulants
- ↓ renal excretion of amantadine: triamterene, hydrochlorothiazide

↑ anticholinergic effect: belladonna, henbane

↑ action/side effects: pheasant's eye, quinine, scopolia root

↓ effect: kava

NURSING CONSIDERATIONS

Assess:

- I&O ratio; report frequency, hesitancy
- CHF, confusion, mottling of skin
- Bowel pattern before, during treatment
- Skin eruptions, photosensitivity after administration of drug
- Respiratory status: rate, character, wheezing, tightness in chest
- Allergies before initiation of treatment, reaction of each medication
- Signs of infection

Administer:

- Before exposure to influenza; continue for 10 days after contact
- At least 4 hr before hs to prevent insomnia
- After meals for better absorption, to decrease GI symptoms
- In divided doses to prevent CNS disturbances: headache, dizziness, fatigue, drowsiness

Perform/provide:

- Storage in tight, dry container

Evaluate:
• Therapeutic response: absence of fever, malaise, cough, dyspnea in infection; tremors, shuffling gait in Parkinson's disease
Teach patient/family:
• To change body position slowly to prevent orthostatic hypotension
• About aspects of drug therapy: need to report dyspnea, weight gain, dizziness, poor concentration, dysuria, behavioral changes
• To avoid hazardous activities if dizziness, blurred vision occurs
• To take drug exactly as prescribed; parkinsonian crisis may occur if drug is discontinued abruptly; do not double dose; if a dose is missed, do not take within 4 hr of next dose; caps may be opened and mixed with food
• To avoid alcohol
Treatment of overdose: Withdraw drug, maintain airway, administer epINEPHrine, aminophylline, O_2, IV corticosteroids, physostigmine

amcinonide topical
See appendix c

amifostine (℞)
(a-mi-foss'teen)
Ethyol
Func. class.: Cytoprotective agent for cisplatin

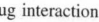

Action: Binds and detoxifies damaging metabolites of cisplatin by converting this drug by alk phosphatase in tissue to an active free thiol compound
Uses: Used to reduce renal toxicity when cisplatin is given in ovarian cancer; reduces xerostomia in radiation therapy for head, neck cancer
Dosage and routes:
Reduction of renal damage with cisplatin
• *Adult:* **IV** 910 mg/m^2 qd, within ½ hr before chemotherapy; may reduce dose to 740 mg/m^2 if higher dose is poorly tolerated
Xerostomia
• *Adult:* **IV** 200 mg/m^2 qd over 3 min as an infusion 15-30 min before radiation therapy
Available forms: Powder for inj 500 mg/vial with 500 mg mannitol
Side effects/adverse reactions:
CNS: Dizziness, somnolence
EENT: Sneezing
INTEG: Flushing, feeling of warmth
CV: Hypotension
GI: Nausea, vomiting, hiccups
MISC: Hypocalcemia, rash, chills
Contraindications: Hypersensitivity to mannitol, aminothiol; hypotension, dehydration, lactation
Precautions: Elderly, CV disease, pregnancy (C), children
Pharmacokinetics: Metabolized to free thiol compound, half-life 8 min, onset 5-8 min
Interactions:
• ↑ hypotension: antihypertensives
NURSING CONSIDERATIONS
Assess:
• For xerostomia: mouth lesions, dry mouth during therapy
• Fluid status before administration; administer antiemetic prior to administration to prevent severe nausea and vomiting; also, dexamethasone 20 mg IV and a serotonin antagonist such as ondansetron, dolasetron, or granisetron
• Calcium levels before and during treatment; calcium supplements may be given for hypocalcemia
• B/P prior to and q5min during infusion; if severe hypotension occurs, give IV 0.9% NaCl to expand fluid volume, place in Trendelenburg position

Administer:

Intermittent IV INF route

• Intermittent inf after reconstituting with 9.5 ml of sterile 0.9% NaCl, further dilute with 0.9% NaCl to a concentration of 5-40 mg/ml, give over 15 min within ½ hr of chemotherapy

Y-site compatibilities: Amikacin, aminophylline, ampicillin, ampicillin/sulbactam, aztreonam, bleomycin, bumetanide, buprenorphine, butorphanol, calcium gluconate, carboplatin, carmustine, cefazolin, cefonicid, cefotaxime, cefotetan, cefoxitin, ceftazidime, ceftizoxime, ceftriaxone, cefuroxime, cimetidine, ciprofloxacin, clindamycin, cyclophosphamide, cytarabine, dacarbazine, dactinomycin, DAUNOrubicin, dexamethasone, diphenhydrAMINE, DOBUTamine, DOPamine, DOXOrubicin, doxycycline, droperidol, enalaprilat, etoposide, famotidine, floxuridine, fluconazole, fludarabine, fluorouracil, furosemide, gallium, gentamicin, granisetron, haloperidol, heparin, hydrocortisone, hydromorphone, idarubicin, ifosfamide, imipenem-cilastatin, leucovorin, lorazepam, magnesium sulfate, mannitol, mechlorethamine, meperidine, mesna, methotrexate, methylPREDNISolone, metoclopramide, metronidazole, mezlocillin, mitomycin, mitoxantrone, morphine, nalbuphine, netilmicin, ondansetron, piperacillin, plicamycin, potassium chloride, promethazine, ranitidine, sodium bicarbonate, streptozocin, teniposide, thiotepa, ticarcillin, ticarcillin/clavulanate, tobramycin, trimethoprim-sulfamethoxazole, trimetrexate, vancomycin, vinBLAStine, vinCRIStine, zidovudine

Additive incompatibilities: Do not mix with other drugs or solutions

Evaluate:

• Therapeutic response: prevention of renal toxicity associated with cisplatin therapy; decreased xerostomia associated with radiation therapy of head, neck cancer

Teach patient/family:

• The reason for the medication and expected results; supine position during infusion

• That side effects may cause severe nausea, vomiting, decreased B/P, chills, dizziness, somnolence, hiccups, sneezing

amikacin (℞)

(am-i-kay′sin)

amikacin sulfate, Amikin

Func. class.: Antiinfective

Chem. class.: Aminoglycoside

Action: Interferes with protein synthesis in bacterial cell by binding to ribosomal subunit, which causes misreading of genetic code; inaccurate peptide sequence forms in protein chain, causing bacterial death

Uses: Severe systemic infections of CNS, respiratory, GI, urinary tract, bone, skin, soft tissues caused by *Staphylococcus, Pseudomonas aeruginosa, Escherichia coli, Enterobacter, Acinetobacter, Providencia, Citrobacter, Serratia, Proteus, Klebsiella* pneumonia

Investigational uses: *Mycobacterium avium* complex (intrathecal or intraventricular) in combination; aerosolization

Dosage and routes:

Severe systemic infections

• *Adult and child:* **IV INF** 15 mg/kg/day in 2-3 divided doses q8-12h in 100-200 ml D_5W over 30-60 min, not to exceed 1.5 g; decreased doses are needed in poor renal function as determined by blood levels, renal function studies; **IM** 15 mg/kg/day

in divided doses q8-12h; qd or extended interval dosing as an alternative dosing regimen
• *Infant:* **IV/IM** 10 mg/kg initially; then 7.5 mg/kg q12h
• *Neonate:* **IV/IM** 10 mg/kg, initially, 7.5 mg/kg q12h
• *Premature neonate:* 10 mg/kg initially, then 7.5 mg/kg q8-12h

Severe urinary tract infections
• *Adult:* **IM** 250 mg q12h

Renal dose
• *Adult:* **IV/IM** 7.5 mg/kg initially, then increased as determined by blood levels, renal function studies

Available forms: Inj 50, 250 mg/ml

Side effects/adverse reactions:
GU: ***Oliguria, hematuria, renal damage, azotemia, renal failure, nephrotoxicity***
CNS: Confusion, depression, numbness, tremors, ***convulsions,*** muscle twitching, ***neurotoxicity,*** dizziness, vertigo, tinnitus
EENT: ***Ototoxicity,*** deafness, visual disturbances
HEMA: ***Agranulocytosis, thrombocytopenia,*** leukopenia, eosinophilia, anemia
GI: Nausea, vomiting, anorexia; increased ALT, AST, bilirubin; hepatomegaly, ***hepatic necrosis,*** splenomegaly
CV: Hypotension or hypertension, palpitations
INTEG: Rash, burning, urticaria, dermatitis, alopecia

Contraindications: Mild to moderate infections, hypersensitivity to aminoglycosides, sulfites

Precautions: Neonates, mild renal disease, pregnancy (D), myasthenia gravis, lactation, hearing deficits, Parkinson's disease, elderly

Do not confuse:
Amikin/Amicar

Pharmacokinetics:
IM: Onset rapid, peak 1-2 hr
IV: Onset immediate, peak 15-30 min; plasma half-life 2-3 hr, prolonged up to 7 hr in infants; not metabolized, excreted unchanged in urine, crosses placental barrier, poor penetration into CSF, removed by hemodialysis

Interactions:
• ↑ neuromuscular blockade, respiratory depression: anesthetics, nondepolarizing neuromuscular blockers
• Inactivation of amikacin: parenteral penicillins, cephalosporins; do not use together
• May ↑ serum trough and peak: indomethacin
• Mask ototoxicity: dimenhydrinate, ethracrynic acid
• Nephrotoxicity: cephalosporins
Do not use acidophilus with anti-infectives
Toxicity: lysine (large amounts)

Lab test interferences:
Increase: BUN, ALT, AST, bilirubin, LDH, alk phosphatase, creatinine
Decrease: Ca, Na, K, Mg

NURSING CONSIDERATIONS

Assess:
• Weight before treatment; calculation of dosage is usually based on ideal body weight but may be calculated on actual body weight
• I&O ratio; urinalysis daily for proteinuria, cells, casts; report sudden change in urine output
• VS during infusion; watch for hypotension, change in pulse
• IV site for thrombophlebitis including pain, redness, swelling q30 min; change site if needed; apply warm compresses to discontinued site
• Serum peak, drawn at 30-60 min

after IV infusion or 60 min after IM injection, trough level drawn just before next dose; peak 20-30 mcg/ml, trough 4-8 mcg/ml; adjust dosage per levels

• Urine pH if drug is used for UTI; urine should be kept alkaline

• Renal impairment by securing urine for CCr, BUN, serum creatinine; lower dosage should be given in renal impairment (CCr <80 ml/min); nephrotoxicity may be reversible if drug stopped at first sign

Deafness by audiometric testing, ringing, roaring in ears, vertigo; assess hearing before, during, after treatment

• Dehydration: high specific gravity, decrease in skin turgor, dry mucous membranes, dark urine

• Overgrowth of infection, including increased temp, malaise, redness, pain, swelling, perineal itching, diarrhea, stomatitis, change in cough, sputum

• C&S before starting treatment to identify organism

• Vestibular dysfunction: nausea, vomiting, dizziness, headache; drug should be discontinued if severe

• Inj sites for redness, swelling, abscesses; use warm compresses at site

Administer:

IM route

• Inj in large muscle mass; rotate inj sites

• Bicarbonate to alkalinize urine if ordered for UTI because drug is most active in alkaline environment

Intermittent IV INF route

• Dilute 500 mg of drug/100-200 ml of IV D_5W, D_5RL, D_5NaCl, or 0.9% NaCl and give over ½-1 hr; flush after administration with D_5W or 0.9% NaCl; solution is clear or pale yellow; discard if precipitate or dark color develop

• In evenly spaced doses to maintain blood level

Additive compatibilities:

• Avoid admixing

Syringe compatibilities: Clindamycin, doxapram

Y-site compatibilities: Acyclovir, amifostine, amiodarone, amsacrine, aztreonam, cefepime, cisatracurium, cyclophosphamide, dexamethasone, diltiazem, enalaprilat, esmolol, filgrastim, fluconazole, fludarabine, foscarnet, furosemide, granisetron, idarubicin, IL-2, labetalol, lorazepam, magnesium sulfate, melphalan, midazolam, morphine, ondansetron, paclitaxel, perphenazine, remifentanil, sargramostim, teniposide, thiotepa, TPN #54, #61, #91, #203, #204, #212, vinorelbine, warfarin, zidovudine

Perform/provide:

• Adequate fluids of 2-3 L/day, unless contraindicated, to prevent irritation of tubules

• Flush of IV line with NS or D_5W after infusion

• Supervised ambulation, other safety measures with vestibular dysfunction

Evaluate:

• Therapeutic response: absence of fever, draining wounds, negative C&S after treatment

Teach patient/family:

• To report headache, dizziness, symptoms for overgrowth of infection, renal impairment

To report loss of hearing, ringing, roaring in ears or feeling of fullness in head

• To report hypersensitivity: rash, itching, trouble breathing, facial edema and notify health care provider

Treatment of hypersensitivity: Hemodialysis, exchange transfusion in the newborn, monitor serum levels of drug, may give ticarcillin or carbenicillin

amiloride (℞)

(a-mill'oh-ride)

amiloride HCl, Midamor

Func. class.: Potassium-sparing diuretic

Chem. class.: Pyrazine

Action: Acts primarily on proximal distal tubule by inhibiting reabsorption of sodium, H_2O, and increasing potassium retention

Uses: Edema in CHF in combination with other diuretics, for hypertension, adjunct with other diuretics to maintain potassium

Dosage and routes:

• *Adult:* **PO** 5 mg qd, may be increased to 10-20 mg qd if needed

Available forms: Tabs 5 mg

Side effects/adverse reactions:

GU: Polyuria, dysuria, urinary frequency, impotence

ELECT: ***Hyperkalemia***

RESP: Cough, dyspnea, shortness of breath

CNS: Headache, dizziness, fatigue, weakness, paresthesias, tremor, depression, anxiety

GI: Nausea, diarrhea, dry mouth, *vomiting, anorexia,* cramps, constipation, abdominal pain, jaundice, bleeding

EENT: Loss of hearing, tinnitus, blurred vision, nasal congestion, increased intraocular pressure

INTEG: Rash, pruritus, alopecia, urticaria

MS: Cramps, joint pain

CV: Orthostatic hypotension, dysrhythmias, angina

HEMA: ***Aplastic anemia, neutropenia***

Contraindications: Anuria, hypersensitivity, hyperkalemia, impaired renal function

Precautions: Dehydration, pregnancy (B), diabetes, acidosis, lactation

Do not confuse:

amiloride/amlodipine

Pharmacokinetics:

PO: 15%-25% absorbed from GI tract; widely distributed; onset 2 hr, peak 6-10 hr, duration 24 hr; excreted in urine, feces, half-life 6-9 hr

Interactions:

• Enhanced action of antihypertensives

• Hyperkalemia: other potassium-sparing diuretics, potassium products, ACE inhibitors, salt substitutes

• ↓ effect of amiloride: NSAIDs

• Lithium toxicity: lithium

• Drug/food: possible hyperkalemia: foods high in potassium

Fatal hypokalemia: arginine

Hypokalemia: bearberry, gossypol

↑ effect: cucumber, dandelion, horsetail, licorice, nettle, pumpkin, Queen Anne's lace

↑ hypotension: khella

Severe photosensitivity St. John's wort

Lab test interferences:

Interference: GTT

NURSING CONSIDERATIONS

Assess:

• Weight, I&O daily to determine fluid loss; effect of drug may be decreased if used qd

• B/P lying, standing; postural hypotension may occur

• Electrolytes: K, Na, Cl; glucose (serum), BUN, CBC, serum creatinine, blood pH, ABGs

• Improvement in CVP q8h

• Rashes, temp elevation qd

• Confusion, especially in elderly; take safety precautions if needed

Administer:

PO route

• In AM to avoid interference with sleep if using drug as a diuretic

• With food; if nausea occurs, absorption may be decreased slightly

Evaluate:

• Therapeutic response: improvement in edema of feet, legs, sacral area daily if medication is being used in CHF

Teach patient/family:

• To take as prescribed; if dose is missed, take when remembered within 1 hr of next dose

• About adverse reactions: muscle cramps, weakness, nausea, dizziness, blurred vision

• To take with food or milk for GI symptoms

• To take early in day to prevent nocturia

• To avoid potassium-rich foods: oranges, bananas; salt substitutes, dried fruits

Treatment of overdose: Lavage if taken orally, monitor electrolytes, administer sodium bicarbonate for potassium >6.5 mEq/L, monitor hydration, CV, renal status

amino acid injection (℞)

(a-mee′noe)

FreAmine, HepatAmine

Func. class.: Nitrogen product

Action: Needed for anabolism to maintain structure, decrease catabolism, promote healing

Uses: Hepatic encephalopathy, cirrhosis, hepatitis, nutritional support in cancer

Dosage and routes:

• *Adult:* **IV** 80-120 g/day; 500 ml of amino acids/500 ml D_{50} given over 24 hr

Available forms: Inj; many strengths, types

Side effects/adverse reactions:

CNS: *Dizziness, headache,* confusion, ***loss of consciousness***

CV: Hypertension, ***CHF, pulmonary edema***

GI: Nausea, vomiting, liver fat deposits, abdominal pain

GU: Glycosuria, osmotic diuresis

ENDO: *Hyperglycemia, rebound hypoglycemia, electrolyte imbalances, hyperosmolar syndrome, hyperosmolar hyperglycemic nonketotic syndrome,* alkalosis, acidosis, hypophosphatemia, hyperammonemia, dehydration, hypocalcemia

INTEG: Chills, flushing, warm feeling, rash, urticaria, extravasation necrosis, phlebitis at inj site

Contraindications: Hypersensitivity, severe electrolyte imbalances, anuria, severe liver damage, maple syrup urine disease, PKU

Precautions: Renal disease, pregnancy (C), lactation, children, diabetes mellitus, CHF

NURSING CONSIDERATIONS

Assess:

• Electrolytes (K, Na, Ca, Cl, Mg), blood glucose, ammonia, phosphate, ketones

• Renal, hepatic studies: BUN, creatinine, ALT, AST, bilirubin

• Injection site for extravasation: redness along vein, edema at site, necrosis, pain, hard tender area; site should be changed immediately

• Respiratory function q4h: auscultate lung fields bilaterally for crackles, respirations, quality, rate, rhythm

• Temp q4h for increased fever, indicating infection; if infection suspected, infusion is discontinued, tubing and solution cultured

◆ For impending hepatic coma: asterixis, confusion, uremic fetor, lethargy

• Hyperammonemia: nausea, vomiting, malaise, tremors, anorexia, convulsions

Administer:

CONT IV route

• Up to 40% protein and dextrose

(up to 12.5%) via peripheral vein; stronger solutions require central IV administration
• TPN only mixed with dextrose to promote protein synthesis
• Immediately after mixing under strict aseptic technique, use infusion pump, in-line filter (0.22 μm) unless mixed with fat emulsion and dextrose (3 in 1)
Using careful monitoring technique; do not speed up infusion; pulmonary edema, glucose overload will result

Additive compatibilities: Amikacin, aminophylline, aztreonam, calcium gluconate, cefamandole, cefazolin, cefepime, cefotaxime, cefoxitin, cefsulodin, ceftazidime, ceftriaxone, cefuroxime, cimetidine, clindamycin, cyanocobalamin, cyclophosphamide, cycloSPORINE, cytarabine, DOPamine, epoetin, erythromycin, famotidine, folic acid, fosphenytoin, furosemide, heparin, insulin (regular), isoproterenol, lidocaine, meperidine, metaraminol, methicillin, methotrexate, methyldopate, methylPREDNISolone, metoclopramide, morphine, nafcillin, netilmicin, nizatidine, norepinephrine, ondansetron, oxacillin, penicillin G potassium, penicillin G sodium, phytonadione, polymyxin B, sodium bicarbonate, tacrolimus, tobramycin, vancomycin

Y-site compatibilities: Amikacin, aminophylline, amoxicillin, ampicillin, ascorbic acid inj, atracurium, azlocillin, aztreonam, bumetanide, buprenorphine, calcium gluconate, carboplatin, cefamandole, cefonicid, cefoperazone, cefotaxime, cefotetan, cefoxitin, ceftazidime, ceftizoxime, ceftriaxone, cefuroxime, cephalothin, cephapirin, chloramphenicol, chlorproMAZINE, cimetidine, clindamycin, clonazepam, dexamethasone, diazepam, digoxin, diphenhydrAMINE, DOBUTamine, DOPamine, doxycycline, droperidol, enalaprilat, epINEPHrine, erythromycin, famotidine, fentanyl, flucloxacillin, fluconazole, folic acid, foscarnet, gentamicin, granisetron, haloperidol, heparin, hydrocortisone, hydromorphone, hydrOXYzine, idarubicin, ifosfamide, IL-2, imipenem/cilastatin, insulin (regular), isoproterenol, kanamycin, leucovorin, levorphanol, lidocaine, lorazepam, magnesium sulfate, mannitol, meperidine, mesna, methicillin, metronidazole, mezlocillin, miconazole, morphine, moxalactam, multivitamins, nafcillin, netilmicin, nitroglycerin, nitroprusside, norepinephrine, octreotide, ofloxacin, ondansetron, oxacillin, paclitaxel, penicillin G, penicillin G potassium, pentobarbital, phenobarbital, piperacillin, potassium chloride, prochlorperazine, ranitidine, salbutamol, sargramostim, tacrolimus, thiotepa, ticarcillin, ticarcillin/clavulanate, tobramycin, trimethoprim-sulfamethoxazole, urokinase, vancomycin, vecuronium, zidovudine

Perform/provide:
• Storage depends on type of solution; consult manufacturer
• Changing dressing and IV tubing to prevent infection q24-48h

Evaluate:
• Therapeutic response: weight gain, decrease in jaundice in liver disorders, increased LOC

Teach patient/family:
• The reason for use of TPN
• If chills, sweating are experienced, report at once
• About infusion pump and blood glucose monitoring

amino acid solution (℞)

Aminees, Aminosyn, Branch Amin, FreAmine III, NeprAmine, Novamine, ProcalAmine, Ren Amin, Travasol, Troph Amine

Func. class.: Nitrogen product

Action: Needed for anabolism to maintain structure, decrease catabolism, promote healing

Uses: Nutritional support in cancer, trauma, intestinal obstruction, short bowel syndrome, severe malabsorption

Dosage and routes:

• *Adult:* **IV** 1-1.5 g/kg/day titrated to patient's needs

• *Child:* **IV** 2-3 g/kg/day titrated to patient's needs

Available forms: Inj, many types, strengths

Side effects/adverse reactions:

CNS: Dizziness, headache, confusion, ***loss of consciousness***

CV: Hypertension, ***CHF, pulmonary edema***

GI: Nausea, vomiting, liver fat deposits, abdominal pain, jaundice

GU: Glycosuria, osmotic diuresis

ENDO: Hyperglycemia, rebound hypoglycemia, electrolyte imbalances, hyperosmolar syndrome, hyperosmolar hyperglycemic nonketotic syndrome, alkalosis, acidosis, hypophosphatemia, hyperammonemia, dehydration, hypocalcemia

INTEG: Chills, flushing, warm feeling, rash, urticaria, extravasation necrosis, phlebitis at injection site

Contraindications: Hypersensitivity, severe electrolyte imbalances, anuria, severe liver damage, maple syrup urine disease, PKU

Precautions: Renal disease, pregnancy (C), lactation, children, diabetes mellitus, CHF

NURSING CONSIDERATIONS

Assess:

• Electrolytes (K, Na, Ca, Cl, Mg), blood glucose, ammonia, phosphate

• Renal, hepatic studies: BUN, creatinine, ALT, AST, bilirubin

• Injection site for extravasation: redness along vein, edema at site, necrosis, pain, hard tender area; site should be changed immediately

• Monitor respiratory function q4h: auscultate lung fields bilaterally for crackles, respirations, quality, rate, rhythm

• Monitor temp q4h for increased fever, indicating infection; if infection suspected, discontinue infusion, culture tubing, bottle

• Urine glucose q6h using Tes-Tape, Clinistix, which are not affected by infusion substances; blood glucose is preferred testing method

• Hyperammonemia: nausea, vomiting, malaise, tremors, anorexia, convulsions

Administer:

CONT IV route

• Up to 40% protein and dextrose (up to 12.5%) via peripheral vein; stronger solutions require central IV administration, use infusion pump

• TPN only mixed with dextrose to promote protein synthesis

• Immediately after mixing in pharmacy under strict aseptic technique using laminar flow hood, use infusion pump, in-line filter (0.22 μm) unless mixed with fat emulsion and dextrose (3 in 1)

⬘ Using careful monitoring technique; do not speed up infusion; pulmonary edema, glucose overload will result

Y-site compatibilities: Cefamandole, cefazolin, cefoperazone, cefotaxime, cefoxitin, cephalothin, cephapirin, chloramphenicol, clindamycin, digoxin, DOBUTamine, DOPamine, doxycycline, erythromycin lactobionate, fat emulsion, foscarnet, furosemide, gentamicin, isoproterenol, kanamycin, lidocaine, meperidine, methicillin, mezlocillin, miconazole, morphine, nafcillin, netilmicin, norepinephrine, oxacillin, penicillin G potassium, piperacillin, sargramostim, ticarcillin, tobramycin, urokinase, vancomycin

Perform/provide:
- Storage depends on type of solution; consult label
- Dressing and IV tubing change q24-48h to prevent infection

Evaluate:
- Therapeutic response: weight gain, decrease in jaundice in liver disorders, increased serum albumin

Teach patient/family:
- The reason for use of TPN
- That any chills, sweating should be reported at once
- About infusion pump and blood glucose monitoring

RARELY USED

aminocaproic acid (℞)

(a-mee-noe-ka-proe'ik)

Amicar, aminocaproic acid, EACA

Func. class.: Hemostatic

Uses: Hemorrhage from hyperfibrinolysis, adjunctive therapy in hemophilia

Dosage and routes:
- *Adult:* **PO/IV** 5 g loading dose, then 1-1.25 g q1h

Contraindications: Hypersensitivity, abnormal bleeding, postpartum bleeding, DIC, upper urinary tract bleeding, new burns

---

RARELY USED

aminoglutethimide (℞)

(a-meen-oh-gloo-teth'i-mide)

Cytadren

Func. class.: Antineoplastic, adrenal steroid inhibitor

Chem. class.: Hormone

Dosage and routes:
- *Adult:* **PO** 250 mg qid at 6 hr intervals, may increase by 250 mg/day q1-2wk, not to exceed 2 g/day

Uses: Suppression of adrenal function in Cushing's syndrome, adrenal cancer

Contraindications: Hypersensitivity, hypothyroidism, pregnancy (D)

RARELY USED

aminolevulinic acid (℞)

Levulan Kerastick

Func. class.: Photochemotherapy

Uses: Face/scalp nonhyperkeratotic actinic keratoses

Dosage and routes:
- *Adult:* **TOP** 1 application of solution and 1 dose of illumination/treatment site × 8 wk

Contraindications: Hypersensitivity to porphyrins

---

aminophylline (℞)

(am-in-off'i-lin)

Phyllocontin, Truphylline

Func. class.: Bronchodilator, spasmolytic

Chem. class.: Xanthine, ethylenediamide

Action: Exact mechanism unknown, relaxes smooth muscle of respiratory system by blocking phosphodiesterase, which increases cAMP; increased cAMP alters intracellular calcium ion movements; produces bronchodilation, increased pulmonary blood flow, relaxation of respiratory tract

Uses: Bronchial asthma, bronchospasm associated with chronic bronchitis, emphysema, bradycardia

Investigational uses: Apnea in infancy for respiratory/myocardial stimulation

Dosage and routes:

- *Adult:* **PO** 6 mg/kg, then 3 mg/kg q6h × 2 doses, then 3 mg/kg q8h maintenance, max 900 mg/day or 13 mg/kg; **PO** in CHF 6 mg/kg, then 2 mg/kg q8h × 2 doses, then 1-2 mg/kg q12h maintenance; **IV** 4.7 mg/kg, then 0.55 mg/kg/hr × 12 hr, then 0.36/kg/hr maintenance; **IV** in CHF 4.7 mg/kg, then 0.39 mg/kg/hr × 12 hr, then 0.08-0.16 mg/kg/hr maintenance
- *Geriatric and in cor pulmonale:* **PO** 6 mg/kg, then 2 mg/kg q6h × 2 doses, then 2 mg/kg q8h maintenance; **IV** 4.7 mg/kg, then 0.47 mg/kg/hr × 12 hr, then 0.24 mg/kg/hr maintenance
- *Child 9-16 yr:* **PO** 6 mg/kg, then 3 mg/kg q4h × 3 doses, then 3 mg/kg q6h maintenance, max 18 mg/kg/day 12-16 yr, or 20 mg/kg/day 9-12 yr; **IV** 4.7 mg/kg, then 0.79 mg/kg/hr × 12 hr, then 0.63 mg/kg/hr maintenance
- *Child 6 mo-9 yr:* **PO** 4 mg/kg q4h × 3 doses, then 4 mg/kg q6h maintenance, max 24 mg/kg/day; **IV** 4.7 mg/kg, then 0.95 mg/kg/hr × 12 hr, then 0.79 mg/kg/hr maintenance
- *Infants 6-52 wk:* Dose (0.2 × age in wk) ÷ 5 × kg = 24 hr dose in mg
- *Neonate—up to 40 wk premature postconception age:* **PO/IV** 1 mg/kg q12h
- *Neonate at birth or 40 wk postconception age:* **PO/IV** over 8 wk postnatal 1-3 mg/kg q6h; 4-8 wk postnatal 1-2 mg/kg q8h; up to 4 wk postnatal 1-2 mg/kg q12h

Hepatic disease

- *Adult:* **PO** 6 mg/kg/ then 2 mg/kg q8h × 2 doses, then 1-2 mg/kg q12h maintenance; **IV** 4.7 mg/kg, then 0.39 mg/kg/hr × 12 hr, then 0.08-0.16 mg/kg/hr maintenance

Available forms: Inj 250 mg/10 ml, 500 mg/20 ml, 100 mg/100 ml in 0.45% NaCl, 200 mg/100 ml in 0.45% NaCl; rect supp 250, 500 mg, oral liq 105 mg/5 ml; tabs 100, 200 mg, tabs con rel 225, 350 mg

Side effects/adverse reactions:

CNS: Anxiety, restlessness, insomnia, *dizziness,* ***seizures,*** headache, light-headedness, muscle twitching

CV: Palpitations, sinus tachycardia, hypotension, flushing, ***dysrhythmias***

GI: Nausea, vomiting, diarrhea, dyspepsia, anal irritation (suppositories), epigastric pain

RESP: Tachypnea, increased respiratory rate

INTEG: Flushing, urticaria, *rectal irritation* (suppositories)

GU: Urinary frequency, SIADH

Contraindications: Hypersensitivity to xanthines, tachydysrhythmias, active peptic ulcer disease

Precautions: Elderly, CHF, cor pulmonale, hepatic disease, diabetes mellitus, hyperthyroidism, hypertension, seizure disorder, irritation of the rectum or lower colon, children, pregnancy (C), lactation, alcoholism

Pharmacokinetics: Well absorbed PO; extended rel well absorbed slowly, rect supp is erratic, rect sol is absorbed quickly; metabolized by liver (caffeine); excreted in urine; crosses placenta; appears in breast milk; half-life 3-12 hr; half-life increased in geriatric patients, hepatic disease, CHF, smokers

PO: Onset ¼ hr, peak 1-2 hr, duration 6-8 hr
PO-ER: Unknown, peak 4-7 hr, duration 8-12 hr
IV: Onset rapid, duration 6-8 hr
REC: Onset erratic, peak 1-2 hr, duration 6-8 hr

Interactions:

• ↑ action of aminophylline, toxicity: cimetidine, nonselective β-blockers, erythromycin, clarithromycin, oral contraceptives, corticosteroids, interferons, fluoroquinolones, disulfiram, mexiletine, fluvoxamine, high doses of allopurinol, influenza vaccines, interferon, benzodiazepines
• Dysrhythmias: halothane
• ↑ elimination: smoking
• ↓ effects of lithium
• May ↑ or ↓ aminophylline levels: carbamazepine, loop diuretics, isoniazid
• ↑ adverse reactions: tetracyclines
• Dose-dependent reversal of: neuromuscular blockade
• ↓ effect of aminophylline: nicotine products, adrenergics, barbiturates, phenytoin, ketoconazole, rifampin
• Drug/food: ↑ effect: xanthines; elimination ↑ by low-carbohydrate, high-protein diet; charcoal-broiled beef; elimination ↓ by high-carbohydrate and low-protein diet
↑ effects: cola tree, guarana, yerba maté, tea (black, green), horsetail, ginseng, Siberian ginseng
↓ effects: St. John's wort

Lab test interferences:

Increase: Plasma free fatty acids

NURSING CONSIDERATIONS

Assess:

• Theophylline blood levels (therapeutic level is 10-20 mcg/ml); toxicity may occur with small increase above 20 mcg/ml, especially elderly
• Monitor I&O; diuresis occurs; dehydration may occur in elderly or children
• Whether theophylline was given recently (24 hr)
• Respiratory rate, rhythm, depth; auscultate lung fields bilaterally; notify prescriber of abnormalities
• Allergic reactions: rash, urticaria; if these occur, drug should be discontinued

Administer:

• Avoid IM injection; pain and tissue damage may occur

PO route

• Avoid giving with food
Do not break, crush, or chew enteric-coated or cont rel tabs

Rectal route

• If patient is unable to take PO; retain rectal dose for ½ hr

IV route

• Only clear sol; flush IV line before dose
• May be diluted for IV INF in 100-200 ml in D_5W, $D_{10}W$, $D_{20}W$, 0.9% NaCl, 0.45% NaCl, LR
• Give loading dose over ½ hr; max rate of inf 25 mg/min, use infusion pump; after loading dose give by cont inf

Additive compatibilities: Amobarbital, bretylium, calcium gluconate, chloramphenicol, cibenzoline, cimetidine, dexamethasone, diphenhydrAMINE, DOPamine, erythromycin lactobionate, esmolol, floxacillin, flumazenil, furosemide, heparin, hydrocortisone, lidocaine, mephentermine, meropenem, methyldopate, metronidazole/sodium bicarbonate, nitroglycerin, pentobarbital, phenobarbital, potassium chloride, ranitidine, secobarbital, sodium bicarbonate, terbutaline

Syringe compatibilities: Heparin, metoclopramide, pentobarbital, thiopental

Y-site compatibilities: Allopurinol, amifostine, amphotericin B, amrinone, aztreonam, ceftazidime, cholesteryl sulfate complex, cimetidine, cladribine, DOXOrubicin liposome, enalaprilat, esmolol, famotidine, filgrastim, fluconazole, fludarabine, foscarnet, gallium, granisetron, heparin sodium with hydrocortisone sodium succinate, labetalol, melphalan, meropenem, netilmicin, paclitaxel, pancuronium, piperacillin/tazobactam, potassium chloride, propofol, ranitidine, remifentanil, sargramostim, tacrolimus, teniposide, thiotepa, tolazoline, vecuronium

Perform/provide:

• Storage of diluted solution for 24 hr if refrigerated

Evaluate:

• Therapeutic response: decreased dyspnea, respiratory stimulation in infancy, clear lung fields bilaterally

Teach patient/family:

• To take doses as prescribed, not to skip dose, not to double dose

• To check OTC medications, current prescription medications for ephedrine; will increase CNS stimulation; not to drink alcohol or caffeine products (tea, coffee, chocolate, colas)

• To avoid hazardous activities; dizziness may occur

• If GI upset occurs, to take drug with 8 oz water; avoid food, since absorption may be decreased

• To remain in bed 15-20 min after rect supp is inserted to avoid removal

⬥ To notify prescriber of toxicity: insomnia, anxiety, nausea, vomiting, rapid pulse, seizures, flushing, headache, diarrhea; notify prescriber immediately

• To notify prescriber of change in smoking habit; a change in dose may be required

• To increase fluids to 2 L/day to decrease secretion viscosity

• To avoid smoking; decreases blood levels and terminal half-life

---

HIGH ALERT

amiodarone (℞)

(a-mee-oh'da-rone)

Cordarone, Pacerone

Func. class.: Antidysrhythmic (class III)

Chem. class.: Iodinated benzofuran derivative

Action: Prolongs duration of action potential and effective refractory period, noncompetitive α- and β-adrenergic inhibition; increases PR and QT intervals, decreases sinus rate, decreases peripheral vascular resistance

Uses: Severe ventricular tachycardia, supraventricular tachycardia, atrial fibrillation, ventricular fibrillation not controlled by first-line agents, cardiac arrest

Dosage and routes:

Ventricular dysrhythmias

• *Adult:* **PO** loading dose 800-1600 mg/day for 1-3 wk; then 600-800 mg/day × 1 mo; maintenance 400 mg/day; **IV** loading dose (first rapid) 150 mg over the first 10 min then slow 360 mg over the next 6 hr; maintenance 540 mg given over the remaining 18 hr, decrease rate of the slow infusion to 0.5 mg/min

• *Child:* **PO** loading dose 10-15 mg/kg/day in 1-2 divided doses for 4-14 days then 5 mg/kg/day (not recommended in children)

• *Child/Infants:* **IV/Intraosseous** 5 mg/kg as a bolus (PALS guidelines)

Perfusion tachycardia

• **IV** 5 mg/kg loading dose given over 20-60 min

Supraventricular tachycardia
• *Adult:* **PO** 600-800 mg/day × 7 days or until desired response, then 400 mg/day × 21 days, then 200-400 mg/day maintenance
• *Child:* **PO** 10 mg/kg/day (800 mg/1.72 m^2/day) × 10 days or until desired response, then 5 mg/kg/day (400 mg/1.72 m^2/day) × 21-28 days, then 2.5 mg/kg/day (200 mg/1.72 m^2/day) (not recommended in children)
Available forms: Tabs 200, 400 mg; inj 50 mg/ml
Side effects/adverse reactions:
CNS: Headache, dizziness, involuntary movement, tremors, peripheral neuropathy, malaise, fatigue, ataxia, paresthesias, insomnia
GI: Nausea, vomiting, diarrhea, abdominal pain, anorexia, constipation, ***hepatotoxicity***
CV: Hypotension, bradycardia, ***sinus arrest, CHF, dysrhythmias, SA node dysfunction***
INTEG: Rash, photosensitivity, blue-gray skin discoloration, alopecia, spontaneous ecchymosis, ***toxic epidermal necrolysis***
EENT: Blurred vision, halos, photophobia, ***corneal microdeposits,*** dry eyes
ENDO: Hyperthyroidism or hypothyroidism
MS: Weakness, pain in extremities
RESP: ***Pulmonary fibrosis,*** pulmonary inflammation, ***ARDS; gasping syndrome if used in neonates***
MISC: Flushing, abnormal taste or smell, edema, abnormal salivation, coagulation abnormalities
Contraindications: Pregnancy (D), lactation, 2nd-, 3rd-degree AV block, bradycardia, severe sinus node dysfunction, neonates, infants
Precautions: Goiter, Hashimoto's thyroiditis, electrolyte imbalances, CHF, severe hepatic, respiratory disease, children

Do not confuse:
amiodarone/amrinone
Cordarone/Inocor
Pharmacokinetics:
PO: Onset 1-3 wk, peak 2-10 hr; half-life 15-100 days; metabolized by liver, excreted by kidneys
Interactions:
• Bradycardia: β-blockers, calcium channel blockers
• ↑ levels of cycloSPORINE, dextromethorphan, digoxin, disopyramide, flecainide, methotrexate, phenytoin, procainamide, quinidine, theophylline
• ↑ anticoagulant effects: warfarin
May ↑ amiodarone effect: aloe, broom, buckthorn, cascara sagrada, Chinese rhubarb, figwort, fumitory, goldenseal, kudzu, licorice, rhubarb, senna
Toxicity/death: aconite
↓ amiodarone effect: coltsfoot
Serotonin effect: horehound
Lab test interferences:
Increase: T_4
NURSING CONSIDERATIONS
Assess:
• I&O ratio; electrolytes (K, Na, Cl); hepatic studies: AST, ALT, bilirubin, alk phosphatase
• Chest x-ray, thyroid function tests
• ECG continuously to determine drug effectiveness, measure PR, QRS, QT intervals, check for PVCs, other dysrhythmias, B/P continuously for hypotension, hypertension
• For dehydration or hypovolemia
• For rebound hypertension after 1-2 hr
• For ARDS, pulmonary fibrosis
• CNS symptoms: confusion, psychosis, numbness, depression, involuntary movements; if these occur, drug should be discontinued
• Hypothyroidism: lethargy, dizziness, constipation, enlarged thyroid gland, edema of extremities, cool, pale skin

• Hyperthyroidism: restlessness, tachycardia, eyelid puffiness, weight loss, frequent urination, menstrual irregularities, dyspnea; warm, moist skin
• Ophthalmic exams
⬥ Pulmonary toxicity: dyspnea, fatigue, cough, fever, chest pain; drug should be discontinued
• Cardiac rate, respiration: rate, rhythm, character, chest pain; start with patient hospitalized and monitored up to 1 wk

Administer:

PO route
• Loading dose with food to decrease nausea

Intermittent IV INF route
• 1000 mg/24 hr during loading/maintenance
• Initial loading: Add 3 ml (150 mg) 100 ml D_5W (1.5 mg/ml) give over 10 min
• Loading inf: Add 18 ml (900 mg) 500 ml D_5W (1.8 mg/ml) give over next 6 hr
• Maintenance inf: Give remainder of loading inf 540 mg over 18 hr (0.5 mg/min)

Continuous inf route
• After 24 hr, give 1-6 mg/ml at 0.5 mg/ml, do not exceed 30 mg/min

Additive compatibilities: DOBUTamine, lidocaine, potassium chloride, procainimide, verapamil

Y-site compatibilities: Amikacin, bretylium, clindamycin, DOBUTamine, DOPamine, doxycycline, erythromycin, esmolol, gentamicin, insulin, isoproterenol, labetalol, lidocaine, metaraminol, metronidazole, midazolam, morphine, nitroglycerin, norepinephrine, penicillin G potassium, phentolamine, phenylephrine, potassium chloride, procainamide, tobramycin, vancomycin

Solution compatibility: D_5W, 0.9% NaCl

Evaluate:
• Therapeutic response: decrease in ventricular tachycardia, supraventricular tachycardia or fibrillation

Teach patient/family:
• To take this drug as directed; avoid missed doses
• To use sunscreen or stay out of sun to prevent burns
• To report side effects immediately
• That skin discoloration is usually reversible
• That dark glasses may be needed for photophobia

Treatment of overdose: O_2, artificial ventilation, ECG, administer dopamine for circulatory depression, administer diazepam or thiopental for convulsions, isoproterenol

amitriptyline (℞)

(a-mee-trip′ti-leen)
amitriptyline HCl, Apo-Amitriptyline✤, Elavil, Endep, Levate✤, Novotriptyn✤

Func. class.: Antidepressant—tricyclic
Chem. class.: Tertiary amine

Action: Blocks reuptake of norepinephrine, serotonin into nerve endings, increasing action of norepinephrine, serotonin in nerve cells

Uses: Major depression

Investigational uses: Chronic pain management, prevention of cluster/migraine headaches, fibromyalgia

Dosage and routes:

Depression
• *Adult:* **PO** 75 mg/day in divided doses, may increase to 150 mg qd, not to exceed 300 mg/day; **IM** 20-30 mg qid, or 80-120 mg hs
• *Geriatric and adolescent:* **PO** 30 mg/day in divided doses, may be increased to 100 mg/day

Cluster/migraine headache
- *Adult:* **PO** 50-150 mg/day

Chronic pain
- *Adult:* **PO** 75-150 mg/day

Fibromyalgia
- *Adult:* **PO** 10-50 mg qhs

Available forms: Tabs 10, 25, 50, 75, 100, 150 mg; inj 10 mg/ml; syr 10 mg/5 ml

Side effects/adverse reactions:

HEMA: ***Agranulocytosis, thrombocytopenia, eosinophilia, leukopenia***

CNS: Dizziness, drowsiness, confusion, headache, anxiety, tremors, stimulation, weakness, insomnia, nightmares, EPS (elderly), increased psychiatric symptoms, ***seizures***

GI: Constipation, dry mouth, weight gain, nausea, vomiting, ***paralytic ileus,*** increased appetite, cramps, epigastric distress, jaundice, ***hepatitis,*** stomatitis

GU: Urinary retention

INTEG: Rash, urticaria, sweating, pruritus, photosensitivity

CV: Orthostatic hypotension, ***ECG changes, tachycardia, hypertension,*** palpitations, ***dysrhythmias***

EENT: Blurred vision, tinnitus, mydriasis, ophthalmoplegia

Contraindications: Hypersensitivity to tricyclics, recovery phase of myocardial infarction, narrow-angle glaucoma

Precautions: Suicidal patients, convulsive disorders, prostatic hypertrophy, schizophrenia, psychosis, severe depression, increased intraocular pressure, narrow-angle glaucoma, urinary retention, cardiac disease, hepatic disease, renal disease, hyperthyroidism, electroshock therapy, elective surgery, child <12 yr, lactation, elderly, pregnancy (C)

Do not confuse:
amitriptyline/nortriptyline
Elavil/Mellaril/Oruvail/Plavix

Pharmacokinetics:

PO/IM: Onset 45 min, peak 2-12 hr, therapeutic response 4-10 days; metabolized by liver; excreted in urine, feces; crosses placenta, excreted in breast milk, half-life 10-46 hr

Interactions:
- ↑ risk of agranulocytosis: Antithyroid agents
- ↑ amitriptyline levels, toxicity: cimetidine, fluoxetine, phenothiazines, oral contraceptives, antidepressants, carbamazepine, IC antidysrhythmics
- ↓ effects of: guanethidine, clonidine, indirect-acting sympathomimetics (epHEDrine)
- ↑ effects of: direct-acting sympathomimetics (epINEPHrine), alcohol, barbiturates, benzodiazepines, CNS depressants, opioids, sedative/hypnotics

Hyperpyretic crisis, convulsions, hypertensive episode: MAOIs

↑ CNS depression: kava, skullcap, hops, chamomile, lavender, valerian

↑ anticholinergic effect: belladonna leaf/root, henbane leaf, jimsonweed, scopolia

↑ action of amitriptyline: scopolia root

Serotonin syndrome: SAM-e, St. John's wort

↑ hypertension: yohimbe

Lab test interferences:

Increase: Serum bilirubin, blood glucose, alk phosphatase

NURSING CONSIDERATIONS

Assess:
- B/P lying, standing; pulse q4h; if systolic B/P drops 20 mm Hg, hold drug, notify prescriber; take vital signs q4h in patients with cardiovascular disease
- Blood studies: CBC, leukocytes, differential, cardiac enzymes if patient is receiving long-term therapy

- Hepatic studies: AST, ALT, bilirubin
- Weight qwk; appetite may increase with drug
- ECG for flattening of T wave, prolongation of QTc interval, bundle branch block, AV block, dysrhythmias in cardiac patients
- EPS primarily in elderly: rigidity, dystonia, akathisia
- Mental status: mood, sensorium, affect, suicidal tendencies; increase in psychiatric symptoms: depression, panic
- Urinary retention, constipation; constipation is most likely to occur in children and elderly
- Withdrawal symptoms: headache, nausea, vomiting, muscle pain, weakness; do not usually occur unless drug was discontinued abruptly
- Alcohol consumption; if alcohol is consumed, hold dose until morning

Administer:

PO route

- Increased fluids, bulk in diet if constipation, urinary retention occur, especially elderly
- With food or milk for GI symptoms
- Crushed if patient is unable to swallow medication whole
- Dosage hs if oversedation occurs during day; may take entire dose hs; elderly may not tolerate once/day dosing

Perform/provide:

- Storage at room temperature; do not freeze
- Assistance with ambulation during beginning therapy, since drowsiness/dizziness occurs
- Gum; hard, sugarless candy; or frequent sips of water for dry mouth

Evaluate:

- Therapeutic response: decrease in depression, absence of suicidal thoughts

Teach patient/family:

- To take medication as directed; do not double dose; that therapeutic effects may take 2-3 wk
- To use caution in driving, other activities requiring alertness because of drowsiness, dizziness, blurred vision; to avoid rising quickly from sitting to standing, especially elderly
- To avoid alcohol ingestion, other CNS depressants
- Not to discontinue medication quickly after long-term use: may cause nausea, headache, malaise
- To wear sunscreen or large hat, since photosensitivity occurs
- That contraception is recommended during treatment

Treatment of overdose: ECG monitoring, lavage, administer anticonvulsant, sodium bicarbonate

amlodipine (℞)

(am-loe'di-peen)

Norvasc

Func. class.: Antianginal, antihypertensive, calcium channel blocker

Chem. class.: Dihydropyridine

Action: Inhibits calcium ion influx across cell membrane during cardiac depolarization; produces relaxation of coronary vascular smooth muscle, peripheral vascular smooth muscle; dilates coronary vascular arteries; increases myocardial oxygen delivery in patients with vasospastic angina

Uses: Chronic stable angina pectoris, hypertension, vasospastic angina (Prinzmetal's angina); may coadminister with other antihypertensives, antianginals

Dosage and routes:

Angina

- *Adult:* **PO** 5-10 mg qd

Hypertension
• *Adult:* **PO** 5 mg qd initially, max 10 mg/dayO

Hepatic dose/elderly
• *Adult:* **PO** 2.5 mg/day; may increase up to 10 mg/day (antihypertensive); 5 mg/day, may increase up to 10 mg/day (antianginal)

Available forms: Tabs 2.5, 5, 10 mg

Side effects/adverse reactions:
CV: Dysrhythmia, edema, bradycardia, hypotension, palpitations, syncope
GI: Nausea, vomiting, diarrhea, gastric upset, constipation, flatulence, anorexia, gingival hyperplasia, dyspepsia
GU: Nocturia, polyuria
INTEG: Rash, pruritus, urticaria, hair loss
CNS: Headache, fatigue, dizziness, asthenia, anxiety, depression, insomnia, paresthesia, somnolence
OTHER: Flushing, sexual difficulties, muscle cramps, cough, weight gain, tinnitus, epistaxis

Contraindications: Sick sinus syndrome, 2nd- or 3rd-degree heart block, hypersensitivity

Precautions: CHF, hypotension, hepatic injury, pregnancy (C), lactation, children, elderly

Do not confuse:
amlodipine/amiloride
Norvasc/Navane

Pharmacokinetics:
PO: Onset not determined, peak 6-12 hr, half-life 30-50 hr, increased in geriatric, hepatic disease; metabolized by liver, excreted in urine (90% as metabolites), protein binding >95%

Interactions:
• ↑ hypotension: alcohol, antihypertensives, nitrates
• Neurotoxicity: lithium
• ↓ antihypertensive effect: NSAIDs
• Drug/food: may ↑ hypotensive effect: grapefruit juice
↑ effects: barberry, betel palm, burdock, goldenseal, khat, khella, lily of the valley, plantain
↓ effect: yohimbe

NURSING CONSIDERATIONS

Assess:
• Cardiac status: B/P, pulse, respiration, ECG; some patients have developed severe angina, acute MI after calcium channel blockers if obstructive CAD is severe
• I&O ratio, weight qd; peripheral edema, dyspnea, jugular vein distension, rales, crackles that are signs of CHF

Administer:

PO route
• Once a day, without regard to meals

Evaluate:
• Therapeutic response: decreased anginal pain, decreased B/P, increased exercise tolerance

Teach patient/family:
• To take drug as prescribed, do not double or skip dose
• To avoid hazardous activities until stabilized on drug, dizziness is no longer a problem
• To avoid OTC drugs unless directed by prescriber
• To comply in all areas of medical regimen: diet, exercise, stress reduction, drug therapy, smoking cessation
• To notify prescriber of irregular heartbeat, shortness of breath, swelling of feet and hands, severe dizziness, constipation, nausea, hypotension
• To use correct technique in monitoring pulse, to contact prescriber if pulse <50 bpm
• To change positions slowly, to prevent orthostatic hypotension
• To continue with good oral hygiene to prevent gingival disease
• To notify all health care providers of this drug use

Treatment of overdose: Defibrillation, β-agonists, IV calcium inotropic agents, diuretics, atropine for AV block, vasopressor for hypotension

RARELY USED

ammonium chloride

(PO-OTC, IV-℞)

(ah-mohn'ee-um klor'ide)

ammonium chloride

Func. class.: Acidifier

Uses: Alkalosis (metabolic), systemic and urinary acidifier, expectorant, diuretic

Dosage and routes:

Alkalosis: *Adult and child:* **IV INF** 0.9-1.3 ml/min of a 2.14% sol, not to exceed 5 ml/min

Acidifier: *Adult:* **PO** 4-12 g/day in divided doses; *Child:* **PO** 75 mg/kg/day in divided doses

Expectorant: *Adult:* **PO** 250-500 mg q2-4h as needed

Contraindications: Hypersensitivity, severe hepatic disease, severe renal disease

amoxapine (℞)

(a-mox'a-peen)

amoxapine, Asendin

Func. class.: Antidepressant

Chem. class.: Dibenzoxazepine derivative—secondary amine

Action: Blocks reuptake of norepinephrine, serotonin into nerve endings, increasing action of norepinephrine, serotonin in nerve cells

Uses: Depression

Dosage and routes:

• *Adult:* **PO** 50 mg tid, may increase to 100 mg tid on 3rd day of therapy; not to exceed 300 mg/day unless lower doses have been given for at least 2 wk, may be given daily dose hs, not to exceed 600 mg/day in hospitalized patients

• *Elderly:* **PO** 25 mg hs, may increase by 25 mg/wk, up to 150 mg/day in divided doses

Available forms: Tabs 25, 50, 100, 150 mg

Side effects/adverse reactions:

HEMA: ***Agranulocytosis, thrombocytopenia, eosinophilia, leukopenia***

CNS: Dizziness, drowsiness, confusion, headache, anxiety, tremors, stimulation, weakness, insomnia, nightmares, EPS (elderly), increased psychiatric symptoms, paresthesia, ***neuroleptic malignant syndrome,*** impairment of sexual functioning

GI: Dry mouth, weight gain, *constipation,* nausea, vomiting, ***paralytic ileus,*** increased appetite, cramps, epigastric distress, jaundice, ***hepatitis,*** stomatitis

GU: Urinary retention, ***acute renal failure***

INTEG: Rash, urticaria, sweating, pruritus, photosensitivity

CV: Orthostatic hypotension, ECG changes, tachycardia, hypertension, palpitations

META: Increased prolactin levels

EENT: Blurred vision, tinnitus, mydriasis, ophthalmoplegia

Contraindications: Hypersensitivity to tricyclics, recovery phase of myocardial infarction, convulsive disorders, prostatic hypertrophy, narrow-angle glaucoma

Precautions: Suicidal patients, severe depression, increased intraocular pressure, urinary retention, cardiac disease, hepatic disease, hyperthyroidism, electroshock therapy, elective surgery, elderly, pregnancy (C)

Do not confuse:

amoxapine/amoxicillin/Amoxil

Pharmacokinetics:
PO: Steady state 2-7 days; metabolized by liver, excreted by kidneys, crosses placenta, half-life 8 hr

Interactions:
• ↑ CNS depression: CNS depressants
• ↓ amoxapine effect: barbiturates
• ↑ amoxapine level: cimetidine, fluoxetine, fluvoxamine, paroxetine, sertraline
• ↑ hypertensive effect: clonidine, epinephrine, norepinephrine
Hyperpyretic crisis, convulsions, hypertensive episode: MAOIs
↑ CNS depression: chamomile, hops, kava, lavender, skullcap, St. John's wort, valerian
↑ anticholinergic effects: belladonna, corkwood, henbane, jimsonweed
↑action of amoxapine: scopolia root

Lab test interferences:
Increase: LFTs, blood glucose
Decrease: WBC, blood glucose

NURSING CONSIDERATIONS

Assess:
• B/P lying, standing; pulse q4h; if systolic B/P drops 20 mm Hg, hold drug, notify prescriber; take vital signs q4h in patients with cardiovascular disease
• Blood studies: CBC, leukocytes, differential, cardiac enzymes if patient is receiving long-term therapy
• Blood level: ther 20-100 ng/ml
• Hepatic studies: AST, ALT, bilirubin
• Weight qwk, appetite may increase with drug
• ECG for flattening of T wave, bundle branch block, AV block, dysrhythmias in cardiac patients
• EPS primarily in elderly: rigidity, dystonia, akathisia
• Mental status: mood, sensorium, affect, suicidal tendencies; increase in psychiatric symptoms: depression, panic; confusion (elderly)
• Urinary retention, constipation; constipation is more likely to occur in children, elderly
• Withdrawal symptoms: headache, nausea, vomiting, muscle pain, weakness; do not usually occur unless drug is discontinued abruptly
• Alcohol consumption; if alcohol is consumed, hold dose until morning

Administer:

PO route
• Increased fluids, bulk in diet if constipation, urinary retention occur, especially in elderly
• Crushed if patient is unable to swallow medication whole, with food or milk for GI symptoms
• Dosage hs if oversedation occurs during day; may take entire dose hs; elderly may not tolerate once/day dosing

Perform/provide:
• Storage at room temperature; do not freeze
• Check to see PO medication swallowed
• Gum, hard candy, or frequent sips of water for dry mouth

Evaluate:
• Therapeutic response: decreased depression, absence of suicidal thoughts

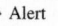

Teach patient/family:
• To take as directed, not to double dose
• That therapeutic effects may take 2-3 wk
• To use caution in driving or other activities requiring alertness because of drowsiness, dizziness, blurred vision
• To avoid alcohol ingestion, other CNS depressants
• Not to discontinue medication quickly after long-term use; may cause nausea, headache, malaise

• To wear sunscreen or large hat, since photosensitivity occurs
Treatment of overdose: ECG monitoring, induce emesis, lavage, activated charcoal, administer anticonvulsant

amoxicillin (℞)

(a-mox-i-sill'in)
amoxicillin, Amoxil, Apo-Amoxi✦, Novamoxin✦, Nu-Amoxi✦, Trimox, Wymox
Func. class.: Antiinfective, antiulcer
Chem. class.: Aminopenicillin

Action: Interferes with cell wall replication of susceptible organisms; the cell wall, rendered osmotically unstable, swells and bursts from osmotic pressure
Uses: Treatment of skin, respiratory, GI, GU infections; otitis media, gonorrhea. For gram-positive cocci *(Staphylococcus aureus, Streptococcus pyogenes, Streptococcus faecalis, Streptococcus pneumoniae),* gram-negative cocci *(Neisseria gonorrhoeae, Neisseria meningitidis),* gram-positive bacilli *(Corynebacterium diphtheriae, Listeria monocytogenes),* gram-negative bacilli *(Haemophilus influenzae, Escherichia coli, Proteus mirabilis, Salmonella);* prophylaxis of bacterial endocarditis; in combination with other drugs used for treatment of *Helicobacter pylori*
Investigational uses: Lyme disease
Dosage and routes:
Systemic infections
• *Adult:* **PO** 750 mg-1.5 g qd in divided doses q8h
• *Child:* **PO** 20-50 mg/kg/day in divided doses q8h
Renal disease
• *Adult:* **PO** CCr 10-50 ml/min dose q12h; CCr <10 ml/min dose q24h
Gonorrhea/urinary tract infections
• *Adult:* **PO** 3 g given with 1 g probenecid as a single dose; followed by tetracycline or erythromycin therapy
Chlamydia trachomatis
• *Adult:* **PO** 500 mg/day × 1 wk
Bacterial endocarditis prophylaxis
• *Child:* **PO** 50 mg/kg/hr before and 25 mg/kg 6 hr after procedure
Helicobacter pylori
• *Adult:* **PO** 1000 mg bid, given with lansoprazole 30 mg bid, clarithromycin 500 mg bid × 2 wk or 1000 mg bid given with omeprazole 20 mg bid, clarithromycin 500 mg bid × 2 wk, or 1000 mg tid given with lansoprazole 30 mg tid × 2 wk
Available forms: Caps 250, 500 mg; chew tabs 125, 200, 250, 400 mg; tabs 500, 875 mg; susp pediatric drops 50 mg/ml; susp 125, 200, 250, 400 mg/5 ml
Side effects/adverse reactions:
HEMA: Anemia, increased bleeding time, ***bone marrow depression, granulocytopenia***
GI: Nausea, vomiting, diarrhea, increased AST, ALT, abdominal pain, glossitis, colitis, ***pseudomembranous colitis***
CNS: Headache, ***seizures***
SYST: ***Anaphylaxis, respiratory distress, serum sickness***
INTEG: Urticaria, rash
Contraindications: Hypersensitivity to penicillins
Precautions: Pregnancy (B), lactation, hypersensitivity to cephalosporins, neonates, renal disease
Do not confuse:
amoxicillin/amoxapine/Amoxil
Trimox/Diamox/Tylox
Wymox/Tylox
Pharmacokinetics:
PO: Peak 2 hr, duration 6-8 hr; half-life 1-1⅓ hr, metabolized in liver, excreted in urine, crosses placenta, enters breast milk

Interactions:

• ↑ amoxicillin level: probenecid

• ↓ effectiveness of oral contraceptives

• ↑ anticoagulant action: warfarin

Do not use with acidophilus

Delayed or reduced absorption: khat; separate by 2 hr

Lab test interferences:

False positive: Urine glucose, urine protein, direct Coombs' test

NURSING CONSIDERATIONS

Assess:

• I&O ratio; report hematuria, oliguria, since penicillin in high doses is nephrotoxic

• Any patient with a compromised renal system, since drug is excreted slowly in poor renal system function; toxicity may occur rapidly

• Hepatic studies: AST, ALT

• Blood studies: WBC, RBC, Hgb and Hct, bleeding time

• Renal studies: urinalysis, protein, blood, BUN, creatinine

• Culture, sensitivity before drug therapy; drug may be given as soon as culture is taken

• Bowel pattern before, during treatment; diarrhea, cramping, blood in stools, report to prescriber, pseudomembranous colitis may occur

• Skin eruptions after administration of penicillin to 1 wk after discontinuing drug

• Respiratory status: rate, character, wheezing, tightness in the chest

• Anaphylaxis: rash, itching, dyspnea, facial/laryngeal edema

Administer:

PO route

• Shake suspension well before each dose, may be used alone or mixed in drinks, use immediately

• Give around the clock, caps may be emptied and mixed with liquids if needed

Perform/provide:

• Adrenaline, suction, tracheostomy set, endotracheal intubation equipment on unit

• Adequate intake of fluids (2 L) during diarrhea episodes

• Scratch test to assess allergy after securing order from prescriber; usually done when penicillin is only drug of choice

• Storage in tight container; after reconstituting, oral suspension refrigerated for 14 days

Evaluate:

• Therapeutic response: absence of infection; prevention of endocarditis, resolution of ulcer symptoms

Teach patient/family:

• That caps may be opened and contents taken with fluids; chewable form is available

• To take as prescribed, not to double dose

• All aspects of drug therapy: need to complete entire course of medication to ensure organism death (10-14 days); culture may be taken after completed course of medication

To report sore throat, fever, fatigue, diarrhea (may indicate superinfection or agranulocytopenia)

• That drug must be taken in equal intervals around the clock to maintain blood levels; take on empty stomach with a full glass of water

• To wear or carry emergency ID if allergic to penicillins

Treatment of anaphylaxis: Withdraw drug, maintain airway, administer epinephrine, aminophylline, O_2, IV corticosteroids

A

amoxicillin/clavulanate potassium (℞)

(a-mox-i-sill'in)

Augmentin, Augmentin ES-600, Augmentin XR, Clavulin✤

Func. class.: Broad-spectrum antiinfective

Chem. class.: Aminopenicillin β-lactamase inhibitor

Action: Interferes with cell wall replication of susceptible organisms; the cell wall, rendered osmotically unstable, swells and bursts from osmotic pressure; combination increases spectrum of activity against β-lactamase–resistant organisms

Uses: Sinus infections, pneumonia, otitis media, skin infection, UTI; effective for strains of *Escherichia coli, Proteus mirabilis, Haemophilus influenzae, Streptococcus faecalis, Streptococcus pneumoniae,* and some β-lactamase–producing organisms

Dosage and routes:

• *Adult:* **PO** 250-500 mg q8h or 500-875 mg q12h depending on severity of infection

• *Child ≤40 kg:* **PO** 20-40 mg/kg/day in divided doses q8h or 25-45 mg/kg/day in divided doses q12h

Renal disease

• *Adult:* **PO** CCr 10-30 ml/min dose q12h; CCr <10 ml/min dose q24h

Available forms: Tabs 250, 500, 875 mg/125 mg clavulanate; chew tabs 125, 200, 250, 400 mg; powder for oral susp 125, 200, 250, 400 mg/5 ml; (XR) ext rel tabs 1000 mg amoxicillin, 62.5 mg clavulanate; (ES) powder for oral susp 600 mg amoxicillin, 42.9 mg clavulanate

Side effects/adverse reactions:

HEMA: Anemia, ***bone marrow depression, granulocytopenia, leukopenia, eosinophilia,*** thrombocytopenic purpura

GI: Nausea, diarrhea, vomiting, increased AST, ALT, abdominal pain, glossitis, colitis, black tongue, ***pseudomembranous colitis***

GU: Oliguria, proteinuria, hematuria, *vaginitis, moniliasis,* ***glomerulonephritis***

CNS: Headache, fever, ***seizures***

META: Hyperkalemia, hypokalemia, alkalosis, hypernatremia

INTEG: Rash, urticaria

SYST: ***Anaphylaxis, respiratory distress, serum sickness, superinfection***

Contraindications: Hypersensitivity to penicillins

Precautions: Pregnancy (B), lactation, hypersensitivity to cephalosporins; neonates, renal disease

Pharmacokinetics:

PO: Peak 2 hr, duration 6-8 hr; half-life 1-1⅓ hr, metabolized in liver, excreted in urine, crosses placenta, excreted in breast milk, removed by hemodialysis

Interactions:

• ↑ amoxicillin levels: probenecid

• ↓ action of: oral contraceptives

• ↑ anticoagulant effect: warfarin

Delayed/reduced absorption: khat; separate by 2 hr

Do not use acidophilus with anti-infectives

Lab test interferences:

False positive: Urine glucose, urine protein, direct Coombs' test

NURSING CONSIDERATIONS

Assess:

• I&O ratio; report hematuria, oliguria since penicillin in high doses is nephrotoxic

• Any patient with a compromised renal system since drug is excreted slowly in poor renal system function; toxicity may occur

• Hepatic studies: AST, ALT

• Blood studies: WBC, RBC, Hgb and Hct, bleeding time
• Renal studies: urinalysis, protein, blood, BUN, creatinine
• Culture, sensitivity before drug therapy; drug may be given as soon as culture is taken
• Bowel pattern before, during treatment; diarrhea, cramping, blood in stools, report to prescriber, pseudomembranous colitis may occur
• Skin eruptions after administration of penicillin to 1 wk after discontinuing drug
• Respiratory status: rate, character, wheezing, tightness in chest
• Anaphylaxis: rash, itching, dyspnea, facial/laryngeal edema

Administer:

PO route

◆ Only as directed, 2 (250 mg tab) not equivalent to 1 (500 mg tab) due to strength of clavulanate
• Shake suspension well before each dose, may be used alone or mixed in drinks, use immediately
• Give around the clock

Perform/provide:
• Adrenaline, suction, tracheostomy set, endotracheal intubation equipment on unit
• Adequate intake of fluids (2 L) during diarrhea episodes
• Scratch test to assess allergy after securing order from prescriber; usually done when penicillin is only drug of choice
• Storage refrigerated for 10 days

Evaluate:
• Therapeutic response: absence of infection

Teach patient/family:
• To take as prescribed, not to double dose
• All aspects of drug therapy: need to complete entire course of medication to ensure organism death (10-14 days); culture may be taken after completed course of medication
◆ To report sore throat, fever, fatigue (may indicate superinfection or agranulocytosis)
• That drug must be taken in equal intervals around the clock to maintain blood levels
• To wear or carry emergency ID if allergic to penicillins
• To notify prescriber of diarrhea, cramping, blood in stools; pseudomembranous colitis may occur
• To use alternative contraceptive measures, if using oral contraceptives

Treatment of hypersensitivity: Withdraw drug, maintain airway, administer epinephrine, aminophylline, O_2, IV corticosteroids for anaphylaxis

amphotericin B deoxycholate
(am-foe-ter′i-sin)
Fungizone

amphotericin B cholesteryl sulfate
Amphotec

amphotericin B lipid based
Abelcet

amphotericin B liposome
AmBisome

Func. class.: Antifungal
Chem. class.: Amphoteric polyene

Action: Increases cell membrane permeability in susceptible organisms by binding sterols; decreases potassium, sodium, and nutrients in cell

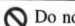

Uses: Histoplasmosis, blastomycosis, coccidioidomycosis, cryptococcosis, aspergillosis, phycomycosis,

candidiasis, sporotrichosis causing severe meningitis, septicemia, skin infections, cryptococcal meningitis in HIV-infected patients
Investigational uses: Candiduria (bladder irrigation)
Dosage and routes:
Deoxycholate
• *Adult:* **IV** Give test dose of 1 mg; then 0.25 mg/kg, increase qd slowly to 0.5 mg/kg, may give 1 mg/kg/day or 1.5 mg/kg qid, alternate-day dosing may be used
• *Child:* **IV** 0.25 mg/kg infused initially, increase by 0.25 mg/kg qod to max of 1 mg/kg/day
• *Adult/child:* **TOP** apply 2-4 × daily
• *Adult/child:* **PO** 1 ml qid
Amphotec
• *Adult/child:* **IV** 3-4 mg/kg/day, max 6 mg/kg/day
Abelcet
• *Adult/child:* **IV** 5 mg/kg/day as a 1 mg/ml inf given 2.5 mg/kg/hr
AmBisome
Fungal infections
• *Adult/child:* **IV** 3-5 mg/kg q24h
Visceral leishmaniasis 3-4 mg/kg q24h days 1-5, decrease dose
Available forms: *Amphotericin deoxycholate* inj 50 mg vial; oral susp 100 mg/ml, cream, ointment, lotion 3%; *amphotericin B cholesteryl* powder for inj 50 mg/20 ml, 100 mg/50 ml; *amphotericin B lipid complex* susp for inj 100 mg/20 ml vial; amphotericin B liposome powder for inj 50 mg vial
Side effects/adverse reactions:
EENT: Tinnitus, deafness, diplopia, blurred vision
INTEG: Burning, irritation, pain, necrosis at inj site with extravasation, flushing, dermatitis, skin rash (topical route)
CNS: Headache, fever, chills, peripheral nerve pain, paresthesias, peripheral neuropathy, ***convulsions,*** dizziness
GU: Hypokalemia, azotemia, hyposthenuria, ***renal tubular acidosis,*** nephrocalcinosis, ***permanent renal impairment, anuria, oliguria***
GI: Nausea, vomiting, anorexia, diarrhea, cramps, ***hemorrhagic gastroenteritis, acute liver failure***
MS: ***Arthralgia, myalgia,*** generalized pain, weakness, weight loss
HEMA: Normochromic, normocytic anemia, ***thrombocytopenia, agranulocytosis, leukopenia, eosinophilia,*** hypokalemia, hyponatremia, hypomagnesemia
Contraindications: Hypersensitivity, severe bone marrow depression
Precautions: Renal disease, pregnancy (B), lactation
Pharmacokinetics:
IV: Peak 1-2 hr, initial half-life 24 hr, metabolized in liver, excreted in urine (metabolites), breast milk, highly bound to plasma proteins; penetrates poorly CSF, bronchial secretions, aqueous humor, muscle, bone
Interactions:
• ↑ nephrotoxicity: other nephrotoxic antibiotics (aminoglycosides, cisplatin, vancomycin, cycloSPORINE, polymyxin B)
• ↑ hypokalemia: corticosteroids, digitalis, skeletal muscle relaxants, thiazides
↑ possibility of nephrotoxicity: gossypol
Do not use acidophilus with anti-infectives

NURSING CONSIDERATIONS
Assess:
• VS q15-30min during first infusion; note changes in pulse, B/P
• I&O ratio; watch for decreasing urinary output, change in specific gravity; discontinue drug to prevent permanent damage to renal tubules
• Blood studies: CBC, K, Na, Ca, Mg q2wk, BUN, creatinine weekly

• Weight weekly; if weight increases over 2 lb/wk, edema is present; renal damage should be considered

For renal toxicity: increasing BUN, serum creatinine; if BUN is >40 mg/dl or if serum creatinine >3 mg/dl, drug may be discontinued or dosage reduced

For hepatotoxicity: increasing AST, ALT, alk phosphatase, bilirubin

• For allergic reaction: dermatitis, rash; drug should be discontinued, antihistamines (mild reaction) or epinephrine (severe reaction) administered

• For hypokalemia: anorexia, drowsiness, weakness, decreased reflexes, dizziness, increased urinary output, increased thirst, paresthesias

• For ototoxicity: tinnitus (ringing, roaring in ears) vertigo, loss of hearing (rare)

Administer:

• Do not confuse three different types

IV route

• Drug only after C&S confirms organism, drug needed to treat condition; make sure drug is used in life-threatening infections

Deoxycholate route

• After diluting 50 mg/10 ml sterile water (no preservatives) (5 mg-1 ml), shake, dilute with 500 ml of D_5W to concentration of 0.1 mg/ml; infuse over 2-6 hr

• Test dose of 1 mg/20 ml D_5W; give over 10-30 min

Intermittent IV INF route

• IV using in-line filter (mean pore diameter >1 micron) using distal veins; check for extravasation, necrosis q8h; use an infusion pump; administer over 6 hr; rapid infusion may result in circulation collapse

Additive compatibilities: Heparin, hydrocortisone, sodium bicarbonate

Syringe compatibilities: Heparin

Y-site compatibilities: Aldesleukin, diltiazem, DOXOrubicin liposome, famotidine, remifentanil, tacrolimus, teniposide, thiotepa, zidovudine

Solution compatibilities: D_5W

IV route

• Reconstitute 50 mg vial/10 ml, 100 mg vial/20 ml sterile water for inj (5 mg/5 ml); swirl or shake gently until dissolved, further dilute with D_5W (0.6 mg/ml); wear gloves while preparing

• Test dose 10 ml of final solution (1.6-8.3 mg) over ½ hr, observe for next ½ hr for reactions

• Give 1 mg/kg/hr using infusion pump, do not give rapidly, may increase infusion, if tolerated

• Additive compatibility: Heparin

Cholesteryl

Liposomal complex

IV route

• Reconstitute with 12 ml sterile water/50 ml vial (4 mg/ml), shake, use 5 micron filter, dilute in D_5W (1-2 mg/ml), give over 2 hr

Lipid complex

IV route

• Shake vial until dissolved, withdraw dose using 18G needle, replace needle from syringe with drug using 5 micron filter needle (use needle for 4 vials or less), empty contents in IV of D_5W (1 mg/ml), give at 2.5 mg/kg/hr, use infusion pump

Perform/provide:

• Acetaminophen and diphenhydramine 30 min prior to infusion to reduce fever, chills, headache

• Storage protected from moisture and light; diluted solution is stable for 24 hr at room temperature

Evaluate:

• Therapeutic response: decreased fever, malaise, rash, negative C&S for infecting organism

A

Teach patient/family:
• That long-term therapy may be needed to clear infection (2 wk-3 mo depending on type of infection)
• To notify prescriber of bleeding, bruising, or soft tissue swelling

amphotericin B topical

See appendix c

ampicillin (℞)

(am-pi-sill'in)
Ampicin✤, Apo-Ampi✤, Marcillin, NovoAmpicillin✤, Nu- Ampi✤, Omnipen, Penbriten✤, Polycillin, Principen, Totacillin
Func. class.: Broad-spectrum antiinfective
Chem. class.: Aminopenicillin

Action: Interferes with cell wall replication of susceptible organisms; the cell wall, rendered osmotically unstable, swells, bursts from osmotic pressure
Uses: Effective for gram-positive cocci *(Staphylococcus aureus, Streptococcus pyogenes, Streptococcus faecalis, Streptococcus pneumoniae),* gram-negative cocci *(Neisseria gonorrhoeae, Neisseria meningitidis),* gram-negative bacilli *(Haemophilus influenzae, Proteus mirabilis, Salmonella, Shigella, Listeria monocytogenes),* gram-positive bacilli
Investigational uses: High-risk for infection in patients having C-section
Dosage and routes:
Systemic infections
• *Adult and child ≥40 kg (88 lb):* **PO** 1-2 g qd in divided doses q6h; **IV/IM** 2-8 g qd in divided doses q4-6h
• *Child <40 kg:* **PO** 25-100 mg/kg/day in divided doses q6h; **IV/IM** 25-50 mg/kg/day in divided doses q8h
Renal disease
• CCr 10-30 ml/min dose q8-12h; CCr 30-50 ml/min q6-8hr; <10 ml/min dose q12h
Bacterial meningitis
• *Adult:* **IV** 8-14 g/day in divided doses q3-4h
• *Child:* **IV** 100-200 mg/kg/day in divided doses q3-4h
Gonorrhea
• *Adult and child ≥ 45 kg (99 lb):* **PO** 3.5 g given with 1 g probenecid as a single dose; **IM/IV** 500 mg q6h (≥40 kg); **IM/IV** 50 mg/kg/day in divided doses q6-8h (<40 kg)
Available forms: Powder for inj 125, 250, 500 mg, 1, 2, 10 g; IV inj 500 mg, 1, 2 g; caps 250, 500 mg; powder for oral susp 125, 250, 500 mg/5 ml
Side effects/adverse reactions:
INTEG: Rash, urticaria
HEMA: Anemia, increased bleeding time, ***bone marrow depression, granulocytopenia***
GI: Nausea, vomiting, diarrhea, ***pseudomembranous colitis***
GU: Oliguria, proteinuria, hematuria, *vaginitis, moniliasis,* ***glomerulonephritis***
CNS: Lethargy, hallucinations, anxiety, depression, twitching, ***coma, seizures***
MISC: ***Anaphylaxis, serum sickness***
Contraindications: Hypersensitivity to penicillins
Precautions: Pregnancy (B), lactation; hypersensitivity to cephalosporins; neonates, renal disease
Do not confuse:
Omnipen/imipenem
Pharmacokinetics:
PO: Peak 2 hr, duration 6-8 hr
IV: Peak 5 min

IM: Peak 1 hr
Half-life 50-110 min; metabolized in liver; excreted in urine, bile, breast milk; crosses placenta, removed by dialysis

Interactions:

• ↑ ampicillin concentrations: probenecid

• ↓ effectiveness of oral contraceptives

• ↑ ampicillin-induced skin rash: allopurinol

Delayed/reduced absorption: khat; separate by 2 hr

Do not use acidophilus with anti-infectives

Lab test interferences:

Decrease: Conjugated estrone in pregnancy, conjugated estrial
Increase: AST, ALT
False positive: Urine glucose, urine protein, direct Coombs'

NURSING CONSIDERATIONS

Assess:

• I&O ratio; report hematuria, oliguria, since penicillin in high doses is nephrotoxic

Any patient with compromised renal system, since drug is excreted slowly in poor renal system function; toxicity may occur

• Hepatic studies: AST, ALT

• Blood studies: WBC, RBC, Hgb and Hct, bleeding time

• Renal studies: urinalysis, protein, blood, BUN, creatinine

• C&S before drug therapy; drug may be taken as soon as culture is taken

• Bowel pattern before, during treatment

• Skin eruptions after administration of penicillin to 1 wk after discontinuing drug

• Respiratory status: rate, character, wheezing, tightness in chest

• Anaphylaxis: rash, itching, dyspnea, facial swelling; stop drug, notify prescriber, have emergency equipment available

Administer:

PO route

• On empty stomach for best absorption (1-2 hr ac or 2-3 hr pc)

• Shake suspension well before each dose

IM route

• Reconstitute by adding 0.9-1.2 ml/125 mg vial; 0.9-1.9 ml/250 mg vial; 1.2-1.8 ml/500 mg vial; 2.4-7.4 ml/1 g vial; 6.8 ml/2 g vial

IV route

• After diluting with sterile H_2O 0.9-1.2 ml/125 mg drug, administer over 3-5 min (up to 500 mg), 10-15 min (>500 mg) by direct IV; may be diluted in 50 ml or more of D_5W, D_5 0.45% NaCl to a concentration of 30 mg/ml or less; IV sol is stable for 1 hr; give at prescribed rate

Additive compatibilities: Clindamycin, erythromycin, floxacillin, furosemide

Syringe compatibilities: Chloramphenicol, heparin, procaine

Y-site compatibilities: Acyclovir, allopurinol, amifostine, aztreonam, cyclophosphamide, DOXOrubicin liposome, enalaprilat, esmolol, famotidine, filgrastim, fludarabine, foscarnet, granisetron, heparin, insulin (regular), labetalol, magnesium sulfate, melphalan, meperidine, morphine, multivitamins, ofloxacin, perphenazine, phytonadione, potassium chloride, propofol, remifentanil, tacrolimus, teniposide, theophylline, thiotepa, tolazoline, vit B/C

Perform/provide:

• Adrenaline, suction, tracheostomy set, endotracheal intubation equipment on unit

• Adequate intake of fluids (2 L) during diarrhea episodes

• Scratch test to assess allergy after securing order from prescriber; usually done when penicillin is only drug of choice
• Storage in tight container; after reconstituting, oral suspension refrigerated for 2 wk or stored at room temperature for 1 wk

Evaluate:
• Therapeutic response: absence of temp, draining wounds, other symptoms of infections

Teach patient/family:
• That tabs may be crushed; caps may be opened and mixed with water
• To take oral ampicillin on empty stomach with full glass of water
• All aspects of drug therapy: need to complete entire course of medication to ensure organism death (10-14 days); culture may be taken after completed course of medication
◆ To report sore throat, fever, fatigue, diarrhea (may indicate superinfection); report rash or other signs of allergy
• That drug must be taken in equal intervals around the clock to maintain blood levels
• To wear or carry emergency ID if allergic to penicillins

Treatment of anaphylaxis: Withdraw drug, maintain airway, administer epinephrine, aminophylline, O_2, IV corticosteroids

ampicillin, sulbactam (℞)

Unasyn

Func. class.: Broad-spectrum antiinfective

Chem. class.: Aminopenicillin with β-lactamase inhibitor

Action: Interferes with cell wall replication of susceptible organisms; the cell wall, rendered osmotically unstable, swells, bursts from osmotic pressure; combination extends spectrum of activity by β-lactamase inhibition

Uses: Skin infections, intraabdominal infections, pneumonia *(Staphylococcus aureus, Escherichia coli, Klebsiella, Proteus mirabilis, Bacteroides fragilis, Haemophilus influenzae, Enterobacter, Acinetobacter calcoaceticus)*, intraabdominal infections *(Enterobacter, Klebsiella, Bacteroides, E. coli)*, gynecologic infections *(E. coli, Bacteroides)*, meningitis, septicemia

Dosage and routes:
• *Adult/child ≥40 kg:* **IM/IV** 1 g ampicillin, 0.5 g sulbactam to 2 g ampicillin and 1 g sulbactam q6h, not to exceed 4 g/day sulbactam
• *Child ≤40 kg:* **IV** 100-200 mg/kg/day (ampicillin component) divided q6h, max 8 g/day

Renal disease
• *Adult ≥40 kg:* **IM/IV** CCr 15-29 ml/min dose q12h; CCr 5-14 ml/min dose q24h

Available forms: Powder for inj 1.5 g (1 g ampicillin, 0.5 g sulbactam), 3 g (2 g ampicillin, 1 g sulbactam), 10 g (10 g ampicillin, 5 g sulbactam)

Side effects/adverse reactions:
HEMA: Anemia, increased bleeding time, ***bone marrow depression, granulocytopenia***
GI: Nausea, vomiting, diarrhea, increased AST, ALT, abdominal pain, glossitis, colitis, ***pseudomembranous colitis***
GU: Oliguria, proteinuria, hematuria, *vaginitis, moniliasis,* ***glomerulonephritis,*** dysuria
CNS: Lethargy, hallucinations, anxiety, depression, twitching, ***coma, seizures***
MISC: ***Anaphylaxis, serum sickness***

Contraindications: Hypersensitiv-

ity to penicillins, ampicillin, or sulbactam

Precautions: Pregnancy (B), lactation, hypersensitivity to cephalosporins, neonates, renal disease

Pharmacokinetics:
IV: Peak 5 min; half-life 50-110 min; little metabolized in liver, 75% to 85% of both drugs excreted in urine, diffuses to breast milk, crosses placenta

Interactions:
- ↓ oral contraceptive effect
- ↑ ampicillin level: probenecid
- Ampicillin-induced skin rash: allopurinol

Herb: Delayed/reduced absorption: khat; separate by 2 hr

Herb: Do not use acidophilus with anti-infectives

Lab test interferences:
False positive: Urine glucose, urine protein

NURSING CONSIDERATIONS

Assess:
- Bowel pattern before, during treatment
- Respiratory status: rate, character, wheezing, tightness in chest
- I&O ratio; report hematuria, oliguria, since penicillin in high doses is nephrotoxic

Alert: Any patient with compromised renal system, since drug is excreted slowly in poor renal system function; toxicity may occur rapidly

- Hepatic studies: AST, ALT if on long-term therapy
- Blood studies: WBC, RBC, Hct, Hgb, bleeding time
- Renal studies: urinalysis, protein, blood, BUN, creatinine
- C&S before drug therapy; drug may be given as soon as culture is taken
- Skin eruptions after administration of ampicillin to 1 wk after discontinuing drug
- Allergies before initiation of treatment; reaction of each medication; report allergies

Administer:

IM route
- Reconstitute by adding 3.2 ml sterile water/1.5 g vial; 6.4 ml/3 g vial, give deep in large muscle

IV route
- After diluting 1.5 g/3.2 ml sterile H_2O for inj or 3 g/6.4 ml (250 mg ampicillin/125 mg sulbactam); allow to stand until foaming stops; may give over 15 min as direct IV; dilute further in 50 ml or more of D_5W, NaCl, administer within 1 hr after reconstitution; give as an intermittent inf over 15-30 min

Additive compatibilities: Aztreonam

Y-site compatibilities: Amifostine, aztreonam, cefepime, enalaprilat, famotidine, filgrastim, fluconazole, fludarabine, gallium, granisetron, heparin, insulin (regular), meperidine, morphine, paclitaxel, remifentanil, tacrolimus, teniposide, theophylline, thiotepa

Perform/provide:
- Adrenaline, suction, tracheostomy set, endotracheal intubation equipment on unit for possible anaphylaxis
- Adequate intake of fluids (2 L) during diarrhea episodes
- Scratch test to assess allergy after securing order from prescriber; usually done when penicillin is only drug choice
- Storage in tight container, out of light

Evaluate:
- Therapeutic response: absence of fever, draining wounds, negative C&S

Teach patient/family:
- That oral contraceptives may be reduced and a nonhormonal contraceptive should be taken while on

this drug if pregnancy is to be prevented
• To report superinfection: vaginal itching, loose, foul-smelling stools, black furry tongue
◆ To report immediately pseudomembranous colitis: fever, diarrhea with pus, blood, or mucus; may occur up to 4 wk after treatment
• To wear or carry emergency ID if allergic to penicillin products

Treatment of anaphylaxis: Withdraw drug, maintain airway, administer epinephrine, aminophylline, O_2, IV corticosteroids

amprenavir (℞)

(am-pren'ah-veer)
Agenerase
Func. class.: Antiretroviral
Chem. class.: Protease inhibitor

Action: Inhibits human immunodeficiency virus (HIV) protease, which prevents maturation of the infectious virus

Uses: HIV in combination with other antiretroviral agents

Research note: One study has documented an increased hypersensitivity to amprenavir in the HIV type 1 virus[2]

Dosage and routes:
Caps and sol are not interchangeable
• *Adult:* **PO** (cap) 1200 mg bid
• *Child 13-16 yr:* **PO** (cap) 1200 mg bid
• *Child 4-12 yr or wt <50 kg:* **PO** Caps: 20 mg/kg qd or 15 mg/kg tid, max 2400 mg; sol: 22.5 mg/kg bid or 17 mg/kg tid qd, max 2800 mg

Amprenavir/Ritonavir regimen
• *Adult:* **PO** 600 mg amprenavir, 100 mg ritonavir bid or 1200 mg amprenavir, 200 mg ritonavir bid

Hepatic dose
• *Adult:* **PO** (Child, Pugh score 5-8) 450 mg bid (caps), 513 mg bid (sol) in combination; (Child, Pugh score 9-12) 300 mg bid (caps), 342 mg bid (sol) in combination

Available forms: Caps 50, 150 mg; oral sol 15 mg/ml

Side effects/adverse reactions:
GI: Diarrhea, abdominal pain, nausea, ***hepatotoxicity***
CNS: Paresthesia, headache
INTEG: Rash, ***Stevens-Johnson syndrome***
HEMA: ***Acute hemolytic anemia***
ENDO: New-onset diabetes, hyperglycemia, exacerbation of preexisting diabetes mellitus, hypertriglyceridemia

Contraindications: Hypersensitivity; oral sol: renal failure

Precautions: Liver disease, pregnancy (C), lactation, children, hemophilia, sulfonamide sensitivity, elderly

Pharmacokinetics: Rapidly absorbed, peak 1-2 hr, 90% protein bound, metabolized in liver, excreted unchanged in urine/feces (minimal), half-life 7-10½ hr

Interactions:
• Toxicity: alprazolam, bepridil, carbamazepine, clozapine, dapsone, diazepam, diltiazem, ergots, erythromycin, flurazepam, itraconazole, loratadine, lovastatin, midazolam, niCARdipine, NIFEdipine, pimozide, triazolam
◆ Serious life-threatening interactions: amiodarone, lidocaine, quinidine, tricyclics, warfarin
• ↑ amprenavir levels: cimetidine, clarithromycin, erythromycin, indinavir, itraconazole, ketoconazole, ritonavir
• ↓ amprenavir levels: antacids, carbamazepine, didanosine, efavirenz, nevirapine, phenobarbital, phenytoin, rifamycins

• ↓ effects of: oral contraceptives, methadone
• Drug/food: ↓ bioavailability after high-fat meal
↓ amprenavir levels: St. John's wort

Lab test interferences:
Increase: Glucose, cholesterol, triglycerides

NURSING CONSIDERATIONS
Assess:
For renal or hepatic failure, pregnancy, or those receiving disulfiram, metronidazole; oral solution contains propylene glycol in greater quantities
• Signs of infection, anemia
• Hepatic studies: ALT, AST
• Bowel pattern before, during treatment; if severe abdominal pain with bleeding occurs, drug should be discontinued; monitor hydration
• Viral load, CD4 count throughout treatment
• Skin eruptions, rash, urticaria, itching
• Allergies before treatment, reaction of each medication; place allergies on chart

Administer:
• Do not interchange caps and oral sol; they are not the same on a mg/mg basis.
• With or without food; avoid high-fat meals

Evaluate:
• Therapeutic response: Increasing CD4 counts; decreased viral load, resolution of symptoms of HIV

Teach patient/family:
• To take as prescribed with or without food, avoid high-fat foods; if dose is missed, take as soon as remembered up to 1 hr before next dose; do not double dose, do not share with others
• That drug must be taken in equal intervals around the clock to maintain blood levels for duration of therapy
• To use a nonhormonal method of contraception during treatment, use condoms
• To notify prescriber if diarrhea, nausea, vomiting, rash occurs
• That drug does not cure AIDs or prevent transmission to others, only controls symptoms

---

RARELY USED

amyl nitrite (℞)
(am'il nye'trite)
amyl nitrite, Amyl Nitrite Aspirols, Amyl Nitrite Vaporole
Func. class.: Coronary vasodilator

Uses: Acute angina pectoris, cyanide poisoning

Dosage and routes:
Angina
• *Adult:* **INH** 0.18-0.3 ml as needed, 1-6 inhalations from 1 cap, may repeat in 3-5 min
Cyanide poisoning
• *Adult:* **INH** 0.3 ml ampule inhaled 15 sec until preparation of sodium nitrite infusion is ready

Investigational uses: Cardiac murmur diagnosis

Contraindications: Hypersensitivity to nitrites, severe anemia, increased intracranial pressure, hypertension, pregnancy (X)

anagrelide (℞)

(a-na'gre-lide)

Agrylin

Func. class.: Antiplatelet

Chem. class.: Imidazo-quinazolinone

Action: Reduces platelet count and prevents early platelet shape changes in response to aggregating agents thus inhibiting platelet aggregation

Uses: Essential thrombocythemia, polycythemia vera, chronic myelogenous leukemia

Dosage and routes:

• *Adult:* **PO** 0.5 mg qid or 1 mg bid, may be adjusted after 1 wk, max 10 mg/day or 2.5 mg single dose

Available forms: Caps 0.5, 1.0 mg

Side effects/adverse reactions:

MS: Asthenia, back pain

RESP: Dyspnea

GU: Dysuria

GI: Diarrhea, abdominal pain, nausea, flatulence, vomiting, anorexia, constipation, pancreatitis

CV: Postural hypotension, tachycardia, palpitations, ***CHF, MI, cardiomyopathy, cardiomegaly, complete heart block, atrial fibrillation,*** dysrhythmia, ***chest pain***

CNS: Headache, dizziness, ***seizures, paresthesia, CVA***

INTEG: Rash

HEMA: ***Anemia, thrombocytopenia, ecchymosis, lymphadenoma***

Contraindications: Hypersensitivity, hypotension

Precautions: Pregnancy (C), lactation, child <16 yr, cardiac, renal, hepatic disease

Pharmacokinetics:

PO: Peak 1 hr, duration >24 hr: metabolized in liver: excreted in feces/urine

Interactions:

• ↓ absorption: sucralfate

• Drug/food: ↓ bioavailability

🍃 Gastric irritation: arginine

🍃 ↓ effect: bilberry, saw palmetto

🍃 ↑ effect: bogbean, dong quai, feverfew, ginger, ginkgo

NURSING CONSIDERATIONS

Assess:

• Platelet counts q2day × 1 wk, and qwk thereafter, response should begin after 1-2 wk; Hgb, WBC

• B/P, pulse during treatment until stable; take B/P lying, standing; orthostatic hypotension is common

• Cardiac status: chest pain, what aggravates or ameliorates condition

Administer:

• On an empty stomach: 1 hr before meals or 2 hr after; give with 8 oz water for better absorption

Perform/provide:

• Storage at room temperature

Evaluate:

• Therapeutic response: decreased platelet count

Teach patient/family:

• That medication is not a cure: may have to be taken continuously in evenly spaced doses only as directed

• That it is necessary to quit smoking to prevent excessive vasoconstriction

• To avoid hazardous activities until stabilized on medication; dizziness may occur

• To rise slowly from sitting or lying to prevent orthostatic hypotension

• Not to use alcohol or OTC medications unless approved by prescriber

• To report cardiac reactions, increased bruising, bleeding

• To use contraception (female, child-bearing age)

anakinra (℞)

(an-ah-kin'rah)

Kineret

Func. class.: Antirheumatic agent (disease modifying), immunomodulator

Chem. class.: Recombinant form of human interleukin-1 receptor antagonist (IL-1Ra)

Action: A form of human interleukin-1 receptor antagonist (IL-1Ra) produced by DNA technology; blocks activity of IL-1, resulting in decreased cartilage degradation and decreased bone resorption

Uses: Reduction in signs and symptoms of moderate to severe active rheumatoid arthritis in patients ≥18 years of age who have not responded to other disease-modifying agents

Dosage and routes:

• *Adult:* **SC** 100 mg qd

Available form: Sol for inj 100 mg/ml

Side effects/adverse reactions:

CNS: Headache

EENT: Sinusitis

GI: Abdominal pain, nausea, diarrhea

INTEG: Rash, *inj site reaction*

HEMA: ***Neutropenia***

MISC: Flulike symptoms

RESP: URI

Contraindications: Hypersensitivity to *Escherichia coli*–derived proteins or this product, sepsis

Precautions: Pregnancy (B), lactation, children, renal impairment, elderly

Pharmacokinetics: Terminal half-life 4-6 hr

Interactions:

• ↑ risk of severe infection: TNF blocking agents, etanercept

• Do not give concurrently with vaccines, immunizations should be brought up to date before treatment

NURSING CONSIDERATIONS

Assess:

• Pain, stiffness, ROM, swelling of joints during treatment

• For inj site pain, swelling; usually occur after 2 inj (4-5 days)

• For infections, stop treatment if present

Administer:

• Do not use if cloudy or discolored or if particulate is present, protect from light

• Do not admix with other sol or medications, do not use filter

Evaluate:

• Therapeutic response: decreased inflammation, pain in joints

Teach patient/family:

• About self-administration if appropriate: inj should be made in thigh, abdomen, upper arm; rotate sites at least 1 inch from old site

• To notify prescriber if pregnancy is planned or suspected, avoid breast-feeding

anastrozole

(an-a-stroh'zole)

Arimidex

Func. class.: Antineoplastic

Chem. class.: Aromatase inhibitor

Action: Lowers serum estradiol concentrations; many breast cancers have strong estrogen receptors

Uses: Advanced breast carcinoma not responsive to other therapy in estrogen-receptor–positive patients (usually postmenopausal)

Dosage and routes:

• *Adult:* **PO** 1 mg qd

Available forms: Tabs 1 mg

Side effects/adverse reactions:

HEMA: ***Leukopenia***

GI: Nausea, vomiting, altered taste

leading to anorexia, diarrhea, constipation, abdominal pain, dry mouth
GU: Vaginal bleeding, vaginal dryness, pelvic pain, pruritus vulvae, UTI
INTEG: Rash, alopecia
CV: Chest pain, hypertension, thrombophlebitis, edema
CNS: Hot flashes, headache, lightheadedness, depression, dizziness, confusion, insomnia, anxiety
RESP: Cough, sinusitis, dyspnea
MS: Bone pain, myalgia, asthenia
Contraindications: Hypersensitivity, pregnancy (D)
Precautions: Leukopenia, thrombocytopenia, lactation, children, elderly, liver disease, renal disease
Pharmacokinetics:
PO: Peak 4-7 hr, half-life 50 hr, excreted in feces, urine
Lab test interferences:
Increase: GGT, AST, ALT, alk phosphatase, cholesterol, LDL

NURSING CONSIDERATIONS

Assess:
- For side effects during treatment

Administer:

PO route
- Give with food

Perform/provide:
- Storage in light-resistant container at room temperature

Evaluate:
- Therapeutic response: decreased tumor size, spread of malignancy

Teach patient/family:
- To report any complaints, side effects to prescriber
- That vaginal bleeding, pruritus, hot flashes are reversible after discontinuing treatment
- To report vaginal bleeding immediately
- That tumor flare—increase in size of tumor, increased bone pain—may occur and will subside rapidly; may take analgesics for pain
- That hair may be lost during treatment; a wig or hairpiece may make patient feel better; new hair may be different in color, texture after completion of therapy

---

HIGH ALERT

anistreplase (℞)

(ah-nis′tre-place)
anisoylated plasminogen, APSAC, Eminase

Func. class.: Thrombolytic enzyme
Chem. class.: Plasminogen activator

Action: Promotes thrombolysis by promoting conversion of plasminogen to plasmin
Uses: Acute MI for lysis of coronary artery thrombi
Dosage and routes:
- *Adult:* **IV INJ** 30 units over 2-5 min as soon as possible after onset of symptoms

Available forms: Powder, lyophilized 30 units/vial
Side effects/adverse reactions:
HEMA: Decreased Hct; ***GI, GU, intracranial, retroperitoneal,*** surface bleeding; ***thrombocytopenia***
INTEG: Rash, urticaria, phlebitis at inj site, itching, flushing
CNS: Headache, fever, sweating, agitation, dizziness, paresthesia, tremor, vertigo, ***intracranial hemorrhage***
GI: Nausea, vomiting
RESP: Altered respirations, dyspnea, ***bronchospasm, lung edema***
MS: Low back pain, arthralgia
CV: Hypotension, ***dysrhythmias,*** conduction disorders
SYST: ***Anaphylaxis (rare)***
Contraindications: Hypersensitivity, active internal bleeding, intraspinal or intracranial surgery, neoplasms of CNS, severe, uncontrolled

hypertension, cerebral embolism/thrombosis/hemorrhage, hypersensitivity to this drug or streptokinase, recent trauma/history of CVA

Precautions: Arterial emboli from left side of heart, pregnancy (C), ulcerative colitis/enteritis, renal disease, hepatic disease, hypocoagulation, COPD, subacute bacterial endocarditis, rheumatic valvular disease, intraarterial diagnostic procedure or surgery (10 days), recent major surgery, lactation, elderly

Pharmacokinetics: Half-life 105 min

Interactions:

- ↑ bleeding potential: aspirin, other NSAIDs, heparin, antiplatelets, abciximab, eptifibatide, tirofiban, clopidogrel, ticlopidine, some cephalosporins, plicamycin, valproic acid, anticoagulants, dipyridamole
- ↓ action of anistreplase: aminocaproic acid, aprotinin, trahexamic acid

↑ risk of bleeding: agrimony, alfalfa, angelica, anise, basil, bay, bilberry, black haw, bogbean, bromelain, buchu, chondroitin, cinchona bark, dong quai, fenugreek, feverfew, garlic, ginger, ginkgo, ginseng, horse chestnut, Irish moss, kelp, kelpware, khella, lovage, lungwort, meadowsweet, motherwort, mugwort, nettle, papaya, parsley (large amts), Pau D'arco, pineapple, poplar, prickly ash, safflower, saw palmetto, tonka bean, tumeric, wintergreen, yarrow

↓ anticoagulant effect: chamomile, coenzyme Q10, flax, glucomannan, goldenseal, guar gum

Lab test interferences:

Increase: PT, APTT, TT

Decrease: Fibrinogen, plasminogen

NURSING CONSIDERATIONS

Assess:

- VS, B/P, pulse, respirations, neurologic signs, temp at least q4h, temp >104° F (40° C) or indicators of internal bleeding, monitor ECG, treat bradycardia, ventricular changes; assess neurologic status, neurologic change may indicate intracranial bleeding; ECG continuously, cardiac enzymes, radionuclide, myocardial scanning/coronary angiography
- Hypersensitivity: fever, rash, itching, chills, facial swelling dyspnea; notify prescriber immediately, stop drug, keep resusciatative equipment nearby; mild reaction may be treated with antihistamines

Bleeding during first hr of treatment (hematuria, hematemesis, bleeding from mucous membranes, epistaxis, ecchymosis), continue to monitor for 24 hr after treatment

- Blood studies (Hct, platelets, PTT, PT, TT, APTT) before starting therapy; PT or APTT must be less than 2 × control before starting therapy; TT or PT q3-4h during treatment

Administer:

IV, direct route

- Reconstitute single-dose vial/5 ml sterile water for inj (not bacteriostatic water), and roll (not shake) to enhance reconstitution; give over 2-5 min by direct IV, give within ½ hr of reconstitution or discard, do not add other meds to vial or syringe; give within 6 hr of thrombi identification for best results
- Cryoprecipitate or fresh frozen plasma if bleeding occurs
- Heparin therapy after thrombolytic therapy is discontinued, TT or APTT less than 2 × control (about 3-4 hr)
- About 10% of patients have high streptococcal antibody titers, requiring increased loading doses

Perform/provide:

- Bed rest during entire course of treatment; handle patient as little as possible during therapy

• Storage of powder in refrigerator; use within 30 min after reconstitution
• Avoid invasive procedures: inj, rectal temperature
• Treat fever with acetaminophen
• Pressure of 30 sec to minor bleeding sites, 30 min to sites of arterial puncture followed by dressing; inform prescriber if hemostasis not attained; apply pressure dressing

Evaluate:
• Therapeutic response: absence of thrombi formation in MI, improved ventricular function

---

HIGH ALERT

antihemophilic factor VIII (AHF) (℞)

(an-tee-hee-moe-fill'ik)
antihemophilic factor, Alphanate, Bioclate, Helixate FS, Hemofil M, Humate-P, Hyate C, Koate-DVI, Kogenate, Kogenate FS, Monoclate-P, Recombinate, ReFacto

Func. class.: Hemostatic
Chem. class.: Factor VIII

Action: Necessary for clotting; activates factor X in conjunction with activated factor IX; transforms prothrombin to thrombin

Uses: Hemophilia A, patients with acquired circulating factor VIII inhibitors, factor VIII deficiency

Dosage and routes:

Massive hemorrhage
• *Adult and child:* **IV** 40-50 units/kg, then 20-25 units/kg q8-12h

Overt bleeding
• *Adult and child:* **IV** 15-25 units/kg, then 8-15 units/kg q8-12h × 4 days

Hemorrhage near vital organs
• *Adult and child:* **IV** 15 units/kg, then 8 units/kg q8h × 2 days, then 4 units/kg q8h × 2 days

Minor hemorrhage
• *Adult and child:* **IV** 8-10 units/kg q24h × 2-3 days or 8 units/kg q12h × 2 days, then q24h × 2 days

Joint bleeding
• *Adult and child:* **IV** 5-10 units/kg q8-12h × 1-2 days

Available forms: Inj 250, 500, 1000, 1500 units/vial (number of units noted on label)

Side effects/adverse reactions:
GI: Nausea, vomiting, abdominal cramps, constipation, diarrhea, anorexia, jaundice, ***viral hepatitis***
INTEG: Rash, flushing, *urticaria,* stinging at inj site
CNS: Headache, *lethargy, chills, fever, flushing*
HEMA: ***Thrombosis, hemolysis, risk of hepatitis B, HIV***
CV: Hypotension, tachycardia
RESP: ***Bronchospasm,*** rhinitis, dyspnea, nosebleeds
MISC: ***Anaphylaxis***

Contraindications: Hypersensitivity; mouse, hamster, bovine protein

Precautions: Neonates/infants, hepatic disease; blood types A, B, AB; pregnancy (C), factor VIII inhibitor

Do not confuse:
Kogenate/Kogenate-2

Pharmacokinetics:
IV: Half-life 4 hr, terminal 15 hr

Interactions:
• Do not admix with other drugs
• ↑ bleeding: salicylates, NSAIDs

NURSING CONSIDERATIONS

Assess:
• Blood studies (coagulation factors assay by % normal: 5% prevents spontaneous hemorrhage, 30%-50% for surgery, 80%-100% for severe hemorrhage)
• I&O, urine color; notify prescriber if urine becomes orange, red

• Pulse: discontinue infusion if significant increase
• Hct, Coombs' test with blood types A, B, AB
• Test for factor VIII inhibitors before starting treatment, may require concomitant antiinhibitor coagulant complex therapy
• Allergy: fever, rash, itching, jaundice; give diphenhydramine HCl (Benadryl), continue therapy if reaction is mild
• Blood group of patient, donors (if applicable; most factor VIII not from specific blood group donors)
◆ Bleeding: ankles, knees, elbows, other joints

Administer:

IV route

• After rotating gently to mix
• Using plastic syringe to reconstitute, and administer; adheres to glass; use another needle as a vent when reconstituting
• After dilution with warm NS, D_5W, LR, give within 3 hr

IV INF route

• Give at ≤2 ml/min if concentration exceeds 34 units/ml or over 3 min if concentration is less than 34 units/ml

Perform/provide:

• Storage in refrigerator; do not freeze; after reconstitution, do not refrigerate; give within 3 hr

Evaluate:

• Therapeutic response: absence of bleeding

Teach patient/family:

• To report any signs of bleeding: gums, under skin, urine, stools, emesis; review methods to prevent bleeding
• To avoid salicylates, NSAIDs (increase bleeding tendencies)
• To prepare, administer factor VIII concentrates at first sign of danger
• To advise health professionals of treatment for hemophilia
• The signs of viral hepatitis, AIDS
• That immunization for hepatitis B may be given first
• To report hives, urticaria, chest tightness, hypotension; may be monoclonal antibody-derived factor VIII
• To be checked q2-3mo for HIV screen
• To carry emergency ID describing disease process

HIGH ALERT

antithrombin III, human (℞)

(an'tee-throm-bin)

ATnativ, Thrombate III

Func. class.: Antithrombin

Chem. class.: Pooled human plasma

Action: Inactivates thrombin and the activated forms of factors IX, X, XI, XII, resulting in inhibition of coagulation

Uses: Hereditary antithrombin III deficiency in connection with surgical or obstetric procedures or for thromboembolism

Dosage and routes: Dosage is individualized; after first dose, antithrombin III level should increase to about 120% of normal; thereafter maintain at levels >80%; this is usually achieved by administering maintenance doses q24h

Available forms: 500 international units in 10 ml; 1000 international units in 20 ml

Side effects/adverse reactions:

SYST: ***Bleeding,*** surface bleeding, ***anaphylaxis,*** vasodilatory effects

CNS: Dizziness, chills, severe lightheadedness

GI: Nausea, cramps, bowel fullness

RESP: Shortness of breath

Precautions: Pregnancy (B), lactation, children
Pharmacokinetics: Biologic half-life 2-5 days
Interactions:
- ↑ anticoagulant effect: heparin
- Do not administer with other drugs in syringe or solutions

NURSING CONSIDERATIONS
Assess:
- AT-III levels bid until stabilized, then qd before dose
- VS, B/P, pulse, respirations, neurologic signs, temp at least q4h, temp 104° F (40° C) or indicators of internal bleeding, cardiac rhythm
- ◆ For child born of parents with hereditary AT-III deficiency, obtain AT-III levels immediately after birth
- ◆ For neurologic changes that may indicate intracranial bleeding
- ◆ Retroperitoneal bleeding: back pain, leg weakness, diminished pulses

Administer:
- Heparin after fibrinogen level is over 100 mg/dl; heparin infusion to increase PTT to 1.5-2 × baseline for 3-7 days

IV route
- After reconstituting 500 international units/10 ml of NS or D_5W; do not shake; rotate to dissolve; allow to warm to room temperature; use within 3 hr of reconstitution; give 50 international units or less/min; do not exceed 100 international units/min using 0.22 or 0.45 microfilter

Evaluate:
- Therapeutic response: absence of thrombi formation

Teach patient/family:
- About drug use and expected results; to report adverse reactions; bleeding, bruising

antithymocyte

See lymphocyte immune globulin

apraclonidine ophthalmic

See appendix c

HIGH ALERT

ardeparin (℞)

(are-de-pear′in)
Normiflo
Func. class.: Anticoagulant
Chem. class.: Low-molecular-weight heparin

Action: Prevents conversion of fibrinogen to fibrin and prothrombin to thrombin by enhancing inhibitory effects of antithrombin III
Uses: Prevention of deep vein thrombosis after knee replacement surgery
Dosage and routes:
- *Adult:* **SC** 50 anti–factor Xa units/kg q12h beginning the evening of the day of knee replacement surgery or the following AM continued until patient is fully ambulatory or 2 wk, whichever is first

Available forms: Inj 5000, 10,000 anti–factor Xa units/0.5 ml
Side effects/adverse reactions:
CNS: ***Intracranial bleeding,*** fever, dizziness, headache
SYST: Hypersensitivity, ***hemorrhage, anaphylaxis*** possible
HEMA: ***Thrombocytopenia,*** anemia
INTEG: Pruritus, superficial wound infection, ecchymosis, rash, inj site reactions
CV: Chest pain
GI: Nausea, vomiting
RESP: Dyspnea

Contraindications: Hypersensitivity to this drug, pork products, heparin, or other anticoagulants; hemophilia, leukemia with bleeding, thrombocytopenic purpura, cerebrovascular hemorrhage, cerebral aneurysm, severe hypertension, other severe cardiac disease
Precautions: Elderly, pregnancy (C), hepatic disease, severe renal disease, blood dyscrasias, subacute bacterial endocarditis, acute nephritis, lactation, child, recent childbirth, peptic ulcer disease, pericarditis, pericardial effusion, recent lumbar puncture, vasculitis, other diseases where bleeding is possible
Pharmacokinetics: Unknown
Interactions:
• ↑ risk of bleeding: aspiration, oral anticoagulants, platelet inhibitors, NSAIDs
May ↑ risk of bleeding: agrimony, alfalfa, angelica, anise, bilberry, black haw, bogbean, bromelain, buchu, chondroitin, cinchona bark, dong quai, fenugreek, feverfew, garlic, ginger, ginkgo, ginseng, horse chestnut, Irish moss, kelp, kelpware, khella, lovage, lungwort, meadowsweet, mother wort, mugwort, nettle, papaya, parsley, Pau D'arco, pineapple, poplar, prickly ash, safflower, saw palmetto, senega, tonka bean, tumeric, wintergreen, yarrow
↓ action: chamomile, coenzyme Q10, flax, glucomannan, goldenseal, guar gum
NURSING CONSIDERATIONS
Assess:
• For blood studies (Hct, occult blood in stools, CBC, platelets, urinalysis) during treatment since bleeding can occur
For bleeding gums, petechiae, ecchymosis, black tarry stools, hematuria, epistaxis, decrease in Hct, B/P; may indicate bleeding, possible hemorrhage; notify prescriber immediately, drug should be discontinued, protamine should be = to dose of drug given; 1 mg protamine = 100 anti–factor Xa units of drug
• For hypersensitivity: fever, skin rash, urticaria; notify prescriber immediately
Administer:
• By SC only; have patient sit or lie down; SC inj may be around the navel in a U-shape, upper outer side of thigh or upper outer quadrangle of the buttocks; rotate inj sites
• Changing needles is not recommended
Evaluate:
• Therapeutic response: absence of deep-vein thrombosis
Teach patient/family:
• To avoid OTC preparations that may cause serious drug interactions unless directed by prescriber; may contain aspirin; other anticoagulants, NSAIDs
• To use soft-bristle toothbrush to avoid bleeding gums, avoid contact sports, use electric razor, avoid IM inj
• To report any signs of bleeding: gums, under skin, urine, stools; unusual bruising, hematoma at inj site
Treatment of overdose: Protamine sulfate 1% given IV

HIGH ALERT

argatroban (℞)

(are-ga-troe′ban)
Acova
Func. class.: Anticoagulant
Chem. class.: Thrombin inhibitor

Action: Direct inhibitor of thrombin that is derived from L-arginine;

it reversibly binds to the thrombin active site

Uses: Thrombosis, prophylaxis or treatment; percutaneous coronary intervention (PCI), anticoagulation prevention/treatment of thrombosis in heparin-induced thrombocytopenia

Dosage and routes:

• *Adult:* **IV:** 2 mcg/kg/min (1 mg/ml) give at 6 ml/hr for 50 kg of weight, at 8 ml/hr for 70 kg of weight, at 11 ml/hr for 90 kg of weight, at 13 ml/hr for 110 kg of weight, at 16 ml/hr for 130 kg of weight

Hepatic dose

• *Adult:* **CONT INF** 0.5 mcg/kg/min, adjust rate based on aPTT

• Heparin-induced thrombocytopenia or heparin-induced thrombocytopenia and thrombosis syndrome

Percutaneous coronary intervention (PCI)

• *Adult:* **IV INF** 25 mcg/kg/min and a bolus of 350 mcg/kg given over 3-5 min, check ACT 5-10 min after bolus is completed; proceed if ACT >300 sec

Available forms: Inj 100 mg/ml

Side effects/adverse reactions:

CV: ***Atrial fibrillation, ventricular tachycardia***

SYST: ***Sepsis***

CNS: Fever

GI: Nausea, vomiting, abdominal pain, diarrhea, GI bleeding

GU: ***Hematuria,*** abnormal kidney function, UTI

HEMA: ***Hemorrhage, thrombocytopenia***

RESP: Pneumonia, dyspnea

Contraindications: Hypersensitivity, overt major bleeding

Precautions: Intracranial bleeding, renal function impairment, lactation, children, hepatic disease, pregnancy (B)

Do not confuse:

argatroban/Aggrastat

Pharmacokinetics: Metabolized in the liver, distributed to extracellular fluid, 54% plasma protein binding, half-life 39-51 min, excreted in feces

Interactions:

• ↑ risk of bleeding: other anticoagulants

• ↑ action of argatroban thrombolytics

↓ argatroban effect: chamomile, coenzyme Q10, flax, glucomannan, goldenseal, guar gum

↑ bleeding risk: agrimony, alfalfa, angelica, anise, bilberry, black haw, bogbean, buchu, chondroitin, dong quai, fenugreek, feverfew, garlic, ginger, ginkgo, ginseng, horse chestnut, Irish moss, kelp, kelpware, khella, lovage, lungwort, meadowsweet, mother wort, mugwort, nettle, papaya, parsley, Pau D'arco, pineapple, poplar, prickly ash, safflower, saw palmetto, senega, turmeric, wintergreen

NURSING CONSIDERATIONS

Assess:

• Obtain baseline in aPTT before treatment; do not start treatment if aPTT ratio ≥2.5, then aPTT 4 hr after initiation of treatment and at least qd thereafter, if aPTT above target, stop inf for 2 hr, then restart at 50%, take aPTT in 4 hr; if below target, increase inf rate by 20%, take aPTT in 4 hr, do not exceed inf rate of 0.21 mg/kg/hr without checking for coagulation abnormalities

• aPTT, which should be 1.5-3 × control

Bleeding gums, petechiae, ecchymosis, black tarry stools, hematuria/epistaxis, B/P, vaginal bleeding and possible hemorrhage

• Fever, skin rash, urticaria

Administer:

• Avoiding all IM inj that may cause bleeding

IV INF route

- Dilute in 0.9% NaCl, D_5, LR to a final conc 1 mg/ml. Dilute each 2.5 ml vial 100-fold by mixing with 250 ml of diluent, mix by repeated inversion of the diluent bag for 1 min; may be slightly hazy
- Dosage adjustment may be made after review of aPTT, not to exceed 10 mcg/kg/min

Evaluate:

- Therapeutic response: absence or decrease of thrombosis

Teach patient/family:

- To use soft-bristle toothbrush to avoid bleeding gums, avoid contact sports, use electric razor, avoid IM inj
- To report any signs of bleeding: gums, under skin, urine, stools

aripiprazole (℞)

(a-rip-ip-pra'zol)

Abilify

Func. class.: Antipsychotic/ neuroleptic

Chem. class.: Benzisoxazole derivative

Action: Exact mechanism unknown; may be mediated through both dopamine type 2 (D_2) and serotonin type 2 ($5\text{-}HT_2$) antagonism

Uses: Schizophrenia

Dosage and routes:

- *Adult:* **PO** 10-15 mg/day; if needed, dosage may be increased to 30 mg qd after 2 wk

Available forms: Tabs 10, 15, 20, 30 mg

Side effects/adverse reactions:

CNS: Drowsiness, insomnia, agitation, anxiety, headache, ***seizures, neuroleptic malignant syndrome***

CV: Orthostatic hypotension, ***tachycardia***

EENT: Blurred vision

GI: Nausea, vomiting, jaundice, weight gain

Contraindications: Hypersensitivity, lactation, seizure disorders

Precautions: Children, renal disease, pregnancy (C), hepatic disease, elderly

Pharmacokinetics:

PO: Extensively metabolized by liver to a major active metabolite, plasma protein binding 90%

Interactions:

- ↑ effects of aripiprazole: CYP 3A4 inhibitors (ketoconazole), CYP 2D6 inhibitors (quinidine, fluoxetine, paroxetine); reduce dose of aripiprazole
- ↑ sedation: other CNS depressants, alcohol
- ↑ EPS: other antipsychotics, lithium
- ↓ effects of aripiprazole: CYP 3A4 inducers (carbamazepine), ↑ dose of aripiprazole

↑ EPS: Betel palm, kava

↑ neuroleptic effect: cola tree, hops, nettle, nutmeg

Lab test interferences:

- Not known

NURSING CONSIDERATIONS

Assess:

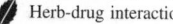

- Mental status before initial administration
- Swallowing of PO medication; check for hoarding or giving of medication to other patients
- I&O ratio; palpate bladder if urinary output is low
- Bilirubin, CBC, LFTs qmo
- Affect, orientation, LOC, reflexes, gait, coordination, sleep pattern disturbances
- B/P standing and lying; also pulse, respirations; take q4h during initial treatment; establish baseline before starting treatment; report drops of 30 mm Hg; watch for ECG changes
- Dizziness, faintness, palpitations, tachycardia on rising

• EPS, including akathisia (inability to sit still, no pattern to movements), tardive dyskinesia (bizarre movements of the jaw, mouth, tongue, extremities), pseudoparkinsonism (rigidity, tremors, pill rolling, shuffling gait)
For neuroleptic malignant syndrome: hyperthermia, increased CPK, altered mental status, muscle rigidity
• Skin turgor qd
• Constipation, urinary retention qd; if these occur, increase bulk and water in diet

Administer:
• Reduced dose in elderly

Perform/provide:
• Decreased stimulus by dimming lights, avoiding loud noises
• Supervised ambulation until patient is stabilized on medication; do not involve in strenuous exercise program because fainting is possible; patient should not stand still for a long time
• Storage in tight, light-resistant container

Evaluate:
• Therapeutic response: decrease in emotional excitement, hallucinations, delusions, paranoia; reorganization of patterns of thought, speech

Teach patient/family:
• That orthostatic hypotension may occur and to rise from sitting or lying position gradually
• To avoid hot tubs, hot showers, tub baths; hypotension may occur
• To avoid abrupt withdrawal of this drug; EPS may result; drug should be withdrawn slowly
• To avoid OTC preparations (cough, hay fever, cold) unless approved by prescriber, since serious drug interactions may occur; avoid use with alcohol, CNS depressants; increased drowsiness may occur
• To avoid hazardous activities if drowsy or dizzy
• Compliance with drug regimen
• To report impaired vision, tremors, muscle twitching, urinary retention
• In hot weather, that heat stroke may occur; take extra precautions to stay cool

Treatment of overdose:
• Lavage if orally ingested; provide airway; *do not induce vomiting*

HIGH ALERT

arsenic trioxide (℞)

Trisenox

Func. class.: Antineoplastic-miscellaneous

Action: Not understood, causes morphological changes and DNA fragmentation

Uses: Acute promyelocytic leukemia

Dosage and routes:

Induction
• *Adult:* **IV** 0.15 mg/kg/day until bone marrow remission, max 60 doses

Consolidation treatment
Wait 3-6 wk after completion of induction
• *Adult:* **IV** 0.15 mg/kg/day × 25 doses over a period of up to 5 wk
• ***Available forms:*** Inj 1 mg/ml

Side effects/adverse reactions:
META: Increased ALT/AST, hyperkalemia, hypokalemia, hypomagnesemia, hyperglycemia
GU: Vaginal hemorrhage, renal failure, incontinence
HEMA: Leukocytosis, anemia, thrombocytopenia, neutropenia, DIC
CV: Hypotension, hypertension, prolonged QT interval, other ECG

changes, chest pain, *tachycardia,* torsades de pointes
GI: Abdominal pain, constipation, diarrhea, dyspepsia, fecal incontinence, GI hemorrhage, dry mouth, *nausea, vomiting, anorexia*
CNS: Anxiety, confusion, insomnia, headache, paresthesia, depression, dizziness, tremor, seizures, agitation, coma, weakness
RESP: ***Pleural effusion,*** dyspnea, cough, epistaxis, hypoxia, sinusitis, wheezing, rales, tachypnea
MISC: Weight gain or decrease, fatigue, severe edema, rigors, herpes simplex/zoster

Contraindications: Hypersensitivity, pregnancy (D)

Precautions: Elderly, lactation, children

Pharmacokinetics: Metabolized in the liver, stored in the liver, kidney, heart, lung, hair, nails, excreted in urine

NURSING CONSIDERATIONS

Assess:

- For APL differentiation syndrome: fever, dyspnea, pulmonary infiltrates, pleural or pericardial effusions, weight gain; this condition can be fatal; give high-dose steroids
- For ECG changes: QT interval prolongation, complete AV block; obtain baseline ECG prior to drug therapy
- Electrolytes: potassium, calcium, magnesium, creatine

Administer:

IV route

- Dilute with 100-250 ml D_5 or 0.9% NaCl immediately after withdrawing from ampule, give over 1-2 hr may give over 4 hr if reactions occur

Evaluate:

Therapeutic response: decrease in malignant cells

Teach patient/family:

- To report planned or suspected pregnancy
- That fertility impairment has not been studied

Treatment of overdose:

- Dimercaprol 3 mg/kg IM q4hr, then 250 mg penicillamine PO, max 4 ×/day (≤1 g/day)

ascorbic acid (vit C) (OTC, ℞)

(a-skor′bic)

Apo-C, ascorbic acid, Ascorbicap, Cebid, Cecon, Cecore-500, Cemill, Cenolate, Cetane, Cevalin, Cevi-Bid, Ce-Vi-Sol, C-Span, Flavorcee, Mega-C/A Plus, Ortho/CS, Sunkist

Func. class.: Vit C—water-soluble vitamin

Action: Needed for wound healing, collagen synthesis, antioxidant, carbohydrate metabolism

Uses: Vit C deficiency, scurvy, delayed wound and bone healing, chronic disease, urine acidification, before gastrectomy, acidification of urine, dietary supplement

Investigational uses: Common cold prevention

Dosage and routes:

- *Child <6 mo:* **PO** 30 mg/day
- ***Dietary supplementation***
- *Adults/child >14 yr:* 50-200 qd
- *Child 11-14 yr:* **PO** 50 mg/day
- *Child 4-10 yr:* **PO** 45 mg/day
- *Child 1-3 yr:* **PO** 40 mg/day
- *Child 6 mo-1 yr:* **PO** 35 mg/day

Scurvy

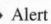

- *Adult:* **PO/SC/IM/IV** 100 mg-500 mg qd × 2 wk, then 50 mg or more qd
- *Child:* **PO/SC/IM/IV** 100-300 mg qd × 2 wk, then 35 mg or more qd

Wound healing/chronic disease/ fracture

• *Adult:* **SC/IM/IV/PO** 200-500 mg qd

• *Child:* **SC/IM/IV/PO** 100-200 mg added doses

Urine acidification

• *Adult:* 4-12 g qd in divided doses

• *Child:* 500 mg q6-8h

Available forms: Tabs 25, 50, 100, 250, 500, 1000, 1500 mg; tabs effervescent 1000 mg; tabs chewable 100, 250, 500 mg; tabs timed release 500, 750, 1000, 1500 mg; caps timed release 500 mg; crys 4 g/tsp; powd 4 g/tsp; liq 35 mg/0.6 ml; sol 100 mg/ml; syr 20 mg/ml, 500 mg/5 ml; inj SC, IM, IV 100, 250, 500 mg/ml

Side effects/adverse reactions:

INTEG: Inflammation at inj site

CNS: Headache, insomnia, dizziness, fatigue, flushing

GI: Nausea, vomiting, diarrhea, anorexia, heartburn, cramps

GU: Polyuria, urine acidification, oxalate or urate renal stones, dysuria

HEMA: ***Hemolytic anemia in patients with G6PD***

Contraindications: Tartrazine, sulfite sensitivity; G-6-PD deficiency

Precautions: Gout, pregnancy (C); diabetes, renal calculi (large doses)

Pharmacokinetics:

PO, INJ: Readily absorbed PO, metabolized in liver, unused amounts excreted in urine (unchanged) and metabolites, crosses placenta, breast milk

Interactions:

• ↓ effects of heparin, warfarin (large doses)

Lab test interferences:

False positive: Negatives in glucose tests

False negative: Occult blood, urine bilirubin, leukocyte determination

NURSING CONSIDERATIONS

Assess:

• I&O ratio

• Ascorbic acid levels throughout treatment if continued deficiency is suspected

• Nutritional status: citrus fruits, vegetables

• Inj sites for inflammation

Administer:

IV, direct route

• Undiluted by direct IV 100 mg over at least 1 min, rapid inf may cause fainting

Intermittent IV INF route

• Diluted with D_5W, D_5NaCl, NS, LR, Ringer's, sodium lactate and given over 15 min

Additive compatibilities: Amikacin, calcium chloride, calcium gluceptate, calcium gluconate, cephalothin, chloramphenicol, chlorproMAZINE, colistimethate, cyanocobalamin, diphenhydrAMINE, heparin, kanamycin, methicillin, methyldopate, penicillin G potassium, polymyxin B, prednisolone, procaine, prochlorperazine, promethazine, verapamil

Syringe compatibilities: Metoclopramide, aminophylline, theophylline

Y-site compatibilities: Warfarin

Evaluate:

• Therapeutic response: absence of anorexia, irritability, pallor, joint pain, hyperkeratosis, petechiae, poor wound healing

Teach patient/family:

⊘ Do not break, crush, or chew ext rel tab or caps

• That caps may be opened and contents mixed with jelly

• The necessary foods in diet, such as citrus fruits

• That smoking decreases vit C levels, not to exceed prescribed dose; increases will be excreted in urine, except timed release

HIGH ALERT

asparaginase (℞)

(a-spare′a-gi-nase)

Elspar, Kidrolase🍁

Func. class.: Antineoplastic

Chem. class.: Escherichia coli enzyme

Action: Indirectly inhibits protein synthesis in tumor cells; without amino acid, DNA, RNA synthesis is halted; asparagine, protein synthesis is halted; G_1 phase of cell cycle specific; a nonvesicant

Uses: Acute lymphocytic leukemia in combination with other antineoplastics

Dosage and routes:

In combination

• *Adult and child:* **IV** 1000 international units/kg/day × 10 days given over 30 min; **IM** 6000 international units/m^2/day

Sole induction

• *Adult and child:* **IV** 200 international units/kg/day × 28 days

Desensitization

• *Adult and child:* Test dose adult/child ID 2 international units **IV/international units** then double dose q10 min, until total dose is administered or reaction occurs

Available forms: Inj 10,000 international units with mannitol

Side effects/adverse reactions:

SYST: ***Anaphylaxis***

HEMA: ***Thrombocytopenia, leukopenia, myelosuppression, anemia, decreased clotting factors (V, VII, VIII, IX), decreased fibrinogen***

GI: Nausea, vomiting, anorexia, diarrhea, weight loss, cramps, stomatitis, ***hepatotoxicity, pancreatitis***

GU: Urinary retention, ***renal failure,*** glycosuria, polyuria, azotemia, uric acid neuropathy, proteinuria

INTEG: *Rash,* urticaria, chills, fever, perspiration

ENDO: Hyperglycemia

RESP: ***Fibrosis, pulmonary infiltrate***

CV: Chest pain

CNS: Neuritis, dizziness, headache, ***coma,*** depression, fatigue, confusion, hallucinations, lethargy, drowsiness, agitation, Parkinson-like syndrome, ***seizures***

Contraindications: Hypersensitivity, infants, pregnancy (C), lactation, pancreatitis

Precautions: Renal disease, hepatic disease

Pharmacokinetics: Half-life 4-9 hr, terminal 1.4-1.8 hr

Interactions:

• ↓ action of: methotrexate
• ↑ toxicity: vincristine, prednisone
• May ↓ response to live virus vaccines

Lab test interferences:

Increase: Uric acid

Decrease: Thyroid function tests

NURSING CONSIDERATIONS

Assess:

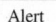

• For signs and symptoms of pancreatitis (nausea, vomiting, severe abdominal pain), anaphylaxis (bronchospasm, dyspnea), cyanosis; more toxic in adults than children
• CBC, differential, platelet count weekly; withhold drug if WBC is <4000 or platelet count is <75,000; notify prescriber of these results
• Pulmonary function tests, chest x-ray studies before, during therapy; chest x-ray film should be obtained q2wk during treatment
• Renal studies: BUN, serum uric acid, ammonia urine CCr, electrolytes before, during therapy
• I&O ratio; report fall in urine output of 30 ml/hr
• Monitor temp q4h; elevated temp may indicate beginning infection

• Hepatic studies before, during therapy (bilirubin, AST, ALT, LDH) as needed or monthly
• RBC, Hct, Hgb, since these may be decreased
• Serum, urine glucose levels
• Bleeding: hematuria, guaiac, bruising or petechiae, mucosa or orifices q8h
◆ Dyspnea, rales, nonproductive cough, chest pain, tachypnea, fatigue, increased pulse, pallor, lethargy, swelling around eyes or lips; anaphylaxis may occur; risk of hypersensitivity increases with repeated dose
• Jaundice of skin and sclera, dark urine, clay-colored stools, itchy skin, abdominal pain, fever, diarrhea
• Local irritation, pain, burning, discoloration at inj site
• Symptoms indicating severe allergic reaction: rash, pruritus, urticaria, purpuric skin lesions, itching, flushing, dyspnea
• Frequency of stools, characteristics: cramping, acidosis; signs of dehydration: rapid respirations, poor skin turgor, decreased urine output, dry skin, restlessness, weakness

Administer:

IM route

• Reconstitute with 2 ml NaCl/10,000 units/vial, refrigerate, use within 8 hr; discard sooner if sol becomes cloudy

IV direct route

• After intradermal skin testing and desensitization, give 0.1 ml (2 international units) intradermally after reconstituting with 5 ml sterile H_2O or 0.9% NaCl for injection; then add 0.1 ml of reconstituted drug to 9.9 ml diluent (20 international units/ml); observe for 1 hr, check for wheal
• Allopurinol or sodium bicarbonate to reduce uric acid levels, alkalinization of urine

Intermittent IV INF route

• Using 21G, 23G, 25G needle; administer by slow IV infusion via Y-tube or 3-way stopcock of flowing D_5W or NS infusion over 30 min after diluting 10,000 international units/5 ml of sterile H_2O or 0.9% NaCl (no preservatives) (2000 international units/ml); use of filter may be necessary if fibers are present

Y-site compatibilities: Methotrexate, sodium bicarbonate

Perform/provide:

• Deep-breathing exercises with patient 3-4 ×/day; place in semi-Fowler's position
• Increase fluid intake to 2-3 L/day to prevent urate deposits, calculi formation
• Brushing of teeth 2-3 ×/day with soft brush or cotton-tipped applicators for stomatitis; use unwaxed dental floss
• Warm compresses at injection site for inflammation

Evaluate:

• Therapeutic response: decreased exacerbations in ALL

Teach patient/family:

• To report any changes in breathing or coughing
• Not to obtain vaccination while taking this drug
• To use contraception, since drug is teratogenic

Treatment of anaphylaxis: Administer epinephrine, diphenhydramine, IV corticosteroids, O_2

aspirin (OTC)

(as'pir-in)

acetylsalicylic acid, Acuprin, Apo-ASA✤, Apo-Asen✤, Arthrinol✤, Arthrisin✤, Artria S.R., A.S.A., Aspergum, Aspirin✤, Aspir-Low, Aspirtab, Astrin✤, Bayer Aspirin, Coryphen✤, Easprin, Ecotrin, 8-Hour Bayer Timed Release, Empirin, Entrophen✤, Halfprin, Norwich Extra-Strength, Novasen✤, PMS-ASA✤, Sloprin, St. Joseph Children's, Supasa✤, Therapy Bayer, ZORprin

Func. class.: Nonopioid analgesic, nonsteroidal antiinflammatory, antipyretic, antiplatelet

Chem. class.: Salicylate

Action: Blocks pain impulses in CNS, reduces inflammation by inhibition of prostaglandin synthesis; antipyretic action results from vasodilation of peripheral vessels; decreases platelet aggregation

Uses: Mild to moderate pain or fever including rheumatoid arthritis, osteoarthritis, thromboembolic disorders; transient ischemic attacks, rheumatic fever, postmyocardial infarction, prophylaxis of MI, ischemic stroke, angina

Investigational uses: Prevention of cataracts (long-term use), prevention of pregnancy loss in women with clotting disorders

Dosage and routes:

Arthritis

- *Adult:* **PO** 2.6-5.2 g/day in divided doses q4-6h
- *Child:* **PO** 90-130 mg/kg/day in divided doses q4-6h

Pain/fever

- *Adult:* **PO/RECT** 325-650 mg q4h prn, not to exceed 4 g/day
- *Child:* **PO/RECT** 40-100 mg/kg/day in divided doses q4-6h prn

Kawasaki disease

- *Child:* **PO** 80-120 mg/kg/day in 4 divided doses, maintenance 3-8 mg/kg/day as a single dose × 8 wk

Acute Rheumatic Fever

- *Adult:* **PO** 5-6 g/day initially
- *Child:* **PO** 100 mg/kg/day × 2 wk, then 75 mg/kg/day × 4-6 wk

Thromboembolic disorders

- *Adult:* **PO** 325-650 mg/day or bid

Transient ischemic attacks

- *Adult:* **PO** 650 mg bid or 350 mg qid

MI, stroke prophylaxis

- *Adult:* **PO** 81-650 mg/day

Available forms: Tabs 81, 162.5, 325, 500, 650, 975 mg; chewable tabs 80, 81 mg; supp 60, 120, 125, 130, 150, 160, 195, 200, 300, 320, 325, 600, 640, 650 mg, 1.2 g; cream; gum 227 mg; dispersible tabs 325, 500 mg, tabs del rel, enteric coated 80, 165, 300, 325, 500, 600, 650, 975 mg; ext rel tab 325, 650, 800 mg, del rel caps 325, 500 mg

Side effects/adverse reactions:

HEMA: ***Thrombocytopenia, agranulocytosis, leukopenia, neutropenia, hemolytic anemia,*** increased pro-time, APTT, bleeding time

CNS: Stimulation, drowsiness, dizziness, confusion, ***seizures,*** headache, flushing, hallucinations, ***coma***

GI: Nausea, vomiting, ***GI bleeding,*** diarrhea, heartburn, anorexia, ***hepatitis***

INTEG: Rash, urticaria, bruising

EENT: Tinnitus, hearing loss

CV: Rapid pulse, pulmonary edema

RESP: Wheezing, hyperpnea

ENDO: Hypoglycemia, hyponatremia, hypokalemia

SYST: ***Reye's syndrome (children), anaphylaxis, laryngeal edema***

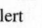

Contraindications: Hypersensitivity to salicylates, tartrazine (FDC yellow dye #5), GI bleeding,

NSAIDs, bleeding disorders, children <12 yr, children with flulike symptoms, pregnancy (D) 3rd trimester, lactation, vit K deficiency, peptic ulcer

Precautions: Anemia, hepatic disease, renal disease, Hodgkin's disease, pre/postoperatively, gastritis, asthmatic patients with nasal polyps or aspirin sensitivity

Pharmacokinetics: Well absorbed PO; enteric metabolized by liver, inactive metabolites excreted by kidneys, crosses placenta, excreted in breast milk; half-life 15-20 min, up to 30 hr in large dose; rectal products may be erratic

PO: Onset 15-30 min, peak 1-2 hr, duration 4-6 hr

REC: Onset slow, duration 4-6 hr

Interactions:

- ↓ effects of aspirin: antacids (high doses), urinary alkalizers, corticosteroids
- ↑ bleeding: alcohol, heparin, plicamycin, cefamandole, thrombolytics, ticlopidine, clopidogrel, tirofiban, eptifibatide
- ↑ effects of warfarin, insulin, methotrexate, thrombolytic agents, penicillins, phenytoin, valproic acid, oral hypoglycemics, sulfonamides
- ↑ salicylate levels: urinary acidifiers, ammonium chloride, nizatidine
- ↑ hypotension: nitroglycemia
- ↓ antihypertensive effect: ACE inhibitors
- ↓ effects of probenecid, spironolactone, sulfinpyrazone, sulfonylamides, NSAIDs, β-blockers, loop diuretics
- Gastric ulcer: steroids, antiinflammatories, NSAIDs
- Drug/food: foods acidifying urine may increase aspirin level

Gastric irritation: arginine, gossypol

↑ risk of bleeding: anise, arnica, bilberry, bogbean, chamomile, chondroitin, clove, fenugreek, feverfew, garlic, ginger, ginkgo, ginseng *(Panax),* horse chestnut, Irish moss, kelpware, licorice, pansy

Lab test interferences:

Increase: Coagulation studies, LFTs, serum uric acid, amylase, CO_2, urinary protein

Decrease: Serum potassium, PBI, cholesterol

Interference: Urine catecholamines, pregnancy test, urine glucose tests (Clinistix, Tes-Tape)

NURSING CONSIDERATIONS

Assess:

- Pain: Character, location, intensity; ROM before and 1 hr after administration
- Fever: Temperature before and 1 hr after administration
- Hepatic studies: AST, ALT, bilirubin, creatinine if patient is on long-term therapy
- Renal studies: BUN, urine creatinine; I&O ratio; decreasing output may indicate renal failure (long-term therapy)
- Blood studies: CBC, Hct, Hgb, PT if patient is on long-term therapy

Hepatotoxicity: dark urine, clay-colored stools, yellowing of skin, sclera, itching, abdominal pain, fever, diarrhea if patient is on long-term therapy

- Allergic reactions: rash, urticaria; if these occur, drug may have to be discontinued; patients with asthma, nasal polyps, allergies: severe allergic reaction may occur
- Ototoxicity: tinnitus, ringing, roaring in ears; audiometric testing needed before, after long-term therapy
- Salicylate level: Therapeutic level 150-300 mcg/ml
- Visual changes: blurring, halos; corneal, retinal damage
- Edema in feet, ankles, legs

• Drug history; many drug interactions

Administer:

PO route

• Crushed or whole; chewable tablets may be chewed

Do not crush enteric product

• With food or milk to decrease gastric symptoms; separate by 2 hr of enteric product

Evaluate:

• Therapeutic response: decreased pain, inflammation, fever

Teach patient/family:

• To report any symptoms of hepatotoxicity, renal toxicity, visual changes, ototoxicity, allergic reactions, bleeding (long-term therapy)

• To take with 8 oz H_2O and sit upright for ½ hr after dose to facilitate drug passing into the stomach

• To avoid if allergic to tartrazine

• Not to exceed recommended dosage; acute poisoning may result

• To read label on other OTC drugs; many contain aspirin or salicylates

• That the therapeutic response takes 2 wk (arthritis); give ½ hr before planned exercise

• To report tinnitus, confusion, diarrhea, sweating, hyperventilation

• To avoid alcohol ingestion; GI bleeding may occur

• That patients who have allergies, nasal polyps, asthma may develop allergic reactions

• To discard tabs if vinegar-like smell is detected

• That medication is not to be given to children or teens with flulike symptoms or chickenpox; Reye's syndrome may develop

Treatment of overdose: Lavage, activated charcoal, monitor electrolytes, VS

atenolol (℞)

(a-ten'oh-lole)

Apo-Atenol♣, atenolol♣, Novo-Atenol♣, Tenormin

Func. class.: Antihypertensive, antianginal

Chem. class.: β-Blocker, β_1, β_2-blocker (high doses)

Action: Competitively blocks stimulation of β-adrenergic receptor within vascular smooth muscle; produces negative chronotropic activity, negative inotropic activity (decreases rate of SA node discharge, increases recovery time), slows conduction of AV node, decreases heart rate, decreases O_2 consumption in myocardium; also decreases renin-aldosterone-angiotensin system at high doses, inhibits β_2 receptors in bronchial system at higher doses

Uses: Mild to moderate hypertension, prophylaxis of angina pectoris; suspected or known myocardial infarction (IV use)

Investigational uses: Dysrhythmia, mitral valve prolapse, pheochromocytoma, hypertrophic cardiomyopathy, vascular headaches, thyrotoxicosis, tremors, alcohol withdrawal

Dosage and routes:

• *Adult:* **IV** 5 mg, repeat in 10 min if initial dose is well tolerated, then start **PO** dose 10 min after last **IV** dose

• *Adult:* **PO** 50 mg qd, increasing q1-2wk to 100 mg qd; may increase to 200 mg qd for angina or up to 100 mg for hypertension

• *Elderly:* **PO** 25 mg/day initially

Renal disease

• *Adult:* **PO** CCr 15-35 ml/min, max 50 mg/day; CCr <15 ml/min max dose 25 mg/day; hemodialysis 25-50 mg after dialysis

MI-Renal dose
• *Adult:* **IV** 5 mg, then 5 mg over 10 min, then after 10 min, give **PO** dose

Available forms: Tabs 25, 50, 100 mg; inj 500 mcg/ml

Side effects/adverse reactions:
CV: ***Profound hypotension, bradycardia, CHF,*** *cold extremities, postural hypotension, 2nd- or 3rd-degree heart block*
CNS: Insomnia, fatigue, dizziness, mental changes, memory loss, hallucinations, depression, lethargy, drowsiness, strange dreams, catatonia
GI: Nausea, diarrhea, vomiting, ***mesenteric arterial thrombosis, ischemic colitis***
INTEG: Rash, fever, alopecia
HEMA: ***Agranulocytosis, thrombocytopenia, purpura***
EENT: Sore throat, dry burning eyes
GU: Impotence
ENDO: Increased hypoglycemic response to insulin
RESP: ***Bronchospasm,*** dyspnea, wheezing

Contraindications: Hypersensitivity to β-blockers, cardiogenic shock, 2nd- or 3rd-degree heart block, sinus bradycardia, cardiac failure, pregnancy (D)

Precautions: Major surgery, lactation, diabetes mellitus, renal disease, thyroid disease, CHF, COPD, asthma, well-compensated heart failure

Do not confuse:
atenolol/albuterol/Altenol
Tenormin/thiamine/Imuran/Trovan

Pharmacokinetics:
IV: Onset rapid, peak 5 min, duration unknown
PO: Peak 2-4 hr, onset 1 hr, duration 24 hr; half-life 6-9 hr, excreted unchanged in urine, feces protein binding 5%-15%

Interactions:
• ↑ hypotension, bradycardia: reserpine, hydralazine, methyldopa, prazosin, anticholinergics, digoxin, diltiazem, verapamil, cardiac glycosides, antihypertensives
• Mutual inhibition: sympathomimetics (cough, cold preparations)
Toxicity/death: aconite
↑ atenolol effect: betel palm, butterbur, cola tree, figwort, fumitory, guarana, hawthorn, jaborandi tree, lily of the valley, motherwort, plantain
↓ atenolol effect: coenzyme Q10, yohimbe

Lab test interferences:
Increase: Blood glucose, BUN, K, triglycerides, uric acid, ANA titer

NURSING CONSIDERATIONS

Assess:
• I&O, weight daily
• B/P, pulse q4h; note rate, rhythm, quality; apical/radial pulse before administration; notify prescriber of any significant changes (<50 bpm)
• Baselines in renal, liver studies before therapy begins

Administer:

PO route
• Drug ac, hs, tablet may be crushed or swallowed whole
• Reduced dosage in renal dysfunction

IV, direct route
• Undiluted over 5 min

IV INF route
• Diluted in 10-50 ml of D_5W, D_5/NaCl, or NS and give as an infusion at prescribed rate

Y-site compatibilities: Meperidine, meropenem, morphine

Perform/provide:
• Storage protected from light, moisture; place in cool environment

Evaluate:
• Therapeutic response: decreased B/P after 1-2 wk

Teach patient/family:

- Not to discontinue drug abruptly, taper over 2 wk
- Not to use OTC products unless directed by prescriber
- To report bradycardia, dizziness, confusion, depression, fever
- To take pulse at home; advise when to notify prescriber
- To limit alcohol, smoking, sodium intake
- To comply with weight control, dietary adjustments, modified exercise program
- To carry emergency ID to identify drug, allergies, conditions being treated
- To avoid hazardous activities if dizziness is present
- That drug may mask symptoms of hypoglycemia in diabetic patients
- To use contraception while taking this drug, pregnancy category (D)

Treatment of overdose: Lavage, IV atropine for bradycardia, IV theophylline for bronchospasm, digitalis, O_2, diuretic for cardiac failure, hemodialysis

atomoxetine (℞)

(at-o-mox'eh-teen)

Strattera

Func. class.: Misc. psychotherapeutic

Action: A selective norepinephrine reuptake inhibitor. May inhibit the presynaptic norepinephrine transporter. Exact mechanism of action is unknown.

Uses: Attention deficit hyperactivity disorder

Dosage and routes:

- *Child ≤70 kg:* **PO** 0.5 mg/kg, increase after 3 days to a target daily dose of 1.2 mg/kg in AM or evenly divided doses AM, late afternoon; max 1.4 mg/kg/day or 100 mg qd, whichever is less
- *Adult/child >70 kg:* **PO** 40 mg qd, increase after 3 days to a target daily dose of 80 mg in AM or evenly divided doses AM, late afternoon; max 100 mg qd

Available forms: Caps 10, 18, 25, 40, 60 mg

Side effects/adverse reactions:

MISC: Cough, rhinorrhea, dermatitis, ear infection

CNS: Insomnia, dizziness, headache, irritability, crying, mood swings, fatigue

GI: Dyspepsia, nausea, anorexia, dry mouth, weight loss, vomiting, diarrhea, constipation

CV: Palpitations, hot flushes

INTEG: ***Exfoliative dermatitis,*** sweating

ENDO: Growth retardation

GU: Urinary hesitancy, retention, dysmenorrhea, erectile disturbance, ejaculation failure, impotence, prostatis, orgasm abnormal

Contraindications: Narrow-angle glaucoma

Precautions: Hypertension, pregnancy (C), lactation, child <6 yr; hepatic, cardiac, or cerebrovascular disease

Pharmacokinetics:

PO: Peak 1-2 hr, metabolized by liver, excreted by kidneys, 98% protein binding

Interactions:

- Hypertensive crisis: MAOIs or within 14 days of MAOIs, vasopressors
- ↑ cardiovascular effects of: albuterol, pressor agents
- ↑ effects of atomoxetine: CYP2D6 inhibitors

NURSING CONSIDERATIONS

Assess:

- VS, B/P; check patients with cardiac disease more often for increased B/P

• Height, growth rate q3mo in children; growth rate may be decreased
• Mental status: mood, sensorium, affect, stimulation, insomnia, aggressiveness
• Appetite, sleep, speech patterns
• For attention span, decreased hyperactivity in ADHD persons

Administer:
• Gum, hard candy, frequent sips of water for dry mouth

Evaluate:
• Therapeutic response: decreased hyperactivity (ADHD)

Teach patient/family:
• To avoid OTC preparations unless approved by prescriber
• To avoid alcohol ingestion
• To avoid hazardous activities until stabilized on medication
• To get needed rest; patients will feel more tired at end of day

atorvastatin (℞)

(a-tore′va-stat-in)
Lipitor
Func. class.: Antilipidemic
Chem. class.: HMG-CoA reductase inhibitor

Action: Inhibits HMG-CoA reductase enzyme, which reduces cholesterol synthesis
Uses: As an adjunct in primary hypercholesterolemia (types Ia, Ib), dysbetalipoproteinemia, elevated triglyceride levels
Dosage and routes:
• *Adult:* **PO** 10 mg qd, usual range 10-80, dosage adjustments may be made in 2-4 wk intervals, max 80 mg/day
Available forms: Tabs 10, 20, 40, 80 mg
Side effects/adverse reactions:
INTEG: Rash, pruritus, alopecia
GI: Abdominal cramps, constipation, diarrhea, flatus, heartburn, dyspepsia, ***liver dysfunction,*** pancreatitis, nausea, increased serum transaminase
EENT: Lens opacities
MS: Arthralgia, myalgia, ***rhabdomyolysis***
CNS: Headache, asthenia
GU: Impotence
RESP: Pharyngitis, sinusitis
MISC: Hypersensitivity
Contraindications: Hypersensitivity, pregnancy (X), lactation, active liver disease
Precautions: Past liver disease, alcoholism, severe acute infections, trauma, severe metabolic disorders, electrolyte imbalance
Pharmacokinetics: Metabolized in liver, highly protein bound, excreted primarily in urine, half-life 14 hr; protein binding 98%
Interactions:
• Risk of possible rhabdomyolysis: azole antifungals, cycloSPORINE, erythromycin, niacin, gemfibrozil, clofibrate
• ↑ serum level of digoxin
• ↑ levels of oral contraceptives
• ↑ levels of atorvastatin: erythromycin
• ↑ effects of warfarin
• ↓ atorvastatin levels: colestipol
↑ effect: glucomannan
↓ effect: gotu kola
Lab test interferences:
• *Increase:* Bilirubin, alk phosphatase
• *Interference:* Thyroid function tests
• Drug/food: possible toxicity when used with grapefruit juice; food increases blood levels

NURSING CONSIDERATIONS
Assess:
• Diet, obtain diet history including fat, cholesterol in diet
• Cholesterol triglyceride levels periodically during treatment

• Hepatic studies q1-2mo during the first 1½ yr of treatment; AST, ALT, LFTs may be increased
• Renal studies in patients with compromised renal system: BUN, I&O ratio, creatinine
• Ophthalmic exam, 1 mo after treatment begins, annually; lens opacities may occur
For muscle pain, tenderness, obtain CPK if these occur, drug may need to be discontinued

Administer:

PO route

• Total daily dose any time of day

Perform/provide:

• Storage in cool environment in tight container protected from light

Evaluate:

• Therapeutic response: decrease in cholesterol to desired level after 8 wk

Teach patient/family:

• That blood work and eye exam will be necessary during treatment
• To report blurred vision, severe GI symptoms, headache, muscle pain, weakness
• That previously prescribed regimen will continue: low-cholesterol diet, exercise program, smoking cessation
• Not to take drug if pregnant
• To stay out of the sun, or use sunscreen, protective clothing to prevent photosensitivity (rare)

atovaquone (℞)

(a-toe′va-kwon)
Mepron
Func. class.: Antiprotozoal
Chem. class.: Aromatic diamide derivative, analog of ubiquinone

Action: Interferes with DNA/RNA synthesis in protozoa
Uses: *Pneumocystis carinii* infections in patients intolerant of trimethoprim-sulfamethoxazole
Dosage and routes:
• *Adult and adolescents 13-16 yr:* **PO** 750 mg with food bid for 21 days
Available forms: 750 mg/5 ml, susp
Side effects/adverse reactions:
CV: Hypotension
HEMA: Anemia, ***leukopenia,*** neutropenia
INTEG: Pruritus, urticaria, *rash*, oral monilia
GI: Nausea, vomiting, diarrhea, anorexia, increased AST and ALT, acute pancreatitis, constipation, abdominal pain
CNS: Dizziness, headache, anxiety, insomnia
META: Hyperkalemia, hypoglycemia, hyponatremia
Contraindications: Hypersensitivity or history of developing life-threatening allergic reactions to any component of the formulation
Precautions: Blood dyscrasias, hepatic disease, diabetes mellitus, pregnancy (C), lactation, children, elderly
Do not confuse:
Mepron (U.S.)/Mepron (meprobamate in Australia)
Pharmacokinetics: Excreted unchanged in feces (94%), highly protein bound (99%)
Interactions:
• Use caution when administering concurrently with other highly plasma protein-bound drugs with narrow therapeutic indices
• ↓ effect of atovaquone: rifampin, rifabutin

NURSING CONSIDERATIONS
Assess:
• Signs of infection, anemia
• Bowel pattern before, during treatment
• Respiratory status: rate, character, wheezing, dyspnea

• Allergies before treatment, reaction of each medication

Administer:

PO route

• With high-fat food because of increased absorption of the drug and higher plasma concentrations

Evaluate:

• Therapeutic response: decreased temp, ability to breathe

Teach patient/family:

• To take with food to increase plasma concentrations

RARELY USED

atracurium (℞)

(a-tra-kyoor′ee-um)

Tracrium

Func. class.: Neuromuscular blocker (nondepolarizing)

Uses: Facilitation of endotracheal intubation, skeletal muscle relaxation during mechanical ventilation, surgery, or general anesthesia

Dosage and routes:

• *Adult and child >2 yr:* **IV BOL** 0.3-0.5 mg/kg, then 0.08-0.10 mg/kg 20-45 min after first dose if needed for prolonged procedures

• *Child, 1 mo-2 yr:* **IV BOL** 0.3-0.4 mg/kg

Contraindications: Hypersensitivity

HIGH ALERT

atropine (℞)

(a′troe-peen)

Atro-Pen

Func. class.: Antidysrhythmic, anticholinergic parasympatholytic, antimuscarinic

Chem. class.: Belladonna alkaloid

Action: Blocks acetylcholine at parasympathetic neuroeffector sites; increases cardiac output, heart rate by blocking vagal stimulation in heart; dries secretions by blocking vagus

Uses: Bradycardia <40-50 bpm, bradydysrhythmia, reversal of anticholinesterase agents, insecticide poisoning, blocking cardiac vagal reflexes, decreasing secretions before surgery, antispasmodic with GU, biliary surgery, bronchodilator

Dosage and routes:

Bradycardia/bradydysrhythmia

• *Adult:* **IV BOL** 0.5-1 mg given q3-5min, not to exceed 2 mg

• *Child:* **IV BOL** 0.01-0.03 mg/kg up to 0.4 mg or 0.3 mg/m^2; may repeat q4-6h; min dose 0.1 mg to avoid paradoxical reaction

Organophosphate poisoning

• *Adult and child:* **IM/IV** 2 mg qh until muscarinic symptoms disappear, may need 6 mg qh

Presurgery

• *Adult/child >20 kg:* **SC/IM/IV** 0.4-0.6 mg before anesthesia

• *Child <20 kg:* **IM/SC** 0.01 mg/kg up to 0.4 mg ½-1 hr preop

Available forms: Inj 0.05, 0.1, 0.3, 0.4, 0.5, 0.8, 1 mg/ml; 2 mg/0.7 ml auto injector; tabs 0.4 mg

Side effects/adverse reactions:

GU: Retention, hesitancy, impotence, dysuria

CNS: Headache, dizziness, involuntary movement, confusion, psychosis, anxiety, coma, flushing, drowsiness, insomnia, weakness; delirium (elderly)
GI: Dry mouth, nausea, vomiting, abdominal pain, anorexia, constipation, ***paralytic ileus,*** abdominal distention, altered taste
CV: Hypotension, paradoxical bradycardia, angina, PVCs, hypertension, ***tachycardia,*** ectopic ventricular beats
INTEG: Rash, urticaria, contact dermatitis, dry skin, flushing
EENT: Blurred vision, photophobia, glaucoma, eye pain, pupil dilation, nasal congestion
MISC: Suppression of lactation, decreased sweating
Contraindications: Hypersensitivity to belladonna alkaloids, angle-closure glaucoma, GI obstructions, myasthenia gravis, thyrotoxicosis, ulcerative colitis, prostatic hypertrophy, tachycardia/tachydysrhythmias, asthma, acute hemorrhage, hepatic disease, myocardial ischemia
Precautions: Pregnancy (C), renal disease, lactation, CHF, tachydysrhythmia, hyperthyroidism, COPD, hepatic disease, child <6 yr, hypertension, elderly, intraabdominal infection, Down syndrome, spastic paralysis, gastric ulcer
Do not confuse:
atropine/Akarpine
Pharmacokinetics: Well absorbed PO, IM, SC; half-life 13-40 hr, excreted by kidneys unchanged (70%-90% in 24 hr); metabolized in liver, 40%-50% crosses placenta, excreted in breast milk
IV: Peak 2-4 min, duration 4-6 hr
IM/SC: Onset 15-50 min; peak 30 min, duration 4-6 hr
PO: Onset ½ hr; peak ½-1 hr; duration 4-6 hr

Interactions:
- $\downarrow$ effect of atropine: antacids
- Mucosal lesions: potassium chloride tab
- $\downarrow$ absorption: ketoconazole, levodopa
- $\uparrow$ anticholinergic effects, tricyclics, amantadine, antiparkinson agents

$\uparrow$ atropine effect: aloe, buckthorn, cascara sagrada, figwort, fumitory, goldenseal, jimsonweed, kudzu, licorice, rhubarb, senna, scopolia
Forms insoluble complex: black root
$\uparrow$ toxicity/death: aconite
$\downarrow$ effect: coltsfoot
Serotonin effect: horehound

NURSING CONSIDERATIONS
Assess:
- I&O ratio; check for urinary retention, daily output
- ECG for ectopic ventricular beats, PVC, tachycardia, in cardiac patients
- For bowel sounds; check for constipation
- Respiratory status: rate, rhythm, cyanosis, wheezing, dyspnea, engorged neck veins
- Increased intraocular pressure: eye pain, nausea, vomiting, blurred vision, increased tearing
- Cardiac rate: rhythm, character, B/P continuously
- Allergic reaction: rash, urticaria

Administer:
PO route
- Increased bulk, water in diet if constipation occurs
- ½ hr ac

IM route
- Atropine flush may occur in children and is not harmful

IV route
- Undiluted or diluted with 10 ml sterile H_2O, give at 0.6 mg/min,

give through Y-tube or 3-way stopcock; do not add to IV sol; may cause paradoxical bradycardia lasting 2 min

Additive compatibilities: DOBUTamine, furosemide, meropenem, netilmicin, sodium bicarbonate, verapamil

Syringe compatibilities: Benzquinamide, butorphanol, chlorproMAZINE, cimetidine, dimenhyDRINATE, diphenhydrAMINE, droperidol, fentanyl, glycopyrrolate, heparin, hydromorphone, hydrOXYzine, meperidine, metoclopramide, midazolam, milrinone, morphine, nalbuphine, pentazocine, perphenazine, prochlorperazine, promazine, promethazine, propiomazine, ranitidine, scopolamine, sufentanil

Y-site compatibilities: Amrinone, etomidate, famotidine, heparin, hydrocortisone, meropenem, nafcillin, potassium chloride, sufentanil, vit B/C

Perform/provide:

- Sugarless hard candy, gum, frequent rinsing of mouth for dryness

Evaluate:

- Therapeutic response: decreased dysrhythmias, increased heart rate, secretions; GI, GU spasms; bronchodilation

Teach patient/family:

- To report blurred vision, chest pain, allergic reactions, constipation, urinary retention
- Not to perform strenuous activity in high temperatures; heat stroke may result
- To take as prescribed; not to skip doses
- Not to operate machinery if drowsiness occurs
- Not to take OTC products without approval of prescriber

Treatment of overdose: O_2, artificial ventilation, ECG; administer dopamine for circulatory depression; administer diazepam or thiopental for convulsions; assess need for antidysrhythmics

atropine ophthalmic

See appendix c

RARELY USED

auranofin (℞)

(au-rane'oh-fin)

Ridaura

Func. class.: Antiinflammatory

Uses: Rheumatoid arthritis; not for first-line therapy

Investigational uses: SLE, psoriatic arthritis, pemphigus

Dosage and routes:

- *Adult:* **PO** 6 mg qd or 3 mg bid; may increase to 9 mg/day after 3 mo

Contraindications: Hypersensitivity to gold, necrotizing enterocolitis, bone marrow aplasia, child <6 yr, lactation, pulmonary fibrosis, exfoliative dermatitis, blood dyscrasias, recent radiation therapy, renal/hepatic disease, marked hypertension, uncontrolled CHF

Do not confuse:

Ridaura/Cardura

RARELY USED

aurothioglucose/gold sodium thiomalate (℞)

(aur-oh-thye-oh-gloo'kose)

Solganal/Aurolate

Func. class.: Antiinflammatory

Uses: Rheumatoid arthritis, psoriatic arthritis

Dosage and routes:

• *Adult:* **IM** 10 mg, then 25 mg qwk × 2-3 wk, then 50 mg/wk until total of 1 g is administered, then 25-50 mg q3-4wk if there is improvement without toxicity (aurothioglucose) total of 800 mg-1 g

• *Adult:* **IM** 10 mg, then 25 mg after 1 wk, then 50 mg qwk for total of 14-20 doses, then 50 mg q2wk × 4, then 50 mg q3wk × 4, then 50 mg qmo for maintenance (gold sodium thiomalate)

• *Child 6-12 yr:* **IM** 1 mg/kg/wk × 20 wk, or ¼ of adult dose (aurothioglucose)

• *Child:* **IM** 1 mg/kg/wk × 20 wk, then q3-4wk if improvement without toxicity (gold sodium thiomalate) not to exceed 2.5 mg

Contraindications: Hypersensitivity to gold, SLE, uncontrolled diabetes mellitus, marked hypertension, recent radiation therapy, CHF, lactation, renal disease, liver disease

azathioprine (℞)

(ay-za-thye'oh-preen)
Imuran

Func. class.: Immunosuppressant

Chem. class.: Purine antagonist

Action: Produces immunosuppression by inhibiting purine synthesis in cells

Uses: Renal transplants to prevent graft rejection, refractory rheumatoid arthritis, refractory ITP, glomerulonephritis, nephrotic syndrome, bone marrow transplant

Investigational uses: Myasthenia gravis, chronic ulcerative colitis, Crohn's disease, Behçet's disease

Dosage and routes:

Prevention of rejection

• *Adult and child:* **PO, IV** 3-5 mg/kg/day, then maintenance (PO) of at least 1-2 mg/kg/day

Refractory rheumatoid arthritis

• *Adult:* **PO** 1/mg/kg/day, may increase dose after 2 mo by 0.5 mg/kg/day, not to exceed 2.5 mg/kg/day

Renal disease

• CCr 10-50 ml/min 75% of dose; CCr <10 ml/min 50% of dose

Available forms: Tabs 50 mg; inj 100 mg

Side effects/adverse reactions:

GI: Nausea, vomiting, stomatitis, esophagitis, ***pancreatitis, hepatotoxicity, jaundice***

HEMA: ***Leukopenia, thrombocytopenia, anemia, pancytopenia***

INTEG: Rash, alopecia

MS: Arthralgia, muscle wasting

MISC: ***Serum sickness,*** Raynaud's symptoms

Contraindications: Hypersensitivity, pregnancy (D), lactation

Precautions: Severe renal disease, severe hepatic disease, elderly

Do not confuse:

Imuran/Imferon/Elmiron/IMDUR/Enduron/Tenormin

Pharmacokinetics: Metabolized in liver, excreted in urine (active metabolite), crosses placenta

Lab test interferences:

Interfere: CBC, diff count

Decrease: Uric acid

Increase: LFTs

Interactions:

• Leukopenia: ACE inhibitors; co-trimoxazole, myelopoiesis

• ↓ immune response: vaccines

• ↓ action of warfarin: warfarin

• ↑ myelosuppression: cycloSPORINE, antineoplastics

• ↑ action of azathioprine: allopurinol

• Do not admix with other drugs

↑ immunosuppression: astragalus, echinacea, melatonin, safflower
↓ immunosuppression: ginseng, maitake, mistletoe, schisandra, St. John's wort, tumeric

NURSING CONSIDERATIONS

Assess:

- For infection: increased temp, WBC; sputum, urine
- For rheumatoid arthritis, pain, mobility, ROM
- I&O, weight qd, report decreasing urine output; toxicity may occur
- Blood studies: Hgb, WBC, platelets during treatment monthly; if leukocytes are <3000/mm^3 or platelets <100,000/mm^3, drug should be discontinued

Hepatotoxicity: dark urine, jaundice, itching, light-colored stools, increased LFTs; drug should be discontinued; hepatic studies: alk phosphatase, AST, ALT, bilirubin

- Arthritis: pain; location, ROM, swelling, before and during treatment

Administer:

- All medications PO if possible, avoiding IM inj, since bleeding may occur

PO route

- With meals to reduce GI upset

IV route

- Prepare in biologic cabinet using gown, gloves, mask
- After diluting 100 mg/10 ml of sterile H_2O for inj; rotate to dissolve; may further dilute with 50 ml or more saline or glucose in saline, give over ½-1 hr
- For several days before transplant surgery

Solution compatibilities: D_5W, NaCl 0.9%, NaCl 0.45%

Evaluate:

- Therapeutic response: absence of graft rejection, immunosuppression in autoimmune disorders

Teach patient/family:

- To take as prescribed, do not miss doses, if dose is missed on qd regimen, skip dose; if on multiple dosing/day, take as soon as remembered
- That therapeutic response may take 3-4 mo in rheumatoid arthritis; to continue with prescribed exercise, rest, other medications
- To report fever, rash, severe diarrhea, chills, sore throat, fatigue, since serious infections may occur
- To use contraceptive measures during treatment, for 12 wk after ending therapy; to avoid vaccinations
- To avoid crowds to reduce risk of infection
- To use soft-bristled toothbrush to prevent bleeding
- That treatment is ongoing to prevent transplant rejection

azelastine nasal agent

See appendix c

azithromycin (℞)

(ay-zi-thro-my′sin)

Zithromax

Func. class.: Antiinfective

Chem. class.: Macrolide (azalide)

Action: Binds to 50S ribosomal subunits of susceptible bacteria and suppresses protein synthesis; much greater spectrum of activity than erythromycin

Uses: Mild to moderate infections of the upper respiratory tract, lower respiratory tract, uncomplicated skin and skin structure infections caused by *Moraxella catarrhalis, Streptococcus pneumoniae, Streptococcus pyogenes, Staphylococcus aureus, Streptococcus agalactiae, Myco-*

plasma pneumoniae, Haemophilus influenzae, Clostridium, Legionella pneumophila; nongonococcal urethritis or cervicitis due to *Chlamydia trachomatis*; in children: acute otitis media (*H. influenzae, M. catarrhalis, S. pneumoniae)* PO; acute pharyngitis/tonsillitis (group A streptococcal) PO; acute skin/soft tissue infections (PO); community-acquired pneumonia *(Chlamydia pneumoniae, H. influenzae, M. pneumoniae, S. pneumoniae)* PO; pharyngitis/tonsillitis *(S. pyogenes);* prophylaxis of disseminated *Mycobacterium avium* complex (MAC)
Investigational uses: Chlamydial infections, gonococcal infections, prophylaxis after sexual assault, bacterial endocarditis prevention
Dosage and routes:
Most infections
• *Adult:* **PO** 500 mg on day 1, then 250 mg qd on days 2-5 for a total dose of 1.5 g
Child 2-15 yr: **PO** 10 mg/kg on day 1, then 5 mg/kg × 4 days
Pharyngitis/tonsillitis
• *Adult:* **PO** 12 mg/kg qd × 5 days
Disseminated MAC infections
• *Adult:* **PO** 600 mg/day in combination with ethambutol
Community-acquired pneumonia
• *Adult:* **PO/IV** 500 mg **IV** q24h × 2 doses, then 500 mg **PO** q24h × 7-10 days
Pelvic inflammatory disease
• *Adult:* **PO/IV** 500 mg **IV** q24h × 2 doses, then 500 mg **PO** q24h × 7-10 days
Cervicitis, chlamydia, chancroid, nongonococcal urethritis
• *Adult:* **PO** 1 g single dose
Gonorrhea
• *Adult:* **PO** 2 g single dose
Endocarditis prophylaxis
• *Adult:* **PO** 500 mg 1 hr prior to procedure
• *Child:* **PO** 15 mg/kg 1 hr prior to procedure
Lower respiratory tract infections, acute skin/soft tissue infections, acute pharyngitis/tonsillitis
• *Child, 3-day regimen:* **PO** 10 mg/kg qd × 3 days
Acute otitis media
• *Child:* **PO** 30 mg/kg as a single dose or 10 mg/kg qd × 3 days or 10 mg/kg as a single dose on day 1 (max 500 mg/day), then 5 mg/kg on days 2-5 (max 250 mg/day)
Prevention of acute otitis media
Child: **PO** 10 mg/kg q wk × 6 mo
Available forms: Tabs 250, 600 mg; powder for inj 500 mg; powder for oral susp 1 g/packet susp 100, 200 mg/5 ml
Side effects/adverse reactions:
INTEG: Rash, urticaria, pruritus, photosensitivity
CV: Palpitations, chest pain
CNS: Dizziness, headache, vertigo, somnolence
GI: Nausea, vomiting, diarrhea, ***hepatotoxicity,*** abdominal pain, stomatitis, heartburn, dyspepsia, flatulence, melena, ***cholestatic jaundice, pseudomembranous colitis***
GU: Vaginitis, moniliasis, nephritis
SYST: ***Angioedema***
Contraindications: Hypersensitivity to azithromycin, erythromycin, or any macrolide
Precautions: Pregnancy (B), lactation; hepatic, renal, cardiac disease; elderly, <6 mo for otitis media, <2 yr for pharyngitis, tonsillitis
Do not confuse:
azithromycin/erythromycin
Zithromax/Zinacef
Pharmacokinetics: *PO:* Peak 2-4 hr, duration 24 hr; *IV:* peak end of inf, duration 24 hr; half-life 11-57 hr, excreted in bile, feces, urine primarily as unchanged drug
Interactions:
• Toxicity; ergotamine

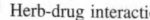

A

• ↑ effects of oral anticoagulants, digoxin, theophylline, methylPREDNISolone, cycloSPORINE, bromocriptine, disopyramide, triazolam, carbamazepine, phenytoin
• ↓ clearance of: triazolam
Dysrhythmias: pimozide; fatal reaction
• ↓ absorption of azithromycin: aluminum, magnesium antacids
Do not use acidophilus with anti-infectives

Lab interferences:
Increase: CPK, ALT, AST, bilirubin, BUN, creatinine, alk phosphatase

NURSING CONSIDERATIONS
Assess:
• I&O ratio; report hematuria, oliguria in renal disease
• Hepatic studies: AST, ALT; CBC with differential
• Renal studies: urinalysis, protein, blood
• C&S before drug therapy; drug may be taken as soon as culture is taken; C&S may be repeated after treatment
• For superinfection: sore throat, mouth, tongue; fever, fatigue, diarrhea, anogenital pruritus
• Bowel pattern before, during treatment
• Respiratory status: rate, character, wheezing, tightness in chest; discontinue drug if these occur

Administer:
PO route
• Susp 1 hr ac or 2 hr pc. Reconstitute 1 g packet for susp with 60 ml water, mix, rinse glass with more water and have patient drink to consume all medication; packets not for pediatric use

IV route
• Reconstitute 500 mg of drug/4.8 ml sterile water for inj (100 mg/ml); shake, dilute with ≥250 ml 0.9% NaCl, 0.45% NaCl, or LR to 1-2 mg/ml; diluted solution is stable for 24 hr or 7 days if refrigerated
• Give 500 mg or more/hr, never give IM or as a bolus

Perform/provide:
• Storage at room temperature

Evaluate:
• Therapeutic response: C&S negative for infection; decreased signs of infection

Teach patient/family:
To report sore throat, fever, fatigue, severe diarrhea, anal, genital itching (may indicate superinfection)
• Not to take aluminum/magnesium-containing antacids simultaneously with this drug (PO)
To notify nurse of diarrhea stools, dark urine, pale stools, yellow discoloration of eyes or skin, severe abdominal pain
• To complete dosage regimen

Treatment of hypersensitivity: Withdraw drug, maintain airway, administer epINEPHrine, aminophylline, O_2, IV corticosteroids

---

RARELY USED

aztreonam (℞)
(az-tree'oh nam)
Azactam
Func. class.: Miscellaneous antibiotic

Uses: Urinary tract infection; septicemia; skin, muscle, bone infection, lower respiratory tract, intra-abdominal infections; and other infections caused by gram-negative organisms

Dosage and routes:
Urinary tract infections
• *Adult:* **IV/IM** 500 mg-1 g q8-12h
Systemic infections
• *Adult:* **IV/IM** 1-2 g q8-12h

• *Child:* **IV/IM** 90-120 mg/kg/day divided q6-8h

Severe systemic infections

• *Adult:* **IV/IM** 2 g q6-8h; do not exceed 8 g/day

Continue treatment for 48 hr after negative culture or until patient is asymptomatic

Contraindications: Hypersensitivity to this drug, penicillins, cephalosporins

RARELY USED

bacitracin (℞)

(bass-i-tray'sin)

BACI-IM, Baciquent, Bacitin✤

Func. class.: Antiinfective, misc.

Uses:

Staphylococcal pneumonia, empyema

Dosage and routes:

• *Infant >2.5 kg:* **IM** 1000 units/kg/day in divided doses q8-12h

• *Infant ≤2.5 kg:* **IM** 900 units/kg/day in divided doses q8-12h

Contraindications: Hypersensitivity, severe renal disease (IM use)

bacitracin ophthalmic

See appendix c

bacitracin topical

See appendix c

baclofen (℞)

(bak'loe-fen)

Lioresal, Lioresal Intrathecal

Func. class.: Skeletal muscle relaxant, central acting

Chem. class.: GABA chlorophenyl derivative

Action: Inhibits synaptic responses in CNS by decreasing GABA, which decreases neurotransmitter function; decreases frequency, severity of muscle spasms

Uses: Spasticity in spinal cord injury, multiple sclerosis

Investigational uses: Pain in trigeminal neuralgia, hiccoughs

Dosage and routes:

• *Adult:* **PO** 5 mg tid × 3 days, then 10 mg tid × 3 days, then 15 mg tid × 3 days, then 20 mg tid × 3 days, then titrated to response, not to exceed 80 mg/day. **IT:** Use implantable intrathecal **INF** pump; use screening trial of 3 separate **BOL** doses if needed (50 mcg/ml, 75 mcg/1.5 ml, 100 mcg/2 ml). Initial: double screening dose that produced result and give over 24 hr: increase by 10%-30% q24h only. Maintenance: 1200-1500 mcg/day; **PO** 5-10 mg tid, taper before discontinuing drug

• *Child >2 yr:* **PO** 10-15 mg/kg/day divided q8h titrate to max 40 mg/day

• *Child ≥8 yr:* as above, max 60 mg/day

• *Child:* **IT** 25-1200 mcg/day infusion, titrated to response in screening phase

Available forms: Tabs 10, 20 mg; intrathecal inj 10 mg/20 ml (500 mcg/ml), 10 mg/5 ml (2000 mcg/ml)

Side effects/adverse reactions:

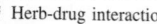

CNS: Dizziness, weakness, fatigue,

drowsiness, headache, *disorientation,* insomnia, paresthesias, tremors, ***seizures*** (IT)
EENT: Nasal congestion, blurred vision, mydriasis, tinnitus
CV: Hypotension, chest pain, palpitations, edema
GI: Nausea, constipation, *vomiting,* increased AST, alk phosphatase, abdominal pain, dry mouth, anorexia
GU: Urinary frequency
INTEG: Rash, pruritus

Contraindications: Hypersensitivity

Precautions: Peptic ulcer disease, renal disease, hepatic disease, stroke, seizure disorder, diabetes mellitus, pregnancy (C), lactation, elderly

Do not confuse:
Lioresal/Lotensin

Pharmacokinetics:
PO: Peak 2-3 hr, duration >8 hr, half-life 2½-4 hr, partially metabolized in liver, excreted in urine (unchanged)
INTRATHECAL: CSF levels with plasma levels 100 times oral route; onset ½-1 hr, peak 4 hr, duration 4-8 hr

Interactions:
- ↑ CNS depression: alcohol, tricyclics, opiates, barbiturates, sedatives, hypnotics, MAOIs
- ↑ CNS depression: chamomile, hops, kava, skullcap, valerian

Lab test interferences:
Increase: AST, alk phosphatase, blood glucose

NURSING CONSIDERATIONS

Assess:
- B/P, weight, blood glucose, and hepatic function periodically
- For increased seizure activity in seizure disorders; this drug decreases seizure threshold
- I&O ratio; check for urinary frequency
- EEG in epileptic patients; poor seizure control has occurred in patients taking this drug
- Allergic reactions: rash, fever, respiratory distress
- Severe weakness, numbness in extremities
- Tolerance: increased need for medication, more frequent requests for medication, increased pain
- CNS depression: dizziness, drowsiness, psychiatric symptoms

Administer:

PO route
- With meals for GI symptoms

IT route
- For screening, dilute to a concentration of 50 mcg/ml with NaCl for inj (preservative-free), give test dose over 1 min; watch for decreasing muscle tone or frequency of spasm; if inadequate, use 2 more test doses q24h; if inadequate response, do not use IT
- Dosage, as individual titration is required
- Do not use IT inj IV, IM, SC, epidural

Additive compatibilities: Morphine

Perform/provide:
- Storage in tight container at room temperature
- Assistance with ambulation if dizziness or drowsiness occurs

Evaluate:
- Therapeutic response: decreased pain, spasticity

Teach patient/family:
- Not to discontinue medication quickly; hallucinations, spasticity, tachycardia will occur; drug should be tapered off over 1-2 wk
- Not to take with alcohol, other CNS depressants
- To avoid hazardous activities if drowsiness or dizziness occurs; rise slowly to prevent orthostatic hypotension
- To avoid using OTC medication:

cough preparations, antihistamines, unless directed by prescriber
• To notify prescriber of nausea, headache, tinnitus, insomnia, confusion, constipation, inadequate, painful urination continues
Treatment of overdose: Induce emesis of conscious patient, lavage, dialysis

balsalazide (℞)

(ball-sal'a-zide)
Colazal
Func. class.: GI antiinflammatory
Chem. class.: Salicylate derivative

Action: Delivered intact to the colon, bioconverted to 4-aminobenzoyl-β-alanine
Uses: Active, mild to moderate ulcerative colitis
Dosage and routes:
• *Adult:* **PO** 2.25 g tid × 8 wk, may take up to 12 wk
Available forms: Tabs 750 mg
Side effects/adverse reactions:
EENT: Dry eyes, rhinitis, sinusitis, watery eyes, blurred vision
SYST: ***Anaphylaxis***
GI: Nausea, vomiting, abdominal pain, diarrhea, rectal bleeding, flatulence, dyspepsia, dry mouth, constipation
CNS: Headache, insomnia, fatigue, fever, dizziness
MS: Arthralgia, back pain, myalgia
Contraindications: Hypersensitivity to salicylates
Precautions: Pregnancy (B), child <14 yr, lactation; pyloric stenosis
Do not confuse:
Colazal/Clozaril
Pharmacokinetics:
PO: Low and variably absorbed, peak 1½ hr, excreted in urine as metabolites, plasma protein binding 99%
Lab test interferences:
False positive: Urinary glucose test
Increase: AST, ALT, GGT, LDH, bilirubin, alk phosphatase
NURSING CONSIDERATIONS
Assess:
• Renal studies: BUN, creatinine, urinalysis (long-term therapy)
• Allergic reaction: rash, dermatitis, urticaria, pruritus, dyspnea, bronchospasm
Administer:
• With food in evenly divided doses
• With resuscitative equipment available; severe allergic reactions may occur
• Total daily dose evenly spaced to minimize GI intolerance
Perform/provide:
• Storage in tight, light-resistant container at room temperature
Evaluate:
• Therapeutic response: absence of fever, mucus in stools, resolution of symptoms of ulcerative colitis
Teach patient/family:
• To notify prescriber if symptoms do not improve, if rash, hives, or respiratory problems occur

HIGH ALERT

basiliximab (℞)

(bas-ih-liks'ih-mab)
Simulect
Func. class.: Immunosuppressant
Chem. class.: Murine/human monoclonal antibody (Interleukin-2) receptor antagonist

Action: Binds to and blocks the IL-2 receptor, which is selectively expressed on the surface of activated

T-lymphocytes; impairs the immune system to antigenic challenges

Uses: Acute allograft rejection in renal transplant patients when used with cycloSPORINE and corticosteroids

Dosage and routes:

• *Adult:* **IV** 20 mg × 2 doses; 1st dose within 2 hr before transplant surgery; 2nd dose given 4 days after transplantation

• *Child 2-15 yr:* **IV** 12 mg/m^2 × 2 doses; 1st dose within 2 hr before transplant surgery; 2nd dose given 4 days after transplantation

Available forms: Powder for inj 20 mg

Side effects/adverse reactions:

INTEG: Acne

CNS: Pyrexia, chills, tremors, headache, insomnia, weakness

META: Acidosis, hypercholesterolemia, hyperuricemia, hyperkalemia, hypocalcemia, hypokalemia, hypophosphatemia

RESP: Dyspnea, wheezing, ***pulmonary edema,*** *cough*

CV: Chest pain, angina, ***cardiac failure***, hypotension, *hypertension, edema*

MS: Arthralgia, myalgia

GI: Vomiting, nausea, diarrhea, constipation, abdominal pain, ***GI bleeding,*** *gingival hyperplasia, stomatitis*

MISC: Infection, moniliasis, ***anaphylaxis***

Contraindications: Hypersensitivity

Precautions: Pregnancy (B), infections, elderly, lactation, children

Pharmacokinetics:

Peak ½ hr (adults) terminal half-life 7 days (adult), 9½ days (children)

Interactions:

• Immunosuppression: other immunosuppressants

↑ Immunosuppression: astragalus, echinacea, melatonin, safflower

↓ immunosuppression: ginseng, maitake, mistletoe, schisandra, St. John's wort, turmeric

Lab test interferences:

Increase: Cholesterol, BUN, uric acid, creatinine, K, Ca, blood glucose, Hgb, Hct

Decrease: Hgb, Hct, platelets, magnesium, phosphate

NURSING CONSIDERATIONS

Assess:

• For infection: increased temp, WBC, sputum, urine

• Blood studies: Hgb, WBC, platelets during treatment qmo; if leukocytes are <3000/mm^3, drug should be discontinued

• Hepatic studies: alk phosphatase, AST, ALT, bilirubin

• Hepatotoxicity: dark urine, jaundice, itching, light-colored stools; drug should be discontinued

Anaphylaxis, hypersensitivity: dyspnea, wheezing, rash, pruritus, hypotension, tachycardia; if severe hypersensitivity reactions occur, drug should not be used again

Administer:

• All medications PO if possible; avoid IM inj, since infection may occur

IV route

• After adding 5 ml sterile water for inj, shake gently to dissolve, reconstitute to a vol of 50 ml with 0.9% NaCl or D_5, gently invert bag, do not shake, give over ½ hr, do not admix

Evaluate:

• Therapeutic response: absence of graft rejection

Teach patient/family:

• To report fever, chills, sore throat, fatigue, since serious infection may occur

• To avoid crowds, persons with known upper respiratory infections

• To use contraception during treatment

beclomethasone (℞)

(be-kloe-meth'a-sone)

Beclodisk♣, Becloforte Inhaler♣, Beclovent, Beclovent Rotocaps♣, QVAR, Vanceril, Vanceril Double Strength

Func. class.: Corticosteroid, synthetic

Chem. class.: Glucocorticoid

Action: Prevents inflammation by depression of migration of polymorphonuclear leukocytes, fibroblasts, reversal of increased capillary permeability and lysosomal stabilization; does not suppress hypothalamus and pituitary function

Uses: Chronic asthma, rhinitis

Dosage and routes:

• *Adult:* **INH** 2-4 puffs tid-qid, not to exceed 20 inhalations/day (42 mcg/actuation); 2 puffs bid, max 10 INH/day (84 mcg/actuation)

• *Child: 6-12 yr:* **INH** 1-2 puffs tid-qid, not to exceed 10 INH/day (42 mcg/actuations); 2 puffs bid, max 5 INH/day (84 mcg/actuations)

Available forms: Aerosol 42, 50, 84, 250 mcg/actuation; INH cap 100, 200 mcg

Side effects/adverse reactions:

CNS: Headache

EENT: Hoarseness, candidal infections of oral cavity, sore throat

GI: Dry mouth, dyspepsia

MISC: ***Angioedema, adrenal insufficiency,*** facial edema, Churg-Strauss syndrome

RESP: ***Bronchospasm,*** wheezing, cough

Contraindications: Hypersensitivity, status asthmaticus (primary treatment), nonasthmatic bronchial disease; bacterial, fungal, viral infections of mouth, throat, lungs; children <12 yr

Do not confuse:

Vanceril/Vancenase

Precautions: Nasal disease/surgery, pregnancy (C), lactation

Pharmacokinetics:

INH: Onset 10 min, excreted in feces, urine (metabolites), half-life 2.8 hr, crosses placenta, metabolized in lungs, liver (by CYP3A), GI system

NURSING CONSIDERATIONS

Assess:

• For fungal infection in mucous membranes

• Adrenal function periodically for HPA axis suppression during prolonged therapy, monitor growth/development

Administer:

• INH with water to decrease possibility of fungal infections

• Titrated dose, use lowest effective dose

Perform/provide:

• Gum, rinsing of mouth for dry mouth

Evaluate:

• Therapeutic response: decreased dyspnea, wheezing, dry rales

Teach patient/family:

• To carry or wear ID as steroid user

• To gargle/rinse mouth after each use to prevent oral fungal infections

• That in times of stress, systemic corticosteroids may be needed to prevent adrenal insufficiency; do not discontinue oral drug abruptly, taper slowly

• To notify prescriber if therapeutic response decreases; dosage adjustment may be needed

• Proper administration technique

• To wash inhaler with warm water and dry after each use

• All aspects of drug usage, including cushingoid symptoms

• The symptoms of adrenal insufficiency: nausea, anorexia, fatigue, dizziness, dyspnea, weakness, joint pain, depression

beclomethasone nasal agent

See appendix c

benazepril (℞)

(ben-aze'uh-pril)

Lotensin

Func. class.: Antihypertensive

Chem. class.: Angiotensin-converting enzyme (ACE) inhibitor

Action: Selectively suppresses renin-angiotensin-aldosterone system; inhibits ACE, preventing conversion of angiotensin I to angiotensin II

Uses: Hypertension, alone or in combination with thiazide diuretics

Dosage and routes:

- *Adult:* **PO** 10 mg qd initially, then 20-40 mg/day divided bid or qd (without a diuretic); 5 mg **PO** qd (with a diuretic)
- *Geriatric:* **PO** 5-10 mg/day initially

Renal dose:

- *Adult:* **PO** CCr <30 ml/min 5 mg **PO** qd, max 40 mg/day

Available forms: Tabs 5, 10, 20, 40 mg

Side effects/adverse reactions:

CV: Hypotension, postural hypotension, syncope, palpitations, angina

GU: Increased BUN, creatinine, decreased libido, impotence, urinary tract infection

INTEG: Rash, flushing, sweating

RESP: Cough, asthma, bronchitis, dyspnea, sinusitis

META: Hyperkalemia, hyponatremia

GI: Nausea, constipation, vomiting, gastritis, melena

CNS: Anxiety, hypertonia, insomnia, paresthesia, headache, dizziness, fatigue

MS: Arthralgia, arthritis, myalgia

MISC: ***Angioedema***

Contraindications: Hypersensitivity to ACE inhibitors, pregnancy (D) 2nd/3rd trimester, lactation, children

Precautions: Impaired renal, liver function, dialysis patients, hypovolemia, blood dyscrasias, CHF, COPD, asthma, elderly, bilateral renal artery stenosis, pregnancy (C) 1st trimester

Do not confuse:

Lotensin/Lioresal

Lotensin/Loniten

Pharmacokinetics:

PO: Peak ½-1 hr, protein binding 97%, half-life 10-11 hr, metabolized by liver (metabolites), excreted in urine

Interactions:

- ↑ hypotension: phenothiazines, nitrates, acute alcohol ingestion: diuretics, other antihypertensives
- ↑ hyperkalemia: potassium-sparing diuretics, potassium supplements
- ↑ serum levels of lithium, digoxin

🌿 ↑ toxicity/death: aconite

🌿 ↑ or ↓ antihypertensive effect: astragalus, cola tree

🌿 ↑ antihypertensive effect: barberry, betony, black catechu, black cohosh, bloodroot, broom, burdock, cat's claw, dandelion, goldenseal, Irish moss, Jamaican dogwood, kelp, khella, mistletoe, parsley

🌿 ↓ antihypertensive effect: coltsfoot, guarana, khat, licorice, pineapple, yohimbe

Lab test interferences:

Increase: AST, ALT, alk phosphatase, bilirubin, uric acid, blood glucose

Positive: ANA titer
False positive: ANA titer

NURSING CONSIDERATIONS

Assess:

• Blood studies: neutrophils, decreased platelets; WBC with diff baseline and q3mo, if neutrophils <1000/mm^3 discontinue treatment
• B/P at peak/trough level of drug, orthostatic hypotension, syncope when used with diuretic
• Renal studies: protein, BUN, creatinine; increased levels may indicate nephrotic syndrome; monitor urine for protein, increased LFTs, uric acid and glucose may be increased
• Potassium levels, although hyperkalemia rarely occurs
• Allergic reactions: rash, fever, pruritus, urticaria; drug should be discontinued if antihistamines fail to help
• Renal symptoms: polyuria, oliguria, frequency, dysuria
• Edema in feet, legs qd, weight qd in CHF

Perform/provide:

• Storage in tight container at 86° F (30° C) or less

Evaluate:

• Therapeutic response: decrease in B/P

Teach patient/family:

• Not to discontinue drug abruptly
• Not to use OTC products (cough, cold, allergy) unless directed by prescriber; do not use salt substitutes containing potassium without consulting prescriber
• The importance of complying with dosage schedule, even if feeling better
• To notify prescriber of pregnancy, drug will need to be discontinued
• To rise slowly to sitting or standing position to minimize orthostatic hypotension
• To notify prescriber of mouth sores, sore throat, fever, swelling of hands or feet, irregular heartbeat, chest pain
• To report excessive perspiration, dehydration, vomiting, diarrhea; may lead to fall in B/P
• That drug may cause dizziness, fainting, light-headedness; may occur during first few days of therapy
• That drug may cause skin rash or impaired perspiration
• How to take B/P, and normal readings for age group

Treatment of overdose: 0.9% NaCl IV INF, hemodialysis

benzocaine topical

See appendix c

RARELY USED

benzonatate (℞)

(ben-zoe′na-tate)
Tessalon Perles
Func. class.: Antitussive, nonopioid

Uses: Nonproductive cough

Dosage and routes:

• *Adult and child:* **PO** 100 mg tid, not to exceed 600 mg/day
• *Child <10 yr:* **PO** 8 mg/kg in 3-6 divided doses

Contraindications: Hypersensitivity

RARELY USED

benzoyl peroxide (OTC)

(ben′zoe-ill per-ox′ide)
Func. class.: Antiacne medication

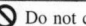

Uses: Mild to moderate acne

Dosage and routes:
• *Adult and child:* **TOP** apply to affected area qd or bid
Contraindications: Hypersensitivity to benzoic acid derivatives

RARELY USED

benzquinamide (℞)
(benz-kwin′a-mide)
Emete-Con
Func. class.: Antiemetic

Uses: To inhibit nausea, vomiting associated with anesthetic, surgery
Dosage and routes:
• *Adult:* **IM** 50 mg or 0.5-1 mg/kg, may be repeated in 1 hr, then q3-4h prn; **IV** 25 mg or 0.2-0.4 mg/kg as a one-time dose
Contraindications: Hypersensitivity, hypertension

benztropine (℞)
(benz′troe-peen)
Apo-Benztropin✤, benztropine mesylate, Cogentin
Func. class.: Cholinergic blocker, antiparkinson agent
Chem. class.: Tertiary amine

Action: Blockade of central acetylcholine receptors
Uses: Parkinson symptoms, EPS associated with neuroleptic drugs, acute dystonic reactions
Dosage and routes:
Drug-induced EPS
• *Adult:* **IM/IV** 1-4 mg qd-bid; give **PO** dose as soon as possible; **PO** 1-2 mg bid/tid, increase by 0.5 mg q5-6 days
• *Child:* **IM/IV** 0.02-0.05 mg/kg/dose 1-2 ×/day
• *Geriatric:* **PO** 0.5 mg qd-bid, increase by 0.5 mg q5-6d
Parkinson symptoms
• *Adult:* **PO** 1-2 mg/day in 1-2 divided doses, increase 0.5 mg q5-6d titrated to patient response, max 6 mg qd
Acute dystonic reactions
• *Adult:* **IM/IV** 1-2 mg, may increase to 1-2 mg bid (PO)
Available forms: Tabs 0.5, 1, 2 mg; inj 1 mg/ml
Side effects/adverse reactions:
MS: Muscular weakness, cramping
INTEG: Rash, urticaria, dermatoses
MISC: Increased temperature, flushing, decreased sweating, hyperthermia, heat stroke, numbness of fingers
CNS: Anxiety, restlessness, irritability, delusions, hallucinations, headache, sedation, depression, incoherence, dizziness, memory loss; confusion, delirium (elderly)
EENT: Blurred vision, photophobia, dilated pupils, difficulty swallowing, dry eyes, mydriasis, increased intraocular tension, angle-closure glaucoma
CV: Palpitations, tachycardia, hypotension, bradycardia
GI: Dryness of mouth, constipation, nausea, vomiting, abdominal distress, ***paralytic ileus,*** epigastric distress
GU: Hesitancy, retention, dysuria
Contraindications: Hypersensitivity, narrow-angle glaucoma, myasthenia gravis, GI/GU obstruction, child <3 yr, peptic ulcer, megacolon, prostate hypertrophy
Precautions: Pregnancy (C), elderly, lactation, tachycardia, liver, kidney disease, drug abuse history, dysrhythmias, hypotension, hypertension, psychiatric patients, children
Pharmacokinetics:
IM/IV: Onset 15 min, duration 6-10 hr

PO: Onset 1 hr, duration 6-10 hr
Interactions:
• ↑ anticholinergic effect: antihistamines, phenothiazines, tricyclics, disopyramide, quinidine
• ↓ absorption: antidiarrheals
↓ benztropine effect: kava, jaborandi, pill-bearing spurge
↑ benztropine effect: butterbur, jimsonweed
↑ constipation: black catechu
NURSING CONSIDERATIONS
Assess:
• I&O ratio; commonly causes decreased urinary output; urinary hesitancy, retention; palpate bladder if retention occurs
• Parkinsonism, EPS: shuffling gait, muscle rigidity, involuntary movements, loss of balance
• Constipation; increase fluids, bulk, exercise if this occurs
• Mental status: affect, mood, CNS depression, worsening of mental symptoms during early therapy
• Use caution in hot weather; drug may increase susceptibility to stroke by decreasing sweating
• For benztropine "buzz" or "high," patients may imitate EPS
Administer:
PO route
• With or after meals to prevent GI upset; may give with fluids other than water
• At hs to avoid daytime drowsiness in patient with parkinsonism
IM route
• Use for dystonic reactions only
IV route
• Undiluted IV (1 mg = 1 ml) give 1 mg/1 min; keep in bed for at least 1 hr after dose
Syringe compatibilities: Metoclopramide
Y-site compatibilities: Fluconazole, tacrolimus
Perform/provide:
• Storage at room temperature
• Hard candy, gum, frequent drinks, to relieve dry mouth
Evaluate:
• Therapeutic response: absence of involuntary movements
Teach patient/family:
• That tabs may be crushed and mixed with food
• Not to discontinue this drug abruptly; to taper off over 1 wk, or withdrawal symptoms may occur (EPS, tremors, insomia, tachycardia, restlessness)
• To avoid driving, other hazardous activities; drowsiness may occur
• To avoid OTC medication: cough, cold preparations with alcohol, antihistamines unless directed by prescriber
• To change positions slowly to prevent orthostatic hypotension
• To use good oral hygiene, frequent sips of water, sugarless gum for dry mouth

bepridil (℞)
(be′pri-dil)
Vascor
Func. class.: Calcium channel blocker, antianginal

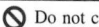

Action: Inhibits calcium ion influx across cell membrane during cardiac depolarization; produces relaxation of coronary vascular smooth muscle, dilates coronary arteries, decreases SA/AV node conduction, inhibits fast sodium inward current, dilates peripheral arteries
Uses: Chronic stable angina, used alone or in combination with β-blockers, nitrates
Dosage and routes:
Angina
• *Adult:* **PO** 200 mg qd, after 10 days may increase dose if needed, max dose 400 mg/day

Available forms: Tabs, film-coated, 200, 300 mg

Side effects/adverse reactions:

CV: ***Dysrhythmia,*** edema, ***CHF,*** bradycardia, hypotension, palpitations, AV block, ***torsades de pointes***

GI: Nausea, vomiting, diarrhea, gastric upset, constipation, increased hepatic studies

GU: Nocturia, polyuria

CNS: Headache, fatigue, drowsiness, dizziness, anxiety, depression, weakness, insomnia, confusion, light-headedness, nervousness

MISC: ***Stevens-Johnson syndrome***

HEMA: ***Agranulocytosis***

Contraindications: Hypersensitivity, sick sinus syndrome, 2nd- or 3rd-degree heart block, Wolff-Parkinson-White syndrome, hypotension less than 90 mm Hg systolic, cardiogenic shock, history of serious ventricular dysrhythmias, uncompensated cardiac insufficiency

Precautions: CHF, hypotension, hepatic injury, pregnancy (C), lactation, children, renal disease, idiopathic hypertropic subaortic stenosis (IHSS), concomitant β-blocker therapy

Do not confuse:

bepridil/Prepidil

Pharmacokinetics: Onset 1 hr, peak 2-3 hr, duration 24 hr, 99% plasma protein bound, half-life 42 hr; completely metabolized in the liver and excreted in urine and feces

Interactions:

- ↑ prolongation of QT, depression of AV node: cardiac glycosides, antidysrhythmics, tricyclics
- ↑ bepridil levels: ritonavir
- ↑ hypotension: fentanyl
- ↑ levels of digoxin

↑ antianginal effect: barbarry, betel palm, burdock, cat's claw, chicory, goldenseal, khat, khella, lily of valley, plantain

- Drug/food: ↑ hypotensive effects: grapefruit juice

↓ effect: yohimbe

Lab test interferences:

Increase: LFTs, aminotransferase, CPK, LDH

NURSING CONSIDERATIONS

Assess:

- Cardiac status: B/P, pulse, respiration, ECG intervals (PR, QRS, QT), dysrhythmias; may increase QT interval, altered T wave
- I&O ratios, weight qd, monitor for CHF: weight gain, jugular vein distention, edema, rales/crackles, dyspnea, restlessness

Administer:

PO route

- Before meals, hs; adjust no more frequently than q10 days; may give with food/fluids to decrease GI upset

Evaluate:

- Therapeutic response: decreased anginal pain, increased activity tolerance

Teach patient/family:

- How to take pulse before taking drug; record or graph should be kept; use demonstration, return demonstration
- To avoid hazardous activities until stabilized on drug, dizziness no longer a problem
- To limit caffeine consumption

⃠ Not to break, crush, or chew tabs

- To avoid OTC drugs unless directed by a prescriber
- The importance of compliance with all areas of medical regimen: diet, exercise, stress reduction, drug therapy
- To notify prescriber of swelling, weight gain, dyspnea, irregular heart beat
- To maintain good oral hygiene to prevent gingival hyperplasia

Treatment of overdose: Defibrillation, atropine for AV block, vasopressor for hypotension

RARELY USED

beractant (℞)

(ber-ak'tant)
Survanta
Func. class.: Natural lung surfactant

Uses: Prevention and treatment (rescue) of respiratory distress syndrome in premature infants
Dosage and routes:
• **INTRATRACHEAL INSTILL:** 4 doses can be administered in the 1st 48 hr of life; give doses no more frequently than q6h; each dose is 100 mg of phospholipids/kg birth weight (4 ml/kg)

betamethasone (℞)

(bay-ta-meth'a-sone)
Betnelan♣, Betnesol♣, Celestone, Cel-U-Jec, Selestoject♣
Func. class.: Corticosteroid, synthetic, long-acting

Action: Decreases inflammation by suppressing migration of polymorphonuclear leukocytes, fibroblasts, reversal of increased capillary permeability and lysosomal stabilization
Uses: Immunosuppression, severe inflammation, prevention of neonatal respiratory distress syndrome (by administration to mother)
Dosage and routes:
• *Adult:* **PO** 0.6-7.2 mg qd; **IM/IV** 0.6-7.2 mg qd in joint or soft tissue (sodium phosphate)
• *Child:* **PO** 17.5 mcg/kg/day in 3 divided doses; **IM** 17.5 mcg/kg/day in 3 divided doses every 3rd day or 5.8-8.75 mcg/kg/day as a single dose (adrenal insufficiency)
• *Child:* **PO** 62.5-250 mcg/kg/day in 3 divided doses; **IM** 20.8-125 mcg/kg/day of the base q12-24h (other uses)
Available forms: Betamethasone: tabs 500; 600 mcg, tabs, effervescent 500 mcg♣, syr 600 mcg/5 ml; ext rel tab 1 mg; sol for inj (phosphate) 3 mg/ml; susp for inj (phosphate/acetate) 6 mg/ml
Side effects/adverse reactions:
INTEG: Acne, poor wound healing, ecchymosis, bruising, petechiae
CNS: Depression, flushing, sweating, headache, ecchymosis, bruising, mood changes
CV: Hypertension, ***circulatory collapse, thrombophlebitis, embolism,*** tachycardia, ***necrotizing angiitis, CHF***
HEMA: ***Thrombocytopenia***
MS: Fractures, osteoporosis, weakness
GI: Diarrhea, nausea, abdominal distention, ***GI hemorrhage,*** *increased appetite,* ***pancreatitis***
EENT: Fungal infections, increased intraocular pressure, blurred vision
Contraindications: Psychosis, hypersensitivity, idiopathic thrombocytopenia, acute glomerulonephritis, amebiasis, fungal infections, nonasthmatic bronchial disease, child <2 yr, AIDS, TB
Precautions: Pregnancy (C), lactation, diabetes mellitus, glaucoma, osteoporosis, seizure disorders, ulcerative colitis, CHF, myasthenia gravis, renal disease, esophagitis, peptic ulcer
Pharmacokinetics:
PO: Onset 1-2 hr, peak 1 hr, duration 3 days
IM/IV: Onset 10 min, peak 4-8 hr, duration 1-1½ days
Metabolized in liver, excreted in urine as steroids, crosses placenta

Interactions:
• ↓ action of betamethasone: barbiturates, rifampin, phenytoin
• ↓ effects of anticoagulants, antidiabetics, insulin, isoniazid, toxoids, vaccines, salicylates
• GI bleeding: NSAIDs, alcohol, salicylates, indomethacin
• Drug/food: grapefruit juice should be avoided
Hypokalemia: aloe, buckthorn, cascara sagrada, Chinese rhubarb, rhubarb, senna
↑ corticosteroid effects: goldenseal, hawthorn, hops, lemon balm, licorice, lily of the valley, mistletoe, perilla, pheasant's eye, squill
↑ hypokalemia: buckthorn, cascara sagrada, Chinese rhubarb
Lab test interferences:
Increase: Cholesterol, sodium, blood glucose, uric acid, calcium, urine glucose
Decrease: Calcium, potassium, T_4, T_3, thyroid ^{131}I uptake test, urine 17-OHCS, 17-KS, PBI
False negative: Skin allergy tests
NURSING CONSIDERATIONS
Assess:
• Potassium, blood glucose, urine glucose while on long-term therapy; hypokalemia and hyperglycemia
• Weight daily; notify prescriber of weekly gain >5 lb
• B/P q4h, pulse; notify prescriber if chest pain occurs
• I&O ratio; be alert for decreasing urinary output and increasing edema
• Plasma cortisol levels during long-term therapy (normal level: 138-635 nmol/L SI units when drawn at 8 AM)
Administer:
PO route
• With food or milk to decrease GI symptoms
IM route
• Inject deeply in large muscle mass, rotate sites, avoid deltoid, use 21G needle
• In one dose in AM to prevent adrenal suppression, avoid SC administration; may damage tissue
IV route
• Only sodium phosphate product; give >1 min; may be given by IV INF in compatible sol
• After shaking suspension (parenteral)
• Titrated dose; use lowest effective dose
Y-site compatibilities: Heparin, hydrocortisone, potassium chloride, vit B/C
Perform/provide:
• Assistance with ambulation in patient with bone tissue disease to prevent fractures
Evaluate:
• Therapeutic response: ease of respirations, decreased inflammation
• Infection: increased temperature, WBC even after withdrawal of medication; drug masks infection symptoms
• Potassium depletion: paresthesias, fatigue, nausea, vomiting, depression, polyuria, dysrhythmias, weakness
• Edema, hypertension, cardiac symptoms
• Mental status: affect, mood, behavioral changes, aggression
Teach patient/family:
• That ID as steroid user should be carried
• To notify prescriber if therapeutic response decreases; dosage adjustment may be needed
Not to discontinue abruptly; adrenal crisis can result
• To avoid OTC products: salicylates, alcohol in cough products, cold preparations unless directed by prescriber

• All aspects of drug usage including cushingoid symptoms
• The symptoms of adrenal insufficiency: nausea, anorexia, fatigue, dizziness, dyspnea, weakness, joint pain

betamethasone topical

See appendix c

betaxolol ophthalmic

See appendix c

bethanechol (℞)

(be-than′e-kole)
bethanechol chloride,
Duvoid, Urebeth, Urecholine
Func. class.: Urinary tract stimulant, cholinergic
Chem. class.: Synthetic choline ester

Action: Stimulates muscarinic Ach receptors directly; mimics effects of parasympathetic nervous system stimulation; stimulates gastric motility, stimulates micturition; increases lower esophageal sphincter pressure
Uses: Urinary retention (postoperative, postpartum), neurogenic atony of bladder with retention
Dosage and routes:
• *Adult:* **PO** 25-50 mg bid-qid; **SC** 5 mg tid-qid prn
• *Child:* **PO** 0.6 mg/kg/day divided in 3-4 doses/day; SC 0.06 mg/kg tid or 0.15 mg/kg qid
Test dose
• *Adult:* **SC** 2.5 mg repeated 15-30 min intervals × 4 doses to determine effective dose
Available forms: Tabs 5, 10, 25, 50 mg; inj 5 mg/ml
Side effects/adverse reactions:
INTEG: Rash, urticaria, flushing, increased sweating
CNS: Dizziness
GI: Nausea, bloody diarrhea, belching, vomiting, cramps, fecal incontinence
CV: Hypotension, bradycardia, orthostatic hypotension, reflex tachycardia, ***cardiac arrest, circulatory collapse***
GU: Urgency
RESP: ***Acute asthma, dyspnea, bronchoconstriction***
EENT: Miosis, increased salivation, lacrimation, blurred vision
Contraindications: Hypersensitivity, severe bradycardia, asthma, severe hypotension, hyperthyroidism, peptic ulcer, parkinsonism, seizure disorders, CAD, COPD, coronary occlusion, mechanical obstruction, peritonitis, recent urinary or GI surgery
Precautions: Hypertension, pregnancy (C), lactation, child <8 yr
Pharmacokinetics:
PO: Onset 30-90 min, peak 1 hr, duration 6 hr
SC: Onset 5-15 min, peak 15-30 min, duration 2 hr, excreted by kidneys
Interactions:
• ↑ action or toxicity: cholinergic agonists, anticholinesterase agents
• Severe hypotension: ganglionic blockers
↓ effects: jimsonweed, scopolia
↑ cholinergic effect: jaborandi tree
Lab test interferences:
Increase: AST, lipase/amylase, bilirubin, BSP
NURSING CONSIDERATIONS
Assess:
• B/P, pulse; observe after parenteral dose for 1 hr
• I&O ratio; check for urinary retention or urge incontinence

• Bradycardia, hypotension, bronchospasm, headache, dizziness, convulsions, respiratory depression; drug should be discontinued if toxicity occurs

Administer:

• To avoid nausea and vomiting, take on an empty stomach

SC route

◆ Parenteral dose by SC route; use of IM, IV may result in cardiac arrest

◆ Only with atropine sulfate available for cholinergic crisis

• Only after all other cholinergics have been discontinued

• Increased doses if tolerance occurs

Perform/provide:

• Storage at room temperature

• Bedpan/urinal if given for urinary retention

• Use of rectal tube if ordered, to increase passage of gas when used for abdominal distention

Evaluate:

• Therapeutic response: absence of urinary retention, abdominal distention

Teach patient/family:

• To take drug exactly as prescribed; 1 hr ac or 2 hr pc

• To make position changes slowly; orthostatic hypotension may occur

Treatment of overdose: Administer atropine 0.6-1.2 mg IV or IM (adult)

bexarotene (℞)

Targretin

Func. class.: Retinoid, 2nd generation

Action: Selectively binds and activates retinoid X receptors (RXRs) that are partially responsible for cellular proliferation and differentiation. Inhibits some tumor cells

Uses: Cutaneous T-cell lymphoma

Investigational uses: Breast cancer

Research note: Bexarotene has been proven effective and safe for refractory advanced-stage cutaneous T-cell lymphoma[3]

Dosage and routes:

• *Adult:* **PO** 300 mg/day/m^2, may increase to 400 mg/day with proper monitoring

Available forms: Cap 75 mg

Side effects/adverse reactions:

CNS: Headache, fatigue, lethargy

GI: Nausea, abdominal pain, diarrhea, ***acute pancreatitis***

INTEG: Rash, asthenia, dry skin

HEMA: ***Leukopenia, neutropenia,*** anemia

SYST: Infection, hypothyroidism

Contraindications: Hypersensitivity to retinoids, pregnancy (X)

Precautions: Lactation, sunburn, hepatic, renal disease, children

Pharmacokinetics: Unknown

Interactions:

• ↑ bexarotene levels: azole antiinfectives, grapefruit juice

• ↓ bexarotene levels: barbiturates, rifampins, phenytoin

• Limit intake of vit A ≤15,000 international units/day

• ↓ action of: tamoxifen, oral contraceptives

• ↑ action of: antidiabetics

NURSING CONSIDERATIONS

Assess:

• Area of body involved, what helps or aggravates condition; cysts, dryness, itching

• Cholesterol, HDL, triglycerides may be elevated

• CBC for leukopenia, neutropenia, anemia

Administer:

• With food

Perform/provide:

• Storage at room temperature

Evaluate:
- Therapeutic response: decrease in size and number of lesions

Teach patient/family:
- To watch for hypoglycemia in diabetic patients on insulin
- To limit vit A intake to ≤15,000 international units/day to avoid toxicity
- To avoid sunlight, sunlamps, or use protective clothing, sunscreen
- To avoid pregnancy while taking this drug and ≥1 mo after discontinuing therapy

bicalutamide (℞)

(bye-kal-u'ta-mide)
Casodex

Func. class.: Antineoplastic hormone

Chem. class.: Nonsteroidal antiandrogen

Action: Binds to cytosol androgen in target tissue, which competitively inhibits the action to androgens

Uses: Prostate cancer in combination with luteinizing hormone–releasing hormone (LHRH) analog

Dosage and routes:
- *Adult:* **PO** 50 mg qd with LHRH

Available forms: Tabs 50 mg

Side effects/adverse reactions:

GI: Diarrhea, constipation, nausea, vomiting, increased liver enzymes, anorexia, dry mouth, melena, abdominal pain

CV: Hot flashes, hypertension, chest pain, ***CHF,*** edema

CNS: Dizziness, paresthesia, insomnia, anxiety, neuropathy, headache

INTEG: Rash, sweating, dry skin, pruritus, alopecia

GU: Nocturia, hematuria, UTI, impotence, gynecomastia, urinary incontinence, frequency, dysuria, retention, urgency, breast tenderness, decreased libido, *hot flashes*

MISC: Infection, anemia, dyspnea, bone pain, headache, asthenia, *back pain,* flulike symptoms

Contraindications: Hypersensitivity, pregnancy (X)

Precautions: Renal, hepatic disease, elderly, lactation

Pharmacokinetics: Well absorbed, peak 31½ hr, metabolized by liver, excreted in urine, feces; half-life 5.8 days

Interactions:
- ↑ anticoagulation: warfarin

Lab test interferences:

Increase: AST, ALT, bilirubin, BUN, creatinine

Decrease: Hgb, WBC

NURSING CONSIDERATIONS

Assess:
- For diarrhea, constipation, nausea, vomiting
- For hot flashes, gynecomastia (assure patient that these are common side effects)
- Prostate specific antigen (PSA), LFTs

Administer:

PO route
- At same time each day, either AM or PM, with/without food
- With LHRH treatment; start at same time for both drugs

Evaluate:
- Therapeutic response: decreased tumor size, decreased spread of malignancy

Teach patient/family:
- To recognize, report signs of anemia, hepatoxicity, renal toxicity
- That hair may be lost, but is reversible after therapy is completed
- Not to use other products, unless approved by prescriber
- To report severe diarrhea
- To use contraception while taking this drug

bimatoprost ophthalmic

See appendix c

biperiden (℞)

(bye-per′i-den)

Akineton

Func. class.: Antiparkinson agent, anticholinergic

Action: Centrally acting competitive anticholinergic

Uses: Parkinson symptoms, EPS secondary to neuroleptic drug therapy

Dosage and routes:

Extrapyramidal symptoms

• *Adult:* **PO** 2 mg qd-tid; **IM/IV** 2 mg q30min, if needed, not to exceed 8 mg/24 hr

• *Child:* **IM** 40 mcg/kg or 1.2 mg/m^2, may repeat q½h

Parkinson symptoms

• *Adult:* **PO** 2 mg tid-qid; max 16 mg/24 hr

Available forms: Tabs 2 mg; inj 5 mg/ml (lactate)

Side effects/adverse reactions:

CNS: Confusion, anxiety, restlessness, irritability, delusions, hallucinations, headache, sedation, depression, incoherence, dizziness, euphoria, tremors, memory loss

EENT: Blurred vision, photophobia, dilated pupils, difficulty swallowing, mydriasis, increased intraocular tension, angle-closure glaucoma

CV: Palpitations, tachycardia, postural hypotension, bradycardia

GI: Dryness of mouth, constipation, nausea, vomiting, abdominal distress, ***paralytic ileus***

GU: Hesitancy, retention, dysuria

INTEG: Rash, urticaria, dermatoses

MISC: Increased temp, flushing, decreased sweating, hyperthermia, ***heat stroke,*** numbness of fingers, weakness, cramping

Contraindications: Hypersensitivity, narrow-angle glaucoma, myasthenia gravis, GI/GU obstruction, megacolon, stenosing peptic ulcers, prostatic hypertrophy

Precautions: Pregnancy (C), elderly, lactation, tachycardia, dysrhythmias, liver or kidney disease, drug abuse, hypotension, hypertension, psychiatric patients, children <8 yr

Pharmacokinetics:

IM/IV: Onset 15 min, duration 6-10 hr

PO: Onset 1 hr, duration 6-10 hr

Interactions:

• ↑ schizophrenic symptoms: haloperidol

• ↑ anticholinergic effect: antihistamines, phenothiazines, amantadine, tricyclics, quinidine

• ↓ biperiden absorption: antacids, antidiarrheals

• ↑ sedation: alcohol

↓ biperiden effect: kava, jaborandi tree, pill-bearing spurge

↑ biperiden effect: butterbur, jimsonweed

↑ constipation: black catechu

NURSING CONSIDERATIONS

Assess:

• I&O ratio; retention commonly causes decreased urinary output

• Parkinsonism, EPS: shuffling gait, muscle rigidity, involuntary movements

• Patient response if anticholinergics are given

• Urinary hesitancy, retention; palpate bladder if retention occurs

• Constipation; increase fluids, bulk, exercise if this occurs

• For tolerance over long-term therapy; dose may have to be increased or changed

• Mental status: affect, mood, CNS depression, worsening of mental symptoms during early therapy

Administer:

PO route

• With or after meals to prevent GI upset; may give with fluids other than water

• At hs to avoid daytime drowsiness in patients with parkinsonism

IM/IV route

• With patient recumbent to prevent postural hypotension, give undiluted 2 mg or less over 1 min or more

Perform/provide:

• Storage at room temperature

• Hard candy, gum, frequent drinks to relieve dry mouth

Evaluate:

• Therapeutic response: absence of involuntary movements

Teach patient/family:

• To use caution in hot weather; drug may increase susceptibility to heat stroke, decreases sweating

• Not to discontinue this drug abruptly; to taper off over 1 wk

• To avoid driving, other hazardous activities; drowsiness may occur

• To avoid OTC medication: cough, cold preparations with alcohol, antihistamines unless directed by prescriber

bisacodyl (℞, OTC)

(bis-a-koe'dill)

Bisac-Evac, Bisaco-Lax, Bisacolax✱, Bisco-Lax, Carter's Little Pills, Dacodyl, Deficol, Dulcagen, Dulcolax, Feen-a-mint, Fleet Laxative, Laxit✱, Modane, Reliable Gentle Laxative, Therelax

Func. class.: Laxative, stimulant

Chem. class.: Diphenylmethane

Action: Acts directly on intestine by increasing motor activity; thought to irritate colonic intramural plexus

Uses: Short-term treatment of constipation, bowel or rectal preparation for surgery, examination

Dosage and routes:

• *Adult ≥12 yr:* **PO** 5-15 mg in PM or AM; may use up to 30 mg for bowel or rectal preparation; **RECT** 10 mg, single dose

• *Child >3 yr:* **PO** 5-10 mg as a single dose; **RECT** 10 mg as a single dose

• *Child <2 yr:* **RECT** 5 mg as a single dose

Available forms: Enteric-coated tabs 5 mg; supp 5, 10 mg; rect sol 10 mg/37 ml; enema 0.33 mg/ml, 10 mg/5 ml; powder for rectal sol/ 1.5 mg bisacodyl/2.5 g tannic acid

Side effects/adverse reactions:

CNS: Muscle weakness

GI: Nausea, vomiting, anorexia, cramps, diarrhea, rectal burning (suppositories)

META: Protein-losing enteropathy, alkalosis, hypokalemia, ***tetany,*** electrolyte, fluid imbalances

Contraindications: Hypersensitivity, rectal fissures, abdominal pain, nausea, vomiting, appendicitis, acute surgical abdomen, ulcerated hemorrhoids, acute hepatitis, fecal impaction, intestinal/biliary tract obstruction

Precautions: Pregnancy (C), lactation

Pharmacokinetics:

PO: Onset 6-10 hr

RECT: Onset 15-60 min

Metabolized by liver; excreted in urine, bile, feces, breast milk

Interactions:

• Gastric irritation: antacids, milk, H_2-blockers, gastric acid pump inhibitors

↑ action: flax, lily of the valley, pheasant's eye, senna, squill

NURSING CONSIDERATIONS

Assess:

• Blood, urine electrolytes if drug is used often by patient

• I&O ratio to identify fluid loss

• Cause of constipation; identify whether fluids, bulk, or exercise missing from lifestyle

• Cramping, rectal bleeding, nausea, vomiting; if these symptoms occur, drug should be discontinued

Administer:

PO route

• Alone only with water for better absorption; do not take within 1 hr of other drugs or within 1 hr of antacids, milk, or cimetidine

• In AM or PM

Evaluate:

• Therapeutic response: decrease in constipation

Teach patient/family:

⊘ To swallow tabs whole; do not break, crush, or chew tabs

• Not to use laxatives for long-term therapy; bowel tone will be lost

• That normal bowel movements do not always occur daily

• Not to use in presence of abdominal pain, nausea, vomiting

• To notify prescriber if constipation is unrelieved or if symptoms of electrolyte imbalance occur: muscle cramps, pain, weakness, dizziness

B

bismuth subsalicylate (OTC)

(bis'muth sub-sal-iss'uh-late)

Bismatrol, Bismatrol Extra Strength, Bismed, Pepto-Bismol, Pepto-Bismol Maximum Strength, Pink Bismuth, PMS-Bismuth Subsalicylate

Func. class.: Antidiarrheal

Chem. class.: Salicylate

Action: Inhibits prostaglandin synthesis responsible for GI hypermotility; stimulates absorption of fluid and electrolytes

Uses: Diarrhea (cause undetermined), prevention of diarrhea when traveling; may be included to treat *Helicobacter pylori*

Dosage and routes:

Antidiarrheal

• *Adult:* **PO** 524 mg q½h or 1048 mg q1h, max 4.2 mg/24 hr

• *Child 9-12 yr:* **PO** 262 mg q½-1hr, max 2.1 mg/24 hr

• *Child 6-9 yr:* **PO** 174.6 mg q½-1hr, max 1.4 mg/24 hr

• *Child 3-6 yr:* **PO** 88 mg q½-1hr, max 704 mg/24 hr

Available forms: Tabs 262 mg; chewable tabs 262, 300 mg; susp 262 mg/15 ml, 524 mg/15 ml

Side effects/adverse reactions:

HEMA: Increased bleeding time

GI: Increased fecal impaction (high doses), dark stools

CNS: Confusion, twitching

EENT: Hearing loss, tinnitus, metallic taste, blue gums, black tongue (chew tabs)

Contraindications: Child <3 yr, history of GI bleeding, renal disease

Precautions: Anticoagulant therapy, immobility

Pharmacokinetics:

PO: Onset 1 hr, peak 2 hr, duration 4 hr

Interactions:

• Salicylate toxicity: salicylates
• ↑ effects of oral anticoagulants, oral antidiabetics
• ↓ absorption of: tetracycline
↑ absorption of bismuth: sarsaparilla
↑ antidiarrheal effect: nutmeg

Lab test interferences:

Interference: Radiographic studies of GI system

NURSING CONSIDERATIONS

Assess:

• Electrolytes (K, Na, Cl) if diarrhea is severe or continues long term; assess skin turgor
• Bowel pattern before drug therapy, after treatment

Administer:

PO route

• Increased fluids to rehydrate the patient
• Shake liquid before using

Evaluate:

• Therapeutic response: decreased diarrhea or absence of diarrhea when traveling

Teach patient/family:

• To chew or dissolve in mouth; do not swallow whole; shake liquid before using
• To avoid other salicylates unless directed by prescriber; not to give to children, possibility of Reye's syndrome
• That stools may turn black; tongue may darken; impaction may occur in debilitated patients
• To stop use if symptoms do not improve within 2 days or become worse, or if diarrhea is accompanied by high fever

bisoprolol (℞)

(bis-oh'pro-lole)
Zebeta
Func. class.: Antihypertensive
Chem. class.: β_1-Blocker

Action: Preferentially and competitively blocks stimulation of β_1-adrenergic receptors within cardiac muscle (decreases rate of SA node discharge, increases recovery time), slows conduction of AV node, decreases heart rate, which decreases O_2 consumption in myocardium; decreases renin-aldosterone-angiotensin system; inhibits β_2-receptors in bronchial and vascular smooth muscle at high doses

Uses: Mild to moderate hypertension

Investigational uses: Stable angina pectoris, stable CHF

Dosage and routes:

• *Adult:* **PO** 5 mg qd; may increase if necessary to 20 mg qd

Renal/hepatic dose:

• *Adult:* **PO** 2.5 mg, titrate upward

Available forms: Tabs 5, 10 mg

Side effects/adverse reactions:

MS: Joint pain, arthralgia

MISC: Facial swelling, weight gain, decreased exercise tolerance

CV: ***Ventricular dysrhythmias, profound hypotension, bradycardia, CHF,*** cold extremities, postural hypotension, ***2nd- or 3rd-degree heart block***

CNS: Vertigo, headache, insomnia, fatigue, dizziness, mental changes, memory loss, hallucinations, depression, lethargy, drowsiness, strange dreams, catatonia, peripheral neuropathy

GI: Nausea, diarrhea, vomiting, ***mesenteric arterial thrombosis,*** isch-

emic colitis, flatulence, gastritis, gastric pain
INTEG: Rash, flushing, alopecia, pruritus, sweating
HEMA: ***Agranulocytosis, thrombocytopenia,*** purpura, eosinophilia
EENT: Sore throat; dry, burning eyes
GU: Impotence, decreased libido
ENDO: Increased hypoglycemic response to insulin
RESP: ***Bronchospasm,*** dyspnea, wheezing, cough, nasal stuffiness

Contraindications: Hypersensitivity to β-blockers, cardiogenic shock, heart block (2nd, 3rd degree), sinus bradycardia, CHF, cardiac failure

Precautions: Major surgery, pregnancy (C), lactation, children, diabetes mellitus, renal or hepatic disease, thyroid disease, COPD, asthma, well-compensated heart failure, aortic or mitral valve disease, peripheral vascular disease, myasthenia gravis

Do not confuse:
Zebeta/Diabeta

Pharmacokinetics:
PO: Peak 2-4 hr; half-life 9-12 hr, 50% excreted unchanged in urine, protein binding 30%; metabolized in liver to inactive metabolites

Interactions:
- ↑ peripheral ischemia: ergots
- ↓ antihypertensive effect: NSAIDs
- Hypotension: reserpine, guanethidine
- Myocardial depression: calcium channel blockers

Toxicity/death: aconite
↑ β-blocking effect: betel palm, butterbur, cola tree, figwort, fumitory, guarana, hawthorn, lily of the valley, motherwort, plantain
↓ β-blocking effect: coenzyme Q10, yohimbe

Lab test interferences:
Increase: AST, ALT, ANA titer, blood glucose, BUN, uric acid, K, lipoprotein
Interference: Glucose/insulin tolerance tests

NURSING CONSIDERATIONS

Assess:
- B/P during beginning treatment, periodically thereafter; pulse q4h: note rate, rhythm, quality
- Apical/radial pulse before administration; notify prescriber of any significant changes (pulse <50 bpm)
- Baselines in renal, hepatic studies before therapy begins
- I&O, weight qd, watch for CHF: increased weight, jugular vein distention, dyspnea, rales, crackles
- Edema in feet, legs daily
- Skin turgor, dryness of mucous membranes for hydration status, especially elderly

Administer:

PO route
- Drug ac, hs, tablet may be crushed or swallowed whole, may give without regard to meals
- Reduced dosage in renal and hepatic dysfunction

Perform/provide:
- Storage protected from light, moisture; place in cool environment

Evaluate:
- Therapeutic response: decreased B/P after 1-2 wk

Teach patient/family:
- Not to discontinue drug abruptly, may cause precipitate angina, evaluate noncompliance
- Not to use OTC products containing α-adrenergic stimulants (such as nasal decongestants, OTC cold preparations) unless directed by prescriber
- To report bradycardia, dizziness, confusion, depression, fever, cold extremities
- To take pulse at home; advise when to notify prescriber
- To avoid alcohol, smoking, sodium intake
- To comply with weight control,

dietary adjustments, modified exercise program

• To carry emergency ID to identify drug taking, allergies

• To avoid hazardous activities if dizziness is present

⬥ To report symptoms of CHF: difficulty breathing, especially on exertion or when lying down, night cough, swelling of extremities

• That if diabetic, may mask signs of hypoglycemia, or alter blood glucose levels

Treatment of overdose: Lavage, IV atropine for bradycardia, IV theophylline for bronchospasm; digitalis, O_2, diuretic for cardiac failure; hemodialysis, IV glucose for hypoglycemia; IV diazepam (or phenytoin) for seizures

RARELY USED

bitolterol (℞)

(bye-tole'ter-ole)

Tornalate

Func. class.: Bronchodilator, adrenergic β_2-agonist

Uses: Asthma, bronchospasm

Dosage and routes:

Inhaler

• *Adult and child >12 yr:* **INH** 2 puffs, wait 1-3 min before 3rd puff if needed, not to exceed 3 **INH** q6h or 2 **INH** q4h

Nebulization

• *Adult and child >12 yr:* **INH** 0.5 ml (1 mg) tid by intermittent flow or 1.25 mg tid by continuous flow, max 8 mg (intermittent), 14 mg (continuous)

Contraindications: Hypersensitivity to bitolterol products

HIGH ALERT

bivalirudin (℞)

(bye-val-i-rue'din)

Angiomax

Func. class.: Anticoagulant

Chem. class.: Thrombin inhibitor

Action: Direct inhibitor of thrombin that is highly specific

Uses: Unstable angina in patients undergoing percutaneous transluminal coronary angioplasty (PTCA)

Dosage and routes:

• *Adult:* **IV BOL** 1 mg/kg, then **IV INF** 2.5 mg/kg/hr for 4 hr; another **IV INF** may be used at 0.2 mg/kg/hr for ≤20 hr; this drug is intended to be used with aspirin (325 mg qd) adjusted to body weight

Renal dose

• *Adult:* **IV** GFR 30-59 ml/min give 80% of dose; GFR 10-29 ml/min give 40% of dose; dialysis-dependent patients (not on dialysis) give 10% of dose

Available forms: Inj, lyophilized 250 mg/vial

Side effects/adverse reactions:

CV: Hypo/hypertension, bradycardia

CNS: Headache, insomnia, anxiety, nervousness

GI: Nausea, vomiting, abdominal pain, dyspepsia

HEMA: ***Hemorrhage***

MS: Back pain

MISC: Pain at inj site, pelvic pain, urinary retention, fever

Contraindications: Hypersensitivity, active bleeding

Precautions: Renal function impairment, elderly, lactation, children, hepatic disease, pregnancy (B)

Pharmacokinetics: Excreted in urine, half-life 25 min

Interactions:

• ↑ bleeding risk: anticoagulants, thrombolytics

↓ anticoagulant effect: chamomile, coenzyme Q10, flax, glucomannan, goldenseal, guar gum

↑ bleeding risk: agrimony, alfalfa, angelica, anise, bilberry, black haw, bogbean, buchu, chondroitin, dong quai, fenugreek, feverfew, garlic, ginger, ginkgo, ginseng, horse chestnut, Irish moss, kelp, kelpware, khella, lovage, lungwort, meadowsweet, motherwort, mugwort, nettle, papaya, parsley (large amts), Pau D'arco, pineapple, poplar, prickly ash, safflower, saw palmetto, senega, tonka bean, turmeric, wintergreen, yarrow

NURSING CONSIDERATIONS

Assess:

Bleeding: check arterial and venous sites, IM inj sites, catheters; all punctures should be minimized; fall in B/P or Hct that may indicate hemorrhage

• Fever, skin rash, urticaria

Administer:

• Prior to PTCA, give with aspirin, 325 mg

IV direct route

• 1 mg/kg as a bolus, then intermittent infusion

• Do not admix before or during administration

Intermittent INF route

• To each 250 mg vial add 5 ml of sterile water for inj, swirl until dissolved, further dilute in 500 ml D_5W or 0.9% NaCl (0.5 mg/ml); give inf after bolus dose at a rate of 2.5 mg/kg/hr (4 hr inf); may give an additional infusion at 0.2 mg/kg/hr

Evaluate

• Therapeutic response: anticoagulation in PTCA

Teach patient/family:

• Reason for drug and expected results

HIGH ALERT

bleomycin (℞)

(blee-oh-mye'sin)

Blenoxane

Func. class.: Antineoplastic, antibiotic

Chem. class.: Glycopeptide

Action: Inhibits synthesis of DNA, RNA, protein; derived from *Streptomyces verticillus;* replication is decreased by binding to DNA, which causes strand splitting; phase specific in the G_2 and M phases; a nonvesicant

Uses: Cancer of head, neck, penis, cervix, vulva of squamous cell origin, Hodgkin's disease, lymphosarcoma, reticulum cell sarcoma, testicular carcinoma, malignant pleural effusion

Dosage and routes:

• *Adult and child:* **SC/IV/IM** 0.25-0.5 units/kg 1-2 times/wk or 10-20 units/m^2, then 1 units/day or 5 units/wk; may also be given by **CONT INF;** do not exceed total dose, 400 units in lifetime

Malignant pleural effusion

• *Adult:* 60 units as a single bolus intrapleural inj; 0.9% NaCl given through a thoracostomy tube following drainage of excess pleural fluid and complete lung expansion, remove after 4 hr

Available forms: Powder for inj, 15 units/vial

Side effects/adverse reactions:

SYST: ***Anaphylaxis,*** radiation recall, Raynaud's phenomenon

GI: Nausea, vomiting, anorexia, sto-

matitis, weight loss, ulceration of mouth, lips

INTEG: Rash, hyperkeratosis, nail changes, alopecia, fever and chills, pruritus, acne, stria, peeling

RESP: ***Fibrosis,*** pneumonitis, wheezing, ***pulmonary toxicity***

CNS: Fever, chills, pain at tumor site, headache, confusion

IDIOSYNCRATIC REACTION: Hypotension, confusion, fever, chills, wheezing

Contraindications: Hypersensitivity, pregnancy (D)

Precautions: Renal, hepatic, respiratory disease

Pharmacokinetics: Half-life 2 hr; when CCr >35 ml/min, half-life is increased in lower clearance; metabolized in liver, 50% excreted in urine (unchanged)

Interactions:

• ↑ toxicity: other antineoplastics, radiation therapy, general anesthesia

Lab test interferences:

Increase: Uric acid

• Decreased serum phenytoin levels: phenytoin

NURSING CONSIDERATIONS

Assess:

• IM test dose in lymphoma

• Pulmonary function tests: chest x-ray film before and during therapy; should be obtained q2wk during treatment

• Temp q4h; fever may indicate beginning infection

• Serum creatinine

• Dyspnea, rales, unproductive cough, chest pain, tachypnea, fatigue, increased pulse, pallor, lethargy

• Effects of alopecia and skin color on body image; discuss feelings about body changes

• Buccal cavity q8h for dryness, sores, ulceration, white patches, oral pain, bleeding, dysphagia

• Local irritation, pain, burning, discoloration at inj site

◆ Symptoms indicating anaphylaxis: rash, pruritus, urticaria, purpuric skin lesions, itching, flushing, wheezing, hypotension; have emergency equipment available

Administer:

• Antiemetic 30-60 min before giving drug to prevent vomiting, continue antiemetics 6-10 hr after treatment

• Topical or systemic analgesics for pain of stomatitis as ordered; antihistamines and antipyretics for fever and chills

IM/SC route

• After reconstituting 15 units/1-5 ml sterile H_2O, D_5W, 0.9% NaCl, or bacteriostatic water for inj, rotate inj sites; do not use products containing benzyl alcohol when giving to neonates

IV direct route

• After reconstituting 15 units or less/5 ml or more of D_5W or 0.9% NaCl; after further diluting with 50-100 ml D_5W or 0.9% NaCl, give 15 units or less/10 min through Y-tube or 3-way stopcock

• In lymphoma, two test doses 2-5 units before initial dose; monitor for anaphylaxis

Intrapleural route

• 60 units/50-100 ml of 0.9% NaCl, administered by MD through thoracotomy tube

Additive compatibilities: Amikacin, cephapirin, dexamethasone, diphenhydrAMINE, fluorouracil, gentamicin, heparin, hydrocortisone, phenytoin, streptomycin, tobramycin, vinBLAStine, vinCRIStine

Solution compatibilities: 0.9% NaCl

Syringe compatibilities: Cisplatin, cyclophosphamide, DOXOrubicin, droperidol, fluorouracil, furosemide, heparin, leucovorin, methotrexate,

metoclopramide, mitomycin, vinBLAStine, vinCRIStine
Y-site compatibilities: Allopurinol, amifostine, aztreonam, cefepime, cisplatin, cyclophosphamide, DOXOrubicin, DOXOrubicin liposome, droperidol, filgrastim, fludarabine, fluorouracil, granisetron, heparin, leucovorin, melphalan, methotrexate, metoclopramide, mitomycin, ondansetron, paclitaxel, piperacillin/tazobactam, sargramostim, teniposide, thiotepa, vinBLAStine, vinCRIStine, vinorelbine
Perform/provide:
• Storage for 2 wk after reconstituting at refrigerated or 24 hr at room temperature; discard unused portions
• Deep-breathing exercises with patient tid-qid; place in semi-Fowler's position
• Liquid diet: carbonated beverage; gelatin may be added if patient is not nauseated or vomiting
• Rinsing of mouth tid-qid with water, club soda; brushing of teeth with baking soda bid-tid with soft brush or cotton-tipped applicators for stomatitis; use unwaxed dental floss
• HOB raised to facilitate breathing
Evaluate:
• Therapeutic response: decrease in size of tumor
Teach patient/family:
• To report any complaints, side effects to nurse or prescriber
• To report any changes in breathing, coughing, fever
• That hair may be lost during treatment, and wig or hairpiece may make patient feel better; that new hair may be different in color, texture
• To avoid foods with citric acid, hot or rough texture
• To report any bleeding, white spots, ulcerations in mouth; to examine mouth qd and report symptoms
• To use contraception during treatment
• Not to receive vaccines during treatment

bosentan (℞)

(boh'sen-tan)
Tracleer
Func. class.: Vasodilator
Chem. class.: Endothelin receptor antagonist

Action: Peripheral vasodilation occurs via antagonism of the effect of endothelin on endothelium and vascular smooth muscle
Uses: Pulmonary arterial hypertension with WHO class III, IV symptoms
Investigational uses: Septic shock to improve microcirculatory blood flow
Dosage and routes:
• *Adult >40 kg/>12 yr:* **PO** 62.5 mg bid × 4 wk, then 125 mg bid
• *Adult <40 kg/>12 yr:* **PO** 62.5 mg bid
Available forms: Tabs 62.5, 125 mg
Side effects/adverse reactions:
CNS: Headache, flushing, fatigue
CV: Hypotension, palpitations, edema of lower limbs
GI: Abnormal hepatic function, dyspepsia, ***hepatotoxicity***
INTEG: Pruritus
MISC: Anemia
Contraindications: Pregnancy (X), hypersensitivity, CVA, CAD
Precautions: Mitral stenosis, elderly, lactation, hepatic function impairment, children
Pharmacokinetics: Is metabolized by CYP2C9, CYP3A4, and possibly CYP2C19, metabolized by the liver, terminal half-life 5 hr, steady state 3-5 days

Interactions:

- ↑ bosentan level: ketoconazole
- Do not coadminister cycloSPORINE A and bosentan; bosentan is ↑, cycloSPORINE is ↓
- Do not coadminister glyBURIDE with bosentan; glyBURIDE is ↓ significantly, bosentan also is ↓, liver enzymes may ↑
- ↓ effects of: simvastatin, other statins, hormonal contraceptives, warfarin

Lab test interferences:

Increase: ALT, AST

Decrease: Hgb, Hct

NURSING CONSIDERATIONS

Assess:

- B/P, pulse during treatment until stable
- Hepatic tests: AST, ALT, bilirubin; liver enzymes may increase; if ALT/AST >3 and ≤5 × ULN, confirm lab value, decrease dose or interrupt treatment and monitor AST/ALT q2wk; if >8 × ULN, stop treatment
- Blood studies: Hct, Hgb may be decreased
- Hepatic involvement: vomiting, jaundice; drug should be discontinued

Perform/provide:

- Storage at room temperature

Evaluate:

- Therapeutic response: decrease in pulmonary hypertension

Teach patient/family:

- To report jaundice, dark urine, joint pain, fatigue, malaise, bruising, easy bleeding; may indicate blood dyscrasias
- To avoid pregnancy; to use nonhormonal form of contraception

HIGH ALERT

bretylium (℞)

(bre-til'ee-um)

Bretylate🍁, bretylium tosylate, Bretylol

Func. class.: Antidysrhythmic (Class III)

Chem. class.: Quaternary ammonium compound

Action: After a transient release of norepinephrine, inhibits further release by postganglionic nerve endings; prolongs duration of action potential and effective refractory period

Uses: Life-threatening ventricular tachycardia, cardioversion, ventricular fibrillation; for short-term use only

Dosage and routes:

Severe ventricular fibrillation

- *Adult:* **IV BOL** 5 mg/kg, over 15-30 sec; increase to 10 mg/kg repeated q15min, up to 30 mg/kg; **IV INF** 1-2 mg/min or give 5-10 mg/kg over 10 min q6h (maintenance)

Ventricular tachycardia

- *Adult:* **IV INF** 500 mg diluted in 50 ml D_5W or NS, infuse over 10-30 min, may repeat in 1 hr, maintain with 1-2 mg/min or 5-10 mg/kg over 10-30 min q6h; **IM** 5-10 mg/kg undiluted; repeat in 1-2 hr if needed; maintain with same dose q6-8h
- *Child:* 2-5 mg/kg/dose

Renal disease

- CCr 10-50 ml/min 25%-50% dose; CCr <10 ml/min avoid use

Available forms: Inj 50 mg/ml; 1, 2, 4 mg/ml prefilled syringes

Side effects/adverse reactions:

CNS: Syncope, dizziness, confusion, psychosis, anxiety

GI: Nausea, vomiting

CV: Hypotension, postural hypoten-

sion, bradycardia, angina, PVCs, substernal pressure, transient hypertension, precipitation of angina
RESP: ***Respiratory depression***
Contraindications: Hypersensitivity, digitalis toxicity, aortic stenosis, pulmonary hypertension
Precautions: Renal disease, pregnancy (C), lactation, children
Do not confuse:
Bretylol/Brevitol
Pharmacokinetics: Well absorbed by IM/IV routes
IV: Onset 5 min, duration 6-24 hr
IM: Onset ½-2 hr, duration 6-24 hr
Half-life 4-17 hr, excreted unchanged by kidneys (70%-80% in 24 hr), not metabolized
Interactions:
- ↑ or ↓ effects of bretylium: quinidine, procainamide, propranolol, other antidysrhythmics
- Hypotension: antihypertensives
- ↑ effects of: sympathomimetics

↑ bretylium action: chronic use of aloe, broom, buckthorn, cascara sagrada, Chinese rhubarb, figwort, fumitory, goldenseal, kudzu, licorice, rhubarb, senna
Toxicity/death: aconite
↓ effect: Coltsfoot
↑ serotonin effect: horehound

NURSING CONSIDERATIONS
Assess:
- ECG continuously to determine drug effectiveness, PVCs, other dysrhythmias
- IV INF rate to avoid causing nausea, vomiting
- For dehydration or hypovolemia
- B/P continuously for hypotension, hypertension; orthostatic hypotension; keep supine until hypotension subsides
- I&O ratio
- If systolic B/P <75 mm Hg, notify prescriber
- For rebound hypertension after 1-2 hr
- Cardiac status: rate, rhythm, character, continuously

Administer:
IM route
- Inj, rotate sites, inject <5 ml in any one site to prevent tissue necrosis, may repeat 1-2 hr

IV direct route
- Undiluted over 15-30 sec (ventricular fibrillation); may repeat in 15-30 min, not to exceed 30 mg/kg/24 hr

Intermittent IV INF route
- Dilute 500 mg of drug/50 ml or more D_5W, 0.9% NaCl, D_5/0.45%, D_5/0.9% NaCl, D_5/LR, give over 15-30 min

CONT IV INF route
- Dilute further; give at 1-2 mg diluted drug/min via infusion pump
- Reduced dosage slowly with ECG monitoring, discontinue over 3-5 days, maintain on oral dysrhythmic

Additive compatibilities: Aminophylline, atracurium, calcium chloride, calcium gluconate, digoxin, dopamine, esmolol, insulin (regular), lidocaine, potassium chloride, quinadine, verapamil
Y-site compatibilities: Amiodarone, amrinone, cisatracurium, diltiazem, DOBUTamine, famotidine, isoproterenol, ranitidine, remifentanil
Perform/provide:
- Place patient in supine position unless otherwise ordered; assist with ambulation
- Have suction equipment available

Evaluate:
- Therapeutic response: absence of ventricular tachycardia, fibrillation

Teach patient/family:
- To make position changes slowly; orthostatic hypotension may occur

Treatment of overdose: O_2, artificial ventilation, ECG; administer dopamine for circulatory depression;

administer diazepam or thiopental for convulsions

brimonidine ophthalmic
See appendix c

brinzolamide ophthalmic
See appendix c

bromocriptine (℞)
(broe-moe-krip'teen)
Alti-Bromocriptine✤, Apo-Bromocriptine✤, Parlodel

Func. class.: Dopamine receptor agonist, antiparkinson agent

Chem. class.: Ergot alkaloid derivative

Action: Inhibits prolactin release by activating postsynaptic DOPamine receptors; activation of striatal DOPamine receptors may be reason for improvement in Parkinson's disease

Uses: Parkinson's disease, amenorrhea/galactorrhea caused by hyperprolactinemia, acromegaly

Investigational uses: Pituitary adenomas, neuroleptic malignant syndrome

Dosage and routes:

Hyperprolactinemia

• *Adult:* **PO** 1.25-2.5 mg with meals; may increase by 2.5 mg q3-7d, usual 5-7.5 mg

Acromegaly

• *Adult:* **PO** 1.25-2.5 mg × 3 days hs; may increase by 1.25-2.5 mg q3-7d; usual range 20-30 mg/day, max 100 mg/day

Parkinson's disease

• *Adult:* **PO** 1.25 mg bid with meals, may increase q2-4wk by 2.5 mg/day, not to exceed 100 mg qd

Pituitary adenoma

• *Adult:* **PO** 1.25 mg bid-tid, may increase over several weeks

Neuroleptic malignant syndrome

• *Adult:* **PO** 5 mg qd, max 20 mg/day

Available forms: Caps 5 mg; tabs 2.5 mg

Side effects/adverse reactions:

EENT: Blurred vision, diplopia, burning eyes, nasal congestion

CNS: Headache, depression, restlessness, anxiety, nervousness, confusion, ***convulsions,*** hallucinations, dizziness, fatigue, drowsiness, abnormal involuntary movements, psychosis

GU: Frequency, retention, incontinence, diuresis

GI: Nausea, vomiting, anorexia, cramps, constipation, diarrhea, dry mouth, GI hemorrhage

INTEG: Rash on face, arms, alopecia; coolness, pallor of fingers, toes

CV: Orthostatic hypotension, decreased B/P, palpitation, extra systole, ***shock,*** dysrhythmias, bradycardia, ***MI***

Contraindications: Hypersensitivity to ergot, severe ischemic disease, severe peripheral vascular disease

Precautions: Lactation, hepatic disease, renal disease, children, pituitary tumors, pregnancy (B)

Do not confuse:
Parlodel/pindolol/Provera

Pharmacokinetics:

PO: Peak 1-3 hr, duration 4-8 hr, 90%-96% protein bound, half-life 3 hr, metabolized by liver (inactive metabolites), 85%-98% of dose excreted in feces

Interactions:

• ↓ action of bromocriptine: phenothiazines, oral contraceptives,

progestins, estrogens, haloperidol, loxapine, methyldopa, metoclopramide, MAOIs, reserpine
• ↑ action of antihypertensives, levodopa
• Disulfiram-like reaction: alcohol
↓ bromocriptine effect: chaste tree fruit, kava
↑ serotonin effect: horehound

Lab test interferences:
Increase: Growth hormone, AST, ALT, CK, BUN, uric acid, alk phosphatase

NURSING CONSIDERATIONS

Assess:
• B/P; establish baseline, compare with other reading; this drug decreases B/P
• Parkinson's symptoms: pill-rolling, shuffling gait, restlessness, tremors, before and during treatment
• For resolution of symptoms of neuroleptic malignant syndrome: decreased temp, seizures, sweating, pulse
• Change in size of soft tissue volume, in acromegaly

Administer:

PO route
• With meal to prevent GI symptoms
• At hs so dizziness, orthostatic hypotension do not occur

Perform/provide:
• Storage at room temperature in tight container

Evaluate:
• Therapeutic response (Parkinson's disease): decreased dyskinesia, decreased slow movements, decreased drooling

Teach patient/family:
• That tabs may be crushed and mixed with food
• To change position slowly to prevent orthostatic hypotension
• To use contraceptives during treatment with this drug; pregnancy may occur; to use methods other than oral contraceptives
• That therapeutic effect for Parkinson's disease may take 2 mo: galactorrhea, amenorrhea
• To avoid hazardous activity if dizziness occurs
• To report symptoms of MI immediately

brompheniramine (℞)

(brome-fen-ir′a-meen)
Bromfenac, brompheniramine, Chlorphed, Dehist, Dimetane, Dimetane Extentabs, Dimetapp Allergy Liqui-Gels, Nasahist-B

Func. class.: Antihistamine
Chem. class.: Alkylamine, H_1-receptor antagonist

Action: Acts on blood vessels, GI, respiratory system by competing with histamine for H_1-receptor site; decreases allergic response by blocking histamine

Uses: Allergy symptoms, rhinitis

Dosage and routes:
• *Adult and child >12 yr:* **PO** 4-8 mg tid-qid, not to exceed 36 mg/day; time rel 8-12 mg bid-tid, not to exceed 36 mg/day; **IM/IV/SC** 10 mg q6-12h, not to exceed 40 mg/day
• *Child 6-12 yr:* **PO** 2 mg tid-qid, not to exceed 12 mg/day; **IM/IV/SC** 0.125 mg/kg
• *Child 2-6 yr:* 1 mg q4-6h, max 6 mg/day

Available forms: Tabs 4 mg; elix 2 mg/5 ml; inj 10 mg/ml; caps 4 mg

Side effects/adverse reactions:
CNS: Dizziness, drowsiness, poor coordination, fatigue, anxiety, euphoria, confusion, paresthesia, neuritis

CV: Hypotension, palpitations, tachycardia
RESP: Increased thick secretions, wheezing, chest tightness
HEMA: ***Thrombocytopenia, agranulocytosis, hemolytic anemia***
GI: Nausea, vomiting, anorexia, constipation, diarrhea
INTEG: Photosensitivity
GU: Retention, dysuria, frequency, impotence
EENT: Blurred vision, dilated pupils, tinnitus, nasal stuffiness, dry nose, throat, mouth

Contraindications: Hypersensitivity to H_1-receptor antagonists, acute asthma attack, lower respiratory tract disease, child <2 yr

Precautions: Increased intraocular pressure, renal disease, cardiac disease, hypertension, bronchial asthma, seizure disorder, stenosed peptic ulcers, hyperthyroidism, prostatic hypertrophy, bladder neck obstruction, pregnancy (C), lactation

Pharmacokinetics:
PO: Peak 2-5 hr, duration to 48 hr; metabolized in liver, excreted by kidneys, excreted in breast milk, half-life 12-34 hr

Interactions:
- ↑ CNS depression: barbiturates, opiates, hypnotics, tricyclics, alcohol
- ↑ anticholinergic effect: MAOIs
- Incompatible with aminophylline, insulins, pentobarbital

↑ effect: hops, Jamaican dogwood, kava, khat, senega
↑ anticholinergic effect: corkwood, henbane leaf

Lab test interferences:
Interfere: Skin allergy tests

NURSING CONSIDERATIONS

Assess:
- Be alert for urinary retention, frequency, dysuria; drug should be discontinued if these occur
- CBC during long-term therapy
- Blood dyscrasias: thrombocytopenia, agranulocytosis (rare) during long-term therapy
- Respiratory status: rate, rhythm, increase in bronchial secretions, wheezing, chest tightness

Administer:

PO route
- With meals if GI symptoms occur; absorption may slightly decrease

IV direct route
- Undiluted or diluted with 10 ml 0.9% NaCl, given over 1 min or more

IV INF route
- Dilute in D_5W, 0.9% NaCl given at prescribed rate

Perform/provide:
- Hard candy, gum, frequent rinsing of mouth for dryness
- Storage in tight container at room temperature

Evaluate:
- Therapeutic response: absence of running or congested nose or rashes

Teach patient/family:

Not to break, crush, or chew sustained release forms
- All aspects of drug use; to notify prescriber if confusion/sedation/hypotension occurs
- To avoid driving, other hazardous activities if drowsiness occurs
- To avoid use of alcohol, other CNS depressants while taking drug

Treatment of overdose: Administer ipecac syrup or lavage, diazepam, vasopressors, barbiturates (short-acting)

budesonide (℞)

(byoo-des'oh-nide)

Entocort EC, Pulmicort, Rhinocort, Rhinocort Aqua

Func. class.: Glucocorticoid

Chem. class.: Nonhalogenated

Action: Prevents inflammation by depression of migration of polymorphonuclear leukocytes, fibroblasts, reversal of increased capillary permeability and lysosomal stabilization; does not suppress hypothalamus and pituitary function

Uses: Rhinitis; prophylaxis for asthma; Crohn's disease

Dosage and routes:

Rhinitis (Rhinocort, Rhinocort Aqua)

• *Adult/child >6 yr:* **SPRAY/INH** 256 mcg qd (2 sprays in each nostril AM, PM or 4 sprays in each nostril, AM)

Asthma

• *Adult and child ≥6 yr:* **INH** 400-600 mcg/day

Crohn's disease

• *Adult:* **PO** 9 mg qd AM × 8 wk

Available forms: Dry powder for INH 200 mcg/metered dose (turbuhaler); inh susp 0.25 mg/2 ml, 0.5 mg/2 ml; cap 3 mg; inhaler 32 mcg micronized/actuation (Rhinocort) 32 mcg/spray (Rhinocort Aqua)

Side effects/adverse reactions:

CNS: Headache, insomnia, hypertonia, syncope

EENT: Sinusitis, pharyngitis, rhinitis, oral candidiasis

GI: Dry mouth, dyspepsia, nausea, vomiting, abdominal pain, oral candidiasis

MISC: Ecchymosis, fever, *hypersensitivity,* flulike symptoms

MS: Back pain, myalgias, fractures

RESP: Nasal irritation, cough, nasal bleeding, *respiratory infections,* ***bronchospasm***

Contraindications: Hypersensitivity, status asthmaticus

Precautions: Pregnancy (C), inhaled form (B); lactation, children, TB, fungal, bacterial, systemic viral infections, ocular herpes simplex, nasal septal ulcers; hepatic disease (caps)

Pharmacokinetics: Unknown

Interactions:

• ↓ budesonide metabolism: ketoconazole

• Avoid using with drugs metabolized by CYP3A4 inhibition

NURSING CONSIDERATIONS

Assess:

• Respiratory status: rate, rhythm, increase in bronchial secretions, wheezing, chest tightness; provide fluids to 2 L/day to decrease thickness of secretions; check for oral candidiasis

• For bronchospasm, stop treatment and give bronchodilator

• With viral infections, corticosteroid use can mask infections

• For increased intraocular pressure, discontinue use if increase occurs

Administer:

INH route (asthma)

• Use scissors to open pouch

• Use Turbuhaler upright to load, prime when using first time, turn grip to the right, then left to click in place; to provide dose turn to right, then to the left, click in place. Place mouthpiece between lips, inhale forcefully, do not exhale through Turbuhaler, rinse after use

PO route (Crohn's disease)

⊘ Caps: whole, do not chew, break

• May repeat 8-wk course if needed; may taper to 6 mg/day for 2 wk before cessation

Perform/provide:
• Storage at 59°-86° F (15°-30° C); keep away from heat, open flame
Evaluate:
• Therapeutic response: absence of asthma, rhinitis
Teach patient/family:
• To notify prescriber of pharyngitis, nasal bleeding
• Not to exceed recommended dose; adrenal suppression may occur
• To carry emergency ID identifying steroid use
• To read and follow package directions
• To prevent exposure to infections, especially viral

bumetanide (℞)

(byoo-met′a-nide)
Bumex
Func. class.: Loop diuretic, antihypertensive
Chem. class.: Sulfonamide derivative

Action: Acts on ascending loop of Henle by inhibiting reabsorption of chloride, sodium
Uses: Edema in CHF, liver disease, renal disease (nephrotic syndrome), pulmonary edema, ascites (nephrotic syndrome), hypertension, anasarca
Investigational uses: May be used alone or as adjunct with antihypertensives such as spironolactone, triamterene
Dosage and routes:
• *Adult:* **PO** 0.5-2.0 mg qd; may give 2nd or 3rd dose at 4-5 hr intervals, not to exceed 10 mg/day; may be given on alternate days or intermittently; **IV/IM** 0.5-1.0 mg; may give 2nd or 3rd dose at 2-3 hr intervals, not to exceed 10 mg/day
• *Child:* **PO/IM/IV** 0.02-0.1 mg/kg q12h, max 10 mg/day

Available forms: Tabs 0.5, 1, 2 mg; inj 0.25 mg/ml
Side effects/adverse reactions:
GU: Polyuria, ***renal failure,*** glycosuria
ELECT: Hypokalemia, hypochloremic alkalosis, hypomagnesemia, hyperuricemia, hypocalcemia, hyponatremia
CNS: Headache, fatigue, weakness, vertigo
GI: Nausea, diarrhea, dry mouth, vomiting, anorexia, cramps, upset stomach, abdominal pain, ***acute pancreatitis, jaundice***
EENT: ***Loss of hearing,*** ear pain, tinnitus, blurred vision
INTEG: Rash, pruritus, purpura, ***Stevens-Johnson syndrome,*** sweating, photosensitivity
MS: Muscular cramps, arthritis, stiffness, tenderness
ENDO: Hyperglycemia
HEMA: ***Thrombocytopenia***
CV: ***Chest pain,*** hypotension, ***circulatory collapse,*** ECG changes, dehydration
Contraindications: Hypersensitivity to sulfonamides, anuria, hepatic coma
Precautions: Dehydration, ascites, severe renal disease, pregnancy (C), hepatic cirrhosis, lactation
Do not confuse:
Bumex/Buprenex/Permax
Pharmacokinetics:
PO: Onset ½-1 hr, peak 1-2 hr, duration 3-6 hr
IM: Onset 40 min, peak 1-2 hr, duration 4-6 hr
IV: Onset 5 min, peak 15-30 min, duration 3-6 hr, excreted by kidneys (50% unchanged), feces (20%), crosses placenta, excreted in breast milk, protein binding >91%; half-life 1-½ hr, 6-15 hr neonates
Interactions:
• ↓ diuretic effect: indomethacin, NSAIDs, probenecid

- Ototoxicity: aminoglycosides
- ↑ toxicity: lithium, digitalis
- ↑ diuresis, electrolyte loss: metolazone
- Hypokalemia: potassium-wasting drugs, corticosteroids
- ↓ antidiabetics effects

↑ effect: aloe, cucumber, dandelion, horsetail, pumpkin, Queen Anne's lace

↑ hypotension: khella

Severe photosensitivity: St. John's wort

Lab test interferences:

Increase: Urinary phosphate

NURSING CONSIDERATIONS

Assess:

- For tinnitus, obtain audiometric testing for long-term IV treatment
- Weight, I&O daily to determine fluid loss; if urinary output decreases or azotemia occurs, drug should be discontinued; the safest dosage schedule is on alternate days
- B/P lying, standing; postural hypotension may occur
- Electrolytes: K, Na, Cl; include BUN, blood sugar, CBC, serum creatinine, blood pH, ABGs, uric acid, Ca, Mg
- Blood glucose if patient is diabetic; blood uric acid levels in those with gout
- Improvement in edema of feet, legs, sacral area daily if medication is being used in CHF
- Signs of metabolic alkalosis: drowsiness, restlessness
- Signs of hypokalemia: postural hypotension, malaise, fatigue, tachycardia, leg cramps, weakness
- Rashes, temp elevation qd
- Confusion, especially in elderly; take safety precautions if needed
- For digitalis toxicity in patients taking digitalis products (anorexia, nausea, vomiting, confusion, paresthesia, muscle cramps); lithium toxicity in those taking lithium

Administer:

- In AM to avoid interference with sleep if using drug as a diuretic
- Potassium replacement if potassium is less than 3.0

PO route

- With food if nausea occurs; absorption may be decreased slightly

IV direct route

- Direct IV undiluted over at least 2 min through Y-tube or 3-way stopcock or heplock

Intermittent IV route

- Dilute in LR, D_5W, 0.9% NaCl (rarely given by this method), give over 12 hr in renal disease

Additive compatibilities: Floxacillin, furosemide

Syringe compatibilities: Doxapram

Y-site compatibilities: Allopurinol, amifostine, aztreonam, cefepime, cisatracurium, cladribine, diltiazem, filgrastim, granisetron, lorazepam, melphalan, meperidine, morphine, piperacillin/tazobactam, propofol, remifentanil, teniposide, thiotepa, vinorelbine

Evaluate:

- Therapeutic response: decreased edema, B/P

Teach patient/family:

- To increase fluid intake to 2-3 L/day unless contraindicated, to take potassium supplement, to rise slowly from lying or sitting position
- To recognize adverse reactions: muscle cramps, weakness, nausea, dizziness
- To take with food or milk for GI symptoms
- To take early in day to prevent nocturia
- To use sunscreen to prevent photosensitivity

Treatment of overdose: Lavage if taken orally; monitor electrolytes; administer dextrose in saline; monitor hydration, CV, renal status

buprenorphine (℞)

(byoo-pre-nor′feen)

Buprenex

Func. class.: Opioid analgesic

Chem. class.: Thebaine derivative

Controlled Substance Schedule V

Action: Depresses pain impulse transmission at the spinal cord level by interacting with opioid receptors

Uses: Moderate to severe pain

Dosage and routes:

- *Adult:* **IM/IV** 0.3 mg q6h prn, reduce dosage in elderly, may repeat after ½ hr; epidural 60-180 mcg over 48 hr
- *Child 2-12 yr:* **IM/IV** 2-6 mcg/kg q4-6h
- *Geriatric:* **PO** 0.15 mg q6h prn

Available forms: Inj 0.3 mg/ml (1 ml vials)

Side effects/adverse reactions:

CNS: Drowsiness, dizziness, confusion, headache, sedation, euphoria, ***increased intracranial pressure,*** amnesia

GI: Nausea, vomiting, anorexia, constipation, cramps, dry mouth

GU: Increased urinary output, dysuria, urinary retention

INTEG: Rash, urticaria, bruising, flushing, diaphoresis, pruritus

EENT: Tinnitus, blurred vision, *miosis,* diplopia

CV: Palpitations, bradycardia, change in B/P, tachycardia

RESP: ***Respiratory depression,*** dyspnea, hypo/hyperventilation

Contraindications: Hypersensitivity

Precautions: Addictive personality, pregnancy (C), lactation, increased intracranial pressure, MI (acute), severe heart disease, respiratory depression, hepatic disease, renal disease, hypothyroidism, Addison's disease, addiction (opioid)

Do not confuse:

Buprenex/Bumex

Pharmacokinetics:

IM: Onset 10-30 min, peak ½ hr, duration 3-4 hr

IV: Onset 1 min, peak 5 min, duration 2-5 hr

Metabolized by liver; excreted by kidneys/feces; crosses placenta; excreted in breast milk; half-life 2½-3½ hr; 96% bound to plasma proteins

Interactions:

- ↑ effect with other CNS depressants: alcohol, opioids, sedative/hypnotics, antipsychotics, skeletal muscle relaxants, MAOIs

↑ CNS depression: Jamaican dogwood, kava, lavender, mistletoe, nettle, pokeweed, poppy, senega, valerian

↑ anticholinergic effect: corkwood

NURSING CONSIDERATIONS

Assess:

- I&O ratio; check for decreasing output; may indicate urinary retention
- CNS changes, dizziness, drowsiness, hallucinations, euphoria, LOC, pupil reaction; withdrawal in opioid-dependent persons; if dependence occurs, within 2 wk of discontinuing drug withdrawal symptoms will occur
- Allergic reactions: rash, urticaria
- Respiratory dysfunction: respiratory depression, character, rate, rhythm; notify prescriber if respirations are <12/min
- Need for pain medication, tolerance; location, intensity, severity

Administer:

IM route

- In deep muscle mass

IV direct route
- Undiluted over 3-5 min (0.3 mg over 2 min), titrate to patient response
- With antiemetic if nausea, vomiting occur
- When pain is beginning to return; determine dosage interval by patient response

Additive compatibilities: Atropine, bupivacaine, diphenhydrAMINE, droperidol, glycopyrrolate, haloperidol, hydrOXYzine, promethazine, scopolamine

Syringe compatibilities: Midazolam

Y-site compatibilities: Allopurinol, amifostine, aztreonam, cefepime, cisatracurium, cladribine, filgrastim, granisetron, melphalan, piperacillin/tazobactam, propofol, remifentanil, teniposide, thiotepa, vinorelbine

Perform/provide:
- Assistance with ambulation if needed

Evaluate:
- Therapeutic response: decrease in pain, absence of grimacing

Teach patient/family:
- To report any symptoms of CNS changes, allergic reactions
- That tolerance may result when used for extended periods
- To avoid hazardous activities

*buPROPion (℞)

(byoo-proe'pee-on)

buPROPion, Wellbutrin, Wellbutrin SR, Zyban

Func. class.: Misc. antidepressant, smoking deterrent

Chem. class.: Aminoketone

Action: Inhibits reuptake of DOPamine, serotonin, norepinephrine

Uses: Depression (Wellbutrin), smoking cessation (Zyban)

Dosage and routes:

Depression
- *Adult:* **PO** 100 mg bid initially, then increase after 3 days to 100 mg tid if needed; may increase after 1 mo to 150 mg tid; **SR** 150 mg bid, initially 150 mg AM, increase to 300 mg/day if initial dose is tolerated
- *Geriatric:* **PO** 50-100 mg/day, may increase by 50-100 mg q3-4 day

Smoking cessation
- *Adult:* **PO** 150 mg bid, begin with 150 mg qd × 3 days, then 300 mg/day; continue for 7-12 wk; not to exceed 300 mg/day

Available forms: Tabs 75, 100 mg; tab sust rel 50, 100, (Zyban) 150, 200 mg

Side effects/adverse reactions:

CNS: Headache, agitation, dizziness, akinesia, bradykinesia, confusion, ***seizures,*** delusions, *insomnia, sedation, tremors*

CV: Dysrhythmias, hypertension, palpitations, *tachycardia,* hypotension, ***complete AV block***

GI: Nausea, vomiting, anorexia, diarrhea, *dry mouth,* increased appetite, *constipation*

GU: Impotence, urinary frequency, retention, *menstrual irregularities*

INTEG: Rash, pruritus, *sweating*

EENT: Blurred vision, auditory disturbance

MISC: Weight loss or gain

Contraindications: Hypersensitivity, eating disorders, seizure disorders

Precautions: Renal and hepatic disease, recent MI, cranial trauma, pregnancy (B), lactation, children <18 yr, elderly, seizure disorder

Do not confuse:
buPROPion/busPIRone
Zyban/Diovan/Zagam

Pharmacokinetics: Onset 2-4 wk, half-life 14 hr; metabolized by liver, steady state 1½-5 wk

Interactions:

◆ ↑ adverse reactions, seizures: levodopa, MAOIs, phenothiazines, antidepressants, benzodiazepines, alcohol, theophylline, systemic steroids

- ↑ buPROPion toxicity: ritonavir
- ↓ buPROPion effect: carbamazepine, cimetidine, phenobarbital, phenytoin or other drugs (CYP450)
- ↑ buPROPion level: cimetidine

Herb: ↑ CNS depression: hops, kava, lavender

Herb: ↑ anticholinergic effect: belladonna, corkwood; jimsonweed

NURSING CONSIDERATIONS

Assess:

- For increased risk of seizures; if patient has excessively used CNS depressants and OTC stimulants, dosage of buPROPion should not be exceeded
- For smoking cessation after 7-12 wk; if progress has not been made, drug should be discontinued
- Mental status: mood, sensorium, affect, suicidal tendencies, increase in psychiatric symptoms

Administer:

PO route

⊘ Do not crush, break, chew sust rel tab

- Increased fluids, bulk in diet if constipation occurs
- With food or milk for GI symptoms
- Sugarless gum, hard candy, or frequent sips of water for dry mouth

Perform/provide:

- Assistance with ambulation during beginning therapy, since sedation occurs
- Safety measures, primarily in elderly

Evaluate:

- Therapeutic response: decreased depression, ability to function in daily activities, ability to sleep throughout the night, smoking cessation

Teach patient/family:

- That therapeutic effects may take 2-4 wk; not to increase dose without prescriber's approval; that treatment for smoking cessation lasts 7-12 wk
- To use caution in driving, other activities requiring alertness; sedation, blurred vision may occur
- To avoid alcohol ingestion, other CNS depressants
- Not to use with nicotine patches unless directed by prescriber, may increase B/P
- To notify prescriber immediately if retention occurs
- That risk of seizures is increased when dose is exceeded, or if patient has seizure disorder
- To notify prescriber if pregnancy is suspected or planned

Treatment of overdose: ECG monitoring; induce emesis, lavage, activated charcoal; administer anticonvulsant

busPIRone (℞)

(byoo-spye′rone)

BuSpar

Func. class.: Antianxiety, sedative

Chem. class.: Azaspirodecanedione

Action: Acts by inhibiting the action of serotonin (5-HT); has shown little potential for abuse, a good choice in substance abuse

Uses: Management and short-term relief of anxiety disorders

Dosage and routes:

- *Adult:* **PO** 5 mg tid; may increase by 5 mg/day q2-3d, not to exceed 60 mg/day

Available forms: Tabs 5, 10, 15, 30 mg

Side effects/adverse reactions:

CNS: Dizziness, headache, depression, stimulation, insomnia, nervousness, light-headedness, numbness, paresthesia, incoordination, nightmares, *tremors,* excitement, involuntary movements, confusion, akathisia

GI: Nausea, dry mouth, diarrhea, constipation, flatulence, increased appetite, rectal bleeding

CV: Tachycardia, palpitations, hypotension, hypertension, ***CVA, CHF, MI***

EENT: Sore throat, tinnitus, blurred vision, nasal congestion; red, itching eyes; change in taste, smell

GU: Frequency, hesitancy, menstrual irregularity, change in libido

MS: Pain, weakness, muscle cramps, spasms

RESP: Hyperventilation, chest congestion, shortness of breath

INTEG: Rash, edema, pruritus, alopecia, dry skin

MISC: Sweating, fatigue, weight gain, fever

Contraindications: Hypersensitivity, child <18 yr

Precautions: Pregnancy (B), lactation, elderly, impaired hepatic/renal function

Do not confuse:

busPIRone/buPROPion

Pharmacokinetics: Half-life 2-3 hr rapidly absorbed, metabolized by liver, excreted in feces

Interactions:

- Drug metabolized by CYP450, 3A4 (erythromycin, itraconazole, nefazodone): ↑ busPIRone
- ↓ busPIRone effects: rifampin
- ↑ B/P: MAOIs; do not use together
- ↑ CNS depression: psychotropic drugs, alcohol (avoid use)

↑ CNS depression: cowslip, kava, Queen Anne's lace, valerian

- Drug/food: ↑ peak concentration of busPIRone: grapefruit juice

NURSING CONSIDERATIONS

Assess:

- B/P (lying, standing), pulse; if systolic B/P drops 20 mm Hg, hold drug, notify prescriber
- CNS reactions, since some reactions may be unpredictable
- Mental status: mood, sensorium, affect, sleeping pattern, drowsiness, dizziness

Administer:

PO route

- With food or milk for GI symptoms
- Crushed if patient unable to swallow medication whole
- Sugarless gum, hard candy, frequent sips of water for dry mouth

Perform/provide:

- Assistance with ambulation during beginning therapy; drowsiness, dizziness occur
- Safety measures if drowsiness occurs
- Check to see PO medication swallowed

Evaluate:

- Therapeutic response: decreased anxiety, restlessness, sleeplessness

Teach patient/family:

- That drug may be taken with food
- To avoid OTC preparations unless approved by prescriber
- To avoid activities requiring alertness, since drowsiness may occur
- To avoid alcohol ingestion, other psychotropic medications, unless directed by prescriber
- Not to discontinue medication abruptly after long-term use; if dose is missed, do not double
- To rise slowly because fainting may occur, especially elderly
- That drowsiness may worsen at beginning of treatment

• That 1-2 wk of therapy may be required before therapeutic effects occur

Treatment of overdose: Gastric lavage, VS, supportive care

HIGH ALERT

busulfan (℞)

(byoo-sul′fan)

Busulfex, Myleran

Func. class.: Antineoplastic alkylating agent

Chem. class.: Nitrosurea

Action: Changes essential cellular ions to covalent bonding with resultant alkylation; this interferes with normal biologic function of DNA; activity is not phase specific; action is due to myelosuppression

Uses: Chronic myelocytic leukemia

Dosage and routes:

• *Adult:* **PO** 4-8 mg/day initially until WBC levels fall to 10,000/mm^3, then drug is stopped until WBC levels raise over 50,000/mm^3, then 1-3 mg/day; **IV** 0.8 mg/kg q6h × 4 days, given with cyclophosphamide

• *Child:* **PO** 0.06-0.12 mg/kg or 1.8-4.6 mg/m^2 day; dose is titrated to maintain WBC levels at 20,000/mm^3

Available forms: Tabs 2 mg; sol for inj 6 mg/ml

Side effects/adverse reactions:

PO route

GI: Anorexia, constipation, diarrhea, dry mouth, nausea, vomiting

RESP: ***Alveolar hemorrhage,*** atelectasis, cough, hemoptysis, hypoxia, pleural effusion, pneumonia, sinusitis, ***pulmonary fibrosis***

CV: Hypotension, thrombosis, chest pain, tachycardia, atrial fibrillation, heart block, pericardial effusion, ***cardiac tamponade*** (high dose with cyclophosphamide)

IV route

CNS: ***Cerebral hemorrhage, coma, seizures,*** *anxiety, depression, dizziness, headache,* encephalopathy, *weakness,* mental changes

EENT: Pharyngitis, epistaxis

HEMA: ***Thrombocytopenia, leukopenia, pancytopenia, severe bone marrow depression***

GI: Nausea, vomiting, *diarrhea, weight loss*

GU: Impotence, sterility, amenorrhea, gynecomastia, ***renal toxicity,*** hyperuremia, adrenal insufficiency–like syndrome

INTEG: Dermatitis, hyperpigmentation, alopecia

RESP: ***Irreversible pulmonary fibrosis,*** pneumonitis

OTHER: ***Chromosomal aberrations***

Contraindications: Radiation, chemotherapy, lactation, pregnancy (3rd trimester) (D), blastic phase of chronic myelocytic leukemia, hypersensitivity

Precautions: Childbearing age women and men, leukopenia, thrombocytopenia, anemia, hepatotoxicity, renal toxicity

Do not confuse:

Myleran/Leukeran

Pharmacokinetics: Well absorbed orally; excreted in urine; crosses placenta; excreted in breast milk, half-life 2.5 hr

Interactions:

• Cardiac tamponade: cyclophosphamide

• ↑ toxicity: other antineoplastics radiation

• ↑ risk of bleeding: anticoagulants, aspirin, acetaminophen, thioguanine

• ↑ antibody response: live virus vaccines

Lab test interferences:

False positive: breast, bladder, cervix, lung cytology tests

NURSING CONSIDERATIONS

Assess:

- CBC, differential, platelet count weekly; withhold drug if WBC is <15,000/mm^3 or platelet count is <150,000/mm^3; notify prescriber of results; institute thrombocytopenia precautions
- Pulmonary function tests, chest x-ray films before, during therapy; chest film should be obtained q2wk during treatment; pulmonary fibrosis may occur up to 10 yr after treatment with busulfan
- Renal studies: BUN, serum uric acid, urine CCr before, during therapy; monitor ALT, alk phosphatase, bilirubin, uric acid before and during treatment
- I&O ratio; report fall in urine output <30 ml/hr
- Monitor for cold, fever, sore throat (may indicate beginning infection)
- Bleeding: hematuria, guaiac, bruising or petechiae, mucosa or orifices q8h, no rectal temps
- Dyspnea, rales, nonproductive cough, chest pain, tachypnea
- Inflammation of mucosa, breaks in skin; use viscous xylocaine for oral pain

Administer:

PO route

- Give at same time qd, on empty stomach

IV route

- Prepared in biologic cabinet, using gloves, gown, mask; dilute with 10 times volume of drug with D_5W or 0.9% NaCl, (0.5 mg/ml). When withdrawing drug, use needle with 5-micron filter provided, remove amount needed, remove filter and inject drug into diluent; always add drug to diluent, not vice versa; stable for 8 hr room temperature (using D_5W) or 12 hr refrigerated
- Give antiemetics before IV route, on schedule
- In those with history of seizures give phenytoin prior to IV route, to prevent seizures (using 0.9% NaCl) give by central venous catheter over 2 hr q6h × 4 days, use infusion pump, do not admix

Perform/provide:

- Comprehensive oral hygiene
- Strict medical asepsis, protective isolation if WBC levels are low
- Increase fluid intake to 2-3 L/day to prevent urate deposits, calculi formation
- Store in tight container

Evaluate:

- Therapeutic response: decreased exacerbations of chronic myelocytic leukemia

Teach patient/family:

- About protective isolation precautions
- To avoid use of products containing aspirin or ibuprofen, razors, commercial mouthwash
- To report signs of anemia (fatigue, headache, irritability, faintness, shortness of breath)
- To report symptoms of bleeding (hematuria, tarry stools)
- That impotence or amenorrhea can occur, are reversible after discontinuing treatment
- To report any changes in breathing or coughing even several months after treatment

butenafine topical

See appendix c

butoconazole vaginal antifungal

See appendix c

butorphanol (℞)

(byoo-tor'fa-nole)

Stadol, Stadol NS

Func. class.: Opioid analgesic

Chem. class.: Opioid antagonist, agonist

Controlled Substance Schedule IV

Action: Depresses pain impulse transmission at the spinal cord level by interacting with opioid receptors

Uses: Moderate to severe pain

Investigational uses: Migraine headache, pain

Dosage and routes:

• *Adult:* **IM** 1-4 mg q3-4h prn; **IV** 0.5-2 mg q3-4h prn; **INTRANASAL,** 1 spray in one nostril q3-4h; may give another dose 1-1½ hr later; repeat if needed q3-4h

Geriatric: **IV** ½ adult dose at 2× the interval; **INTRANASAL,** may repeat q1-2h

Severe pain

• *Adult:* **INTRANASAL** 1 spray in each nostril q3-4h

Renal disease

• CCr 10-50 ml/min 75% dose; CCr <10 ml/min 50% dose

Available forms: Inj 1, 2 mg/ml; nasal spray 10 mg/ml

Side effects/adverse reactions:

CNS: Drowsiness, dizziness, confusion, headache, sedation, euphoria, weakness, hallucinations

GI: Nausea, vomiting, anorexia, constipation, cramps

GU: Increased urinary output, dysuria, urinary retention

INTEG: Rash, urticaria, bruising, flushing, diaphoresis, pruritus

EENT: Tinnitus, blurred vision, miosis, diplopia, nasal congestion

CV: Palpitations, bradycardia, hypotension

RESP: ***Respiratory depression,*** pulmonary hypertension

Contraindications: Hypersensitivity to this drug or preservative, addiction (opioid), CHF, myocardial infarction

Precautions: Addictive personality, pregnancy (C), lactation, increased intracranial pressure, respiratory depression, hepatic disease, renal disease, child <18 yr

Do not confuse:

Stadol/Haldol/sotalol

Pharmacokinetics:

IM: Onset 10-30 min, peak ½ hr, duration 3-4 hr

IV: Onset 1 min, peak 5 min, duration 2-4 hr

INTRANASAL: Onset within 15 min, peak 1-2 hr, duration 4-5 hr

Metabolized by liver; excreted by kidneys; crosses placenta; excreted in breast milk; half-life 2½-3½ hr

Interactions:

• ↑ CNS effects: alcohol, opioids, sedative/hypnotics, antipsychotics, skeletal muscle relaxants

Severe, fatal reactions: MAOIs

↑ anticholinergic effect: corkwood

↑ CNS depression: chamomile, Jamaican dogwood, kava, lavender, mistletoe, nettle, pokewood, poppy, senega, skullcap, valerian

NURSING CONSIDERATIONS

Assess:

• For decreasing output; may indicate urinary retention

For withdrawal symptoms in opioid-dependent patients: pulmonary embolus, vascular occlusion, abscesses, ulcerations

• CNS changes: dizziness, drowsiness, hallucinations, euphoria, LOC, pupil reaction

• Allergic reactions: rash, urticaria

• Respiratory dysfunction: respiratory depression, character, rate,

rhythm; notify prescriber if respirations are <10/min
• Need for pain medication, physical dependence
Administer:
• With antiemetic if nausea, vomiting occur
• When pain is beginning to return; determine dosage interval by patient response
IM route
• Deeply in large muscle mass
IV route
• Undiluted at a rate of <2 mg/>3-5 min, titrate to patient response
Syringe compatibilities: Atropine, chlorproMAZINE, cimetidine, diphenhydrAMINE, droperidol, fentanyl, hydrOXYzine, meperidine, methotrimerprazine, metoclopramide, midazolam, morphine, pentazocine, perphenazine, prochlorperazine, promethazine, scopolamine, thiethylperazine
Y-site compatibilities: Allopurinol, amifostine, aztreonam, cefepime, cisatracurium, cladribine, DOXOrubicin liposome, enalaprilat, esmolol, filgrastim, fludarabine, granisetron, labetalol, melphalan, paclitaxel, piperacillin/tazobactam, propofol, remifentanil, sargramostim, tenoposide, thiotepa, vinorelbine
Perform/provide:
• Storage in light-resistant container at room temperature
• Assistance with ambulation
• Safety measures: night-light, call bell within easy reach, especially elderly
Evaluate:
• Therapeutic response: decrease in pain
Teach patient/family:
• To report any symptoms of CNS changes, allergic reactions
• That physical dependency may result when used for extended periods
• That withdrawal symptoms may occur: nausea, vomiting, cramps, fever, faintness, anorexia
Treatment of overdose: Naloxone HCl (Narcan) 0.2-0.8 mg IV, O_2, IV fluids,vasopressors

C

RARELY USED

cabergoline (℞)

(ka-bear′joe-leen)
Dostinex
Func. class.: Dopamine receptor/agonist

Uses: Reduced prolactin/secretion in postpartum lactation
Dosage and routes:
Hyperprolactinemic indications
• *Adult:* **PO** 0.25 mg 2×/wk, may increase by 0.25 mg 2×/wk at 4 wk intervals, max 1 mg 2×/wk; maintenance therapy may be needed for 6 mo
Contraindications: Hypersensitivity, uncontrolled hypertension

calcifediol (℞)

(kal-si-fe-dye′ole)
Calderol
Func. class.: Vit D analog, 25-hydroxyvitamin D_3, fat soluble vitamin
Chem. class.: Sterol

Action: Increases intestinal absorption of calcium for bones; increases renal tubular absorption of phosphate; increases mobilization of calcium from bones, bone resorption
Uses: Metabolic bone disease with chronic renal failure, osteopenia, osteomalacia, hypocalcemia
Dosage and routes:
• *Adult:* **PO** 300-350 mcg qwk divided into qd or qod doses; may

increase q4wk or 20-100 mcg/day or 20-200 mcg/day qod
• *Supplement Elderly:* **PO** 20 mcg qd

Available forms: Caps 20, 50 mcg

Side effects/adverse reactions:
EENT: Tinnitus, conjunctivitis, photophobia, rhinorrhea
CNS: Drowsiness, headache, vertigo, fever, lethargy
GI: Nausea, diarrhea, vomiting, jaundice, anorexia, dry mouth, constipation, cramps, metallic taste, thirst
MS: Myalgia, arthralgia, decreased bone development, weakness
GU: Polyuria, hypercalciuria, hyperphosphatemia, hematuria
CV: Dysrhythmias

Contraindications: Hypersensitivity, hyperphosphatemia, hypercalcemia, vit D toxicity

Precautions: Pregnancy (C), renal calculi, lactation, CV disease, elderly

Pharmacokinetics: Absorbed by the small intestine; stored in liver and fat deposits, activated in kidneys, excreted in bile and feces; peak 4 hr, duration 15-20 days; half-life 12-22 days

Interactions:
• ↓ absorption of calcifediol: cholestyramine, colestipol, mineral oil, fat-soluble vitamins
• Hypercalcemia: thiazide diuretics, calcium supplements
• Cardiac dysrhythmias: cardiac glycosides
• ↓ effect of this drug: corticosteroids
• Hypermagnesemia: magnesium antacids
• ↑ metabolism of vit D: phenytoin
• Toxicity: other vit D products
• Drug/food: dairy products, other high-calcium foods may cause hypercalcemia

Lab test interferences:
False increase: Cholesterol
Interfere: Alk phosphatase, electrolytes

NURSING CONSIDERATIONS

Assess:
• BUN, urinary calcium, AST, ALT, cholesterol, creatinine, uric acid, chloride, magnesium, electrolytes, urine pH, phosphate; may increase; calcium should be kept at 9-10 mg/dl, vit D 50-135 international units/dl, phosphate 70 mg/dl, alk phosphatase may be decreased
• For increased blood level, since toxic reactions may occur rapidly
• For dry mouth, metallic taste, polyuria, bone pain, muscle weakness, headache, fatigue, tinnitus, change in LOC, irregular pulse, dysrhythmias, increased respirations, anorexia, nausea, vomiting, cramps, diarrhea, constipation; may indicate hypercalcemia
• Renal status: decreased urinary output (oliguria, anuria), edema in extremities, weight gain 5 lb, periorbital edema
• Nutritional status, diet for sources of vit D (milk, some seafood), calcium (dairy products, dark green vegetables), phosphates (dairy products)

Administer:

PO route
• May be taken without regard to food
⃠ Do not break, crush, or chew caps
• May be increased q4wk depending on blood level

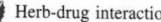

Perform/provide:
• Storage in tight, light-resistant container at room temperature
• Restriction of sodium, potassium if required; ensure adequate calcium intake
• Restriction of fluids if required for chronic renal failure

Evaluate:
- Therapeutic response: calcium levels 9-10 mg/dl, decreasing symptoms of bone disease

Teach patient/family:
- The symptoms of hypercalcemia
- About foods rich in calcium
- To advise prescriber of all other medications, supplements taken

calcitonin (human) (℞)

(kal-sih-toh'nin)
Cibacalcin

calcitonin (salmon) (℞)

Calcimir, Miacalcin, Miacalcin Nasal Spray, Osteocalcin, Salmonine
Func. class.: Parathyroid agents (calcium regulator)
Chem. class.: Polypeptide hormone

Action: Decreases bone resorption, blood calcium levels; increases deposits of calcium in bones; opposes parathyroid hormone
Uses: Paget's disease, postmenopausal osteoporosis, hypercalcemia
Dosage and routes:
Human
Paget's disease
- *Adult:* **SC** 0.5 mg/day initially; may require 0.5 mg bid × 6 mo, then decrease until symptoms reappear

Salmon
Postmenopausal osteoporosis
- *Adult:* **SC/IM** 100 international units/day; **NASAL** 200 international units (1 spray) qd alternating nostrils qd, activate pump before 1st dose

Paget's disease
- *Adult:* **SC/IM** 100 international units qd, maintenance 50-100 international units qd or qod

Hypercalcemia
- *Adult:* **SC/IM** 4 international units/kg q12h, increase to 8 international units/kg q6h if response is unsatisfactory

Available forms: *Human:* **INJ** (SC) 500 mg vial; *salmon:* **INJ** 100 international units, 200 international units/ml, **NASAL** spray 200 international units/actuation
Side effects/adverse reactions:
INTEG: Rash, flushing, pruritus of earlobes, edema of feet, reaction at inj site
CNS: Headache, tetany, chills, weakness, dizziness, fever
GU: Diuresis, nocturia, urine sediment, frequency
GI: Nausea, diarrhea, vomiting, anorexia, abdominal pain, salty taste, epigastric pain
MS: Swelling, tingling of hands
CV: Chest pressure
EENT: Nasal congestion, eye pain
RESP: Dyspnea
SYST: ***Anaphylaxis***
Contraindications: Hypersensitivity
Precautions: Renal disease, children, lactation, osteogenic sarcoma, pregnancy (C), pernicious anemia
Pharmacokinetics:
IM/SC: Onset 15 min, peak 4 hr, duration 8-24 hr; metabolized by kidneys, excreted as inactive metabolites via kidneys

NURSING CONSIDERATIONS
Assess:
- GI symptoms, polyuria, flushing, head swelling, tingling, headache; may indicate hypercalcemia
- Nutritional status; diet for sources of vit D (milk, some seafood), calcium (dairy products, dark green vegetables), phosphates
- BUN, creatinine, uric acid, chloride, electrolytes, urine pH, urinary calcium, magnesium, phosphate, urinalysis (calcium should be kept at

9-10 mg/dl, vit D 50-135 international units/dl), alk phosphatase baseline, q3-6mo
• Increased drug level, since toxic reactions occur rapidly; have calcium chloride on hand if calcium level drops too low; check for tetany
• Urine for sediment
Administer:
SC route (Human)
• By SC route only; rotate inj sites; use within 6 hr of reconstitution; give hs to minimize nausea, vomiting
IM route (Salmon)
• After test dose of 10 international units/ml, 0.1 ml intradermally; watch 15 min; give only with epINEPHrine and emergency meds available
• IM inj slowly in deep muscle mass; rotate sites
Perform/provide:
• Storage at <77° F (25° C); protect from light
Evaluate:
• Therapeutic response: calcium levels 9-10 mg/dl, decreasing symptoms of Paget's disease
Teach patient/family:
• The method of inj if patient will be responsible for self-medication
• To report difficulty swallowing or any change in side effects to prescriber immediately
Nasal
• To use alternating nostrils for nasal spray

calcitriol (℞)
(kal-sih-try'ole)
Calcijex, Rocaltrol (1,25-dihydroxycholecalciferol), vitamin D_3
Func. class.: Parathyroid agent (calcium regulator)
Chem. class.: Vit D hormone

Action: Increases intestinal absorption of calcium, provides calcium for bones, increases renal tubular resorption of phosphate
Uses: Hypocalcemia in chronic renal disease, hyperparathyroidism pseudohypoparathyroidism
Dosage and routes:
• *Adult:* **IV** 0.5 mcg tid, initially; may increase by 0.25-0.5 mcg/dose q2-4wk; 0.5-3 mcg tid maintenance
Predialysis
• ***Adult:*** **PO** 0.25 mcg/day, max 0.5 mcg/day
• *Child:* **PO** 0.25 mcg/day, max 0.5 mcg/day
• *Child <3 yr:* **PO** 10-15 mcg/kg/day
Hypocalcemia during chronic dialysis
• *Adult:* **PO** 0.5-3 mcg/day
• *Child:* **PO** 0.25-2 mcg/day
Renal osteodystrophy
• *Adult:* **PO** 0.25 mcg qod-3 mcg/day
• *Child:* **PO** 0.014-0.041 mcg/kg/day
Hypoparathyroidism
• *Adult:* **PO** 0.25-2.7 mcg/day
• *Child:* **PO** 0.04-0.08 mcg/kg/day
Available forms: Caps 0.25, 0.5 mcg; inj 1 mcg, 2 mcg/ml
Side effects/adverse reactions:
CNS: Drowsiness, headache, vertigo, fever, lethargy
GI: Nausea, diarrhea, vomiting, jaundice, anorexia, dry mouth, constipation, cramps, metallic taste

MS: Myalgia, arthralgia, decreased bone development, weakness
GU: Polyuria, hypercalciuria, hyperphosphatemia, hematuria, thirst
EENT: Blurred vision, photophobia
CV: Palpitations
Contraindications: Hypersensitivity, hyperphosphatemia, hypercalcemia, vit D toxicity
Precautions: Pregnancy (C), renal calculi, lactation, CV disease
Do not confuse:
calcitriol/Calciferol
Pharmacokinetics:
PO: Absorbed readily from GI tract, peak 10-12 hr, duration 3-5 days, half-life 3-6 hr; undergoes hepatic recycling, excreted in bile
Interactions:
• ↓ absorption of calcitriol: cholestyramine, mineral oil, fat-soluble vitamins
• Hypercalcemia: thiazide diuretics, calcium supplements
• Cardiac dysrhythmias: cardiac glycosides, verapamil
• Hypermagnesemia: magnesium antacids
• ↑ metabolism of vit D: phenytoin
• Toxicity: other vit D products
• Drug/food: large amounts of high-calcium foods may cause hypercalcemia
Lab test interferences:
False increase: Cholesterol
Interfere: Alk phosphatase, electrolytes
NURSING CONSIDERATIONS
Assess:
• BUN, urinary calcium, AST, ALT, cholesterol, creatinine, albumin, uric acid, chloride, magnesium, electrolytes, urine pH, phosphate; may increase calcium, should be kept at 9-10 mg/dl, vit D 50-135 international units/dl, phosphate 70 mg/dl
• Alk phosphatase; may be decreased
• For increased drug level, since toxic reactions may occur rapidly
• For dry mouth, metallic taste, polyuria, bone pain, muscle weakness, headache, fatigue, change in LOC, dysrhythmias, increased respirations, anorexia, nausea, vomiting, cramps, diarrhea, constipation; may indicate hypercalcemia
• Renal status: decreased urinary output (oliguria, anuria), edema in extremities, weight gain 5-7 lb, periorbital edema
• Nutritional status, diet for sources of vit D (milk, some seafood); calcium (dairy products, dark green vegetables), phosphates (dairy products) must be avoided
Administer:
PO route
• Give without regard to meals
IV route
• Give by direct IV over 1 min
Perform/provide:
• Storage protected from light, heat, moisture
• Restriction of sodium, potassium if required
• Restriction of fluids if required for chronic renal failure
Evaluate:
• Therapeutic response: calcium 9-10 mg/dl, decreasing symptoms of hypocalcemia, hypoparathyroidism
Teach patient/family:
• The symptoms of hypercalcemia
• About foods rich in calcium
• To avoid products with sodium: cured meats, dairy products, cold cuts, olives, beets, pickles, soups, meat tenderizers in chronic renal failure
• To avoid products with potassium: oranges, bananas, dried fruit, peas, dark green leafy vegetables, milk, melons, beans in chronic renal failure
• To avoid OTC products contain-

ing calcium, potassium, or sodium in chronic renal failure

- To avoid all preparations containing vit D
- To monitor weight weekly

Not to break, crush, or chew caps

calcium carbonate

(PO-OTC, IV-℞)

Alka-Mints, Amitone, Apo-Cal, BioCal, Calcarb, Calci-Chew, Calci-Mix, Calcilac, Calcite, Calglycine, Cal-Plus, Calsan, Caltrate 600, Caltrate Jr., Chooz, Dicarbosil, Equilet, Gencalc, Liquid-Cal, Liquid-Cal-600, Maalox Antacid Caplets, Mallamint, Mylanta Lozenges, Nephro-Calci, Nu-Cal, Os-Cal 500, Oysco 500, Oystercal 500, Oyst-Cal 500, Rolaids Calcium Rich, Titralac, Tums, Tums E-X Extra Strength

Func. class.: Antacid, calcium supplement

Chem. class.: Calcium product

Action: Neutralizes gastric acidity

Uses: Antacid, calcium supplement; not suitable for chronic therapy, hyperphosphatemia, hypertension in pregnancy, osteoporosis, prevention, treatment of hypocalcemia, hyperparathyroidism

Dosage and routes:

Antacid

- *Adult:* **PO** 0.5-1.5 g or 2 pieces of gum 1 hr pc and hs

Prevention of hypocalcemia, depletion, osteoporosis

- *Adult:* **PO** 1-2 g qd

Hyperphosphatemia

- *Adult:* **PO** 1 g or more in divided doses

Hypertension in pregnancy

- *Adult:* **PO** 500 mg tid during 3rd trimester

Available forms: Chewable tabs 350, 420, 450, 500, 750, 1000, 1250 mg; tabs 500, 600, 650, 1000, 1250 mg; gum 300, 450, 500 mg; susp 1250 mg/5 ml; lozenges 600 mg; caps 1250 mg; powder 6.5 g/packet

Side effects/adverse reactions:

GI: Constipation, anorexia, nausea, vomiting, flatulence, diarrhea, rebound hyperacidity, eructation

Contraindications: Hypersensitivity, hypercalcemia, hyperparathyroidism, bone tumors

Precautions: Elderly, fluid restriction, decreased GI motility, GI obstruction, dehydration, renal disease, pregnancy (C), lactation

Pharmacokinetics: $\frac{1}{3}$ of dose absorbed by small intestine, onset 20 min, duration 20-180 min, excreted in feces and urine, crosses placenta

Interactions:

- ↑ plasma levels of quinidine, amphetamines
- ↓ levels of salicylates, calcium channel blockers, ketoconazole, tetracyclines, iron salts, quinolone antibiotics

↑ action/side effects: lily of the valley, pheasant's eye, shark cartilage, squill

Lab test interferences:

False increase: chloride

False positive: benzodiazepines

False decrease: magnesium, oxylate, lipase

NURSING CONSIDERATIONS

Assess:

- Calcium (serum, urine), calcium should be 8.5-10.5 mg/dl, urine calcium should be 150 mg/day, monitor weekly

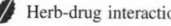

Milk-alkali syndrome: nausea, vomiting, disorientation, headache

- Constipation; increase bulk in the diet if needed

• Hypercalcemia: headache, nausea, vomiting, confusion

Administer:

PO route

• As antacid 1 hr pc and hs
• As supplement 1½ hr pc and hs
• Only with regular tablets or capsules; do not give with enteric-coated tablets
• Laxatives or stool softeners if constipation occurs

Evaluate:

• Therapeutic response: absence of pain, decreased acidity

Teach patient/family:

• To increase fluids to 2 L unless contraindicated, to add bulk to diet for constipation, notify prescriber of constipation
• Not to switch antacids unless directed by prescriber, not to use as antacid for >2 wk without approval by prescriber
• That therapeutic dose recommendations are figured as elemental calcium

calcium chloride
calcium gluceptate
calcium gluconate
calcium lactate (℞)

Func. class.: Electrolyte replacement—calcium product

Action: Cation needed for maintenance of nervous, muscular, skeletal function, enzyme reactions, normal cardiac contractility, coagulation of blood; affects secretory activity of endocrine, exocrine glands

Uses: Prevention and treatment of hypocalcemia, hypermagnesemia, hypoparathyroidism, neonatal tetany, cardiac toxicity caused by hyperkalemia, lead colic, hyperphosphatemia, vit D deficiency, osteoporosis prophylaxis, calcium antagonist toxicity (calcium channel blocker toxicity)

Dosage and routes:

Calcium gluceptate

• *Adult:* **IV** 5-20 ml; **IM** 2-5 ml

Calcium chloride

• *Adult:* **IV** 500 mg-1 g q1-3d as indicated by serum calcium levels, give at <1 ml/min; **IV** 200-800 mg injected in ventricle of heart
• *Child:* **IV** 25 mg/kg over several min

Calcium gluconate

• *Adult:* **PO** 0.5-2 g bid-qid; **IV** 0.5-2 g at 0.5 ml/min (10% solution); max **IV** dose 3 g
• *Child:* **PO/IV** 500 mg/kg/day in divided doses

Calcium lactate

• *Adult:* **PO** 325 mg-1.3 g tid with meals
• *Child:* **PO** 500 mg/kg/day in divided doses

Available forms: Many; check product listings

Side effects/adverse reactions:

INTEG: Pain, burning at IV site, severe venous thrombosis, necrosis, extravasation

HYPERCALCEMIA: Drowsiness, lethargy, muscle weakness, headache, constipation, ***coma,*** anorexia, nausea, vomiting, polyuria, thirst

CV: Shortened QT, heart block, hypotension, bradycardia, ***dysrhythmias; cardiac arrest (IV)***

GI: Vomiting, nausea, constipation

Contraindications: Hypercalcemia, digitalis toxicity, ventricular fibrillation, renal calculi

Precautions: Pregnancy (C), lactation, children, renal disease, respiratory disease, cor pulmonale, digitalized patient, respiratory failure

Pharmacokinetics: Crosses placenta, enters breast milk, excreted via urine and feces; half-life unknown

PO: Onset, peak, duration unknown; absorption (PO) from GI tract
IV: Onset immediate, duration ½-2 hr

Interactions:

• ↑ dysrhythmias: digitalis glycosides
• ↓ effects of: atenolol, verapamil
• ↑ toxicity: verapamil
• milk-alkali syndrome: antacids
• ↓ absorption of: fluoroquinolones, tetracyclines, iron salts, phenytoin, when calcium is taken ***PO***
• ↑ hypercalcemia: thiazide diuretics
↑ action/side effects: lily of the valley, pheasant's eye, shark cartilage, squill

Lab test interferences:
Increase: 11-OHCS
False decrease: Magnesium
Decrease: 17-OHCS

NURSING CONSIDERATIONS

Assess:

• ECG for decreased QT and T wave inversion: hypercalcemia, drug should be reduced or discontinued, consider cardiac monitoring
• Calcium levels during treatment (8.5-11.5 g/dl is normal level)
• Cardiac status: rate, rhythm, CVP, (PWP, PAWP if being monitored directly)

Administer:

PO route

• With or following meals to enhance absorption

IM route

• IM inj may cause severe burning, necrosis, tissue sloughing; warm sol to body temp before administering (only gluconate/gluceptate)

IV route

• Undiluted or diluted with equal amounts of NS to a 5% sol for inj, give 0.5-1 ml/min
• Through small-bore needle into large vein; if extravasation occurs, necrosis will result (IV)

Calcium chloride

Additive compatibilities: Amikacin, amphotericin B, ampicillin, ascorbic acid, bretylium, ceftriaxone, cephapirin, chloramphenicol, DOPamine, hydrocortisone, isoproterenol, lidocaine, methicillin, norepinephrine, penicillin G potassium, penicillin G sodium, pentobarbital, phenobarbital, verapamil, vit B/C

Syringe compatibilities: Milrinone

Y-site compatibilities: Amrinone, DOBUTamine, epINEPHrine, esmolol, morphine, paclitaxel

Calcium gluceptate

Additive compatibilities: Ascorbic acid inj, isoproterenol, lidocaine, norepinephrine, phytonadione, sodium bicarbonate

Calcium gluconate

Additive compatibilities: Amikacin, aminophylline, ascorbic acid injection, bretylium, cephapirin, chloramphenicol, cisatracurium, corticotropin, dimenhyDRINATE, DOXOrubicin liposome, erythromycin, furosemide, heparin, hydrocortisone, lidocaine, magnesium sulfate, methicillin, norepinephrine, penicillin G potassium, penicillin G sodium, phenobarbital, potassium chloride, remifentanil, tobramycin, vancomycin, verapamil, vit B/C

Syringe compatibilities: Aldesleukin, allopurinol, amifostine, aztreonam, cefazolin, cefepime, ciprofloxacin, cladribine, DOBUTamine, enalaprilat, epINEPHrine, famotidine, filgrastim, granisetron, heparin/hydrocortisone, labetalol, melphalan, midazolam, netilmicin, piperacillin/tazobactam, potassium chloride, prochlorperazine, propofol, sargramostim, tacrolimus, teniposide, thiotepa, tolazoline, vinorelbine, vit B/C

Perform/provide:
• Seizure precautions: padded side rails, decreased stimuli (noise, light); place airway suction equipment, padded mouth gag if Ca levels are low
• Store at room temperature

Evaluate:
• Therapeutic response: decreased twitching, paresthesias, muscle spasms, absence of tremors, convulsions, dysrhythmias, dyspnea, laryngospasm, negative Chvostek's sign, negative Trousseau's sign

Teach patient/family:
• To remain recumbent ½ hr after IV dose
• To add foods high in vit D
• To add calcium-rich foods to diet: dairy products, shellfish, dark green leafy vegetables; decrease oxalate-rich and zinc-rich foods: nuts, legumes, chocolate, spinach, soy
• To prevent injuries, avoid immobilization

calcium polycarbophil (OTC)

(pol-ee-kar′boe-fil)
Equalactin, Fiberall, FiberCon, Fiber-Lax, Mitrolan
Func. class.: Laxative
Chem. class.: Bulk-forming

Action: Attracts water, expands in intestine to increase peristalsis; also absorbs excess water in stool; decreases diarrhea

Uses: Constipation, irritable bowel syndrome (diarrhea), acute, nonspecific diarrhea

Dosage and routes:
• *Adult:* **PO** 1 g qd-qid prn, not to exceed 6 g/24 hr
• *Child 6-12 yr:* **PO** 500 mg bid prn, not to exceed 3 g/24 hr
• *Child 3-6 yr:* **PO** 500 mg bid prn, not to exceed 1.5 g/24 hr

Available forms: Chew tabs 500, 1000 mg; tabs 500 mg

Side effects/adverse reactions:
GI: ***Obstruction,*** abdominal distention, flatus, laxative dependence

Contraindications: Hypersensitivity, GI obstruction

Precautions: Pregnancy (C), lactation

Pharmacokinetics:
PO: Onset 12-24 min, peak 1-3 days

Interactions:
↑ action/side effects: flax, lily of the valley, pheasant's eye, senna, squill

NURSING CONSIDERATIONS

Assess:
• Cause of constipation; identify whether fluids, bulk, or exercise is missing from lifestyle
• Cramping, rectal bleeding, nausea, vomiting; if these symptoms occur, drug should be discontinued

Administer:

PO route
• Alone for better absorption; do not take within 1 hr of other drugs
• In morning or evening (oral dose)

Evaluate:
• Therapeutic response: decreased constipation

Teach patient/family:
• Not to use laxatives for long-term therapy; laxative dependence will result
• That normal bowel movements do not always occur daily
• Not to use in presence of abdominal pain, nausea, vomiting
• To notify prescriber if constipation is unrelieved or if symptoms of electrolyte imbalance occur: muscle cramps, pain, weakness, dizziness
• To chew thoroughly (chew tab) and follow with 6-8 oz water

RARELY USED

calfactant (℞)

(cal-fak'tant)

Infasurf

Func. class.: Natural lung surfactant extract

Uses: Prevention and treatment (rescue) of respiratory distress syndrome in premature infants

Dosage and routes:

• Newborn: **INTRATRACHEAL INSTILL:** 3 ml/kg of birth wt, given as 2 doses of 1.5 ml/kg, repeat doses of 3 ml/kg of birth wt until up to 3 doses 12 hr apart have been given

candesartan (℞)

(can-deh-sar'tan)

Atacand

Func. class.: Antihypertensive

Chem. class.: Angiotensin II receptor (type AT_1)

Action: Blocks the vasoconstrictor and aldosterone-secreting effects of angiotensin II; selectively blocks the binding of angiotensin II to the AT_1 receptor found in tissues

Uses: Hypertension, alone or in combination

Dosage and routes:

• *Adult:* **PO,** single agent 16 mg qd initially in patients who are not volume depleted, range 8-32 mg/day; with diuretic, or volume depletion 2-32 mg/day as single dose or divided bid

Renal disease

• Adult: **PO** Give lowest possible dose

Available forms: Tabs 4, 8, 16, 32 mg

Side effects/adverse reactions:

CNS: Dizziness, fatigue, headache

GI: Diarrhea, nausea, abdominal pain, vomiting

MS: Arthralgia, pain

RESP: Cough, upper respiratory infection

SYST: ***Angioedema***

CV: Chest pain, peripheral edema

EENT: Sinusitis, rhinitis, pharyngitis

GU: ***Renal failure***

Contraindications: Hypersensitivity, pregnancy (D) 2nd/3rd trimesters

Precautions: Hypersensitivity to ACE inhibitors; pregnancy (C) 1st trimester, lactation; children; elderly

Pharmacokinetics: Extensively metabolized, excreted in urine and feces

Interactions:

↓ effect: coltsfoot, guarana, khat, licorice

↑ or ↓ effect: astragalus, cola tree

Toxicity/death: aconite

↑ effect: barberry, betony, black catechu, black cohosh, bloodroot, broom, burdock, cats claw, dandelion, goldenseal, Irish moss, Jamaican dogwood, kelp, khella, mistletoe, parsley, Queen Anne's lace, Rue

NURSING CONSIDERATIONS

Assess:

• For angioedema: facial swelling, difficulty breathing (rare)

• For pregnancy, this drug can cause fetal death when given in pregnancy

• Response and adverse reactions especially in renal disease

• B/P, pulse q4h; note rate, rhythm, quality; electrolytes: K, Na, Cl; baselines in renal, hepatic studies before therapy begins

Administer:

• Without regard to meals

Evaluate:

• Therapeutic response: decreased B/P

Teach patient/family:

• To comply with dosage schedule, even if feeling better
• To notify prescriber of mouth sores, fever, swelling of hands or feet, irregular heartbeat, chest pain
• That excessive perspiration, dehydration, vomiting, diarrhea may lead to fall in blood pressure; to consult prescriber if these occur
• That drug may cause dizziness, fainting; light-headedness may occur
• To rise slowly to sitting or standing position to minimize orthostatic hypotension
• To notify prescriber immediately if pregnant; not to use during lactation
• To avoid all OTC medications, unless approved by prescriber; to inform all health-care providers of medication use
• To use proper technique for obtaining B/P and acceptable parameters

capecitabine (℞)

(cap-eh-sit′ah-bean)

Xeloda

Func. class.: Antineoplastic, antimetabolite

Chem. class.: Fluoropyrimidine carbamate

Action: Competes with physiologic substrate of DNA synthesis, thus interfering with cell replication in the S phase of cell cycle (before mitosis); drug is converted to 5-FU

Uses: Metastatic breast, colorectal cancer

Dosage and routes:

• *Adult:* **PO** 2500 mg/m^2/day in 2 divided doses q12h at end of meal × 2 wk, then 1 wk rest period; given in 3 wk cycles; may be combined with Docetaxel, when capecitabine dose is lowered

Available forms: Tabs 150, 500 mg

Side effects/adverse reactions:

HEMA: ***Neutropenia, lymphopenia, thrombocytopenia, myelosuppression,*** anemia

GI: Nausea, vomiting, anorexia, diarrhea, stomatitis, abdominal pain, constipation, anorexia, dyspepsia, ***intestinal obstruction***

OTHER: Hyperbilirubinemia, eye irritation, pyrexia, edema, myalgia, limb pain, *pyrexia*, dehydration

INTEG: Hand and foot syndrome, dermatitis, nail disorder

CNS: Dizziness, headache, *paresthesia, fatigue,* insomnia

Contraindications: Hypersensitivity to 5-FU, infants, pregnancy (D), severe renal impairment (CCr <30 ml/min)

Precautions: Renal disease, hepatic disease, lactation, children, elderly

Do not confuse:

Xeloda/Xenical

Pharmacokinetics: Readily absorbed, peak 1½ hr; food decreases absorption; extensively metabolized in the liver; elimination half-life 45 min

Interactions:

• ↑ toxicity: leucovorin
• ↑ capecitabine levels: antacids
• ↑ risk of bleeding: warfarin
• ↑ phenytoin level: phenytoin

NURSING CONSIDERATIONS

Assess:

• CBC (RBC, Hct, Hgb), differential, platelet count weekly; withhold drug if WBC is <4000/mm^3, platelet count is <75,000/mm^3, or RBC, Hct, Hgb low; notify prescriber of these results
• Renal studies: BUN, serum uric acid, urine creatinine clearance, electrolytes before and during therapy
• Monitor temp q4h; fever may in-

dicate beginning infection; no rectal temps
• Hepatic studies before and during therapy: bilirubin, ALT, AST, alk phosphatase, as needed or monthly
• Bleeding: hematuria, heme-positive stools, bruising or petechiae, mucosa or orifices q8h
• Dyspnea, rales, unproductive cough, chest pain, tachypnea, fatigue, increased pulse, pallor, lethargy; personality changes, with high doses
• For hand and foot syndrome: paresthesia, tingling, painful/painless swelling, blistering, erythema with severe pain of hands or feet
• For toxicity: severe diarrhea, nausea, vomiting, stomatitis
• Buccal cavity q8h for dryness, sores or ulceration, white patches, oral pain, bleeding, dysphagia
• GI symptoms: frequency of stools, cramping, if severe diarrhea occurs, fluid and electrolytes may need to be given

Administer:
• Antiemetic 30-60 min before giving drug and prn

Perform/provide:
• Rinsing of mouth tid-qid with water, club soda; brushing of teeth bid-tid with soft brush or cotton-tipped applicators for stomatitis; use unwaxed dental floss

Evaluate:
• Therapeutic response: decreased tumor size, spread of malignancy

Teach patient/family:
• To avoid foods with citric acid, hot or rough texture if stomatitis is present
• To avoid pregnancy while on this drug; to avoid using while lactating
• Not to double dose, if dose is missed
◆ To immediately report severe diarrhea, vomiting, stomatitis, fever over 100° F (37.8° C), hand and foot syndrome, anorexia
• To report signs of infection: increased temp, sore throat, flulike symptoms
• To report signs of anemia: fatigue, headache, faintness, shortness of breath, irritability
• To report bleeding; to avoid use of razors, commercial mouthwash

captopril (℞)
(kap′toe-pril)
Capoten, Novo-Captoril ♣
Func. class.: Antihypertensive
Chem. class.: Angiotensin-converting enzyme inhibitor (ACE)

Action: Selectively suppresses renin-angiotensin-aldosterone system; inhibits ACE; preventing conversion of angiotensin I to angiotensin II

Uses: Hypertension, CHF, left ventricular dysfunction after MI, diabetic nephropathy

Dosage and routes:

Malignant hypertension
• *Adult:* **PO** 25 mg increasing q2h until desired response, not to exceed 450 mg/day

Hypertension
• *Adult:* **PO** initial dose: 25 mg bid-tid; may increase to 50 mg bid-tid at 1-2 wk intervals; usual range: 25-150 mg bid-tid; max 450 mg
• *Child:* **PO** 0.3-0.5 mg/kg/dose, titrate up to 6 mg/kg/day in 2-4 divided doses
• *Neonate:* **PO** 10 mcg (0.01 mg)/kg bid-tid, may increase as needed

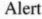

CHF
• *Adult:* **PO** 12.5 mg bid-tid; may increase to 50 mg bid-tid; after 14 days, may increase to 150 mg tid if needed

LVD after MI
• *Adult:* **PO** 50 mg tid, may begin treatment 3 days after MI; give 6.25 mg as a single dose, then 12.5 mg tid, increase to 25 mg tid for several days, then to 50 mg tid
Diabetic nephropathy
• *Adult:* **PO** 25 mg tid
Renal dose
• *Adult:* **PO** 6.25-12.5 mg bid-tid
• *Child:* **PO** 150 mcg (0.15)/kg tid
Available forms: Tabs 12.5, 25, 50, 100 mg
Side effects/adverse reactions:
CV: Hypotension, postural hypotension, *tachycardia,* angina
GU: Impotence, dysuria, nocturia, proteinuria, ***nephrotic syndrome, acute reversible renal failure,*** polyuria, oliguria, urinary frequency
HEMA: ***Neutropenia, agranulocytosis, pancytopenia, thrombocytopenia,*** anemia
INT: Rash, *angioedema*
RESP: ***Bronchospasm,*** *dyspnea, cough*
GI: Loss of taste, increased LFTs
CNS: Fever, chills
MISC: ***Angioedema,*** hyperkalemia
Contraindications: Hypersensitivity, lactation, heart block, children, potassium-sparing diuretics, bilateral renal artery stenosis, pregnancy (D) 2nd/3rd trimester
Precautions: Dialysis patients, hypovolemia, leukemia, scleroderma, SLE, blood dyscrasias, CHF, diabetes mellitus, renal disease, thyroid disease, COPD, asthma, pregnancy (C), 1st trimester
Do not confuse:
captopril/Capitrol/carvedilol
Pharmacokinetics:
PO: Peak 1 hr; duration 6-12 hr; half-life <2 hr, increased in renal disease; metabolized by liver (metabolites), excreted in urine; crosses placenta; excreted in breast milk, small amounts

Interactions:
• ↑ hypotension: diuretics, other antihypertensives, phenothiazines, nitrates, acute alcohol ingestion
• ↓ captopril effect: antacids, NSAIDs
• Possible toxicity: lithium, digoxin
• Hypoglycemia: insulin, oral antidiabetics
• Do not use with potassium-sparing diuretics, sympathomimetics, potassium supplements
↑ toxicity/death: aconite
↑ or ↓ antihypertensive effect: astragalus, cola tree
↑ antihypertensive effect: barberry, betony, black catechu, black cohosh, bloodroot, broom, burdock, cat's claw, dandelion, goldenseal, Irish moss, Jamaican dogwood, kelp, khella, mistletoe, parsley
↓ antihypertensive effect: coltsfoot, guarana, khat, licorice
Lab test interferences:
False positive: Urine acetone, ANA titer
Increase: AST, ALT, alk phosphatase, bilirubin, uric acid, glucose

NURSING CONSIDERATIONS
Assess:
• Blood studies: decreased platelets; WBC with diff baseline and periodically q3mo, if neutrophils <1000/mm^3, discontinue treatment
• B/P, pulse rates baseline, frequently
• Renal studies: protein, BUN, creatinine; watch for raised levels that may indicate nephrotic syndrome
• Baselines in renal, hepatic studies before therapy begins and periodically, increased LFTs, uric acid and glucose may be increased
• Edema in feet, legs daily, weight daily in CHF
• Allergic reaction: rash, fever, pruritus, urticaria; discontinue drug if antihistamines fail to help
• Symptoms of CHF: edema, dyspnea, wet rales, B/P

Administer:
- 1 hr ac or 2 hr pc
- May crush tab and dissolve in water, give within ½ hr, make sure tab is completely dissolved

Perform/provide:
- Storage in tight container at 86° F (30° C) or less

Evaluate:
- Therapeutic response: decrease in B/P in hypertension, edema, moist rales (CHF)

Teach patient/family:
- That tabs may be crushed and mixed with food; to take 1 hr before meals or 2 hr pc; not to discontinue drug abruptly
- Not to use OTC products (cough, cold, or allergy) unless directed by prescriber
- To avoid sunlight or wear sunscreen if in sunlight; photosensitivity may occur
- To comply with dosage schedule, even if feeling better
- To rise slowly to sitting or standing position to minimize orthostatic hypotension
- To notify prescriber of mouth sores, sore throat, fever, swelling of hands or feet, irregular heartbeat, chest pain, signs of angioedema
- That excessive perspiration, dehydration, vomiting; diarrhea may lead to fall in blood pressure; consult prescriber if these occur
- That dizziness, fainting, lightheadedness may occur during first few days of therapy
- That skin rash or impaired perspiration may occur
- How to take B/P and when to notify prescriber
- To report if pregnancy is suspected or planned

Treatment of overdose: 0.9% NaCl IV/INF; hemodialysis

carbachol ophthalmic

See appendix c

carbamazepine (℞)

(kar-ba-maz′e-peen)

Apo-Carbamazepine🍁, Atretol, Carbatrol, Epitol, Novo-Carbamaz🍁, Tegretol, Tegretol CR🍁, Tegretol-XR

Func. class.: Anticonvulsant

Chem. class.: Iminostilbene derivative

Action: Exact mechanism unknown; apppears to decrease polysynaptic responses and block post-tetanic potentiation

Uses: Tonic-clonic, complex-partial, mixed seizures; trigeminal neuralgia

Investigational uses: Diabetes insipidus, bipolar disorder, neurogenic pain, schizophrenia, psychotic behavior with dementia, rectal administration, diabetic neuropathy, restless leg syndrome

Dosage and routes:

Seizures
- *Adult and child >12 yr:* **PO** 200 mg bid, may be increased by 200 mg/day in divided doses q6-8h; maintenance 800-1200 mg/day maximum 1600 mg/day (adult); max child 12-15 yr 1000 mg/day; max child >15 yr 1200 mg/day; adjustment is needed to minimum dose to control seizures; ext rel give bid; rectal administration of oral susp 200 mg/10 ml or 6 mg/kg as a single dose
- *Child 6-12 yr:* **PO** tabs 100 mg bid or susp 50 mg qid; may increase by <100 mg qwk; max 1000 mg/day ext rel tabs qd-bid
- *Child <6 yr:* **PO** 10-20 mg/kg/

day in 2-3 divided doses, may increase qwk

Trigeminal neuralgia

• *Adult:* **PO** 100 mg bid with meals; may increase 100 mg q12h until pain subsides, not to exceed 1200 mg/day; maintenance is 200-400 mg bid

Available forms: Tabs, chewable 100, 200 mg; tabs 200 mg; ext-rel tabs 100, 200, 400 mg; oral susp 100 mg/5 ml; ext rel caps 200, 300 mg

Side effects/adverse reactions:

HEMA: ***Thrombocytopenia, leukopenia, agranulocytosis, leukocytosis, aplastic anemia, eosinophilia,*** increased PT

ENDO: SIADH (elderly)

CNS: Drowsiness, dizziness, unsteadiness, confusion, fatigue, ***paralysis,*** headache, hallucinations, ***worsening of seizures***, speech disturbance

GI: Nausea, constipation, diarrhea, anorexia, vomiting, abdominal pain, stomatitis, glossitis, increased liver enzymes, ***hepatitis***

INTEG: Rash, ***Stevens-Johnson syndrome,*** urticaria, photosensitivity

EENT: Tinnitus, dry mouth, blurred vision, diplopia, nystagmus, conjunctivitis

CV: ***Hypertension, CHF, dysrhythmias, AV block,*** hypotension, aggravation of cardiac artery disease

RESP: Pulmonary hypersensitivity (fever, dyspnea, pneumonitis)

GU: Frequency, retention, albuminuria, glycosuria, impotence, increased BUN, ***renal failure***

Contraindications: Hypersensitivity to carbamazepine or tricyclics, bone marrow depression, concomitant use of MAOIs

Precautions: Glaucoma, hepatic disease, renal disease, cardiac disease, psychosis, pregnancy (D), lactation, child <6 yr

Do not confuse:

Tegretol/Toradol

Pharmacokinetics:

PO: Onset slow, peak 4-8 hr; metabolized by liver; excreted in urine, feces; crosses placenta, blood-brain barrier; excreted in breast milk; half-life 14-16 hr, protein binding 76%

Interactions:

• CNS toxicity: lithium

• ↑ carbamazepine levels: cimetidine, clarithromycin, danazol, diltiazem, erythromycin, fluoxetine, fluvoxamine, isoniazid, propoxyphene, valproic acid, verapamil

• ↓ effects of benzodiazepines, doxycycline, felbamate, haloperidol, oral contraceptives, phenobarbital, phenytoin, primidone, theophylline, thyroid hormones, warfarin

• ↑ effects of desmopressin, lithium, lypressin, vasopressin

• ↓ carbamazepine levels: cisplatin, DOXOrubicin, felbamate, rifampin, phenobarbital, phenytoin, primidone, theophylline

Fatal reaction: MAOIs

• Drug/food: ↑ peak concentration of carbamazepine: grapefruit juice

↓ carbamazepine metabolism, increased levels: quinine, ginkgo

↓ anticonvulsant effect: ginseng, santonica

NURSING CONSIDERATIONS

Assess:

• For seizures: character, location, duration, intensity, frequency, presence of aura

• For trigeminal neuralgia: facial pain including location, duration, intensity, character, activity that stimulates pain

• Renal studies: urinalysis, BUN, urine creatinine q3mo

Blood studies: RBC, Hct, Hgb, reticulocyte counts qwk for 4 wk then qmo; if myelosuppression occurs, drug should be discontinued

• Hepatic studies: ALT, AST, bilirubin

• Drug levels during initial treat-

ment or when changing dose; should remain at 4-12 mcg/ml; anorexia may indicate increased blood levels
• Mental status: mood, sensorium, affect, behavioral changes; if mental status changes, notify prescriber
• Eye problems: need for ophthalmic examinations before, during, after treatment (slit lamp, fundoscopy, tonometry)
• Allergic reaction: purpura, red, raised rash; if these occur, drug should be discontinued
Blood dyscrasias: fever, sore throat, bruising, rash, jaundice
Toxicity: bone marrow depression, nausea, vomiting, ataxia, diplopia, cardiovascular collapse, Stevens-Johnson syndrome

Administer:

PO route

• With food, milk to decrease GI symptoms
Do not crush, break, or chew ext rel tab; chewable tabs: tell patient to chew tab, not swallow it whole; ext rel cap may be opened and mixed with food
• Shake oral susp before use
• Mix an equal amount of water, D_5W, 0.9% NaCl when giving by NG tube, flush tube with 100 ml of above sol

Perform/provide:

• Storage at room temperature
• Hard candy, gum, frequent rinsing for dry mouth

Evaluate:

• Therapeutic response: decreased seizure activity, document on patient's chart

Teach patient/family:

• To carry emergency ID stating patient's name, drugs taken, condition, prescriber's name, phone number
• To avoid driving, other activities that require alertness usually the first 3 days of treatment
• Not to discontinue medication quickly after long-term use
• To report immediately chills, rash, light-colored stools, dark urine, yellowing of skin and eyes, abdominal pain, sore throat, mouth ulcers, bruising, blurred vision, dizziness
• That urine may turn pink to brown

Treatment of overdose: Lavage, VS

carbidopa-levodopa (℞)

(kar-bi-doe′pa) (lee-voe-doe′pa)
carbidopa/levodopa,
Sinemet, Sinemet CR

Func. class.: Antiparkinson agent

Chem. class.: Catecholamine

Action: Decarboxylation of levodopa to periphery is inhibited by carbidopa; more levodopa is made available for transport to brain and conversion to DOPamine in the brain

Uses: Parkinson's disease, parkinsonism resulting from carbon monoxide, chronic manganese intoxication, cerebral arteriosclerosis, restless leg syndrome

Dosage and routes:

Beginning therapy for those not taking levodopa

• *Adult:* **PO** 10 mg carbidopa/100 mg levodopa tid-qid or 25 mg carbidopa/100 mg levodopa tid, may increase qd to desired response

For those not taking levodopa ER

50 mg carbidopa/200 mg levodopa bid

For those taking levodopa ER

Begin treatment with 10% more levodopa/day given q4-8h, may increase or decrease dose q3d

For those taking levodopa <1.5 g/day

• *Adult:* **PO** 25 mg carbidopa/100

mg levodopa tid-qid, may increase qd to desired response

For those taking levodopa >1.5 g/day

• *Adult:* **PO** 25 mg carbidopa/250 mg levodopa tid-qid, may increase qd to desired response

Available forms: Tabs 10/100, 25/100, 25 mg carbidopa/250 mg levodopa; ext rel tab: 25 mg/100 mg, 50 mg/200 mg carbidopa/levodopa (Sinemet CR)

Side effects/adverse reactions:

HEMA: ***Hemolytic anemia, leukopenia, agranulocytosis***

CNS: Involuntary choreiform movements, hand tremors, fatigue, headache, anxiety, twitching, numbness, weakness, confusion, agitation, insomnia, nightmares, psychosis, hallucination, hypomania, severe depression, dizziness

GI: Nausea, vomiting, anorexia, abdominal distress, dry mouth, flatulence, dysphagia, bitter taste, diarrhea, constipation

INTEG: Rash, sweating, alopecia

CV: Orthostatic hypotension, tachycardia, hypertension, palpitation

EENT: Blurred vision, diplopia, dilated pupils

MISC: Urinary retention, incontinence, weight change, dark urine

Contraindications: Hypersensitivity, narrow-angle glaucoma, malignant melanoma, history of malignant melanoma or undiagnosed skin lesions resembling melanoma

Precautions: Renal disease, wide-angle glaucoma, cardiac disease, hepatic disease, respiratory disease, MI with dysrhythmias, convulsions, peptic ulcer, pregnancy (C), lactation

Pharmacokinetics:

PO: Peak 1-3 hr, excreted in urine (metabolites)

Interactions:

• Hypertensive crisis: MAOIs

• ↓ effects of levodopa: anticholinergics, hydantoins, papaverine, pyridoxine, benzodiazepines

• ↑ effects of levodopa: antacids, metoclopramide

• Drug/food: ↑ pyridoxine will ↓ levodopa effect

• ↓ absorption of levodopa: protein

↓ action, increased EPS: Indian snakeroot

↑ Parkinson symptoms: kava, octacosanol

Lab test interferences:

Increase: BUN, AST, ALT, bilirubin, alk phosphatase, LDH

False positive: Urine ketones (dipstick), Coombs' test

False negative: Urine glucose

False increase: Uric acid, urine protein

Decrease: VMA, BUN, creatinine

NURSING CONSIDERATIONS

Assess:

• For Parkinson's symptoms: tremors, pill rolling, drooling, akinesia, rigidity before and during treatment

• B/P, respiration; orthostatic B/P

• Mental status: affect, mood, behavioral changes, depression, complete suicide assessment

• Muscle twitching, blepharospasm that may indicate toxicity

• Renal, liver, hematopoietic tests, also for diabetes, acromegaly if on long-term therapy

Administer:

PO route

• Drug until NPO before surgery

• Adjust dosage to response

• With meals if GI symptoms occur; limit protein taken with drug

• Only after MAOIs have been discontinued for 2 wk; if previously on levodopa, discontinue for at least 8 hr before change to carbidopa-levodopa

Evaluate:

• Therapeutic response: decrease in akathisia, improved mood

Teach patient/family:

- Not to crush or chew cont rel tabs; may be broken in half
- To change positions slowly to prevent orthostatic hypotension
- To report side effects: twitching, eye spasms; indicate overdose
- To use drug exactly as prescribed; if discontinued abruptly, parkinsonian crisis may occur; prescriber may recommend drug-free holidays
- That urine, sweat may darken
- To use physical activities to maintain mobility, lessen spasms
- That improvement may not occur for 3-4 mo

HIGH ALERT

carboplatin (℞)

(kar-boe-pla′-tin)

Paraplatin, Paraplatin-AQ

Func. class.: Antineoplastic alkylating agent

Chem. class.: Platinum coordination compound

Action: Produces interstrand DNA cross-links and, to a lesser extent, DNA-protein cross-links; activity is not cell cycle phase specific

Uses: Initial treatment of advanced ovarian cancer in combination with other agents; palliative treatment of ovarian carcinoma recurrent after treatment with other antineoplastic agents

Dosage and routes (single agent):

- *Adult:* **IV INF** initially 300 mg/m^2 given with cyclophosphamide, q4-6wk; refractory tumors 360 mg/m^2 single dose, may repeat q4wk, as needed

Renal dose

CCr 41-59 ml/min 250 mg/m^2, CCr 16-40 ml/min 200 mg/m^2

Available forms: Inj 50, 150, 450 mg/vial

Side effects/adverse reactions:

EENT: Tinnitus, hearing loss, *vestibular toxicity,* visual changes

HEMA: ***Thrombocytopenia, leukopenia, pancytopenia, neutropenia, anemia,*** bleeding

CV: Cardiac abnormalities

GI: Severe nausea, vomiting, diarrhea, weight loss, mucositis, anorexia, constipation, taste change

GU: ***Renal tubular damage,*** renal insufficiency, impotence, sterility, amenorrhea, gynecomastia

INTEG: Alopecia, dermatitis, rash, erythema, pruritus, urticaria

CNS: ***Seizures, central neurotoxicity,*** peripheral neuropathy, dizziness, confusion

META: Hypomagnesemia, hypocalcemia, hypokalemia, hyponatremia, hyperuremia

SYST: ***Anaphylaxis***

Contraindications: Hypersensitivity to this drug, platinum products, mannitol; severe bone marrow depression, significant bleeding, pregnancy (D)

Precautions: Radiation therapy within 1 mo, chemotherapy within 1 mo, lactation, liver disease

Do not confuse:

carboplatin/cisplatin

Paraplatin/Platinol

Pharmacokinetics: Initial half-life 1-2 hr, postdistribution half-life 2½-6 hr, not bound to plasma proteins, excreted by the kidneys

Interactions:

- ↑ nephrotoxicity or ototoxicity: aminoglycosides
- ↑ risk of bleeding: aspirin
- ↑ toxicity: radiation, bone marrow suppressants
- ↑ myelosuppression: myelosuppressives
- ↓: phenytoin levels: phenytoin; antibody reaction: live virus vaccines

Lab test interferences:
Increase: AST, BUN, alk phosphatase, bilirubin, creatinine

NURSING CONSIDERATIONS

Assess:

- CBC, differential, platelet count weekly; withhold drug if neutrophil count is <2000/mm^3 or platelet count is <100,000/mm^3; notify prescriber of results
- Renal studies: BUN, creatinine, serum uric acid, urine CCr before and during therapy; I&O ratio; report fall in urine output to <30 ml/hr
- Monitor temp q4h (may indicate beginning of infection)
- Hepatic studies tests before and during therapy (bilirubin, AST, ALT, LDH) as needed or monthly; jaundice of skin, sclera, dark urine, clay-colored stools, itchy skin, abdominal pain, fever, diarrhea
- For anaphylaxis: hypotension, rash, pruritus, wheezing, tachycardia; notify prescriber after discontinuing drug, resuscitation equipment should be available
- Bleeding; hematuria, stool guaiac, bruising or petechiae, mucosa or orifices q8h
- Dyspnea, rales, unproductive cough, chest pain, tachypnea
- Effects of alopecia on body image; discuss feelings about body changes

Administer:

- Antiemetic 30-60 min before giving drug and prn for vomiting

IV route

- After diluting 10 mg/ml of sterile water for inj, D_5W, NS (10 mg/ml); then further dilute with the same sol 1-4 mg/ml; give over 15 min or more (Intermittent INF)
- IV INF over 5-6 hr; do not use needles or IV administration sets containing aluminum; may cause precipitate or loss of potency
- Diuretic (furosemide 40 mg IV) after infusion

Additive compatibilities: Cisplatin, etoposide, floxuridine, ifosfamide, ifosfamide/etoposide, paclitaxel

Solution compatibilities: D_5/0.2% NaCl, D_5/0.45% NaCl, D_5/0.9% NaCl, 0.9% NaCl, D_5W, sterile water for inj

Y-site compatibilities: Allopurinol, amifostine, aztreonam, cefepime, cladribine, DOXOrubicin liposome, filgrastim, fludarabine, granisetron, melphalan, ondansetron, paclitaxel, piperacillin/tazobactam, propofol, sargramostim, teniposide, thiotepa, vinorelbine

Perform/provide:

- Storage protected from light at room temperature; reconstituted sol stable for 8 hr at room temperature

Evaluate:

- Therapeutic response: decreasing size of tumor, spread of malignancy

Teach patient/family:

- To report ringing/roaring in the ears, numbness, tingling in face, extremities, weight gain
- That impotence or amenorrhea can occur; reversible after treatment is discontinued, to notify prescriber if pregnancy is suspected or planned; contraception should be used if patient is fertile
- Not to breastfeed during treatment
- To avoid OTC drugs with aspirin, NSAIDs, alcohol or receiving vaccinations during treatment
- To notify prescriber immediately of fever, fatigue, sore throat, and bleeding, bruising, chills, back pain, blood in stools, dyspnea
- That hair may be lost during treatment; a wig or hairpiece may make patient feel better; new hair may be different in color, texture
- To avoid crowds, persons with

known infections; avoid use of razors, stiff-bristle toothbrush

carboprost (℞)

(kar'boe-prost)

Hemabate, Prostin/15M✱

Func. class.: Oxytocic, abortifacient

Chem. class.: Prostaglandin

Action: Stimulates uterine contractions, causing complete abortion in approximately 16 hr

Uses: Abortion at 13-20 wk gestation, postpartum hemorrhage caused by uterine atony not controlled by other methods

Dosage and routes:

To induce abortion

• *Adult:* **IM** 250 mcg, then 250 mcg q1½-3½ h, may increase to 500 mcg if no response, not to exceed 12 mg total dose

Postpartum hemorrhage

• *Adult:* **IM** 250 mcg, repeat at 15-90 min intervals; max total dosage 2 mg

Available forms: Inj 250 mcg/ml

Side effects/adverse reactions:

CNS: Fever, chills, headache

GI: Nausea, vomiting, diarrhea

Contraindications: Hypersensitivity, severe hepatic disease, severe renal disease, PID, respiratory disease, cardiac disease

Precautions: Asthma, anemia, jaundice, diabetes mellitus, convulsive disorders, past uterine surgery, pregnancy (C)

Pharmacokinetics: Onset 15 min, peak 2 hr; metabolized in lungs, liver; excreted in urine (metabolites)

Interactions:

• ↑ action: other oxytocics

NURSING CONSIDERATIONS

Assess:

• B/P, pulse; watch for change that may indicate hemorrhage

• Respiratory rate, rhythm, depth; notify prescriber of abnormalities

• For length, duration of contraction; notify prescriber of contractions lasting over 1 min or absence of contractions

• For incomplete abortion, pregnancy must be terminated by another method; drug is teratogenic

Administer:

• In deep muscle mass; rotate inj sites if additional doses are given

Evaluate:

• Therapeutic response: expulsion of fetus, control of bleeding

Teach patient/family:

• To report increased blood loss, abdominal cramps, increased temp, foul-smelling lochia

carisoprodol (℞)

(kar-eye-soe-proe'dole)

carisoprodol, Soma, Vanadom

Func. class.: Skeletal muscle relaxant, central acting

Chem. class.: Meprobamate congener

Action: Depresses CNS by blocking interneuronal activity in descending reticular formation, spinal cord, producing sedation

Uses: Relieving pain, stiffness in musculoskeletal disorders

Dosage and routes:

• *Adult and child >12 yr:* **PO** 350 mg tid and hs

• *Child 6-12 yr:* **PO** 6.25 mg/kg qid

Available forms: Tabs 350 mg

Side effects/adverse reactions:

CNS: Dizziness, weakness, drowsiness, headache, tremor, depression, insomnia, ataxia, irritability

EENT: Diplopia, temporary loss of vision
HEMA: Eosinophilia
RESP: Asthmatic attacks
CV: Postural hypotension, tachycardia
GI: Nausea, vomiting, hiccups, epigastric discomfort
INTEG: Rash, pruritus, fever, facial flushing, ***erythema multiforme***
SYST: ***Angioedema, anaphylaxis***
Contraindications: Hypersensitivity, child <12 yr, intermittent porphyria
Precautions: Renal disease, hepatic disease, addictive personality, pregnancy (C), elderly, lactation
Do not confuse:
Soma/Soma Compound
Pharmacokinetics:
PO: Onset ½ hr, peak 4 hr, duration 4-6 hr; metabolized by liver; excreted in urine; crosses placenta; excreted in breast milk (large amounts); half-life 8 hr
Interactions:
• ↑ CNS depression: alcohol, tricyclics, opioids, barbiturates, sedatives, hypnotics
↑ CNS depression: chamomile, kava, skullcap, valerian
Lab test interferences:
Increase: AST, alk phosphatase blood glucose
NURSING CONSIDERATIONS
Assess:
• Pain, stiffness, mobility, activities of daily living baseline and throughout treatment
• ECG in seizure patients; poor seizure control has occurred with patients taking this drug
• Idiosyncratic reaction (weakness, dizziness, blurred vision, confusion, euphoria), anaphylaxis within a few min or hr of 1st to 4th dose
• Allergic reactions: rash, fever, respiratory distress
• CNS depression: dizziness, drowsiness, psychiatric symptoms
Administer:
PO route
• With meals for GI symptoms
Perform/provide:
• Storage in tight container at room temperature
• Assistance with ambulation if dizziness, drowsiness occurs, especially elderly
Evaluate:
• Therapeutic response: decreased pain, spasticity
Teach patient/family:
• Not to take with alcohol, other CNS depressants
• To avoid hazardous activities if drowsiness, dizziness occur
• To avoid using OTC medication: cough preparations, antihistamines, unless directed by prescriber
Treatment of overdose: Induce emesis of conscious patient, lavage, dialysis

---

HIGH ALERT

carmustine (℞)

(kar-mus′teen)
BiCNU, BCNU, Gliadel
Func. class.: Antineoplastic alkylating agent
Chem. class.: Nitrosourea

Action: Alkylates DNA, RNA; is able to inhibit enzymes that allow synthesis of amino acids in proteins; activity is not cell cycle phase specific
Uses: Brain tumors such as glioblastoma, medulloblastoma, astrocytoma, ependymoma, metastatic brain tumors; multiple myeloma (with predniSONE), Hodgkin's disease, other lymphomas; GI, breast, bronchogenic, renal carcinomas, other lymphomas; wafer, as adjunct

to surgery/radiation in newly diagnosed high-grade malignant glioma patients; in recurrent glioblastoma multiforme patients as an adjunct to surgery

Investigational uses: Primary cutaneous T cell lymphoma, malignant melanoma

Dosage and routes:

• *Adult:* **IV** 75-100 mg/m^2 over 1-2 hr × 2 days or 150-200 mg/m^2 × 1 dose q6-8wk or 40 mg/m^2/day × 5 days q6wk; if WBC is 3000-3999/mm^3 give 50% of dose; if WBC is 2000-2999/mm^3 and platelets are 25,000-75,000/mm^3 give 25% of dose; withhold dose if WBC is <2000/mm^3 and platelets are <25,000/mm^3

• *Adult:* **INTRACAVITARY** wafer: 8 inserted into resection cavity

Available forms: Powder for inj 100 mg; wafer 7.7 mg (intracavitary)

Side effects/adverse reactions:

HEMA: ***Thrombocytopenia, leukopenia, myelosuppression, anemia***

GI: Nausea, vomiting, anorexia, stomatitis, ***hepatotoxicity***

GU: Azotemia, ***renal failure***

INTEG: Burning, hyperpigmentation at inj site

RESP: ***Fibrosis, pulmonary infiltrate***

Contraindications: Hypersensitivity, leukopenia, thrombocytopenia

Precautions: Pregnancy (D), lactation

Pharmacokinetics: Degraded within 15 min; crosses blood-brain barrier; 70% excreted in urine within 96 hr; 10% excreted as CO_2; fate of 20% is unknown

Interactions:

• ↑ toxicity: other antineoplastics, radiation, cimetidine

• Risk of bleeding: aspirin, anticoagulants

• Myelosuppression: myelosuppressive agents

• ↓ effects of: digoxin, phenytoin

• ↑ adverse reactions, ↓ antibody reaction: live vaccines

NURSING CONSIDERATIONS

Assess:

• CBC, differential, platelet count weekly; withhold drug if WBC is <4000 or platelet count is <100,000; notify prescriber of results

• Hepatic studies: AST, ALT, bilirubin

• Pulmonary function tests, chest x-ray films before, during therapy; chest film should be obtained q2wk during treatment; monitor for dyspnea, cough, pulmonary fibrosis; infiltrate occurs after high doses or several low-dose courses

• Renal studies: BUN, serum uric acid, urine CCr before, during therapy; I&O ratio; report fall in urine output of 30 ml/hr

• Monitor for cold, cough, fever (may indicate beginning infection)

• Bleeding: hematuria, guaiac, bruising, petechiae, mucosa, orifices q8h

Administer:

• Blood transfusions or RBC colony-stimulating factors to counter anemia

• Antiemetic 30-60 min before giving drug to prevent vomiting

• All medications PO, if possible, avoid IM inj if platelets are <100,000/mm^3

Wafer route

• Foil pouches may be kept at room temperature for 6 hr if unopened

⊘ If wafers are broken in several pieces, they should not be used

IV route

• Prepare in biologic cabinet wearing gown, gloves, mask; avoid contact with skin

• After diluting 100 mg drug/3 ml ethyl alcohol (provided); then further dilute 27 ml sterile H_2O for inj;

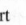

then dilute with 100-500 ml 0.9% NaCl or D_5W, give over 1 hr or more, reduce rate if discomfort is felt; use only glass containers
• Flush IV line after carmustine with 10 ml 0.9% NaCl to prevent irritation at site
Y-site compatibilities: Amifostine, aztreonam, cefepime, filgrastim, fludarabine, granisetron, melphalan, ondansetron, piperacillin/tazobactam, sargramostim, teniposide, thiotepa, vinorelbine
Perform/provide:
• Storage of reconstituted sol in refrigerator for 24 hr, or room temperature for 8 hr
• Rinsing of mouth tid-qid with water or club soda; use of sponge brush for stomatitis
• Warm compresses at inj site for inflammation; reduce flow rate if patient complains of burning at infusion site
Evaluate:
• Therapeutic response: decreasing size of tumor, spread of malignancy
Teach patient/family:
• To report any changes in breathing or coughing, avoid smoking
• To avoid foods with citric acid, hot or rough texture if stomatitis is present; to report any bleeding, white spots, ulceration in mouth to prescriber; tell patient to examine mouth qd
• To avoid use of aspirin, ibuprofen, razors, commercial mouthwash
• To report signs of anemia (fatigue, irritability, shortness of breath, faintness); to report signs of infection (sore throat, fever)
• To use contraception during treatment
• Not to receive vaccinations during treatment

carteolol (℞)

(kar-tee'oh-lole)
Cartrol
Func. class.: Antihypertensive, antianginal
Chem. class.: Nonselective β-blocker
See ophthalmics, Appendix C

Action: Produces fall in B/P without reflex tachycardia or significant reduction in heart rate through mixture of α-blocking, β-blocking effects and intrinsic sympathomimetic activity; elevated plasma renins are reduced
Uses: Mild to moderate hypertension, ophthalmic, intraocular, open-angle glaucoma
Dosage and routes:
• *Adult:* **PO** 2.5 mg qd initially, may gradually increase to desired response, max 10 mg/day
Renal dose
• *Adult:* **PO** CCr >60 ml/min give dose q24h; CCr 20-60 ml/min give dose q48h; CCr <20 ml/min give dose q72h
Available forms: Tabs 2.5, 5 mg
Side effects/adverse reactions:
CV: Orthostatic hypotension, ***bradycardia, CHF, chest pain, ventricular dysrhythmias, AV block, peripheral vascular insufficiency,*** palpitations
CNS: Dizziness, mental changes, drowsiness, fatigue, headache, catatonia, depression, anxiety, nightmares, paresthesia, lethargy, insomnia, decreased concentration
GI: Nausea, vomiting, diarrhea, dry mouth, flatulence, constipation, anorexia
INTEG: Rash, alopecia, urticaria, pruritus, fever
HEMA: ***Agranulocytosis, thrombocytopenic purpura (rare)***

EENT: Tinnitus, visual changes, sore throat, double vision, dry, burning eyes
GU: Impotence, dysuria, ejaculatory failure, urinary retention
RESP: ***Bronchospasm,*** dyspnea, wheezing, nasal stuffiness, pharyngitis
MS: Joint pain, arthralgia, muscle cramps, pain
OTHER: Facial swelling, decreased exercise tolerance, weight change, Raynaud's disease, lupus-like syndrome

Contraindications: Hypersensitivity to β-blockers, cardiogenic shock, heart block (2nd or 3rd degree), sinus bradycardia, bronchial asthma

Precautions: Major surgery, pregnancy (C), lactation, CHF, diabetes mellitus, renal disease, thyroid disease, COPD, well-compensated heart failure, nonallergic bronchospasm

Do not confuse:
carteolol/carvedilol

Pharmacokinetics:
PO: Onset 1-2 hr, peak 2-4 hr, duration 8-12 hr, half-life 6-8 hr; metabolized by liver (metabolites inactive); excreted in urine, bile; crosses placenta; excreted in breast milk

Interactions:
- ↓ carteolol effect: thyroid agents
- ↑ myocardial depression: phenytoin (IV), verapamil
- ↑ hypertension: MAOIs, amphetamines
- ↓ CV effect: DOPamine, DOBUTamine
- ↓ antihypertensive effect: NSAIDs
- ↑ hypotension: other antihypertensives, clonidine, nitrates, general anesthetics, alcohol (large amts)
- ↑ hypoglycemic effect: insulin, oral antidiabetics
- ↓ bronchodilating effects of theophylline, β-agonists
- ↑ effect: betel palm, butterbur, cola tree, figwort, fumitory, guarana, hawthorn, jaborandi tree, lily of the valley, motherwort, plantain
- ↓ effect: coenzyme Q10, yohimbe

Lab test interferences:
Increase: ANA titer, blood glucose, BUN, uric acid, potassium, lipoprotein, triglyceride

NURSING CONSIDERATIONS

Assess:
- I&O, weight daily; edema in feet, legs daily, jugular vein distention, dyspnea, rales, crackles
- B/P, pulse q4h; note rate, rhythm, quality; apical/radial pulse before administration; notify prescriber of any significant changes
- Baselines in renal, hepatic studies before therapy begins
- Skin turgor, dryness of mucous membranes for hydration status
- Blood glucose in those taking insulin/oral antidiabetics

Administer:

PO route
- Drug ac, hs; tablet may be crushed or swallowed whole

Perform/provide:
- Storage in dry area at room temperature; do not freeze

Evaluate:
- Therapeutic response: decreased B/P after 1-2 wk

Teach patient/family:
- Not to discontinue drug abruptly; taper over 2 wk or may precipitate hypertension, dysrhythmias, myocardial ischemia
- Not to use OTC products containing α-adrenergic stimulants (nasal decongestants, OTC cold preparations) unless directed by prescriber
- To report bradycardia, dizziness, confusion, depression, fever
- To take pulse, B/P at home, advise when to notify prescriber

• To avoid alcohol, smoking, sodium intake
• To comply with weight control, dietary adjustments, modified exercise program
• To carry emergency ID to identify drug being taken, allergies
• To avoid hazardous activities if dizziness is present
• To report symptoms of CHF: difficulty breathing, especially on exertion or when lying down, night cough, swelling of extremities
• To take medication hs to minimize orthostatic hypotension

Treatment of overdose: Lavage, IV atropine for bradycardia, IV theophylline for bronchospasm, digitalis, O_2, diuretic for cardiac failure; administer vasopressor (norepINEPHrine) for hypotension, isoproterenol for heart block

carteolol ophthalmic

See appendix c

carvedilol (℞)

(kar-ved'i-lole)

Coreg

Func. class.: Antihypertensive, α/β-adrenergic blocker

Action: A mixture of nonselective α/β-adrenergic blocking activity; decreases cardiac output, exercise-induced tachycardia, reflex orthostatic tachycardia; causes vasodilation, reduction in peripheral vascular resistance

Uses: Essential hypertension alone or in combination with other antihypertensives, CHF

Investigational uses: Angina pectoris, idiopathic cardiomyopathy

Dosage and routes:

Essential hypertension

• *Adult:* **PO** 6.25 mg bid × 7-14 days; if tolerated well, then increase to 12.5 mg bid × 7-14 days; if tolerated well, may be increased (if needed) to 25 mg bid; not to exceed 50 mg qd

Congestive heart failure

• *Adult:* **PO** 3.125 mg bid × 2 wk; if tolerated well, give 6.25 mg bid × 2 wk, then double q2wk to max dose, 25 mg bid <85 kg or 50 mg bid >85 kg

Angina pectoris

• *Adult:* **PO** 25-50 mg bid

Idiopathic cardiomyopathy

• *Adult:* **PO** 6.25-25 mg bid

Available forms: Tabs 3.125, 6.25, 12.5, 25 mg

Side effects/adverse reactions:

CNS: Dizziness, fatigue, weakness, somnolence, insomnia, ataxia, hyperesthesia, paresthesia, vertigo, depression

GI: Diarrhea, abdominal pain, increased alk phosphatase, ALT/AST

*CV: **Bradycardia,** postural hypotension,* dependent edema, peripheral edema, ***AV block,*** extrasystoles, hypertension, hypotension, palpitations, peripheral ischemia, ***CHF, pulmonary edema***

GU: Decreased libido, *impotence*

RESP: Rhinitis, pharyngitis, dyspnea

MISC: Fatigue, injury, back pain, UTI, viral infection, hypertriglyceridemia, ***thrombocytopenia,*** *hyperglycemia*

Contraindications: Hypersensitivity, bronchial asthma, class IV decompensated cardiac failure, 2nd- or 3rd-degree heart block, cardiogenic shock, severe bradycardia, pulmonary edema

Precautions: Cardiac failure, hepatic injury, peripheral vascular disease, anesthesia, major surgery, diabetes mellitus, thyrotoxicosis, elderly, pregnancy (C), lactation, children, emphysema, chronic bronchitis, renal disease

Pharmacokinetics: Readily and extensively absorbed PO, >98% protein binding, extensively metabolized by liver, excreted through bile into feces, terminal half-life 7-10 hr with increases in elderly, hepatic disease

Do not confuse:
carvedilol/captopril/carteolol

Interactions:

- ↑ hypoglycemia: antidiabetic agents
- ↓ heart rate, B/P: clonidine
- ↑ concentrations of digoxin
- ↑ toxicity of carvedilol: cimetidine, other antihypertensives, nitrates, acute alcohol ingestion
- ↓ carvedilol levels: rifampin, NSAIDs, thyroid medications
- Conduction disturbances: calcium channel blockers
- Bradycardia, hypotension: MAOIs, reserpine

↑ toxicity/death: aconite

↑ or ↓ antihypertensive effect: astragalus, cola tree

↑ antihypertensive effect: barberry, betony, black catechu, black cohosh, bloodroot, broom, burdock, cat's claw, dandelion, goldenseal, Irish moss, Jamaican dogwood, kelp, khella, mistletoe, parsley

↓ antihypertensive effect: coltsfoot, guarana, khat, licorice

NURSING CONSIDERATIONS

Assess:

Renal studies, including protein, BUN, creatinine; watch for increased levels that may indicate nephrotic syndrome; obtain baselines in renal, hepatic studies before beginning treatment; I&O, weight daily

- Hepatic studies, jaundice; if LFTs are elevated, drug should be discontinued
- B/P during beginning treatment, periodically thereafter; pulse q4h, note rate, rhythm, quality; apical/radial pulse before administration; notify prescriber of significant changes
- Edema in feet, legs daily, fluid overload: dyspnea, weight gain, jugular vein distention, fatigue, rales, crackles

Administer:

PO route

- Pulse: if <50 bpm, hold drug, call prescriber
- Drug ac, hs; tablets may be crushed or swallowed whole
- Reduced dosage in renal dysfunction; may give with food

Evaluate:

- Therapeutic response: decreased B/P in hypertension

Teach patient/family:

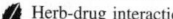

- To comply with dosage schedule, even if feeling better, that improvement may take several wk
- To rise slowly to sitting or standing position to minimize orthostatic hypotension
- To report bradycardia, dizziness, confusion, depression, fever, weight gain, SOB, cold extremities, rash, sore throat, bleeding, or bruising
- To take pulse, B/P at home; advise when to notify prescriber
- Not to discontinue drug abruptly, taper over 1-2 wk
- To avoid hazardous activities until stabilized on medication; dizziness may occur
- To avoid all OTC medications unless approved by prescriber
- To carry emergency ID with drug name, prescriber at all times
- To inform all health care providers of drugs, supplements taken

cascara sagrada/ cascara sagrada aromatic fluid extract/ cascara sagrada fluid extract (OTC)

(kas-kar′a)

Func. class.: Laxative

Chem. class.: Anthraquinone

Action: Direct chemical irritation in colon; increases propulsion of stool

Uses: Constipation; bowel or rectal preparation for surgery or examination

Dosage and routes:

- *Adult:* **PO** 325 mg hs; **FLUID** 1 ml qd; **AROMATIC FLUID** 5 ml qd
- *Child 2-12 yr:* **PO/FLUID/AROMATIC FLUID** ½ adult dose
- *Child <2 yr:* **PO/FLUID/AROMATIC FLUID** ¼ adult dose

Available forms: Tabs 325 mg; fluid extract 1 g/ml; aromatic fluid extract 1 g/ml

Side effects/adverse reactions:

GI: Nausea, vomiting, anorexia, cramps, diarrhea

META: Hypocalcemia, enteropathy, alkalosis, hypokalemia, ***tetany***

Contraindications: Hypersensitivity, GI bleeding, obstruction, CHF, lactation, abdominal pain, nausea/vomiting, appendicitis, acute surgical abdomen, alcoholics (aromatic form)

Precautions: Pregnancy (C)

Pharmacokinetics:

PO: Peak 6-12 hr; metabolized by liver; excreted in urine, feces, breast milk

Interactions:

- ↓ absorption of: antibiotics, digitalis, nitrofurantoin, salicylates, tetracyclines, oral anticoagulants

↑ action/side effects: flax, lily of the valley, pheasant's eye, senna, squill

NURSING CONSIDERATIONS

Assess:

- Monitor blood, urine electrolytes if drug is used often by patient; check I&O ratio to identify fluid loss
- Cause of constipation; identify whether fluids, bulk, or exercise missing from lifestyle
- Cramping, rectal bleeding, nausea, vomiting; if these symptoms occur, drug should be discontinued

Administer:

- Alone for better absorption; do not take within 1 hr of other drugs or within 1 hr of antacids, milk
- In morning or evening (oral dose)

Evaluate:

- Therapeutic response: decrease in constipation

Teach patient/family:

⊘ To swallow tabs whole; do not break, crush, or chew

- Not to use laxatives for long-term therapy; bowel tone will be lost
- That normal bowel movements do not always occur daily
- Not to use in presence of abdominal pain, nausea, vomiting
- To notify prescriber if constipation unrelieved or of symptoms of electrolyte imbalance: muscle cramps, pain, weakness, dizziness

cefaclor
See cephalosporins—2nd generation

cefadroxil
cefazolin
See cephalosporins—1st generation

cefdinir
See cephalosporins—3rd generation

cefditoren
See cephalosporins—2nd generation

cefepime
cefixime
See cephalosporins—3rd generation

cefamandole
cefmetazole
cefonicid
See cephalosporins—2nd generation

cefoperazone
cefotaxime
See cephalosporins—3rd generation

cefotetan
cefoxitin
See cephalosporins—2nd generation

cefpodoxime
See cephalosporins—3rd generation

cefprozil
See cephalosporins—2nd generation

ceftazidime
ceftibuten
ceftizoxime
ceftriaxone
See cephalosporins—3rd generation

cefuroxime
See cephalosporins—2nd generation

celecoxib (℞)

(sel-eh-cox′ib)
Celebrex
Func. class.: Nonsteroidal anti-inflammatory, antirheumatic
Chem. class.: COX-2 inhibitor

Action: Inhibits prostaglandin synthesis by decreasing enzyme needed for biosynthesis; analgesic, antiinflammatory, antipyretic properties
Uses: Acute, chronic rheumatoid arthritis, osteoarthritis, familial adenomatous polyposis (FAP), acute pain, primary dysmenorrhea
Investigational uses: Colorectal polyps
Dosage and routes:
Acute pain/primary dysmenorrhea
• *Adult:* **PO** 400 mg initially, then 200 mg if needed on first day, then 200 mg bid prn on subsequent days
Osteoarthritis
• *Adult:* **PO** 200 mg/day as a single dose or 100 mg bid
Rheumatoid arthritis
• *Adult:* **PO** 100-200 mg bid
Familial adenomatous polyposis (FAP)
• *Adult:* **PO** 400 mg bid
Colorectal polyps
• *Adult:* **PO** 400 mg bid × 6 mo
Hepatic disease (Child-Pugh class II)
• *Adult:* **PO** reduce dose by 50%
Available forms: Caps 100, 200 mg
Side effects/adverse reactions:
CNS: Fatigue, anxiety, depression, nervousness, paresthesia, dizziness, insomnia
CV: ***Tachycardia,*** angina, ***MI,*** palpitations, dysrhythmias, hypertension, fluid retention
EENT: Tinnitus, hearing loss, blurred vision, glaucoma, cataract, conjunctivitis, eye pain
GI: Nausea, anorexia, vomiting, con-

stipation, dry mouth, diverticulitis, gastritis, gastroenteritis, hemorrhoids, hiatal hernia, stomatitis, ***GI bleeding***
GU: ***Nephrotoxicity:*** *dysuria,* ***hematuria, oliguria, azotemia,*** cystitis, UTI
HEMA: ***Blood dyscrasias,*** epistaxis, bruising, anemia
INTEG: Purpura, rash, pruritus, sweating, erythema, petechiae, photosensitivity, alopecia
RESP: Pharyngitis, shortness of breath, pneumonia, coughing
Contraindications: Hypersensitivity to aspirin, iodides, other NSAIDs, sulfonamides, 3rd trimester of pregnancy, asthma triad, asthma
Precautions: Pregnancy 1st/2nd trimester (C), 3rd trimester (D), lactation, bleeding, GI, cardiac, renal, hepatic, disorders, hypersensitivity to other antiinflammatory agents, glucocorticoids, anticoagulants, geriatrics, hypertension, severe dehydration, children <18 yr
Do not confuse:
Celebrex/Celexa/Cerebra/Cerebyx
Pharmacokinetics: Well absorbed, crosses placenta, bound to plasma proteins, metabolized in liver, excreted by kidneys, peak 3 hr
Interactions:
- ↑ effect of: anticoagulants
- ↓ effect of: aspirin, ACE inhibitors, thiazide diuretics, furosemide
- ↑ adverse reactions: glucocorticoids, NSAIDs, aspirin
- ↑ toxicity: lithium, anti-neoplastics
- ↑ celecoxib blood level: fluconazole

↑ celecoxib effect: bearberry, bilberry
↑ gastric irritation: arginine, gossypol
↑ bleeding risk: bogbean, saw palmetto, turmeric
Severe photosensitivity: St. John's wort

NURSING CONSIDERATIONS
Assess:
- For pain of rheumatoid arthritis, osteoarthritis; check ROM, inflammation of joints, characteristics of pain
- FAP clients for decreasing number of polyps
- Blood counts during therapy; watch for decreasing platelets; if low, therapy may need to be discontinued, restarted after hematologic recovery

For blood dyscrasias (thrombocytopenia): bruising, fatigue, bleeding, poor healing
Administer:
PO route
- With food or milk to decrease gastric symptoms, do not increase dose

Do not crush, dissolve, or chew caps
Evaluate:
- Therapeutic response: decreased pain, inflammation in arthritic conditions; decreased number of polyps

Teach patient/family:
- To check with prescriber to determine when drug should be discontinued prior to surgery
- That drug must be continued for prescribed time to be effective; to avoid other NSAIDs, aspirin, sulfonamides
- To notify prescriber if pregnancy is planned or suspected

To notify prescriber of GI symptoms: black, tarry stools; cramping or rash; edema of extremities, weight gain
To report bleeding, bruising, fatigue, malaise since blood dyscrasias do occur
To take with a full glass of water to enhance absorption; do not crush, break, or chew

cephalexin

See cephalosporins—1st generation

CEPHALOSPORINS—1ST GENERATION

cefadroxil (℞)
(sef-a-drox'ill)
cefadroxil, Duricef

cefazolin (℞)
(sef-a'zoe-lin)
Ancef, cefazolin, Kefzol

cephalexin (℞)
(sef-a-lex'in)
Apo-Cephalex♣, Biocef, cephalexin, Keflex, Keftab, Novo-Lexin♣, Nu-Cephalex♣

cephapirin (℞)
(sef-a-pye'rin)
Cefadyl, cephapirin

cephradine (℞)
(sef'ra-deen)
cephradine, Velosef

Func. class.: Antiinfective
Chem. class.: Cephalosporin (1st generation)

Action: Inhibits bacterial cell wall synthesis, rendering cell wall osmotically unstable, leading to cell death by binding to cell wall membrane

Uses:
cefadroxil: Gram-negative bacilli: *Escherichia coli, Proteus mirabilis, Klebsiella* (UTI only); gram-positive organisms: *Streptococcus pneumoniae, Streptococcus pyogenes, Staphylococcus aureus;* upper, lower respiratory tract, urinary tract, skin infections, otitis media; tonsillitis; and UTIs
cefazolin: Gram-negative bacilli: *Haemophilus influenzae, Escherichia coli, Proteus mirabilis, Klebsiella;* gram-positive organisms: *Staphylococcus aureus;* upper, lower respiratory tract, urinary tract, skin infections, bone, joint, biliary, genital infections, endocarditis, surgical prophylaxis, septicemia
cephalexin: Gram-negative bacilli: *Haemophilus influenzae, Escherichia coli, Proteus mirabilis, Klebsiella;* gram-positive organisms: *Streptococcus pneumoniae, Streptococcus pyogenes, Staphylococcus aureus;* upper, lower respiratory tract, urinary tract, skin, bone infections, otitis media
cephapirin: Gram-negative bacilli: *Haemophilus influenzae, Escherichia coli, Proteus mirabilis, Klebsiella;* gram-positive organisms: *Streptococcus pneumoniae, Streptococcus viridans, Staphylococcus aureus;* lower respiratory tract, skin infections, endocarditis, bacterial peritonitis
cephradine: Gram-negative bacilli: *Haemophilus influenzae, Escherichia coli, Proteus mirabilis, Klebsiella;* gram-positive organisms: *Streptococcus pneumoniae, Streptococcus pyogenes, Staphylococcus aureus;* serious respiratory tract, skin infections, urinary tract infections, otitis media

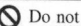

Dosage and routes:
cefadroxil
• *Adult:* **PO** 1-2 g qd or q12h in divided doses, give a loading dose of 1 g initially
• *Child:* **PO** 30 mg/kg/day in divided doses bid
Renal dose: CCr 25-50 ml/min 500 mg q12h; CCr 10-24 ml/min 500 mg q24h; CCr <10 ml/min 500 mg q36h
Available forms: Caps 500 mg; tabs 1 g; oral susp 125, 250, 500 mg/5 ml
cefazolin
Life-threatening infections
• *Adult:* **IM/IV** 1-2 g q6h

• *Child >1 mo:* **IM/IV** 100 mg/kg in 3-4 divided doses
Mild/moderate infections
• *Adult:* **IM/IV** 250 mg-1 g q8h
• *Child >1 mo:* **IM/IV** 25-50 mg/kg in 3-4 equal doses
Renal dose: CCr 35-54 ml/min: 250-1000 mg q12h; CCr 10-34 ml/min: 50% of dose q12h; CCr <10 ml/min: 50% of dose q18-24h
Available forms: Inj 250, 500 mg, 1, 5, 10, 20 g; infusion 500 mg, 1 g/50 ml vial
cephalexin
Moderate infections
• *Adult:* **PO** 250-500 mg q6h
• *Child:* **PO** 25-50 mg/kg/day in 4 equal doses
Moderate skin infections
• *Adult:* **PO** 500 mg q12h
Endocarditis prophylaxis
• 2 g 1 hr before procedure
Severe infections
• *Adult:* **PO** 500 mg-1 g q6h
• *Child:* **PO** 50-100 mg/kg/day in 4 equal doses
Renal dose: CCr <40 ml/min give q8-12h; CCr 5-10 ml/min give q12h; CCr <5 ml/min give q24h
Available forms: Caps 250, 500 mg; tabs 250, 500 mg, 1 g; oral susp 125, 250 mg/5ml
cephapirin
• *Adult:* **IM/IV** 500 mg-1 g q4-6h
• *Child:* **IM/IV** 40-80 mg/kg/day in divided doses q6h or 10-20 mg/kg q6h
Renal dose: CCr <10 ml/min give q12h
Available forms: Powder for inj 500 mg, 1, 2, 20 g; IV only 1, 2, 4 g
cephradine
• *Adult:* **PO** 250 mg-1 g q6-12h
• *Child >1 yr:* **PO** 6-12 mg/kg q6h
Renal dose: CCr >20 ml/min 500 mg q6h; CCr 5-20 ml/min 250 mg q6h
Available forms: Caps 250, 500 mg; oral susp 125, 250 mg/5ml

Side effects/adverse reactions:
CNS: Headache, dizziness, weakness, paresthesia, fever, chills, ***seizures*** (high doses)
GI: Nausea, vomiting, *diarrhea, anorexia,* pain, glossitis, bleeding; increased AST, ALT, bilirubin, LDH, alk phosphatase; abdominal pain, ***pseudomembranous colitis***
GU: Proteinuria, vaginitis, pruritus, candidiasis, increased BUN, ***nephrotoxicity, renal failure***
HEMA: ***Leukopenia, thrombocytopenia, agranulocytosis,*** anemia, ***neutropenia, lymphocytosis, eosinophilia, pancytopenia, hemolytic anemia***
INTEG: Rash, urticaria, dermatitis
SYST: ***Anaphylaxis, serum sickness,*** superinfection
RESP: Dyspnea
Contraindications: Hypersensitivity to cephalosporins, infants <1 mo
Precautions: Hypersensitivity to penicillins, pregnancy (B), lactation, renal disease
Do not confuse:
cephalexin/cefaclor
cephapirin/cephradine
Kefzol/Cefzil
Pharmacokinetics:
cefadroxil: Peak 1-1½ hr, duration 12-24 hr, half-life 1-2 hr; 20% bound by plasma proteins; crosses placenta; excreted in breast milk
cefazolin
IM: Peak ½-2 hr, duration 6-12 hr, half-life 1½-2¼ hr
IV: Peak 10 min, duration 6-12 hr; eliminated unchanged in urine; 70%-86% protein bound
cephalexin: Peak 1 hr, duration 6-12 hr, half-life 30-72 min; 5%-15% bound by plasma proteins; 90%-100% eliminated unchanged in urine; crosses placenta; excreted in breast milk
cephapirin
IV: Peak 5 min, duration 4-6 hr

IM: Peak 30 min, duration 4-6 hr
Half-life 21-47 min; 44%-50% bound by plasma proteins; 40%-70% eliminated unchanged in urine; crosses placenta; excreted in breast milk; metabolized in liver
cephradine: Peak 1-2 hr, duration 6-12 hr, half-life 0.75-1.5 hr; 20% bound by plasma proteins; 80%-90% eliminated unchanged in urine; crosses placenta; excreted in breast milk

Interactions:
- ↑ toxicity: aminoglycosides, loop diuretics, probenecid

Do not use acidophilus with anti-infectives

Lab test interferences:
Increase: AST, ALT, alk phosphatase, LDH, BUN, creatinine, bilirubin
False positive: Urinary protein, direct Coombs' test, urine glucose
Interference: Cross-matching

NURSING CONSIDERATIONS

Assess:
- Sensitivity to penicillin and other cephalosporins

Nephrotoxicity: increased BUN, creatinine
- I&O daily
- Blood studies: AST, ALT, CBC, Hct, bilirubin, LDH, alk phosphatase, Coombs' test monthly if patient is on long-term therapy
- Electrolytes: K, Na, Cl monthly if patient is on long-term therapy
- Bowel pattern qd; if severe diarrhea occurs, drug should be discontinued; may indicate pseudomembranous colitis
- Urine output: if decreasing, notify prescriber; may indicate nephrotoxicity

Anaphylaxis: rash, urticaria, pruritus, chills, fever, joint pain; angioedema; may occur few days after therapy begins; discontinue drug, notify prescriber immediately, keep emergency equipment nearby
- Bleeding: ecchymosis, bleeding gums, hematuria, stool guaiac daily

Overgrowth of infection: perineal itching, fever, malaise, redness, pain, swelling, drainage, rash, diarrhea, change in cough, sputum

Administer:

cefadroxil
- For 10-14 days to ensure organism death, prevent superinfection
- With food if needed for GI symptoms
- Shake susp, refrigerate, discard after 2 wk
- After C&S completed

cefazolin
- IV; check for irritation, extravasation often; dilute in 10 ml sterile H_2O for inj and run over 3-5 min; may be further diluted with 50-100 ml of NS, D_5W sol and run over ½-1 hr by Y-tube or 3-way stopcock
- For 10-14 days to ensure organism death, prevent superinfection
- After C&S completed

Additive compatibilities: Aztreonam, clindamycin, famotidine, fluconazole, metronidazole, verapamil
Syringe compatibilities: Heparin, vit B
Y-site compatibilities: Acyclovir, allopurinol, amifostine, atracurium, aztreonam, calcium gluconate, cyclophosphamide, diltiazem, DOXOrubicin liposome, enalaprilat, esmolol, famotidine, filgrastim, fluconazole, fludarabine, foscarnet, heparin, hydromorphone, insulin (regular), labetalol, lidocaine, magnesium sulfate, melphalan, meperidine, midazolam, morphine, multivitamins, ondansetron, perphenazine, pancuronium, remifentanil, sargramostim, tacrolimus, teniposide, theophylline, thiotepa, vecuronium, vit B/C, warfarin

cephalexin
• Shake susp, refrigerate, discard after 2 wk
• For 10-14 days to ensure organism death, prevent superinfection
• With food if needed for GI symptoms
• After C&S

cephapirin
• IV after diluting 1 g or less/10 ml or more NS, D_5W, or bacteriostatic H_2O for inj; give 1 g or less/5 min or more; may be further diluted in 50-100 ml of D_5W, NS; run over 15 min; discontinue primary IV during administration; may also be given by continuous infusion, store refrigerated 96 hr, room temperature 24 hr
• For 10-14 days to ensure organism death, prevent superinfection
• After C&S

Additive compatibilities: Bleomycin, calcium chloride, calcium gluconate, chloramphenicol, diphenhydrAMINE, ergonovine, heparin, hydrocortisone, metaraminol, oxacillin, penicillin G potassium, pentobarbital, phenobarbital, phytonadione, potassium chloride, sodium bicarbonate, succinylcholine, verapamil, vit B, warfarin

Y-site compatibilities: Acyclovir, cyclophosphamide, famotidine, heparin, hydrocortisone, hydromorphone, magnesium sulfate, meperidine, morphine, multivitamins, perphenazine, potassium chloride, vit B/C

cephradine
• Shake suspension well before each dose
• For 10-14 days to ensure organism death, prevent superinfection
• With food if needed for GI symptoms
• After C&S

Evaluate:
• Therapeutic response: decreased symptoms of infection, negative C&S

Teach patient/family:
• Not to drink alcohol or use meds with alcohol: reaction may occur
• To use yogurt or buttermilk to maintain intestinal flora, decrease diarrhea
• To take all medication prescribed for length of time ordered
◆ To report sore throat, bruising, bleeding, joint pain (may indicate blood dyscrasias [rare]); diarrhea with mucus, blood, may indicate pseudomembranous colitis

Treatment of anaphylaxis: EpINEPHrine, antihistamines; resuscitate if needed

CEPHALOSPORINS—2ND GENERATION

cefaclor (℞)
(sef'a-klor)
Ceclor
cefamandole (℞)
(sef-a-man'dole)
Mandol
cefditoren pivoxil (℞)
(sef-dit'oh-ren pih-vox'il)
Spectracef
cefmetazole (℞)
(sef-met'a-zole)
Zefazone
cefonicid (℞)
(se-fon'i-sid)
Monocid
cefotetan (℞)
(sef'oh-tee-tan)
Cefotan
cefoxitin (℞)
(se-fox'i-tin)
Mefoxin
cefprozil (℞)
(sef-proe'zill)
Cefzil
cefuroxime (℞)
(sef-yoor-ox'eem)
Ceftin, cefuroxime, Kefurox, Zinacef
loracarbef (℞)
(lor-a-kar'beff)
Lorabid
Func. class.: Antiinfective
Chem. class.: Cephalosporin (2nd generation)

Action: Inhibits bacterial cell wall synthesis, rendering cell wall osmotically unstable, leading to cell death by binding to cell wall membrane

Uses:
cefaclor: Gram-negative bacilli: *Haemophilus influenzae, Escherichia coli, Proteus mirabilis, Klebsiella;* gram-positive organisms: *Streptococcus pneumoniae, Streptococcus pyogenes, Staphylococcus aureus;* respiratory tract, urinary tract, skin, bone, joint infections, otitis media
cefamandole: Gram-negative bacilli: *Haemophilus influenzae, Escherichia coli, Proteus mirabilis, Klebsiella;* gram-positive organisms: *Streptococcus pneumoniae, Streptococcus pyogenes, Staphylococcus aureus;* upper, lower respiratory tract, urinary tract, skin infections, peritonitis, septicemia, surgical prophylaxis
cefditoren pivoxil: Acute bacterial exacerbation of chronic bronchitis caused by *Haemophilus influenzae, Haemophilus parainfluenzae, Streptococcus pneumoniae, Moraxella catarrhalis*; pharyngitis/tonsillitis caused by *Streptococcus pyogenes*; uncomplicated skin and skin structure infections caused by *Staphylococcus aureus, S. pyogenes*
cefmetazole: Gram-negative bacilli: *Haemophilus influenzae, Escherichia coli, Proteus, Klebsiella, Bacteroides fragilis;* gram-positive organisms: *Streptococcus pneumoniae, Streptococcus pyogenes, Staphylococcus aureus;* anaerobes, including *Clostridium;* infections of lower respiratory tract, urinary tract, skin, bone, intraabdominal infections
cefonicid: Gram-negative bacilli: *Haemophilus influenzae, Escherichia coli, Proteus mirabilis, Klebsiella;* gram-positive organisms: *Streptococcus pneumoniae, Streptococcus pyogenes, Staphylococcus aureus;* lower respiratory tract, urinary tract, skin infections, otitis media, peritonitis, septicemia
cefotetan: Gram-negative organisms: *Haemophilus influenzae, Esch-*

erichia coli, Enterobacter aerogenes, Proteus mirabilis, Klebsiella, Citrobacter, Enterobacter, Salmonella, Shigella, Acinetobacter, Bacteroides fragilis, Neisseria, Serratia; gram-positive organisms: *Streptococcus pneumoniae, Streptococcus pyogenes, Staphylococcus aureus;* upper, lower, serious respiratory tract, urinary tract, skin, bone, joint, gynecologic, gonococcal, intraabdominal infections

cefoxitin: Gram-negative bacilli: *Haemophilus influenzae, Escherichia coli, Proteus, Klebsiella, Bacteroides fragilis, Neisseria gonorrhoeae;* gram-positive organisms: *Streptococcus pneumoniae, Streptococcus pyogenes, Staphylococcus aureus;* anaerobes including *Clostridium,* lower respiratory tract, urinary tract, skin, bone, gynecologic, gonococcal infections, septicemia, peritonitis

cefprozil: Pharyngitis/tonsillitis, otitis media, secondary bacterial infection of acute bronchitis, and acute bacterial exacerbation of chronic bronchitis and uncomplicated skin and skin structure infections; acute sinusitis

cefuroxime: Gram-negative bacilli: *Haemophilus influenzae, Escherichia coli, Neisseria, Proteus mirabilis, Klebsiella;* gram-positive organisms: *Streptococcus pneumoniae, Streptococcus pyogenes, Staphylococcus aureus;* serious lower respiratory tract, urinary tract, skin, bone, joint, gonococcal infections, septicemia, meningitis

loracarbef: Gram-negative bacilli: *Haemophilus influenzae, Escherichia coli, Proteus mirabilis, Klebsiella;* gram-positive organisms: *Streptococcus pneumoniae, Streptococcus pyogenes, Staphylococcus aureus;* upper and lower respiratory tract, urinary tract, skin infections, otitis media, pharyngitis, tonsillitis

Dosage and routes:

cefaclor

• *Adult:* **PO** 250-500 mg q8h, not to exceed 4 g/day or 375-500 mg (ext rel) q12h × 7-10 days

• *Child >1 mo:* **PO** 20-40 mg/kg qd in divided doses q8h, or total daily dose may be divided and given q12h, not to exceed 1 g/day

Acute bacterial exacerbations of chronic bronchitis or acute bronchitis

• *Adult:* 500 mg/12 hr × 1 wk (ext rel)

Pharyngitis/tonsillitis

• *Adult:* 375 mg/12 hr × 10 days (ext rel)

Available forms: Caps 250, 500 mg; oral susp 125, 187, 250, 375 mg/5 ml; tabs, ext rel 375, 500 mg

cefamandole

• *Adult:* **IM/IV** 500 mg-1 g q4-8h; may give up to 2 g q4h for severe infections

• *Child >1 mo:* **IM/IV** 8.3-16.7 mg/kg q4h, not to exceed adult dose

• Dosage reduction indicated in renal impairment (CCr <50 ml/min)

Available forms: Inj 1, 2, 10 g

cefditoren pivoxil

Acute bacterial exacerbation of chronic bronchitis

• *Adult:* **PO** 400 mg bid × 10 days

Pharyngitis/tonsillitis

• *Adult:* **PO** 200 mg bid × 10 days

Uncomplicated skin and skin structure infections

• *Adult:* **PO** 200 mg bid × 10 days

Renal dose

• CCr 30-49 ml/min give ≤200 mg bid × 10 days

• CCr <30 ml/min give 200 mg qd × 10 days

Available form: Tabs 200 mg

cefmetazole

Renal dose: CCr <50 ml/min 1-2 g

q12h; CCr 10-29 ml/min 1-2 g q24h; CCr <10 ml/min 1-2 g q48h

• *Adult:* **IV** 2 g divided q6-12h × 5-14 days

Available forms: Powder for inj 1, 2 g/vial

cefonicid

Life-threatening infections

• *Adult:* **IM/IV BOL** or **INF** 0.5-2 g/24 hr; divide in two doses if giving 2 g

• Dosage reduction indicated in renal impairment

Available forms: Inj 500 mg, 1, 10 g

cefotetan

Renal dose: CCr 10-30 ml/min give q24h; CCr <10 ml/min give q48h

• *Adult:* **IV/IM** 1-2 g q12h × 5-10 days

Perioperative prophylaxis

• *Adult:* **IV** 1-2 g ½-1 hr before surgery

Available forms: Inj 1, 2, 10 g

cefoxitin

Renal dose: CCr <50 ml/min give q8-12h; CCr 10-29 ml/min give q24h; CCr <10 ml/min give q24-48h

• *Adult:* **IM/IV** 1-2 g q6-8h

• Dosage reduction indicated in renal impairment (CCr <50 ml/min)

Uncomplicated gonorrhea: 2 g IM as single dose with 1 g **PO** probenecid at same time

Severe infections

• *Adult:* **IM/IV** 2 g q4h

• *Child ≥3 mo:* **IM/IV** 80-160 mg/kg/day divided q4-6h; max 12 g/day

Available forms: Powder for inj 1, 2, 10 g

cefprozil

Renal dose: CCr <30 ml/min 50% of dose

Upper respiratory infections

• *Adult:* **PO** 500 mg q24h × 10 days

Otitis media

• *Child 6 mo-12 yr:* **PO** 15 mg/kg q12h × 10 days

Lower respiratory infections

• *Adult:* **PO** 500 mg q12h × 10 days

Skin/skin structure infections

• *Adult:* **PO** 250-500 mg q12h × 10 days

Available forms: Tabs 250, 500 mg; susp 125, 250 mg/5 ml

cefuroxime

• *Adult and child:* **PO** 250 mg q12h; may increase to 500 mg q12h in serious infections

• *Adult:* **IM/IV** 750 mg-1.5 g q8h for 5-10 days

Urinary tract infections

• *Adult:* **PO** 125 mg q12h; may increase to 250 mg q12h if needed

Otitis media

• *Child <2 yr:* **PO** 125 mg bid

• *Child >2 yr:* **PO** 250 mg bid

Surgical prophylaxis

• *Adult:* **IV** 1.5 g ½-1 hr preop

Severe infections

• *Adult:* **IM/IV** 1.5 g q6h; may give up to 3 g q8h for bacterial meningitis

• *Child >3 mo:* **IM/IV** 50-100 mg/kg/day; may give up to 200-240 mg/kg/day **IV** in divided doses for bacterial meningitis (not recommended)

• Dosage reduction indicated in severe renal impairment (CCr <20 ml/min)

Uncomplicated gonorrhea

• *Adult:* 1.5 g **IM** as single dose with oral probenecid in 2 separate sites

Available forms: Tabs 125, 250, 500 mg; inj 150, 750 mg, 1.5, 7.5 g; inj 750 mg; 1.5 g powder; susp 125, 250 mg/5 ml

loracarbef

Renal dose: CCr 10-49 ml/min 50% of dose; CCr <10 ml/min q3-5 days

• *Adult and child >13:* **PO** 200-400 mg q12h

• *Child <12 yr:* **PO** 15-30 mg/kg/day in 2 divided doses q12h

Available forms: Caps 200, 400 mg; 100, 200 mg/5 ml oral susp

Side effects/adverse reactions:
CNS: Dizziness, headache, fatigue, paresthesia, fever, chills, confusion
GI: Diarrhea, nausea, vomiting, anorexia, dysgeusia, glossitis, bleeding; increased AST, ALT, bilirubin, LDH, alk phosphatase; abdominal pain, loose stools, flatulence, heartburn, stomach cramps, colitis, jaundice, ***pseudomembranous colitis***
INTEG: Rash, urticaria, dermatitis, ***Stevens-Johnson syndrome***
GU: Vaginitis, pruritus, candidiasis, increased BUN, ***nephrotoxicity, renal failure,*** pyuria, dysuria, reversible interstitial nephritis
HEMA: ***Leukopenia, thrombocytopenia, agranulocytosis,*** anemia, ***neutropenia, lymphocytosis, eosinophilia, pancytopenia, hemolytic anemia, leukocytosis, granulocytopenia***
RESP: Dyspnea
SYST: ***Anaphylaxis, serum sickness,*** superinfection
Contraindications: Hypersensitivity to cephalosporins or related antibiotics, seizures
Precautions: Pregnancy (B), lactation, children, renal disease
Do not confuse:
cefaclor/cephalexin
Cefotan/Ceftin
cefprozil/Cefazolin
cefprozil/cefuroxime
Cefzil/Ceftin
Cefzil/Kefzol
Pharmacokinetics:
cefaclor:
PO: Peak ½-1 hr, ext rel peak 1½-2½ hr, half-life 36-54 min; 25% bound by plasma proteins; 60%-85% eliminated unchanged in urine in 8 hr; crosses placenta; excreted in breast milk (low concentrations)
cefamandole: Peak 1-1½ hr, half-life ½-1 hr; 60%-75% bound by plasma proteins; crosses placenta; excreted in breast milk; poor penetration into CSF
cefditoren pivoxil: Peak 1-1½ hr, half-life ½-1 hr; 60%-75% bound by plasma proteins; crosses placenta; excreted in breast milk; poor penetration into CSF
cefmetazole
IM: Peak 30-45 min; 68% bound by plasma proteins, excreted by kidneys; half-life 1-3 hr
cefonicid
IV: Onset 5 min
IM: Peak 1 hr
Half-life 4½ hr; excreted in breast milk (small amounts); 98% protein bound; poor penetration in CSF
cefotetan
IV/IM: Peak 1½-3 hr; half-life 3-5 hr, 70%-90% bound by plasma proteins, 50%-80% eliminated unchanged in urine, crosses placenta, excreted in breast milk
cefoxitin
IV: Peak 3 min
IM: Peak 15-60 min
Half-life 1 hr, 55%-75% bound by plasma proteins, 90%-100% eliminated unchanged in urine; crosses placenta, blood-brain barrier; eliminated in breast milk, not metabolized
cefprozil
PO: Peak 6-10 hr; plasma protein binding 99%; elimination half-life 25 hr; extensively metabolized to an active metabolite
cefuroxime: 65% excreted unchanged in urine, half-life 1-2 hr in normal renal function
loracarbef
PO: Peak 1 hr, half-life 1 hr; excreted in urine as unchanged drug
Interactions:
• Bleeding (cefamandole, cefmetazole, cefotetan) anticoagulants, thrombolytics, NSAIDs, antiplatelets, plicamycin, valproic acid

• ↑ effect/toxicity: aminoglycosides, furosemide, probenecid
• Disulfiram-like reaction: alcohol
Bleeding may occur (cefamandole, cefmetazole, cefotetan): angelica, anise, arnica, bogbean, boldo, celery, chamomile, clove, fenugreek, feverfew, garlic, ginger, ginkgo, ginseng *(Panax),* horse chestnut, horseradish, licorice, meadowsweet, prickly ash, onion, papain, passion flower, poplar, red clover, turmeric, willow
Do not use acidophilus with anti-infectives

Lab test interferences:
False increase: Creatinine (serum urine), urinary 17-KS
False positive: Urinary protein, direct Coombs' test, urine glucose testing (Clinitest)
Interference: Cross-matching

NURSING CONSIDERATIONS

Assess:
Nephrotoxicity: increased BUN, creatinine
• I&O ratio
• Blood studies: AST, ALT, CBC, Hct, bilirubin, LDH, alk phosphatase, Coombs' test qmo if patient is on long-term therapy
• Electrolytes: K, Na, Cl qmo if patient is on long-term therapy
• Bowel pattern qd; if severe diarrhea occurs, drug should be discontinued; may indicate pseudomembranous colitis
• Urine output; if decreasing, notify prescriber (may indicate nephrotoxicity)
Anaphylaxis: rash, flushing, urticaria, pruritus, dyspnea, discontinue drug, notify prescriber, have emergency equipment available
• Bleeding: ecchymosis, bleeding gums, hematuria, stool guaiac daily
Overgrowth of infection: perineal itching, fever, malaise, redness, pain, swelling, drainage, rash, diarrhea, change in cough, sputum

Administer:
cefaclor
• Shake susp, refrigerate, discard after 2 wk
• For 10-14 days to ensure organism death, prevent superinfection
• With food if needed for GI symptoms
• After C&S completed
Do not break, crush, or chew ext rel tabs

cefamandole
• IV; check often for irritation, extravasation; dilute 1 g or less of drug/10 ml or more normal saline or sterile H_2O for inj; run over 3-5 min; may be further diluted with 100 ml of compatible sol and run over 15-30 min via Y-tube or 3-way stopcock; may also be diluted in 1 L compatible sol, run over prescribed rate
• For 10-14 days to ensure organism death, prevent superinfection
• After C&S completed

Additive compatibilities: Clindamycin, floxacillin, furosemide, metronidazole, verapamil
Syringe compatibilities: Heparin
Y-site compatibilities: Acyclovir, cyclophosphamide, hydromorphone, magnesium sulfate, meperidine, morphine, perphenazine

cefditoren pivoxil
• For 10 days to ensure organism death, prevent superinfection
• With food if needed for GI symptoms
• After C&S completed

cefmetazole
• For 10-14 days to ensure organism death, prevent superinfection
• After C&S completed

Solution compatibilities: D_5W, 0.9% NaCl
Additive compatibilities: Clindamycin, famotidine, KCl

• IV after diluting 3.7 or 10 ml sterile H_2O for inj, 2 g/7 or 15 ml, shake, let stand until clear, run over 3-5 min; may be further diluted in 50-100 ml of D_5W, NS, LR to 1-20 mg/ml and run over ½-1 hr by Y-tube or 3-way stopcock

cefonicid

• IV direct dilute 0.5 g/2 ml or 1 g/2.5 ml sterile H_2O for inj and give by Y-tube or 3-way stopcock over 3-5 min

• IV Intermittent INF may be further diluted in 50-100 ml D_5W, NS and given over 30 min; slight yellowing of sol does not affect potency

• IV; check for irritation, extravasation often

Additive compatibilities: Clindamycin

Y-site compatibilities: Acyclovir, amifostine, aztreonam, teniposide, thiotepa

cefotetan

• IV direct after diluting 1 g/10 ml sterile H_2O for inj and give over 3-5 min; may be diluted further with 50-100 ml of normal saline or D_5W, shake; run over ½-1 hr by Y-tube or 3-way stopcock; discontinue primary inf during administration

• May be stored 96 hr refrigerated or 24 hr room temperature

Y-site compatibilities: Allopurinol, amifostine, aztreonam, diltiazem, famotidine, filgrastim, fluconazole, fludarabine, heparin, insulin (regular), melphalan, meperidine, morphine, paclitaxel, remifentanil, sargramostim, tacrolimus, teniposide, theophylline, thiotepa

cefoxitin

• IV after diluting 1 g or less/10 ml or more D_5W, NS and give over 3-5 min; may be diluted further with 50-100 ml of normal saline or D_5W; run over ½-1 hr by Y-tube or 3-way stopcock; discontinue primary inf during administration; by cont inf at prescribed rate; may store 96 hr refrigerated or 24 hr room temperature

• For 10-14 days to ensure organism death, prevent superinfection

• After C&S completed

Additive compatibilities: Amikacin, cimetidine, clindamycin, gentamicin, kanamycin, multivitamins, sodium bicarbonate, tobramycin, verapamil, vit B/C

Syringe compatibilities: Heparin, insulin

Y-site compatibilities: Acyclovir, amifostine, amphotericin B cholesteryl sulfate complex, aztreonam, cyclophosphamide, diltiazem, doxorubicin liposome, famotidine, fluconazole, foscarnet, hydromorphone, magnesium sulfate, meperidine, morphine, ondansetron, perphenazine, remifentanil, teniposide, thiotepa

cefprozil

• For 10-14 days to ensure organism death, prevent superinfection

• After C&S

• Refrigerate/shake susp prior to use

cefuroxime

• For 10-14 days to ensure organism death, prevent superinfection

• With food if needed for GI symptoms

• After C&S

Additive compatibilities: Clindamycin, floxacillin, furosemide, metronidazole, netilmicin

Y-site compatibilities: Acyclovir, allopurinol, amifostine, atracurium, aztreonam, cyclophosphamide, diltiazem, famotidine, fludarabine, foscarnet, hydromorphone, melphalan, meperidine, morphine, ondansetron, pancuronium, perphenazine, remifentanil, sargramostim, tacrolimus, teniposide, thiotepa, vecuronium

loracarbef
• Oral susp should be shaken before giving; store for 2 wk at room temperature, discard after 2 wk
• 1 hr before or 2 hr after a meal
• After C&S is completed
• For 7 days to ensure organism death, prevent superinfection

Evaluate:
• Therapeutic response: negative C&S

Teach patient/family:
• If diabetic, to use blood glucose testing
• Not to drink alcohol or take meds with alcohol or reaction may occur
• To complete full course of drug therapy, to report persistent diarrhea
• To take on an empty stomach 1 hr before or 2 hr after a meal
Not to break, crush, or chew caps
• To use yogurt or buttermilk to maintain intestinal flora, decrease diarrhea
• To notify prescriber if breastfeeding or of any side effects
To report sore throat, bruising, bleeding, joint pain (may indicate blood dyscrasias [rare]); diarrhea with mucus, blood, may indicate pseudomembranous colitis
• Cefditoren can be taken with oral contraceptives

Treatment of anaphylaxis: EpINEPHrine, antihistamines; resuscitate if needed

CEPHALOSPORINS—3RD GENERATION

cefdinir (℞)
(sef'dih-ner)
Omnicef

cefepime (℞)
(sef'e-peem)
Maxipime

cefixime (℞)
(sef-icks'ime)
Suprax

cefoperazone (℞)
(sef-oh-per'a-zone)
Cefobid

cefotaxime (℞)
(sef-oh-taks'eem)
Claforan

cefpodoxime (℞)
(sef-poe-docks'eem)
Vantin

ceftazidime (℞)
(sef'tay-zi-deem)
Ceptaz, Fortaz, Tazicef, Tazidime

ceftibuten (℞)
(sef-ti-byoo'tin)
Cedax

ceftizoxime (℞)
(sef-ti-zox'eem)
Cefizox

ceftriaxone (℞)
(sef-try-ax'one)
Rocephin

Func. class.: Broad-spectrum antibiotic

Chem. class.: Cephalosporin (3rd generation)

Action: Inhibits bacterial cell wall synthesis, rendering cell wall osmotically unstable, leading to cell death

Uses:
cefdinir: Gram-negative bacilli: *Haemophilus influenzae, Haemoph-*

ilus parainfluenzae, Moraxella catarrhalis; gram-positive organisms: *Streptococcus pneumoniae, Streptococcus pyogenes, Staphylococcus aureus*, acute exacerbations of chronic bronchitis

cefepime: Gram-negative bacilli: *Escherichia coli, Proteus, Klebsiella;* gram-positive organisms: *Streptococcus pneumoniae, Streptococcus pyogenes, Staphylococcus aureus;* lower respiratory tract, urinary tract, skin, bone infections

cefixime: Uncomplicated UTI *(Escherichia coli, Proteus mirabilis)*, pharyngitis and tonsillitis *(Streptococcus pyogenes)*, otitis media *(Haemophilus influenzae), Moraxella catarrhalis,* acute bronchitis, and acute exacerbations of chronic bronchitis *(Streptococcus pneumoniae, H. influenzae)*

cefoperazone: Gram-negative bacilli: *Haemophilus influenzae, Escherichia coli, Proteus mirabilis, Klebsiella, Enterobacter, Serratia, Citrobacter, Providencia, Proteus aeruginosa;* lower respiratory tract, urinary tract, skin, bone infections, bacterial septicemia, peritonitis, PID

cefotaxime: Gram-negative organisms: *Haemophilus influenzae, Escherichia coli, Neisseria gonorrhoeae, Neisseria meningitidis, Proteus mirabilis, Klebsiella, Citrobacter, Serratia, Salmonella, Shigella;* gram-positive organisms: *Streptococcus pneumoniae, Streptococcus pyogenes, Staphylococcus aureus;* serious lower respiratory tract, urinary tract, skin, bone, gonococcal infections; bacteremia, septicemia, meningitis

cefpodoxime: Gram-negative bacilli: *Neisseria gonorrhoeae, Haemophilus influenzae, Escherichia coli, Proteus mirabilis, Klebsiella;* gram-positive organisms: *Streptococcus pneumoniae, Streptococcus pyogenes, Staphylococcus aureus;* upper and lower respiratory tract, urinary tract, skin infections; otitis media, sexually transmitted diseases

ceftazidime: Gram-negative organisms: *Haemophilus influenzae, Escherichia coli, Enterobacter aerogenes, Pseudomonas aeruginosa, Proteus mirabilis, Klebsiella, Citrobacter, Enterobacter, Salmonella, Shigella, Acinetobacter, Bacteroides fragilis, Neisseria, Serratia;* gram-positive organisms: *Streptococcus pneumoniae, Streptococcus pyogenes, Staphylococcus aureus;* serious upper/lower respiratory tract, urinary tract, skin, gynecologic, bone, joint, intraabdominal infections; septicemia, meningitis

ceftibuten: Pharyngitis/tonsillitis, otitis media, secondary bacterial infection of acute bronchitis

ceftizoxime: Gram-negative bacilli: *Haemophilus influenzae, Escherichia coli, Enterobacter aerogenes, Proteus mirabilis, Klebsiella, Enterobacter;* gram-positive organisms: *Streptococcus pneumoniae, Streptococcus pyogenes, Staphylococcus aureus;* serious lower respiratory tract, urinary tract, skin, intraabdominal infections, septicemia, meningitis, bone and joint infections, PID caused by *Neisseria gonorrhoeae*

ceftriaxone: Gram-negative bacilli: *Haemophilus influenzae, Escherichia coli, Enterobacter aerogenes, Proteus mirabilis, Klebsiella, Citrobacter, Enterobacter, Salmonella, Shigella, Acinetobacter, Bacteroides fragilis, Neisseria, Serratia;* gram-positive organisms: *Streptococcus pneumoniae, Streptococcus pyogenes, Staphylococcus aureus;* serious lower respiratory tract, urinary tract, skin, gonococcal, intraabdominal infections, septicemia, meningitis, bone, joint infections

Dosage and routes:
cefdinir
Uncomplicated skin and skin structure infections/community-acquired pneumonia
• *Adult and child ≥13 yr:* **PO** 300 mg q12h × 10 days
• *Child 6 mo-12 yr:* **PO** 7 mg/kg q12h or 14 mg/kg q24h × 10 days, max 60 mg qd
Acute exacerbations of chronic bronchitis/acute maxillary sinusitis
• *Adult and child ≥13 yr:* **PO** 300 mg q12h or 600 mg q24h × 10 days or 300 mg bid × 5 days in some infections
Pharyngitis/tonsillitis
• *Adult and child ≥13 yr:* **PO** 300 mg q12h or 600 mg q24h × 10 days
• *Child 6 mo-12 yr:* **PO** 7 mg/kg q12h × 5-10 days or 14 mg/kg q24h × 10 days
Renal dose
• CCr <30 ml/min 300 mg qd (adult); 7 mg/kg qd (child)
Available forms: Caps 300 mg; susp: 125 mg/5 ml
cefepime
Urinary tract infections (mild to moderate)
• *Adult:* **IV/IM** 0.5-1 g q12h × 7-10 days
Urinary tract infections (severe)
• *Adult:* **IV** 2 g q12h × 10 days
Pneumonia (moderate to severe)
• *Adult:* **IV** 1-2 g q12h × 10 days
• Dosage reduction indicated in renal impairment (CCr <50 ml/min)
Uncomplicated gonorrhea
• **IM** 2 g as a single dose with 1 g **PO** probenecid at the same time
Available forms: Powder for inj 500 mg, 1, 2 g
cefixime
Renal dose: CCr 21-60 ml/min give 75% of dose; CCr <20 ml/min give 50% of dose
• *Adult:* **PO** 400 mg qd as a single dose or 200 mg q12h
• *Child >50 kg or >12 yr:* **PO** use adult dosage
• *Child <50 kg or <12 yr:* **PO** 8 mg/kg/day as a single dose or 4 mg/kg q12h
Available forms: Tabs 200, 400 mg; powder for oral susp 100 mg/5 ml
cefoperazone
Hepatic dose: give 50% of dose
Mild/Moderate infections
• *Adult:* **IM/IV** 1-2 g q12h
Severe infections
• *Adult:* **IM/IV** 6-12 g/day divided in 2-4 equal doses
Available forms: Inj 1, 2 g
cefotaxime
• *Adult:* **IM/IV** 1-2 g q12h as a single dose
• *Child 1 mo-12 yr:* **IM/IV** 50-180 mg/kg/day divided q6h
Severe infections
• *Adult:* **IM/IV** 2 g q4h, not to exceed 12 g/day
• *Child 1 mo-12 yr:* **IM/IV** 50 mg/kg q6h
Uncomplicated gonorrhea
• *Adult:* **IM** 1 g
Dosage reduction indicated for severe renal impairment (CCr <30 ml/min)
Available forms: Powder for inj 1, 2, 10 g; frozen inj 20, 40 mg/ml
cefpodoxime
• Reduce dose in renal disease
• *Adult >13 yr: Pneumonia:* 200 mg q12h for 14 days; *uncomplicated gonorrhea:* 200 mg single dose; *skin and skin structure:* 400 mg q12h for 7-14 days; *pharyngitis and tonsillitis:* 100 mg q12h for 10 days; *uncomplicated UTI:* 100 mg q12h for 7 days; dosing interval increased in presence of severe renal impairment
• *Child 5 mo-12 yr: acute otitis media:* 5 mg/kg q12h for 10 days; *pharyngitis/tonsillitis:* 5 mg/kg q12h

(max 100 mg/dose or 200 mg/day) × 5-10 days
Available forms: Tabs 100, 200 mg/granules for susp 50, 100 mg/5 ml
ceftazidime
Renal dose: CCr <50 ml/min give q12h; CCr 10-30 ml/min give q24h; CCr <10 ml/min give q48h
• *Adult:* **IV/IM** 1-2 g q8-12h × 5-10 days
• *Child:* **IV** 30-50 mg/kg q8h not to exceed 6 g/day
• *Neonate:* **IV** 30-50 mg/kg q12h
Available forms: Inj 500 mg, 1, 2, 6 g
ceftibuten
Renal dose: CCr <50 ml/min give 200 mg q24h; CCr 5-20 ml/min give 100 mg q24h
• *Adult:* **PO** 400 mg qd × 10 days
• *Child 6 mo-12 yr:* **PO** 9 mg/kg qd × 10 days
Available forms: Caps 400 mg; susp 90, 180 mg/5 ml
ceftizoxime
Renal dose: CCr <80 ml/min give 500-1500 mg q8h; CCr 10-49 ml/min give 250-1000 mg q12h
• *Adult:* **IM/IV** 1-2 g q8-12h, may give up to 4 g q8h in life-threatening infections
• *Child >6 mo:* **IM/IV** 50 mg/kg q6-8h
PID
• *Adult:* **IV** 2 g q8h, may increase to 4 g q8h in severe infections
Available forms: Powder for inj 500 mg, 1, 2, 10 g; premixed 1 g, 2 g/50 ml
ceftriaxone
• *Adult:* **IM/IV** 1-2 g qd, max 2 g q12h
• *Child:* **IM/IV** 50-75 mg/kg/day in equal doses q12h
Uncomplicated gonorrhea
• *Adult:* 250 mg **IM** as single dose
• Reduce dosage in severe renal impairment (CCr <10 ml/min)
Meningitis
• *Adult and child:* **IM/IV** 100 mg/kg/day in equal doses q12h, max 4 g/day
Surgical prophylaxis
• *Adult:* **IV** 1 g ½-2 hr preop
Available forms: Inj 500 mg, 1, 2, 10 g

Side effects/adverse reactions:
CNS: Headache, dizziness, weakness, paresthesia, fever, chills, ***seizures***
GI: Nausea, vomiting, diarrhea, anorexia, pain, glossitis, ***bleeding;*** increased AST, ALT, bilirubin, LDH, alk phosphatase; abdominal pain, ***pseudomembranous colitis***
GU: ***Proteinuria,*** vaginitis, pruritus, candidiasis, increased BUN, ***nephrotoxicity, renal failure***
HEMA: ***Leukopenia, thrombocytopenia, agranulocytosis,*** anemia, ***neutropenia, lymphocytosis, eosinophilia, pancytopenia, hemolytic anemia***
INTEG: Rash, urticaria, dermatitis
RESP: Dyspnea
SYST: ***Anaphylaxis, serum sickness***

Contraindications: Hypersensitivity to cephalosporins, infants <1 mo

Precautions: Hypersensitivity to penicillins, pregnancy (B), lactation, renal disease, children

Do not confuse:
Vantin/Ventolin
ceftazidime/ceftizoxime

Pharmacokinetics:
cefdinir
Unchanged in urine; crosses placenta, blood-brain barrier; eliminated in breast milk; not metabolized
cefepime
Peak 79 min, half-life 2 hr, 20% bound by plasma proteins, 90% excreted unchanged in urine; crosses placenta, blood-brain barrier; excreted in breast milk; not metabolized
cefixime
PO: Peak 1-2 hr, half-life 3-4 hr,

65% bound by plasma proteins, 50% eliminated unchanged in urine; crosses placenta; excreted in breast milk

cefoperazone

IV: Onset 5 min, peak 5-20 min, duration 6-8 hr

IM: Peak 1-2 hr, duration 6-8 hr

Half-life 2 hr; 70%-75% is eliminated unchanged in bile; 20%-30% unchanged in urine; excreted in breast milk (small amounts)

cefotaxime

IV: Onset 5 min

IM: Onset 30 min

Half-life 1 hr; 35%-65% is bound by plasma proteins; 40%-65% is eliminated unchanged in urine in 24 hr; 25% metabolized to active metabolites; excreted in breast milk (small amounts)

cefpodoxime

Half-life 2-3 hr; 25% bound by plasma proteins; 30% eliminated unchanged in urine in 8 hr; crosses placenta; excreted in breast milk

ceftazidime

IV/IM: Peak 1 hr, half-life ½-1 hr, 90% bound by plasma proteins, 80% eliminated unchanged in urine, crosses placenta, excreted in breast milk

ceftibuten

PO: Peak 6-10 hr; plasma protein binding 99%; elimination half-life 25 hr; extensively metabolized to an active metabolite

ceftizoxime

IV: Onset 5 min

IM: Peak 1 hr

Half-life 5-8 hr; 90% bound by plasma proteins; 36%-60% eliminated unchanged in urine; crosses placenta; excreted in breast milk

ceftriaxone

IV: Onset 5 min

IM: Peak 1 hr

Half-life 5-8 hr, 90% bound by plasma proteins; 35%-60% eliminated unchanged in urine; crosses placenta; excreted in breast milk

Interactions:

- Bleeding: anticoagulants, thrombolytics, plicamycin, valproic acid, NSAIDs
- ↓ absorption of cefdinir: iron
- ↑ toxicity: aminoglycosides, furosemide, probenecid

Bleeding (cefoperazone): angelica, anise, arnica, bogbean, boldo, celery, chamomile, clove, fenugreek, feverfew, garlic, ginger, gingko, ginseng *(Panax)*, horse chestnut, horseradish, licorice, meadowsweet, prickly ash, onion, papain, passion flower, poplar, red clover, turmeric, willow

Do not use acidophilus with anti-infectives

Lab test interferences:

False: ↑ creatinine (serum urine) ↑ urinary 17-ks

Increase: ALT, AST, alk phosphatase, LDH, bilirubin, BUN, creatinine

False positive: Urinary protein, direct Coombs' test, urine glucose

Interference: Cross-matching

NURSING CONSIDERATIONS

Assess:

- Sensitivity to penicillin, other cephalosporins

Nephrotoxicity: increased BUN, creatinine; urine output: if decreasing, notify prescriber; may indicate nephrotoxicity

- Blood studies: AST, ALT, CBC, Hct, bilirubin, LDH, alk phosphatase, Coombs' test monthly if patient is on long-term therapy
- Electrolytes: K, Na, Cl monthly if patient is on long-term therapy
- Bowel pattern qd; if severe diarrhea occurs, drug should be discontinued; may indicate pseudomembranous colitis
- IV site for extravasation, phlebitis; change site q72h

Anaphylaxis: rash, urticaria, pruritus, chills, fever, joint pain, angioedema; may occur few days after therapy begins
• Bleeding: ecchymosis, bleeding gums, hematuria, stool guaiac
Overgrowth of infection: perineal itching, fever, malaise, redness, pain, swelling, drainage, rash, diarrhea, change in cough, sputum

Administer:

cefdinir
• Oral susp after adding 39 ml water to the 60 ml bottle; 65 ml water to the 120 ml bottle; discard unused portion after 10 days
• After C&S completed

cefepime
• IV after diluting in 50-100 ml or more D_5, NS and give over 30 min
• For 7-10 days to ensure organism death, prevent superinfection

Solution compatibilities: 0.9% NaCl, D_5, D_5W, 0.5%, 10% lidocaine, bacteriostatic water for inj with parabens/benzyl alcohol

Y-site compatibilities: Doxorubicin liposome

cefixime
• For 10-14 days to ensure organism death, prevent superinfection

cefoperazone
• IV after diluting 1 g/ml sterile H_2O for inj, or 0.9% NaCl; shake, give over 3-5 min; each g may be further diluted with 20-40 ml D_5W, NS given over 30 min or as a cont inf over 6-24 hr to a concentration no greater than 25 mg/ml
• IM for concentration >250 mg/ml, dilute in sterile water, then lidocaine, inject deeply
• For 10-14 days to ensure organism death, prevent superinfection

Additive compatibilities: Cimetidine, clindamycin, furosemide

Syringe compatibilities: Heparin

Y-site compatibilities: Acyclovir, allopurinol, aztreonam, cyclophosphamide, enalaprilat, esmolol, famotidine, foscarnet, fludarabine, hydromorphone, magnesium sulfate, melphalan, morphine, teniposide, thiotepa

cefotaxime
• IV after diluting 1 g/10 ml D_5W, NS, sterile H_2O for inj and give over 3-5 min by Y-tube or 3-way stopcock; may be diluted further with 50-100 ml of normal saline or D_5W; run over ½-1 hr; discontinue primary inf during administration; or may be diluted in larger vol of sol and given as a cont inf over 6-24 hr
• For 10-14 days to ensure organism death, prevent superinfection

Additive compatibilities: Clindamycin, metronidazole, verapamil

Syringe compatibilities: Heparin, ofloxacin

Y-site compatibilities: Acyclovir, amifostine, aztreonam, cyclophosphamide, diltiazem, famotidine, fludarabine, hydromorphone, lorazepam, magnesium sulfate, melphalan, meperidine, midazolam, morphine, ondansetron, perphenazine, sargramostim, teniposide, thiotepa, tolazoline, vinorelbine

cefpodoxime
• For 10-14 days to ensure organism death, prevent superinfection
• With food to enhance absorption

Y-site compatibilities: Famotidine, fluconazole, fludarabine, insulin (regular), meperidine, morphine, sargramostim

ceftazidime
• IV after diluting 1 g/10 ml sterile H_2O for inj, shake, invert needle, push plunger, insert needle through stopper and keep in sol, expel bubbles and give over 3-5 min; may be diluted further with 50-100 ml of normal saline or D_5W; run over ½-1 hr, give through Y-tube or 3-way stopcock, discontinue primary inf during administration; store for 96

hr refrigerated, 24 hr room temperature

• For 5-10 days to ensure organism death, prevent superinfection

Syringe compatibilities: Hydromorphone

Additive compatibilities: Ciprofloxacin, clindamycin, fluconazole, metronidazole, ofloxacin

Y-site compatibilities: Acyclovir, allopurinol, amifostine, aztreonam, ciprofloxacin, diltiazem, enalaprilat, esmolol, famotidine, filgrastim, fludarabine, foscarnet, granisetron, heparin, hydromorphone, labetalol, meperidine, melphalan, morphine, ondansetron, paclitaxel, ranitidine, remifentanil, tacrolimus, teniposide, theophylline, thiotepa, vinorelbine, zidovudine

ceftibuten

• For 10 days to ensure organism death, prevent superinfection

ceftizoxime

• IV after diluting 1 g/10 ml sterile water, shake and give over 3-5 min; may be diluted further with 50-100 ml NS or D_5W give through Y-tube or 3-way stopcock; run over ½-1 hr

• For 10-14 days to ensure organism death, prevent superinfection

Additive compatibilities: Clindamycin

Y-site compatibilities: Acyclovir, allopurinol, amphotericin B cholesteryl sulfate complex, aztreonam, DOXOrubicin liposome, enalaprilat, esmolol, famotidine, fludarabine, foscarnet, hydromorphone, labetalol, melphalan, meperidine, morphine, ondansetron, remifentanil, sargramostim, teniposide, vinorelbine

ceftriaxone

• For 10-14 days to ensure organism death, prevent superinfection

• IV after diluting 250 mg/2.4 ml D_5W, H_2O for inj, 0.9% NaCl; may be further diluted with 50-100 ml NS, D_5W, $D_{10}W$, shake; run over ½-1 hr

Additive compatibilities: Amino acids or sodium bicarbonate, metronidazole

Y-site compatibilities: Acyclovir, allopurinol, aztreonam, cisatracurium, diltiazem, DOXOrubicin liposome, fludarabine, foscarnet, heparin, melphalan, meperidine, methotrexate, morphine, paclitaxel, remifentanil, sargramostim, tacrolimus, teniposide, theophylline, vinorelbine, warfarin, zidovudine

Evaluate:

• Therapeutic response: decreased symptoms of infection; negative C&S

Teach patient/family:

• If diabetic, to check blood glucose

◆ To report sore throat, bruising, bleeding, joint pain; may indicate blood dyscrasias (rare); diarrhea with mucus, blood, may indicate pseudomembranous colitis

• To report persistent diarrhea

Treatment of anaphylaxis: EpINEPHrine, antihistamines; resuscitate if needed

cephalothin
cephapirin
cephradine

See cephalosporins—1st generation

cetirizine (℞)

(se-teer'i-zeen)

Zyrtec

Func. class.: Antihistamine (2nd generation, peripherally selective)

Chem. class.: Piperazine, H_1-histamine antagonist

Action: Acts on blood vessels, GI, respiratory system by competing with histamine for H_1-receptor site; decreases allergic response by blocking pharmacologic effects of histamine; minimal anticholinergic action

Uses: Rhinitis, allergy symptoms

Dosage and routes:

- *Adult and child ≥6 yr:* **PO** 5-10 mg qd
- *Child 2-6:* **PO** 2.5 mg qd, may increase to 5 mg qd or 2.5 mg bid
- *Geriatric:* **PO** 5 mg qd, may increase to 10 mg/day

Renal/hepatic dose: CCr 11-31 ml/min 5 mg qd

Available forms: Tabs 5, 10 mg; syr 5 mg/5 ml

Side effects/adverse reactions:

RESP: Thickening of bronchial secretions, dry nose, throat

GI: Dry mouth

CNS: Headache, stimulation, *drowsiness,* sedation, *fatigue,* confusion, blurred vision, tinnitus, restlessness, tremors, paradoxical excitation in children or elderly

INTEG: Rash, eczema, photosensitivity, urticaria

Contraindications: Hypersensitivity to this drug or hydrOXYzine, newborn or premature infants, lactation, severe hepatic disease

Precautions: Pregnancy (B), elderly, children, respiratory disease, narrow-angle glaucoma, prostatic hypertrophy, bladder neck obstruction, asthma

Do not confuse:

Zyrtec/Xanax/Zantac

Pharmacokinetics:

Onset ½ hr, peak 1-2 hr, duration 24 hr, protein binding 93%, half-life 8.3 hr, decreased in children, increased in hepatic/renal disease

Interactions:

- ↑ CNS depression: alcohol, other CNS depressants
- ↑ anticholinergic/sedative effect: MAOIs
- Drug/food: food ↓ absorption by 1.7 hr

↑ effect: hops, Jamaican dogwood, kava, senega, valerian

↑ anticholinergic effect: corkwood

Lab test interferences:

False negative: Skin allergy tests

NURSING CONSIDERATIONS

Assess:

- Allergy symptoms: pruritus, urticaria, watering eyes, baseline and during treatment
- Respiratory status: rate, rhythm, increase in bronchial secretions, wheezing, chest tightness

Administer:

- Without regard to meals

Perform/provide:

- Hard candy, gum, frequent rinsing of mouth for dryness
- Storage in tight, light-resistant container

Evaluate:

- Therapeutic response: absence of running or congested nose or rashes

Teach patient/family:

- All aspects of drug use; to notify prescriber if confusion, sedation, hypotension occur
- To avoid driving, other hazardous activity if drowsiness occurs
- To avoid alcohol, other CNS depressants
- That drug is not recommended during lactation
- To avoid exposure to sunlight; burns may occur
- To use sugarless gum, candy, frequent sips of water to minimize dry mouth

Treatment of overdose: Administer ipecac syrup or lavage, diazepam, vasopressors, barbiturates (short-acting)

cetrorelix (℞)

(set-roe-ree'lix)

Cetrotide

Func. class.: Gonadotropin-releasing hormone antagonist

Chem. class.: Synthetic decapeptide

Action: Inhibitor of pituitary gonadotropin secretion; initially increases LH and FSH, induces a rapid suppression of gonadotropin secretion

Uses: For inhibition of premature LH surges in women undergoing controlled ovarian hyperstimulation

Dosage and routes:

Single-dose regimen

• *Adult:* **SC** 3 mg when serum estradiol level is at appropriate stimulation response, usually on stimulation day 7; if hCG has not been given withiin 4 days after inj of 3 mg cetrorelix, give 0.25 mg qd until day of hCG administration

Multiple-dose regimen

• *Adult:* **SC** 0.25 mg is given on stimulation day 5 (either morning or evening) or 6 (morning) and continued qd until day hCG is given

Available forms: Inj 0.25, 3 mg

Side effects/adverse reactions:

CNS: Headache

ENDO: Ovarian hyperstimulation syndrome, abdominal pain (gyn)

GI: Nausea

INTEG: Pain on inj; local site reactions

SYST: ***Fetal death***

Contraindications: Hypersensitivity, pregnancy (X), latex allergy, lactation

Pharmacokinetics: Excreted in feces/urine, half-life depends on dosage, metabolized to metabolites, protein binding 86%

NURSING CONSIDERATIONS

Assess:

• For suspected pregnancy, drug should not be used

• For latex allergy, drug should not be used

• For ALT, AST, GGT, alk phosphatase

Administer:

• SC using abdomen, around navel or upper thigh, swab inj area with disinfectant, clean a 2 in circle and allow to dry, pinch up area between thumb and finger, insert needle 45-90 degrees to surface; if positioned correctly, no blood will be drawn back into syringe, reposition needle without removing it

• Do not administer if patient is pregnant

Perform/provide:

• Protection from light

Evaluate:

• Therapeutic response: pregnancy

Teach patient/family:

• To report abdominal pain, vaginal bleeding

• To teach self-administration technique if needed

chloral hydrate (℞)

(klor-al hye'drate)

Aquachloral, chloral hydrate, Novo-Chlorhydrate✱, PMS-chloral hydrate✱

Func. class.: Sedative/hypnotic

Chem. class.: Chloral derivative

Controlled Substance Schedule IV (USA), Schedule F (Canada)

Action: Reduction product trichloroethanol produces mild cerebral depression, which causes sleep

Uses: Sedation, short-term treatment of insomnia

Dosage and routes:

Sedation

• *Adult:* **PO/RECT** 250 mg tid pc

• *Child:* **PO** 25-50 mg/kg tid, not to exceed 500 mg tid
Insomnia
• *Adult:* **PO/RECT** 500 mg-1 g ½ hr before hs
• *Child:* **PO/RECT** 50-75 mg/kg (one dose)
Procedure sedation
• *Child:* **PO/RECT** 25-50 mg/kg, not to exceed 100 mg/kg or 2 g
Renal disease
• CCr <50 ml/min avoid use
Available forms: Caps 250, 500, 650 mg; syr 250, 500 mg/5 ml; supp 325, 500 mg
Side effects/adverse reactions:
HEMA: ***Eosinophilia, leukopenia***
CNS: Drowsiness, dizziness, stimulation, nightmares, ataxia, hangover (rare), light-headedness, headache, paranoia
GI: Nausea, vomiting, flatulence, diarrhea, unpleasant taste, ***gastric necrosis***
INTEG: Rash, urticaria, ***angioedema,*** fever, purpura, eczema
CV: Hypotension, ***dysrhythmias***
RESP: ***Depression***
Contraindications: Hypersensitivity to this drug or triclofos, severe renal disease, severe hepatic disease, GI disorders (oral forms), gastritis
Precautions: Severe cardiac disease, depression, suicidal individuals, asthma, intermittent porphyria, pregnancy (C), lactation, elderly
Pharmacokinetics:
PO: Onset 30 min-1 hr, duration 4-8 hr
RECT: Onset slow, duration 4-8 hr; metabolized by liver; excreted by kidneys (inactive metabolite) and feces; crosses placenta; excreted in breast milk; metabolite is highly protein bound
Interactions:
• ↑ action: oral anticoagulants, furosemide
• ↓ effects of: phenytoin
• ↑ action of both drugs: alcohol, CNS depressants
↑ sedative effect: catnip, chamomile, clary, cowslip, hops, kava, lavender, mistletoe, nettle, pokeweed, poppy, Queen Anne's lace, senega, skullcap, valerian
↑ hypotension: black cohosh
Lab test interferences:
Interference: Urine catecholamines, urinary 17-OHCS

NURSING CONSIDERATIONS
Assess:
• Mental status: mood, sensorium, affect, memory (long-, short-term)
• Physical dependency: more frequent requests for medication, tremors, anxiety, pinpoint pupils
• Respiratory dysfunction: respiratory depression, character, rate, rhythm; hold drug if respirations <10/min or if pupils dilated (rare)
• History of substance abuse, cardiac disease, gastritis
Administer:
• ½-1 hr before hs for sleeplessness
On empty stomach with full glass of water or juice for best absorption and to decrease corrosion (do not break, crush, or chew); after meals to decrease GI symptoms if using for sedation
Perform/provide:
• Assistance with ambulation after receiving dose, especially elderly
• Safety measure: night-light, call bell within easy reach
• Check to see PO medication swallowed
• Check dose of syrup carefully, fatal overdoses have occurred
• Storage in dark container, suppositories in refrigerator
Evaluate:
• Therapeutic response: ability to sleep at night, decreased amount of early morning awakening if taking drug for insomnia

Teach patient/family:
- To avoid driving, other activities requiring alertness
- To avoid alcohol ingestion, CNS depressants; serious CNS depression may result
- Not to discontinue medication quickly after long-term use; drug should be tapered over 1-2 wk
- That effects may take 2 nights for benefits to be noticed

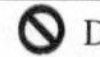 Not to break, crush, or chew caps
- Alternative measures to improve sleep (reading, exercise several hours before hs, warm bath, warm milk, TV, self-hypnosis, deep breathing)

Treatment of overdose: Lavage, activated charcoal; monitor electrolytes, vital signs

chlorambucil (℞)

(klor-am′byoo-sil)

Leukeran

Func. class.: Antineoplastic alkylating agent

Chem. class.: Nitrogen mustard

Action: Alkylates DNA, RNA; inhibits enzymes that allow synthesis of amino acids in proteins; activity is not cell cycle phase specific

Uses: Chronic lymphocytic leukemia, Hodgkin's disease, other lymphomas, macroglobulinemia, nephrotic syndrome, breast carcinoma, choreocarcinoma, ovarian carcinoma

Dosage and routes:
- *Adult:* **PO** 0.1-0.2 mg/kg/day for 3-6 wk initially, then 2-6 mg/day; maintenance 0.2 mg/kg for 2-4 wk; course may be repeated at 2-4 wk intervals, or 0.4 mg/kg (12 mg/m^2) 2 × /wk, may increase by 0.1 mg/kg (3 mg/m^2) q2wk, adjust as needed
- *Geriatric:* **PO** initially ≤2-4 mg/day
- *Child:* **PO** 0.1-0.2 mg/kg/day (4.5 mg/m^2/day) in divided doses or 4.5 mg/m^2/day as 1 dose or in divided doses

Available forms: Tabs 2 mg

Side effects/adverse reactions:

CNS: ***Seizures***

HEMA: ***Thrombocytopenia, leukopenia, pancytopenia*** (prolonged use), ***permanent bone marrow depression***

GI: Nausea, vomiting, diarrhea, weight loss, ***hepatoxicity,*** *jaundice*

GU: Hyperuremia

INTEG: Alopecia (rare), dermatitis, rash, ***Stevens-Johnson syndrome***

RESP: ***Fibrosis, pneumonitis***

Contraindications: Radiation therapy within 1 mo, chemotherapy within 1 mo, thrombocytopenia, recent smallpox vaccination, pregnancy (D), lactation

Precautions: *Pneumococcus* vaccination

Do not confuse:

Leukeran/leucovorin

Leukeran/Leukine

Pharmacokinetics: Well absorbed orally; metabolized in liver; excreted in urine; half-life 2 hr

Interactions:
- ↑ toxicity: other antineoplastics, radiation
- ↑ risk of bleeding: anticoagulants, salicylates

NURSING CONSIDERATIONS

Assess:
- Bleeding: hematuria, guaiac, bruising or petechiae, mucosa or orifices q8h
- Jaundice of skin, sclera, dark urine, clay-colored stools, itchy skin, abdominal pain, fever, diarrhea
- Dyspnea, rales, unproductive cough, chest pain, tachypnea
- Effects of alopecia on body image; discuss feelings about body changes (rare)

• CBC, differential, platelet count weekly; withhold drug if WBC is <2000 or granulocyte count is <1000/mm^3; notify prescriber of results
• Pulmonary function tests, chest x-ray films before, during therapy; chest film should be obtained q2wk during treatment
• Renal studies: BUN, serum uric acid, urine CCr before, during therapy; I&O ratio; report urine output of <30 ml/hr
• Monitor temp q4h (may indicate beginning infection)
• Hepatic studies before, during therapy (bilirubin, AST, ALT, LDH) as needed or monthly

Administer:

PO route

• All drugs PO if possible, avoid IM inj when platelets <100,000/mm^3
• Antacid before oral agent; give drug 2 hr after evening meal, before bedtime or 1 hr before breakfast
• Antiemetic 30-60 min before giving drug to prevent vomiting
• Allopurinol to maintain uric acid levels, alkalinization of urine; increase fluid intake to 2-3 L/day to prevent urate deposits, calculi formation

Perform/provide:

• Storage in tight container

Evaluate:

• Therapeutic response: decreased size of tumor, spread of malignancy

Teach patient/family:

• To report signs of infection: increased temperature, sore throat, flu-like symptoms
• To report signs of anemia: fatigue, headache, faintness, shortness of breath, irritability
• To report bleeding; avoid use of razors, commercial mouthwash
• To avoid use of aspirin products, ibuprofen
• To avoid vaccinations during treatment
• To use contraception during and several months after completion of therapy, may cause irreversible gonadal suppression
• To report any changes in breathing or coughing
• To drink 2-3 L of fluid qd unless contraindicated

chloramphenicol (℞)

(klor-am-fen'i-kole)
chloramphenicol,
Chloromycetin,
Pentamycetin ✤

Func. class.: Antiinfective, misc
Chem. class.: Dichloroacetic acid derivative

Action: Binds to 50S ribosomal subunit, which interferes with or inhibits protein synthesis

Uses: Infections caused by *Haemophilus influenzae, Salmonella typhi, Rickettsia, Neisseria,* mycoplasma; not to be used if less toxic drugs can be used

Dosage and routes:

• *Adult and child:* **PO/IV** 50-75 mg/kg/day in divided doses q6h, 100 mg/kg/day (for meningitis only) max 4 g/day
• *Premature infants and neonates:* **IV/PO** 25 mg/kg/day in divided doses q12-24h

Available forms: Inj 1 g; caps 250 mg

Side effects/adverse reactions:

HEMA: ***Anemia, thrombocytopenia, aplastic anemia, granulocytopenia, leukopenia*** (rare)
EENT: Optic neuritis, blindness
GI: Nausea, vomiting, diarrhea, abdominal pain, xerostomia, glossitis, colitis, pruritus ani

INTEG: Itching, urticaria, contact dermatitis, rash
CV: ***Gray syndrome in newborns: failure to feed, pallor, cyanosis, abdominal distention, irregular respiration, vasomotor collapse***
CNS: Headache, *depression,* confusion, peripheral neuritis
Contraindications: Hypersensitivity, severe renal disease, severe hepatic disease, minor infections
Precautions: Hepatic disease, renal disease, infants, children, bone marrow depression (drug-induced), pregnancy (C), lactation
Pharmacokinetics:
PO/IV: Peak 1-2 hr, duration 8 hr, half-life 1½-4 hr; conjugated in liver; excreted in urine (up to 15% as free drug, up to 80% in neonates), excreted in breast milk, feces; crosses placenta
Interactions:
• ↑ action of: barbiturates, anticoagulants, hydantoins, iron products, antidiabetics
• ↓ action of: vit B_{12}, folic acid, penicillins, rifampin
• Do not use acidophilus with anti-infectives

NURSING CONSIDERATIONS
Assess:
• Signs of infection, anemia
Any patient with compromised renal system; drug is excreted slowly in poor renal system function; toxicity may occur rapidly
• Hepatic studies: AST, ALT
• Blood studies: WBC, RBC, Hct, Hgb, platelets, serum iron, reticulocytes; drug should be discontinued if bone marrow is depressed
• Renal studies: urinalysis, protein, blood, BUN, creatinine
• C&S before drug therapy; may be given as soon as culture is taken
• Drug level in impaired hepatic, renal systems; peak 15-20 mg/ml 3 hr after dose, trough 5-10 mg/ml prior to next dose
• Bowel pattern before, during treatment
• Skin eruptions, itching, dermatitis after administration
• Allergies before treatment, reaction of each medication
Neonates for beginning Gray syndrome: cyanosis, abdominal distention, irregular respiration, failure to feed; drug should be discontinued immediately
Administer:
• Oral form on empty stomach with full glass of water
• IM route not recommended
IV route
• After diluting 1 g/10 ml of sterile H_2O for inj or D_5W (10% sol); give >1 min; may be further diluted in 50-100 ml of D_5W; give through Y-tube, 3-way stopcock, or additive inf set; run over ½-1 hr
Additive compatibilities: Amikacin, aminophylline, ascorbic acid, calcium chloride or gluconate, cephalothin, cephapirin, colistimethate, corticotropin, cyanocobalamin, dimenhyDRINATE, DOPamine, epHEDrine, heparin, hydrocortisone, kanamycin, lidocaine, magnesium sulfate, metaraminol, methicillin, methyldopate, methylPREDNISolone, metronidazole, nafcillin, oxacillin, oxytocin, penicillin G potassium, penicillin G sodium, pentobarbital, phenylephrine, phytonadione, plasma protein fraction, potassium chloride, promazine, ranitidine, sodium bicarbonate, thiopental, verapamil, vit B/C
Syringe compatibilities: Ampicillin, cloxacillin, heparin, methicillin, penicillin G sodium
Y-site compatibilities: Acyclovir, cyclophosphamide, enalaprilat, esmolol, foscarnet, hydromorphone,

labetalol, magnesium sulfate, meperidine, morphine, perphenazine, tacrolimus

Perform/provide:

• Storage of capsules in tight container at room temperature, reconstituted sol at room temperature 30 days

Evaluate:

• Therapeutic response: decreased symptoms of infection

Teach patient/family:

• All aspects of drug therapy: the need to complete entire course to ensure organism death (10-14 days); culture may be taken after complete course of medication

🚫 Not to break, crush, or chew caps

• To report sore throat, fever, fatigue, unusual bleeding, bruising; could indicate bone marrow depression (may occur weeks or months after termination of drug)

• That drug must be taken in equal intervals around clock to maintain blood levels

Treatment of hypersensitivity: Withdraw drug, maintain airway, administer epINEPHrine, aminophylline, O_2, IV corticosteroids

chloramphenicol ophthalmic

See appendix c

chloramphenicol otic

See appendix c

chloramphenicol topical

See appendix c

chlordiazepoxide (℞)

(klor-dye-az-e-pox′ide)

Apo-Chlordiazepoxide♣, chlordiazepoxide HCl♣, Libritabs, Librium, Novopoxide♣

Func. class.: Antianxiety

Chem. class.: Benzodiazepine

Controlled Substance Schedule IV

Action: Potentiates the actions of GABA, especially in the limbic system, reticular formation

Uses: Short-term management of anxiety, acute alcohol withdrawal, preoperatively for relaxation

Dosage and routes:

Mild anxiety

• *Adult:* **PO** 5-10 mg tid-qid

• *Child >6 yr:* **PO** 5 mg bid-qid, not to exceed 10 mg bid-tid

Severe anxiety

• *Adult:* **PO** 20-25 mg tid-qid

Preoperatively

• *Adult:* **PO** 5-10 mg tid-qid on day before surgery; **IM** 50-100 mg 1 hr before surgery

Alcohol withdrawal

• *Adult:* **PO/IM/IV** 50-100 mg, not to exceed 300 mg/day

Available forms: Caps 5, 10, 25 mg; tabs 5, 10, 25 mg; inj 100 mg ampule

Side effects/adverse reactions:

CNS: Dizziness, drowsiness, confusion, headache, anxiety, tremors, stimulation, fatigue, depression, insomnia, hallucinations

GI: Constipation, dry mouth, nausea, vomiting, anorexia, diarrhea

INTEG: Rash, dermatitis, itching

CV: Orthostatic hypotension, ***ECG changes, tachycardia,*** hypotension

EENT: Blurred vision, tinnitus, mydriasis

Contraindications: Hypersensitivity to benzodiazepines, narrow-angle glaucoma, psychosis, pregnancy (D), lactation, child <6 yr

Precautions: Elderly, debilitated, hepatic disease, renal disease

Do not confuse:

Librium/Librax

Pharmacokinetics:

PO: Onset 30 min, peak within 2 hr, duration 4-6 hr; metabolized by liver, excreted by kidneys; crosses placenta, excreted in breast milk; half-life 5-30 hr (increased in elderly)

Interactions:

• ↑ CNS depression: CNS depressants, alcohol

• ↑ chlordiazepoxide: cimetidine, disulfiram, fluoxetine, isoniazid, ketoconazole, metoprolol, oral contraceptives, propranolol, valproic acid

• ↓ action of: levodopa

• ↓ action of chlordiazepoxide: barbiturates, rifamycins

↑ effect: cowslip, kava, Queen Anne's lace, valerian

Lab test interferences:

False increase: 17-OHCS

False positive: Pregnancy test (some methods)

NURSING CONSIDERATIONS

Assess:

• B/P (lying, standing), pulse; if systolic B/P drops 20 mm Hg, hold drug, notify prescriber

• Blood studies: CBC during long-term therapy; blood dyscrasias have occurred rarely

• Hepatic studies: AST, ALT, bilirubin, creatinine, LDH, alk phosphatase during long-term therapy

• I&O; may indicate renal dysfunction

• For ataxia, oversedation in elderly, debilitated patients

• Mental status: mood, sensorium, affect, sleeping pattern, drowsiness, dizziness

• Physical dependency, withdrawal symptoms: headache, nausea, vomiting, muscle pain, weakness after long-term use

• Suicidal tendencies, paradoxic reactions such as excitement, stimulation, acute rage

• For pregnancy; drug should be avoided during pregnancy

Administer:

PO route

• With food or milk for GI symptoms

• Crushed if patient is unable to swallow medication whole

IM route

• Add 2 ml diluent to powder, rotate until clear, use immediately

• Preferred route is IM

IV route

• 5 ml NS/100 mg powder; agitate ampule gently; give through Y-tube or 3-way stopcock; give 100 mg or less ≥1 min; do not use IM diluent for IV use

• Keep powder from light; refrigerate, mix when ready to use

Solution compatibilities: D_5W, 0.9% NaCl

Y-site compatibilities: Heparin, hydrocortisone, potassium chloride, vit B/C

Perform/provide:

• Assistance with ambulation during beginning therapy, since drowsiness/dizziness occurs

• Check to see PO medication has been swallowed if patient is depressed, suicidal

• Sugarless gum, hard candy, frequent sips of water for dry mouth

Evaluate:

• Therapeutic response: decreased anxiety, restlessness, sleeplessness

Teach patient/family:

• That drug may be taken with food

• Not to use drug for everyday stress or use longer than 4 mo, unless directed by prescriber

• Not to take more than prescribed amount; may be habit forming

• To avoid OTC preparations unless approved by prescriber

• To avoid driving, activities that require alertness; drowsiness may occur
• To avoid alcohol ingestion, other psychotropic medications, unless directed by prescriber
• Not to discontinue medication abruptly after long-term use; may precipitate seizures
• To rise slowly or fainting may occur, especially elderly
• That drowsiness may be worse at beginning of treatment
• To notify prescriber if pregnancy is suspected or planned

Treatment of overdose: Lavage, VS, supportive care, give flumazenil

chloroquine (℞)

(klor'oh-kwin)

Aralen HCl, Aralen Phosphate, chloroquine phosphate

Func. class.: Antimalarial

Chem. class.: Synthetic 4-aminoquinoline derivative

Action: Inhibits parasite replications, transcription of DNA to RNA by forming complexes with DNA of parasite

Uses: Malaria of *Plasmodium vivax, P. malariae, P. ovale, P. falciparum* (some strains), amebiasis

Dosage and routes:

Malaria suppression

• *Adult and child:* **PO** 5 mg base/kg/wk on same day of week, not to exceed 300 mg base; treatment should begin 1-2 wk before exposure and for 8 wk after; if treatment begins after exposure, 600 mg base for adult and 10 mg base/kg for children in 2 divided doses 6 hr apart

Extraintestinal amebiasis

• *Adult:* **IM** 160-200 mg base qd × 10-12 days or **PO** (HCl) 600 mg base qd × 2 days, then 300 mg base qd × 2-3 wk (phosphate)
• *Child:* **IM/PO** 10 mg/kg qd (HCl) × 2-3 wk, not to exceed 300 mg/day

Available forms: Tabs 250 mg (150 mg base), 500 mg (300 mg base) phosphate; inj 50 mg (40 mg base)/ml HCl

Side effects/adverse reactions:

CV: Hypotension, ***heart block, asystole with syncope,*** ECG changes

INTEG: Pruritus, pigmentary changes, skin eruptions, lichen planus–like eruptions, eczema, ***exfoliative dermatitis***

CNS: Headache, stimulation, fatigue, ***convulsion,*** psychosis

EENT: Blurred vision, corneal changes, retinal changes, difficulty focusing, tinnitus, vertigo, deafness, photophobia, corneal edema

GI: Nausea, vomiting, anorexia, diarrhea, cramps

HEMA: ***Thrombocytopenia, agranulocytosis, hemolytic anemia, leukopenia***

Contraindications: Hypersensitivity, retinal field changes

Precautions: Pregnancy (C), children, blood dyscrasias, severe GI disease, neurologic disease, alcoholism, hepatic disease, G6PD deficiency, psoriasis, eczema, lactation

Pharmacokinetics: Metabolized in liver; excreted in urine, feces, breast milk; crosses placenta

PO: Peak 1-3 hr, half-life 3-5 days

IM: Peak 30 min

Interactions:

• ↓ action of chloroquine: magnesium, aluminum compounds, kaolin
• Reduced oral clearance and metabolism of chloroquine: cimetidine

NURSING CONSIDERATIONS

Assess:

• Ophthalmic test if long-term treatment or dosage >150 mg/day

- Hepatic studies qwk: AST, ALT, bilirubin
- Blood studies: CBC, since blood dyscrasias occur
- ECG during therapy; watch for depression of T waves, widening of QRS complex
- Allergic reactions: pruritus, rash, urticaria
- Blood dyscrasias: malaise, fever, bruising, bleeding (rare)
- For ototoxicity (tinnitus, vertigo, change in hearing); audiometric testing should be done before, after treatment

◆For toxicity: blurring vision; difficulty focusing; headache; dizziness; decreased knee, ankle reflexes, seizures, CV collapse; drug should be discontinued immediately

Administer:

- IM after aspirating to avoid injection into blood system, which may cause hypotension, asystole, heart block; rotate inj sites

PO route

- Before or after meals at same time each day to maintain drug level

Additive compatibilities: Promethazine

Perform/provide:

- Storage in tight, light-resistant container at room temperature; keep injection in cool environment

Evaluate:

- Therapeutic response: decreased symptoms of infection

Teach patient/family:

- To use sunglasses in bright sunlight to decrease photophobia
- That urine may turn rust or brown color
- To report hearing, visual problems, fever, fatigue, bruising, bleeding, which may indicate blood dyscrasias

Treatment of overdose: Induce vomiting, gastric lavage, administer barbiturate (ultrashort-acting), vasopressor; tracheostomy may be necessary

chlorothiazide (℞)

(klor-oh-thye'a-zide)

Diuril

Func. class.: Diuretic

Chem. class.: Thiazide; sulfonamide derivative

Action: Acts on distal tubule and thick ascending limb of the loop of Henle by increasing excretion of water, sodium, chloride, potassium, magnesium

Uses: Edema, hypertension, diuresis

Dosage and routes:

Edema, hypertension

- *Adult:* **PO/IV** 500 mg-2 g qd may divide bid

Diuresis

- *Adult:* **IV** 250 mg q6-12h
- *Child >6 mo:* **PO** 10-20 mg/kg/day may divide bid
- *Child <6 mo:* **PO** up to 40 mg/kg/day in 2 doses

Available forms: Tabs 250, 500 mg; inj 500 mg; oral susp 250 mg/5 ml

Side effects/adverse reactions:

CNS: Paresthesia, anxiety, depression, headache, *dizziness, fatigue, weakness,* insomnia

CV: Irregular pulse, orthostatic hypotension, palpitations, volume depletion

EENT: Blurred vision

ELECT: Hypokalemia, hypercalcemia, hyponatremia, hypochloremia, hypophosphatemia, hypomagnesemia

GI: Nausea, vomiting, anorexia, constipation, diarrhea, cramps, pancreatitis, GI irritation, ***hepatitis***

GU: Urinary frequency, polyuria, ***uremia,*** glucosuria, hematuria

HEMA: ***Aplastic anemia, hemolytic anemia, leukopenia, agranulocytosis, thrombocytopenia, neutropenia***
INTEG: Rash, urticaria, purpura, photosensitivity, fever, alopecia
META: Hyperglycemia, *hyperuricemia,* increased creatinine, BUN

Contraindications: Hypersensitivity to thiazides or sulfonamides, hepatic coma, anuria, renal decompensation, lactation

Precautions: Hypokalemia, renal disease, hepatic disease, gout, COPD, SLE, diabetes mellitus, elderly, hyperlipidemia, pregnancy (B)

Do not confuse:
chlorothiazide/chlorproMAZINE, chlorthalidone, chlorproPAMIDE

Pharmacokinetics: Not well absorbed PO
PO: Onset 2 hr, peak 4 hr, duration 6-12 hr; crosses placenta, excreted in breast milk, excreted unchanged by kidneys; half-life 2 hr

Interactions:
- ↑ toxicity: lithium, nondepolarizing skeletal muscle relaxants, digitalis, allopurinol
- ↑ hypotension: other antihypertensives, alcohol, nitrates
- ↓ absorption of thiazides: cholestyramine, colestipol
- ↓ diuretic action: NSAIDs
- Hypokalemia: ticarcillin, glucocorticoids, amphotericin, mezlocillin, piperacillin

Hypokalemia: chronic use aloe, buckthorn, cascara sagrada, Chinese rhubarb, gossypol, licorice, nettle, senna

Severe photosensitivity: St. John's wort

↑ diuretic effect: aloe, cucumber, dandelion, horsetail, pumpkin, Queen Anne's lace

Lab test interferences:
False negative: Phentolamine and tyramine tests
Interference: Urine steroid tests
Increase: BSP retention, Ca, amylase, parathyroid test
Decrease: PBI, PSP

NURSING CONSIDERATIONS

Assess:
- Weight, I&O daily to determine fluid loss; effect of drug may be decreased if used qd
- Rate, depth, rhythm of respirations; effect of exertion
- B/P lying, standing; postural hypotension may occur, especially in elderly
- Electrolytes: K, Na, Cl; include BUN, blood glucose, CBC, serum creatinine, blood pH, ABGs, uric acid, Ca, Mg
- Glucose in urine if patient is diabetic
- Signs of metabolic alkalosis: drowsiness, restlessness
- Rashes, temp elevation qd
- Confusion, especially in elderly; take safety precautions if needed

Administer:
- In AM to avoid interference with sleep if using drug as a diuretic
- Potassium replacement if potassium less than 3 mg/dl
- With food if nausea occurs; absorption may be decreased slightly; tablets may be crushed
- After shaking suspension

IV route
- After diluting 0.5 g/18 ml or more of sterile water for inj; may be diluted further with 0.9% NaCl, D_5W, check for extravasation; give over 5 min (0.5 g/5 min)

Additive compatibilities: Cimetidine, lidocaine, nafcillin, ranitidine, sodium bicarbonate

Evaluate:
- Therapeutic response: improvement in edema of feet, legs, sacral area daily if medication is being used for CHF; decreased B/P; increased urinary output

Teach patient/family:

- To rise slowly from lying or sitting position; orthostatic hypotension may occur
- To notify prescriber of muscle weakness, cramps, nausea, dizziness
- That drug may be taken with food or milk; to take at same time each day; not to double dose; dehydration may occur
- That blood sugar may be increased in diabetics
- To take early in day to avoid nocturia
- To use sunscreen; use protective clothing to prevent photosensitivity
- To weigh weekly and notify prescriber of change of >3 lb
- To eat diet high in potassium if recommended by prescriber; teach high-potassium foods
- Not to take OTC medications without consulting prescriber

Treatment of overdose: Lavage if taken orally; monitor electrolytes; administer dextrose in saline; monitor hydration, CV, renal status

chlorpheniramine (OTC, ℞)

(klor-fen-ir'a-meen)

Aller-Chlor, Chlo-Amine, Chlorate, chlorpheniramine maleate, Chlor-Trimeton, Chlor-Tripolon ♣, GenAllerate, Novo-Pheniram ♣, Pedia Care Allergy Formula, Phenetron, Teldrin

Func. class.: Antihistamine (1st generation, nonselective)

Chem. class.: Alkylamine, H_1-receptor antagonist

Action: Acts on blood vessels, GI system, respiratory system, by competing with histamine for H_1-receptor site; decreases allergic response by blocking histamine

Uses: Allergy symptoms, rhinitis

Dosage and routes:

- *Adult and child ≥12 yr:* **PO** 2-4 mg tid-qid, not to exceed 24 mg/day; **TIME-REL** 8-12 mg bid-tid, not to exceed 24 mg/day; **IM/IV/SC** 5-40 mg/day, max 40 mg/day
- *Child 6-12 yr:* **PO** 2 mg q4-6h, not to exceed 12 mg/day; **SUS REL** 8 mg hs or qd, **SUS REL** not recommended for child <6 yr; SC 87.5 mcg/kg or 2.5 mg/m^2 q6h
- *Child 2-5 yr:* **PO** 1 mg q4-6h, not to exceed 4 mg/day

Available forms: Tabs, chewable 2 mg; tabs 4, 8, 12 mg; tabs, time-rel 8, 12 mg; caps, time-rel 8, 12 mg; syr 1 mg/5 ml, 2 mg/5 ml, 2.5 mg/5 ml; inj 10, 100 mg/ml

Side effects/adverse reactions:

CNS: Dizziness, drowsiness, poor coordination, fatigue, anxiety, euphoria, confusion, paresthesia, neuritis

RESP: Increased thick secretions, wheezing, chest tightness

HEMA: ***Thrombocytopenia, agranulocytosis, hemolytic anemia***

GI: Nausea, anorexia, diarrhea

INTEG: Photosensitivity

GU: Retention, dysuria, urinary frequency

EENT: Blurred vision, dilated pupils, tinnitus, nasal stuffiness, dry nose, throat, mouth

Contraindications: Hypersensitivity to H_1-receptor antagonists, acute asthma attack, lower respiratory tract disease, stenosed peptic ulcers, bladder neck obstruction

Precautions: Increased intraocular pressure, renal disease, cardiac disease, hypertension, bronchial asthma, seizure disorder, hyperthyroidism, prostatic hypertrophy, pregnancy (B), lactation, elderly

Do not confuse:
Teldrin/Tedral

Pharmacokinetics:
PO: Onset ½ hr, duration 4-12 hr; *PO-ER:* Duration 8-24 hr; *SC/IM/IV:* duration 4-12 hr; detoxified in liver; excreted by kidneys (metabolites/free drug); half-life 12-15 hr

Interactions:
- ↑ CNS depression: barbiturates, opiates, hypnotics, tricyclics, alcohol
- ↑ effect of chlorpheniramine: MAOIs
- ↑ anticholinergic action: atropine, phenothiazines, quinidine, haloperidol

↑ effect: hops, Jamaican dogwood, kava, khat, senega

↑ anticholinergic effect: corkwood, henbane leaf

Lab test interferences:
False negative: Skin allergy tests

NURSING CONSIDERATIONS

Assess:
- Be alert for urinary retention, frequency, dysuria; drug should be discontinued
- Respiratory status: rate, rhythm, increase in bronchial secretions, wheezing, chest tightness

Administer:

PO route
- With meals for GI symptoms; absorption may slightly decrease

IV route
- Undiluted at ≥10 mg/1 min
- The 100 mg/ml form is not to be used IV; for IM/SC use

Perform/provide:
- Hard candy, gum, frequent rinsing of mouth for dryness
- Storage in tight container at room temperature

Evaluate:
- Therapeutic response: absence of running, congested nose, rashes

Teach patient/family:
- Not to break, crush, or chew sustained-release forms
- All aspects of drug use; to notify prescriber of confusion/sedation/hypotension, difficulty voiding
- To avoid driving, other hazardous activity if drowsiness occurs, especially elderly
- To avoid concurrent use of alcohol, other CNS depressants

Treatment of overdose: Administer ipecac syrup or lavage, diazepam, vasopressors, barbiturates (short-acting)

*chlorproMAZINE (℞)

(klor-proe'ma-zeen)
Chlorpromanyl✤, chlorproMAZINE HCl, Largactil✤, Novo-Chlorpromazine✤, Thorazine, Thor-Prom

Func. class.: Antipsychotic/neuroleptic/antiemetic

Chem. class.: Phenothiazine-aliphatic

Action: Depresses cerebral cortex, hypothalamus, limbic system, which control activity aggression; blocks neurotransmission produced by DOPamine at synapse; exhibits a strong α-adrenergic, anticholinergic blocking action; mechanism for antipsychotic effects is unclear

Uses: Psychotic disorders, mania, schizophrenia, anxiety, intractable hiccups in adults, nausea, vomiting; preoperatively for relaxation; acute intermittent porphyria, behavioral problems in children, nonpsychotic, demented patients, Tourette's syndrome

Investigational uses: Vascular headache

Dosage and routes:

Psychosis
- *Adult:* **PO** 10-50 mg q1-4h initially, then increase up to 2 g/day if

necessary; **IM** 10-50 mg q1-4h, usual dose 300-800 mg/day
• *Geriatric:* 10-25 mg qd-bid, increase by 10-25 mg/day q4-7 days, max 800 mg/day
• *Child>6 mo:* **PO** 0.5 mg/kg q4-6h; **IM** 0.5 mg/kg q6-8h; **RECT** 1 mg/kg q6-8h

Nausea and vomiting
• *Adult:* **PO** 10-25 mg q4-6h prn; **IM** 25-50 mg q3h prn; **RECT** 50-100 mg q6-8h prn, not to exceed 400 mg/day; **IV** 25-50 mg qd-qid
• *Child ≥6 mo:* **PO** 0.55 mg/kg q4-6h; **IM** q6-8h; **RECT** 1.1 mg/kg q6-8h; max **IM** ≤5 yr or ≤22.7 kg 40 mg; max **IM** 5-10 yr or 22.7-45.5 kg, 75 mg

Intractable hiccups
• *Adult:* **PO** 25-50 mg tid-qid; **IM** 25-50 mg (only if PO dose does not work); **IV** 25-50 mg in 500-1000 ml **NS** (only for severe hiccups)

Available forms: Tabs 10, 25, 50, 100, 200 mg; sus-rel caps 30, 75, 150, 200, 300 mg; syr 10, 25, 100 mg/5 ml; conc 30, 40, 100 mg/ml; supp 25, 100 mg; inj 25 mg/ml

Side effects/adverse reactions:
CV: Orthostatic hypotension, hypertension, ***cardiac arrest,*** ECG changes, ***tachycardia***
EENT: Blurred vision, glaucoma, dry eyes
GI: Dry mouth, nausea, vomiting, anorexia, constipation, diarrhea, jaundice, weight gain
GU: Urinary retention, enuresis, impotence, amenorrhea, gynecomastia, breast engorgement
HEMA: Anemia, ***leukopenia, leukocytosis, agranulocytosis***
INTEG: Rash, photosensitivity, dermatitis
RESP: ***Laryngospasm,*** dyspnea, ***respiratory depression***
CNS: EPS: pseudoparkinsonism, akathisia, dystonia, tardive dyskinesia, seizures, *headache,* ***neuroleptic malignant syndrome,*** dizziness

Contraindications: Hypersensitivity, circulatory collapse, liver damage, cerebral arteriosclerosis, coronary disease, severe hypertension/hypotension, blood dyscrasias, coma, child <6 mo, brain damage, bone marrow depression, alcohol/barbiturate withdrawal, narrow-angle glaucoma

Precautions: Pregnancy (C), lactation, seizure disorders, hypertension, hepatic disease, cardiac disease, elderly, prostatic enlargement

Do not confuse:
chlorproMAZINE/chlorproPAMIDE
chlorproMAZINE/prochlorperazine

Pharmacokinetics:
PO: Absorption variable, widely distributed; onset erratic 30-60 min, duration 4-6 hr
PO-ER: Onset 30-60 min, peak unknown, duration 10-12 hr
REC: Onset erratic, duration 3 hr
IM: Well absorbed; peak 15-20 min, duration 4-8 hr
IV: Onset 5 min, peak 10 min, duration unknown
Metabolized by liver, excreted in urine (metabolites), crosses placenta, enters breast milk; 95% bound to plasma proteins; elimination half-life 10-30 hr

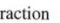

Interactions:
• Lowered seizure threshold: anticonvulsants
• Oversedation: other CNS depressants, alcohol, barbiturate anesthetics, antihistamines, sedatives/hypnotics, antidepressants
• Toxicity: epINEPHrine
• ↓ absorption: aluminum hydroxide, magnesium hydroxide antacids
• ↓ antiparkinson activity: levodopa, bromocriptine

- ↓ serum chlorproMAZINE: lithium, barbiturates
- ↓ anticoagulant effect: warfarin
- ↑ effects of both drugs: β-adrenergic blockers, alcohol
- ↑ anticholinergic effects: anticholinergics, antidepressants, antiparkinsonian agents
- Agranulocystosis: antithyroid agents
- ↑ valproic acid level

↑ action: cola tree, hops, nettle, nutmeg

↑ anticholinergic effect: henbane leaf

↑ EPS: betel palm, kava

Lab test interferences:

Increase: Hepatic studies, cardiac enzymes, cholesterol, blood glucose, prolactin, bilirubin, PBI, cholinesterase, ^{131}I, alk phosphatase, leukocytes, granulocytes, platelets

Decrease: Hormones (blood and urine)

False positive: Pregnancy tests, PKU

False negative: Urinary steroids, 17-OHCS

NURSING CONSIDERATIONS

Assess:

- Mental status: orientation, mood, behavior, presence and type of hallucinations before initial administration and monthly
- Any potentially reversible causes of behavior problems in the elderly before and during therapy
- Swallowing of PO medication; check for hoarding or giving of medication to other patients
- I&O ratio; palpate bladder if low urinary output occurs, especially in elderly
- Bilirubin, CBC, LFTs, ocular exam; agranulocytosis may occur, monthly
- Urinalysis recommended before, during prolonged therapy
- Affect, orientation, LOC, reflexes, gait, coordination, sleep pattern disturbances
- B/P sitting, standing, lying; take pulse and respirations q4h during initial treatment; establish baseline before starting treatment; report drops of 30 mm Hg; obtain baseline ECG, Q-wave and T-wave changes
- Dizziness, faintness, palpitations, tachycardia on rising

For neuroleptic malignant syndrome: hyperpyrexia, muscle rigidity, increased CPK, altered mental status, for acute dystonia (check chewing, swallowing, eyes, pin rolling)

- EPS including akathisia (inability to sit still, no pattern to movements), tardive dyskinesia (bizarre movements of the jaw, mouth, tongue, extremities), pseudoparkinsonism (rigidity, tremors, pill rolling, shuffling gait)
- Skin turgor daily
- Constipation, urinary retention daily; increase bulk, H_2O in diet

Administer:

- IM, inject in deep muscle mass, do not give SC
- Rectal after placing in refrigerator for ½ hr if too soft to insert
- Antiparkinsonian agent for EPS if ordered

PO route

- With full glass of water, milk; or with food to decrease GI upset
- Drug in liquid form mixed in glass of juice or cola if hoarding is suspected
- Periodically attempt dosage reduction in behavioral problems

IV route

- After diluting 1 mg/1 ml with NS, give 1 mg or less/2 min or more; may be further diluted in 500-1000 ml of NS

Additive compatibilities: Ascorbic acid, ethacrynate, netilmicin, theophylline, vit B/C

Syringe compatibilities: Atropine, benztropine, butorphanol, diphenhydrAMINE, doxapram, droperidol, fentanyl, glycopyrrolate, hydromorphone, hydrOXYzine, meperidine, metoclopramide, midazolam, morphine, pentazocine, perphenazine, prochlorperazine, promazine, promethazine, scopolamine

Y-site compatibilities: Amsacrine, cisatracurium, cisplatin, cladribine, cyclophosphamide, cytarabine, DOXOrubicin, DOXOrubicin liposome, famotidine, filgrastim, fluconazole, granisetron, heparin, hydrocortisone, ondansetron, potassium chloride, propofol, teniposide, thiotepa, vinorelbine, vit B/C

Perform/provide:
• Supervised ambulation until stabilized on medication; do not involve in strenuous exercise program because fainting is possible; patient should not stand still for long periods
• Increased fluids and roughage to prevent constipation
• Candy, gum, sips of water for dry mouth
• Storage in tight, light-resistant container, oral sol in amber bottle

Evaluate:
• Therapeutic response: decrease in emotional excitement, hallucinations, delusions, paranoia, reorganization of patterns of thought, speech, increase in target behaviors

Teach patient/family:
• To use good oral hygiene; frequent rinsing of mouth, sugarless gum, candy, ice chips for dry mouth
• To avoid hazardous activities until drug response is determined
⊘ Not to break, crush, or chew time-rel caps
• That orthostatic hypotension occurs often and to rise gradually from sitting or lying position
• To remain lying down for at least 30 min after IM inj
• To avoid hot tubs, hot showers, tub baths, since hypotension may occur; that in hot weather, heat stroke may occur; take extra precautions to stay cool
• To avoid abrupt withdrawal of this drug or EPS may result; drug should be withdrawn slowly
• To avoid OTC preparations (cough, hay fever, cold) unless approved by prescriber, since serious drug interactions may occur; avoid use with alcohol, CNS depressants; increased drowsiness may occur
• To use a sunscreen and sunglasses to prevent burns
• To take antacids 2 hr before or after this drug
• To report sore throat, malaise, fever, bleeding, mouth sores; CBC should be drawn and drug discontinued
• Contraceptive measures
• That urine may turn pink or red

Treatment of overdose: Lavage if orally ingested; provide airway; *do not induce vomiting or use epinephrine*

RARELY USED

*chlorproPAMIDE (Rx)

(klor-proe'pa-mide)
Chloronase ✱, ChlorproPAMIDE, Diabinese, Novopropamide ✱
Functional class.: Antidiabetic

Uses: Stable adult-onset diabetes mellitus (type 2) NIDDM

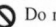

Dosage and routes:
• *Adult:* **PO** 100-250 mg qd, ini-

tially, then 100-500 mg maintenance according to response; not to exceed 750 mg/day

Contraindications: Hypersensitivity to sulfonylureas, juvenile or brittle diabetes, pregnancy (D), lactation, renal failure

chlorthalidone (℞)

(klor-thal'i-done)

Apo-Chlorthalidone♣, chlorthalidone, Hygroton, Thalitone, Uridon♣

Func. class.: Diuretic

Chem. class.: Thiazide-like phthalimidine derivative

Action: Acts on distal tubule and thick ascending limb of the loop of Henle by increasing excretion of water, sodium, chloride, potassium, magnesium, bicarbonate, possible arteriolar dilation

Uses: Edema, hypertension, diuresis, edema in CHF, nephrotic syndrome

Dosage and routes:

- *Adult:* **PO** 25-200 mg/day or 100 mg every other day
- *Geriatric:* **PO** 12.5 mg qd, initially
- *Child:* **PO** 2 mg/kg or 60 mg/m^2 3 ×/wk

Available forms: Tabs 25, 50, 100 mg

Side effects/adverse reactions:

GU: Urinary frequency, polyuria, ***uremia,*** glucosuria, impotence

CNS: Paresthesia, headache, *dizziness, fatigue, weakness*

GI: Nausea, vomiting, anorexia, constipation, diarrhea, cramps, pancreatitis, GI irritation, ***hepatitis***

EENT: Blurred vision

INTEG: Rash, urticaria, purpura, photosensitivity, fever

META: Hyperglycemia, hyperuremia, increased creatinine, BUN, gout

HEMA: ***Aplastic anemia, hemolytic anemia, leukopenia, agranulocytosis, thrombocytopenia, neutropenia***

CV: Irregular pulse, orthostatic hypotension, palpitations, volume depletion

ELECT: Hypokalemia, hypomagnesemia, hypercalcemia, hyponatremia, hypochloremia

Contraindications: Hypersensitivity to thiazides or sulfonamides, anuria, renal decompensation, lactation

Precautions: Hypokalemia, renal disease, pregnancy (B), hepatic disease, gout, diabetes mellitus, elderly, hyperlipidemia

Do not confuse:

Uridon/Vicodin

Hygroton/Regroton

Pharmacokinetics:

PO: Onset 2 hr, peak 6 hr, duration 24-72 hr; excreted unchanged by kidneys; crosses placenta; enters breast milk; half-life 40 hr

Interactions:

- ↑ toxicity of: lithium, nondepolarizing skeletal muscle relaxants, allopurinol
- ↓ absorption of thiazides: cholestyramine, colestipol
- Hyperglycemia, hypotension: diazoxide
- ↑ hypotensive effect: alcohol
- Hypokalemia: glucocorticoids, amphotericin B

Potassium deficiency: chronic use of buckthorn, cascara sagrada, Chinese rhubarb, gossypol, licorice, nettle, senna

↑ hypotension: cucumber, dandelion, khella, horsetail, pumpkin, Queen Anne's lace

Severe photosensitivity: St. John's Wort

Lab test interferences:

Increase: BSP retention, calcium,

cholesterol, triglycerides, amylase
Decrease: PBI, PSP, parathyroid test

NURSING CONSIDERATIONS

Assess:

- Weight, I&O daily to determine fluid loss; effect of drug may be decreased if used qd
- Rate, depth, rhythm of respiration, effect of exertion, B/P lying, standing; postural hypotension may occur
- Electrolytes: K, Mg, Na, Cl; include BUN, blood glucose, CBC, serum creatinine, blood pH, ABGs, uric acid, Ca
- Blood glucose levels if patient is diabetic
- Signs of metabolic alkalosis: drowsiness, restlessness
- Signs of hypokalemia: postural hypotension, malaise, fatigue, tachycardia, leg cramps, weakness
- Rashes, temp elevation qd
- Confusion, especially in elderly; take safety precautions if needed

Administer:

- In AM to avoid interference with sleep if using drug as a diuretic
- Potassium replacement if potassium less than 3 mg/dl
- With food if nausea occurs; absorption may be decreased slightly

Evaluate:

- Therapeutic response: improvement in edema of feet, legs, sacral area daily if medication used in CHF

Teach patient/family:

- To rise slowly from lying or sitting position
- To notify prescriber of muscle weakness, cramps, nausea, dizziness
- That drug may be taken with food or milk
- That blood glucose may be increased in diabetics
- To use sunscreen to protect against photosensitivity
- To take early in day to avoid nocturia

Treatment of overdose: Lavage if taken orally, monitor electrolytes, administer dextrose in NS, monitor hydration, CV, renal status

chlorzoxazone (℞)

(klor-zox'a-zone)

EZE-DS, chlorzoxazone, Paraflex, Parafon Forte DSC, Relaxazone, Remular, Remular-S, Strifon Forte DSC

Func. class.: Skeletal muscle relaxant, central acting

Chem. class.: Benzoxazole derivative

Action: Inhibits multisynaptic reflex arcs causing skeletal muscle relaxation

Uses: Relieving pain, spasm in musculoskeletal conditions

Dosage and routes:

- *Adult:* **PO** 250-750 mg tid-qid
- *Child:* **PO** 20 mg/kg/day in divided doses bid-tid

Available forms: Tabs 250, 500 mg

Side effects/adverse reactions:

GU: Urine discoloration
HEMA: ***Granulocytopenia, anemia***
CNS: Dizziness, drowsiness, headache, insomnia, stimulation, malaise
GI: Nausea, vomiting, anorexia, diarrhea, constipation, ***GI bleeding***
INTEG: Rash, pruritus, petechiae, ecchymoses, ***angioedema***
SYST: ***Anaphylaxis, angioedema***

Contraindications: Hypersensitivity, impaired hepatic function

Precautions: Pregnancy (unknown), lactation, hepatic disease, elderly

Do not confuse:

Parafon Forte DSC/Fam-Pren Forte

Pharmacokinetics:

PO: Onset 1 hr, peak 1-2 hr, duration 3-4 hr, half-life 1 hr; metabolized in liver; excreted in urine (metabolites)

Interactions:

• ↑ CNS depression: alcohol, tricyclics, opiates, barbiturates, sedatives, hypnotics

May ↑ CNS depression: kava

NURSING CONSIDERATIONS

Assess:

• Blood studies: CBC, WBC, differential for blood dyscrasias if on long-term therapy

• Allergic reactions: rash, fever, respiratory distress

• CNS depression: dizziness, drowsiness, psychiatric symptoms

Administer:

• With meals for GI symptoms

Perform/provide:

• Storage in tight container at room temperature

Evaluate:

• Therapeutic response: decreased pain, spasticity

Teach patient/family:

• Not to discontinue abruptly; insomnia, nausea, headache, spasticity, tachycardia will occur; drug should be tapered over 1-2 wk

• Not to take with alcohol, other CNS depressants; take with food

• To avoid hazardous activities if drowsiness, dizziness occurs

• To avoid using OTC medication: cough preparations, antihistamines, unless directed by prescriber

• That urine may be orange or purple

Treatment of overdose: Gastric lavage or induce emesis, then administer activated charcoal; use other supportive treatment as necessary; monitor cardiac function

cholestyramine (℞)

(koe-less-tir'a-meen)

LoCHOLEST, LoCHOLEST Light, Prevalite, Questran, Questran Light

Func. class.: Antilipemic

Chem. class.: Bile acid sequestrant

Action: Absorbs, combines with bile acids to form insoluble complex that is excreted through feces; loss of bile acids lowers cholesterol levels

Uses: Primary hypercholesterolemia, pruritus associated with biliary obstruction

Investigational uses: Diarrhea caused by excess bile acid

Dosage and routes:

• *Adult:* **PO** 4 g qd or bid, max 24 g/day

• *Child:* **PO** 240 mg/kg/day in 3 divided doses with food or drink, max 8 g/day

Available forms: Powder for susp 4 g cholestyramine/packet or scoop

Side effects/adverse reactions:

CNS: Headache, dizziness, drowsiness, vertigo, tinnitus, anxiety

MS: Muscle, joint pain

GI: Constipation, abdominal pain, nausea, fecal impaction, hemorrhoids, flatulence, vomiting, steatorrhea, peptic ulcer

INTEG: Rash, irritation of perianal area, tongue, skin

HEMA: ***Bleeding,*** increased PT

META: Decreased vit A, D, K, red cell folate content; ***hyperchloremic acidosis***

Contraindications: Hypersensitivity, biliary obstruction

Precautions: Pregnancy (C), lactation, children

Pharmacokinetics:

PO: Excreted in feces, LDL lowered

in 4-7 days, serum cholesterol lowered in 1 mo

Interactions:

- ↓ absorption of: warfarin, thiazides, cardiac glycosides; propranolol, corticosteroids, iron, thyroid hormones, fat-soluble vitamins, clindamycin, penicillin G, tetracyclines, clofibrate, gemfibrozil, glipiZIDE, phenytoin, Vit A, D, E, K

↑ effect: glucomannan

↓ gotu kola

Lab test interferences:

Interfere: cholecystography

Increase: AST, ALT, alk phosphatase

Decrease: Sodium, potassium

NURSING CONSIDERATIONS

Assess:

- Cardiac glycoside level, if both drugs are being administered
- For signs of vit A, D, K deficiency
- Fasting LDL, HDL, total cholesterol, triglyceride levels, electrolytes if on extended therapy
- Bowel pattern daily; increase bulk, H_2O in diet for constipation

Administer:

- Drug qd or bid; give all other medications 1 hr before cholestyramine or 4-6 hr after cholestyramine to avoid poor absorption
- Drug mixed with applesauce or stirred into beverage (2-6 oz), let stand for 2 min; do not take dry, avoid inhaling powder
- Supplemental doses of vit A, D, K, if levels are low

Evaluate:

- Therapeutic response: decreased cholesterol level (hyperlipidemia); diarrhea, pruritus (excess bile acids)

Teach patient/family:

The symptoms of hypoprothrombinemia: bleeding mucous membranes, dark tarry stools, hematuria, petechiae; report immediately

- The importance of compliance
- That risk factors should be decreased: high-fat diet, smoking, alcohol consumption, absence of exercise

choline salicylate (℞)

(koe'leen sa-liss'ih-late)

Arthropan, choline/magnesium salicylates CMT, Tricosal, Trilisate

Func. class.: Nonopioid analgesic

Chem. class.: Salicylate

Action: Blocks pain impulses in CNS that occur in response to inhibition of prostaglandin synthesis; antipyretic action results from inhibition of hypothalamic heat-regulating center to produce vasodilation to allow heat dissipation

Uses: Mild to moderate pain or fever including arthritis, juvenile rheumatoid arthritis

Dosage and routes:

Choline salicylate

- *Adult and child >12 yr:* **PO** 870-1740 mg qid; max 6×/day

Pain/fever

- *Adult:* **PO** 435-870 mg q3-4h prn

Choline/magnesium salicylates

- *Adult:* **PO** 2-3 g salicylate/day divided bid-tid
- *Child >37 kg:* **PO** 2.2 g of salicylate/day divided bid
- *Child <37 kg:* **PO** 50 mg of salicylate/kg/day divided bid

Available forms: Choline salicylate liq 870 mg/5 ml; choline/magnesium salicylate tabs 500, 750, 1000 mg; liq 500 mg/5 ml

Side effects/adverse reactions:

HEMA: ***Thrombocytopenia, agranulocytosis, leukopenia, neutropenia, hemolytic anemia,*** increased PT

CNS: Stimulation, drowsiness, diz-

ziness, confusion, ***convulsion,*** headache, flushing, hallucinations, ***coma***
GI: Nausea, vomiting, GI bleeding, diarrhea, heartburn, anorexia, ***hepatitis, hepatotoxicity***
INTEG: Rash, urticaria, bruising, sweating
EENT: Tinnitus, hearing loss
CV: Rapid pulse, pulmonary edema
RESP: Wheezing, hyperpnea, hyperventilation
ENDO: Hypoglycemia, hyponatremia, hypokalemia

Contraindications: Hypersensitivity to salicylates, GI bleeding, bleeding disorders, children <3 yr, vit K deficiency, children with flulike symptoms

Precautions: Anemia, hepatic disease, renal disease, Hodgkin's disease, pregnancy (C), lactation

Pharmacokinetics:
Absorbed via GI tract, onset 15-30 min; metabolized by liver; crosses placenta; excreted in breast milk, by kidneys, half-life 2-3 hr, large doses 15-30 hr

Interactions:
- ↓ effects of aspirin: antacids (high doses), steroids, urinary alkalizers, corticosteroids
- ↑ bleeding: alcohol, heparin, plicamycin, cefamandole
- ↑ effects of warfarin, insulin, methotrexate, thrombolytic agents, penicillins, phenytoin, valproic acid, oral hypoglycemics, sulfonamides
- ↑ salicylate levels: urinary acidifiers, ammonium chloride, nizatidine
- ↓ effects of probenecid, spironolactone, sulfinpyrazone, sulfonylamides, NSAIDs, β-blockers
- Gastric ulcer: steroids, antiinflammatories, NSAIDs

↑ bleeding risk: bilberry, bogbean, chondroitin, horse chestnut, Irish moss, kelpware, pansy

Lab test interferences:
Increase: Coagulation studies, LFTs, serum uric acid, amylase, CO_2, urinary protein
Decrease: Serum K, PBI, cholesterol
Interference: Urine catecholamines, pregnancy test

NURSING CONSIDERATIONS

Assess:
- Pain: location, intensity, character baseline and 1-2 hr after dose
- Hepatic studies: AST, ALT, bilirubin, creatinine (long-term therapy)
- Renal studies: BUN, urine creatinine (long-term therapy)
- Blood studies: CBC, Hct, Hgb, PT (long-term therapy)
- I&O ratio; decreasing output may indicate renal failure (long-term therapy)

Hepatotoxicity: dark urine; clay-colored stools; yellowing of skin, sclera; itching; abdominal pain; fever; diarrhea (long-term therapy)
- Allergic reactions: rash, urticaria; drug may have to be discontinued
- Renal dysfunction: decreased urine output
- Ototoxicity: tinnitus, ringing, roaring in ears; audiometric testing needed before, after long-term therapy
- Visual changes: blurring, halos, corneal, retinal damage
- Edema in feet, ankles, legs
- Drug history; many interactions

Administer:
- Mixed with fruit juice, carbonated beverage, water

Evaluate:
- Therapeutic response: decreased pain, fever, stiffness of joints

Teach patient/family:
- To report any symptoms of hepatotoxicity, renal toxicity, visual changes, ototoxicity, allergic reactions, bleeding (long-term therapy)

• Not to exceed recommended dosage; acute poisoning may result
• To read label on other OTC drugs; many contain aspirin
• That therapeutic response takes 2 wk (arthritis)
• To avoid alcohol ingestion; GI bleeding may occur
• That if anticoagulants are given with this drug, this drug should be decreased 2 wk before surgery

Treatment of overdose: Lavage, activated charcoal, monitor electrolytes, VS

ciclopirox topical

See appendix c

cidofovir (℞)

(si-doh-foh'veer)

Vistide

Func. class.: Antiviral

Chem. class.: Nucleotide analog

Action: Suppresses cytomegalovirus (CMV) replication by selective inhibition of viral DNA synthesis

Uses: CMV retinitis in patients with HIV, used with probenecid

Dosage and routes:

• Dilute in 100 ml 0.9% saline sol before administration; probenecid must be given **PO** 2 g 3 hr prior to the cidofovir infusion and 1 g at 2 and 8 hr after ending the cidofovir infusion; give 1 L of 0.9% saline sol **IV** with each **INF** of cidofovir, give saline **INF** over 1-2 hr period immediately prior to cidofovir; patient should be given a 2nd L if the patient can tolerate the fluid load (2nd L given at time of cidofovir or immediately afterward and should be given over a 1-3 hr period)

Renal dose

• CCr <50 ml/min reduce dose

Induction

• *Adult:* **IV INF** initially, 5 mg/kg given over 1 hr at a constant rate qwk × 2 consecutive wk; then **IV INF** 5 mg/kg given over 1 hr q2wk

Available forms: Inj 75 mg/ml

Side effects/adverse reactions:

CNS: Fever, chills, ***coma,*** confusion, abnormal thought, *dizziness*, bizarre dreams, *headache*, psychosis, tremors, somnolence, paresthesia, *amnesia, anxiety, insomnia,* ***seizures***

CV: Dysrhythmias, hypertension/hypotension

EENT: Retinal detachment in CMV retinitis

GI: Abnormal LFTs, *nausea, vomiting, anorexia, diarrhea*, abdominal pain, ***hemorrhage***

GU: ***Hematuria,*** increased creatinine, BUN, ***nephrotoxicity***

HEMA: ***Granulocytopenia, thrombocytopenia, irreversible neutropenia, anemia, eosinophilia***

INTEG: Rash, alopecia, pruritus, acne, urticaria, pain at inj site, phlebitis

RESP: Dyspnea

Contraindications: Hypersensitivity to this drug or probenecid, sulfa drugs

Precautions: Preexisting cytopenias, renal function impairment, pregnancy (C), lactation, children <6 mo, elderly, platelet count <25,000/mm^3

Pharmacokinetics: Unknown

Interactions:

• Nephrotoxicity: amphotericin B, foscarnet, aminoglycosides, pentamidine IV, NSAIDs

NURSING CONSIDERATIONS

Assess:

• Culture before treatment is initiated; cultures of blood, urine, and throat may all be taken; CMV is not

confirmed by this method; the diagnosis is made by an ophthalmic exam
• Renal, hepatic, increased hemopoietic studies and BUN; serum creatinine, AST, ALT, creatinine, CCr, A-G ratio, baseline and drip treatment, blood counts should be done q2wk; watch for decreasing granulocytes, Hgb; if low, therapy may have to be discontinued and restarted after hematologic recovery; blood transfusions may be required
• For GI symptoms: severe nausea, vomiting, diarrhea; severe symptoms may necessitate discontinuing drug
• Electrolytes and minerals: calcium, phosphorus, magnesium, sodium, potassium; watch closely for tetany during first administration
• For symptoms of blood dyscrasias (anemia, granulocytopenia); bruising, fatigue, bleeding, poor healing
• Allergic reactions: flushing, rash, urticaria, pruritus
• For leukopenia, neutropenia, thrombocytopenia: WBCs, platelets q2d during 2×/day dosing and qwk thereafter; check for leukopenias, with qd WBC count in patients with prior leukopenia, with other nucleoside analogs, or for whom leukopenia counts are <1000 cells/mm^3 at start of treatment
• Monitor serum creatinine or CCr at least q2wk; give only to those with creatinine levels ≤1.5 mg/dl, CCr >55 ml/min, urine protein <100 mg/dl

Administer:

IV route

• Mix under strict aseptic conditions using gloves, gown, and mask, and using precautions for antineoplastic
• After diluting in 100 ml 0.9% NaCl
• Slowly; do not give by bolus IV, SC inj
• Use diluted sol within 12 hr, do not refrigerate or freeze; do not use sol with particulate matter or discoloration

Evaluate:

• Therapeutic response: decreased symptoms of CMV

Teach patient/family:

• To notify prescriber if sore throat, swollen lymph nodes, malaise, fever occur; may indicate other infections
• To report perioral tingling, numbness in extremities, and paresthesias
• That serious drug interactions may occur if OTC products are ingested; check first with prescriber
• That drug is not a cure, but will control symptoms
• That regular ophthalmic exams must be continued
• That major toxicities may necessitate discontinuing drug
• To use contraception during treatment and that infertility may occur; men should use barrier contraception for 90 days after treatment

Treatment of overdose: Discontinue drug; use hemodialysis, and increase hydration

cilostazol (℞)

(sih-los'tah-zol)

Pletal

Func. class.: Platelet aggregation inhibitor

Chem. class.: Quinolinone derivative

Action: Inhibits cellular phosphodiesterase; reversibly inhibits platelet aggregation induced by thrombin, ADP, collagen, arachidonic acid, epINEPHrine, and sheer stress

Uses: Intermittent claudication

Dosage and routes:

• *Adult:* **PO** 100 mg bid taken ≥30

min ac or 2 hr pc breakfast and dinner or 50 mg bid if using drugs that inhibit CYP3A4 and CYP2C19; 12 wk of treatment may be needed for beneficial effect

Available forms: Tabs 50, 100 mg

Side effects/adverse reactions:

CNS: Dizziness, headache

CV: Palpitations, tachycardia, nodal dysrhythmia, postural hypotension

GI: Nausea, vomiting, *diarrhea,* GI discomfort, colitis, cholelithiasis, ulcer, esophagitis, gastritis, anorexia, *flatulence, dyspepsia*

HEMA: ***Bleeding (epistaxis, hematuria, retinal hemorrhage, GI bleeding), thrombocytopenia,*** anemia, polycythemia

INTEG: Rash, urticaria, dry skin

GU: Cystitis, frequency, vaginitis, ***vaginal hemorrhage,*** hematuria

EENT: Blindness, diplopia, ear pain, tinnitus, retinal hemorrhage

MISC: Back pain, headache, infection, myalgia, peripheral edema, chills, fever, malaise, diabetes mellitus

RESP: Cough, pharyngitis, rhinitis, asthma, pneumonia

Contraindications: Hypersensitivity, CHF

Precautions: Past liver disease, renal disease, elderly, pregnancy (C), lactation, children, increased bleeding risk, low platelet count, platelet dysfunction, active bleeding

Do not confuse:

Pletal/Plendil

Pharmacokinetics: 95%-98% protein binding, metabolism-hepatic extensively by cytochrome P450 enzymes, excreted urine (74%), feces (20%), half-life 11-13 hr

Interactions:

• ↑ bleeding tendencies: anticoagulants

• ↑ cilostazol levels: diltiazem, erythromycin, omeprazole; exercise caution when coadministering with fluvoxamine, fluoxetine, nefazodone, ketoconazole, itraconazole, fluconazole and reduce dose to 50 mg bid

• Drug/food: do not use with grapefruit juice

↑ bleeding risk: agrimony, alfalfa, angelica, anise, bilberry, black haw, bogbean, buchu, chondroitin, dong quai, fenugreek, feverfew, garlic, ginger, ginkgo, ginseng, horse chestnut, Irish moss, kelp, kelpware, khella, lovage, lungwort, meadowsweet, motherwort, mugwort, nettle, papaya, parsley (large amt), Pau D'arco, pineapple, poplar, prickly ash, safflower, saw palmetto, senega, tonka bean, turmeric, wintergreen, yarrow

↓ action: chamomile, coenzyme Q10, flax, glucomannan, goldenseal

NURSING CONSIDERATIONS

Assess:

• For underlying CV disease since CV risk is great; for CV lesions with repeated oral administration

• For congestive heart failure

• Blood studies: CBC q2 wk, Hct, Hgb, PT

Administer:

• Give bid 1 hr ac or 2 hr pc; do not give with grapefruit juice

Evaluate:

• Therapeutic response: improved walking distance and duration, decreased pain

Teach patient/family:

• To report any unusual bleeding

• To report side effects such as diarrhea, skin rashes, subcutaneous bleeding

• That effects may take 2-4 wk, treatment of up to 12 wk may be required for necessary effect

• About potential risk for patients with CHF

• To take 1 hr ac or 2 hr pc

• That reading the patient package insert is necessary

cimetidine (OTC, ℞)

(sye-met'i-deen)

Apo-Cimetidine♣, cimetidine, Novo-Cimetidine♣, Peptol♣, Tagamet, Tagamet HB

Func. class.: H_2-histamine receptor antagonist

Chem. class.: Imidazole derivative

Action: Inhibits histamine at H_2-receptor site in the gastric parietal cells, which inhibits gastric acid secretion

Uses: Short-term treatment of duodenal and gastric ulcers and maintenance; management of GERD and Zollinger-Ellison syndrome

Investigational uses: Prevention of aspiration pneumonitis, stress ulcers, upper GI bleeding, herpes infection, hirsutism, cutaneous/nongenital warts, weight loss

Dosage and routes:

Treatment of active ulcers

• *Adult:* **PO** 300 mg qid with meals, hs × 8 wk or 400 mg bid, 800 mg hs; after 8 wk give hs dose only; **IV BOL** 300 mg/20 ml 0.9% NaCl over 1-2 min q6h; **IV INF** 300 mg/50 ml D_5W over 15-20 min; **IM** 300 mg q6h, not to exceed 2400 mg/day

• *Child:* **PO** 20-40 mg/kg/day; **IM/IV** 5-10 mg/kg q6-8h

Prophylaxis of duodenal ulcer

• *Adult and child >16 yr:* 400 mg hs

GERD

• *Adult:* **PO** 800-1600 mg/day in divided doses

Hypersecretory conditions (Zollinger-Ellison syndrome)

• *Adult:* **PO/IM/IV** 300-600 mg q6h; may increase to 12 g/day if needed

Upper GI bleeding prophylaxis

• *Adult:* **IV** 50 mg/hr; lowered in renal disease

Aspiration pneumonitis prophylaxis

• *Adult:* **IM/IV** 300 mg **IM** 1 hr before anesthesia, then 300 mg **IV** q4h until patient is alert, max 2400 mg/day

Hirsutism

• *Adult:* **PO** 300 mg qid × 5 days or 1600 mg qd up to 6 mo

Warts

• *Adult:* **PO** 400-800 mg tid × 12 wk or 30-40 mg/kg/day given tid × 3 mo

Weight loss

• *Adult:* **PO** 200-400 mg tid × 8-12 wk

Renal disease

• CCr 20-40 ml/min 300 mg q8h; CCr <20 ml/min 300 mg q12h

Available forms: Tabs 100, 200, 300, 400, 800 mg; liq 200, 300 mg/5 ml; inj 300 mg/2 ml, 300 mg/50 ml 0.9% NaCl

Side effects/adverse reactions:

CNS: Confusion, headache, depression, dizziness, anxiety, weakness, psychosis, tremors, ***convulsions***

CV: Bradycardia, tachycardia, ***dysrhythmias***

GI: Diarrhea, abdominal cramps, ***paralytic ileus, jaundice***

GU: Gynecomastia, galactorrhea, impotence, increase in BUN, creatinine

HEMA: ***Agranulocytosis, thrombocytopenia, neutropenia, aplastic anemia, increase in PT***

INTEG: Urticaria, rash, alopecia, sweating, flushing, ***exfoliative dermatitis***

Contraindications: Hypersensitivity

Precautions: Pregnancy (B), lactation, child <16 yr, organic brain syndrome, hepatic disease, renal disease, elderly

Pharmacokinetics: Well absorbed (PO, IM)

IM/IV: Onset 10 min, peak ½ hr, duration 4-5 hr

PO: Peak 1-1½ hr, half-life 1½-2 hr; 30%-40% metabolized by liver, excreted in urine unchanged, crosses placenta, enters breast milk

Interactions:

- ↑ toxicity due to CYP450 pathway: benzodiazepines, β-blockers, calcium channel blockers, carbamazepine, chloroquine, lidocaine, metronidazole, moricizine, phenytoin, quinidine, quinine, sulfonylureas, theophylline, tricyclics, valproic acid, warfarin
- ↓ absorption of cimetidine: antacids, sucralfate
- ↓ absorption: ketoconazole

Lab test interferences:

Increase: Alk phosphatase, AST, creatinine, prolactin

False positive: Gastroccult, hemoccult

False negative: Skin tests

NURSING CONSIDERATIONS

Assess:

- Gastric pH (5 or more should be maintained), also epigastric pain and duration, intensity; aggravating, ameliorating factors
- I&O ratio, BUN, creatinine, CBC with differential periodically

Administer:

- With meals for prolonged drug effect; antacids 1 hr before or 1 hr after cimetidine

IV route

- After diluting 300 mg/20 ml of 0.9% NaCl for inj; give ≥5 min; may be diluted 300 mg/50 ml of D_5W; run over 15-20 min; or total daily dose (900 mg) diluted in 100-1000 ml D_5W given over 24 hr

Additive compatibilities: AcetaZOLAMIDE, amikacin, aminophylline, atracurium, cefoperazone, cefoxitin, chlorothiazide, clindamycin, colistimethate, dexamethasone, digoxin, epINEPHrine, erythromycin, ethacrynate, floxacillin, flumazenil, furosemide, gentamicin, insulin (regular), isoproterenol, lidocaine, lincomycin, meropenem, metaraminol, methylPREDNISolone, norepinephrine, nitroprusside, penicillin G potassium, phytonadione, polymyxin B, potassium chloride, protamine, quinidine, tacrolimus, vancomycin, verapamil, vit B/C

Syringe compatibilities: Atropine, butorphanol, cephalothin, diazepam, diphenhydrAMINE, doxapram, droperidol, fentanyl, glycopyrrolate, heparin, hydromorphone, hydrOXYzine, lorazepam, meperidine, midazolam, morphine, nafcillin, nalbuphine, penicillin G sodium, pentazocine, perphenazine, prochlorperazine, promazine, promethazine, scopolamine

Y-site compatibilities: Acyclovir, amifostine, aminophylline, amrinone, atracurium, aztreonam, cisatracurium, cisplatin, cladribine, cyclophosphamide, cytarabine, diltiazem, DOXOrubicin, DOXOrubicin liposome, enalaprilat, esmolol, filgrastim, fluconazole, fludarabine, foscarnet, gallium, granisetron, haloperidol, heparin, hetastarch, idarubicin, labetalol, melphalan, meropenem, methotrexate, midazolam, ondansetron, paclitaxel, pancuronium, piperacillin/tazobactam, propofol, remifentanil, sargramostim, tacrolimus, teniposide, theophylline, thiotepa, tolazoline, vecuronium, vinorelbine, zidovudine

Perform/provide:

- Storage of diluted sol at room temperature up to 48 hr

Evaluate:

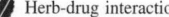

- Therapeutic response: decreased

pain in abdomen; healing of ulcers, absence of gastroesophageal reflux, gastric pH 5

Teach patient/family:

• That gynecomastia, impotence may occur, are reversible

• To avoid driving, other hazardous activities until patient is stabilized on this medication; drowsiness or dizziness may occur

• To avoid black pepper, caffeine, alcohol, harsh spices, extremes in temperature of food

• To avoid OTC preparations: aspirin, cough, cold preparations; condition may worsen

• That smoking decreases the effectiveness of the drug

• That drug must be taken exactly as prescribed and continued for prescribed time to be effective; doses not to be doubled

• To report bruising, fatigue, malaise; blood dyscrasias may occur

• To report to prescriber diarrhea, black tarry stools, sore throat, rash

ciprofloxacin (℞)

(sip-ro-floks′a-sin)

Cipro, Cipro IV

Func. class.: Broad-spectrum antiinfective

Chem. class.: Fluoroquinolone

Action: Interferes with conversion of intermediate DNA fragments into high-molecular-weight DNA in bacteria; DNA gyrase inhibitor

Uses: Infection caused by susceptible *Escherichia coli, Enterobacter cloacae, Proteus mirabilis, Klebsiella pneumoniae, Proteus vulgaris, Citrobacter freundii, Serratia marcescens, Pseudomonas aeruginosa, Staphylococcus aureus, Staphylococcus epidermidis, Enterobacter, Campylobacter jejuni, Salmonella;* chronic bacterial prostatitis, acute sinusitis, postexposure inhalation anthrax

Dosage and routes:

Uncomplicated urinary tract infections

• *Adult:* **PO** 250 mg q12h; **IV** 200 mg q12h

Complicated/severe urinary tract infections

• *Adult:* **PO** 500 mg q12h; **IV** 400 mg q12h

Respiratory, bone, skin, joint infections

• *Adult:* **PO** 500-750 mg q12h; **IV** 400 mg q12h

Renal disease

• CCr 30-50 ml/min **PO** 250-500 mg q12h; CCr 5-29 ml/min **PO** 250-500 mg q18h; **IV** 200-400 mg q18-24h

Available forms: Tabs 250, 500, 750 mg; inj 200 mg/20 ml, 400 mg/40 ml, 200 mg/100 ml D_5, 400 mg/200 ml D_5; oral susp 250, 500 mg/5 ml

Side effects/adverse reactions:

CNS: Headache, dizziness, fatigue, insomnia, depression, *restlessness,* ***seizures,*** confusion

GI: Nausea, diarrhea, increased ALT, AST, dry mouth, flatulence, heartburn, *vomiting*, oral candidiasis, dysphagia, ***pseudomembranous colitis***

INTEG: Rash, pruritus, urticaria, photosensitivity, flushing, fever, chills

MS: Tremor, arthralgia, tendon rupture

MISC: ***Anaphylaxis, Stevens-Johnson syndrome***

Contraindications: Hypersensitivity to quinolones

Precautions: Pregnancy (C), lactation, children, renal disease, epilepsy

Do not confuse:

ciprofloxacin/cephalexin

Pharmacokinetics:

PO: Peak 1 hr, half-life 3-4 hr; excreted in urine as active drug, metabolites

Interactions:

- ↓ ciproflaxin absorption: antacids containing magnesium, aluminum; zinc, iron, sucralfate, enteral feedings, calcium
- Nephrotoxicity: cycloSPORINE
- ↑ ciprofloxacin levels: probenecid; monitor for toxicity
- ↑ levels of: theophylline, warfarin, monitor blood levels
- Drug/food: ↑ effect of: caffeine; ↓ absorption: dairy products, food

Possible toxicity: yerba maté

↓ effect: fennel

Do not use acidophilus with anti-infectives

Lab test interferences:

Increase: AST, ALT, BUN, creatinine, LDH, bilirubin, alk phosphatase, glucose proteinuria, albuminuria

Decrease: WBC, glucose

NURSING CONSIDERATIONS

Assess:

- CNS symptoms: headache, dizziness, fatigue, insomnia, depression
- Renal, hepatic studies: BUN, creatinine, AST, ALT
- I&O ratio, urine pH <5.5 is ideal

Anaphylaxis: fever, flushing, rash, urticaria, pruritus, dyspnea

Administer:

- 2 hr before or 2 hr after antacids, zinc, iron, calcium

IV route

- Over 1 hr as an INF, comes in premixed plastic INF container or diluted 20 or 40 ml vial to a final conc of 0.5-2 mg/ml of NS or D_5W; give through Y-tube or 3-way stopcock
- After clean-catch urine for C&S

Additive compatibilities: Amikacin, aztreonam, ceftazidime, cycloSPORINE, gentamicin, metronidazole, netilmicin, piperacillin, potassium acetate, potassium chloride, potassium phosphates, prednisoLONE, promethazine, propofol, ranitidine, Ringer's, sodium chloride, tobramycin, vit B/C

Y-site compatibilities: Amifostine, amino acids, aztreonam, calcium gluconate, ceftazidime, cisatracurium, digoxin, diltiazem, diphenhydrAMINE, DOBUTamine, DOPamine, DOXOrubicin liposome, gallium, gentamicin, granisetron, hydrOXYzine, lidocaine, lorazepam, metoclopramide, midazolam, midodrine, piperacillin, potassium acetate, potassium chloride, potassium phosphates, prednisoLONE, promethazine, propofol, ranitidine, remifentanil, Ringer's, sodium chloride, tacrolimus, teniposide, thiotepa, tobramycin, verapamil

Perform/provide:

- Limited intake of alkaline foods, drugs: milk, dairy products, alkaline antacids, sodium bicarbonate

Evaluate:

- Therapeutic response: decreased pain, frequency, urgency, C&S; absence of infection

Teach patient/family:

- Not to take any products containing magnesium or calcium (such as antacids), iron, or aluminum with this drug or within 2 hr of drug
- That photosensitivity may occur; patient should avoid sunlight or use sunscreen to prevent burns
- That fluids must be increased to 3 L/day to avoid crystallization in kidneys
- If dizziness occurs, to ambulate, perform activities with assistance
- To complete full course of drug therapy, not to double or miss doses
- To contact prescriber if adverse reaction occurs or if inflammation or pain in tendon occurs
- To use frequent rinsing of mouth, sugarless candy or gum for dry mouth
- Not to use theophylline with this product, will cause toxicity, con-

tact prescriber if taking theophylline

ciprofloxacin ophthalmic

See appendix c

HIGH ALERT

cisplatin (℞)

(sis'pla-tin)

Platinol✦, Platinol-AQ

Func. class.: Antineoplastic alkylating agent

Chem. class.: Inorganic heavy metal

Action: Alkylates DNA, RNA; inhibits enzymes that allow synthesis of amino acids in proteins; activity is not cell cycle phase specific

Uses: Advanced bladder cancer, adjunctive in metastatic testicular cancer, adjunctive in metastatic ovarian cancer, head, neck cancer, esophagus, prostate, lung and cervical cancer, lymphoma

Dosage and routes:

Dosage protocols may vary

Testicular cancer

• *Adult:* **IV** 20 mg/m^2 qd × 5 days, repeat q3wk for 3 cycles or more, depending on response

Bladder cancer

• *Adult:* **IV** 50-70 mg/m^2 q3-4wk

Metastatic ovarian cancer

• *Adult:* **IV** 100 mg/m^2 q4wk or 50 mg/m^2 q3wk with cyclophosphamide; mix with 2 L NaCl and 37.5 g mannitol over 6 hr

Available forms: Inj 0.5✦, 1 mg/ml; powder for inj 10, 50 mg vials

Side effects/adverse reactions:

EENT: Tinnitus, hearing loss, vestibular toxicity

HEMA: ***Thrombocytopenia, leukopenia, pancytopenia***

CV: Cardiac abnormalities

GI: Severe nausea, vomiting, diarrhea, weight loss

GU: ***Renal tubular damage,*** renal insufficiency, impotence, sterility, amenorrhea, gynecomastia, hyperuremia

INTEG: Alopecia, dermatitis

CNS: ***Seizures,*** peripheral neuropathy

RESP: ***Fibrosis***

META: Hypomagnesemia, hypocalcemia, hypokalemia, hypophosphatemia

SYST: ***Anaphylaxis***

Contraindications: Radiation therapy or chemotherapy within 1 mo, thrombocytopenia, recent smallpox vaccination, pregnancy (D)

Precautions: Pneumococcus vaccination, lactation

Do not confuse:

cisplatin/carboplatin

Platinol/Paraplatin

Pharmacokinetics: Absorption complete, metabolized in liver, excreted in urine; half-life 30-100 hr, accumulates in body tissues for several months, enters breast milk

Interactions:

• Risk of bleeding: aspirin, NSAIDs, alcohol

• Ototoxicity: bumetanide, ethacrynic acid, furosemide

• ↓ antibody response: live virus vaccines

• ↑ myelosuppression: myelosuppressive agents, radiation

• ↑ nephrotoxicity: aminoglycosides, loop diuretics

• ↓ effects of: phenytoin

Lab test interferences:

Positive: Coombs' test

Increase: Uric acid, BUN, creatinine

Decrease: CCr, calcium, phosphate, potassium, magnesium

NURSING CONSIDERATIONS

Assess:

For bone marrow depression

• CBC, differential, platelet count weekly; withhold drug if WBC is <4000 or platelet count is <100,000; notify prescriber of results

• Renal studies: BUN, creatinine, serum uric acid, urine CCr before, electrolytes during therapy; dose should not be given if BUN <25 mg/dl; creatinine <1.5 mg/dl; I&O ratio; report fall in urine output of <30 ml/hr

• For anaphylaxis: wheezing, tachycardia, facial swelling, fainting; discontinue drug and report to prescriber; resuscitation equipment should be nearby

• Monitor temp q4h (may indicate beginning infection)

• Hepatic studies before, during therapy (bilirubin, AST, ALT, LDH) as needed or monthly

• Bleeding: hematuria, guaiac, bruising or petechiae, mucosa or orifices q8h; obtain prescription for viscous lidocaine (Xylocaine)

• Effects of alopecia on body image; discuss feelings about body changes

• Jaundice of skin, sclera; dark urine; clay-colored stools; itchy skin; abdominal pain; fever; diarrhea

• Edema in feet, joint pain, stomach pain, shaking

Administer:

IV route

• Do not use aluminum equipment during any preparation or administration, will form precipitate; do not refrigerate unopened powder or solution, protect from sunlight

• Prepare in biologic cabinet using gown, gloves, mask, do not allow drug to come in contact with skin, use soap and water if contact occurs

• For intermittent inf, dilute 10 mg/10 ml or 50 mg/50 ml sterile H_2O for inj; withdraw prescribed dose, dilute ½ dose with 1000 ml D_5 0.2 NaCl or D_5 0.45 NaCl with 37.5 g mannitol; IV INF is given over 3-4 hr; use a 0.45 μm filter; total dose 2 L over 6-8 hr; check site for irritation, phlebitis

• For continuous inf give over 24 hr × 5 days

• Hydrate patient with 0.9% NaCl over 8-12 hr before treatment

• Epinephrine, antihistamines, corticosteroids for hypersensitivity reaction

• Antiemetic 30-60 min before giving drug and prn

• Allopurinol to maintain uric acid levels, alkalinization of urine

• Diuretic (furosemide 40 mg IV) or mannitol after infusion

Additive compatibilities: Carboplatin, cyclophosphamide with etoposide, etoposide, etoposide with floxuridine, floxuridine, floxuridine with leucovorin, hydroxyzine, ifosfamide, ifosfamide with etoposide, leucovorin, magnesium sulfate, mannitol, ondansetron

Solution compatibilities: D_5/0.225% NaCl, D_5/0.45% NaCl, D_5/0.9% NaCl, D_5/0.45% NaCl with mannitol 1.875%, D_5/0.33% NaCl with KCl 20 mEq and mannitol 1.875%, 0.9% NaCl, 0.45% NaCl, 0.3% NaCl, 0.225% NaCl

Syringe compatibilities: Bleomycin, cyclophosphamide, doxapram, DOXOrubicin, droperidol, fluorouracil, furosemide, heparin, leucovorin, methotrexate, metoclopramide, mitomycin, vinBLAStine, vinCRIStine

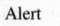

Y-site compatibilities: Allopurinol, aztreonam, bleomycin, chlorproMAZINE, cimetidine, cladribine, cyclophosphamide, dexamethasone, diphenhydrAMINE, DOXOrubicin, DOXOrubicin liposome, droperidol, famotidine, filgrastim, fludarabine, fluorouracil, furosemide, ganciclovir, granisetron, heparin, hydromorphone, leucovorin, lorazepam, melphalan, methotrexate, methylPREDNISolone, metoclopramide, mitomycin, morphine, ondansetron, paclitaxel, prochlorperazine, promethazine, propofol, ranitidine, sargramostim, teniposide, vinBLAStine, vinCRIStine, vinorelbine

Perform/provide:
- Comprehensive oral hygiene
- All medications PO, if possible, avoid IM inj when platelets <100,000/mm^3
- Increase fluid intake to 2-3 L/day to prevent urate deposits, calculi formation; promote elimination of drug

Evaluate:
- Therapeutic response: decreased tumor size, spread of malignancy

Teach patient/family:
- To report signs of infection: increased temp, sore throat, flulike symptoms
- To report signs of anemia: fatigue, headache, faintness, shortness of breath, irritability
- To report bleeding, bruising, petechiae: avoid use of razors, commercial mouthwash
- To avoid aspirin, ibuprofen, NSAIDs, alcohol; may cause GI bleeding
- To report any complaints or side effects to nurse or prescriber
- That impotence or amenorrhea can occur; reversible after discontinuing treatment
- To report any changes in breathing, coughing
- That hair may be lost during treatment; a wig or hairpiece may make patient feel better; new hair may be different in color, texture
- To report numbness, tingling in face or extremities, poor hearing or joint pain, swelling
- Not to receive vaccinations during treatment
- To use contraception during treatment and 4 mo after; this drug may cause infertility

C

citalopram (℞)

(sigh-tal'oh-pram)

Celexa

Func. class.: Antidepressant

Chem. class.: Selective serotonin reuptake inhibitor (SSRI)

Action: Inhibits CNS neuron uptake of serotonin but not of norepinephrine; weak inhibitor of CYP450 enzyme system, making it more appealing than other drugs

Uses:
Major depressive disorder

Investigational uses: Fibromyalgia, premenstrual disorders, panic disorder, social phobia, impulsive aggression in children, obsessive-compulsive disorder in adolescents, treatment of psychotic symptoms in nondepressed demented patients

Dosage and routes:

Depression
- *Adult:* **PO** 20 mg qd AM or PM, may increase if needed to 40 mg/day after 1 wk; maintenance: after 6-8 wk of initial treatment, continue for 24 wk (32 wk total), reevaluate long-term usefulness (max 60 mg/day)

Fibromyalgia
- *Adult:* **PO** 20 mg qd × 4 wk; increase dose to 40 mg qd × 4 wk

Hepatic dose/Elderly
- *Adult:* **PO** 20 mg/day, may increase to 40 mg/day if no response

Panic disorder
- *Adult:* **PO** 20-30 mg/day

Premenstrual dysphoria, social phobia, impulsive aggression in children
- *Adult:* **PO** 20-40 mg/day, used in-

termittently in premenstrual dysphoria

Available forms: Tabs 10, 20, 40 mg; oral sol 2 mg (as base)/ml

Side effects/adverse reactions:

CNS: Headache, nervousness, insomnia, drowsiness, anxiety, tremor, dizziness, fatigue, sedation, poor concentration, abnormal dreams, agitation, ***convulsions,*** apathy, euphoria, hallucinations, delusions, psychosis, ***suicidal attempts***

GI: Nausea, diarrhea, dry mouth, anorexia, dyspepsia, constipation, cramps, vomiting, taste changes, flatulence, decreased appetite

INTEG: Sweating, rash, pruritus, acne, alopecia, urticaria

RESP: Infection, pharyngitis, nasal congestion, sinus headache, sinusitis, cough, dyspnea, bronchitis, asthma, hyperventilation, pneumonia

CV: Hot flashes, palpitations, angina pectoris, ***hemorrhage,*** hypertension, tachycardia, 1st-degree AV block, bradycardia, *MI,* thrombophlebitis

MS: Pain, arthritis, twitching

GU: Dysmenorrhea, decreased libido, urinary frequency, UTI, amenorrhea, cystitis, impotence, urine retention

EENT: Visual changes, ear/eye pain, photophobia, tinnitus

SYST: Asthenia, viral infection, fever, allergy, chills

Contraindications: Hypersensitivity

Precautions: Pregnancy (C), lactation, children, elderly

Do not confuse:

Celexa/Celebrex/Cerebyx/Cerebra

Pharmacokinetics:

PO: Metabolized in liver; excreted in urine; steady state 28-35 days; peak 2-4 hr; half-life 35 hr

Interactions:

- ↑ effect of tricyclics, use cautiously
- ↑ CNS effects: CNS depressants

Fatal reactions: do not use with MAOIs

- ↑ citalopram levels: macrolides, azole antifungals
- ↑ plasma levels of: β-blockers
- ↓ citalopram levels: carbamazepine
- ↑ serotonergic effects: lithium

Serotonin syndrome: St. John's wort, SAM-e; fatal reaction may occur; do not use concurrently

↑ CNS stimulation: yohimbe

Lab test interferences:

- *Increase:* Serum bilirubin, blood glucose, alk phosphatase
- *Decrease:* VMA, 5-HIAA
- *False increase:* Urinary catecholamines

NURSING CONSIDERATIONS

Assess:

- Mental status: mood, sensorium, affect, suicidal tendencies, increase in psychiatric symptoms, depression, panic
- B/P (lying/standing), pulse q4h; if systolic B/P drops 20 mm Hg, hold drug, notify prescriber; take vital signs q4h in patients with cardiovascular disease
- Weight qwk; appetite may decrease or increase with drug
- ECG for flattening of T wave, bundle branch, AV block, dysrhythmias in cardiac patients
- Alcohol consumption; if alcohol is consumed, hold dose until AM

Administer:

- With food or milk for GI symptoms
- Crushed if patient is unable to swallow medication whole
- Dosages hs if oversedation occurs during the day; may take entire dose hs

Perform/provide:
- Storage at room temperature; do not freeze
- Assistance with ambulation during therapy, since drowsiness, dizziness occur
- Safety measures primarily in elderly
- Check to see if PO medication swallowed
- Sugarless gum, hard candy, frequent sips of water for dry mouth

Evaluate:
- Therapeutic response: decreased depression

Teach patient/family:
- That therapeutic effect may take 2-3 wk
- To use caution in driving, other activities requiring alertness because of drowsiness, dizziness, blurred vision
- To avoid alcohol ingestion, other CNS depressants
- To notify prescriber if pregnant or plan to become pregnant or breast-feed

RARELY USED

cladribine (CdA) (℞)

(kla′dri-been)

Leustatin

Func. class.: Antineoplastic antiinfective

Uses: Treatment of active hairy cell leukemia; may be useful in chronic lymphocytic leukemia, non-Hodgkin's lymphomas, acute myeloid leukemia, autoimmune hemolytic anemia

Dosage and routes:
- *Adult:* **IV** 0.09 mg/kg diluted with 0.9% NaCl qs to 100 ml; pass through 0.22 μm microfilter, given for 1 wk

Contraindications: Hypersensitivity, lactation

C

clarithromycin (℞)

(klare-ith′row-my-sin)

Biaxin, Biaxin XL

Func. class.: Antiinfective

Chem. class.: Macrolide

Action: Binds to 50S ribosomal subunits of susceptible bacteria and suppresses protein synthesis

Uses: Mild to moderate infections of the upper respiratory tract, lower respiratory tract, uncomplicated skin and skin structure infections caused by *Streptococcus pneumoniae, Mycoplasma pneumoniae, Legionella pneumophila, Moraxella catarrhalis, Neisseria gonorrhoeae, Corynebacterium diphtheriae, Listeria monocytogenes, Haemophilus influenzae, Streptococcus pyogenes, Staphlococcus aureus, Mycobacterium avium (MAC)* complex infection in AIDS patients, *Mycobacterium intracellulare, Helicobacter pylori* in combination with omeprazole

Dosage and routes:
- *Adult:* **PO** 250-500 mg q12h for 7-14 days; 500 mg q12h continues for *M. avium* complex (MAC)
- *Child:* **PO** 15 mg/kg/day (max 1000 mg) divided q12h × 10 days

H. pylori *infection*
- *Adult:* **PO** 500 mg qd plus omeprazole 2 × 20 mg q AM (day 1-14), then omeprazole 20 mg q AM (days 15-28)

Acute maxillary sinusitis/acute bacterial bronchitis
- *Adult:* **PO** 500 mg q12h × 10 days

Available forms: Tabs 250, 500 mg; granules for oral susp 125 mg/5 ml, 250 mg/5 ml; ext rel tab

Side effects/adverse reactions:
INTEG: Rash, urticaria, pruritus, ***Stevens-Johnson syndrome***
CV: ***Ventricular dysrhythmias***
HEMA: Leukopenia, thrombocytopenia, increased INR
GI: Nausea, vomiting, diarrhea, ***hepatotoxicity,*** *abdominal pain,* stomatitis, heartburn, anorexia, *abnormal taste,* ***pseudomembranous colitis***
GU: Vaginitis, moniliasis
MISC: Headache

Contraindications: Hypersensitivity to this drug or macrolide antibiotics

Precautions: Pregnancy (C), lactation, hepatic, renal disease, elderly

Pharmacokinetics: Peak 2 hr, duration 12 hr, half-life 4-6 hr; metabolized by liver; excreted in bile, feces

Interactions:
- Dysrhythmias: cisapride, pimozide
- ↑ clarithromycin levels: fluconazole
- ↑ oral anticoagulants effect: digoxin, theophylline, carbamazepine
- ↓ action: zidovudine

Do not use acidophilus with anti-infectives

Lab test interferences:
Increase: 17-OHCS/17-KS, AST, ALT, BUN, creatinine, LDH, total bilirubin
Decrease: Folate assay, WBC

NURSING CONSIDERATIONS
Assess:
- Renal, hepatic studies; report hematuria, oliguria
- C&S before drug therapy; drug may be given as soon as culture is taken; C&S may be repeated after treatment
- Bowel pattern before, during treatment
- Skin eruptions, itching
- Respiratory status: rate, character, wheezing, tightness in chest; discontinue drug
- Allergies before treatment, reaction of each medication

Administer:
- Adequate intake of fluids (2 L) during diarrhea episodes
- q12h to maintain serum level

Perform/provide:
- Storage at room temperature

Evaluate:
- Therapeutic response: C&S negative for infection

Teach patient/family:
- To take with full glass H_2O; may give with food to decrease GI symptoms

Not to crush tabs

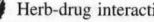

To report sore throat, fever, fatigue; may indicate superinfection

To notify nurse of diarrhea, dark urine, pale stools, yellow discoloration of eyes or skin, severe abdominal pain

- To take at evenly spaced intervals; complete dosage regimen
- To notify prescriber if pregnancy is suspected or planned

Treatment of hypersensitivity: Withdraw drug, maintain airway, administer epINEPHrine, aminophylline, O_2, IV corticosteroids

clindamycin HCl (℞)

(klin-da-my'sin)

Cleocin HCl

clindamycin palmitate (℞)

Cleocin Pediatric, Dalacin C Palmitate

clindamycin phosphate (℞)

Cleocin Phosphate, Dalacin C, Dalacin C Phosphate

Func. class.: Antiinfective, misc.

Chem. class.: Lincomycin derivative

Action: Binds to 50S subunit of bacterial ribosomes, suppresses protein synthesis

Uses: Infections caused by staphylococci, streptococci, *Rickettsia, Fusobacterium, Actinomyces, Peptococcus, Bacteroides, Pneumocystis carinii*

Dosage and routes:

- *Adult:* **PO** 150-450 mg q6h, max 1.8 g/day; **IM/IV** 1.2-1.8 g/day in 2-4 divided doses, not to exceed 4800 mg/day
- *Child >1 mo:* **PO** 8-25 mg/kg/day in divided doses q6-8h; **IM/IV** 20-40 mg/kg/day in divided doses q6-8h (3-4 equal doses)
- *Child <1 mo:* 15-20 mg/kg/day divided q6-8h
- ***PID:*** *Adult:* **IV** 600 mg qid plus gentamicin or 900 mg q8h

Bacterial endocarditis prophylaxis

- *Adult:* 600 mg 1 hr prior to procedure

Available forms:

Phosphate: inj 150, 300, 600 mg base/4 ml; 900 mg base/ml; inj INF in D_5 300 mg, 600 mg, 900 mg; HCl: caps 75, 150, 300 mg; palmitate: oral sol 75 mg/ml

Side effects/adverse reactions:

HEMA: ***Leukopenia, eosinophilia, agranulocytosis, thrombocytopenia, polyarthritis***

GI: Nausea, vomiting, abdominal pain, diarrhea, ***pseudomembranous colitis,*** anorexia, weight loss, increased AST, ALT, bilirubin, alk phosphatase; jaundice

GU: Vaginitis, urinary frequency

INTEG: Rash, urticaria, pruritus, erythema, pain, abscess at inj site

Contraindications: Hypersensitivity to this drug or lincomycin, tartrazine dye; ulcerative colitis/enteritis

Precautions: Renal disease, liver disease, GI disease, elderly, pregnancy (B), lactation, tartrazine sensitivity

Pharmacokinetics:

PO: Peak 45 min, duration 6 hr

IM: Peak 3 hr, duration 8-12 hr; half-life 2½ hr; metabolized in liver; excreted in urine, bile, feces as inactive metabolites; crosses placenta; excreted in breast milk

Interactions:

- ↓ absorption: kaolin
- May block clindamycin effect: erythromycin
- ↑ neuromuscular blockade: neuromuscular blockers

Do not use acidophilus with antiinfectives

Lab test interferences:

Increase: Alk phosphatase, bilirubin, CPK, AST, ALT

NURSING CONSIDERATIONS

Assess:

- Hepatic studies: AST, ALT if on long-term therapy
- Blood studies: WBC, RBC, Hct, Hgb, platelets, serum iron, reticulocytes; drug should be discontinued if bone marrow depression occurs

• C&S before drug therapy; drug may be given as soon as culture is taken
• B/P, pulse in patient receiving drug parenterally
• Bowel pattern before, during treatment; if severe diarrhea occurs, drug should be discontinued; may indicate pseudomembranous colitis
• Skin eruptions, itching, dermatitis after administration
• Respiratory status: rate, character, wheezing, tightness in chest
• Allergies before treatment, reaction of each medication

Administer:

• IM deep inj; rotate sites
• Orally with at least 8 oz H_2O

IV route

• By infusion only; do not administer bolus dose; dilute 300 mg or less/50 ml or more of D_5W, NS; may be further diluted in greater amounts of D_5W, NS and given as a cont inf in acute PID; give first dose 10 mg/min over ½ hr, then 0.75 mg/min; increased rates may be used to keep serum blood levels higher; run >10 min; no more than 1200 mg in a single 1-hr inf

Additive compatibilities: Amikacin, ampicillin, aztreonam, cefamandole, cefazolin, cefepime, cefonicid, cefoperazone, cefotaxime, cefoxitin, ceftazidime, ceftizoxime, cefuroxime, cephalothin, cimetidine, fluconazole, heparin, hydrocortisone, kanamycin, methylPREDNISolone, metoclopramide, metronidazole, netilmicin, ofloxacin, penicillin G, piperacillin, potassium chloride, sodium bicarbonate, tobramycin, verapamil, vit B/C

Syringe compatibilities: Amikacin, aztreonam, gentamicin, heparin

Y-site compatibilities: Amifostine, amiodarone, amphotericin B cholesteryl, amsacrine, aztreonam, cefpirome, cisatracurium, cyclophosphamide, diltiazem, DOXOrubicin liposome, enalaprilat, esmolol, fludarabine, foscarnet, granisetron, heparin, hydromorphone, labetalol, magnesium sulfate, melphalan, meperidine, midazolam, morphine, multivitamins, ondansetron, perphenazine, piperacillin/tazobactam, propofol, remifentanil, sargramostim, tacrolimus, teniposide, theophylline, thiotepa, vinorelbine, vit B/C, zidovudine

Perform/provide:

• Storage at room temperature (caps) up to 2 wk (reconstituted)
• EpINEPHrine, suction, tracheostomy set, endotracheal intubation equipment on unit
• Adequate intake of fluids (2 L) during diarrhea episodes

Evaluate:

• Therapeutic response: decreased temp, negative C&S

Teach patient/family:

• To take oral drug with full glass H_2O; may give with food to reduce GI symptoms; antiperistaltic drugs may worsen diarrhea
• All aspects of drug therapy: need to complete entire course of medication to ensure organism death (10-14 days); culture may be taken after medication course completed
◆ To report sore throat, fever, fatigue; may indicate superinfection
⊘ Not to break, crush, or chew caps
• That drug must be taken in equal intervals around clock to maintain blood levels
• To notify nurse or prescriber of diarrhea

Treatment of hypersensitivity: Withdraw drug; maintain airway; administer epINEPHrine, aminophylline, O_2, IV corticosteroids

clioquinol topical
See appendix c

clobetasol topical
See appendix c

clocortolone topical
See appendix c

RARELY USED

clofazimine (℞)
(kloe-fa'zi-meen)
Lamprene
Func. class.: Leprostatic

Uses: Lepromatous leprosy, dapsone-resistant leprosy, lepromatous leprosy complicated by erythema nodosum leprosum
Dosage and routes:
Erythema nodosum leprosum
• *Adult:* **PO:** 100-200 mg qd × 3 mo, then taper dosage to 100 mg when disease is controlled; do not exceed 200 mg/day
Dapsone-resistant leprosy
• *Adult:* **PO:** 100 mg/day in combination with at least one other antileprosy drug × 3 yr, then 100 mg qd clofazimine (only)
Contraindications: Hypersensitivity to this drug

C

*clomiPHENE (℞)
(kloe'mi-feen)
Clomid, clomiphene citrate, Milophene, Serophene
Func. class.: Ovulation stimulant
Chem. class.: Nonsteroidal antiestrogenic

Action: Increases LH, FSH release from the pituitary, which increases maturation of ovarian follicle, ovulation, development of corpus luteum
Uses: Female infertility (ovulatory failure)
Dosage and routes:
• *Adult:* **PO** 50-100 mg qd × 5 days or 50-100 mg qd beginning on day 5 of cycle; may be repeated until conception occurs or 3 cycles of therapy have been completed
Available forms: Tabs 50 mg
Side effects/adverse reactions:
CV: Vasomotor flushing, phlebitis, ***deep-vein thrombosis***
EENT: Blurred vision, diplopia, photophobia
CNS: Headache, depression, restlessness, anxiety, nervousness, fatigue, insomnia, dizziness, flushing
GI: Nausea, vomiting, constipation, abdominal pain, bloating
INTEG: Rash, dermatitis, urticaria, alopecia
GU: Polyuria, urinary frequency, birth defects, spontaneous abortions, multiple ovulation, breast pain, oliguria, abnormal uterine bleeding
Contraindications: Hypersensitivity, pregnancy (X), hepatic disease, undiagnosed uterine bleeding, uncontrolled thyroid or adrenal dysfunction, intracranial lesion, ovarian cysts
Precautions: Hypertension, depression, convulsions, diabetes mellitus

Do not confuse:
clomiPHENE/clomiPRAMINE
Pharmacokinetics: Metabolized in liver, excreted in feces
Lab test interferences:
Increase: FSH/LH, BSP, thyroxine, TBG

NURSING CONSIDERATIONS
Administer:
• After discontinuing estrogen therapy
• At same time qd to maintain drug level
Evaluate:
• Therapeutic response: fertility
Teach patient/family:
• That multiple births are common
• To notify prescriber immediately if low abdominal pain occurs; may indicate ovarian cyst, cyst rupture
• To notify prescriber of photophobia, blurred vision, diplopia
• That if dose is missed, to double at next time; if more than one dose is missed, to call prescriber
• That response usually occurs 4-10 days after last day of treatment
• The method for taking, recording basal body temp to determine whether ovulation has occurred
• If ovulation can be determined (there is a slight decrease in temp, then a sharp increase for ovulation), to attempt coitus 3 days before and qod until after ovulation
• If pregnancy is suspected, to notify prescriber immediately

*clomiPRAMINE (℞)
(kloe-mip′ra-meen)
Anafranil
Func. class.: Antidepressant, tricyclic
Chem. class.: Tertiary amine

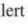

Action: Potentiates serotonin and norepinephrine; also increases dopamine metabolism; moderate anticholinergic effect
Uses: Obsessive-compulsive disorder, depression, dysphoria, phobias, anxiety, agoraphobia
Dosage and routes:
Obsessive-compulsive disorder
• *Adult:* **PO** 25 mg hs and increase gradually over 4 wk to 75-250 mg/day in divided doses
• *Child 10-18 yr:* **PO** 25-50 mg/day gradually increased; or 3 mg/kg/day, whichever is smaller, not to exceed 200 mg/day
Depression
• *Adult:* **PO** 50-150 mg/day in a single or divided dose
Anxiety/agoraphobia
• *Adult:* **PO** 25-75 mg/day
Available forms: Caps 25, 50, 75 mg
Side effects/adverse reactions:
HEMA: ***Agranulocytosis, neutropenia, pancytopenia***
CV: Hypotension, tachycardia, ***cardiac arrest***
CNS: Dizziness, tremors, mania, ***seizures,*** aggressiveness, EPS, drowsiness, headache
ENDO: Galactorrhea, hyperprolactinemia
META: Hyponatremia
GI: Constipation, dry mouth, nausea, dyspepsia, weight gain
GU: Delayed ejaculation, anorgasmia, urinary retention, decreased libido
EENT: Blurred vision
INTEG: Diaphoresis, photosensitivity
Contraindications: Hypersensitivity, immediate post-MI
Precautions: Seizures, suicidal patients, elderly, pregnancy (C), lactation, cardiac disease
Do not confuse:
clomiPRAMINE/clomiPHENE/desipramine/Norpramin
Pharmacokinetics: Onset ≥2 wk,

peak 2-6 hr; extensively bound to tissue and plasma proteins; demethylated in liver; active metabolites excreted in urine; half-life: 19-37 hr; steady state 1-2 wk

Interactions:

• ↓ clomiPRAMINE levels: barbiturates, carbamazepine, phenytoin

• ↑ clomiPRAMINE levels: cimetidine, fluoxetine, fluvoxamine, sertraline; do not use together

• ↑ hypertensive effect: clonidine, epINEPHrine, norepinephrine

• ↑ CNS depression: alcohol, CNS depressants

• Hypertensive crisis, convulsions, hypertensive episode: MAOIs

↑ CNS depression: hops, kava, lavender

↑ anticholinergic effect: belladonna, corkwood, henbane, jimsonweed

↑ clomiPRAMINE action: scopolia root

Serotonin syndrome: SAM-e, St. John's wort; do not use concurrently

Lab test interferences:

Increase: Prolactin, TBG

Decrease: Serum thyroid hormone

NURSING CONSIDERATIONS

Assess:

• B/P (lying, standing), pulse q4h; if systolic B/P drops 20 mm Hg, withhold drug, notify prescriber; take vital signs q4h in patients with cardiovascular disease

• ECG for flattening of T wave, QTc prolongation, bundle branch block, AV block, dysrhythmias in cardiac patients

• Blood studies: CBC, leukocytes, differential, cardiac enzymes if patient is receiving long-term therapy

• Hepatic studies: AST, ALT, bilirubin

• Mental status: mood, sensorium, affect, suicidal tendencies; increase in psychiatric symptoms: depression, panic, frequency of obsessive-compulsive behaviors

• Urinary retention, constipation; constipation more likely in children

• Withdrawal symptoms: headache, nausea, vomiting, muscle pain, weakness; not usual unless drug discontinued abruptly

• Alcohol consumption; if alcohol consumed, withhold dose until AM

Administer:

• Increased fluids, bulk in diet for constipation, especially elderly

• With food or milk for GI symptoms

Perform/provide:

• Storage in tight container at room temperature; do not freeze

• Assistance with ambulation during beginning therapy, since drowsiness/dizziness occurs

• Safety measures, primarily in elderly

• Checking to see PO medication swallowed

• Gum, hard candy, or frequent sips of water for dry mouth

Evaluate:

• Therapeutic response: decreased anxiety, depression

Teach patient/family:

🚫 Not to break, crush, or chew caps

• That the effects may take 2-3 wk

• To use caution in driving, other activities requiring alertness because of drowsiness, dizziness, blurred vision

• To avoid alcohol ingestion, other CNS depressants

• Not to discontinue medication quickly after long-term use; may cause nausea, headache, malaise

• To wear sunscreen, protective clothing to prevent photosensitivity

• To notify prescriber if pregnancy is planned or suspected

Treatment of overdose: ECG monitoring; induce emesis; lavage, activated charcoal; anticonvulsant

clonazepam (℞)

(kloe-na'zi-pam)
Klonopin, Rivotril♣, Syn-Clonazepam♣

Func. class.: Anticonvulsant
Chem. class.: Benzodiazepine derivative

Controlled Substance Schedule IV

Action: Inhibits spike, wave formation in absence seizures (petit mal), decreases amplitude, frequency, duration, spread of discharge in minor motor seizures

Uses: Absence, atypical absence, akinetic, myoclonic seizures, Lennox-Gastaut syndrome

Investigational uses: Parkinsonian dysarthrosis, acute manic episodes, adjunction schizophrenia, neuralgias, multifocal tic disorders, restless leg syndrome, rectal administration

Dosage and routes:

- *Adult:* **PO** not to exceed 1.5 mg/day in 3 divided doses; may be increased 0.5-1 mg q3d until desired response, not to exceed 20 mg/day; rectal 0.02 mg/kg
- *Child <10 yr or <30 kg:* **PO** 0.01-0.03 mg/kg/day in divided doses q8h, not to exceed 0.05 mg/kg/day; may be increased 0.25-0.5 mg q3d until desired response, not to exceed 0.1-0.2 mg/kg/day; rectal 0.05-0.1 mg/kg

Available forms: Tabs 0.5, 1, 2 mg; oral susp; IV sol

Side effects/adverse reactions:

HEMA: ***Thrombocytopenia, leukocytosis, eosinophilia***

CNS: Drowsiness, dizziness, confusion, behavioral changes, tremors, insomnia, headache, suicidal tendencies, slurred speech

GI: Nausea, constipation, polyphagia, anorexia, xerostomia, diarrhea, gastritis, sore gums

INTEG: Rash, alopecia, hirsutism

EENT: Increased salivation, nystagmus, diplopia, abnormal eye movements

RESP: ***Respiratory depression,*** dyspnea, congestion

CV: Palpitations, bradycardia, tachycardia

GU: Dysuria, enuresis, nocturia, retention, libido changes

Contraindications: Hypersensitivity to benzodiazepines, acute narrow-angle glaucoma, psychosis, severe liver disease

Precautions: Open-angle glaucoma, chronic respiratory disease, lactation, renal, hepatic disease, elderly, pregnancy (C)

Do not confuse:
clonazepam/lorazepam/clorazepate
Klonopin/clonidine

Pharmacokinetics:

PO: Peak 1-2 hr; metabolized by liver; excreted in urine; half-life 18-50 hr, duration 6-12 hr

Interactions:

- ↑ CNS depression: alcohol, barbiturates, opiates, antidepressants, other anticonvulsants, general anesthetics, hypnotics, sedatives
- ↓ clonazepam effect: carbamazepine, phenobarbital, phenytoin

↑ CNS depression: kava
↑ clonazepam effect: ginkgo
↓ clonazepam effect: ginseng, santonica

Lab test interferences:

Increase: AST, alk phosphatase

NURSING CONSIDERATIONS

Assess:

- Blood level: ther level 20-80 ng/ml
- Renal studies: urinalysis, BUN, urine creatinine

• Blood studies: RBC, Hct, Hgb, reticulocyte counts qwk for 4 wk, then qmo
• Hepatic studies: ALT, AST, bilirubin, creatinine
• Drug levels during initial treatment (therapeutic 20-80 ng/ml)
• Signs of physical withdrawal if medication suddenly discontinued
• Mental status: mood, sensorium, affect, oversedation, behavioral changes; if mental status changes, notify prescriber
• Eye problems: need for ophthalmic exam before, during, after treatment (slit lamp, fundoscopy, tonometry)
• Allergic reaction: red, raised rash; drug should be discontinued
◆ Blood dyscrasias: fever, sore throat, bruising, rash, jaundice
• Toxicity: bone marrow depression, nausea, vomiting, ataxia, diplopia, cardiovascular collapse

Administer:
• With food, milk for GI symptoms

Oral suspension
• May use rectally (1 mg/ml of clonazepam with 1 ml of water); use plastic tube (volume 2.2-3.3 ml)

IV solution
• May use rectally 1 ml syringe inserted 3 cm into rectum

Perform/provide:
• Storage at room temperature
• Assistance with ambulation during early part of treatment; dizziness occurs, especially elderly

Evaluate:
• Therapeutic response: decreased seizure activity, document on patient's chart

Teach patient/family:
• To carry emergency ID bracelet stating name, drugs taken, condition, prescriber's name, phone number
• To avoid driving, other activities that require alertness
• To avoid alcohol ingestion, CNS depressants; increased sedation may occur
• Not to discontinue medication quickly after long-term use; taper off over several wk

Treatment of overdose: Lavage, activated charcoal, monitor electrolytes, VS, administer vasopressors

clonidine (℞)

(klon'i-deen)

Catapres, Catapres-TTS, clonidine HCl, Dixarit♣, Duraclon

Func. class.: Antihypertensive, centrally acting analgesic

Chem. class.: Central α-adrenergic agonist

Action: Inhibits sympathetic vasomotor center in CNS, which reduces impulses in sympathetic nervous system; blood pressure, pulse rate, cardiac output decrease, prevents pain signal transmission in CNS by α-adrenergic receptor stimulation of the spinal cord

Uses: Mild to moderate hypertension, used alone or in combination; severe pain in cancer patients

Investigational uses: Opioid withdrawal, prevention of vascular headaches, treatment of menopausal symptoms, dysmenorrhea, attention deficit hyperactivity disorder

Dosage and routes:

Hypertension
• *Adult:* **PO/TRANS** 0.1 mg bid, then increase by 0.1-0.2 mg/day at weekly intervals, until desired response; range 0.2-0.6 mg/day in divided doses
• *Geriatric:* **PO** 0.1 mg hs, may increase gradually
• *Child:* 5-10 mcg/kg/day in divided doses q8-12h, max 0.9 mg/day

Opioid withdrawal (unlabeled use)
• *Adult:* **PO** 0.3-1.2 mg/day; may decrease by 50% × 3 days then decrease by 0.1-0.2 mg/day or discontinue
Severe pain
• *Adult:* **CONT EPIDURAL INF** 30 mcg/hr
• *Child:* **CONT EPIDURAL INF** 0.5 mcg/kg/hr, then titrate to response
ADHD (unlabeled use)
• *Child:* 5 mcg/kg/day × 8 wk
Menopausal symptoms (unlabeled use)
• *Adult:* **TD** 0.1 mg patch q1wk; **PO** 0.05-0.4 mg qd
Available forms: Tabs 0.025✤, 0.1, 0.2, 0.3 mg; TRANS 2.5, 5, 7.5 mg delivering 0.1, 0.2, 0.3 mg/24 hr, respectively; inj 100, 500 mcg/ml
Side effects/adverse reactions:
CNS: Drowsiness, sedation, headache, fatigue, nightmares, insomnia, mental changes, anxiety, depression, hallucinations, delirium
CV: Orthostatic hypotension, palpitations, ***CHF,*** ECG abnormalities
EENT: Taste change, parotid pain
ENDO: Hyperglycemia
GI: Nausea, vomiting, malaise, constipation, *dry mouth*
GU: Impotence, dysuria, nocturia, gynecomastia
INTEG: Rash, alopecia, facial pallor, pruritus, hives, edema, burning papules, excoriation (transdermal patches)
MS: Muscle, joint pain; leg cramps
MISC: Withdrawal symptoms
Contraindications: Hypersensitivity; (epidural) bleeding disorders, anticoagulants
Precautions: MI (recent), diabetes mellitus, chronic renal failure, Raynaud's disease, thyroid disease, depression, COPD, child <12 yr (transdermal), asthma, pregnancy (C), lactation, elderly, noncompliant patients
Do not confuse:
clonidine/Klonopin/clonazepam
Catapres/Cataflam/Catarase
Pharmacokinetics: Absorbed well
PO: Onset ½ to 1 hr, peak 2-4 hr, duration 8-12 hr; half-life 12-21 hr
TD: Onset 3 days, duration 1 wk; metabolized by liver (metabolites), excreted in urine (30% unchanged, inactive metabolites), feces; crosses blood-brain barrier, excreted in breast milk
Interactions:
• ↑ CNS depression: opiates, sedatives, hypnotics, anesthetics, alcohol
• ↓ hypotensive effects: tricyclics, MAOIs, appetite suppressants, amphetamines, prazosin
• ↑ hypotensive effects: diuretics, other antihypertensive nitrates
• AV block: verapamil
• ↓ effect of: levodopa
• Life-threatening elevations of B/P: tricyclics, β-blockers
• Toxicity/death: aconite
↓ antihypertensive effect: astragalus, capsicum peppers, cola tree, coltsfoot, khat, guarana, licorice
↑ antihypertensive effect: barberry, betony, black catechu, black cohosh, bloodroot, broom, burdock, cat's claw, dandelion, goldenseal, Irish moss, Jamaican dogwood, kelp, khella, mistletoe, parsley, Queen Anne's lace, rue
Lab test interferences:
Increase: Blood glucose
Decrease: VMA, urinary catecholamines, aldosterone
NURSING CONSIDERATIONS
Assess:
• Blood studies: neutrophils, decreased platelets
• Renal studies: protein, BUN, creatinine; increased levels may indicate nephrotic syndrome

- Baselines in renal, hepatic studies before therapy begins; potassium levels, although hyperkalemia rare
- B/P, pulse if used for hypertension, report significant changes
- For opiate withdrawal including fever, diarrhea, nausea, vomiting, cramps, insomnia, shivering, dilated pupils
- Pain: location, intensity, character; alleviating, aggravating factors, baseline and frequently
- Edema in feet, legs daily; monitor I&O; check for falling output
- Allergic reaction: rash, fever, pruritus, urticaria; drug should be discontinued if antihistamines fail to help
- Allergic reaction from patches: rash, urticaria, angioedema; should not continue to use
- Symptoms of CHF: edema, dyspnea, wet rales, B/P
- Renal symptoms: polyuria, oliguria, frequency

Administer:

- PO: give last dose at hs
- Transdermal patch qwk; apply to site without hair; best absorption over chest or upper arm; rotate sites with each application; clean site before application; apply firmly, especially around edges

Perform/provide:

- Storage of patches in cool environment, tablets in tight container

Evaluate:

- Therapeutic response: decrease in B/P in hypertension, decrease in withdrawal symptoms (opioid), decrease in pain

Teach patient/family:

- To avoid hazardous activities, since drug may cause drowsiness
- To notify all health care providers of medication use
- Not to discontinue drug abruptly or withdrawal symptoms may occur: anxiety, increased B/P, headache, insomnia, increased pulse, tremors, nausea, sweating
- Not to use OTC (cough, cold, or allergy) products unless directed by prescriber
- To comply with dosage schedule even if feeling better
- To rise slowly to sitting or standing position to minimize orthostatic hypotension, especially elderly
- To notify prescriber of mouth sores, sore throat, fever, swelling of hands, feet, irregular heartbeat, chest pain, signs of angioedema
- About excessive perspiration, dehydration, vomiting; diarrhea may lead to fall in blood pressure; consult prescriber if these occur
- That drug may cause dizziness, fainting; light-headedness may occur during first few days of therapy
- That drug may cause dry mouth; use hard candy, saliva product, or frequent rinsing of mouth
- That compliance is necessary; not to skip or stop drug unless directed by prescriber
- That drug may cause skin rash or impaired perspiration
- To use patch; patch comes in two parts: drug patch and overlay to keep patch in place
- That response may take 2-3 days if drug is given transdermally; instruct on administration of patch

Treatment of overdose: Supportive treatment; administer tolazoline, atropine, DOPamine prn

clopidogrel (℞)

(klo-pid′oh-grel)

Plavix

Func. class.: Platelet aggregation inhibitor

Chem. class.: Thienopyridine derivative

Action: Inhibits first and second phases of ADP-induced effects in platelet aggregation

Uses: Reducing the risk of stroke, MI, peripheral arterial disease in high-risk patients, acute coronary syndrome

Dosage and routes:

Recent MI, stroke, peripheral arterial disease

• *Adult:* **PO** 75 mg qd with or without food

Acute coronary syndrome

• *Adult:* **PO** 300 mg then 75 mg qd

Available forms: Tabs 75 mg

Side effects/adverse reactions:

INTEG: Rash, pruritus

GI: Nausea, vomiting, diarrhea, GI discomfort, ***GI bleeding***

HEMA: Epistaxis, purpura, ***bleeding, neutropenia***

CV: Edema, hypertension

CNS: Headache, dizziness, depression, syncope, hypesthesia, neuralgia

MS: Arthralgia, back pain

RESP: Upper respiratory tract infection, dyspnea, rhinitis, bronchitis, cough

MISC: UTI, hypercholesterolemia, chest pain, fatigue, ***intracranial hemorrhage***

Contraindications: Hypersensitivity, active bleeding

Precautions: Past hepatic disease, pregnancy (B), lactation, children, increased bleeding risk, neutropenia, agranulocytosis

Do not confuse:

Plavix/Paxil/Elavil

Pharmacokinetics: Rapidly absorbed, peak 1-3 hr, metabolized by liver, excreted in urine, feces, half-life 8 hr, plasma protein binding 95%

Interactions:

• ↑ bleeding risk; anticoagulants, aspirin, NSAIDs, abciximab, eptifibatide, tirofiban, thrombolytics, ticlopidine

• ↑ action of: some NSAIDs, phenytoin, TOLBUTamide, tamoxifen, torsemide, fluvastatin, warfarin

↓ clopidogrel effect: bilberry, saw palmetto

↑ clopidogrel effect: bogbean, dong quai, feverfew, ginger, ginkgo

↑ gastric irritation: arginine

NURSING CONSIDERATIONS

Assess:

• For symptoms of stroke, MI during treatment

• Hepatic studies: AST, ALT, bilirubin, creatinine (long-term therapy)

• Blood studies: CBC, Hct, Hgb, PT, cholesterol (long-term therapy)

Administer:

• With food to decrease gastric symptoms

Evaluate:

• Therapeutic response: absence of stroke, MI

Teach patient/family:

• That blood work will be necessary during treatment

• To report any unusual bruising, bleeding to prescriber, that it may take longer to stop bleeding

• To take with food or just after eating to minimize GI discomfort

• To report diarrhea, skin rashes, subcutaneous bleeding, chills, fever, sore throat

• To tell all health care providers that clopidogrel is used

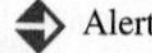 Alert  Herb-drug interaction ⃠ Do not crush *"Tall Man" lettering

clorazepate (℞)

(klor-az′e-pate)

Apo-Clorazepate♣, clorazepate, Gen-XENE, Novo-Clopate♣, Tranxene, Tranxene-SD

Func. class.: Antianxiety, anticonvulsant, sedative/hypnotic

Chem. class.: Benzodiazepine

Controlled Substance Schedule IV

Action: Potentiates the actions of GABA, especially in limbic system, reticular formation

Uses: Anxiety, acute alcohol withdrawal, adjunct in seizure disorders

Dosage and routes:

Anxiety

• *Adult:* **PO** 15-60 mg/day or 7.5-15 mg 2-4×/day or 11.25-22.5 mg at hs

• *Geriatric:* **PO** 7.5 mg qd-bid

Alcohol withdrawal

• *Adult:* **PO** 30 mg then 30-60 mg in divided doses; day 2, 45-90 mg in divided doses; day 3, 22.5-45 mg in divided doses; day 4, 15-30 mg in divided doses; then reduce daily dose to 7.5-15 mg

Seizure disorders

• *Adult and child >12 yr:* **PO** 7.5 mg tid; may increase by 7.5 mg/wk or less, not to exceed 90 mg/day

• *Child 9-12 yr:* **PO** 3.75-7.5 mg bid; may increase by 3.75 mg/wk or less, not to exceed 60 mg/day

Available forms: Caps 3.75, 7.5, 15 mg; tabs 3.75, 7.5, 15 mg

Side effects/adverse reactions:

CNS: Dizziness, drowsiness, confusion, headache, anxiety, tremors, stimulation, fatigue, depression, insomnia, hallucinations, lethargy

GI: Constipation, dry mouth, nausea, vomiting, anorexia, diarrhea

INTEG: Rash, dermatitis, itching

*CV: Orthostatic hypotension, **ECG changes, tachycardia,*** hypotension, chest pain

EENT: Blurred vision, tinnitus, mydriasis

Contraindications: Hypersensitivity to benzodiazepines, narrow-angle glaucoma, psychosis, pregnancy (D), lactation, child <9 yr

Precautions: Elderly, debilitated, hepatic disease, renal disease

Do not confuse:

clorazepate/clonazepam

Pharmacokinetics:

PO: Onset 1 hr, peak 1-2 hr, duration up to 24 hr; metabolized by liver, excreted by kidneys; crosses placenta, breast milk; half-life 30-100 hr

Interactions:

• ↑ clorazepate effects: CNS depressants, alcohol, valproic acid, antidepressants, MAOIs, cimetidine, oral contraceptives, disulfiram, fluoxetine, isoniazid, ketoconazole, propoxyphene, some β-blockers

• ↓ clorazepate action: rifampin, barbiturates

↑ CNS depression: catnip, chamomile, clary, cowslip, kava, mistletoe, nettle, pokeweed, poppy, Queen Anne's lace, senega, valerian

↑ hypotension: black cohosh

Lab test interferences:

Increase: AST, ALT

Decrease: Hct

NURSING CONSIDERATIONS

Assess:

• B/P (lying, standing), pulse; if systolic B/P drops 20 mm Hg, hold drug, notify prescriber

• Blood studies: CBC during long-term therapy; blood dyscrasias have occurred rarely

• Hepatic studies: AST, ALT, bilirubin, creatinine, LDH, alk phosphatase

• I&O; may indicate renal dysfunction

• Mental status: mood, sensorium, affect, sleeping pattern, drowsiness, dizziness; for delirium, tremors, hallucination in alcohol withdrawal
• Physical dependency, withdrawal symptoms: headache, nausea, vomiting, muscle pain, weakness after long-term use
• Suicidal tendencies, anxiety level
• Seizures: location, duration, intensity

Administer:
• With food, milk for GI symptoms
• Crushed if patient cannot swallow whole (tab only)

Perform/provide:
• Assistance with ambulation during beginning therapy because of drowsiness/dizziness, especially elderly
• Safety measures, including side rails
• Check to see PO medication has been swallowed
• Sugarless gum, hard candy, frequent sips of water for dry mouth

Evaluate:
• Therapeutic response: decreased anxiety, restlessness, insomnia

Teach patient/family:
• That drug may be taken with food
• That drug is not to be used for everyday stress or used longer than 4 mo unless directed by prescriber; not to take more than prescribed amount; may be habit forming
⊘ Not to break, crush, or chew caps
• To avoid OTC preparations unless approved by prescriber
• To avoid driving, activities that require alertness; drowsiness may occur, especially in elderly
• To avoid alcohol ingestion, other psychotropic medications, unless directed by prescriber
• Not to discontinue medication abruptly after long-term use
• To rise slowly because fainting may occur
• That drowsiness may worsen at beginning of treatment

Treatment of overdose: Lavage, VS, supportive care, flumazenil

clotrimazole topical

See appendix c

clotrimazole vaginal antifungal

See appendix c

cloxacillin (℞)

(klox-a-sill′in)

Apo-Cloxi✦, cloxacillin, Cloxapen, Novo-Cloxin✦, Nu-Clox✦, Orbenin✦

Func. class.: Broad-spectrum antiinfective

Chem. class.: Penicillinase-resistant penicillin

Action: Interferes with cell wall replication of susceptible organisms; the cell wall, rendered osmotically unstable, swells, bursts from osmotic pressure, resists the penicillinase action that inactivates penicillin

Uses: Gram-positive cocci *(Staphylococcus aureus, Streptococcus pyogenes, Streptococcus pneumoniae),* penicillinase-producing staphylococci

Dosage and routes:
• *Adult:* **PO** 1-4 g/day in divided doses q6h
• *Child:* **PO** 50-100 mg/kg in divided doses q6h, max 4 g/day

Available forms: Caps 250, 500 mg; oral sol 125 mg/5 ml

Side effects/adverse reactions:
HEMA: Anemia, increased bleeding

time, ***bone marrow depression, granulocytopenia***
GI: Nausea, vomiting, diarrhea, increased AST, ALT, abdominal pain, glossitis, colitis, ***pseudomembranous colitis***
GU: ***Oliguria, proteinuria,*** hematuria, *vaginitis, moniliasis,* ***glomerulonephritis***
CNS: Lethargy, hallucinations, anxiety, depression, twitching, ***coma, seizures***
SYST: ***Anaphylaxis, serum sickness***
Contraindications: Hypersensitivity to penicillins; neonates, severe renal, hepatic disease
Precautions: Pregnancy (B), lactation, hypersensitivity to cephalosporins
Pharmacokinetics:
PO: Peak 1 hr, duration 6 hr; half-life 30-60 min; metabolized in liver; excreted in urine, bile, breast milk; crosses placenta, poor penetration in CSF
Interactions:
• ↑ cloxacillin concentrations: probenecid
• ↑ action of anticoagulants
• Food/drug: citric juices/food ↓s absorption of cloxacillin
↓ absorption: khat
Do not use acidophilus with anti-infectives
Lab test interferences:
False positive: Urine glucose, urine protein
Decrease: Uric acid
NURSING CONSIDERATIONS
Assess:
Anaphylaxis: pruritus, rash, dyspnea, laryngeal edema; have emergency equipment available; skin eruptions after administration of penicillin to 1 wk after discontinuing drug
• For infection: temp, draining wounds, WBC, sputum, urine, stool before and during treatment
• I&O ratio; report hematuria, oliguria, since penicillin in high doses is nephrotoxic
Any patient with compromised renal system, since drug is excreted slowly in poor renal system function; toxicity may occur rapidly
• Hepatic studies: AST, ALT
• Blood studies: WBC, RBC, Hgb, Hct, bleeding time
• Renal studies: urinalysis, protein, blood
• C&S before drug therapy; drug may be taken as soon as culture is taken
• Bowel pattern before, during treatment, report diarrhea
Administer:
• After C&S completed
• Shake suspension well before each dose
Perform/provide:
• Adrenaline, suction, tracheostomy set, endotracheal intubation equipment on unit
• Adequate intake of fluids (2 L) during diarrhea episodes
• Scratch test to assess allergy after securing order from prescriber; usually done when penicillin is only drug of choice
• Storage in tight container; after reconstituting, store in refrigerator for 2 wk, room temperature 3 days
Evaluate:
• Therapeutic response: absence of fever, draining wounds
Teach patient/family:
Not to break, crush, or chew caps
• All aspects of drug therapy, including need to complete entire course of medication to ensure organism death (10-14 days); culture may be taken after course of medication completed
• To report sore throat, fever, fatigue (may indicate superinfection)

• To wear or carry emergency ID if allergic to penicillins
• To notify prescriber of diarrhea, fever
• To take on an empty stomach with a full glass of water

Treatment of overdose: Withdraw drug; maintain airway; administer epINEPHrine, aminophylline, O_2, IV corticosteroids for anaphylaxis

clozapine (℞)

(kloz'a-peen)
clozapine, Clozaril
Func. class.: Antipsychotic
Chem. class.: Tricyclic dibenzodiazepine derivative

Action: Interferes with DOPamine receptor binding with lack of extrapyramidal symptoms; also acts as an adrenergic, cholinergic, histaminergic, serotonergic antagonist

Uses: Management of psychotic symptoms in schizophrenic patients for whom other antipsychotics have failed

Dosage and routes:
• *Adult:* **PO** 25 mg qd or bid; may increase by 25-50 mg/day; normal range 300-450 mg/day after 2 wk; do not increase dose more than 2 × per wk; do not exceed 900 mg/day; use lowest dose to control symptoms

Available forms: Tabs 25, 100 mg

Side effects/adverse reactions:
CNS: ***Neuroleptic malignant syndrome,*** *sedation, salivation, dizziness, headache, tremors, sleep problems, akinesia, fever,* ***seizures,*** *sweating, akathisia, confusion, fatigue, insomnia,* depression, slurred speech, anxiety, agitation
GI: Drooling or excessive salivation, constipation, nausea, abdominal discomfort, vomiting, diarrhea, anorexia, weight gain, dry mouth, heartburn
MS: Weakness; pain in back, neck, legs; spasm
CV: Tachycardia, hypotension, hypertension, chest pain, ECG changes, orthostatic hypotension
GU: Urinary abnormalities, incontinence, ejaculation dysfunction, frequency, urgency, retention, dysuria
RESP: Dyspnea, nasal congestion, throat discomfort
HEMA: ***Leukopenia, neutropenia, agranulocytosis, eosinophilia, thrombocytopenia***
EENT: Blurred vision

Contraindications: Hypersensitivity, myeloproliferative disorders, severe granulocytopenia (WBC <3500 before therapy), CNS depression, coma

Precautions: Pregnancy (B); lactation; children <16; hepatic, renal, cardiac disease; seizures; prostatic enlargement; elderly, narrow-angle glaucoma

Do not confuse:
Clozaril/Clinoril/Colazal

Pharmacokinetics: Steady state 2.5 hr; 95% protein bound; completely metabolized by liver; excreted in urine and feces (metabolites); half-life 8-12 hr

Interactions:
• ↓ effect of: phenytoin
• ↑ anticholinergic effect: anticholinergics
• ↑ hypotension: antihypertensives, nitrates, large quantities of alcohol
• ↑ CNS depression: CNS depressants, psychoactives, alcohol
• ↑ bone marrow suppression: antineoplastics, other drugs suppressing bone marrow
• ↑ clozapine level: cimetidine, erythromycin
• ↑ plasma concentration: warfarin, digoxin, other highly protein-bound drugs

• Drug/food: ↓ clozapine level: caffeine

↑ CNS depression: kava, St. John's wort

↑ EPS: betel palm, kava

↑ clozapine action: cola tree, hops, nettle, nutmeg

Lab test interferences:

Increase: LFTs, cardiac enzymes, cholesterol, blood glucose, bilirubin, PBI, cholinesterase, ^{131}I

False positive: Pregnancy tests, PKU

False negative: Urinary steroids, 17-OHCS

NURSING CONSIDERATIONS

Assess:

• Swallowing of PO medication; check for hoarding or giving of medication to other patients
• I&O ratio; obtain baseline before treatment begins; palpate bladder if low urinary output occurs
• Bilirubin, CBC, LFTs monthly; discontinue treatment if WBC <3000/mm^3 or ANC <1500/mm^3 test qwk; may resume when normal; if WBC <2000/mm^3 or ANC <1000/mm^3 discontinue
• Urinalysis is recommended before, during prolonged therapy
• Affect, orientation, LOC, reflexes, gait, coordination, sleep pattern disturbances
• B/P standing and lying; take pulse and respirations q4h during initial treatment; establish baseline before starting treatment; report drops of 30 mm Hg
• Dizziness, faintness, palpitations, tachycardia on rising
• EPS including akathisia (inability to sit still, no pattern to movements), tardive dyskinesia (bizarre movements of the jaw, mouth, tongue, extremities), pseudoparkinsonism (rigidity, tremors, pill rolling, shuffling gait)
• For neuroleptic malignant syndrome: tachycardia, seizures, fever, dyspnea, diaphoresis, increased or decreased B/P, notify prescriber immediately
• Skin turgor daily
• Constipation, urinary retention daily; if these occur, increase bulk, water in diet, especially elderly

Perform/provide:

• Decreased sensory input by dimming lights, avoiding loud noises
• Supervised ambulation until stabilized on medication; do not involve in strenuous exercise program because fainting is possible; patient should not stand still for long periods
• Storage in tight, light-resistant container

Evaluate:

• Therapeutic response: decrease in emotional excitement, hallucinations, delusions, paranoia, reorganization of patterns of thought, speech

Teach patient/family:

• About symptoms of agranulocytosis and need for blood tests qwk for 6 mo, then q2wk; report flulike symptoms
• That orthostatic hypotension often occurs, and to rise gradually from sitting or lying position
• To avoid hot tubs, hot showers, tub baths; hypotension may occur
• To avoid abrupt withdrawal of this drug because EPS may result; drug should be withdrawn slowly
• To avoid OTC preparations (cough, hay fever, cold) unless approved by prescriber, since serious drug interactions may occur; avoid use with alcohol or CNS depressants, increased drowsiness may occur
• About compliance with drug regimen
• About EPS and necessity for meticulous oral hygiene, since oral candidiasis may occur

• To report sore throat, malaise, fever, bleeding, mouth sores; if these occur, CBC should be drawn and drug discontinued
• That heat stroke may occur in hot weather; take extra precautions to stay cool
• To avoid driving, other hazardous activities; seizures may occur
• To notify prescriber if pregnant or if pregnancy is intended

Treatment of overdose: Lavage, activated charcoal; provide an airway; do not induce vomiting

HIGH ALERT

coagulation factor VIIa, recombinant

(℞)

NovoSeven

Func. class.: Antihemophilic

Action: Promotes hemostasis by activating the intrinsic pathway of coagulation

Uses: Bleeding in hemophilia A or B, with inhibitors to factor VIII or IX

Research note: One study concluded that a high-fat meal does not activate blood coagulation factor VII

Dosage and routes:

• *Adult:* **IV BOL** 90 mcg/kg q2h until hemostasis occurs, or until therapy is deemed to be inadequate; posthemostatic doses q3-6h may be required

Available forms: Lyophilized powder, 1.2 mg/vial (1200 mcg/vial), 4.8 mg/vial (4800 mcg/vial) recombinant human coagulation factor VIIa (rFVIIa)

Side effects/adverse reactions:

CNS: Fever, headache

SYST: ***Hemorrhage NOS, hemarthrosis, fibrinogen plasma decreased,*** hypertension, bradycardia, ***DIC, coagulation disorder, thrombosis***

INTEG: Pain, redness at inj site, pruritus, purpura, rash

Contraindications: Hypersensitivity to this product or mouse, hamster, or bovine products

Precautions: Pregnancy (C), lactation, children

Pharmacokinetics: Half-life 2.3 hr

Interactions:

• Do not use with activated prothrombin complex concentrates or prothrombin complex concentrate

NURSING CONSIDERATIONS

Assess:

• VS, B/P, pulse, respirations, neurologic signs, temp at least q4h, temp 104° F (40° C) or indicators of internal bleeding, cardiac rhythm
• PT, aPTT, plasma FVII clotting
• For thrombosis, dose should be reduced or stopped

Administer:

IV route

• Bring to room temperature; for 1.2 mg vial/2.2 ml sterile water for inj; 4.8 mg vial/8.5 ml sterile water for inj
• Remove caps from stop, cleanse stopper with alcohol, allow to dry, draw back plunger of sterile syringe and allow air into syringe, insert needle of syringe into sterile water for inj, inject the air and withdraw amount required, insert syringe needle with diluent into drug vial, aim to side so liquid runs down vial wall, gently swirl until dissolved, use within 3 hr, give by bol over 3-5 min
• Do not admix, keep refrigerated until ready to use, avoid sunlight

Evaluate:

• Therapeutic response: hemostasis

codeine (℞)

(koe'deen)

Paveral✦

Func. class.: Opiate analgesic, antitussive

Chem. class.: Opiate, phenathrene derivative

Controlled Substance Schedule II, III, IV, V (depends on route)

Action: Depresses pain impulse transmission at the spinal cord level by interacting with opioid receptors, decreases cough reflex, GI motility

Uses: Moderate to severe pain, nonproductive cough

Investigational uses: Diarrhea

Dosage and routes:

Pain

• *Adult:* **PO** 15-60 mg q4h prn; **IM/SC** 15-60 mg q4h prn

• *Child:* **PO** 3 mg/kg/day in divided doses q4h prn

Cough

• *Adult:* **PO** 10-20 mg q4-6h, not to exceed 120 mg/day

• *Child:* **PO** 1-1.5 mg/kg/day in 4 divided doses, not to exceed 60 mg/day

Diarrhea

• *Adult:* **PO** 30 mg; may repeat qid prn

Renal disease

• CCr 10-50 ml/min 75% of dose; CCr <10 ml/min 50% of dose

Available forms: Inj 30, 60 mg/ml; tabs 15, 30, 60 mg; oral sol 10 mg/5 ml, 15 mg/5 ml

Side effects/adverse reactions:

CNS: Drowsiness, sedation, dizziness, agitation, dependency, lethargy, restlessness, euphoria, ***seizures***

GI: Nausea, vomiting, anorexia, constipation

RESP: ***Respiratory depression, respiratory paralysis***

CV: Bradycardia, palpitations, orthostatic hypotension, tachycardia, ***circulatory collapse***

GU: Urinary retention

INTEG: Flushing, rash, urticaria, pruritus

SYST: ***Anaphylaxis***

Contraindications: Hypersensitivity to opiates, respiratory depression, increased intracranial pressure, seizure disorders, severe respiratory disorders

Precautions: Elderly, cardiac dysrhythmias, pregnancy (C), lactation, prostatic hypertrophy

Do not confuse:

codeine/Lodine/Iodine/Cardene

Pharmacokinetics: Onset 10-30 min, peak ½-1 hr, duration 4-6 hr; metabolized by liver; excreted by kidneys, in breast milk; crosses placenta; half-life 3 hr

Interactions:

• ↑ CNS depression: alcohol, opiates, sedative/hypnotics, antipsychotics, skeletal muscle relaxants

• ↑ toxicity: MAOIs, use cautiously

(herb) ↑ CNS depression: Jamaican dogwood, kava, lavender, mistletoe, nettle, pokeweed, poppy, senega, valerian

(herb) ↑ anticholinergic effect: corkwood

Lab test interferences:

Increase: Lipase, amylase

NURSING CONSIDERATIONS

Assess:

• I&O ratio; check for decreasing output; may indicate urinary retention, especially elderly

• GI function: nausea, vomiting, constipation

• By using pain-scoring method

• For productive cough

• Cough: type, duration, ability to raise secretion

• CNS changes, dizziness, drowsiness, hallucinations, euphoria, LOC, pupil reaction

• Allergic reactions: rash, urticaria

• Respiratory dysfunction: respiratory depression, character, rate, rhythm; notify prescriber if respirations are <10/min, shallow
• Need for pain medication, tolerance

Administer:

IV route

• Give slowly by direct inj
• With antiemetic for nausea, vomiting
• When pain is beginning to return; determine dosage interval by patient response

Syringe compatibilities: Glycopyrrolate, hydrOXYzine

Y-site compatibilities: Cefmetazole

Perform/provide:

• Storage in light-resistant container at room temperature
• Assistance with ambulation if needed
• Safety measures: top side rails, night-light, call bell

Evaluate:

• Therapeutic response: decrease in pain, absence of grimacing, decreased cough; decreased diarrhea

Teach patient/family:

• To report any symptoms of CNS changes, allergic reactions
• That physical dependency may result after extended periods
• To change position slowly; orthostatic hypotension may occur
• To avoid hazardous activities if drowsiness, dizziness occurs
• To avoid alcohol, other CNS depressants unless directed by prescriber

colchicine (℞)

(kol′chi-seen)

Func. class.: Antigout agent
Chem. class.: Colchicum autumnale alkaloid

Action: Inhibits microtubule formation of lactic acid in leukocytes, which decreases phagocytosis and inflammation in joints

Uses: Gout, gouty arthritis (prevention, treatment); to arrest progression of neurologic disability in multiple sclerosis

Investigational uses: Hepatic cirrhosis, familial Mediterranean fever, pericarditis

Dosage and routes:

Prevention

• *Adult:* **PO** 0.6-1.8 mg qd depending on severity; **IV** 0.5-1 mg 1-2 × day

Treatment

• *Adult:* **PO** 0.6-1.2 mg, then 0.5-1.2 mg q1h, until pain decreases or side effects occur; **IV** 2 mg, then 0.5 mg q6h until response, max 4 mg total

Available forms: Tabs 0.6 mg; inj 0.5 mg/ml

Side effects/adverse reactions:

MISC: Myopathy, alopecia, reversible azoospermia, peripheral neuritis
GU: Hematuria, ***oliguria, renal damage***
HEMA: ***Agranulocytosis, thrombocytopenia, aplastic anemia, pancytopenia***
GI: Nausea, vomiting, anorexia, malaise, metallic taste, cramps, peptic ulcer, diarrhea
INTEG: Chills, dermatitis, pruritus, purpura, erythema

Contraindications: Hypersensitivity; serious GI, renal, hepatic, cardiac disorders; pregnancy (D) IV

Precautions: Blood dyscrasias, pregnancy (C) PO, hepatic disease, elderly, lactation, children

Pharmacokinetics:

PO: Peak ½-2 hr, half-life 20 min; deacetylates in liver; excreted in feces (metabolites/active drug)

Interactions:

- Toxicity: cycloSPORINE
- ↑ GI effects: NSAIDs
- ↑ bone marrow depression: radiation, bone marrow depressants, cycloSPORINE
- ↓ action of vit B_{12}, may cause reversible malabsorption

Lab test interferences:

Increase: Alk phosphatase, AST
False positive: Urine, RBC, Hgb
Interfere: Urinary 17-hydroxycorticosteroids

NURSING CONSIDERATIONS

Assess:

- I&O ratio; observe for decrease in urinary output
- CBC, platelets, reticulocytes before, during therapy (q3mo), may cause aplastic anemia, agranulocytosis, decreased platelets
- For toxicity: weakness, abdominal pain, nausea, vomiting, diarrhea; drug should be discontinued

Administer:

PO route

- With food for GI symptoms

IV route

- Do not give IM or SC
- Do not dilute in D_5W, or change in IV line that contains D_5W
- Give over 2-5 min
- Wait ≥1 wk after giving a full course of IV colchicine before giving subsequent doses

Evaluate:

- Therapeutic response: decreased stone formation on x-ray, decreased pain in kidney region, absence of hematuria, decreased pain in joints

Teach patient/family:

- To avoid alcohol, OTC preparations that contain alcohol
- To report any pain, redness, or hard area, usually in legs; rash, sore throat, fever, bleeding, bruising, weakness, numbness, tingling
- The importance of complying with medical regimen (diet, weight loss, drug therapy); the possibility of bone marrow depression occurring

Treatment of overdose: D/C medication, may need opioids to treat diarrhea

colesevelam (℞)

(coal-see-vel′am)
Welchol
Func. class.: Antilipemic
Chem. class.: Bile acid sequestrant

Action: Absorbs, combines with bile acids to form insoluble complex that is excreted through feces; loss of bile acids lowers cholesterol levels

Uses: Elevated LDL cholesterol, alone or in combination with HMG-CoA reductase inhibitor

Dosage and routes:

- *Adult:* **PO** Monotherapy: 3 625-mg tabs bid with meals or 6 tabs qd with a meal; may increase to 7 tabs if needed
- Combination therapy: 3 tabs bid with meals or 6 tabs qd with a meal given with an HMG-CoA reductase inhibitor

Available forms: Tabs 625 mg

Side effects/adverse reactions:

CNS: Headache, dizziness, drowsiness, vertigo, tinnitus
MS: Muscle, joint pain
GI: Constipation, abdominal pain, nausea, fecal impaction, hemorrhoids, flatulence, vomiting, steatorrhea, peptic ulcer

INTEG: Rash, irritation of perianal area, tongue, skin
META: Decreased vit A, D, K; ***hyperchloremic acidosis***
HEMA: Decreased red cell folate content; ***bleeding,*** increased PT
Contraindications: Hypersensitivity, biliary obstruction
Precautions: Pregnancy (C), lactation, children
Pharmacokinetics:
PO: Excreted in feces, LDL decreased in 4-7 days
Interactions:
• ↓ absorption of: gemfibrozil, glipiZIDE, phenytoin, propranolol, warfarin, thiazides, digitalis, penicillin G, tetracyclines, corticosteroids, iron, thyroid, clindamycin, fat-soluble vitamins
↓ antilipidemic effect: gotu kola
↑ effect: glucomannan
Lab test interferences:
Increase: LFTs, Cl, PO_4
NURSING CONSIDERATIONS
Assess:
• Cardiac glycoside level, if both drugs are being administered
• For signs of vit A, D, K deficiency
• Fasting LDL, HDL, total cholesterol, triglyceride levels, electrolytes if on extended therapy
• Bowel pattern daily; increase bulk, H_2O in diet for constipation
Administer:
• Drug qd or bid with meals; give all other medications 1 hr before colesevelam or 4 hr after colesevelam to avoid poor absorption take with liquid
• Supplemental doses of vit A, D, K, if levels are low
Evaluate:
• Therapeutic response: decreased cholesterol level (hyperlipidemia); diarrhea, pruritus (excess bile acids)
Teach patient/family:
The symptoms of hypoprothrombinemia: bleeding mucous membranes, dark tarry stools, hematuria, petechiae; report immediately
• The importance of compliance; toxicity may result if doses missed
• That risk factors should be decreased: high-fat diet, smoking, alcohol consumption, absence of exercise
• Not to discontinue suddenly

colestipol (℞)

(koe-les'ti-pole)
Colestid
Func. class.: Antilipemic
Chem. class.: Bile acid sequestrant

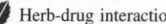

Action: Absorbs, combines with bile acids to form insoluble complex excreted through feces; loss of bile acids lowers cholesterol levels
Uses: Primary hypercholesterolemia, xanthomas
Investigational uses: Digitalis toxicity
Dosage and routes:
• *Adult:* **PO** tabs 2 g qd-bid, may increase q1mo, max 16 g/day; granules: 5 g qd-bid, may increase q1mo, max 30 g/day
Available forms: Granules 300 g, 450, 500 g bottles, 5, 7.5 g packets; tabs 1 g
Side effects/adverse reactions:
GI: Constipation, abdominal pain, nausea, fecal impaction, hemorrhoids, flatulence, vomiting, steatorrhea, peptic ulcer
INTEG: Rash, irritation of perianal area, tongue, skin
HEMA: ***Bleeding, increased PT***
META: Decreased vit A, D, K, red folate content; ***hyperchloremic acidosis***
Contraindications: Hypersensitivity, biliary obstruction

Precautions: Pregnancy (B), lactation, children, bleeding disorders
Pharmacokinetics:
PO: Onset 24-48 hr, peak/duration 30 days, excreted in feces
Interactions:
• ↓ action of: thiazides, digitalis, warfarin, penicillin G, gemfibrozil, glipiZIDE, propranolol, phenytoin, TOLBUTamide, tetracycline, corticosteroids, iron, thyroid agents, clindamycin, fat-soluble vitamins
↑ lipidemic effect: glucomannan
↓ lipidemic effect: gotu kola
Lab test interferences:
Increase: AST, ALT, alk phosphatase, chloride, PO_4
Decrease: Na, K, Ca
NURSING CONSIDERATIONS
Assess:
• Cardiac glycoside levels, if both drugs are being administered
• For signs of vit A, D, K deficiency
• Serum cholesterol, triglyceride levels, electrolytes (extended therapy)
• Bowel pattern daily; increase bulk, water in diet if constipation develops
Administer:
• Drug qd or bid; give all other medications 1 hr before colestipol or 4 hr after colestipol to avoid poor absorption
• Drug mixed in applesauce or stirred into beverage (2-6 oz); do not take dry; let stand for 2 min
Tabs should be swallowed whole; do not break, crush, or chew
• Supplemental doses of vit A, D, K if levels are low
Evaluate:
• Therapeutic response: decreased triglycerides
Teach patient/family:
The symptoms of hypoprothrombinemia: bleeding mucous membranes; dark, tarry stools; hematuria, petechiae; report immediately
• That compliance is needed; not to miss or double doses
• That risk factors should be decreased: high-fat diet, smoking, alcohol consumption, absence of exercise

RARELY USED

corticotropin (ACTH) (℞)

(kor-ti-koe-troe′pin)
H.P. Acthar Gel
Func. class.: Pituitary hormone

Uses: Testing adrenocortical function, treatment of adrenal insufficiency caused by administration of corticosteroids (long term), multiple sclerosis, infantile spasms
Dosage and routes:
Acute exacerbations of multiple sclerosis
• *Adult:* **IM** 80-120 units/day × 14-21 days
Infantile spasms
• *Infant:* **IM Gel** 20 units/day × 2 wks, increase if needed
Contraindications: Hypersensitivity, scleroderma, osteoporosis, CHF, peptic ulcer disease, hypertension, systemic fungal infections, smallpox vaccination, recent surgery, ocular herpes simplex, primary adrenocortical insufficiency/hyperfunction

cortisone (℞)

(kor′ti-sone)

Cortone✤, Cortone Acetate

Func. class.: Corticosteroid, synthetic

Chem. class.: Glucocorticoid, short-acting

Action: Decreases inflammation by suppression of migration of polymorphonuclear leukocytes, fibroblasts, reversal of increased capillary permeability and lysosomal stabilization

Uses: Inflammation, severe allergy, adrenal insufficiency, collagen disorders; respiratory, dermatologic, rheumatic disorders

Dosage and routes:

• *Adult:* **PO/IM** 25-300 mg qd or q2d, titrated to response

• *Child:* **PO** 2.5-10 mg/kg/day; **IM** 1-5 mg/kg/day

Available forms: Tabs 5, 10, 25 mg; inj 50 mg/ml

Side effects/adverse reactions:

INTEG: Acne, poor wound healing, ecchymosis, bruising, petechiae

CNS: Depression, flushing, sweating, headache, mood changes

*CV: Hypertension, **circulatory collapse, thrombophlebitis, embolism,*** tachycardia, ***necrotizing angiitis, CHF,*** edema

HEMA: ***Thrombocytopenia***

MS: Fractures, osteoporosis, weakness, loss of muscle mass

GI: Diarrhea, nausea, abdominal distention, ***GI hemorrhage,*** increased appetite, ***pancreatitis***

EENT: Fungal infections, increased intraocular pressure, blurred vision

META: Sodium, fluid retention, potassium loss

Contraindications: Psychosis, hypersensitivity, idiopathic thrombocytopenia, acute glomerulonephritis, amebiasis, fungal infections, nonasthmatic bronchial disease, pregnancy (D), child <2 yr, AIDS, TB

Precautions: Lactation, diabetes mellitus, glaucoma, osteoporosis, seizure disorders, ulcerative colitis, CHF, myasthenia gravis, renal disease, esophagitis, peptic ulcer

Pharmacokinetics:

PO: Peak 2 hr, duration 1½ days

IM: Peak 20-48 hr, duration 1½ days

Interactions:

• ↓ cortisone action: barbiturates, rifampin, phenytoin, theophylline

• ↑ GI symptoms: salicylates, indomethacin, NSAIDs

• ↓ effects of anticoagulants, antidiabetics, toxoids, vaccines, salicylates

• ↑ side effects: alcohol, salicylates, indomethacin, potassium-wasting diuretics

• ↑ action of cortisone: salicylates, estrogens, indomethacin, oral contraceptives, ketoconazole, macrolide antiinfectives

Potassium deficiency: aloe, buckthorn, cascara sagrada, Chinese rhubarb, rhubarb, senna

↑ steroid effect: aloe, licorice, perilla

Lab test interferences:

Increase: Cholesterol, Na, blood glucose, uric acid, Ca, urine glucose

Decrease: Ca, K, T_4, T_3, thyroid ^{131}I uptake test, urine 17-OHCS, 17-KS, PBI

False negative: Skin allergy tests

NURSING CONSIDERATIONS

Assess:

• Potassium, blood, urine glucose while on long-term therapy; hypokalemia and hyperglycemia

• Weight daily; notify prescriber of weekly gain >5 lb

• B/P q4h, pulse; notify prescriber if chest pain occurs

• I&O ratio; be alert for decreasing urinary output and increasing edema
• Plasma cortisol levels during long-term therapy (normal level: 138-635 nmol/L SI units if drawn at 8 AM)
• Infection: fever, WBC even after withdrawal of medication; drug masks infection
• Potassium depletion: paresthesias, fatigue, nausea, vomiting, depression, polyuria, dysrhythmias, weakness
• Edema, hypertension, cardiac symptoms
• Mental status: affect, mood, behavioral changes, aggression

Administer:
• After shaking suspension (parenteral)
• Titrated dose; use lowest effective dose
• IM inj deeply in large mass; rotate sites; avoid deltoid; use a 21G needle
• In one dose in AM to prevent adrenal suppression; avoid SC administration; tissue may be damaged; never administer by IV route
• With food or milk to decrease GI symptoms

Perform/provide:
• Assistance with ambulation in patient with bone tissue disease to prevent fractures

Evaluate:
• Therapeutic response: ease of respirations, decreased inflammation

Teach patient/family:
• That medical ID as steroid user should be carried at all times
• To notify prescriber if therapeutic response decreases; dosage adjustment may be needed
◆ Not to discontinue abruptly or adrenal crisis can result
• To avoid OTC products: salicylates, alcohol in cough products, cold preparations unless directed by prescriber
• All aspects of drug usage, including cushingoid symptoms
• The symptoms of adrenal insufficiency: nausea, anorexia, fatigue, dizziness, dyspnea, weakness, joint pain
• Avoid exposure to chickenpox and measles
• To take PO dose in AM with food or fluid (milk)

RARELY USED

cosyntropin (℞)
(koe-sin-troe'pin)
Cortrosyn, Synacthen ✦, Tetracosactrin
Func. class.: Pituitary hormone

Uses: Testing adrenocortical function

Dosage and routes:
• *Adult and child >2 yr:* **IM/IV** 0.25-1 mg between blood sampling; *Child <2 yr:* **IM/IV** 0.125 mg

Contraindications: Hypersensitivity

cromolyn (OTC, ℞)
(kroe'moe-lin)
Gastrocrom Intal, Nasalcrom, Rynacrom ✦
Func. class.: Antiasthmatic
Chem. class.: Mast cell stabilizer

Action: Stabilizes the membrane of the sensitized mast cell, preventing release of chemical mediators after an antigen-IgE interaction

Uses: Severe perennial bronchial asthma, prevention of exercise-induced bronchospasm, acute bron-

chospasm induced by environmental pollutants, mastocytosis
Investigational uses: Allergic rhinitis, chronic urticarial angioedema
Dosage and routes:
Allergic rhinitis
• *Adult and child >2 yr:* **NASAL SOL** 1 spray in each nostril tid-qid, not to exceed 6 doses/day
Bronchospasm
• *Adult and child >2 yr:* **INH** 20 mg <1 hr before exercise
Bronchial asthma
• *Adult and child >2 yr:* **INH** 20 mg qid; **NEB** 20 mg qid by nebulization
• *Adult and child ≥13 yr:* oral conc 2 amp 4×/day ½ hr ac and hs, may increase after 2-3 wk, max 40 mg/kg/day, reduce after dose to lowest dose
• *Child 2-12 yr:* oral conc 1 amp 4×/day ½ hr ac and hs, may increase after 2-3 wk, reduce dose to lowest possible dose
Systemic mastocytosis
• *Adult and child >12 yr:* **PO** 200 mg qid ½ hr ac and hs
• *Child 2-12 yr:* **PO** 100 mg qid ½ ac and hs
Available forms: Nasal sol 5.2 mg/metered spray (40 mg/ml); neb sol 20 mg/2 ml; aerosol 800 mcg/actuation; oral conc 100 mg/5 ml
Oral conc
CV: Tachycardia, PVCs, palpitations
CNS: Dizziness, headache, paresthesia, migraine, seizures, psychosis, anxiety, depression, hallucinations, insomnia
INTEG: Pruritus, rash, flushing, photosensitivity
GI: Diarrhea, nausea, abdominal pain, constipation, dyspepsia, stomatitis, vomiting
HEMA: Polycythemia, neutropenia, pancytopenia
Side effects/adverse reactions:
EENT: Throat irritation, cough, nasal congestion, burning eyes, nasal stinging, sneezing
CNS: Headache, dizziness, neuritis
GU: Urinary frequency, dysuria
GI: Nausea, vomiting, anorexia, dry mouth, bitter taste
INTEG: Rash, urticaria, angioedema
MS: Joint pain/swelling
Contraindications: Hypersensitivity to this drug or lactose, status asthmaticus, acute asthma
Precautions: Pregnancy (B), lactation, renal disease, hepatic disease, safety not established; child <5 yr (aerosol); <2 yr (nebulizer); <2 yr (nasal sol); oral <2 yr
Do not confuse:
Nasalcrom/Nasalide
Pharmacokinetics: Excreted unchanged in feces; half-life 80 min
NURSING CONSIDERATIONS
Assess:
• Eosinophil count during treatment
• Respiratory status: rate, rhythm, characteristics, cough, wheezing, dyspnea
Administer:
• For oral conc: break open ampule, squeeze contents in glass of water, stir, drink
Perform/provide:
• Gargle, sip of water to decrease irritation in throat
Evaluate:
• Therapeutic response: decrease in asthmatic symptoms; congested, runny nose
Teach patient/family:
Nasal sol
• Blow nose, hold pump between fingers, if first use spray in air until fine mist occurs, insert nozzle in nostril, spray and breathe in through nose, repeat in other nostril
Aerosol
• Take cover off mouthpiece, shake gently, breathe out slowly, place mouthpiece in mouth, close mouth around it, tilt head back, breathe in

as the inhaler is depressed, remove, hold breath, then breathe out slowly

Inhalation

- Do not swallow sol
- Empty ampule into power driven nebulizer as directed. Do not combine different meds.

Oral

- To take ½ hr before meals and hs

RARELY USED

crotamiton (℞)

(kroe-tam'i-ton)

Func. class.: Scabicide

Uses: Scabies, pruritus

Dosage and routes:

Scabies:

- *Adult and child:* **CREAM** wash area with soap, water; remove visible crusts, apply cream, apply another coat in 24 hr, remove with soap, water in 48 hr

Pruritus: Massage into affected area, repeat as necessary

Contraindications: Hypersensitivity, skin inflammation, abrasions, breaks in skin, mucous membranes

C

cyanocobalamin (vit B_{12}) (OTC, ℞)

(sye-an-oh-koe-bal'a-min)

Alphamin, Anacobin✤, Bedoz✤, Cobex, Cobolin-M, Crystamine, Crysti-1000, Cyanabin✤, Cyanoject, Cyomin, Ener-B, Hydrobexan, Hydro Cobex, Hydro-Crysti-12

hydroxocobalamin

Hydroxycobal, LA-12, Nascobal, Neuroforte-R, Rubesol-1000, Rubramin PC, Shovite, Vibal LA, Vibral, Vitamin B_{12}

Func. class.: Vit B_{12}, water-soluble vitamin

Action: Needed for adequate nerve functioning, protein and carbohydrate metabolism, normal growth, RBC development, cell reproduction

Uses: Vit B_{12} deficiency, pernicious anemia, vit B_{12} malabsorption syndrome, Schilling test, increased requirements with pregnancy, thyrotoxicosis, hemolytic anemia, hemorrhage, renal and hepatic disease

Dosage and routes:

Cyanocobalamin

- *Adult:* **PO** up to 1000 mcg/day **SC/IM** 30-100 mcg/day × 1 wk, then 100-200 mcg/mo

Schilling test

- *Adult and child:* **IM** 1000 mcg in one dose
- Child: **PO** up to 1000 mcg/day **SC/IM** 30-50 mcg/day × 2 wk, then 100 mcg/mo; nasal 500 mcg qwk

Hydroxocobalamin

- *Adult:* **SC/IM** 30-50 mcg/day × 5-10 days, then 100-200 mcg/mo

• *Child:* **SC/IM** 30-50 mcg/day × 5-10 days, then 100 mcg/mo
Available forms: Cyanocobalamin: tabs 25, 50, 100, 250, 500, 1000, 5000 mcg; ext rel tabs: 100, 200, 500, 1000 mcg; lozenges: 100, 250, 500 mcg; nasal jel 500 mcg/spray; inj 100, 1000 mcg/ml; hydroxocobalamin: inj 1000 mcg/ml
Side effects/adverse reactions:
CNS: Flushing, optic nerve atrophy
GI: Diarrhea
CV: ***CHF,*** peripheral vascular thrombosis, ***pulmonary edema***
INTEG: Itching, rash, pain at inj site
META: Hypokalemia
SYST: ***Anaphylactic shock***
Contraindications: Hypersensitivity, optic nerve atrophy
Precautions: Pregnancy (A), lactation, children
Pharmacokinetics: Gastric intrinsic factor must be present for absorption to occur; stored in liver, kidneys, stomach; 50%-90% excreted in urine; crosses placenta, excreted in breast milk
Interactions:
• ↓ absorption: aminoglycosides, anticonvulsants, colchicine, chloramphenicol, aminosalicylic acid, potassium preparations, cimetidine
• ↑ absorption: predniSONE
↓ Vit B_{12} absorption: goldenseal
Lab test interferences:
False positive: Intrinsic factor
NURSING CONSIDERATIONS
Assess:
• For vit B_{12} deficiency: red, beefy tongue, psychosis, pallor, neuropathy
• GI function: diarrhea, constipation
• Potassium levels during beginning treatment in megaloblastic anemia; q6mo in pernicious anemia; folic acid, plasma vit B_{12} (after 1 wk), reticulocyte counts
• Nutritional status: egg yolks, fish, organ meats, dairy products, clams, oysters: good sources of vit B_{12}
• For pulmonary edema, worsening of CHF in cardiac patients
Administer:
PO route
• With fruit juice to disguise taste; immediately after mixing
• With meals if possible for better absorption
Nasal route
• Avoid use within 1 hr of hot fluids/food
IM route
• By IM inj for pernicious anemia for life unless contraindicated
IV route
• IV route not recommended but may be admixed in TPN solution
Additive compatibilities: Ascorbic acid, chloramphenicol, metaraminol, vit B/C
Solution compatibilities: Dextrose/Ringer's or lactated Ringer's combinations, dextrose/saline combinations, D_5W, $D_{10}W$, 0.45% NaCl, Ringer's or lactated Ringer's sol
Y-site compatibilities: Heparin, hydrocortisone, potassium chloride, vit B/C
Perform/provide:
• Protection from light and heat
Evaluate:
• Therapeutic response: decreased anorexia, dyspnea on exertion, palpitations, paresthesias, psychosis, visual disturbances
Teach patient/family:
• That treatment must continue for life for pernicious anemia
• To eat well-balanced diet
• To avoid contact with persons with infection; infections common
Treatment of overdose: Discontinue drug

cyclobenzaprine (℞)

(sye-kloe-ben′za-preen)
cyclobenzaprine HCl,
cycloflex, Flexeril

Func. class.: Skeletal muscle relaxant, central acting

Chem. class.: Tricyclic amine salt

Action: Unknown; may be related to antidepressant effects
Uses: Adjunct for relief of muscle spasm and pain in musculoskeletal conditions
Dosage and routes:
Muscloskeletal disorders
• *Adult:* **PO** 10 mg tid × 1 wk, not to exceed 60 mg/day × 3 wk
• *Child:* 20-40 mg/kg/day in 2-4 divided doses
Fibromyalgia
• *Adult:* **PO** 10-40 mg hs
Available forms: Tabs 10 mg
Side effects/adverse reactions:
CNS: Dizziness, weakness, drowsiness, headache, tremor, depression, insomnia, confusion, paresthesia
EENT: Diplopia, temporary loss of vision
CV: Postural hypotension, tachycardia, ***dysrhythmias***
GI: Nausea, vomiting, hiccups, dry mouth, constipation
INTEG: Rash, pruritus, fever, facial flushing, sweating
GU: Urinary retention, frequency, change in libido
Contraindications: Acute recovery phase of myocardial infarction, dysrhythmias, heart block, CHF, hypersensitivity, child <12 yr, intermittent porphyria, thyroid disease
Precautions: Renal disease, hepatic disease, addictive personality, pregnancy (B), lactation, elderly

Do not confuse:
cyclobenzaprine/cyproheptadine
Pharmacokinetics:
PO: Onset 1 hr, peak 3-8 hr, duration 12-24 hr, half-life 1-3 days; metabolized by liver; excreted in urine; crosses placenta; excreted in breast milk
Interactions:
• ↑ CNS depression: alcohol, tricyclics, opiates, barbiturates, sedatives, hypnotics
• Do not use within 14 days of MAOI
↑ CNS depression: kava

NURSING CONSIDERATIONS
Assess:
• For pain: location, duration, mobility, stiffness, baseline and periodically
• Blood studies: CBC, WBC, differential for blood dyscrasias
• Hepatic studies: AST, ALT, alk phosphatase; hepatitis may occur
• ECG in epileptic patients; poor seizure control has occurred
• Allergic reactions: rash, fever, respiratory distress
• Severe weakness, numbness in extremities
• Psychologic dependency: increased need for medication, more frequent requests for medication, increased pain
• CNS depression: dizziness, drowsiness, psychiatric symptoms
Administer:
• With meals for GI symptoms
Perform/provide:
• Storage in tight container at room temperature
• Assistance with ambulation if dizziness, drowsiness occur, especially elderly
Evaluate:
• Therapeutic response: decreased pain, spasticity; muscle spasms of acute, painful musculoskeletal con-

ditions generally short term; long-term therapy seldom warranted

Teach patient/family:

- Not to discontinue medication abruptly; insomnia, nausea, headache, spasticity, tachycardia will occur; drug should be tapered off over 1-2 wk
- Not to take with alcohol, other CNS depressants
- To avoid hazardous activities if drowsiness/dizziness occurs
- To avoid using OTC medication: cough preparations, antihistamines, unless directed by prescriber
- To use gum, frequent sips of water for dry mouth

Treatment of overdose: Empty stomach with emesis, gastric lavage, then administer activated charcoal; use anticonvulsants if indicated; monitor cardiac function

cyclopentolate ophthalmic

See appendix c

HIGH ALERT

cyclophosphamide (℞)

(sye-kloe-foss'fa-mide)

Cytoxan, Neosar, Procytox🍁

Func. class.: Antineoplastic alkylating agent

Chem. class.: Nitrogen mustard

Action: Alkylates DNA, RNA; inhibits enzymes that allow synthesis of amino acids in proteins; is also responsible for cross-linking DNA strands; activity is not cell cycle phase specific

Uses: Hodgkin's disease; lymphomas; leukemia; cancer of female reproductive tract, breast; lung, prostate; multiple myeloma; neuroblastoma; retinoblastoma; Ewing's sarcoma

Dosage and routes:

- *Adult:* **PO** initially 1-5 mg/kg over 2-5 days, maintenance is 1-5 mg/kg; **IV** initially 40-50 mg/kg in divided doses over 2-5 days, maintenance 10-15 mg/kg q7-10d, or 3-5 mg/kg q3d
- *Child:* **PO/IV** 2-8 mg/kg or 60-250 mg/m^2 in divided doses for 6 or more days; maintenance 10-15 mg/kg q7-10d or 30 mg/kg q3-4wk; dose should be reduced by half when bone marrow depression occurs

Renal disease

- CCr 25-50 ml/min 50% of dose; CCr <25 ml/min avoid use

Available forms: Inj 100, 200, 500, 750 mg, 1, 2 g; tabs 25, 50 mg

Side effects/adverse reactions:

CV: ***Cardiotoxicity*** (high doses)

HEMA: ***Thrombocytopenia, leukopenia, pancytopenia; myelosuppression***

GI: Nausea, vomiting, diarrhea, weight loss, colitis, ***hepatotoxicity***

GU: ***Hemorrhagic cystitis,*** *hematuria, neoplasms, amenorrhea, azoospermia, sterility, ovarian fibrosis*

INTEG: Alopecia, dermatitis

RESP: ***Fibrosis***

ENDO: Syndrome of inappropriate antidiuretic hormone (SIADH), gonadal suppression

CNS: Headache, dizziness

META: Hyperuricemia

MISC: Secondary neoplasms

Contraindications: Lactation, pregnancy (D)

Precautions: Radiation therapy

Do not confuse:

cyclophosphamide/cycloSPORINE

Cytoxan/Cytosar/Cytotec/Centoxin/cytarabine

Pharmacokinetics: Metabolized by liver; excreted in urine; half-life

4-6½ hr; 50% bound to plasma proteins

Interactions:

- ↑ cyclophosphamide toxicity: barbiturates
- Potentiation of neuromuscular blockade: succinylcholine
- ↑ bone marrow depression: allopurinol, thiazides
- ↑ hypoglycemia: insulin
- ↓ digoxin levels: digoxin
- ↓ cyclophosphamide effect: chloramphenicol, corticosteroids
- ↓ antibody response: live virus vaccines
- ↑ action of: warfarin

Lab test interferences:

Increase: Uric acid

False positive: Pap smear

False negative: PPD, mumps, trichophytin, *Candida*

Decrease: Pseudocholinesterase

NURSING CONSIDERATIONS

Assess:

- For hemorrhagic cystitis; renal studies: BUN, serum uric acid, urine CCr before, during therapy; I&O ratio; report fall in urine output <30 ml/hr
- CBC, differential, platelet count baseline, weekly; withhold drug if WBC is <2500 or platelet count is <75,000; notify prescriber of results
- Pulmonary function tests, chest x-ray films before, during therapy; chest film should be obtained q2wk during treatment
- Monitor temp q4h (elevated temp may indicate beginning infection)
- Hepatic studies before, during therapy (bilirubin, AST, ALT, LDH) as needed or monthly
- Bleeding: hematuria, guaiac, bruising or petechiae, mucosa or orifices q8h
- Dyspnea, rales, unproductive cough, chest pain, tachypnea
- Effects of alopecia on body image, discuss feelings about body changes
- Jaundice of skin, sclera; dark urine; clay-colored stools; itchy skin; abdominal pain; fever; diarrhea
- Buccal cavity q8h for dryness, sores or ulceration, white patches, oral pain, bleeding, dysphagia; obtain prescription for viscous lidocaine (Xylocaine)

⬦ Symptoms indicating severe allergic reaction: rash, pruritus, urticaria, purpuric skin lesions, itching, flushing

Administer:

- In AM so drug can be eliminated before hs
- Fluids IV or PO before chemotherapy to hydrate patient
- Antacid before oral agent, give after evening meal, before bedtime
- Antiemetic 30-60 min before giving drug and prn
- Allopurinol or sodium bicarbonate to maintain uric acid levels, alkalinization of urine

IV route

- IV after diluting 100 mg/5 ml of sterile H_2O or bacteriostatic H_2O; shake; let stand until clear; may be further diluted in up to 250 ml D_5 or NS; give 100 mg or less/min through 3-way stopcock of glucose or saline inf
- Using 21, 23, 25G needle; check site for irritation, phlebitis

Additive compatibilities: Cisplatin with etoposide, fluorouracil, hydrOXYzine, methotrexate, methotrexate/fluorouracil, mitoxantrone, ondansetron

Solution compatibilities: Amino acids 4.25%/D_{25}, D_5/0.9% NaCl, D_5W, 0.9% NaCl

Syringe compatibilities: Bleomycin, cisplatin, doxapram, DOXOrubicin, droperidol, fluorouracil, furosemide, heparin, leucovorin, methotrexate, metoclopramide, mitomycin, vinBLAStine, vinCRIStine

Y-site compatibilities: Allopurinol, amifostine, amikacin, ampicillin, azlocillin, aztreonam, bleomycin, cefamandole, cefazolin, cefepime, cefoperazone, cefotaxime, cefoxitin, cefuroxime, cephalothin, cephapirin, chloramphenicol, chlorproMAZINE, cimetidine, cisplatin, cladribine, clindamycin, dexamethasone, diphenhydramine, DOXOrubicin, DOXOrubicin liposome, doxycycline, droperidol, erythromycin, famotidine, filgrastim, fludarabine, fluorouracil, furosemide, gallium, ganciclovir, gentamicin, granisetron, heparin, hydromorphone, idarubicin, kanamycin, leucovorin, lorazepam, melphalan, methotrexate, methylPREDNISolone, metoclopramide, metronidazole, mezlocillin, minocycline, mitomycin, morphine, moxalactam, nafcillin, ondansetron, oxacillin, paclitaxel, penicillin G potassium, piperacillin, piperacillin/tazobactam, prochlorperazine, promethazine, propofol, ranitidine, sargramostim, sodium bicarbonate, teniposide, thiotepa, ticarcillin, ticarcillin-clavulanate, tobramycin, trimethoprim - sulfamethoxazole, vancomycin, vinBLAStine, vinCRIStine, vinorelbine

Perform/provide:

- Storage in tight container at room temperature
- Strict medical asepsis, protective isolation if WBC levels are low
- Increase fluid intake to 2-3 L/day to prevent urate deposits, calculi formation, reduce incidence of hemorrhagic cystitis
- Diet low in purines: organ meats (kidney, liver), dried beans, peas to maintain alkaline urine
- Rinsing of mouth tid-qid with water, club soda; brushing of teeth bid-tid with soft brush or cotton-tipped applicators for stomatitis; use unwaxed dental floss
- Warm compresses at injection site for inflammation

Evaluate:

- Therapeutic response: decreased tumor size, spread of malignancy

Teach patient/family:

- About protective isolation
- That amenorrhea can occur; reversible after stopping treatment
- To report any changes in breathing or coughing
- That hair may be lost during treatment; a wig or hairpiece may make patient feel better; new hair may be different in color, texture
- To avoid foods with citric acid, hot or rough texture
- To report any bleeding, white spots, ulcerations in mouth to prescriber; tell patient to examine mouth qd
- To report signs of infection: increased temperature, sore throat, flu-like symptoms
- To report signs of anemia: fatigue, headache, faintness, shortness of breath, irritability
- To report bleeding (bruising, hematuria, petechiae): avoid use of razors, commercial mouthwash
- To avoid use of aspirin products, ibuprofen
- To avoid vaccinations during therapy

*cycloSPORINE (℞)

(sye'kloe-spor-een)

Neoral, Sandimmune, SangCya

Func. class.: Immunosuppressant

Chem. class.: Fungus-derived peptide

Action: Produces immunosuppression by inhibiting lymphocytes (T)

Uses: Organ transplants (liver, kidney, heart) to prevent rejection, rheumatoid arthritis, psoriasis

Investigational uses: Recalcitrant ulcerative colitis

Dosage and routes:

Prevention of transplant rejection

• *Adult and child:* **PO** 15 mg/kg several hr before surgery, daily for 2 wk, reduce dosage by 2.5 mg/kg/wk to 5-10 mg/kg/day; **IV** 5-6 mg/kg several hr before surgery, daily, switch to PO form as soon as possible

Rheumatoid arthritis

• *Adult:* **PO** 2.5 mg/kg/day divided bid, may increase 0.5-0.75 mg/kg/day after 8-12 wk, max 4 mg/kg/day

Psoriasis

• *Adult:* **PO** 2.5 mg/kg/day divided bid, × 4 wk, then increase by 0.5 mg/kg/day q2wk, max 4 mg/kg/day

Available forms: Microemulsion oral sol (Neoral) 100 mg/ml; microemulsion soft gel cap (Neoral) 25, 100 mg; soft gel caps 25, 100 mg; oral sol 100 mg/ml; inj 50 mg/ml

Side effects/adverse reactions:

GI: Nausea, vomiting, diarrhea, *oral Candida, gum hyperplasia,* ***hepatotoxicity,*** pancreatitis

INTEG: Rash, acne, *hirsutism*

CNS: Tremors, headache, ***seizures***

GU: ***Albuminuria, hematuria, proteinuria, renal failure***

META: Hyperkalemia, hypomagnesemia, hyperlipidemia, hyperuricemia

MISC: Infection

Do not confuse:

cycloSPORINE/CycloSERINE

cycloSPORINE/cyclophosphamide

Contraindications: Hypersensitivity

Precautions: Severe renal disease, severe hepatic disease, pregnancy (C)

Pharmacokinetics: Peak 4 hr, highly protein bound, half-life (biphasic) 1.2 hr, 25 hr; metabolized in liver; excreted in feces; crosses placenta; excreted in breast milk

Interactions:

• ↑ levels of: digoxin, etoposide

• ↑ action, toxicity of cycloSPORINE: amiodarone, amphotericin B, androgens, azole antifungals, calcium channel blockers, carvedilol, cimetidine, colchicine, corticosteroids, foscarnet, imipenem-cilastatin, ketoconazole, macrolides, metoclopramide, oral contraceptives, NSAIDs, melphalan, fluconazole

• ↓ cycloSPORINE action: carbamazepine, phenobarbital, phenytoin, rifamycins, sulfamethoxazole-trimethoprim

• ↓ antibody reaction: live virus vaccines

• Do not use with tacrolimus

• ↓ absorption of neoral products

• Drug/food: Slowed metabolism of drug: grapefruit juice

↓ immunosuppressant effect: ginseng, maitake, mistletoe, schisandra, St. John's wort, turmeric

↑ immunosuppressant effect: safflower

NURSING CONSIDERATIONS
Assess:
• Renal studies: BUN, creatinine at least monthly during treatment, 3 mo after treatment
• Hepatic studies: alk phosphatase, AST, ALT, bilirubin
• Drug blood level during treatment
• Hepatotoxicity: dark urine, jaundice, itching, light-colored stools; drug should be discontinued
• For nephrotoxicity: 6 wk post op, acute tubular necrosis, CyA trough level >200 ng/ml, gradual rise in creatinine (0.15 mg/dl/day), creatinine plateau <25% above baseline, intracapsular pressure <40 mm Hg
Administer:
PO route
• Use pipette provided to draw up oral sol; may mix with milk or juice, wipe pipette, do not wash
• For several days before transplant surgery
• With corticosteroids
• With meals for GI upset or in chocolate milk
• With oral antifungal for *Candida* infections
• Microemulsion products (Neoral) and other products are not interchangeable
IV route
• After diluting each 50 mg/20-100 ml of 0.9% NaCl or D_5W; run over 2-6 hr, may give as a continuous inf over 24 hr; use an infusion pump, glass inf bottles only
Additive compatibilities: Ciprofloxacin
Solution compatibilities: D_5W, NaCl 0.9%
Y-site compatibilities: Cefmetazole, propofol, sargramostim
Evaluate:
• Therapeutic response: absence of rejection
Teach patient/family:
• To report fever, chills, sore throat, fatigue, since serious infections may occur; tremors, bleeding gums, increased B/P
• To use contraceptive measures during treatment, for 12 wk after ending therapy
⊘ Not to break, crush, or chew caps

cyproheptadine (℞)
(si-proe-hep'ta-deen)
cyproheptadine HCl,
Periactin, PMS-Cyproheptadine✦
Func. class.: Antihistamine, H_1-receptor antagonist
Chem. class.: Piperidine

Action: Acts on blood vessels, GI, respiratory system by competing with histamine for H_1-receptor site; decreases allergic response by blocking histamine
Uses: Allergy symptoms, rhinitis, pruritus, cold, urticaria
Investigational uses: Appetite stimulant, management of vascular headache, nightmares, posttraumatic stress disorder
Dosage and routes:
• *Adult:* **PO** 4 mg tid-qid, not to exceed 0.5 mg/kg/day
• *Child 7-14 yr:* **PO** 4 mg bid-tid, not to exceed 16 mg/day
• *Child 2-6 yr:* **PO** 2 mg bid-tid, not to exceed 12 mg/day
Nightmares, posttraumatic stress disorder
• *Adult:* **PO** 4-12 mg qhs, max 32 mg
Available forms: Tabs 4 mg; syr 2 mg/5 ml
Side effects/adverse reactions:
HEMA: ***Hemolytic anemia, leukopenia, thrombocytosis, agranulocytosis***
SYST: ***Anaphylactic shock***
CNS: *Dizziness, drowsiness,* poor co-

ordination, fatigue, anxiety, euphoria, confusion, paresthesia, neuritis
CV: Hypotension, palpitations, tachycardia
RESP: Increased thick secretions, wheezing, chest tightness
GI: Constipation, dry mouth, nausea, vomiting, anorexia, diarrhea, weight gain, increased appetite
INTEG: Rash, urticaria, photosensitivity
GU: Retention, dysuria, frequency
EENT: Blurred vision, dilated pupils; tinnitus; nasal stuffiness; dry nose, throat, mouth
Contraindications: Hypersensitivity to H_1-receptor antagonist, acute asthma attack, lower respiratory tract disease
Precautions: Increased intraocular pressure, renal disease, cardiac disease, hypertension, bronchial asthma, seizure disorder, stenosed peptic ulcers, hyperthyroidism, prostatic hypertrophy, bladder neck obstruction, pregnancy (B), lactation, elderly
Do not confuse:
cyproheptadine/cyclobenzaprine
Pharmacokinetics:
PO: Duration 4-6 hr; metabolized in liver; excreted by kidneys; excreted in breast milk
Interactions:
• ↑ CNS depression: barbiturates, opiates, hypnotics, tricyclics, alcohol
• ↑ effect of cyproheptadine: MAOIs
↑ CNS depression: hops, Jamaican dogwood, kava, khat, senega
↑ anticholinergic effect: corkwood, henbane
Lab test interferences:
False negative: Skin allergy tests
NURSING CONSIDERATIONS
Assess:
• I&O ratio; be alert for urinary retention, frequency, dysuria; drug should be discontinued
• CBC during long-term therapy
• Respiratory status: rate, rhythm, increase in bronchial secretions, wheezing, chest tightness
• Cardiac status: palpitations, increased pulse, hypotension
Administer:
• With meals for GI symptoms; absorption may slightly decrease
Perform/provide:
• Hard candy, gum, frequent rinsing of mouth for dryness
• Storage in airtight container at room temperature
Evaluate:
• Therapeutic response: absence of running or congested nose, rashes
Teach patient/family:
• All aspects of drug use; to notify prescriber of confusion, sedation, hypotension
• That this drug decreases anticoagulant (oral) effect
• To avoid driving, other hazardous activity if drowsiness occurs, especially elderly
• To avoid concurrent use of alcohol, other CNS depressants
Treatment of overdose: Ipecac syrup or lavage, diazepam, vasopressors, barbiturates (short-acting)

HIGH ALERT

cytarabine (℞)

(sye-tare'a-been)
Ara-C, Cytosar♣, Cytosar-U, cytosine arabinoside, DepoCyt
Func. class.: Antineoplastic, antimetabolite
Chem. class.: Pyrimidine nucleoside

Action: Competes with physiologic substrate of DNA synthesis, thus interfering with cell replication in the

S phase of the cell cycle (before mitosis)

Uses: Acute myelocytic leukemia, acute lymphocytic leukemia, chronic myelocytic leukemia, lymphomatous meningitis (IT), and in combination for non-Hodgkin's lymphomas in children

Dosage and routes:

Acute myelocytic leukemia

• *Adult:* **IV INF** 200 mg/m²/day × 5 days q2wk as single agent or 2-6 mg/kg/day (100-200 mg/m²/day) as single dose or 2-3 divided doses for 5-10 days until remission, used in combination; maintenance 70-200 mg/m²/day for 2-5 days qmo; **SC** maintenance 1 mg/kg q1-2×/wk

Lymphomatous meningitis

Liposomal (DepoCyt)

• *Adult* **IT:** 50 mg q14d × 2 doses (wk 1, 3) then 50 mg q14d × 3 doses (wk 5, 7, 9) followed by 1 dose wk 13; then 50 mg q28d × 4 doses (wk 17, 21, 25, 29); if neurotoxicity occurs, reduce dose to 25 mg, if it persists, discontinue use

In combination

• *Child:* **IV INF** 100 mg/m²/day × 5-10 days

Available forms: Powder for inj 100, 500 mg, 1, 2 g; liposomal for intrathecal use 10 mg/ml

Side effects/adverse reactions:

HEMA: Thrombophlebitis, bleeding, ***thrombocytopenia, leukopenia, myelosuppression, anemia***

META: Hyperuricemia

GI: Nausea, vomiting, anorexia, diarrhea, stomatitis, ***hepatotoxicity,*** abdominal pain, hematemesis, ***GI hemorrhage***

EENT: Sore throat, conjunctivitis

GU: Urinary retention, ***renal failure, hyperuricemia***

INTEG: Rash, fever, freckling, cellulitis

RESP: ***Pneumonia,*** dyspnea, ***pulmonary edema*** (high doses)

CV: Chest pain, ***cardiopathy***

CNS: Neuritis, dizziness, headache, personality changes, ataxia, mechanical dysphasia, ***coma; chemical arachnoiditis*** (IT)

SYST: ***Anaphylaxis***

CYTARABINE SYNDROME: Fever, myalgia, bone pain, chest pain, *rash,* conjunctivitis, malaise (6-12 hr after administration)

Contraindications: Hypersensitivity, infants, pregnancy (D)

Precautions: Renal disease, hepatic disease, lactation

Do not confuse:

Cytosar/Cytoxan/Cytovene

Cytosar/Cytovene

Pharmacokinetics:

INTRATHECAL: Half-life 100-236 hr; metabolized in liver; excreted in urine (primarily inactive metabolite); crosses blood-brain barrier, placenta

IV/SC: Distribution half-life 10 min, elimination half-life 1-3 hr

Interactions:

• ↑ toxicity, bone marrow depression: radiation or other antineoplastics

• ↓ effects of: oral digoxin

NURSING CONSIDERATIONS

Assess:

• CBC (RBC, Hct, Hgb), differential, platelet count weekly; withhold drug if WBC is <1000/mm³, platelet count is <50,000/mm³, or RBC, Hct, Hgb low; notify prescriber of these results

• Renal studies: BUN, serum uric acid, urine CCr, electrolytes before and during therapy

• I&O ratio; report fall in urine output to <30 ml/hr

• Monitor temp q4h; fever may indicate beginning infection; no rectal temps

• Hepatic studies before and during therapy: bilirubin, ALT, AST, alk phosphatase, as needed or monthly;

check for jaundice of skin, sclera; dark urine; clay-colored stools; pruritus; abdominal pain; fever; diarrhea

• Blood uric acid during therapy

◆ For anaphylaxis: rash, pruritus, facial swelling, dyspnea; resuscitation equipment should be nearby

◆ Chemical arachnoiditis (IT): headache, nausea, vomiting, fever; neck ridigity pain, meningism, CSF pleocytosis; may be decreased by dexamethasone

• Cytarabine syndrome 6-12 hr after inf: fever, myalgia, bone pain, chest pain, rash, conjunctivitis, malaise; corticosteroids may be ordered

• Bleeding: hematuria, heme-positive stools, bruising or petechiae, mucosa or orifices q8h

◆ Dyspnea, rales, unproductive cough, chest pain, tachypnea, fatigue, increased pulse, pallor, lethargy; personality changes, with high doses; pulmonary edema may be fatal (rare)

• Buccal cavity q8h for dryness, sores or ulceration, white patches, oral pain, bleeding, dysphagia

• Local irritation, pain, burning, discoloration at inj site

• GI symptoms: frequency of stools, cramping, antispasmodic may be used

• Acidosis, signs of dehydration: rapid respirations, poor skin turgor, decreased urine output, dry skin, restlessness, weakness

Administer:

• Antiemetic 30-60 min before giving drug and prn

• Allopurinol to maintain uric acid levels and alkalinization of the urine

• Topical or systemic analgesics for pain

IT route

• Liposomal: withdraw drug immediately before use; use within 4 hr, do not save unused portions, or use in-line filter; give directly into CSF by intraventricular reservoir or by direct inj into lumbar site

• Give slowly over 1-5 min, follow with lumbar puncture, instruct patient to lie flat, give dexamethasone 4 mg bid PO or IV × 5 days beginning on day of liposomal inj

IV route

• After diluting 100 mg/5 ml of sterile H_2O for inj; given by direct IV over 1-3 min through free-flowing tubing (IV); may be further diluted in 50-100 ml NS or D_5W, given over 30 min to 24 hr depending on dose; also may be given by continuous inf

Additive compatibilities: Corticotropin, DAUNOrubicin with etoposide, etoposide, hydrOXYzine, lincomycin, mitoxantrone, ondansetron, potassium chloride, prednisoLONE, sodium bicarbonate, vinCRIStine

Solution compatibilities: Amino acids, D_5/LR, D_5/0.2% NaCl, D_5/0.9% NaCl, D_{10}/0.9% NaCl, D_5W, invert sugar 10% in electrolyte #1, Ringer's LR, 0.9% NaCl, sodium lactate ⅙ mol/L, TPN #57

Syringe compatibilities: Metoclopramide

Y-site compatibilities: Amifostine, amsacrine, aztreonam, cefepime, chlorproMAZINE, cimetidine, cladribine, dexamethasone, diphenhydrAMINE, DOXOrubicin liposome, droperidol, famitodine, filgrastim, fludarabine, gentamicin, granisetron, heparin, hydrocortisone, hydromorphone, idarubicin, lorazepam, melphalan, methotrexate, methylPREDNISolone, metoclopramide, morphine, ondansetron, paclitaxel, piperacillin/tazobactam, prochlorperazine, promethazine, propofol, ranitidine, sargramostim, sodium bicarbonate, teniposide, thiotepa, vinorelbine

Perform/provide:

• Strict medical asepsis and protective isolation if WBC levels are low

• Increase fluid intake to 2-3 L/day to prevent urate deposits and calculi formation, unless contraindicated

• Diet low in purines: absence of organ meats (kidney, liver), dried beans, peas to prevent increased urate deposits

• Rinsing of mouth tid-qid with water, club soda; brushing of teeth bid-tid with soft brush or cotton-tipped applicators for stomatitis; use unwaxed dental floss

Evaluate:

• Therapeutic response: decreased tumor size, spread of malignancy

Teach patient/family:

• To report any coughing, chest pain, changes in breathing; may indicate beginning pneumonia, pulmonary edema

• To avoid foods with citric acid, hot or rough texture if stomatitis is present, use sponge brush and rinse with water after each meal; to report stomatitis: any bleeding, white spots, ulcerations in mouth; tell patient to examine mouth qd, report any symptoms

• To report signs of infection: increased temp, sore throat, flulike symptoms; avoid crowds, persons with infections

• To report signs of anemia: fatigue, headache, faintness, shortness of breath, irritability

• To report bleeding; avoid use of razors, commercial mouthwash, salicylates, NSAIDs

• To use thrombocytopenia precautions

• To take fluids to 3 L/day to prevent renal damage

• To use contraception during treatment and 4 mo thereafter

• To avoid receiving vaccines during treatment

• To continue using dexamethasone with IT administration, that fever, headache, nausea, vomiting are likely to occur

HIGH ALERT

dacarbazine (℞)

(da-kar′ba-zeen)

dacarbazine, DTIC✦, DTIC-Dome

Func. class.: Antineoplastic alkylating agent

Chem. class.: Cytotoxic triazine

Action: Alkylates DNA, RNA; inhibits enzymes that allow synthesis of amino acids in proteins; also responsible for cross-linking DNA strands; activity is not cell cycle phase specific

Uses: Hodgkin's disease, sarcomas, neuroblastoma, malignant melanoma

Dosage and routes:

Malignant melanoma

• *Adult:* **IV** 2-4.5 mg/kg or 250 mg/m^2 qd × 5 days; repeat q3wk depending on response

Hodgkin's disease

• *Adult:* IV 150 mg/m^2 qd × 5 days with other agents, repeat q4wk; or 375 mg/m^2 on day 1 when given in combination, repeat q15d

Available forms: Inj 100, 200 mg

Side effects/adverse reactions:

HEMA: ***Thrombocytopenia, leukopenia,*** anemia

GI: Nausea, anorexia, vomiting, ***hepatotoxicity*** (rare)

CNS: Facial paresthesia, flushing, fever, malaise

INTEG: Alopecia, dermatitis, pain at inj site
SYST: ***Anaphylaxis***
Contraindications: Lactation
Precautions: Radiation therapy, pregnancy (1st trimester) (C)
Pharmacokinetics: Metabolized by liver; excreted in urine; half-life 35 min, terminal 5 hr, 5% protein bound
Interactions:
• ↓ dacarbazine effect: phenytoin, phenobarbital
• Toxicity, bone marrow suppression: bone marrow suppressants, radiation, other antineoplastics
• Bleeding: salicylates, anticoagulants
• ↑ adverse reaction ↓ antibody reaction: live virus vaccines
• ↑ nephrotoxicity: aminoglycosides
• ↑ ototoxicity: loop diuretics

NURSING CONSIDERATIONS

Assess:
• CBC, differential, platelet count weekly; withhold drug if WBC <4000 or platelet count <75,000; notify prescriber of results
• Monitor temp q4h (may indicate beginning infection)
• Hepatic studies before, during therapy (bilirubin, AST, ALT, LDH) as needed or monthly
• Bleeding: hematuria, guaiac, bruising or petechiae, mucosa or orifices q8h
• Effects of alopecia on body image, discuss feelings about body changes
• Jaundice of skin, sclera; dark urine; clay-colored stools; itchy skin; abdominal pain; fever; diarrhea
• Inflammation of mucosa, breaks in skin
Administer:
• Antiemetic 30-60 min before giving drug to prevent vomiting
• Antibiotics for prophylaxis of infection
IV route
• After diluting 100 mg/9.9 ml of sterile H_2O for inj (10 mg/ml), give by direct IV over 1 min through Y-tube or 3-way stopcock; may be further diluted in 50-250 ml D_5W or NS for inj, given as an inf over ½ hr
• Watch for extravasation; give Na thiosulfate 10% 4 ml plus sterile H_2O 5 ml, 3-5 ml SC if needed
Additive compatibilities: Bleomycin, carmustine, cyclophosphamide, cytarabine, dactinomycin, DOXOrubicin, fluorouracil, mercaptopurine, methotrexate, ondansetron, vinBLAStine
Additive incompatibilities: Hydrocortisone sodium succinate, cysteine
Y-site compatibilities: Amifostine, aztreonam, filgrastim, fludarabine, granisetron, melphalan, ondansetron, paclitaxel, sargramostim, teniposide, thiotepa, vinorelbine
Perform/provide:
• Storage in light-resistant container, dry area
• Strict medical asepsis, protective isolation if WBC levels are low
• Increase fluid intake to 2-3 L/day to prevent urate deposits, calculi formation
• Warm compresses at infusion site for inflammation
Evaluate:
• Therapeutic response: decreased tumor size, spread of malignancy
Teach patient/family:
• That patient should avoid prolonged exposure to sun
• That hair may be lost during treatment; a wig or hairpiece may make the patient feel better; new hair may be different in color, texture
• To report signs of infection: fever, sore throat, flulike symptoms
• To report signs of anemia: fatigue, headache, faintness, shortness of breath, irritability

• To report bleeding; avoid use of razors, commercial mouthwash
• To avoid use of aspirin products or ibuprofen
• To use contraceptives during and for several months after therapy

HIGH ALERT

daclizumab (℞)

(dah-kliz′uh-mab)

Zenapax

Func. class.: Immunosuppressant

Chem. class.: Humanized IgG1 monoclonal antibody

Action: Binds to the IL-2 (interleukin-2) receptor antagonist

Uses: Acute allograft rejection in renal transplant patients

Dosage and routes:

• *Adult:* **IV** 1 mg/kg as part of a regimen that includes cyclosporine and corticosteroids, mix calculated vol with 50 ml of 0.9% NaCl and give via peripheral/central vein over 15 min

Available forms: Inj 25 mg/ml

Side effects/adverse reactions:

CNS: Chills, tremors, headache, prickly sensation

RESP: Dyspnea, wheezing, ***pulmonary edema,*** coughing, atelectasis, congestion, hypoxia

GI: Vomiting, nausea, diarrhea, constipation, abdominal pain, pyrosis

CV: Hypertension, ***tachycardia, thrombosis,*** bleeding

GU: Oliguria, dysuria, ***renal tubular necrosis,*** renal damage, ***hydronephrosis***

INTEG: Impaired wound healing

Contraindications: Hypersensitivity

Precautions: Pregnancy (C), child <2 yr, lactation, elderly

Interactions:

↓ immunosuppressant effect: ginseng, maitake, mistletoe, schisandra, St. John's wort, turmeric

↑ immunosuppressant effect: safflower

NURSING CONSIDERATIONS

Assess:

• Blood studies: Hgb, WBC, platelets during treatment qmo; if leukocytes are $<3000/mm^3$, drug should be discontinued
• Hepatic studies: alk phosphatase, AST, ALT, bilirubin
• Hepatotoxicity: dark urine, jaundice, itching, light-colored stools; drug should be discontinued
• For anaphylaxis, have corticosteroids, epinephrine available

Administer:

• All other medications PO if possible
• Avoid IM inj, since infection may occur
• Protect undiluted sol from direct light; should be used with drugs for immunosuppression

Solution compatibilities: 0.9% NaCl

Evaluate:

• Therapeutic response: absence of graft rejection

Teach patient/family:

• To report fever, chills, sore throat, fatigue, since serious infection may occur
• To use contraception (women) before, during, and for 4 mo after treatment
• To avoid vaccinations during treatment
• To increase fluid intake during treatment

HIGH ALERT

dactinomycin (℞)

(dak-ti-noe-mye'sin)

Cosmegen

Func. class.: Antineoplastic, antibiotic

Action: Inhibits DNA, RNA, protein synthesis; derived from *Streptomyces parvullus;* replication is decreased by binding to DNA, which causes strand splitting; cell cycle nonspecific; a vesicant

Uses: Sarcomas, melanomas, trophoblastic tumors in women, testicular cancer, Wilms' tumor, rhabdomyosarcoma

Dosage and routes:

• *Adult:* **IV** 500 mcg/m^2/day × 5 days; stop drug for 2-4 wk; then repeat cycle

• *Child:* **IV** 15 mcg/kg/day × 5 days, not to exceed 500 mcg/day; stop drug until bone marrow recovery, then repeat cycle

Available forms: Inj 0.5 mg/vial

Side effects/adverse reactions:

HEMA: ***Thrombocytopenia, leukopenia, aplastic anemia***

GI: Nausea, vomiting, anorexia, stomatitis, ***hepatotoxicity,*** abdominal pain, diarrhea

INTEG: Rash, alopecia, pain at injection site, folliculitis, acne, desquamation, ***extravasation***

EENT: Chelitis, dysphagia, esophagitis

CNS: Malaise, fatigue, lethargy, fever

MS: Myalgia

Contraindications: Hypersensitivity, herpes infection, child <6 mo

Precautions: Renal disease, hepatic disease, pregnancy (C), lactation, bone marrow depression

Pharmacokinetics: Half-life 36 hr; IV onset 2-5 min; concentrates in kidneys, liver, spleen; does not cross blood-brain barrier; excreted in feces and urine

Interactions:

• ↑ toxicity: other antineoplastics, radiation

Lab test interferences:

Increase: Uric acid

NURSING CONSIDERATIONS

Assess:

• CBC, differential, platelet count weekly; withhold drug if WBC is <4000/mm^3 or platelet count is <75,000/mm^3; notify prescriber

• Renal studies: BUN, serum uric acid, urine CCr, electrolytes before, during therapy

• I&O ratio; report fall in urine output to <30 ml/hr

• Monitor temp q4h; fever may indicate beginning infection

• Hepatic studies before, during therapy: bilirubin, AST, ALT, alk phosphatase, as needed or monthly; check for jaundice of skin, sclera; dark urine; clay-colored stools; itchy skin; abdominal pain; fever; diarrhea

• Bleeding: hematuria, guaiac stools, bruising, petechiae, mucosa or orifices q8h

• Food preferences; list likes, dislikes

• Effects of alopecia on body image; discuss feelings about body changes

• Inflammation of mucosa, breaks in skin

• Buccal cavity q8h for dryness, sores, ulceration, white patches, oral pain, bleeding, dysphagia

◆ Symptoms indicating severe allergic reaction: rash, pruritus, urticaria, purpuric skin lesions, itching, flushing

• GI symptoms: frequency of stools, cramping, nausea, vomiting, anorexia

• Acidosis, signs of dehydration: rapid respirations, poor skin turgor, decreased urine output, dry skin, restlessness, weakness, sunken eyeball in children

Administer:

- Antiemetic 30-60 min before giving drug to prevent vomiting

IV route

- After diluting 0.5 mg/1.1 ml of sterile H_2O for inj without preservative; use 2.2 ml (0.25 mg/ml), give by direct IV at 0.5 mg or less/min through Y-tube or 3-way stopcock if inf in progress; may be further diluted if required in 50 ml D_5W or NS for infusion; run over 10-15 min; change needles between reconstitution and direct IV administration
- Hydrocortisone, sodium thiosulfate to infiltration area, and ice compress after stopping infusion

Y-site compatibilities: Allopurinol, amifostine, aztreonam, cefepime, fludarabine, granisetron, melphalan, ondansetron, sargramostim, teniposide, thiotepa, vinorelbine

Perform/provide:

- Strict hand-washing technique, gloves and protective covering
- Liquid diet: carbonated beverages; gelatin may be added if patient is not nauseated or vomiting
- Rinsing of mouth tid-qid with water, club soda; brushing of teeth bid-qid with soft brush or cotton-tipped applicators for stomatitis; use unwaxed dental floss to prevent injury
- Storage in cool, dark environment; do not expose to bright light or freeze

Evaluate:

- Therapeutic response: decreased tumor size, spread of malignancy

Teach patient/family:

- That contraception is needed during treatment and for 4-6 mo after discontinuing therapy
- To avoid vaccinations without order by prescriber
- That hair may be lost during treatment after 1-2 wk and that wig or hairpiece may make patient feel better; that new hair may be different in color, texture
- To avoid foods with citric acid, hot or rough texture when stomatitis is present
- To report any bleeding, white spots, ulcerations in mouth to prescriber; tell patient to examine mouth qd
- To avoid crowds, persons with known infection when granulocyte count is low
- To increase fluids to 3 L/day

HIGH ALERT

dalteparin (℞)

(dahl'ta-pear-in)

Fragmin

Func. class.: Anticoagulant

Chem. class.: Low molecular weight heparin

Action: Prevents conversion of fibrinogen to fibrin and prothrombin to thrombin by enhancing inhibitory effects of antithrombin III

Uses: Unstable angina/non-Q-wave MI; prevention of deep vein thrombosis in abdominal surgery, hip replacement patients

Investigational uses: Systemic anticoagulation in venous/arterial thromboembolic complications

Dosage and routes:

Hip replacement surgery/DVT prophylaxis

- *Adult:* **SC** 2500 international units 2 hr prior to surgery and 2nd dose in the evening the day of surgery, then 5000 international units SC 1st postop day and qd 5-10 days

Unstable angina/non-Q-wave MI

- *Adult:* **SC** 120 international units/

kg, do not exceed 10,000 international units q12h with concurrent aspirin, continue until stable

Systemic anticoagulation

• *Adult:* **SC** 200 international units/kg qd or 100 international units/kg bid

DVT, prophylaxis for abdominal surgery

• *Adult:* **SC** 2500 international units qd, 1-2 hr prior to abdominal surgery and repeat qd × 5-10 days; in high-risk patients 5000 international units may be used

Available forms: Prefilled syringes, 2500, 5000 international units/0.2 ml; 10,000 international units multidose vials; 7500 international units/0.3 ml, 10,000 international units/ml

Side effects/adverse reactions:

CNS: ***Intracranial bleeding***

SYST: Hypersensitivity, ***hemorrhage, anaphylaxis*** possible

HEMA: ***Thrombocytopenia***

INTEG: Pruritus, superficial wound infection

Contraindications: Hypersensitivity to this drug, heparin, or pork products, benzyl alcohol; hemophilia, leukemia with bleeding, thrombocytopenic purpura, cerebrovascular hemorrhage, cerebral aneurysm, severe hypertension, other severe cardiac disease, those undergoing regional anesthesia for unstable angina, non–Q wave MI

Precautions: Elderly, pregnancy (B), hepatic disease, severe renal disease, blood dyscrasias, subacute bacterial endocarditis, acute nephritis, lactation, children, recent childbirth, peptic ulcer disease, pericarditis, pericardial effusion, recent lumbar puncture, vasculitis, other diseases where bleeding is possible

Pharmacokinetics: 87% absorbed, excreted by kidneys, elimination half-life 3-5 hr, peak 4 hr, onset and duration unknown

Interactions:

• ↑ risk of bleeding: aspirin, oral anticoagulants, platelet inhibitors, NSAIDs, thrombolytics

↑ bleeding risk: agrimony, alfalfa, angelica, anise, bilberry, black haw, bogbean, bromelain, buchu, chondroitin, cinchona bark, dong quai, fenugreek, feverfew, garlic, ginger, ginkgo, ginseng, horse chestnut, Irish moss, kelp, kelpware, khella, lovage, lungwort, meadowsweet, motherwort, mugwort, nettle, papaya, parsley (large amts), pau d'arco, pineapple, poplar, prickly ash, safflower, saw palmetto, senega, tonka bean, turmeric, wintergreen, yarrow

↓ anticoagulant action: chamomile, coenzyme Q10, flax, glucomannan, goldenseal, guar gum

NURSING CONSIDERATIONS

Assess:

• For blood studies (Hct, CBC, platelets, occult blood in stools) during treatment since bleeding can occur

For bleeding gums, petechiae, ecchymosis, black tarry stools, hematuria, epistaxis, decrease in Hct, B/P; may indicate bleeding, possible hemorrhage; notify prescriber immediately, drug should be discontinued

• For hypersensitivity: fever, skin rash, urticaria; notify prescriber immediately

• For needed dosage change q1-2wk; dose may need to be decreased if bleeding occurs

Administer:

• Cannot be used interchangeably (unit for unit) with unfractionated heparin or LMWHs

• Do not give IM or IV drug route; approved is SC only; do not mix with other inj or sol

• By SC only; have patient sit or lie down; SC inj may be 2 in from umbilicus in a U-shape, upper outer

side of thigh, around navel, or upper outer quadrangle of the buttocks; rotate inj sites
- Changing needles is not recommended; change inj site qd; use at same time of day

Evaluate:
- Therapeutic response: absence of deep-vein thrombosis

Teach patient/family:
- To avoid OTC preparations that contain aspirin; other anticoagulants, serious drug interaction may occur
- To use soft-bristle toothbrush to avoid bleeding gums, avoid contact sports, use electric razor, avoid IM inj
- To report any signs of bleeding: gums, under skin, urine, stools; unusual bruising

Treatment of overdose: Protamine sulfate 1% given IV; 1 mg protamine/100 anti-Xa international units of dalteparin given

---

HIGH ALERT

danaparoid (℞)

(dan-a-pair′oid)

Orgaran

Func. class.: Anticoagulant, antithrombotic

Chem. class.: Glycosaminoglycan

Action: Prevents conversion of fibrinogen to fibrin and prothrombin to thrombin by enhancing inhibitory effects of antithrombin III

Uses: Prevention of vein thrombosis in hemodialysis, stroke, elective surgery for malignancy or total hip replacement, hip fracture surgery

Dosage and routes:

Prevention of venous thrombosis
- *Adult:* **SC** 750 anti–factor-Xa units bid × 7-10 days, begin 1-4 hr presurgery and restart 2 hr after surgery; use lower dose in renal failure

Hemodialysis
- *Adult:* **SC** 2400-4800 anti-Xa units given predialysis

Available forms: Inj 750 anti-Xa units/0.6 ml

Side effects/adverse reactions:

SYST: Hypersensitivity, ***hemorrhage***

HEMA: ***Thrombocytopenia***

INTEG: Rash, pruritus, inj site pain

CV: ***Hemorrhage,*** peripheral edema

CNS: Insomnia, headache

GI: Nausea, vomiting, constipation

MS: Asthenia

Contraindications: Hypersensitivity to this drug, sulfites, pork; hemophilia, leukemia with bleeding, thrombocytopenia, purpura, cerebrovascular hemorrhage, cerebral aneurysm, other severe cardiac disease

Precautions: Hypersensitivity to heparin, severe hypertension, elderly, pregnancy (B), severe renal disease, blood dyscrasias, subacute bacterial endocarditis, acute nephritis, lactation, children, recent childbirth, peptic ulcer disease, pericarditis, pericardial effusion, recent lumbar puncture, vasculitis, other diseases where bleeding is possible

Pharmacokinetics: 100% absorbed, excreted by kidneys, half-life 24 hr, peak 4 hr

Interactions:
- ↑ bleeding risk: aspirin, oral anticoagulants, platelet inhibitors, NSAIDs, penicillin, dextran

↑ bleeding risk: agrimony, alfalfa, angelica, anise, bilberry, black haw, bogbean, bromelain, buchu, chondroitin, cinchona bark, dong quai, fenugreek, feverfew, garlic, ginger, ginkgo, ginseng, horse chestnut, Irish moss, kelp, kelpware, khella, lovage, lungwort, meadowsweet, motherwort, mugwort, nettle, papaya, parsley (large amts), pau d'arco, pineapple, poplar, prickly ash, safflower, saw palmetto, senega, tonka bean, turmeric, wintergreen, yarrow

↓ anticoagulant action: chamomile, coenzyme Q10, flax, glucomannan, goldenseal, guar gum

NURSING CONSIDERATIONS

Assess:

• For blood studies (Hct, CBC, occult blood in stools) during treatment since bleeding can occur; aPTT, ACT, anti–factor-Xa test, platelets

• For bleeding gums, petechiae, ecchymosis, black tarry stools, hematuria, epistaxis, decrease in Hct, B/P; may indicate bleeding, possible hemorrhage; notify prescriber immediately, drug should be discontinued

• For hypersensitivity: fever, skin, rash, urticaria; notify prescriber immediately

• For needed dosage change q1-2wk; dose may need to be decreased if bleeding occurs

Administer:

• Cannot be used interchangeably (unit for unit) with heparin, LMWHs, or heparinoids

• By SC only, have patient sit or lie down; SC inj may be around the navel in a U-shape, upper outer side of thigh or upper outer quadrangle of the buttocks; rotate inj sites

• Changing needles is not recommended

Evaluate:

• Therapeutic response: absence of deep-vein thrombosis

Teach patient/family:

• To avoid OTC preparations that may cause serious drug interactions unless directed by prescriber; may contain aspirin, other anticoagulants

• To use soft-bristle toothbrush to avoid bleeding gums, avoid contact sports, use electric razor, avoid IM inj

• To report any signs of bleeding: gums, under skin, urine, stools; unusual bruising

Treatment of overdose: Discontinue drug, protamine sulfate 1% given IV; 1 mg protamine/100 anti–factors-Xa international units of danaparoid given

danazol (℞)

(da′na-zole)

Cyclomen✱, danazol, Danocrine

Func. class.: Androgen, anabolic steroid

Chem. class.: α-Ethinyl testosterone derivative

Action: Atrophy of endometrial tissue; decreases FSH, LH, which are controlled by pituitary; this leads to amenorrhea/anovulation

Uses: Endometriosis, prevention of hereditary angioedema, fibrocystic breast disease

Dosage and routes:

Endometriosis

• *Adult:* **PO** 100-500 mg bid uninterrupted for 3-9 mo

Fibrocystic breast disease

• *Adult:* **PO** 100-400 mg qd in 2 divided doses × 2-6 mo

Hereditary angioedema prevention

• *Adult:* **PO** 200 mg bid-tid until desired response, then decrease dose to 100 mg at 1-3 mo intervals

Available forms: Caps 50, 100, 200 mg

Side effects/adverse reactions:

INTEG: Rash, *acneiform lesions,* oily hair, skin, flushing, sweating, acne vulgaris, alopecia, *hirsutism,* pruritus

CNS: Dizziness, headache, fatigue, tremors, paresthesias, flushing, sweating, anxiety, *lability,* insomnia

MS: Cramps, spasms, joint swelling

CV: Increased B/P

GU: Hematuria, *amenorrhea,* atrophic vaginitis, decreased libido, *decreased breast size,* clitoral hypertrophy, testicular atrophy

GI: Nausea, vomiting, constipation, *weight gain,* ***cholestatic jaundice***

EENT: Conjunctival edema, nasal congestion, voice weakness

ENDO: Abnormal GTT

Contraindications: Severe renal, severe cardiac, severe hepatic disease, hypersensitivity, genital bleeding (abnormal), pregnancy (X), children

Precautions: Migraine headaches, seizure disorders

Do not confuse:

danazol/Dantrium

Interactions:

• ↑ action: anticoagulants, oral antidiabetics, insulin, corticosteroids

• Nephrotoxicity: cycloSPORINE

Lab test interferences:

Increase: Cholesterol

Decrease: Cholesterol, T_4, T_3, thyroid ^{131}I uptake test, 17-KS, PBI

Interference: GTT

NURSING CONSIDERATIONS

Assess:

• For pain before and after treatment in endometriosis, fibrocystic breast disease; tenderness, nodules in fibrocystic breast disease

• Potassium, blood, urine glucose while on long-term therapy; LFTs, periodically, semen volume, sperm count, motility in hereditary angioedema

• Weight daily; notify prescriber if weekly weight gain is >5 lb; drug should be decreased or discontinued

• I&O ratio; be alert for decreasing urinary output, increasing edema

• Edema, hypertension, cardiac symptoms, jaundice

• Mental status: affect, mood, behavioral changes, aggression, sleep disorders, depression, anxiety, lability

• Signs of virilization: deepening of voice, decreased libido, facial hair that may not be reversible

• Hypercalcemia: GI symptoms, polydipsia, polyuria, increased calcium levels above 11 mg/dl, loss of muscle tone

Administer:

• Start treatment during menstruation in endometriosis, fibrocystic breast disease

• With food or milk to decrease GI symptoms (i.e., nausea, vomiting, anorexia, dyspepsia)

Perform/provide:

• Storage in airtight container at room temperature; do not freeze

Evaluate:

• Therapeutic response: decreased pain in endometriosis; decreased size, pain in fibrocystic breast disease

Teach patient/family:

⊘ Not to break, crush, or chew caps

• To notify prescriber if therapeutic response decreases

• Not to discontinue medication abruptly; to taper over several wk

• To report menstrual irregularities; that amenorrhea usually occurs but menstruation resumes 2-3 mo after termination of therapy without medical intervention

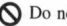

• About routine breast self-exam and to report any increase in nodule size

• That drug should induce anovulation; reversible within 60-90 days after drug is discontinued and treatment will need to be resumed
• That endometriosis tends to recur after drug is discontinued
• To use nonhormonal contraception
• That virilization may occur, to notify prescriber
• To use sunscreen or stay out of the sun to prevent burns

dantrolene (℞)

(dan′troe-leen)
Dantrium
Func. class.: Skeletal muscle relaxant, direct acting
Chem. class.: Hydantoin

Action: Interferes with intracellular release of calcium from the sarcoplasmic reticulum necessary to initiate contraction; slows catabolism in malignant hyperthermia
Uses: Spasticity in multiple sclerosis, stroke, spinal cord injury, cerebral palsy, malignant hyperthermia
Dosage and routes:
Spasticity
• *Adult:* **PO** 25 mg/day; may increase by 25-100 mg bid-qid, not to exceed 400 mg/day × 1 wk
• *Child:* **PO** 1 mg/kg/day given in divided doses bid-tid; dosage may increase gradually, not to exceed 100 mg qid
Prevention of malignant hyperthermia
• *Adult and child:* **PO** 4-8 mg/kg/day in 3-4 divided doses × 1-2 days prior to procedures, give last dose 4 hr preop; **IV** 2.5 mg/kg prior to anesthesia
Malignant hyperthermia
• *Adult and child:* **IV** 1 mg/kg, may repeat to total dose of 10 mg/kg; **PO** 4-8 mg/kg/day in 4 divided doses × 3 days to prevent further hyperthermia; post-crisis follow-up 4-8 mg/kg/day for 1-3 days
Available forms: Caps 25, 50, 100 mg; powder for inj 20 mg/vial
Side effects/adverse reactions:
CNS: Dizziness, weakness, fatigue, drowsiness, headache, disorientation, insomnia, paresthesias, tremors, ***seizures***
EENT: Nasal congestion, blurred vision, mydriasis
HEMA: ***Eosinophilia***
CV: Hypotension, chest pain, palpitations
GI: ***Hepatic injury***, *nausea,* constipation, vomiting, increased AST, alk phosphatase, abdominal pain, dry mouth, anorexia, hepatitis, dyspepsia
GU: Urinary frequency, nocturia, impotence, crystalluria
INTEG: Rash, pruritus, photosensitivity
Contraindications: Hypersensitivity, compromised pulmonary function, active hepatic disease, impaired myocardial function
Precautions: Peptic ulcer disease, renal disease, hepatic disease, stroke, seizure disorder, diabetes mellitus, pregnancy (C), lactation, elderly
Do not confuse:
Dantrium/danazol
Pharmacokinetics:
PO: Peak 5 hr; highly protein bound; half-life 8 hr; metabolized in liver; excreted in urine (metabolites)
Interactions:
• Dysrhythmias: verapamil
• ↑ CNS depression: alcohol, tricyclics, opiates, barbiturates, sedatives, hypnotics, antihistamines
• Hepatotoxicity: estrogens, other hepatotoxics
• Considered incompatible in sol or syringe; compatibility unknown

NURSING CONSIDERATIONS

Assess:

- For increased seizure activity, ECG in epilepsy patient; poor seizure control has occurred
- I&O ratio; check for urinary retention, frequency, hesitancy, especially elderly
- Hepatic function by frequent determination of AST, ALT, bilirubin, alk phosphatase, GGTP; renal function studies, BUN, creatinine, CBC
- Allergic reactions: rash, fever, respiratory distress
- Severe weakness, numbness in extremities; prescriber should be notified and drug discontinued
- Tolerance: increased need for medication, more frequent requests for medication, increased pain
- CNS depression: dizziness, drowsiness, insomnia, psychiatric symptoms

Signs of hepatotoxicity: jaundice, yellow sclera, pain in abdomen, nausea, fever; prescriber should be notified, drug should be discontinued

Administer:

PO route

- With meals for GI symptoms, caps may be opened and mixed with food/liquid

IV route

- IV after diluting 20 mg/60 ml sterile H_2O for inj without bacteriostatic agent (333 mcg/ml); shake until clear; give by rapid IV push through Y-tube or 3-way stopcock; follow by prescribed doses immediately; may also give by intermittent inf over 1 hr prior to anesthesia

Perform/provide:

- Storage in tight container at room temperature; protect diluted sol from light, use within 6 hr
- Gum, frequent sips of water for dry mouth
- Assistance with ambulation if dizziness/drowsiness occurs

Evaluate:

- Therapeutic response: decreased pain, spasticity

Teach patient/family:

- Not to discontinue medication quickly; hallucinations, spasticity, tachycardia will occur; drug should be tapered off over 1-2 wk; notify prescriber of abdominal pain, jaundiced sclera, clay-colored stools, change in color of urine
- Not to take with alcohol, other CNS depressants
- That if improvement does not occur within 6 wk, prescriber may discontinue
- To avoid hazardous activities if drowsiness, dizziness occurs
- To avoid using OTC medication: cough preparations, antihistamines, unless directed by prescriber

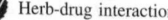

Not to break, crush, or chew caps

- To use sunscreen or stay out of the sun to prevent burns

Treatment of overdose: Induce emesis of conscious patient; lavage, dialysis

dapiprazole ophthalmic

See appendix c

RARELY USED

dapsone (DDS) (℞)

(dap'sone)

Avlosulfon✤, Dapsone

Func. class.: Leprostatic

Uses: Hansen's disease, PCP (*Pneumocystis carinii* pneumonia), malaria, dermatitis herpetiformis

Dosage and routes:
Hansen's disease
• *Adult:* **PO** 100 mg qd with rifampin 600 mg qd × 6 mo, then dapsone alone for 3-10 yr
• *Child:* **PO** 1-2 mg/kg/day
PCP
• *Adult:* **PO** 50-100 mg/day usually given with trimethoprim 20 mg/kg/day in 4 divided doses for 3 wk
• *Child:* **PO** 2 mg/kg/day
Contraindications: Hypersensitivity to sulfones, severe anemia

darbepoetin alfa (℞)

(dar'bee-poh'eh-tin al'fah)
Aranesp
Func. class.: Hematopoietic agent
Chem. class.: Recombinant human erythropoietin

Action: Stimulates erythropoiesis by the same mechanism as endogenous erythropoietin; in response to hypoxia, erythropoietin is produced in the kidney and released into the bloodstream, where it interacts with progenitor stem cells to increase red cell production
Uses: Anemia associated with chronic renal failure, in patients on and not on dialysis and anemia in nonmyeloid malignancies receiving coadministered chemotherapy
Dosage and routes:
Correction of anemia
• *Adult:* **SC/IV** 0.45 mcg/kg as a single inj, titrate not to exceed a target Hgb of 12 g/dl
Epoetin alfa to darbepoetin conversion
• *Adult:* **SC/IV** estimate starting dose based on weekly epoetin alfa dose; because of longer serum half-life, darbepoetin must be administered less frequently than epoetin alfa; if epoetin was given 2-3×/wk, give darbepoetin 1×/wk; if epoetin was given 1×/wk, give darbepoetin 1×q2wk; do not increase doses more often than 1×/mo
Available forms: Sol for inj 25, 40, 60, 100, 150, 200, 300, 500 mcg/ml
Side effects/adverse reactions:
CNS: ***Seizures***, sweating, headache, dizziness, ***stroke***
CV: Hypertension, hypotension, ***cardiac arrest,*** *angina pectoris,* ***thrombosis, CHF, acute MI, dysrhythmias,*** chest pain, transient ischemic attacks
GI: Diarrhea, vomiting, nausea, abdominal pain, constipation
MISC: Infection, fatigue, fever, ***death,*** *fluid overload,* ***vascular access hemorrhage***
MS: Bone pain, myalgia, limb pain, back pain
RESP: URI, dyspnea, cough, bronchitis
SYST: Allergic reactions, ***anaphylaxis***
Contraindications: Hypersensitivity to mammalian cell-derived products or human albumin, uncontrolled hypertension
Precautions: Seizure disorder, porphyria, pregnancy (C), hypertension, lactation, children
Pharmacokinetics: IV: Onset of increased reticulocyte count 1-6 wk; distributed to vascular space; absorption slow and rate-limiting; terminal half-life 49 hr; peak concentration at 34 hr; increased Hgb levels not generally observed until 2-6 wk after treatment initiated
Interactions:
Unknown

NURSING CONSIDERATIONS
Assess:
⬥ Serious allergic reactions: rash, urticaria; if anaphylaxis occurs, stop drug, administer emergency treatment (rare)

• Renal studies: urinalysis, protein, blood, BUN, creatinine
• Blood studies: ferritin, transferrin qmo; transferrin sat ≥20%, ferritin ≥100 ng/ml; Hgb 2×/wk until stabilized in target range (30%-33%), then at regular intervals; those with endogenous erythropoietin levels of <500 units/L respond to this agent
• B/P; check for rising B/P as Hgb rises, antihypertensives may be needed
• CV status: hypertension may occur rapidly leading to hypertensive encephalopathy
• I&O; report drop in output to <50 ml/hr
• For seizures if Hgb is increased within 2 wk by 4 pts
• CNS symptoms: sweating, pain in long bones
• Dialysis patients: thrill, bruit of shunts, monitor for circulation impairment

Administer:

IV/SC route

• Without shaking; check for discoloration, particulate matter, do not use if present; do not dilute, do not mix with other drugs or solutions, discard unused portion, do not pool unused portions

Evaluate:

• Therapeutic response: increase in reticulocyte count, Hgb/Hct; increased appetite, enhanced sense of well-being

Teach patient/family:

• To avoid driving or hazardous activity during beginning of treatment
• To monitor B/P, Hgb
• To take iron supplements, vit B_{12}, folic acid as directed
• To report side effects to prescriber, to comply with treatment regimen
• Home administration procedures, if appropriate

HIGH ALERT

*DAUNOrubicin (℞)

(daw-noe-roo′bi-sin)

Cerubidine

*DAUNOrubicin citrate liposome

DaunoXome

Func. class.: Antineoplastic, anti-infective

Chem. class.: Anthracycline glycoside

Action: Inhibits DNA synthesis, primarily; derived from *Streptomyces coerulorubidus;* replication is decreased by binding to DNA, which causes strand splitting; cell cycle specific (S phase); a vesicant

Uses: Myelogenous, monocytic leukemia, acute nonlymphocytic leukemia, Ewing's sarcoma, Wilms' tumor, neuroblastoma, rhabdomyosarcoma; DAUNOrubicin citrate liposome: advanced Kaposi's sarcoma in HIV

Dosage and routes:

Use decreased dose for those >60 yr of age

DAUNOrubicin

Single agent

• *Adult:* **IV** 60 mg/m^2/day × 3-5 days q4wk

In combination

• *Adult:* **IV** 45 mg/m^2/day × 3 days, then 2 days of subsequent courses in combination
• *Child:* **IV** 25-60 mg/m^2 depending on cycle

DAUNOrubicin citrate liposome

• *Adult:* **IV** 40 mg/m^2 q2wk

Renal dose

• *Adult:* **IV** serum Cr >3 mg/dl reduce dose by 50%

Hepatic dose

• *Adult:* **IV** serum bilirubin 1.2-3 mg/dl reduce dose by 25%; bilirubin >3 mg/dl reduce dose by 50%

Available forms: Inj 20 mg powder/vial, sol for inj 5 mg/ml; liposome: dispersion for inj 2 mg/ml

Side effects/adverse reactions:

DAUNOrubicin

HEMA: ***Thrombocytopenia, leukopenia, anemia***

GI: Nausea, vomiting, anorexia, mucositis, ***hepatotoxicity***

GU: Impotence, sterility, amenorrhea, gynecomastia, hyperuricemia

INTEG: Rash, ***extravasation,*** dermatitis, reversible alopecia, cellulitis, thrombophlebitis at inj site

CV: ***Dysrhythmias, CHF, pericarditis, myocarditis,*** peripheral edema

CNS: Fever, chills

SYST: ***Anaphylaxis***

DAUNOrubicin citrate liposome

CV: Chest pain, edema

GI: Cramps, diarrhea, constipation, stomatitis

INTEG: Sweating, pruritus

MS: Arthralgia, back pain

CNS: Fatigue, headache, depression, insomnia, dizziness, malaise, neuropathy

Contraindications: Hypersensitivity, pregnancy (D), lactation, systemic infections, cardiac disease

Precautions: Renal, hepatic disease; gout; bone marrow depression

Pharmacokinetics: Half-life 18½ hr, liposome 55½ hr; metabolized by liver; crosses placenta; excreted in breast milk, urine, bile

Do not confuse:

DAUNOrubicin/DOXOrubicin

Interactions:

- ↑ bleeding risk: NSAIDs, salicylates
- ↑ toxicity: other antineoplastics, radiation, cyclophosphamide
- ↓ antibody reaction: live virus vaccines

Lab test interferences:

Increase: Uric acid

NURSING CONSIDERATIONS

Assess:

- CBC, differential, platelet count weekly, leukocyte nadir within 2 wk after administration, recovery within 3 wk; do not administer if absolute granulocyte count is <750/mm^3 (liposome)
- Blood, urine uric acid levels baseline and during therapy
- Renal studies: BUN, urine CCr, electrolytes baseline, before each dose
- I&O ratio; report fall in urine output to <30 ml/hr
- Monitor temp q4h; fever may indicate beginning infection
- Hepatic studies baseline, before each dose: bilirubin, AST, ALT, alk phosphatase; check for jaundice of skin, sclera; dark urine; clay-colored stools; itchy skin; abdominal pain; fever; diarrhea
- Chest x-ray, echocardiography, radionuclide angiography, ECG; watch for ST-T wave changes, low QRS and T, possible dysrhythmias (sinus tachycardia, heart block, PVCs); watch for CHF (jugular vein distention, weight gain, edema, rales or crackles), may occur after 2-6 mo of treatment
- Bleeding: hematuria, guaiac stools, bruising or petechiae, mucosa or orifices q8h
- Effects of alopecia on body image; discuss feelings about body changes
- Buccal cavity q8h for dryness, sores or ulceration, white patches, oral pain, bleeding, dysphagia
- Local irritation, pain, burning at inj site
- GI symptoms: frequency of stools, cramping
- Acidosis, signs of dehydration: rapid respirations, poor skin turgor, decreased urine output, dry skin, restlessness, weakness

Administer:
• Antiemetic 30-60 min before giving drug and 6-10 hr after treatment to prevent vomiting
• Allopurinol or sodium bicarbonate to reduce uric acid levels, alkalinization of urine

IV route (Cerubidine)
• After diluting 20 mg/4 ml sterile H_2O for inj (5 mg/ml), rotate, further dilute in 10-15 ml 0.9% NaCl; give over 3-5 min by direct IV through Y-tube or 3-way stopcock of inf of D_5 or 0.9% NaCl; or dilute in 50 ml 0.9% NaCl and give over 10-15 min; or dilute in 100 ml and give over 30 min
• Hydrocortisone for extravasation; apply ice compress after stopping infusion

Additive compatibilities: Cytarabine/etoposide, hydrocortisone; not recommended for admixing

Solution compatibilities: $D_{3.3}$/0.3% NaCl, D_5W, Normosol R, Ringer's, 0.9% NaCl

Y-site compatibilities: Amifostine, filgrastim, granisetron, melphalan, methotrexate, ondansetron, sodium bicarbonate, teniposide, thiotepa, vinorelbine

IV route (DaunoXome)
• Dilute with D_5W to (1 mg/ml) give over 60 min, do not use in-line filter, reconstituted sol may be stored ≤6 hr refrigerated; do not admix

Perform/provide:
• Increased fluid intake to 2-3 L/day to prevent urate and calculi formation
• Diet low in purines: absence of organ meats (kidney, liver), dried beans, peas to reduce uric acid level
• Rinsing of mouth tid-qid with water, club soda; brushing of teeth bid-qid with soft brush or cotton-tipped applicators for stomatitis; use unwaxed dental floss

Evaluate:
• Therapeutic response: decreased tumor size, spread of malignancy

Teach patient/family:
• To report signs of infection, bleeding, bruising, shortness of breath, swelling, change in heart rate
• That hair may be lost during treatment and wig or hairpiece may make patient feel better; tell patient that new hair may be different in color, texture
• To avoid pregnancy while on this drug, and 4 mo thereafter
• To avoid foods with citric acid, hot or rough texture
• To report any bleeding, white spots, ulcerations in mouth; tell patient to examine mouth qd
• That urine and other body fluids may be red-orange for 48 hr
• To avoid vaccines while taking this drug
• To avoid crowds, those with known infections
• To avoid alcohol, aspirin, NSAIDs

RARELY USED

deferoxamine (℞)

(de-fer-ox'a-meen)

Desferal

Func. class.: Heavy metal antagonist

Uses: Acute, chronic iron intoxication, hemochromatosis, hemosiderosis

Dosage and routes:

Acute iron toxicity
• *Adult and child:* **IM/IV** 1 g, then 500 mg q4h × 2 doses, then 500 mg q4-12h × 2 doses, not to exceed 15 mg/kg/hr or 6 g/24 hr

Chronic iron toxicity
• *Adult and child:* **IM** 500 mg-1 g/day plus **IV INF** 2 g given by

separate line with each blood transfusion, not to exceed 15 mg/kg/hr or 6 g/24 hr; **SC** 1-2 g over 8-24 hr by SC inf pump
Contraindications: Hypersensitivity, anuria, severe renal disease, child <3 yr
Do not confuse:
deferoxamine/cefuroxime

delavirdine (℞)

(de-la-veer′deen)
Rescriptor
Func class.: Antiretroviral
Chem. class.: Nonnucleoside reverse transcriptase inhibitor (NNRTI)

Action: Binds directly to reverse transcriptase and blocks RNA, DNA, causing a disruption of the enzyme's site
Uses: HIV-1 in combination with other antiretrovirals
Dosage and routes:
- *Adult and child ≥16 yr:* 400 mg tid

Available forms: Tabs 100, 200 mg
Side effects/adverse reactions:
CNS: Headache, fatigue
GI: Diarrhea, abdominal pain, nausea, anorexia, vomiting, dyspepsia, ***hepatotoxicity***
GU: ***Nephrotoxicity***
HEMA: ***Neutropenia, leukopenia, thrombocytopenia, anemia, granulocytopenia***
INTEG: Rash
MS: Pain, myalgia
Contraindications: Hypersensitivity to this drug or atevirdine
Precautions: Liver disease, pregnancy (C), lactation, children, renal disease, myleosuppression
Pharmocokinetics:
Highly protein bound, half-life 2-11 hr, peak 1 hr, duration 8 hr, extensively metabolized
Interactions:
- ↑ levels of: alprazolam, clarithromycin, dapsone, ergots, felodipine, midazolam, nifedipine, indinavir, amprenavir, saquinavir
- ↓ delavirdine levels: antacids, anticonvulsants, rifamycins, protease inhibitors
- ↓ action of: oral contraceptives
- ↑ delavirdine levels: fluoxetine, ketoconazole
- ↑ levels of both drugs: quinidine, warfarin, clarithromycin

◆ Serious life-threatening adverse reaction: amphetamines, ergots, benzodiazepines, calcium channel blockers, sedative/hypnotics, antidysrhythmics, sildenafil, pimozide, cisapride

NURSING CONSIDERATIONS
Assess:
- For signs of infection, anemia
- Hepatic studies: ALT, AST; renal studies
- C&S before drug therapy; drug may be taken as soon as culture is taken; repeat C&S after treatment; determine the presence of other sexually transmitted disease
- Bowel pattern before, during treatment; if severe abdominal pain with bleeding occurs, drug should be discontinued; monitor hydration
- For skin eruptions; rash, urticaria, itching
- For allergies before treatment, reaction to each medication; place allergies on chart
- Plasma delavirdine concentrations (trough 10 micromolar)
- CBC, blood chemistry, plasma HIV RNA, absolute CD4+/CD8+/ cell counts/%, serum β-2 microglobulin, serum ICD+24 antigen levels
- For signs of delavirdine toxicity: severe nausea/vomiting, maculopapular rash

Administer:

• Dispersion by adding 4 tab/3-4 oz water, let stand, stir, swallow, rinse glass, swallow; use only 100 mg tabs for dispersion

Evaluate:

• Therapeutic response: increased CD4 cell count, decreased viral load, improvement in symptoms of HIV

Teach patient/family:

• To take as prescribed; if dose is missed, take as soon as remembered up to 1 hr before next dose; do not double dose

• That tabs may be dissolved in ½ cup of water, stir, when dissolved, drink right away, rinse cup with water, and drink that to get all medication

• To make sure health care provider knows of all the medications being taken

• That if severe rash, mouth sores, swelling, aching muscles/joints, or eye redness occur, stop taking and notify health care provider

• Not to breastfeed if taking this drug

demecarium ophthalmic

See appendix c

RARELY USED

demeclocycline (℞)

(dem-e-kloe-sye′kleen)

Declomycin

Func. class.: Antiinfective

Uses: Uncommon gram-positive/gram-negative bacteria, protozoa, *Rickettsia, Mycoplasma, Haemophilus ducreyi, Yersinia pestis, Campylobacter fetus, Chlamydia trachomatis,* psittacosis, granuloma inguinale

Dosage and routes:

• *Adult:* **PO** 150 mg q6h or 300 mg q12h

• *Child >8 yr:* **PO** 6-12 mg/kg/day in divided doses q6-12h

Gonorrhea

• *Adult:* **PO** 600 mg, then 300 mg q12h × 4 days, total 3 g

Contraindications: Hypersensitivity to tetracyclines, children <8 yr, pregnancy (D)

denileukin diftitox (℞)

(den-ih-loo′kin dif′tih-tox)

Ontak

Func. class.: Antineoplastic—misc.

Action: A recombinant DNA-derived cytotoxic protein; inhibits cellular protein synthesis

Uses: Cutaneous T-cell lymphoma that expresses CD25 component of the IL-2 receptor

Research note: Research has concluded that denileukin is effective for cutaneous T-cell lymphoma[6]

Dosage and routes:

• *Adult:* **IV** 9-18 mcg/kg/day given for 5 days q21 days, given over ≥15 min

Available forms: Sol for inj, frozen 150 mcg/ml

Side effects/adverse reactions:

CNS: Dizziness, paresthesia, nervousness, confusion, insomnia

CV: Hypotension, vasodilation, tachycardia, thrombosis, hypertension, dysrhythmias

GI: Nausea, anorexia, vomiting, diarrhea, constipation, dyspepsia, dysphagia

GU: Hematuria, albuminuria, pyuria, creatinine increase

HEMA: ***Thrombocytopenia, leukopenia,*** anemia

INTEG: Rash, pruritus, sweating
META: Hypoalbuminemia, edema, hypocalcemia, weight decrease, dehydration, hypokalemia
MISC: Fever, chills, asthenia, infection, pain, headache, chest pain, flu-like symptoms
MS: Myalgia, arthralgia
RESP: Dyspnea, cough, pharyngitis, rhinitis

Contraindications: Hypersensitivity to denileukin, diphtheria toxin, IL-2

Precautions: Radiation therapy, pregnancy (C), lactation, elderly, children

Pharmacokinetics: Concentrates in liver/kidneys; metabolized by proteolytic degradation

Interactions:

- ↑ bone marrow depression: radiation, other antineoplastics
- ↓ antibody reaction: live vaccines

NURSING CONSIDERATIONS

Assess:

- CBC, differential, platelet count weekly; withhold drug if WBC $<4000/mm^3$ or platelet count $<75{,}000/mm^3$; notify prescriber of results
- Monitor temp q4h (may indicate beginning infection)
- Hepatic studies before, during therapy (bilirubin, AST, ALT, LDH) as needed or monthly
- Bleeding: hematuria, guaiac, bruising or petechiae, mucosa or orifices q8h
- Jaundice of skin, sclera; dark urine; clay-colored stools; itchy skin; abdominal pain; fever; diarrhea
- For vascular leak syndrome after 2 wk of treatment, hypotension, edema, hypoalbuminemia; monitor weight, B/P, serum albumin, edema
- Obtain CD25 expression on skin biopsy samples

Administer:

- Antiemetic 30-60 min before giving drug to prevent vomiting
- Antibiotics for prophylaxis of infection

IV route

- Prepare and hold sol in plastic syringes or soft plastic IV bags only
- Draw calculated dose from vial, inject into empty IV infusion bag, for each 1 ml of drug removed from vial, no more than 9 ml of sterile saline without preservative should be added to IV bag; infuse over ≥15 min; do not give by bolus; do not admix with other drugs; do not use a filter
- Use within 6 hr, discard unused portions

Perform/provide:

- Storage in light-resistant container, dry area
- Warm compresses at infusion site for inflammation

Evaluate:

- Therapeutic response: decreased tumor size, spread of malignancy

Teach patient/family:

- To report signs of infection: fever, sore throat, flulike symptoms
- To report signs of anemia: fatigue, headache, faintness, shortness of breath, irritability
- To report bleeding; avoid use of razors, commercial mouthwash
- To avoid use of aspirin products or ibuprofen

RARELY USED

desipramine

(dess-ip'ra-meen)

desipramine HCl, Norpramin, Pertofrane

Func. class.: Antidepressant, tricyclic

Uses: Depression

Dosage and routes:

• *Adult:* **PO** 75-150 mg/day in divided doses; may increase to 300 mg/day or may give daily dose hs

• *Adolescent and elderly:* **PO** 25-50 mg/day, may increase to 100 mg/day

Contraindications: Hypersensitivity to tricyclics, recovery phase of myocardial infarction, narrow-angle glaucoma, convulsive disorders, prostatic hypertrophy, child <12 yr

desloratadine (℞)

(des'lor-at'ah-deen)

Clarinex

Func. class.: Antihistamine, 2nd generation

Chem. class.: Selective histamine (H_1)-receptor antagonist

Action: Binds to peripheral histamine receptors, providing antihistamine action without sedation

Uses: Seasonal allergic rhinitis

Dosage and routes:

• *Adult and child ≥12 yr:* **PO** 5 mg qd

Hepatic/renal dose

• *Adult:* **PO** 5 mg qod

Available form: Tabs 5 mg

Side effects/adverse reactions:

CNS: Sedation (more common with increased doses), headache

Contraindications: Hypersensitivity, acute asthma attacks, lower respiratory tract disease

Precautions: Pregnancy (C), bronchial asthma, liver or renal impairment

Pharmacokinetics: Peak 1½ hr, elimination half-life 8½-28 hr; metabolized in liver to active metabolites, excreted in urine

Interactions:

• None significant

NURSING CONSIDERATIONS

Assess:

• Allergy: hives, rash, rhinitis; monitor respiratory status

Administer:

• Without regard to meals

Perform/provide:

• Storage in tight container at room temperature

Evaluate:

• Therapeutic response: absence of running or congested nose, other allergy symptoms

Teach patient/family:

• To avoid driving, other hazardous activities if drowsiness occurs; observe caution until drug's effects on the patient are known

• That drug may cause photosensitivity; use sunscreen or stay out of the sun to prevent burns

desmopressin (℞)

(des-moe-press'in)

DDAVP, Stimate

Func. class.: Pituitary hormone

Chem. class.: Synthetic antidiuretic hormone

Action: Promotes reabsorption of water by action on renal tubular epithelium; causes smooth muscle constriction, increase in plasma factor VIII levels, which increases platelet aggregation resulting in vasopressor effect, similar to vasopressin

Uses: Hemophilia A, von Willebrand's disease type 1, nonnephrogenic diabetes insipidus, symptoms of polyuria/polydipsia caused by pituitary dysfunction, nocturnal enuresis

Dosage and routes:

Primary nocturnal enuresis

• *Adult and child ≥6 yr:* **INTRANASAL** 20 mcg (10 mcg in each nostril) hs, may increase to 40 mcg; **PO** 0.2 mg hs, may be increased to max 0.6 mg hs

Diabetes insipidus

• *Adult:* **INTRANASAL** 0.1-0.4 ml qd in divided doses (1-4 sprays with pump); **IV/SC** 0.5-1 ml qd in divided doses

• *Child 3 mo to 12 yr:* **INTRANASAL** 0.05-0.3 ml qd in divided doses

Hemophilia/von Willebrand's disease

• *Adult and child >3 mo:* **IV** 0.3 mcg/kg in NaCl over 15-30 min; may repeat if needed

Antihemorrhagic

• *Adult and child >3 mo:* **IV** 0.3 mcg/kg

• *Adult and child <50 kg:* **INTRANASAL** 1 spray in one nostril

• *Adult and child >50 kg:* 1 spray each nostril

Available forms: Inj 4, 15 mcg/ml, Rhihal Tube del 2.5 mg/vial (0.1 mg/ml); tabs 0.1, 0.2 mg; nasal spray pump 10 mcg/spray (0.1 mg/ml); nasal sol 1.5 mg/ml (150 mcg/dose)

Side effects/adverse reactions:

EENT: Nasal irritation, congestion, rhinitis

CNS: Drowsiness, headache, lethargy, flushing

GU: Vulval pain

GI: Nausea, heartburn, cramps

CV: Increased B/P

SYST: ***Anaphylaxis (IV)***

Contraindications: Hypersensitivity, nephrogenic diabetes insipidus

Precautions: Pregnancy (B), CAD, lactation, hypertension

Pharmacokinetics:

NASAL: Onset 1 hr, peak 1-4 hr, duration 8-20 hr, half-life 8 min, 76 min (terminal)

PO: Onset 1 hr, peak 4-7 hr

IV: Onset 1 min, peak ½ hr, duration more than 3 hr

Interactions:

• ↑ antidiuretic action: carbamazepine, chlorpropamide, clofibrate

• ↓ antidiuretic action: lithium, alcohol, demeclocycline, heparin, large doses of epinephrine

NURSING CONSIDERATIONS

Assess:

• Pulse, B/P when giving IV or SC

• I&O ratio, weight daily; check for edema in extremities; if water retention is severe, diuretic may be prescribed

• Water intoxication: lethargy, behavioral changes, disorientation, neuromuscular excitability

• Intranasal use: nausea, congestion, cramps, headache; usually decreased with decreased dose

◆ For severe allergic reaction including anaphylaxis (IV route)

• For nasal mucosa changes: congestion, edema, discharge, scarring (nasal route)

• Urine vol/osmolality and plasma osmolality (diabetes insipidus)

• Factor VIII coagulant activity before using for hemostasis

Administer:

• Undiluted over 1 min in diabetes insipidus

• Diluted, one single dose/50 ml of 0.9% NaCl (adult and child >10 kg), a single dose/10 ml as an IV inf over 15-30 min in von Willebrand's disease or hemophilia A

Perform/provide:

• Storage in refrigerator or cool environment

Evaluate:

• Therapeutic response: absence of severe thirst, decreased urine output, decreased osmolality

Teach patient/family:

• The proper technique for nasal instillation: to insert tube into nostril to instill drug

• To avoid OTC products: cough, hay fever products, since these preparations may contain epinephrine, decrease drug response; do not use with alcohol, adverse reactions may occur

• To wear emergency ID specifying therapy

• That if dose is missed, take when remembered up to 1 hr before next dose; do not double dose

desonide topical

See appendix c

desoximetasone topical

See appendix c

desoxyephedrine nasal agent

See appendix c

dexamethasone (℞)

(dex-ah-meth'a-sone)

Decadron, Deronil ♣ Dexasone ♣, Dexon, Hexadrol, Mymethasone

dexamethasone acetate (℞)

Dalalone DP, Dalalone LA, Decadron-LA, Decaject-LA, Dexacen LA-8, Dexasone-LA, Dexone LA, Solurex-LA

dexamethasone sodium phosphate (℞)

Dalalone, Decadron Phosphate, Decaject, Dexacen-4, Dexone, Hexadrol Phosphate, Solurex

Func. class.: Corticosteroid

Chem. class.: Glucocorticoid, long-acting

Action: Decreases inflammation by suppression of migration of polymorphonuclear leukocytes, fibroblasts, reversal of increased capillary permeability and lysosomal stabilization

Uses: Inflammation, allergies, neoplasms, cerebral edema, septic shock, collagen disorders

Dosage and routes:

Inflammation

• *Adult:* **PO** 0.75-9 mg/day in divided doses q6-12h or phosphate **IM** 0.5-9 mg/day; or acetate **IM** 4-16 mg q1-3wk

• *Child:* **PO** 0.08-0.3 mg/kg/day in divided doses q6-12h

Shock (Phosphate)

• *Adult:* **IV** single dose 1-6 mg/kg or **IV** 40 mg q2-6h as needed up to 72h

Cerebral edema

• *Adult:* ***(Phosphate)*** **IV** 10 mg, then 4-6 mg **IM** q6h × 2-4 days, then taper over 1 wk

• *Child:* **PO** 0.2 mg/kg/day in divided doses

Adrenocortical insufficiency

• *Child:* 23.3 mcg/kg/day in 3 divided doses

Supression test

• *Adult:* **PO** 1 mg at 11 PM or 0.5 mg q6h × 48 hr

Available forms: dexamethasone: Tabs 0.25, 0.5, 0.75, 1, 1.5, 2, 4, 6 mg; elix 0.5 mg/5 ml; oral sol 0.5 mg/5 ml, 1 mg/1 ml; inj acetate 8, 16 mg/ml; inj phosphate 4, 10, 20, 24 mg/ml

Side effects/adverse reactions:

INTEG: Acne, poor wound healing, ecchymosis, petechiae, hirsutism

CNS: Depression, flushing, sweating, headache, mood changes, euphoria, psychosis, ***seizures,*** insomnia

CV: Hypertension, ***circulatory collapse, thrombophlebitis, embolism,*** tachycardia, edema

HEMA: ***Thrombocytopenia***

MS: Fractures, osteoporosis, weakness

GI: Diarrhea, nausea, abdominal distention, ***GI hemorrhage,*** *increased appetite,* ***pancreatitis***

EENT: Fungal infections, increased intraocular pressure, blurred vision

ENDO: HPA suppression, hyperglycemia, sodium, fluid retention

META: Hypokalemia

Contraindications: Psychosis, hypersensitivity, idiopathic thrombocytopenia, acute glomerulonephritis, amebiasis, fungal infections, nonasthmatic bronchial disease, child <2 yr, AIDS, TB

Precautions: Pregnancy (C), lactation, diabetes mellitus, glaucoma, osteoporosis, seizure disorders, ulcerative colitis, CHF, myasthenia gravis, renal disease, peptic ulcer, esophagitis

Do not confuse:

Decadron/Percodan

Pharmacokinetics:

PO: Onset 1 hr, peak 1-2 hr, duration 2½ days

IM: (acetate) Peak 8 hr, duration 6 days

Half-life 3-4½ hr

Interactions:

• ↓ dexamethasone action: cholestyramine, colestipol, barbiturates, rifampin, epHEDrine, phenytoin, theophylline, antacids

• ↓ anticoagulants effects, anticonvulsants, antidiabetics, ambenonium, neostigmine, isoniazid, toxoids, vaccines, anticholinesterases, salicylates, somatrem

• ↑ side effects: alcohol, salicylates, indomethacin, amphotericin B, digitalis, cycloSPORINE, diuretics

• ↑ dexamethasone action: salicylates, estrogens, indomethacin, oral contraceptives, ketoconazole, macrolide antiinfectives

↑ corticosteroid effect: aloe, licorice, perilla

Potassium deficiency: aloe, buckthorn, cascara sagrada, Chinese rhubarb, senna

Lab test interferences:

Increase: Cholesterol, sodium, blood glucose, uric acid, calcium, urine glucose

Decrease: Calcium, K, T_4, T_3, thyroid ^{131}I uptake test, urine 17-OHCS, 17-KS, PBI

False negative: Skin allergy tests

NURSING CONSIDERATIONS

Assess:

• Potassium, blood, urine glucose while on long-term therapy; hypokalemia and hyperglycemia

• Weight daily; notify prescriber of weekly gain >5 lb

• B/P q4h, pulse; notify prescriber of chest pain

• I&O ratio; be alert for decreasing urinary output, increasing edema

- Plasma cortisol levels during long-term therapy (normal: 138-635 nmol/L SI units when drawn at 8 AM)
- Infection: fever, WBC even after withdrawal of medication; drug masks infection
- Potassium depletion: paresthesias, fatigue, nausea, vomiting, depression, polyuria, dysrhythmias, weakness
- Edema, hypertension, cardiac symptoms
- Mental status: affect, mood, behavioral changes, aggression

Administer:

- Titrated dose; use lowest effective dose
- IM inj deeply in large muscle mass; rotate sites; avoid deltoid; use 21G needle
- In one dose in AM to prevent adrenal suppression; avoid SC administration, may damage tissue
- With food or milk to decrease GI symptoms

IV route

- Undiluted direct over 1 min or less or diluted with 0.9% NaCl or D_5W and give as an IV inf at prescribed rate
- After shaking suspension (parenteral); do not give suspension IV

Dexamethasone sodium phosphate

Additive compatibilities: Aminophylline, bleomycin, cimetidine, floxacillin, furosemide, granisetron, lidocaine, meropenem, mitomycin, nafcillin, netilmicin, ondansetron, prochlorperazine, ranitidine, verapamil

Syringe compatibilities: Granisetron, metoclopramide, ranitidine, sufentanil

Y-site compatibilities: Acyclovir, allopurinol, amifostine, amikacin, amphotericin B cholesteryl, amsacrine, aztreonam, cefepime, cefpirome, cisatracurium, cisplatin, cladribine, cyclophosphamide, cytarabine, DOXOrubicin, DOXOrubicin liposome, famotidine, filgrastim, fluconazole, fludarabine, foscarnet, granisetron, heparin, lorazepam, melphalan, meperidine, meropenem, morphine, ondansetron, paclitaxel, piperacillin/tazobactam, potassium chloride, propofol, remifentanil, sargramostim, sodium bicarbonate, sufentanil, tacrolimus, teniposide, theophylline, thiotepa, vinorelbine, vit B/C, zidovudine

Perform/provide:

- Assistance with ambulation in patient with bone tissue disease to prevent fractures

Evaluate:

- Therapeutic response: ease of respirations, decreased inflammation

Teach patient/family:

- That ID as steroid user should be carried
- To contact prescriber if surgery, trauma, stress occurs; dose may need to be adjusted
- To notify prescriber if therapeutic response decreases; dosage adjustment may be needed
- Not to discontinue abruptly or adrenal crisis can result
- Symptoms of adrenal insufficiency: nausea, anorexia, fatigue, dizziness, dyspnea, weakness, joint pain
- To avoid OTC products: salicylates, alcohol in cough products, cold preparations unless directed by prescriber
- To teach patient all aspects of drug usage, including cushingoid symptoms; to notify health care provider of infection
- Avoid exposure to chickenpox or measles, persons with infection

dexamethasone nasal agent

See appendix c

dexamethasone ophthalmic

See appendix c

dexamethasone topical

See appendix c

dexmedetomidine

Precedex

Func. class.: Sedative, α_2 adrenoceptor agonist

Action: Produces α_2 activity seen at low and moderate doses, also α_1 at high doses

Uses: Sedation in mechanically ventilated, intubated patients ICU

Research note: One study has concluded that more research is needed before wider applications of this drug can be pursued[7]

Dosage and routes:

- *Adult:* **IV** loading dose of 1 mcg/kg over 10 min then 0.2-0.7 mcg/kg/hr, do not use for more than 24 hr

Available forms: Inj 100 mcg/ml

Side effects/adverse reactions:

GI: Nausea, thirst

GU: Oliguria

CV: Bradycardia, hypotension, hypertension, ***atrial fibrillation, infarction***

RESP: Pulmonary edema, pleural effusion, hypoxia

HEMA: Leukocytosis, anemia

Contraindications: Hypersensitivity

Precautions: Elderly, respiratory depression, severe respiratory disorders, cardiac dysrhythmias, pregnancy (C), lactation, children, renal disease

Pharmacokinetics: Rapid distribution, excreted in urine; metabolized in liver

Interactions:

- ↑ CNS depression: alcohol, opioids, sedative/hypnotics, antipsychotics, skeletal muscle relaxants, inhalational anesthetics

NURSING CONSIDERATIONS

Assess:

- Injection site: phlebitis, burning, stinging
- ECG for changes: atrial fibrillation
- CNS changes: movement, jerking, tremors, dizziness, LOC, pupil reaction
- Respiratory dysfunction: respiratory depression, character, rate, rhythm; notify prescriber if respirations are <10/min

Administer:

IV route

- After diluting with D_5W 0.9% NaCl, withdraw 2 ml of drug and add to 48 ml of 0.9% NaCl to a total of 50 ml, shake to mix well
- Only with resuscitative equipment available
- Only by qualified persons trained in ICU sedation

Solution compatibilities: LR, D_5W, 0.9% NaCl, 20% mannitol

Additive compatibilities: Thiopental, etomidate, vecuronium, pancuronium, succinylcholine, atracurium, mivacurium, glycopyrrolate, phenylephrine, atropine, midazolam, morphine, fentanyl

Perform/provide:

- Safety measures: side rails, nightlight, call bell within easy reach

Evaluate:

- Therapeutic response: induction of anesthesia

dexmethylphenidate (℞)

(dex′meth-ul-fen′ih-dayt)

Focalin

Func. class.: Central nervous system (CNS) stimulant

Controlled Substance Schedule II

Action: Increases release of norepinephrine and dopamine into the extraneuronal space, also blocks reuptake of norepinephrine and dopamine into the presynaptic neuron; mode of action in treating attention deficit hyperactivity disorder (ADHD) is unknown

Uses: ADHD

Dosage and routes:

- *Child >6 yr:* **PO** 2.5 mg bid with doses at least 4 hr apart, gradually increase to a maximum of 20 mg/day (10 mg bid); for those taking methylphenidate, use ½ of methylphenidate dose initially, then increase as needed to a maximum of 20 mg/day

Available forms: Tabs 2.5, 5, 10 mg

Side effects/adverse reactions:

CNS: Dizziness, headache, drowsiness, ***toxic psychosis, neuroleptic malignant syndrome (rare)***, Gilles de la Tourette's syndrome

CV: Palpitations, B/P changes, angina, ***dysrhythmias***

GI: Nausea, anorexia, abnormal liver function, ***hepatic coma***, abdominal pain

INTEG: ***Exfoliative dermatitis***, urticaria, rash, erythema multiforme

HEMA: ***Leukopenia, anemia, thrombocytopenic purpura***

MISC: Fever, arthralgia, scalp hair loss

Contraindications: Hypersensitivity to methylphenidate, anxiety, history of Gilles de la Tourette's syndrome; children <6 yr, glaucoma, concurrent treatment with MAOIs or within 14 days of discontinuing treatment with MAOIs

Precautions: Hypertension, depression, pregnancy (C), seizures, lactation, drug abuse, psychosis, cardiovascular disorders

Pharmacokinetics: Readily absorbed, peak 1-1½ hr, elimination half-life 2.2 hr, onset ½-1 hr, duration 4 hr, metabolized by liver, excreted by kidneys

Interactions:

- Hypertensive crisis: MAOIs or within 14 days of MAOIs, vasopressors
- ↑ sympathomimetic effect: decongestants, vasoconstrictors
- ↓ effects of: antihypertensives
- ↑ effects of: anticonvulsants, tricyclics, SSRIs, coumarin anticoagulants (warfarin)

↑ stimulant effect: horsetail, yohimbe

Synergistic effect: melatonin

NURSING CONSIDERATIONS

Assess:

- VS, B/P; may reverse antihypertensives; check patients with cardiac disease more often for increased B/P
- CBC, urinalysis in diabetes; blood glucose, urine glucose; insulin changes may have to be made, because eating will decrease
- Height, growth rate q3mo in children; growth rate may be decreased
- Mental status: mood, sensorium, affect, stimulation, insomnia, aggressiveness

Withdrawal symptoms: headache, nausea, vomiting, muscle pain, weakness

- Appetite, sleep, speech patterns
- For attention span, decreased hyperactivity in persons with ADHD

Administer:

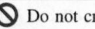

- Twice daily at least 4 hr apart
- Without regard to meals

Evaluate:
• Therapeutic response: decreased hyperactivity or ability to stay awake
Teach patient/family:
• To decrease caffeine consumption (coffee, tea, cola, chocolate); may increase irritability, stimulation
• To avoid OTC preparations unless approved by prescriber
• To taper off drug over several wk to avoid depression, increased sleeping, lethargy
• To avoid alcohol ingestion
• To avoid hazardous activities until stabilized on medication
• To get needed rest; patients will feel more tired at end of day
Treatment of overdose: Administer fluids; hemodialysis or peritoneal dialysis; antihypertensive for increased B/P; administer short-acting barbiturate before lavage

dextran 40 (℞)

(deks'tran)
Dextran 40, Gentran 40, LMD 10%, Rheomacrodex
Func. class.: Plasma volume expander
Chem. class.: Low molecular weight polysaccharide

Action: Similar to human albumin, which expands plasma volume by drawing fluid from interstitial space to intravascular space
Uses: Expand plasma volume, prophylaxis of embolism, thrombosis
Dosage and routes:
Shock
• *Adult:* **IV INF** 500 ml over 15-30 min, total dose in 24 hr not to exceed 20 ml/kg; subsequent doses given slowly; if given >24 hr, not to exceed 10 ml/kg/day; not to exceed therapy >5 days
Thrombosis/embolism
• *Adult:* **IV INF** 500-1000 ml, then 500 ml/day × 3 days, then 500 ml q2-3 days × 2 wk if needed
Available forms: 10% dextran 40/D_5W, 10% dextran 40/0.9% NaCl
Side effects/adverse reactions:
HEMA: Decreased hematocrit, platelet function; ***increased bleeding/coagulation times***
INTEG: Rash, urticaria, pruritus, ***angioedema,*** chills, fever, flushing
RESP: Wheezing, dyspnea, ***bronchospasm, pulmonary edema***
CV: Hypotension, ***cardiac arrest***
GU: ***Osmotic nephrosis, renal failure, stasis,*** hyponatremia
GI: Nausea, vomiting, increased AST, ALT
SYST: ***Anaphylaxis***
Contraindications: Hypersensitivity, renal failure, CHF (severe), extreme dehydration
Precautions: Active hemorrhage, pregnancy (C)
Pharmacokinetics:
IV: Expands blood vol 1-2 × amount infused; excreted in urine and feces
Interactions:
• Incompatible with chlortetracycline, phytonadione, promethazine
Lab test interferences:
False increase: Blood glucose, urinary protein, bilirubin, total protein
Interference: Rh test, blood typing/crossmatching
NURSING CONSIDERATIONS
Assess:
• VS q5min × 30 min; Hgb/Hct, if falling by 30%, notify prescriber
• CVP during infusion (5-10 cm H_2O—normal range)
• Urine output q1h; watch for increase in urinary output (common); if output does not increase, decrease or discontinue infusion

• I&O ratio and specific gravity, urine osmolarity; if specific gravity is very low, renal clearance is low; drug should be discontinued
• Allergy: rash, urticaria, pruritus, wheezing, dyspnea, bronchospasm, drug should be discontinued immediately
◆ Circulatory overload: increased pulse, respirations, SOB, wheezing, chest tightness, chest pain
• Dehydration after infusion: decreased output, decreased specific gravity of urine, increased temp, poor skin turgor, increased specific gravity, dry skin

Administer:

IV route

• After prescribed dilution; may give inital 500 mg at 15-30 min; distribute remainder of daily dose over 8-24 hr
• After crossmatch is drawn, if blood is to be given also
• D_5W sol in heart failure patients as ordered

Additive compatibilities: Cloxacillin

Y-site compatibilities: Enalaprilat, famotidine

Perform/provide:

• Storage at constant temperature (15°-30° C [59°-86° F]); discard unused portions, protect from freezing

Evaluate:

• Therapeutic response: increased plasma volume

dextran 70/75 (℞)

(deks'tran)

Dextran 75, Gentran 70, Gentran 75, Macrodex

Func. class.: Plasma volume expander

Chem. class.: High-molecular-weight polysaccharide

Action: Similar to human albumin, which expands plasma volume by drawing fluid from interstitial spaces to intravascular space

Uses: Expand plasma volume in hypovolemic shock or impending shock

Dosage and routes:

• *Adult:* **IV INF** 500-1000 ml not to exceed 20-40 ml/min, not to exceed 10 ml/kg/24 hr if therapy >24 hr

Available forms: 70/75 dextran in 0.9% NaCl, $D_5\%$

Side effects/adverse reactions:

HEMA: Decreased hematocrit, platelet function; ***increased bleeding/coagulation times***

INTEG: Rash, urticaria, pruritus, ***angioedema,*** chills, fever, flushing

RESP: Wheezing, dyspnea, ***bronchospasm, pulmonary edema***

CV: Hypotension, ***cardiac arrest***

GU: ***Osmotic nephrosis, renal failure, stasis,*** hypernatremia

GI: Nausea, vomiting, increased AST, ALT

SYST: ***Anaphylaxis***

Contraindications: Hypersensitivity, renal failure, CHF (severe), extreme dehydration

Precautions: Active hemorrhage, pregnancy (C)

Pharmacokinetics:

IV: Onset within mins, duration 12 hr, expands blood vol 1-2 × amount infused; excreted in urine, feces

Lab test interferences:
False increase: Blood glucose, urinary protein, bilirubin, total protein
Interference: Rh test, blood typing/crossmatching

NURSING CONSIDERATIONS

Assess:
- VS q5min × 30 min; Hgb/Hct, if falling by 30%, notify prescriber
- CVP during infusion (5-10 cm H_2O—normal range)
- Urine output q1h; watch for increase in urinary output (common); if output does not increase, decrease or discontinue infusion
- I&O ratio and specific gravity, urine osmolarity; if specific gravity is very low, renal clearance is low; drug should be discontinued
- Allergy: rash, urticaria, pruritus, wheezing, dyspnea, bronchospasm; drug should be discontinued immediately
- ◆ Circulatory overload: increased pulse, respirations, SOB, wheezing, chest tightness, chest pain
- Dehydration after infusion: decreased output, increased temp, poor skin turgor, increased specific gravity, dry skin

Administer:
- After prescribed dilution, may give inital 500 mg at 20-40 ml/min, reduce flow to lowest rate
- After crossmatch is drawn, if blood is to be given also
- D_5W sol in heart failure patients as ordered

Perform/provide:
- Storage at constant temperature (<25° C [77° F]); discard unused portions; do not use unless clear

Evaluate:
- Therapeutic response: increased plasma volume

dextroamphetamine (℞)

(dex-troe-am-fet'a-meen)
Dexedrine, dextroamphetamine, Dextrostat
Func. class.: Cerebral stimulant
Chem. class.: Amphetamine

Controlled Substance Schedule II

Action: Increases release of norepinephrine, DOPamine in cerebral cortex to reticular activating system

Uses: Narcolepsy, attention deficit disorder with hyperactivity (ADHD)

Dosage and routes:

Narcolepsy
- *Adult:* **PO** 5-60 mg qd in divided doses
- *Child >12 yr:* **PO** 10 mg qd increasing by 10 mg/day at weekly intervals
- *Child 6-12 yr:* **PO** 5 mg qd increasing by 5 mg/wk (max 60 mg/day)

ADHD
- *Adult:* **PO** 5-60 mg/day in divided doses
- *Child >6 yr:* **PO** 5 mg qd-bid increasing by 5 mg/day at weekly intervals
- *Child 3-6 yr:* **PO** 2.5 mg qd increasing by 2.5 mg/day at weekly intervals

Available forms: Tabs 5, 10 mg; caps sus rel 5, 10, 15 mg

Side effects/adverse reactions:
CNS: Hyperactivity, insomnia, restlessness, talkativeness, dizziness, headache, chills, stimulation, dysphoria, irritability, aggressiveness, tremor, dependence, addiction
GI: Anorexia, dry mouth, diarrhea, constipation, weight loss, metallic taste
GU: Impotence, change in libido
CV: Palpitations, tachycardia, hy-

pertension, decrease in heart rate, ***dysrhythmias***
INTEG: Urticaria

Contraindications: Hypersensitivity to sympathomimetic amines, hyperthyroidism, hypertension, glaucoma, severe arteriosclerosis, drug abuse, cardiovascular disease, anxiety

Precautions: Gilles de la Tourette's disorder, pregnancy (C), lactation, child <3 yr

Pharmacokinetics:
PO: Onset 30 min, peak 1-3 hr, duration 4-20 hr; metabolized by liver; urine excretion pH dependent; crosses placenta, breast milk; half-life 10-30 hr

Interactions:
Hypertensive crisis: MAOIs or within 14 days of MAOIs
• Delayed absorption of: barbiturates, phenytoin
• ↑ dextroamphetamine effect: acetaZOLAMIDE, antacids, sodium bicarbonate
• ↑ CNS effect: haloperidol, tricyclics, phenothiazines
• ↓ dextroamphetamine effect: ascorbic acid, ammonium chloride
• ↓ effect of: adrenergic blockers, antidiabetics
• Drug/food: ↑ amine effect: caffeine
↓ stimulant effect: eucalyptus
↑ stimulant effect: khat
serotonin syndrome: St. John's wort

NURSING CONSIDERATIONS

Assess:
• VS, B/P; this drug may reverse antihypertensives; check patients with cardiac disease often
• CBC, urinalysis; in diabetes: blood glucose, urine glucose; insulin changes may be required, since eating will decrease
• Height, growth rate in children; growth rate may be decreased
• Mental status: mood, sensorium, affect, stimulation, insomnia, irritability
• Tolerance or dependency: an increased amount may be used to get same effect; will develop after long-term use
• Overdose: pain, fever, dehydration, insomnia, hyperactivity

Administer:
• At least 6 hr before hs to avoid sleeplessness

Perform/provide:
• Gum, hard candy, frequent sips of water for dry mouth

Evaluate:
• Therapeutic response: increased CNS stimulation, decreased drowsiness

Teach patient/family:
Not to break, crush, or chew sus rel forms
• To decrease caffeine consumption (coffee, tea, cola, chocolate); may increase irritability, stimulation
• To avoid OTC preparations unless approved by prescriber
• To taper drug over several wk; depression, increased sleeping, lethargy
• To avoid alcohol ingestion
• To avoid hazardous activities until stabilized on medication
• To get needed rest; patient will feel more tired at end of day

Treatment of overdose: Administer fluids, hemodialysis or peritoneal dialysis; antihypertensive for increased B/P, ammonium Cl for increased excretion

dextromethorphan (OTC)

(dex-troe-meth-or'fan)

Balminil DM♣, Benylin DM♣, Broncho-Grippol-DM♣, Children's Hold, Creo-Terpin, Delsym, dextromethorphan, Hold DM, Koffex♣, Neo-DM♣, Orex DM♣, Pertussin, Pertussin ES, Robidex♣, Robitussin Cough Calmers, Robitussin Pediatric, Sedatuss♣, St. Joseph Cough Suppressant, Scot-Tussin DM, Sucrets Cough Control, Suppress, Vicks Formula 44

Func. class.: Antitussive, nonopioid

Chem. class.: Levorphanol derivative

Action: Depresses cough center in medulla by direct effect

Uses: Nonproductive cough

Investigational uses: Neuropathy

Dosage and routes:

- *Adult and child ≥12 yr:* **PO** 10-20 mg q4h, or 30 mg q6-8h, not to exceed 120 mg/day; **SUS-REL LIQ** 60 mg q12h, not to exceed 120 mg/day
- *Child 6-12 yr:* **PO** 5-10 mg q4h; **SUS-REL LIQ** 30 mg bid, not to exceed 60 mg/day
- *Child 2-6 yr:* **PO** 2.5-5 mg q4h, or 7.5 mg q6-8h, not to exceed 30 mg/day

Neuropathy

- *Adult:* **PO** doses vary widely

Available forms: Loz 2.5, 5, 7.5, 15 mg; sol; liq 3.5 mg, 7.5, 15 mg/5 ml, 3.5, 5, 7.5, 10, 15 mg/5 ml; syr 15 mg/15 ml, 10 mg/5 ml; sus action liq equivalent to 30 mg/5 ml; caps 30 mg; ext rel susp 30 mg/5 ml

Side effects/adverse reactions:

CNS: Dizziness, sedation

GI: Nausea

Contraindications: Hypersensitivity, asthma/emphysema, productive cough

Precautions: Nausea/vomiting, fever, persistent headache, pregnancy (C)

Pharmacokinetics:

PO: Onset 15-30 min, duration 3-6 hr

SUS: Duration 12 hr

Interactions:

- Do not give with MAOIs or within 2 wk of MAOIs
- ↑ CNS depression: alcohol, antidepressants, antihistamines, opioids, sedative/hypnotics
- ↑ adverse reactions: amiodarone, fluoxetine, quinidine

NURSING CONSIDERATIONS

Assess:

- Cough: type, frequency, character, including sputum

Administer:

- Decreased dose to elderly patients; metabolism may be slowed

Perform/provide:

- Increased fluids to liquefy secretions
- Humidification of patient's room

Evaluate:

- Therapeutic response: absence of cough

Teach patient/family:

- To avoid driving, other hazardous activities until patient is stabilized on this medication
- To avoid smoking, smoke-filled rooms, perfumes, dust, environmental pollutants, cleaners that increase cough
- To avoid alcohol, CNS depressants
- To notify prescriber if cough persists over a few days

dextrose (D-glucose) (℞)

Glucose, Glutose, Insta-Glucose

Func. class.: Caloric

Action: Needed for adequate utilization of amino acids; decreases protein, nitrogen loss; prevents ketosis

Uses: Increases intake of calories; increases fluids in patients unable to take adequate fluids, calories orally; acute hypoglycemia

Dosage and routes:

• *Adult and child:* **IV** depends on individual requirements

Available forms: Inj 2.5%, 5%, 10%, 20%, 30%, 40%, 50%, 60%, 70%; oral gel 40%; chew tab 5 g

Side effects/adverse reactions:

CNS: Confusion, ***loss of consciousness,*** dizziness

CV: Hypertension, ***CHF, pulmonary edema***

GU: Glycosuria, osmotic diuresis

ENDO: Hyperglycemia, rebound hypoglycemia, hyperosmolar syndrome, hyperglycemic nonketotic syndrome

INTEG: Chills, flushing, warm feeling, rash, urticaria, extravasation necrosis

Contraindications: Hyperglycemia, delirium tremens, hemorrhage (cranial/spinal), CHF

Precautions: Renal, hepatic, cardiac disease, diabetes mellitus

Interactions:

• ↑ fluid retention/electrolyte excretion: corticosteroids

NURSING CONSIDERATIONS

Assess:

• Electrolytes (K, Na, Ca, Cl, Mg), blood glucose, ammonia, phosphate

• Injection site for extravasation: redness along vein, edema at site, necrosis, pain; hard, tender area; site should be changed immediately

• Monitor temp q4h for increased fever, indicating infection; if infection suspected, infusion is discontinued, tubing, bottle, catheter tip cultured

• Serum glucose in patients receiving hypotonic glucose 50% and over

• Nutritional status: calorie count by dietitian

Administer:

• Only (4%) protein and dextrose (up to 12.5%) via peripheral vein; stronger sol: central IV administration

• May be given undiluted via prepared sol; give 10% sol, 5 ml/15 sec; 10% sol, 1000 ml/3 hr or more; 20% sol, 500 ml/½-1 hr; 50% sol, 10 ml/min; control rate, rapid infusions may cause fluid shifts

• Oral glucose preparations (gel, chew tabs) are to be used in conscious patients only; check serum blood glucose after first dose

• After changing IV catheter, dressing q24h with aseptic technique

Evaluate:

• Therapeutic response: increased weight

Teach patient/family:

• The reason for dextrose infusion

• To review hypoglycemia/hyperglycemia symptoms

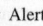

• To review blood glucose monitoring procedure

diazepam (℞)

(dye-az′-e-pam)

Apo-Diazepam✤, Diastat, Diazemuls✤, diazepam, Novodiapam✤, PMS-Diazepam✤, Valium, Valrelease, Vivol✤

Func. class.: Antianxiety, anticonvulsant, skeletal muscle relaxant, central acting

Chem. class.: Benzodiazepine

Controlled Substance Schedule IV

Action: Potentiates the actions of GABA, especially in limbic system, reticular formation; enhances presympathetic inhibition, inhibits spinal polysynaptic afferent paths

Uses: Anxiety, acute alcohol withdrawal, adjunct in seizure disorders; preoperatively as a relaxant, skeletal muscle relaxation; rectally for acute repetitive seizures

Investigational uses: Panic attacks

Dosage and routes:

Anxiety/convulsive disorders

• *Adult:* **PO** 2-10 mg bid-qid; **EXT REL** 15-30 mg qd

• *Geriatric:* **PO** 1-2 mg qd-bid, increase slowly as needed

• *Child >6 mo:* **PO** 1-2.5 mg tid-qid

Muscle relaxation

• *Adult:* **PO** 2-10 mg tid-qid or ext rel 15-30 mg qd; **IV/IM** 5-10 mg repeat in 2-4 hr

• *Geriatric:* **PO** 2-5 mg bid-qid; **IV/IM** 2-5 mg, may repeat in 2-4 hr

Tetanic muscle spasms

• *Child >5 yr:* **IM/IV** 5-10 mg q3-4h prn

• *Infant >30 days:* **IM/IV** 1-2 mg q3-4h prn

Status epilepticus

• *Adult:* **IV/IM** 5-10 mg, 2 mg/min, may repeat q10-15min, not to exceed 30 mg; may repeat in 2-4 hr if seizures reappear

• *Child 1 mo-5 yr:* **IV/IM** 0.2-0.5 mg slowly q2-5min up to 5 mg

• *Child >5 yr:* **IV/IM** 1 mg q2-5min max 10 mg, may repeat in 2-4 hr

• *Adult:* **RECT** 0.2 mg/kg, may repeat 4-12 hr later

• *Child 6-11 yr:* **RECT** 0.3 mg/kg, may repeat 4-12 hr later

• *Child 2-5 yr:* **RECT** 0.5 mg/kg, may repeat 4-12 hr later

Alcohol withdrawal

• *Adult:* **PO** 10 mg tid-qid in 1st 24 hr, then 5 mg tid-qid; **IV/IM** 10 mg, then 5-10 mg after 3 hr

Available forms: Tabs 2, 5, 10 mg; caps ext rel 15 mg; inj emulsified 5 mg/ml; oral sol 5 mg/5 ml; gel, rectal delivery system 2.5, 5, 10, 15, 20 mg, twin packs

Side effects/adverse reactions:

HEMA: ***Neutropenia***

RESP: ***Respiratory depression***

CNS: Dizziness, drowsiness, confusion, headache, anxiety, tremors, stimulation, fatigue, depression, insomnia, hallucinations

CV: Orthostatic hypotension, ***ECG changes, tachycardia,*** hypotension

EENT: Blurred vision, tinnitus, mydriasis, nystagmus

GI: Constipation, dry mouth, nausea, vomiting, anorexia, diarrhea

INTEG: Rash, dermatitis, itching

Contraindications: Hypersensitivity to benzodiazepines, narrow-angle glaucoma, psychosis, pregnancy (D), lactation, coma, respiratory depression

Precautions: Elderly, debilitated, hepatic disease, renal disease, addiction, child <6 mo

Do not confuse:

diazepam/Ditropan/lorazepam

Pharmacokinetics:

PO: Rapidly absorbed; onset ½ hr, duration 2-3 hr

IM: Onset 15-30 min, duration 1-1½ hr; absorption slow and erratic

IV: Onset immediate, duration 15 min–1 hr

Metabolized by liver, excreted by kidneys, crosses placenta, excreted in breast milk, crosses the blood-brain barrier; half-life 20-50 hr, more reliable by mouth

Interactions:

• ↑ toxicity: barbiturates, SSRIs, cimetidine, CNS depressants, valproic acid

• ↓ diazepam metabolism: oral contraceptives, valproic acid, disulfiram, isoniazid, propranolol

• ↑ CNS depression: CNS depressants, alcohol

↑ diazepam action: cowslip, goldenseal, kava, melatonin, mistletoe, pokeweed, poppy, Queen Anne's lace, valerian

↓ diazepam effect: cola tree

Lab test interferences:

Increase: AST/ALT, serum bilirubin

False increase: 17-OHCS

Decrease: RAIU

NURSING CONSIDERATIONS

Assess:

• B/P (lying, standing), pulse; respiratory rate; if systolic B/P drops 20 mm Hg, hold drug, notify prescriber; respirations q5-15min if given IV

• Blood studies: CBC during long-term therapy; blood dyscrasias (rare)

• Degree of anxiety; what precipitates anxiety and whether drug controls symptoms

• For alcohol withdrawal symptoms, including hallucinations (visual, auditory), delirium, irritability, agitation, fine to coarse tremors

• For seizure control and type, duration, intensity of convulsions

• Hepatic studies: AST, ALT, bilirubin, creatinine, LDH, alk phosphatase

• IV site for thrombosis or phlebitis, which may occur rapidly

• Mental status: mood, sensorium, affect, sleeping pattern, drowsiness, dizziness

• Physical dependency, withdrawal symptoms: headache, nausea, vomiting, muscle pain, weakness after long-term use

• Suicidal tendencies

Administer:

• With food or milk for GI symptoms; crushed if patient is unable to swallow medication whole; do not crush ext rel capsules

• Sugarless gum, hard candy, frequent sips of water for dry mouth

• Reduced opioid dose by ⅓ if given concomitantly with diazepam

IV route

• Into large vein; give IV 5 mg or less/1 min or total dose over 3 min or more (children, infants); continuous infusion is not recommended

Additive compatibilities: Netilmicin, verapamil

Syringe compatibilities: Cimetidine

Y-site compatibilities: Cefmetazole, DOBUTamine, nafcillin, quinidine, sufentanil

Sterile emulsion for INJ

• Use IV only, within 6 hr, flush line after use and after 6 hr

Rectal route

• Do not use more than 5 ×/mo or for an episode q5d

Perform/provide:

• Assistance with ambulation during beginning therapy, for drowsiness, dizziness, safety measures

• Check to see PO medication has been swallowed

Evaluate:

• Therapeutic response: decreased anxiety, restlessness, insomnia

Teach patient/family:

• That drug may be taken with food

• That drug is not to be used for everyday stress or used longer than 4 mo unless directed by prescriber;

no more than prescribed amount; may be habit forming
• To avoid OTC preparations unless approved by prescriber
• To avoid driving, activities that require alertness; drowsiness may occur
• To avoid alcohol, other psychotropic medications unless directed by prescriber; that smoking may decrease diazepam effect
• Not to discontinue medication abruptly after long-term use
• To rise slowly or fainting may occur, especially in elderly
• That drowsiness may worsen at beginning of treatment
• To avoid use during pregnancy
⊘ Not to break, crush, or chew ext rel caps

Treatment of overdose: Lavage, VS, supportive care, flumazenil

diazoxide (℞)

(dye-az-ox′ide)
diazoxide parenteral,
Hyperstat IV
Func. class.: Antihypertensive
Chem. class.: Vasodilator

Action: Vasodilates arteriolar smooth muscle by direct relaxation; a reduction in blood pressure with concomitant increases in heart rate, cardiac output; reduces release of insulin from the pancreas

Uses: Hypertensive crisis when urgent decrease of diastolic pressure required; increase blood glucose levels in hyperinsulinism

Dosage and routes:

Hypoglycemia
• *Adult and child:* **PO** 3-8 mg/kg/day in 2-3 divided doses q8-12h
• *Infants and neonates:* **PO** 8-15 mg/kg/day in 2-3 divided doses 8-12h

Hypertension
• *Adult:* **IV BOL** 1-3 mg/kg rapidly up to a max of 150 mg in a single injection; dose may be repeated at 5-15 min intervals until desired response is achieved; give IV in 30 sec or less
• *Child:* **IV BOL** 1-2 mg/kg rapidly; administration same as adult, not to exceed 150 mg

Available forms: Caps 50 mg; oral susp 50 mg/ml; inj 15 mg/ml, 300 mg/20 ml

Side effects/adverse reactions:
CV: ***Hypotension,*** T-wave changes, angina pectoris, palpitations, ***supraventricular tachycardia, edema,*** rebound hypertension, ***shock, MI***
CNS: Headache, sleepiness, euphoria, anxiety, EPS, confusion, tinnitus, blurred vision, dizziness, weakness, ***seizures, cerebral ischemia, paralysis***
GI: Nausea, vomiting, dry mouth
INTEG: Rash
HEMA: Decreased Hgb, Hct, ***thrombocytopenia***
GU: Breast tenderness; increased BUN, fluid, electrolyte imbalances; Na, water retention
ENDO: Hyperglycemia in diabetics, transient hyperglycemia in nondiabetics, increased uric acid

Contraindications: Hypersensitivity to thiazides, sulfonamides, hypertension of aortic coarctation or AV shunt, pheochromocytoma, dissecting aortic aneurysm

Precautions: Tachycardia, fluid, electrolyte imbalances, pregnancy (C), lactation, impaired cerebral or cardiac circulation, children

Pharmacokinetics:
IV: Onset 1-2 min, peak 5 min, duration 3-12 hr; *PO:* onset 1 hr, peak 8-12 hr, duration 8 hr, half-life 20-36 hr, excreted slowly in urine, crosses blood-brain barrier, placenta; highly protein bound (>90%)

Interactions:
- Severe hypotension: antihypertensives
- ↑ hyperuricemic, antihypertensive effects of diazoxide: thiazide diuretics
- Hyperglycemia: sulfonylureas
- ↓ anticonvulsant effect: hydantoins

Toxicity/death: aconite

NURSING CONSIDERATIONS

Assess:
- B/P q5min until stabilized, then q1h × 2 hr, then q4h
- Pulse, jugular venous distention q4h
- Electrolytes, blood studies: K, Na, Cl, CO_2, CBC, serum glucose
- Weight daily, I&O
- Edema in feet, legs daily
- Skin turgor, mucous membranes for hydration status
- Rales, dyspnea, orthopnea
- IV site for extravasation
- Signs of CHF: dyspnea, edema, wet rales
- Postural hypotension, take B/P sitting, standing

Administer:
- Undiluted; give over ½ min or less
- To patient in recumbent position; keep in that position for 1 hr after administration

Syringe compatibilities: Heparin

Perform/provide:
- Store protected from light

Evaluate:
- Therapeutic response: decreased B/P, primarily diastolic pressure

Treatment of overdose: DOPamine, or norepinephrine for hypotension, Trendelenburg maneuver

dibucaine topical

See appendix c

diclofenac ophthalmic

See appendix c

diclofenac potassium (℞)

(dye-kloe'fen-ak)

Cataflam, Voltaren Rapide✤

diclofenac sodium

Apo-Dilo✤, Novo-Difenac✤, Nu-Diclo, Voltaren, Voltaren-XR

Func. class.: Nonsteroidal antiinflammatory (NSAIDs), nonopioid analgesic

Chem. class.: Phenylacetic acid

Action: Inhibits prostaglandin synthesis by decreasing enzyme needed for biosynthesis; analgesic, antiinflammatory, antipyretic

Uses: Acute, chronic rheumatoid arthritis, osteoarthritis; ankylosing spondylitis, analgesia, primary dysmenorrhea

Dosage and routes:

Osteoarthritis
- *Adult:* **PO** 100-150 mg/day in 2-3 divided doses

Rheumatoid arthritis
- *Adult:* **PO** 100-200 mg/day in 2-4 divided doses (potassium); 50 mg tid-qid, then reduce to lowest dose needed (25 mg tid) (sodium)

Ankylosing spondylitis
- *Adult:* **PO** 100-125 mg/day in 4-5 divided doses, give 25 mg qid and 25 mg hs if needed (potassium)

Analgesia/primary dysmenorrhea
- *Adult:* **PO** 50 mg tid, max 150 mg/day (potassium)

Available forms: Potassium: tabs 50, 75 mg; sodium: tabs delayed rel (enteric-coated) 25, 50, 75 mg; ext rel tabs 75, 100 mg; supp 50, 100 mg

Side effects/adverse reactions:
SYST: ***Anaphylaxis***
GI: Nausea, anorexia, vomiting, diarrhea, ***jaundice, cholestatic hepatitis,*** constipation, flatulence, cramps, dry mouth, peptic ulcer, GI bleeding, ***hepatotoxicity***
CNS: Dizziness, headache, drowsiness, fatigue, tremors, confusion, insomnia, anxiety, depression, nervousness, paresthesia, muscle weakness
CV: ***CHF,*** tachycardia, peripheral edema, palpitations, ***dysrhythmias,*** hypotension, hypertension, fluid retention
INTEG: Purpura, rash, pruritus, sweating, erythema, petechiae, photosensitivity, alopecia
GU: ***Nephrotoxicity: dysuria, hematuria, oliguria, azotemia, cystitis, UTI***
HEMA: ***Blood dyscrasias,*** epistaxis, bruising
EENT: Tinnitus, hearing loss, blurred vision, ***laryngeal edema***
RESP: Dyspnea, hemoptysis, pharyngitis, ***bronchospasm,*** rhinitis, shortness of breath

Contraindications: Hypersensitivity to aspirin, iodides, other nonsteroidal antiinflammatory agents, asthma

Precautions: Pregnancy (B) 1st trimester, not recommended in 2nd half of pregnancy, lactation, children, bleeding disorders, GI disorders, cardiac disorders, hypersensitivity to other antiinflammatory agents, CCr <30 ml/min

Do not confuse:
Cataflam/Catapres

Pharmacokinetics:
PO: Peak 2-3 hr, elimination half-life 1-2 hr, 90% bound to plasma proteins, metabolized in liver to metabolite, excreted in urine

Interactions:
- ↓ antihypertensive effect: β-blockers, diuretics
- ↑ anticoagulant effect: anticoagulants
- ↑ toxicity: phenytoin, lithium, cycloSPORINE, methotrexate
- ↑ GI side effects: aspirin, other NSAIDs
- Hyperkalemia: potassium-sparing diuretics
- Need for dosage adjustment: antidiabetics

↑ bleeding risk: bogbean, chondroitin, saw palmetto, turmeric
Severe photosensitivity: St. John's wort
↑gastric irritation: arginine, gossypol
↑ NSAIDs effect: bearberry, bilberry

NURSING CONSIDERATIONS
Assess:
- For pain: location, character, aggravating, alleviating factors, ROM, before and 1 hr after dose
- Blood counts during therapy; watch for decreasing platelets; if low, therapy may need to be discontinued, restarted after hematologic recovery
- For clients with asthma, aspirin hypersensitivity, nasal polyps; may develop hypersensitivity
- LFTs (may be elevated) and uric acid (may be decreased—serum; increased—urine) periodically; also BUN, creatinine, electrolytes (may be elevated)

Blood dyscrasias (thrombocytopenia): bruising, fatigue, bleeding, poor healing

Evaluate:
- Therapeutic response: decreased inflammation in joints, decreased inflammation after cataract surgery

Teach patient/family:
- That drug must be continued for prescribed time to be effective; to

contact prescriber prior to surgery as when to discontinue this drug
- To report bleeding, bruising, fatigue, malaise; blood dyscrasias do occur

Not to break, crush, or chew enteric products
- To avoid aspirin, alcoholic beverages, NSAIDs, acetaminophen, or other OTC medications unless approved by prescriber
- To take with food, milk, or antacids to avoid GI upset, to swallow whole
- To use caution when driving; drowsiness, dizziness may occur
- To take with a full glass of water to enhance absorption, remain upright for ½ hr; if dose is missed, take as soon as remembered within 2 hr if taking 1-2 ×/day, do not double doses
- To report hepatotoxicity: flulike symptoms, nausea, vomiting, jaundice, pruritus, lethargy
- To use sunscreen to prevent photosensitivity

dicloxacillin (℞)

(dye-klox-a-sill′-in)
dicloxacillin sodium, Dycill, Dynapen, Pathocil
Func. class.: Antiinfective
Chem. class.: Penicillinase-resistant penicillin

Action: Interferes with cell wall replication of susceptible organisms; osmotically unstable cell wall swells, bursts from osmotic pressure

Uses: Effective for gram-positive cocci *(Staphylococcus aureus, Streptococcus pyogenes, S. viridans, S. faecalis, S. bovis, S. pneumoniae),* infections caused by penicillinase-producing *Staphylococcus*

Dosage and routes:
- *Adult/child ≥40 kg:* **PO** 0.5-4 g/day in divided doses q6h, max 4 g/day
- *Child ≤40 kg:* **PO** 12.5-50 mg/kg in divided doses q6h, max 4 g/day

Available forms: Caps 125, 250, 500 mg; powder for oral susp 62.5 mg/5 ml

Side effects/adverse reactions:
HEMA: Anemia, increased bleeding time, ***bone marrow depression, granulocytopenia***
GI: Nausea, vomiting, diarrhea, increased AST, ALT, abdominal pain, glossitis, ***pseudomembranous colitis***
GU: ***Oliguria, proteinuria, hematuria,*** *vaginitis, moniliasis,* ***glomerulonephritis***
CNS: Lethargy, hallucinations, anxiety, depression, twitching, ***coma, convulsions***
SYST: ***Anaphylaxis***

Contraindications: Hypersensitivity to penicillins; neonates

Precautions: Hypersensitivity to cephalosporins, pregnancy (B), lactation, severe renal or hepatic disease

Do not confuse:
Pathocil/Bactocil

Pharmacokinetics:
PO: Peak 1 hr, duration 4-6 hr, half-life 30-60 min; metabolized in liver; excreted in urine, bile, breast milk; crosses placenta

Interactions:
- ↑ dicloxacillin concentrations: aspirin, probenecid, oral contraceptives
- ↓ anticoagulant effect
- Food/drug: citric juices/food ↓ absorption of dicloxacillin

↓ absorption: khat, separate by 2 hr

Do not use acidophilus with anti-infectives

Lab test interferences:
False positive: Urine glucose, urine protein

NURSING CONSIDERATIONS

Assess:
• I&O ratio; report hematuria, oliguria, since penicillin in high doses is nephrotoxic
◆ Any patient with compromised renal system, since drug is excreted slowly in poor renal system function; toxicity may occur rapidly
• Blood studies: WBC, RBC, Hgb, Hct, bleeding time
• Renal studies: urinalysis, protein, blood
• C&S before drug therapy; drug may be given as soon as culture is taken
• WBC and differential, ALT, AST, BUN, creatinine for patients on long-term therapy
• Bowel pattern before, during treatment
• Anaphylaxis: pruritus, rash, dyspnea, laryngeal edema; have emergency equipment available; skin eruptions after administration of penicillin to 1 wk after discontinuing drug
• For infection: temp, draining wounds, WBC, sputum, urine, stool, before, during treatment

Administer:
• Drug after C&S
• On an empty stomach with a full glass of water
• Susp after shaking well before each dose

Perform/provide:
• Adrenalin, suction, tracheostomy set, endotracheal intubation equipment
• Adequate fluid intake (2 L) during diarrhea episodes
• Scratch test to assess allergy after securing order from prescriber; usually done when penicillin is only drug of choice
• Storage in tight container; after reconstituting, store in refrigerator up to 2 wk

Evaluate:
• Therapeutic response: absence of fever, draining wounds

Teach patient/family:
• All aspects of drug therapy, including need to complete course of medication to ensure organism death (10-14 days); culture may be taken after completed course
• To report sore throat, fever, fatigue; may indicate superinfection
⊘ Not to break, crush, or chew caps
• To wear or carry emergency ID if allergic to penicillins
• To notify prescriber of diarrhea, fever

Treatment of anaphylaxis: Withdraw drug; maintain airway; administer epINEPHrine, aminophylline, O_2, IV corticosteroids

RARELY USED

dicyclomine (℞)

(dye-sye'kloe-meen)
Antispas, Bentyl, Bentylol♣, Byclomine, Dibent, dicyclomine HCL, Dilomine, Di-Spaz, Formulex♣, Lomine♣, Neoquess, Or-Tyl, Spasmoject

Func. class.: Gastrointestinal anticholinergic

Uses: Treatment of peptic ulcer disease in combination with other drugs; infant colic, urinary incontinence

Dosage and routes:
• *Adult:* **PO** 10-20 mg tid-qid; **IM** 20 mg q4-6h
• *Child >2 yr:* **PO** 10 mg tid-qid
• *Child 6 mo-2 yr:* **PO** 5 mg tid-qid

Contraindications: Hypersensitivity to anticholinergics, narrow-angle glaucoma, GI obstruction, myasthenia gravis, paralytic ileus, GI atony, toxic megacolon

didanosine (℞)

(dye-dan'oh-seen)

ddI, dideoxyinosine, Videx, Videx EC

Func. class.: Antiretroviral

Chem. class.: Nucleoside reverse transcriptase inhibitor

Action: Nucleoside analog incorporating into cellular DNA by viral reverse transcriptase, thereby terminating the cellular DNA chain

Uses: HIV infection in combination with other antiretrovirals

Dosage and routes:

• Reduce dosage CCr <60 ml/min

• *Adult:* **PO** >60 kg, 200 mg bid tabs, or 250 mg bid buffered powder; caps, del rel 400 mg qd; <60 kg, 125 mg bid tabs, or 167 mg bid buffered powder; caps, del rel 250 mg qd

• *Child:* **PO** tabs 90-120 mg/m^2 q12h; buffered powder packets 112.5-150 mg/m^2 q12h; **PO** (child BSA 1.1-1.4 m^2) tab 100 mg q8-12h; recon pedi powder 125 mg q8-12h; **PO** (child BSA 0.8-1 m^2) tabs 75 mg q8-12h; recon pedi powder 94 mg q8-12h; **PO** (child BSA 0.5-0.7 m^2) tabs 50 mg q8-12h; recon pedi powder 62 mg q8-12h; **PO** (child BSA <0.4 m^2) tabs 25 mg q8-12h; recon pedi powder 31 mg q8-12h

Available forms: Tabs, buffered, chewable/dispersible 25, 50, 100, 150 mg; powder for oral sol, buffered 100, 167, 250, 375 mg/packet; powder for oral sol, pedi 10 mg, 20 mg/ml; caps, del rel 125, 200, 250, 400

Side effects/adverse reactions:

GI: ***Pancreatitis,*** *diarrhea, nausea,* vomiting, *abdominal pain,* constipation, stomatitis, dyspepsia, liver abnormalities, flatulence, taste perversion, dry mouth, oral thrush, melena, increased ALT, AST, alk phosphatase, amylase, ***hepatic failure***

GU: Increased bilirubin, uric acid

CNS: ***Peripheral neuropathy, seizures,*** confusion, *anxiety,* hypertonia, abnormal thinking, asthenia, *insomnia,* ***CNS depression,*** pain, dizziness, chills, fever

RESP: Cough, pneumonia, dyspnea, asthma, epistaxis, hypoventilation, sinusitis

INTEG: Rash, pruritus, alopecia, ecchymosis, hemorrhage, petechiae, sweating

MS: Myalgia, arthritis, myopathy, muscular atrophy

CV: Hypertension, vasodilation, dysrhythmia, syncope, ***CHF,*** palpitation

EENT: Ear pain, otitis, photophobia, visual impairment, retinal depigmentation

HEMA: ***Leukopenia, granulocytopenia, thrombocytopenia, anemia***

SYST: ***Lactic acidosis, anaphylaxis***

Contraindications: Hypersensitivity

Precautions: Renal, hepatic disease, pregnancy (B), lactation, children, sodium-restricted diets, elevated amylase, preexistant peripheral neuropathy, phenylketonuria, hyperuricemia

Pharmacokinetics:

PO: Peak 0.67 hr; del rel 2 hr; elimination half-life 1.62 hr, extensive metabolism is thought to occur; administration within 5 min of food will decrease absorption

Interactions:
• ↑ didanosine level: allopurinol, tenofovir, adjust dose as needed
• ↓ absorption: ketoconazole, dapsone
• ↑ side effects from: magnesium, aluminum antacids
• ↓ concentrations of: fluoroquinolones, other antiretrovirals, itraconazole, tetracyclines
• Drug/food: any food ↓ rate of absorption
• Do not use with acidic juices

NURSING CONSIDERATIONS
Assess:
• Peripheral neuropathy: tingling or pain in hands and feet, distal numbness; onset usually occurs 2-6 mo after beginning treatment, may persist if drug is not discontinued
◆Pancreatitis: abdominal pain, nausea, vomiting, elevated liver enzymes; drug should be discontinued, since condition can be fatal
• For anaphylaxis, lactic acidosis
• Children by dilated retinal exam q6mo to rule out retinal depigmentation
• CBC, differential, platelet count qmo; withhold drug if WBC is <4000 or platelet count is <75,000; notify prescriber of results; alk phosphatase, monitor amylase; viral load, CD4 count
• Renal studies: BUN, serum uric acid, urine CCr before, during therapy
• Temp q4h, may indicate beginning infection
• Hepatic studies before, during therapy (bilirubin, AST, ALT) as needed or qmo

Administer:
• Pediatric powder for oral sol after preparation by pharmacist; dilution is required using purified USP water, then antacid (10 mg/ml), refrigerate, shake before use
• On an empty stomach ≥30 min, ac or 2 hr pc
• Adjust dose in renal impairment

Perform/provide:
• Cleanup of powdered products; use wet mop or damp sponge
• Storage of tabs, caps in tightly closed bottle at room temperature; store oral sol after dissolving at room temperature ≤4 hr

Evaluate:
• Therapeutic response: absence of infection; symptoms of HIV

Teach patient/family:
• To avoid use with alcohol
• To report numbness/tingling in extremities
• To take on an empty stomach; not to take dapsone at same time as ddI; do not mix powder with fruit juice; chew tab or crush and dissolve in water; drink powder immediately after mixing
• To report signs of infection: increased temp, sore throat, flulike symptoms
• To report signs of anemia: fatigue, headache, faintness, shortness of breath, irritability
• To report bleeding; avoid use of razors, commercial mouthwash
• That hair may be lost during therapy (rare); a wig or hairpiece may make patient feel better

---

RARELY USED

dienestrol (℞)
(dye-en-ess'trole)
DV, Ortho Dienestrol
Func. class.: Estrogen

Uses: Atrophic vaginitis, kraurosis vulvae

Dosage and routes:
• *Adult:* **VAG CREAM** 1-2 appli-

cations qd × 2 wk, then ½ dose × 2 wk, then 1 application
Contraindications: Breast cancer, thromboembolic disorders, reproductive cancer, genital bleeding (abnormal, undiagnosed), pregnancy (X), lactation

diflorasone topical

See appendix c

RARELY USED

diflunisal (℞)

(dye-floo'ni-sal)
diflunisal, Dolobid
Func. class.: Nonsteroidal anti-inflammatory/analgesic (non-opioid)

Uses: Mild to moderate pain or fever including arthritis; 3-4 times more potent than aspirin
Dosage and routes:
• *Adult:* **PO** loading dose 1 g; then 500-1000 mg/day in 2 divided doses, q12h, not to exceed 1500 mg/day
• *Geriatric:* ½ adult dose
Contraindications: Hypersensitivity to salicylates, GI bleeding, bleeding disorders, children <12 yr, vit K deficiency

HIGH ALERT

digoxin (℞)

(di-jox'in)
digoxin, Lanoxicaps, Lanoxin
Func. class.: Cardiac glycoside, inotropic, antidysrhythmic
Chem. class.: Digitalis preparation

Action: Inhibits the sodium-potassium ATPase, which makes more calcium available for contractile proteins, resulting in increased cardiac output; increases force of contraction (+ inotropic effect); decreases heart rate (chronotropic effect); decreases AV conduction speed
Uses: CHF, atrial fibrillation, atrial flutter, atrial tachycardia, cardiogenic shock, paroxysmal atrial tachycardia, rapid digitalization in these disorders
Dosage and routes:
• *Adult:* **IV** *digitalizing dose* 0.6-1.0 mg given as 50% of the dose initially, additional fractions given at 4-8 hr intervals; **PO digitalizing dose** 0.75-1.25 mg given as 50% of the dose initially, additional fractions given at 4-8 hr intervals; **maintenance** 0.063-0.5 mg/day (tabs), or 0.350-0.5 mg/day (gelatin cap)
• *Child>10 yr:* **IV digitalizing dose** 8-12 mcg/kg given as 50% of the dose initially, additional fractions given at 4-8 hr intervals; **PO digitalizing dose** 0.01-0.015 mg/kg given as 50% of the dose initially, additional fractions given at 6-8 hr intervals; **maintenance** 25%-35% of the loading dose qd as a single dose
• *Child 5-10 yr:* **IV digitalizing dose** 0.015-0.03 mg/kg given as 50% of the dose initially, additional fractions given at 4-8 hr intervals; **PO digitalizing dose** 0.02-0.035 mg/kg given as 50% of the dose initially, additional fractions given at 6-8 hr intervals; **maintenance** 25%-35% of the loading dose qd in 2 divided doses
• *Child 2-5 yr:* **IV digitalizing dose** 0.025-0.035 mg/kg given as 50% of the dose initially, additional fractions given at 4-8 hr intervals; **PO digitalizing dose** 0.03-0.04 mg/kg given as 50% of the dose initially, additional fractions given at 6-8 hr intervals; **maintenance** 25%-35%

of the loading dose qd in 2 divided doses

• *Child 1-2 yr:* **IV digitalizing dose** 0.03-0.05 mg/kg given as 50% of the dose initially, additional fractions given at 4-8 hr intervals; **PO digitalizing dose** 0.035-0.06 mg/kg given as 50% of the dose initially, additional fractions given at 4-8 hr intervals; **maintenance** 25%-35% of the loading dose qd in 2 divided doses

• *Infants:* **IV digitalizing dose** 0.02-0.03 mg/kg given as 50% of the dose initially, additional fractions given at 4-8 hr intervals; **PO digitalizing dose** 0.025-0.035 mg/kg given as 50% of the dose initially, additional fractions given at 6-8 hr intervals; **maintenance** 25%-35% of the loading dose qd in 2 divided doses

• *Infants, premature:* **IV digitalizing dose** 0.015-0.025 mg/kg given as 50% of the dose initially, additional fractions given at 4-8 hr intervals; **PO digitalizing dose** 0.02-0.03 mg/kg given as 50% of the dose initially, additional fractions given at 6-8 hr intervals; **maintenance** 20%-30% of the loading dose qd in 2 divided doses

Available forms: Caps 0.05, 0.1, 0.2 mg; elix 0.05 mg/ml; tabs 0.125, 0.25, 0.5 mg; inj 0.5✤, 0.25 mg/ml: pediatric inj 0.1 mg/ml

Side effects/adverse reactions:

CNS: Headache, drowsiness, apathy, confusion, disorientation, fatigue, depression, hallucinations

CV: ***Dysrhythmias,*** *hypotension,* bradycardia, ***AV block***

EENT: Blurred vision, yellow-green halos, photophobia, diplopia

GI: Nausea, vomiting, anorexia, abdominal pain, diarrhea

Contraindications: Hypersensitivity to digitalis, ventricular fibrillation, ventricular tachycardia, carotid sinus syndrome, 2nd- or 3rd-degree heart block

Precautions: Renal disease, acute MI, AV block, severe respiratory disease, hypothyroidism, elderly, pregnancy (C), sinus nodal disease, lactation, hypokalemia

Do not confuse:

Lanoxin/Lasix/Lonox

Lanoxin/Lomotil

Lanoxin/Xanax/Levoxine

Pharmacokinetics:

PO: Onset ½-2 hr, peak 6-8 hr, duration 3-4 days

IV: Onset 5-30 min, peak 1-5 hr, duration variable

Half-life 1.5 days, excreted in urine

Interactions:

• ↓ digoxin absorption: antacids kaolin/pectin

• Hypercalcemia, hypomagnesemia, digitalis toxicity: thiazides, parenteral calcium

• Hypokalemia, digitalis toxicity: diuretics, amphotericin B, carbenicillin, ticarcillin, corticosteroids

• ↓ digoxin level: thyroid agents, cholestyramine, colestipol, metoclopramide

• ↑ digoxin levels: propantheline, quinidine, verapamil, amiodarone, anticholinergics, diltiazem, NIFEdipine

• ↑ bradycardia: β-adrenergic blockers, antidysrythmics

• ↑ cardiac dysrhythmia risk: sympathomimetics

↑ digoxin action: aloe, betel palm, broom, buckthorn, cascara sagrada, castor, Chinese rhubarb, figwort, fumitory, hawthorn, khat, kudzu, licorice, lily of the valley, Mayapple, mistletoe, motherwort, night-blooming cereus, oleander, pheasant's eye, purple foxglove, Queen Anne's lace, rhubarb, rue, senna, Siberian ginseng, squill, yellow dock

Bradycardia: Indian snakeroot
Cardiac toxicity: aconite, hawthorn, horsetail
↓ digoxin absorption: psyllium
↑ hypokalemia: cocoa, coffee, cola, guarana, horsetail, licorice, yerba maté
↓ digoxin effect: beth root, goldenseal
Forms insoluble complex: blackroot

Lab test interferences:
Increase: CPK

NURSING CONSIDERATIONS

Assess:
- Apical pulse for 1 min before giving drug; if pulse <60 in adult or <90 in an infant, take again in 1 hr; if <60 in adult, call prescriber; note rate, rhythm, character; monitor ECG continuously during parenteral loading dose
- Electrolytes: K, Na, Cl, Mg, Ca; renal function studies: BUN, creatinine; blood studies: ALT, AST, bilirubin, Hct, Hgb before initiating treatment and periodically thereafter
- I&O ratio, daily weights; monitor turgor, lung sounds, edema
- Monitor drug levels (therapeutic level 0.5-2 ng/ml)
- Cardiac status: apical pulse, character, rate, rhythm

Administer:

PO route
- PO with or without food; may crush tabs, mix with food/fluids
- Potassium supplements if ordered for potassium levels <3, or foods high in potassium: bananas, orange juice

IV route
- Undiluted or 1 ml of drug/4 ml sterile H_2O, D_5, or NS; give >5 min through Y-tube or 3-way stopcock; during digitalization close monitoring is necessary

Additive compatibilities: Bretylium, cimetidine, floxacillin, furosemide, lidocaine, ranitidine, verapamil

Syringe compatibilities: Heparin, milrinone

Y-site compatibilities: Amrinone, cefmetazole, ciprofloxacin, cisatracurium, diltiazem, famotidine, meperidine, meropenem, midazolam, milrinone, morphine, potassium chloride, propofol, remifentanil, tacrolimus, vit B/C

Perform/provide:
- Storage protected from light

Evaluate:
- Therapeutic response: decreased weight, edema, pulse, respiration, rales; increased urine output; serum digoxin level (0.5-2 ng/ml)

Teach patient/family:
- Not to stop drug abruptly; teach all aspects of drug, to take exactly as ordered; how to monitor heart rate
- To avoid OTC medications, since many adverse drug interactions may occur; do not take antacid at same time
- To notify prescriber of loss of appetite, lower stomach pain, diarrhea, weakness, drowsiness, headache, blurred or yellow vision, rash, depression, toxicity
- The toxic symptoms of this drug and when to notify prescriber
- To maintain a sodium-restricted diet as ordered

Not to break, crush, or chew caps
- To report shortness of breath, difficulty breathing, weight gain, edema, persistent cough

Treatment of overdose: Discontinue drug; give potassium; monitor ECG; give adrenergic-blocking agent, digoxin immune FAB

digoxin immune FAB (ovine) (℞)

(di-jox′in im-myoon′ FAB)

Digibind, DigiFab

Func. class.: Antidote—digoxin specific

Action: Antibody fragments bind to free digoxin or digitoxin to reverse toxicity by not allowing digoxin or digitoxin to bind to sites of action

Uses: Life-threatening digoxin toxicity

Dosage and routes:

Digoxin toxicity (known amount) (tabs, oral sol, IM)

• *Adult/child:* **IV** dose (mg) = dose ingested (mg) × 0.8/1000 × 38; if ingested amount is unknown, give 760 mg **IV**

Toxicity (known amount) (cap, IV)

• *Adult/child:* **IV** dose = dose ingested (mg)/0.5 × 38

Toxicity (known amount) by serum digoxin concentrations (SDCs)

• *Adult/child:* **IV** SDC (nanograms/ml) × kg of weight/100 × 38

Skin test

• *Adult:* **ID** 9.5 mcg

Available forms: Inj 38 mg/vial (binds 0.5 mg digoxin), 40 mg/vial (binds 0.5 mg digoxin)

Side effects/adverse reactions:

CV: ***CHF,*** ventricular rate increase, ***atrial fibrillation,*** low cardiac output

RESP: ***Impaired respiratory function, rapid respiratory rate***

META: ***Hypokalemia***

MISC: ***Anaphylaxis*** (rare)

INTEG: Hypersensitivity, allergic reactions, facial swelling, redness

Contraindications: Mild digoxin toxicity, hypersensitivity to this product or papain

Precautions: Children, lactation, elderly, cardiac disease, renal disease, pregnancy (C), allergy to ovine proteins

Pharmacokinetics:

IV: Peaks after completion of infusion, onset 30 min (variable); not known if crosses placenta, breast milk; half-life biphasic—14-20 hr; prolonged in renal disease; excreted by kidneys

Interactions:

• Considered incompatible with all drugs in syringe or sol

Lab test interferences:

Interference: Immunoassay digoxin

NURSING CONSIDERATIONS

Assess:

• Hypokalemia: ST depression, flat T waves, presence of U wave, ventricular dysrhythmia; potassium levels may decrease rapidly

• CHF: Dyspnea, rales, peripheral edema, weight gain >5 lbs

Administer:

• Test doses have proven to be ineffective in the general population; only use test dose in those with known allergies or those previously treated with digoxin immune FAB

• For test dose dilute 0.1 ml or reconstituted drug (9.5 mg/ml) in 9.9 ml sterile isotonic saline, inj 0.1 ml (1 : 100 dilution) ID and observe for wheal with erythema; read in 20 min

• For scratch test place 1 gtt of sol on skin and make a scratch through the drop with a sterile needle; read in 20 min

• After diluting 38 mg/4 ml of sterile H_2O for inj 10 mg/ml mix; may be further diluted with normal saline, sol should be clear, colorless

• By bolus if cardiac arrest is imminent or IV over 30 min using a 0.22 μm filter

Perform/provide:

• Storage of reconstituted sol for up to 4 hr in refrigerator

• Do not freeze DigiFab

Evaluate:
• Therapeutic response: correction of digoxin toxicity; check digoxin levels 0.5-2 ng/ml; digitoxin level 9-25 ng/ml

Teach patient/family:
• The purpose of medication; to report delayed hypersensitivity; fever, chills, itching, swelling, dyspnea

dihydroergotamine (℞)

(dye-hye-droe-er-got'a-meen)
D.H.E. 45,
Dihydroergotamine-Sandoz✤

Func. class.: α-Adrenergic blocker

Chem. class.: Ergot alkaloid (dihydrogenated)

Action: Constricts smooth muscle in periphery, cranial blood vessels; inhibits norepinephrine uptake

Uses: Vascular headache (migraine or histamine)

Dosage and routes:
• *Adult:* **IM/IV** 1 mg; may repeat q1-2h if needed, not to exceed 3 mg/day or 6 mg/wk

Available forms: Inj 1 mg/ml

Side effects/adverse reactions:

CNS: Numbness in fingers, toes, general weakness

CV: Transient tachycardia, chest pain, bradycardia, increase or decrease in B/P, *gangrene*

GI: Nausea, vomiting

MS: Muscle pain

Contraindications: Hypersensitivity to ergot preparations, occlusion (peripheral vascular), CAD, hepatic disease, pregnancy (X), renal disease, peptic ulcer, hypertension, lactation, children, uremia

Pharmacokinetics:

IM: Onset 15-30 min, peak 2 hr, duration 3-4 hr

IV: Onset 5 min, peak 45 min, duration 3-4 hr; half-life 1.3-4 hr

Interactions:
• Ergot toxicity symptoms: macrolide antiinfectives
• ↑ vasoconstriction: β-blockers
• Incompatible with any drug in syringe or sol

🌿 ↓ alpha blocking effect: Butcher's broom, capsicum peppers

🌿 Toxicity: yohimbe

NURSING CONSIDERATIONS

Assess:
• Weight daily, check for peripheral edema in feet, legs
• For stress level, activity, recreation, coping mechanisms
• Neurologic status: LOC, blurring vision, nausea, vomiting, tingling in extremities that precedes headache
• Ingestion of tyramine (pickled products, beer, wine, aged cheese), food additives, preservatives, colorings, artificial sweeteners, chocolate, caffeine; may precipitate these headaches

Administer:
• IV undiluted; give over 3 min
• At beginning of headache; dose must be titrated to patient response
• Only to women who are not pregnant; harm to fetus may occur

Perform/provide:
• Storage in dark area; do not use discolored solutions
• Quiet, calm environment with decreased stimulation for noise, bright light, excessive talking

Evaluate:
• Therapeutic response: decrease in frequency, severity of headache

Teach patient/family:
• Not to use OTC medications; serious drug interactions may occur
• To report side effects: increased vasoconstriction starting with cold extremities, then paresthesia, weakness
• That an increase in headaches may

occur when this drug is discontinued after long-term use

- To keep drug out of reach of children; death may occur
- Not to use during pregnancy

dihydrotachysterol (℞)

(dye-hye-droh-tak-iss'ter-ole)

DHT Intensol✦, Hytakerol

Func. class.: Parathyroid agent (calcium regulator)

Chem. class.: Vit D analog

Action: Increases intestinal absorption of calcium for bones, increases renal tubular absorption of phosphate; regulates calcium levels by regulating calcitonin, parathyroid hormone

Uses: Renal osteodystrophy, hypoparathyroidism, pseudohypoparathyroidism, familial hypophosphatemia, postoperative tetany

Dosage and routes:

Hypophosphatemia

- *Adult and child:* **PO** 0.5-2 mg qd, maintenance 0.2-1.5 mg qd

Hypoparathyroidism/pseudohypoparathyroidism

- *Adult:* **PO** 0.8-2.4 mg qd × 4 days, maintenance 0.2-2 mg qd regulated by serum calcium levels
- *Neonates:* **PO** 0.05-0.1 mg/day
- *Infants, young child:* **PO** 0.1-0.5 mg/day
- *Older child:* **PO** 0.5-1 mg/day

Renal osteodystrophy

- *Adult:* **PO** 0.25-0.375 mg/day
- *Child:* **PO** 0.125-0.5 mg/day

Rickets (Vit. D–resistant)

- *Child:* **PO** 0.25-1 mg/day

Available forms: Tabs 0.125, 0.2, 0.4 mg; caps 0.125 mg; oral sol 0.2, 0.25 mg/5 ml, 0.2 mg/ml✦ (Intensol)

Side effects/adverse reactions:

EENT: Tinnitus

CNS: Drowsiness, headache, vertigo, fever, lethargy, depression

GI: Nausea, diarrhea, vomiting, jaundice, anorexia, dry mouth, constipation, cramps, metallic taste, thirst

MS: Myalgia, arthralgia, decreased bone development, weakness, ataxia

GU: Polyuria, hypercalciuria, hyperphosphatemia, hematuria, nocturia, renal calculi

CV: ***Dysrhythmias,*** hypertension

Contraindications: Hypersensitivity, renal disease, hyperphosphatemia, hypercalcemia

Precautions: Pregnancy (C), renal calculi, lactation, CV disease

Pharmacokinetics:

PO: Onset 2 wk; readily absorbed from small intestine; metabolized by liver, excreted in feces (active/inactive)

Interactions:

- ↓ dihydrotachysterol absorption: cholestyramine, colestipol mineral oil
- Hypercalcemia: thiazide diuretics, calcium supplements
- Cardiac dysrhythmias: cardiac glycosides, verapamil
- ↓ dihydrotachysterol effect: corticosteroids, phenytoin, barbiturates

Lab test interferences:

False increase: Cholesterol

NURSING CONSIDERATIONS

Assess:

- BUN, urinary Ca, AST, ALT, cholesterol, creatinine, alk phosphatase, uric acid, chlorine, magnesium, electrolytes, urine pH, phosphate; may increase calcium, should be kept at 9-10 mg/dl, vit D 50-135 international units/dl, phosphate 70 mg/dl
- Alk phosphatase: may be decreased
- For increased blood level, since toxic reactions may occur rapidly
- For dry mouth, metallic taste, polyuria, bone pain, muscle weakness,

headache, fatigue, tinnitus, change in LOC, irregular pulse, dysrhythmias, increased respirations, anorexia, nausea, vomiting, cramps, diarrhea, constipation; may indicate hypercalcemia

• Renal status: decreased urinary output (oliguria, anuria), edema in extremities, weight gain >5 lb, periorbital edema

• Nutritional status, diet for sources of vit D (milk, some seafood), calcium (dairy products, dark green vegetables), phosphates (dairy products) must be avoided

Administer:

• PO, may be increased q4wk depending on blood level

Perform/provide:

• Storage in tight, light-resistant containers at room temperature

• Restriction of sodium, potassium if required

• Restriction of fluids if required for chronic renal failure

Evaluate:

• Therapeutic response: prevention of bone deficiencies

Teach patient/family:

• The symptoms of hypercalcemia

• About foods rich in calcium, vit D

⊘ Not to break, crush, or chew caps

HIGH ALERT

diltiazem (℞)

(dil-tye′a-zem)

Apo-Diltiaz✱, Cardizem, Cardizem CD, Cardizem SR, Dilacor-XR, Diltia XR, diltiazem, Tiazac

Func. class.: Calcium channel blocker

Chem. class.: Benzothiazepine

Action: Inhibits calcium ion influx across cell membrane during cardiac depolarization; produces relaxation of coronary vascular smooth muscle, dilates coronary arteries, slows SA/AV node conduction times, dilates peripheral arteries

Uses: Angina pectoris due to coronary insufficiency, hypertension, coronary artery spasm; parenteral: atrial fibrillation, flutter, paroxysmal supraventricular tachycardia

Dosage and routes:

Hypertension

• *Adult:* **PO** 60-120 mg bid (sus rel), max 360 mg/day, or 180-240 mg (ext rel) qd

Prinzmetal's or variant angina, chronic stable angina

• *Adult:* **PO** 30 mg qid, increasing dose gradually to 180-360 mg/day in divided doses or 60-120 mg bid; may increase to 240-360 mg/day or 120 or 180 mg ext rel **PO** qd

Atrial fibrillation/flutter, paroxysmal supraventricular tachycardia

• *Adult:* **IV BOL** 0.25 mg/kg over 2 min initially, then 0.35 mg/kg may be given after 15 min; if no response, may give **CONT INF** 5-15 mg/hr for up to 24 hr

Available forms: Tabs 30, 60, 90, 120 mg; caps ext rel 60, 90, 120, 180, 240, 300, 360, 420 mg; cap, sus rel 60, 90, 120, 180, 240, 300, 360, 420 mg; inj 5 mg/ml (5, 10 ml); inj 25 mg; inj for IV only 100 mg

Side effects/adverse reactions:

CV: ***Dysrhythmia,*** *edema,* ***CHF,*** bradycardia, hypotension, palpitations, ***heart block***

DI: Increased effects, toxicity: theophylline

GI: Nausea, vomiting, diarrhea, gastric upset, *constipation*, increased LFTs

RESP: Rhinitis, dyspnea, pharyngitis

GU: Nocturia, polyuria, ***acute renal failure***

INTEG: Rash, pruritus, flushing, photosensitivity
CNS: Headache, fatigue, drowsiness, dizziness, depression, weakness, insomnia, tremor, paresthesia
Contraindications: Sick sinus syndrome, 2nd- or 3rd-degree heart block, hypotension less than 90 mm Hg systolic, acute MI, pulmonary congestion
Precautions: CHF, hypotension, hepatic injury, pregnancy (C), lactation, children, renal disease
Do not confuse:
Cardiazem CD/Cardiazem SR
Cardiazem/Cardene
Cardiazem SR/Cardene SR
Pharmacokinetics: Onset 30-60 min; peak 2-3 hr immediate rel; 10-14 hr ext rel, 6-11 hr sus rel; half-life 3½-9 hr; metabolized by liver; excreted in urine (96% as metabolites)
Interactions:
• ↑ effects of: β-blockers, digoxin, lithium, carbamazepine, cyclosporine, anesthetics, HMG CO-A reductase inhibitors
• ↑ effects of diltiazem: cimetidine
• Drug/food: ↑ hypotensive effects: grapefruit juice
↑ diltiazem effect: barberry, betel palm, burdock, goldenseal, khat, khella, lily of the valley, plantain
↓ diltiazem effect: yohimbe
NURSING CONSIDERATIONS
Assess:
• Cardiac status: B/P, pulse, respiration, ECG and intervals PR, QRS, QT; if systolic B/P <90 mm Hg or HR <60 bpm, hold dose, notify prescriber
Administer:
• Before meals, hs (PO)
IV route
• IV undiluted over 2 min or diluted 125 mg/100 ml, 250 mg/250 ml of D_5W, 0.9% NaCl, D_5/0.45% NaCl, give 10 mg/hr, may increase by 5 mg/hr to 15 mg/hr, continue infusion up to 24 hr
Y-site compatibilities: Albumin, amikacin, amphotericin B, aztreonam, bretylium, bumetanide, cefazolin, cefotaxime, cefotetan, cefoxitin, ceftazidime, ceftriaxone, cefuroxime, cimetidine, ciprofloxacin, clindamycin, digoxin, DOBUTamine, DOPamine, doxycycline, epINEPHrine, erythromycin, esmolol, fentanyl, fluconazole, gentamicin, hetastarch, hydromorphone, imipenem-cilastatin, labetalol, lidocaine, lorazepam, meperidine, metoclopramide, metronidazole, midazolam, milrinone, morphine, multivitamins, niCARdipine, nitroglycerin, norepinephrine, oxacillin, penicillin G potassium, pentamidine, piperacillin, potassium chloride, potassium phosphates, ranitidine, sodium nitroprusside, theophylline, ticarcillin, ticarcillin/clavulanate, tobramycin, trimethoprim-sulfamethoxazole, vancomycin, vecuronium
Perform/provide:
• Storage in tight container at room temperature
Evaluate:
• Therapeutic response: decreased anginal pain, decreased B/P
Teach patient/family:
• How to take pulse before taking drug; record or graph should be kept
• To avoid hazardous activities until stabilized on drug, dizziness is no longer a problem
• To limit caffeine consumption
• To avoid OTC drugs unless directed by prescriber
• The importance of complying with all areas of medical regimen: diet, exercise, stress reduction, drug therapy
⊘ Not to break, crush, or chew sus rel caps or tabs

D

To report dizziness, shortness of breath, palpitations
- Not to discontinue abruptly
- To take with a full glass of water

Treatment of overdose: Atropine for AV block, vasopressor for hypotension

* dimenhyDRINATE (OTC, ℞)

(dye-men-hye'dri-nate)

Apo-Dimenhydrinate, Calm-X, Children's Dramamine, dimenhyDRINATE, Dimetabs, Dinate, Dramamine, Dramanate, Dymenate, Gravol, Gravol L/A, Hydrate, Nauseatol, Novo-Dimenate, PMS-Dimenhydrinate, Travamine, Triptone Caplets

Func. class.: Antiemetic, antihistamine, anticholinergic

Chem. class.: H_1-Receptor antagonist, ethanolamine derivative

Action: Vestibular stimulation is decreased

Uses: Motion sickness, nausea, vomiting

Dosage and routes:
- *Adult:* **PO** 50-100 mg q4h; **IM/IV** 50 mg q4h as needed
- *Child:* **IM/PO** 5 mg/kg divided in 4 equal doses

Available forms: Tabs 50 mg; inj 50 mg/ml; elixir 15 mg/5 ml; chew tabs 50 mg

Side effects/adverse reactions:

CNS: Drowsiness, restlessness, headache, dizziness, insomnia, confusion, nervousness, tingling, vertigo

GI: Nausea, anorexia, vomiting, *constipation*

CV: Hypertension, *hypotension*, palpitation

INTEG: Rash, urticaria, fever, chills, flushing

EENT: Dry mouth, blurred vision, diplopia, nasal congestion, photosensitivity

MISC: ***Anaphylaxis***

Contraindications: Hypersensitivity to opioids, shock

Precautions: Children, cardiac dysrhythmias, elderly, asthma, pregnancy (B), lactation, prostatic hypertrophy, bladder-neck obstruction, narrow-angle glaucoma, stenosing peptic ulcer, pyloroduodenal obstruction

Do not confuse:
dimenhyDRINATE/
diphenhydrAMINE

Pharmacokinetics:

IM/PO: Duration 4-6 hr

Interactions:
- ↑ effect: alcohol, other CNS depressants

↑ anticholinergic effect: corkwood, henbane

↑ effect: hops, Jamaican dogwood, khat, senega

Lab test interferences:

False negative: Allergy skin testing

NURSING CONSIDERATIONS

Assess:
- VS, B/P; check patients with cardiac disease more often
- Signs of toxicity of other drugs or masking of symptoms of disease: brain tumor, intestinal obstruction
- Observe for drowsiness, dizziness

Administer:
- IM inj in large muscle mass; aspirate to avoid IV administration
- Tablets may be swallowed whole, chewed, or allowed to dissolve

IV route
- After diluting 50 mg/10 ml of NaCl inj; give 50 mg or less over 2 min

Additive compatibilities: Amika-

cin, calcium gluconate, chloramphenicol, corticotropin, erythromycin, heparin, hydrOXYzine, methicillin, norepinephrine, penicillin G potassium, pentobarbital, phenobarbital, potassium chloride, prochlorperazine, vancomycin, vit B/C
Syringe compatibilities: Atropine, diphenhydrAMINE, droperidol, fentanyl, heparin, hydromorphone, meperidine, metoclopramide, morphine, pentazocine, perphenazine, ranitidine, scopolamine
Y-site compatibilities: Acyclovir
• Therapeutic response: absence of nausea, vomiting
Teach patient/family:
• That a false-negative result may occur with skin testing; these procedures should not be scheduled for 4 days after discontinuing use
• To avoid hazardous activities, activities requiring alertness; dizziness may occur; instruct patient to request assistance with ambulation
• To avoid alcohol, other depressants

RARELY USED

dimercaprol (℞)

(dye-mer-cap'role)
BAL in Oil, British Anti-Lewisite♣, dimercaptopropanol
Func. class.: Heavy metal antagonist

Uses: Arsenic, gold, mercury, lead poisoning
Dosage and routes:
Severe gold/arsenic poisoning
• *Adult:* **IM** 3 mg/kg q4h × 2 days then qid × 1 day, then bid × 10 days
Mild gold/arsenic poisoning
• *Adult:* **IM** 2.5 mg/kg qid × 2 days, then bid × 1 day, then qd × 10 days
Acute lead poisoning
• *Adult:* **IM** 4 mg/kg, then q4h with edetate calcium disodium 12.5 mg/kg **IM,** not to exceed 5 mg/kg/dose
Mercury poisoning
• *Adult:* **IM** 5 mg/kg, then 2.5 mg/kg/day or bid × 10 days
Contraindications: Hypersensitivity, anuria, hepatic insufficiency, poisoning of other metals (iron, cadmium, selenium), severe renal disease, child <3 yr, pregnancy (D)

dinoprostone (℞)

(dye-noe-prost'one)
Cervidil Vaginal Insert, Prepidil, Endocervical Gel, Prostin E Vaginal Suppository
Func. class.: Oxytocic, abortifacient
Chem. class.: Prostaglandin E_2

Action: Stimulates uterine contractions, causing abortion; acts within 30 hr for complete abortion
Uses: Abortion during 2nd trimester, benign hydatidiform mole, expulsion of uterine contents in fetal deaths to 28 wk, missed abortion, to efface and dilate the cervix in pregnancy at term
Dosage and routes:
Abortifacient
• *Adult:* **VAG SUPP** 20 mg, repeat q3-5h until abortion occurs, max dose is 240 mg
Cervical ripening
• *Adult:* **GEL** warm to room temperature, choose correct length shielded catheter (10 or 20 mm), fill catheter by pushing plunger; patient should remain recumbent for 15-30 min; insert one 10 mg insert
Available forms: Vag supp 20 mg;

gel 0.5 mg/3 g (prefilled syringe); 10 mg insert

Side effects/adverse reactions:

CNS: Headache, dizziness, chills, fever

CV: Hypotension, ***dysrhythmias***

GI: Nausea, vomiting, diarrhea

GU: Vaginitis, vaginal pain, vulvitis, vaginismus

INTEG: Rash, skin color changes

MS: Leg cramps, joint swelling, weakness

EENT: Blurred vision

INSERT: Uterine hyperstimulation, fever, nausea, vomiting, diarrhea, abdominal pain

GEL: Uterine contractile abnormality, GI side effects, back pain, fever

FETAL: Bradycardia (i.e., deceleration)

SUPPOSITORY: ***Uterine rupture, anaphylaxis***

Contraindications: Hypersensitivity, uterine fibrosis, cervical stenosis, pelvic surgery, pelvic inflammatory disease, respiratory disease

Precautions: Hepatic disease, renal disease, cardiac disease, asthma, anemia, jaundice, diabetes mellitus, convulsive disorders, hypertension, hypotension, pregnancy (C)

Do not confuse:

Prepidil/bepridil

Interactions

- ↑ effect: other oxytocics
- ↓ oxytocic effect: alcohol

Pharmacokinetics:

SUPP: Onset 10 min, duration 2-3 hr; metabolized in spleen, kidney, lungs; excreted in urine

NURSING CONSIDERATIONS

Assess:

- Dilation, effacement of cervix and uterine contraction, fetal heart tones, check for contractions over 1 min
- For fever that occurs ½ hr after suppository insertion (abortion)
- Respiratory rate, rhythm, depth; notify prescriber of abnormalities, pulse, B/P, temp
- Vaginal discharge: check for itching, irritation; indicates vaginal infection
- For fever, chills: increase fluids or give tepid sponge bath or blanket

Administer:

- By gel: after warming to room temp, remove seal from end of syringe, and remove the protective end cap and insert into plunger stopper assembly; make sure patient is in dorsal position

Antiemetic/antidiarrheal before administration of this drug

Evaluate:

- Therapeutic response: expulsion of fetus

Teach patient/family:

- To remain supine for 10-15 min after insertion of supp 2 hr after insert, 15-30 min after gel
- To report excessive cramping, bleeding, chills, fever
- Some methods of pain, comfort control

* diphenhydrAMINE (OTC, ℞)

(dye-fen-hye'dra-meen)

Allerdryl✦, AllerMax✦, Allermed, Banophen, Benadryl, Benadryl 25, Benadryl Kapseals, Benahist 10, Benahist 50, Ben-Allergin-50, Benoject-10, Benoject-50, Benylin Cough, Bydramine, Compoz, Diphenadryl, Diphen Cough, Diphenhist, diphenhydrAMINE HCl, Dormin, Genahist, Hydramine, Hydramyn, Hydril, Hyrexin-50, Insomnal✦, Nidryl, Nighttime Sleep Aid, Nordryl, Nordryl Cough, Nytol, Phendry, Siladryl, Sleep-Eze 3, Sominex 2, Tusstat, Twilite, Uni-Bent Cough, Wehdryl

Func. class.: Antihistamine (1st generation, nonselective)

Chem. class.: Ethanolamine derivative, H_1-receptor antagonist

Action: Acts on blood vessels, GI, respiratory system by competing with histamine for H_1-receptor site; decreases allergic response by blocking histamine

Uses: Allergy symptoms, rhinitis, motion sickness, antiparkinsonism, nighttime sedation, infant colic, nonproductive cough

Dosage and routes:

• *Adult:* **PO** 25-50 mg q4-6h, not to exceed 400 mg/day; **IM/IV** 10-50 mg, not to exceed 400 mg/day

• *Child >12 kg:* **PO/IM/IV** 5 mg/kg/day in 4 divided doses, not to exceed 300 mg/day

Nighttime sleep aid

• *Adult and child ≥12 yr:* **PO** 25-50 mg hs

Antitussive (syrup only)

• *Adult and child ≥12 yr:* 25 mg q4h, max 100 mg/24 hr

• *Child 6-12 yr:* 12.5 mg q4h, max 50 mg/24 hr

• *Child 2-6 yr:* 6.25 mg q4h, max 25 mg/24 hr

Renal disease

• CCr 10-50 ml/min dose q6-12h; CCr <10 ml/min dose q12-18h

Available forms: Caps 25, 50 mg; tabs 25, 50 mg; chew tabs 25 mg; elix 12.5 mg/5 ml; syr 12.5 mg/5 ml; inj 10, 50 mg/ml

Side effects/adverse reactions:

CNS: Dizziness, drowsiness, poor coordination, fatigue, anxiety, euphoria, confusion, paresthesia, neuritis, ***seizures***

RESP: Increased thick secretions, wheezing, chest tightness

HEMA: ***Thrombocytopenia, agranulocytosis, hemolytic anemia***

GI: Nausea, anorexia, diarrhea

INTEG: Photosensitivity

GU: Retention, dysuria, frequency

EENT: Blurred vision, dilated pupils, tinnitus, nasal stuffiness, dry nose, throat, mouth

MISC: ***Anaphylaxis***

Contraindications: Hypersensitivity to H_1-receptor antagonist, acute asthma attack, lower respiratory tract disease

Precautions: Increased intraocular pressure, renal disease, cardiac disease, hypertension, bronchial asthma, seizure disorder, stenosed peptic ulcers, hyperthyroidism, prostatic hypertrophy, bladder neck obstruction, pregnancy (B), lactation

Do not confuse:

diphenhydrAMINE/dicyclomine
diphenhydrAMINE/dimenhyDRINATE

Pharmacokinetics:

PO: Peak 1-3 hr, duration 4-7 hr

IM: Onset ½ hr, peak 1-4 hr, duration 4-7 hr; *IV:* Onset immediate, duration 4-7 hr; metabolized in liver, excreted by kidneys; crosses placenta, excreted in breast milk; half-life 2-7 hr

Interactions:

• ↑ CNS depression: barbiturates, opiates, hypnotics, tricyclics, alcohol

• ↑ diphenhydrAMINE effect: MAOIs

↑ anticholinergic effect: corkwood, henbane

↑ effect: hops, Jamaican dogwood, khat, senega

Lab test interferences:

False negatives: Skin allergy tests

NURSING CONSIDERATIONS

Assess:

• Be alert for urinary retention, frequency, dysuria; drug should be discontinued

• CBC during long-term therapy; blood dyscrasias may occur

• Respiratory status: rate, rhythm, increase in bronchial secretions, wheezing, chest tightness

Administer:

• With meals for GI symptoms; absorption may slightly decrease

• Deep IM in large muscle; rotate site

• hs only if using for sleep aid

IV route

• Undiluted; give 25 mg/1 min

Additive compatibilities: Amikacin, aminophylline, ascorbic acid, bleomycin, cephapirin, erythromycin, hydrocortisone, lidocaine, methicillin, methyldopate, nafcillin, netilmicin, penicillin G potassium, penicillin G sodium, polymyxin B, vit B/C

Syringe compatibilities: Atropine, butorphanol, chlorproMAZINE, cimetidine, dimenhyDRINATE, droperidol, fentanyl, fluphenazine, glycopyrrolate, hydromorphone, hydrOXYzine, meperidine, metoclopramide, midazolam, morphine, nalbuphine, pentazocine, perphenazine, prochlorperazine, promazine, promethazine, ranitidine, scopolamine, sufentanil, thiothixene

Y-site compatibilities: Acyclovir, aldesleukin, amifostine, amsacrine, aztreonam, ciprofloxacin, cisatracurium, cisplatin, cladribine, cyclophosphamide, cytarabine, DOXOrubicin, DOXOrubicin liposome, famotidine, filgrastim, fluconazole, fludarabine, gallium, granisetron, heparin, hydrocortisone, idarubicin, melphalan, meperidine, meropenem, methotrexate, ondansetron, paclitaxel, piperacillin/tazobactam, potassium chloride, propofol, remifentanil, sargramostim, sufentanil, tacrolimus teniposide, thiotepa, vinorelbine, vit B/C

Perform/provide:

• Hard candy, gum, frequent rinsing of mouth for dryness

• Storage in tight container at room temperature

Evaluate:

• Therapeutic response: absence of running or congested nose or rashes, improved sleep

Teach patient/family:

• All aspects of drug use; to notify prescriber of confusion, sedation, hypotension

• To avoid driving, other hazardous activity if drowsiness occurs

• That photosensitivity may occur

• To avoid concurrent use of alcohol, other CNS depressants

Treatment of overdose: Administer ipecac syrup or lavage, diazepam, vasopressors, barbiturates (short-acting)

diphenoxylate/ atropine (℞)

(dye-fen-ox'ee-late a'troe-peen)

Logene, Lomanate, Lomotil, Lonox

Func. class.: Antidiarrheal

Chem. class.: Phenylpiperidine derivative opiate agonist

Controlled Substance Schedule IV (US)

Action: Inhibits gastric motility by acting on mucosal receptors responsible for peristalsis

Uses: Acute nonspecific and acute exacerbations of chronic functional diarrhea

Dosage and routes:

• *Adult:* **PO** 5 mg qid titrated to patient response needed, not to exceed 8 tabs/24 hr

• *Child 2-12 yr:* **PO** 0.3-0.4 mg/kg/ day in divided dose

Available forms: Tabs 2.5 mg with atropine 0.025 mg; liquid 2.5 mg with atropine 0.025 mg/5 ml

Side effects/adverse reactions:

RESP: ***Respiratory depression***

MISC: ***Anaphylaxis, angioedema***

CNS: Dizziness, drowsiness, lightheadedness, headache, fatigue, nervousness, insomnia, confusion

GI: Nausea, vomiting, dry mouth, epigastric distress, constipation, ***paralytic ileus***

EENT: Burning eyes, blurred vision

Contraindications: Hypersensitivity, pseudomembranous enterocolitis, jaundice, glaucoma, child <2 yr, severe electrolyte imbalances, diarrhea associated with organisms that penetrate intestinal mucosa

Precautions: Hepatic disease, renal disease, ulcerative colitis, pregnancy (C), lactation, severe liver disease

Do not confuse:

Lomotil/Lamictal/Lamasil

Lomotil/Lanoxin

Lomotil/Lasix

Pharmacokinetics:

PO: Onset 40-60 min, peak 2 hr, duration 3-4 hr, terminal half-life 12-14 hr; metabolized in liver to inactive metabolite; excreted in urine, feces

Interactions:

• Do not use with MAOIs; hypertensive crisis may occur

• ↑ action of: alcohol, opioids, barbiturates, other CNS depressants, anticholinergics

• ↑ antidiarrheal action: nutmeg

NURSING CONSIDERATIONS

Assess:

• Electrolytes (K, Na, Cl) if on long-term therapy

• Bowel pattern before; for rebound constipation after termination of medication; bowel sounds

• Response after 48 hr; if none, drug should be discontinued

• Abdominal distention, toxic megacolon, which may occur in ulcerative colitis

• Hepatic studies if on long-term therapy

Administer:

• For 48 hr only; if no response, drug should be discontinued

Evaluate:

• Therapeutic response: decreased diarrhea

Teach patient/family:

• To avoid OTC products unless directed by prescriber (may contain alcohol); do not use alcohol or CNS depressants

• Not to exceed recommended dose

• That drug may be habit forming

• Not to engage in hazardous activities; drowsiness may occur, not to use for longer than 48 hr for acute diarrhea

dipivefrin ophthalmic

See appendix c

dipyridamole (℞)

(dye-peer-id′a-mole)

Apo-Dipyridamole, dipyridamole, Novo-Dipiradol, Persantine, Persantine IV

Func. class.: Coronary vasodilator, antiplatelet agent

Chem. class.: Nonnitrate

Action: Inhibits adenosine uptake, which produces coronary vasodilation; increases oxygen saturation in coronary tissues, coronary blood flow; acts on small resistance vessels with little effect on vascular resistance; may increase development of collateral circulation; decreases platelet aggregation by the inhibition of phosphodiesterase (an enzyme)

Uses: Prevention of transient ischemic attacks, inhibition of platelet adhesion to prevent myocardial reinfarction, thromboembolism, with warfarin in prosthetic heart valves, prevention of coronary bypass graft occlusion with aspirin; IV form used to evaluate coronary artery disease; used as alternative to exercise in thallium myocardial perfusion imaging to evaluate coronary artery disease

Dosage and routes:

TIA

• *Adult:* **PO** 50 mg tid, 1 hr ac, not to exceed 400 mg qd

Inhibition of platelet adhesion

• *Adult:* **PO** 50-75 mg qid in combination with aspirin or warfarin thallium myocardial perfusion imaging

• *Adult:* **IV** 570 mcg/kg

Available forms: Tabs 25, 50, 75 mg; inj 10 mg/2 ml

Side effects/adverse reactions:

CV: Postural hypotension; IV: ***MI***

CNS: Headache, dizziness, weakness, fainting, syncope; IV: transient cerebral ischemia, weakness

RESP: IV: ***Bronchospasm***

GI: Nausea, vomiting, anorexia, diarrhea

INTEG: Rash, flushing

Contraindications: Hypersensitivity

Precautions: Pregnancy (B), lactation, hypotension

Pharmacokinetics:

PO: Peak 1.25 hr, duration 6 hr; therapeutic response may take several months; metabolized in liver; excreted in bile; undergoes enterohepatic recirculation

Interactions:

• Prevention of coronary vasodilation: theophylline

• ↑ bleeding risk: NSAIDs, cefamandole, cefotetan, cefoperazone, plicamycin, valproic acid, sulfinpyrazole, anticoagulants, thrombolytics

↓ antiplatelet effect: bilberry, saw palmetto

Gastric irritation: arginine

↑ antiplatelet effect: bogbean, dong quai, feverfew, ginger, ginkgo

NURSING CONSIDERATIONS

Assess:

• B/P, pulse during treatment until stable; take B/P lying, standing; orthostatic hypotension is common

• Cardiac status: chest pain, what aggravates or ameliorates condition

Administer:

IV route

• IV after diluting to at least 1:2 ratio using D_5W, 0.45% NaCl, or 0.9% NaCl to a total vol of 20-50 ml; give over 4 min; do not give undiluted

PO route
• On an empty stomach: 1 hr before meals or 2 hr after; give with 8 oz water for better absorption
Perform/provide:
• Storage at room temperature
Evaluate:
• Therapeutic response: decreased chest pain (angina), decreased platelet adhesion
Teach patient/family:
• That medication is not a cure; may have to be taken continuously in evenly spaced doses only as directed
• To avoid hazardous activities until stabilized on medication; dizziness may occur
• To rise slowly from sitting or lying to prevent orthostatic hypotension
• Not to use alcohol or OTC medications unless approved by prescriber
Treatment of overdose: Administer IV phenylephrine

dirithromycin (℞)
(dye-rith-roe-mye'sin)
Dynabac
Func. class.: Antiinfective
Chem. class.: Macrolide

Action: Binds to 50S ribosomal subunits of susceptible bacteria, suppresses protein synthesis
Uses: Infections of the respiratory tract caused by *Moraxella catarrhalis, Streptococcus* sp. *(S. pneumoniae, S. agalactiae, S. viridans), Legionella pneumophilia, Mycoplasma pneumoniae, Streptococcus pyogenes, Staphylococcus aureus, Bordetella pertussis*
Dosage and routes:
• *Adult:* **PO** 500 mg qd, given for 7-14 days depending on infections
Available forms: Tabs, enteric coated 250 mg

Side effects/adverse reactions:
GI: Abdominal pain, nausea, diarrhea, vomiting, dyspepsia, GI disorders, flatulence, abnormal stools, anorexia, constipation, ***pseudomembranous colitis***
CNS: Headache, dizziness, insomnia
HEMA: Increased platelet count, increased eosinophils
RESP: Cough, dyspnea
INTEG: Pruritus, urticaria
Contraindications: Hypersensitivity to this drug or any other macrolide, or erythromycin, bacteremias
Precautions: Pregnancy (C), lactation, children, hepatic, renal disease
Do not confuse:
Dynabac/DynaCirc
Pharmacokinetics: Rapidly absorbed, widely distributed, no hepatic metabolism, excreted in bile, feces (up to 97%), plasma half-life 8 hr, terminal 44 hr
Interactions:
• Absorption of dirithromycin slightly enhanced: antacids, H_2-antagonists
• May alter effect of: theophylline
• Drug/food: ↑ absorption with food
Do not use acidophilus with antiinfectives

NURSING CONSIDERATIONS
Assess:
• Report hematuria, oliguria
• Hepatic studies: AST, ALT if on long-term therapy
• Renal studies: Urinalysis, protein, blood if on long-term therapy
• C&S before drug therapy; drug may be given as soon as culture is taken; C&S may be repeated after treatment
• Bowel pattern before, during treatment; pseudomembranous colitis may occur
• Skin eruptions, itching

• Respiratory status: rate, character, wheezing, tightness in chest; discontinue drug

Administer:

• Adequate intake of fluids (2 L) during diarrhea episodes

Whole; do not break, crush, or chew tablets

• With food or within 1 hr of food at same time each day

Perform/provide:

• Storage at room temperature, in tight container

Evaluate:

• Therapeutic response: C&S negative for infection

Teach patient/family:

• To take with full glass of water; to give with food

• To report sore throat, fever, fatigue; may indicate superinfection

• To notify prescriber of diarrhea stools, dark urine, pale stools, jaundiced eyes or skin, severe abdominal pain

• To take at evenly spaced intervals; complete dosage regimen

Treatment of hypersensitivity: Withdraw drug, maintain airway, administer epinephrine, aminophylline, O_2, IV corticosteroids

disopyramide (℞)

(dye-soe-peer′a-mide)

disopyramide, Norpace, Norpace CR, Rhythmodan

Func. class.: Antidysrhythmic (Class IA)

Chem. class.: Nonnitrate

Action: Prolongs duration of action potential and effective refractory period; reduces disparity in refractory period between normal and infarcted myocardium; prevents increased myocardial excitability and conduction contractility

Uses: PVCs, ventricular tachycardia, supraventricular tachycardia, atrial flutter, fibrillation

Investigational uses: Supraventricular tachycardia (prevention, treatment)

Dosage and routes:

Renal disease

• CCr 30-40 ml/min dose q8h; CCr 15-30 ml/min dose q12h; CCr <15 ml/min dose q24h

• *Adult:* **PO** 100-200 mg q6h, **CONT REL CAPS** 200-400 mg q12h

• *Child 12-18 yr:* **PO** 6-15 mg/kg/day, in divided doses q6h

• *Child 4-12 yr:* **PO** 10-15 mg/kg/day in divided doses q6h

• *Child 1-4 yr:* **PO** 10-20 mg/kg/day in divided doses q6h

• *Child <1 yr:* **PO** 10-30 mg/kg/day, in divided doses q6h

Available forms: Caps 100, 150 mg; cont rel caps 100, 150 mg; tabs, sus rel 250 mg

Side effects/adverse reactions:

GU: Urinary retention, hesitancy, impotence

CNS: Headache, dizziness, psychosis, fatigue, depression, paresthesias, insomnia

GI: Dry mouth, constipation, nausea, anorexia, flatulence, diarrhea, vomiting

CV: Hypotension, bradycardia, angina, PVCs, tachycardia, increased QRS, QT segments, ***cardiac arrest,*** edema, weight gain, AV block, ***CHF,*** syncope, chest pain

META: Hypoglycemia, hypokalemia

INTEG: Rash, pruritus, urticaria

MS: Weakness, pain in extremities

EENT: Blurred vision; dry nose, throat, eyes; narrow-angle glaucoma

HEMA: ***Thrombocytopenia, agranulocytosis,*** anemia (rare), decreased Hgb, Hct

Contraindications: Hypersensitiv-

ity, 2nd- or 3rd-degree block, cardiogenic shock, CHF (uncompensated), sick sinus syndrome, QT prolongation

Precautions: Pregnancy (C), lactation, diabetes mellitus, renal disease, children, hepatic disease, myasthenia gravis, narrow-angle glaucoma, cardiomyopathy, conduction abnormalities, potassium imbalance

Pharmacokinetics:

PO: Peak 30 min-3 hr, duration 6-12 hr; half-life 4-10 hr; metabolized in liver; excreted in feces, urine, breast milk; crosses placenta

Interactions:

• ↑ disopyramide effect: quinidine, procainamide, propranolol, lidocaine, atenolol, other antidysrhythmics, erythromycin

• ↑ side effects, urinary retention: anticholinergics

• ↓ disopyramide effect: phenytoin, rifampin, phenobarbital

↑ action: aloe, broom, buckthorn, cascara sagrada, Chinese rhubarb, figwort, fumitory, goldenseal, kudzu, licorice, senna

↓ antiarrhythmic action: coltsfoot

↑ serotonin effect: horehound

Toxicity/death: aconite

Lab test interferences:

Increase: Liver enzymes, lipids, BUN, creatinine

Decrease: Hgb/Hct, blood glucose

NURSING CONSIDERATIONS

Assess:

• Apical pulse for 1 min; if less than 60, check again in 1 hr; if still less than 60, notify prescriber

• ECG; check for increased QT, widening QRS; drug should be discontinued

• Weight daily; a rapid weight gain should be reported

• For dehydration or hypovolemia, I&O ratio, electrolytes (Na, K, Cl)

• Renal, hepatic studies (AST, ALT, bilirubin, BUN, creatinine) during treatment

• Diabetics for signs of hypoglycemia (rare)

• B/P continuously for hypotension, hypertension

• For rebound hypertension after 1-2 hr

• Constipation: increased bulk in diet, water, stool softeners, or laxatives needed

• Cardiac rate, respiration: rate, rhythm, character

• Urinary hesitancy, frequency, or a change in I&O ratio; check for edema daily; check for toxicity

Administer:

⊘ Do not break, crush, or chew sus rel cap; give 1 hr before or 2 hr after meals

• Sugar-free gum, frequent sips of water for dry mouth

• Reduced dosage slowly with ECG monitoring

Evaluate:

• Therapeutic response: decreased dysrhythmias

Teach patient/family:

• To take drug exactly as prescribed; if dose is missed, take within 3-4 hr of next dose; do not double dose

• To avoid alcohol, or severe hypotension may occur; to avoid OTC drugs, or serious drug interactions may occur

• To make position change slowly during early therapy to prevent orthostatic hypotension

• To avoid hazardous activities if dizziness or blurred vision occurs

• The importance of complying with drug regimen; tell patient that this drug does not cure condition

Treatment of overdose: O_2, artificial ventilation, ECG, dopamine for circulatory depression, diazepam or thiopental for convulsions, gastric lavage

RARELY USED

disulfiram (℞)

(dye-sul'fi-ram)

Antabuse, disulfiram

Func. class.: Alcohol deterrent

Uses: Chronic alcoholism (as adjunct)

Dosage and routes:

• *Adult:* **PO** 250-500 mg qd × 1-2 wk, then 125-500 mg qd until fully socially recovered

Contraindications: Hypersensitivity, alcohol intoxication, psychoses, CV disease, pregnancy (X), lactation

*DOBUTamine (℞)

(doe-byoo'ta-meen)

DOBUTamine, Dobutrex

Func. class.: Adrenergic direct-acting β_1-agonist, cardiac stimulant

Chem. class.: Catecholamine

Action: Causes increased contractility, increased cardiac output without marked increase in heart rate by acting on β_1-receptors in heart; minor α and β_2 effects

Uses: Cardiac decompensation due to organic heart disease or cardiac surgery

Investigational uses: Cardiogenic shock in children; congenital heart disease in children undergoing cardiac cath

Dosage and routes:

• *Adult:* **IV INF** 2.5-10 mcg/kg/min; may increase to 40 mcg/kg/min if needed

• *Child:* **IV INF** 5-20 mcg/kg/min over 10 min for cardiac cath

Available forms: Inj 12.5 mg/ml

Side effects/adverse reactions:

CNS: Anxiety, headache, dizziness

CV: Palpitations, tachycardia, hypertension, hypotension, PVCs, angina

GI: Heartburn, nausea, vomiting

MS: Muscle cramps (leg)

Contraindications: Hypersensitivity, idiopathic hypertrophic subaortic stenosis

Precautions: Pregnancy (B), lactation, children, hypertension

Do not confuse:

DOBUTamine/DOPamine

Dobutrex/Diamox

Pharmacokinetics:

IV: Onset 1-2 min, peak 10 min, half-life 2 min; metabolized in liver (inactive metabolites); excreted in urine

Interactions:

• Severe hypertension: guanethidine

• Dysrhythmias: general anesthetics, bretylium

• ↓ DOBUTamine action: other β-blockers

• ↑ pressor effect, dysrhythmias: tricyclics, MAOIs, oxytocics

NURSING CONSIDERATIONS

Assess:

• Hypovolemia; if present, correct first; administer cardiac glycoside before DOBUTamine

• Oxygenation/perfusion deficit (check B/P, chest pain, dizziness, loss of consciousness)

• Heart failure: S_3 gallop, dyspnea, neck vein distention, bibasilar crackles in patients with CHF, cardiomyopathy

• ECG during administration continuously; if B/P increases, drug is decreased; CVP or PWP, cardiac output during infusion

• Serum electrolytes, urine output

◆ Sulfite sensitivity, which may be life-threatening

Administer:

IV route

• Diluting each 250 mg/10 ml of sterile H_2O or D_5W for inj; may be further diluted in 50 ml or more given at prescribed rate; should be gradually increased to desired rate; use a CVP catheter or large peripheral vein, use inf pump, titrate to patient response

• Change IV site q48h

• Plasma expanders for hypovolemia

Additive compatibilities: Amiodarone, atracurium, atropine, DOPamine, enalaprilat, epINEPHrine, flumazenil, hydralazine, isoproterenol, lidocaine, meperidine, meropenem, metaraminol, morphine, nitroglycerin, norepinephrine, phentolamine, phenylephrine, procainamide, propranolol, ranitidine

Syringe compatibilities: Heparin, ranitidine

Y-site compatibilities: Amifostine, amiodarone, amrinone, atracurium, aztreonam, bretylium, calcium chloride, calcium gluconate, ciprofloxacin, cisatracurium, cladribine, diazepam, diltiazem, DOPamine, doxorubicin liposome, enalaprilat, epINEPHrine, famotidine, fentanyl, fluconazole, granisetron, haloperidol, hydromorphone, insulin (regular), labetalol, lidocaine, lorazepam, magnesium sulfate, meperidine, milrinone, morphine, niCARdipine, nitroglycerin, norepinephrine, pancuronium, potassium chloride, propofol, ranitidine, remifentanil, sodium nitroprusside, streptokinase, tacrolimus, theophylline, thiotepa, tolazoline, vecuronium, verapamil, zidovudine

Perform/provide:

• Storage of reconstituted solution for 24 hr if refrigerated

Evaluate:

• Therapeutic response: increased B/P with stabilization, increased urine output

Teach patient/family:

• The reason for drug administration; to report dyspnea, chest pain, numbness of extremities, headache, IV site discomfort

Treatment of overdose: Administer a β_1-adrenergic blocker; reduce IV or discontinue, ensure oxygenation/ventilation; for severe tachydysrhythmias (ventricular) give lidocaine or propranolol

docosanol topical

See appendix c

docusate calcium (OTC)

(dok'yoo-sate cal'see-um)

DC Softgels, Pro-Cal-Sof, Sulfalax Calcium, Surfak

docusate sodium (OTC)

Colace, Correctol Extra Gentle, Dialose, Diocto, Dioeze, Disonate, Di-Sosul, DOK, DOS, D-S-S, Ex-Lax, Modane, Regulax SS, Regulex♣, Silace

Func. class.: Laxative, emollient

Chem. class.: Anionic surfactant

Action: Increases water, fat penetration in intestine; allows for easier passage of stool

Uses: To soften stools

Dosage and routes:

• *Adult:* **PO** 50-300 mg qd (sodium) or 240 mg (calcium or potassium) prn; **ENEMA** 5 ml (sodium)

• *Child >12 yr:* **ENEMA** 2 ml (sodium)

• *Child 6-12 yr:* **PO** 40-120 mg qd (sodium)
• *Child 3-6 yr:* **PO** 20-60 mg qd (sodium)
• *Child <3 yr:* **PO** 10-40 mg qd (sodium)

Available forms: *Calcium:* caps 50, 240 mg; *sodium:* caps 50, 100, 240, 250 mg; tabs 50, 100 mg; syr 20 mg/5 ml, 50, 60/15 ml; liq 150 mg/15 ml; oral sol 10, 50 mg/ml; enema 283 mg/3.9 cap

Side effects/adverse reactions:
GI: Nausea, anorexia, cramps, diarrhea
INTEG: Rash
EENT: Bitter taste, throat irritation

Contraindications: Hypersensitivity, obstruction, fecal impaction, nausea/vomiting

Precautions: Pregnancy (C), lactation

Pharmacokinetics: Onset 24-72 hr

Interactions:
• Toxicity: mineral oil
↑ laxative action: flax, senna

NURSING CONSIDERATIONS

Assess:
• Cause of constipation; identify whether fluids, bulk, or exercise are missing from lifestyle
• Cramping, rectal bleeding, nausea, vomiting; if these symptoms occur, drug should be discontinued

Administer:
• In milk, fruit juice to decrease bitter taste
• In morning or evening (oral dose)

Perform/provide:
• Storage in cool environment; do not freeze

Evaluate:
• Therapeutic response: decrease in constipation

Teach patient/family:
To swallow tabs whole; do not break, crush, or chew
• That normal bowel movements do not always occur daily
• Not to use in presence of abdominal pain, nausea, vomiting
• To notify prescriber if constipation unrelieved or if symptoms of electrolyte imbalance occur: muscle cramps, pain, weakness, dizziness, excessive thirst
• Inform patient that drug may take up to 3 days to soften stools
• Take oral prep with a full glass of water unless on fluid restrictions and increase fluid intake

dofetilide (℞)

Tikosyn

Func. class.: Antidysrhythmic (Class III)

Action: Blocks cardiac ion channel carrying the rapid component of delayed potassium current, no effect on sodium channels

Uses: Atrial fibrillation, flutter, maintenance of normal sinus rhythm

Research note: One study has concluded that dofetilide can be used in structural heart disease to maintain sinus rhythm[8]

Dosage and routes:
• *Adult:* **PO** 125-500 mcg bid depending on CCr, may be adjusted q2-3h to get appropriate increase in QTc

Renal dose
• CCr >60 ml/min 500 mcg bid; CCr 40-60 ml/min 250 mcg bid; CCr 20-40 ml/min 125 mcg bid; CCr <20 ml/min do not use

Available forms: Caps 125, 250, 500 mcg

Side effects/adverse reactions:
CNS: Syncope, dizziness, headache
GI: Nausea, vomiting, severe diarrhea, anorexia
CV: Hypotension, postural hypotension, bradycardia, angina, PVCs, substernal pressure, transient hypertension, precipitation of angina

Contraindications: Hypersensitivity, digitalis toxicity, aortic stenosis, pulmonary hypertension, children, QT syndromes, severe renal disease
Precautions: Renal disease, pregnancy (C), lactation
Pharmacokinetics: Well absorbed, max plasma conc 2-3 hr, steady state 2-3 days, half-life 10 hr, metabolized by liver, excreted by kidneys
Interactions:
- ↑ hypokalemia: potassium-depleting diuretics
- Do not use with cimetidine, ketoconazole, verapamil, prochlorperazine, trimethoprim-sulfamethizole, amiloride, metformin, megestrol, triamterene

NURSING CONSIDERATIONS
Assess:
- ECG continuously to determine drug effectiveness, PVCs, other dysrhythmias; renal function, QTc q3mo; this drug is only available to facilities that have been educated in this administration, patient must be hospitalized
- B/P continuously for hypotension, hypertension; orthostatic hypotension; keep supine until hypotension subsides
- Cardiac status: rate, rhythm, character, continuously

Administer:
PO route
- For 3 days hospitalized
- Give dofetilide after withholding class I or III antidysrhythmic for 3 half-lives of dofetilide

Perform/provide:
- Place patient in supine position unless otherwise ordered; assist with ambulation

Evaluate:
- Therapeutic response: control in atrial fibrillation

Teach patient/family:
- To make position changes slowly; orthostatic hypotension may occur
- Notify prescriber if fast heartbeats with fainting or dizziness occur
- Notify all prescribers of all medications and supplements taken
- That if dose is missed, do not double, take next dose at usual time

D

dolasetron (℞)
(do-la′se-tron)
Anzemet
Func. class.: Antiemetic
Chem. class.: 5-HT3 receptor antagonist

Action: Prevents nausea, vomiting by blocking serotonin peripherally, centrally, and in the small intestine
Uses: Prevention of nausea, vomiting associated with cancer chemotherapy, radiotherapy, and prevention of postoperative nausea, vomiting
Investigational uses: Radiotherapy-induced nausea/vomiting
Dosage and routes:
Prevention of nausea/vomiting of cancer chemotherapy
- *Adult and child 2-16 yr:* **IV** 1.8 mg/kg as a single dose, ½ hr prior to chemotherapy
- *Adult:* **PO** 100 mg 1 hr prior to chemotherapy
- *Child 2-16 yr:* **PO** 1.8 mg/kg/hr prior to chemotherapy; max 100 mg

Prevention of postoperative nausea/vomiting
- *Adult:* **IV** 12.5 mg as a single dose, 15 min before cessation of anesthesia; **PO** 100 mg 2 hr before surgery (prevention only)
- *Child 2-16 yr:* **IV** 0.35 mg/kg as a single dose, 15 min before cessation of anesthesia; **PO** 1.2 mg/kg 2 hr before surgery (prevention only)

Available forms: Tabs 50, 100 mg; inj 20 mg/ml (12.5 mg/0.625 ml)

Side effects/adverse reactions:
GI: Diarrhea, constipation, increased AST, ALT, abdominal pain, anorexia
CNS: Headache, dizziness, fatigue, drowsiness
MISC: Rash, ***bronchospasm***
GU: Urinary retention, oliguria
CV: ***Dysrhythmias,*** ECG changes, hypotension, tachycardia, hypertension, bradycardia
Contraindications: Hypertensivity
Precautions: Pregnancy (B), lactation, children, elderly
Pharmacokinetics: Unknown
Interactions:
- Dysrhythmias: antidysrhythmics
- ↑ dolasetron levels: cimetidine
- ↓ dolasetron levels: rifampin

NURSING CONSIDERATIONS
Assess:
- For absence of nausea, vomiting during chemotherapy
- For hypersensitivity reaction: rash, bronchospasm
- For cardiac conduction conditions, electrolyte imbalances, or dysrhythmias

Administer:
- By inj 100 mg/½ min or less or diluted in 50 ml compatible sol; give over 15 min

Perform/provide:
- Storage at room temperature 48 hr after dilution

Evaluate:
- Therapeutic response: absence of nausea, vomiting during cancer chemotherapy

Teach patient/family:
- To report diarrhea, constipation, nausea, vomiting, rash, or changes in respirations
- Not to mix product for oral administration in juice until immediately before administration
- May cause headache, use analgesic

donepezil (℞)
(don-ep-ee'zill)
Aricept
Func. class.: Reversible cholinesterase inhibitor

Action: Elevates acetylcholine concentrations (cerebral cortex) by slowing degradation of acetylcholine released in cholinergic neurons; does not alter underlying dementia
Uses: Treatment of mild to moderate dementia in Alzheimer's disease
Dosage and routes:
- *Adult:* **PO** 5 mg qd hs; may increase to 10 mg qd after 4-6wk

Available forms: Tabs 5, 10 mg
Side effects/adverse reactions:
CNS: Dizziness, *insomnia,* somnolence, *headache,* fatigue, abnormal dreams, syncope, ***seizures***
GI: Nausea, vomiting, anorexia; *diarrhea*
GU: Urinary frequency, UTI, incontinence
INTEG: Rash, flushing
RESP: Rhinitis, URI, cough, pharyngitis
CV: ***Atrial fibrillation,*** hypotension or hypertension
MS: Cramps, arthritis
Contraindications: Hypersensitivity to this drug or piperidine derivatives
Precautions: Sick sinus syndrome, history of ulcers, GI bleeding, hepatic disease, bladder obstruction, asthma, pregnancy (C), lactation, children, seizures, asthma, COPD
Pharmacokinetics: Well absorbed PO, metabolized to metabolites, elimination half-life 10 hr single dose, 70 hr multiple dosing
Interactions:
- ↓ action of: anticholinergics

• Synergistic effect: succinylcholine, cholinesterase inhibitors, cholinergic agonists
• ↑ gastric acid secretions: NSAIDs
• ↓ donepezil effect: carbamazepine, dexamethasone, phenytoin, phenobarbital, rifampin

NURSING CONSIDERATIONS

Assess:
• B/P: hypotension, hypertension
• Mental status: affect, mood, behavioral changes, depression, complete suicide assessment
• GI status: nausea, vomiting, anorexia, diarrhea
• GU status: urinary frequency, incontinence

Administer:
• Between meals; may be given with meals for GI symptoms
• Dosage adjusted to response no more than q6wk

Perform/provide:
• Assistance with ambulation during beginning therapy; dizziness, ataxia may occur

Evaluate:
• Therapeutic response: decrease in confusion, improved mood

Teach patient/family:
• To report side effects: twitching, nausea, vomiting, sweating; indicates overdose
• To use drug exactly as prescribed; at regular intervals, preferably between meals; may be taken with meals for GI upset
• To notify prescriber of nausea, vomiting, diarrhea (dose increase or beginning treatment), or rash
• Not to increase or abruptly decrease dose; serious consequences may result
• That drug is not a cure, relieves symptoms

Treatment of overdose: Withdraw drug, administer tertiary anticholinergics, provide supportive care

HIGH ALERT

*DOPamine (℞)

(doe′pa-meen)

dopamine HCl, Intropin, Revimine✤

Func. class.: Adrenergic

Chem. class.: Catecholamine

Action: Causes increased cardiac output; acts on β_1- and α-receptors, causing vasoconstriction in blood vessels; low dose causes renal and mesenteric vasodilation; β_1 stimulation produces inotropic effects with increased cardiac output

Uses: Shock; increased perfusion; hypotension

Unlabeled uses: COPD, RDS in infants

Dosage and routes:

Shock
• *Adult:* **IV INF** 2-5 mcg/kg/min, not to exceed 50 mcg/kg/min, titrate to patient's response
• *Child:* **IV** 5-20 mcg/kg/min adjust depending on response

COPD
• *Adult:* **IV** 4 mcg/kg/min

CHF
• *Adult:* **IV** 2-5 mcg/kg/min

RDS
• *Infant:* **IV** 5 mcg/kg/min

Available forms: Inj 40 mg, 80 mg, 160 mg/ml conc for IV inf; 0.8, 1.6, 3.2 mg/ml in D_5W

Side effects/adverse reactions:

CNS: Headache

CV: Palpitations, tachycardia, hypertension, ectopic beats, angina, wide QRS complex, peripheral vasoconstriction

GI: Nausea, vomiting, diarrhea

INTEG: Necrosis, tissue sloughing with extravasation, ***gangrene***

RESP: Dyspnea

Contraindications: Hypersensitiv-

ity, ventricular fibrillation, tachydysrhythmias, pheochromocytoma

Precautions: Pregnancy (C), lactation, arterial embolism, peripheral vascular disease

Do not confuse:

DOPamine/DOBUTamine

Pharmacokinetics:

IV: Onset 5 min, duration <10 min; metabolized in liver, kidney, plasma, excreted in urine (metabolites), half-life 2 min

Interactions:

- Do not use within 2 wk of MAOIs, phenytoin; hypertensive crisis may result
- Dysrhythmias: general anesthetics
- Severe hypertension: ergots
- ↓ DOPamine action: β-blockers, α-blockers
- ↑ B/P: oxytocics
- ↑ pressor effect: tricyclics, MAOIs

Lab test interferences:

Increase: Urinary catecholamine, serum glucose

NURSING CONSIDERATIONS

Assess:

- Hypovolemia; if present, correct first
- Oxygenation/perfusion deficit (check B/P, chest pain, dizziness, loss of consciousness)
- Heart failure: S_3 gallop, dyspnea, neck vein distention, bibasilar crackles in patients with CHF, cardiomyopathy
- I&O ratio: if urine output decreases, without decrease in B/P, drug may need to be reduced
- ECG during administration continuously; if B/P increases, drug should be decreased
- B/P and pulse q5min after parenteral route
- CVP or PWP during infusion if possible
- Paresthesias and coldness of extremities; peripheral blood flow may decrease
- Injection site: tissue sloughing; if this occurs, administer phentolamine mixed with NS

Administer:

IV route

- Plasma expanders or whole blood for hypovolemia
- IV after diluting 200-400 mg/250-500 ml of D_5W, D_5 0.45% NaCl, D_5 0.9% NaCl, D_5LR, LR
- Parenteral IV dose slowly; after reconstituting, use infusion pump; flush line before infusing; infuse as secondary IV line

Additive compatibilities: Aminophylline, atracurium, bretylium, calcium chloride, cephalothin, chloramphenicol, DOBUTamine, enalaprilat, flumazenil, heparin, hydrocortisone, kanamycin, lidocaine, meropenem, methylPREDNISolone, nitroglycerin, oxacillin, potassium chloride, ranitidine, verapamil

Syringe compatibilities: Doxapram, heparin, ranitidine

Y-site compatibilities: Aldesleukin, amifostine, amiodarone, amrinone, atracurium, aztreonam, cefmetazole, cefpirome, ciprofloxacin, cisatracurium, cladribine, diltiazem, DOBUTamine, doxorubicin liposome, enalaprilat, epINEPHrine, esmolol, famotidine, fentanyl, fluconazole, foscarnet, granisetron, haloperidol, heparin, hydrocortisone, hydromorphone, labetalol, lidocaine, lorazepam, meperidine, methylPREDNISolone, metronidazole, midazolam, milrinone, morphine, niCARdipine, nitroglycerin, norepinephrine, ondansetron, pancuronium, piperacillin/tazobactam, potassium chloride, propofol, ranitidine, remifentanil, sargramostim, sodium nitroprusside, streptokinase, tacrolimus, theophylline, thiotepa, tolazoline, vecuronium, verapamil, vit B/C, warfarin, zidovudine

Perform/provide:
- Storage of reconstituted sol for up to 24 hr if refrigerated
- Do not use discolored sol; protect from light

Evaluate:
- Therapeutic response: increased B/P with stabilization; increased urine output

Teach patient/family:
- The reason for drug administration

Treatment of overdose: Discontinue IV, may give a short-acting α-adrenergic blocker

RARELY USED

dornase alfa (℞)

(door′nace alfa)

Pulmozyme

Func. class.: Cystic fibrosis agent (orphan drug)

Uses: Management of cystic fibrosis

Dosage and routes:
- *Adult/child >5 yr:* **INH** 2.5 mg qd by nebulizer

Contraindications: Hypersensitivity to this drug or Chinese hamster ovary cell products
- About all aspects of drug; avoid smoking, smoke-filled rooms, persons with respiratory infections

dorzolamide ophthalmic

See appendix c

RARELY USED/HIGH ALERT

doxacurium (℞)

(dox-a-cure′ee-um)

Nuromax

Func. class.: Neuromuscular blocker (nondepolarizing)

Uses: Facilitation of endotracheal intubation, skeletal muscle relaxation during mechanical ventilation, surgery, or general anesthesia

Dosage and routes:
- *Adult:* **IV** 0.05 mg/kg; 0.08 mg/kg is used for prolonged neuromuscular blockade; maintenance 0.025 mg/kg
- *Child 2-12 yr:* **IV** 0.03-0.05 mg/kg; may decrease for maintenance dose

Contraindications: Hypersensitivity, neonates

doxapram (℞)

(dox′a-pram)

Dopram

Func. class.: Analeptic

Action: Respiratory stimulation through activation of peripheral carotid chemoreceptor; with higher doses, medullary respiratory centers are stimulated; with progressive CNS stimulation

Uses: Chronic obstructive pulmonary disease (COPD), postanesthesia respiratory depression, prevention of acute hypercapnia, drug-induced CNS depression

Investigational uses:
- Treatment of apnea in premature infants when methylxanthines have failed

Dosage and routes:

Postanesthesia
- *Adult:* **IV** inj 0.5-1 mg/kg, not to

exceed 1.5 mg/kg total as a single injection; **IV INF** 250 mg in 250 ml sol, not to exceed 4 mg/kg; run at 1-3 mg/min

Drug-induced CNS depression

• *Adult:* **IV** priming dose of 2 mg/kg, repeated in 5 min; repeat q1-2h till patient awakes; **IV INF** priming dose 2 mg/kg at 1-3 mg/min, not to exceed 3 g/day

COPD (Hypercapnia)

• *Adult:* **IV INF** 1-2 mg/min, not to exceed 3 mg/min for no longer than 2 hr

Apnea of premature infant

• *Infant:* **IV** 1-1.5 mg/kg/hr loading dose followed by infusion of 0.5-2.5 mg/kg/hr

Available forms: Inj 20 mg/ml

Side effects/adverse reactions:

CNS: ***Convulsions,*** (clonus/generalized), *headache,* restlessness, dizziness, confusion, paresthesias, flushing, sweating, bilateral Babinski's sign, rigidity, depression

GI: Nausea, vomiting, diarrhea, desire to defecate

GU: Retention, incontinence, elevation of BUN, albuminuria

CV: Chest pain, hypertension, change in heart rate, lowered T waves, tachycardia, ***dysrhythmias***

INTEG: Pruritus, irritation at inj site

EENT: Pupil dilation, sneezing

RESP: ***Laryngospasm, bronchospasm,*** rebound hypoventilation, dyspnea, cough, tachypnea, hiccups

Contraindications: Hypersensitivity, seizure disorders, severe hypertension, severe bronchial asthma, severe dyspnea, severe cardiac disorders, pneumothorax, pulmonary embolism, severe respiratory disease

Precautions: Bronchial asthma, pheochromocytoma, severe tachycardia, dysrhythmias, pregnancy (B), hypertension, lactation, children

Pharmacokinetics:

IV: Onset 20-40 sec, peak 1-2 min, duration 5-10 min; metabolized by liver; excreted by kidneys (metabolites); half-life 2.5-4 hr

Interactions:

• Synergistic pressor effect: MAOIs, sympathomimetics

• Cardiac dysrhythmias: halothane, cyclopropane, enflurane; delay use of doxapram for at least 10 min after inhalation anesthetics

NURSING CONSIDERATIONS

Assess:

• BP, heart rate, deep tendon reflexes, ABGs, LOC before administration, q30min

• Po_2, Pco_2, O_2 saturation during treatment

• Hypertension, dysrhythmias, tachycardia, dyspnea, skeletal muscle hyperactivity; may indicate overdosage; discontinue drug

• Respiratory stimulation: increased rate, abnormal rhythm

• Extravasation; change IV site q48h

Administer:

IV route

• Undiluted or diluted with equal parts of sterile H_2O for inj; may be diluted 250 mg/250 ml of D_5W, $D_{10}W$ and run as infusion

• IV undiluted over 5 min; IV inf at 1-3 mg/min; adjust for desired respiratory response, using infusion pump IV; if an inf is used after initial dose, start at 1-3 mg/min depending on patient response; D/C after 2 hr; wait 1-2 hr and repeat

• Only after adequate airway is established

• After O_2, IV barbiturates, resuscitative equipment available

Syringe compatibilities: Amikacin, bumetadine, chlorproMAZINE, cimetidine, cisplatin, cyclophosphamide, DOPamine, doxycycline, epINEPHrine, hydrOXYzine, imipramine, isoniazid, lincomycin, methotrexate, netilmicin, phytonadione, pyridoxine, terbutaline, thiamine, tobramycin, vinCRIStine

Perform/provide:

- Placing patient in Sims' position to prevent aspiration of vomitus
- Discontinue infusion if side effects occur; narrow margin of safety

Evaluate:

- Therapeutic response: increased breathing capacity

Teach patient/family:

- Purpose of medication

doxazosin (℞)

(dox-ay'zoe-sin)

Cardura

Func. class.: Peripheral α_1-adrenergic blocker

Chem. class.: Quinazoline

Action: Peripheral blood vessels are dilated, peripheral resistance lowered; reduction in blood pressure results from α_1-adrenergic receptors being blocked

Uses: Hypertension, urinary outflow obstruction, symptoms of benign prostatic hyperplasia

Investigational uses: CHF with digoxin and diuretics

Dosage and routes:

BPH

- *Adult:* **PO** 1 mg qd, increase in stepwise manner to 2, 4, 8 mg qd as needed at 1-2 wk intervals, max 8 mg

Hypertension

- *Adult:* **PO** 1 mg qd, increasing up to 16 mg qd if required; usual range 4-16 mg/day
- *Geriatric:* **PO** 0.5 mg qhs, gradually increase

Available forms: Tabs 1, 2, 4, 8 mg

Side effects/adverse reactions:

CV: Palpitations, *orthostatic hypotension,* tachycardia, edema, ***dysrhythmias,*** chest pain

CNS: Dizziness, headache, drowsiness, anxiety, depression, vertigo, weakness, fatigue, asthenia

GI: Nausea, vomiting, diarrhea, constipation, abdominal pain

GU: Incontinence, polyuria

EENT: Epistaxis, tinnitus, dry mouth, red sclera, pharyngitis, rhinitis

Contraindications: Hypersensitivity to quinazolines

Precautions: Pregnancy (C), children, lactation, hepatic disease

Do not confuse:

Cardura/Coumadin/Cardene

Cardura/Ridaura

Pharmacokinetics:

PO: Onset 2 hr, peak 2-6 hr, duration 6-12 hr; half-life 22 hr; metabolized in liver; excreted via bile/feces (<63%) and in urine (9%); extensively protein bound (98%)

Interactions:

- ↑ hypotensive effects: β-blockers, verapamil
- ↓ hypotensive effects: indomethacin, NSAIDs
- ↓ antihypertensive effects of clonidine

↑ doxazosin effect: angelica

↓ doxazosin effect: butcher's broom, capsicum peppers

Toxicity: yohimbe

NURSING CONSIDERATIONS

Assess:

- B/P (lying, standing) and pulse 2-6 hr after each dose and with each increase; postural effects may occur, rales, dyspnea, orthopnea with B/P; pulse, jugular venous distention q4h
- BUN, uric acid if on long-term therapy
- I&O, weight daily
- Edema in feet, legs daily
- Skin turgor, dryness of mucous membranes for hydration status

Administer:

- Tablets broken, crushed or chewed; if chewed, will be bitter

Perform/provide:
• Storage in tight container in cool environment
Evaluate:
• Therapeutic response: decreased B/P; decreased symptoms of BPH
Teach patient/family:
• That fainting occasionally occurs after first dose; do not drive or operate machinery for 4 hr after first dose or after dosage increase or take first dose hs
• To take 1st dose at hs to decrease orthostatic B/P changes
Treatment of overdose: Administer volume expanders or vasopressors; discontinue drug; place in supine position

doxepin (℞)

(dox′e-pin)
Adepin, doxepin HCl, Novo-Doxepin♣, Sinequan, Sinequan Concentrate, Triadapin♣, Zonolon Topical Cream
Func. class.: Antidepressant, tricyclic
Chem. class.: Dibenzoxepin, tertiary amine

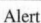

Action: Blocks reuptake of norepinephrine, serotonin into nerve endings, increasing action of norepinephrine, serotonin in nerve cells
Uses: Major depression, anxiety
Investigational uses: Chronic pain management, topical pruritus
Dosage and routes:
Depression/anxiety
• *Adult:* **PO** 25-75 mg/day, may increase to 300 mg/day for severely ill
• *Geriatric:* **PO** 10-25 mg hs, increase qwk by 10-25 mg to desired dose
Pruritus
• *Adult:* **PO** 10 mg hs, may increase to 25 mg hs; **TOP** apply thin film qid at least 3 hr apart
Available forms: Caps 10, 25, 50, 75, 100, 150 mg; oral conc 10 mg/ml; cream 5%
Side effects/adverse reactions:
HEMA: ***Agranulocytosis, thrombocytopenia, eosinophilia, leukopenia***
CNS: Dizziness, drowsiness, confusion, headache, anxiety, tremors, stimulation, weakness, insomnia, nightmares, EPS (elderly), increased psychiatric symptoms, paresthesia
GI: Diarrhea, dry mouth, nausea, vomiting, ***paralytic ileus,*** increased appetite, cramps, epigastric distress, jaundice, ***hepatitis,*** stomatitis, constipation
GU: Urinary retention, ***acute renal failure***
INTEG: Rash, urticaria, sweating, pruritus, photosensitivity
CV: Orthostatic hypotension, ECG changes, tachycardia, ***hypertension,*** palpitations, ***dysrhythmias***
EENT: Blurred vision, tinnitus, mydriasis, ophthalmoplegia, glossitis
Contraindications: Hypersensitivity to tricyclics, urinary retention, narrow-angle glaucoma, prostatic hypertrophy
Precautions: Suicidal patients, elderly, pregnancy (C), UK-PO lactation, seizures
Do not confuse:
Sinequan/Serentil/Sarafem
Pharmacokinetics:
PO: Steady state 2-8 days; metabolized by liver; excreted by kidneys; crosses placenta; excreted in breast milk; half-life 8-24 hr
Interactions:
• ↑ hypertensive action: clonidine, epINEPHrine, norepinephrine

• ↑ doxepin effect: cimetidine, fluoxetine, sertraline
• ↑ CNS depression: other CNS depressants
• Hyperpyretic crisis, convulsions, hypertensive episode: MAOI
↑ anticholinergic effect: belladonna, corkwood, jimsonweed, henbane
↑ doxepin action: hops, kava, lavender, scopolia
Serotonin syndrome: SAM-e, St. John's wort
↑ hypertension: yohimbe

Lab test interferences:
Increase: Serum bilirubin, blood glucose, alk phosphatase

NURSING CONSIDERATIONS

Assess:
• B/P (lying, standing), pulse q4h; if systolic B/P drops 20 mm Hg, hold drug, notify prescriber; take vital signs q4h in patients with cardiovascular disease
• Blood studies: CBC, leukocytes, differential, cardiac enzymes if patient is receiving long-term therapy
• Hepatic studies: AST, ALT, bilirubin
• Weight qwk; appetite may increase with drug
• ECG for flattening of T wave, bundle branch block, AV block, dysrhythmias in cardiac patients; drug should be discontinued gradually several days before surgery
• EPS primarily in elderly: rigidity, dystonia, akathisia
• Mental status: mood, sensorium, affect, suicidal tendencies, increase in psychiatric symptoms: depression, panic
• Urinary retention, constipation; constipation most likely in children, elderly
• Withdrawal symptoms: headache, nausea, vomiting, muscle pain, weakness; not usual unless drug is discontinued abruptly
• Alcohol consumption; if alcohol is consumed, hold dose until morning

Administer:
• Oral conc should be diluted with 120 ml of water, milk, orange, grapefruit juice, tomato, prune, pineapple juice; do not mix with grape juice
• Increased fluids, bulk in diet for constipation
• With food, milk for GI symptoms, do not give with carbonated beverages
• Dosage hs for oversedation during day; may take entire dose hs; elderly may not tolerate qd dosing
• Gum, hard candy, or frequent sips of water for dry mouth
• Topically by applying to affected area, rub slightly

Perform/provide:
• Storage in tight container protected from direct sunlight
• Assistance with ambulation during beginning therapy, since drowsiness/dizziness occurs
• Safety measures primarily for elderly
• Checking to see PO medication swallowed

Evaluate:
• Therapeutic response: decreased anxiety, depression

Teach patient/family:
• That therapeutic effect (depressions) may take 2-3 wk, antianxiety effects sooner
• To use caution in driving, other activities requiring alertness, because of drowsiness, dizziness, blurred vision
• To avoid alcohol ingestion, other CNS depressants
• Not to discontinue medication quickly after long-term use; may cause nausea, headache, malaise

• To wear sunscreen or large hat, since photosensitivity occurs
• To report immediately urinary retention

Treatment of overdose: ECG monitoring; lavage, activated charcoal; administer anticonvulsant, sodium bicarbonate

doxercalciferol (℞)

Hectorol

Func. class.: Parathyroid agent (calcium regulator)
Chem. class.: Vit D hormone

Action: Synthetic vit D analog, reduces parathyroid hormone

Uses: To lower high parathyroid hormone levels in patients undergoing chronic kidney dialysis, postmenopausal osteoporosis, prostate cancer

Dosage and routes:
• *Adult:* **PO** 10 mcg 3×/wk at dialysis
• *Adults:* **IV** 4 mcg × 3/wk at end of dialysis, max 18 mcg/dose

Available forms: Caps 2.5 mcg; inj 2 mcg/ml

Side effects/adverse reactions:
CNS: Drowsiness, headache, lethargy
GI: Nausea, diarrhea, vomiting, anorexia, dry mouth, constipation, cramps, metallic taste
MS: Myalgia, arthralgia, decreased bone development
GU: Polyuria, hypercalciuria, hyperphosphatemia, hematuria
RESP: SOB

Contraindications: Hypersensitivity, hyperphosphatemia, hypercalcemia, vit D toxicity

Precautions: Pregnancy (C), renal calculi, lactation, CV disease

Pharmacokinetics: Metabolism in liver, terminal half-life 96 hr

Interactions:
• ↓ absorption of doxercalciferol: cholestyramine, magnesium antacids, mineral oil, do not use together

NURSING CONSIDERATIONS

Assess:
• BUN, urinary calcium, AST, ALT, cholesterol, creatinine, albumin, uric acid, chloride, magnesium, electrolytes, urine pH, phosphate; may increase calcium, should be kept at 9-10 mg/dl, vit D 50-135 international units/dl, phosphate 70 mg/dl
• Alk phosphatase; may be decreased
• For increased drug level, since toxic reactions may occur rapidly
• For dry mouth, metallic taste, polyuria, bone pain, muscle weakness, headache, fatigue, change in LOC, dysrhythmias, increased respirations, anorexia, nausea, vomiting, cramps, diarrhea, constipation; may indicate hypercalcemia
• Renal status: decreased urinary output (oliguria, anuria), edema in extremities, weight gain 5-7 lb, periorbital edema
• Nutritional status, diet for sources of vit D (milk, some seafood); calcium (dairy products, dark green vegetables), phosphates (dairy products) must be avoided

Perform/provide:
• Storage protected from light, heat, moisture
• Restriction of sodium, potassium if required
• Restriction of fluids if required for chronic renal failure

Evaluate:
• Therapeutic response: calcium 9-10 mg/dl, decreasing symptoms of hypocalcemia, hypoparathyroidism

Teach patient/family:
• The symptoms of hypercalcemia
• About foods rich in calcium
• To avoid products with sodium: cured meats, dairy products, cold

cuts, olives, beets, pickles, soups, meat tenderizers in chronic renal failure
• To avoid products with potassium: oranges, bananas, dried fruit, peas, dark green leafy vegetables, milk, melons, beans in chronic renal failure
• To avoid OTC products containing calcium, potassium, or sodium in chronic renal failure
• To avoid all preparations containing vit D
• To monitor weight weekly
⊘ Not to break, crush, or chew caps

HIGH ALERT

*DOXOrubicin (℞)

(dox-oh-roo'bi-sin)

Adriamycin PFS, Adriamycin RDF, Rubex

*DOXOrubicin liposome (℞)

Doxil

Func. class.: Antineoplastic, antibiotic

Chem. class.: Anthracycline glycoside

Action: Inhibits DNA synthesis primarily; derived from *Streptomyces peucetius;* replication is decreased by binding to DNA, which causes strand splitting; active throughout entire cell cycle; a vesicant

Uses: Wilms' tumor; bladder, breast, cervical, head, neck, liver, lung, ovarian, prostatic, stomach, testicular, thyroid cancer; Hodgkin's disease; acute lymphoblastic leukemia; myeloblastic leukemia; neuroblastomas; lymphomas; sarcomas

Dosage and routes:

DOXOrubicin

• *Adult:* **IV** 60-75 mg/m^2 q3wk, or 30 mg/m^2 on days 1-3 of 4-wk cycle, not to exceed 550 mg/m^2 cumulative dose; Doxil: Adult **IV** 20 mg/m^2 q3wk
• *Child:* **IV** 30 mg/m^2/day × 3 days, may repeat q4wk

DOXOrubicin liposome

• *Adult:* **IV** 20 mg/m^2 q3wk

Available forms: Inj 10, 20, 50, 100, 150 mg; Doxil: liposomal dispersion for inj: 20 mg/ml

Side effects/adverse reactions:

HEMA: ***Thrombocytopenia, leukopenia, anemia***

GI: Nausea, vomiting, anorexia, mucositis, ***hepatotoxicity***

GU: Impotence, sterility, amenorrhea, gynecomastia, hyperuricemia

INTEG: Rash, necrosis at inj site, dermatitis, reversible alopecia, cellulitis, thrombophlebitis at inj site

CV: Increased B/P, ***sinus tachycardia, PVCs,*** chest pain, ***bradycardia, extrasystoles***

Contraindications: Hypersensitivity, pregnancy (1st trimester) (D), lactation, systemic infections, cardiac disorders

Precautions: Renal, hepatic, cardiac disease; gout, bone marrow depression (severe)

Do not confuse:
Adriamycin/Aredia
Adriamycin/Indamycin
DOXOrubicin/idamycin
DOXOrubicin/DAUNOrubicin

Pharmacokinetics: Triphasic pattern of elimination; half-life 12 min, 3⅓ hr, 29⅔ hr; metabolized by liver; crosses placenta; excreted in urine, bile, breast milk

Interactions:
• ↑ toxicity: other antineoplastics or radiation, mercaptopurine
• ↑ hemorrhagic cystitis risk

• Cardiac toxicity: cyclophosphamide
• ↓ antibody response: live virus vaccine

Lab test interferences:
Increase: Uric acid

NURSING CONSIDERATIONS
Assess:
• CBC, differential, platelet count weekly; withhold drug if WBC is <4000/mm^3 or platelet count is <75,000/mm^3; notify prescriber of these results
• Blood, urine uric acid levels
• Renal studies: BUN, serum uric acid, urine CCr, electrolytes before, during therapy
• I&O ratio; report fall in urine output to <30 ml/hr
• Monitor temp q4h; fever may indicate beginning infection
• Hepatic studies before, during therapy: bilirubin, AST, ALT, alk phosphatase as needed or monthly; check for jaundice of skin and sclera, dark urine, clay-colored stools, itchy skin, abdominal pain, fever, diarrhea
• ECG; watch for ST-T wave changes, low QRS and T, possible dysrhythmias (sinus tachycardia, heart block, PVCs); signs of irreversible cardiomyopathy
• Bleeding: hematuria, guaiac, bruising, or petechiae, mucosa or orifices q8h
• Effects of alopecia on body image; discuss feelings about body changes
• Inflammation of mucosa, breaks in skin
• Buccal cavity q8h for dryness, sores, ulceration, white patches, oral pain, bleeding, dysphagia
• Alkalosis if severe vomiting is present
• Local irritation, pain, burning at inj site
• GI symptoms: frequency of stools, cramping
• Acidosis, signs of dehydration: rapid respirations, poor skin turgor, decreased urine output, dry skin, restlessness, weakness
• Cardiac status: B/P, pulse, character, rhythm, rate, ABGs, ECG

Administer:
• Antiemetic 30-60 min before giving drug to prevent vomiting
• Allopurinol or sodium bicarbonate to maintain uric acid levels, alkalinization of urine
• Topical or systemic analgesics for pain
• Transfusion for anemia
• Antispasmodic for GI symptoms

IV route
Do not interchange DOXOrubicin with DOXOrubicin liposome
• Hydrocortisone, dexamethasone, or sodium bicarbonate (1 mEq/1 ml) for extravasation; apply ice compresses
• IV after diluting 10 mg/5 ml of NaCl for inj; another 5 ml of diluent/10 mg is recommended; shake; give over 3-5 min; give through Y-tube of free-flowing 5% dextrose INF or NS

Additive compatibilities: Ondansetron

Syringe compatibilities: Bleomycin, cisplatin, cyclophosphamide, droperidol, leucovorin, methotrexate, metoclopramide, mitomycin, vincristine

Y-site compatibilities: Amifostine, aztreonam, bleomycin, chlorproMAZINE, cimetidine, cisplatin, cladribine, cyclophosphamide, dexamethasone, diphenhydrAMINE, droperidol, famotidine, filgrastim, fludarabine, fluorouracil, granisetron, hydromorphone, leucovorin, lorazepam, melphalan, methotrexate, methylPREDNISolone, metoclopramide, mitomycin, morphine, ondansetron, paclitaxel, prochlorperazine, promethazine, propofol, ranitidine, sargramostim, sodium bicarbonate, teniposide, thiotepa, vinBLAStine, vinCRIStine, vinorelbine

• IV liposome inj (Doxil): dilute dose up to 90 mg/250 ml D_5W, give over ½ hr; do not admix with other sol or meds

Perform/provide:

• Liquid diet: carbonated beverages, geletin may be added if patient is not nauseated or vomiting

• Increased fluid intake to 2-3 L/day to prevent urate, calculi formation

• Rinsing of mouth tid-qid with water, club soda; brushing of teeth bid-tid with soft brush or cotton-tipped applicators for stomatitis; use unwaxed dental floss

• Storage at room temperature for 24 hr after reconstituting or 48 hr refrigerated

Evaluate:

• Therapeutic response: decreased tumor size, spread of malignancy

Teach patient/family:

• To add 2-3L of fluids unless contraindicated prior to and for 24-48 hr after, to decrease possible hemorrhagic cystitis

• To report any complaints, side effects to nurse or prescriber

• That hair may be lost during treatment and wig or hairpiece may make patient feel better; tell patient that new hair may be different in color, texture

• To avoid foods with citric acid, hot or rough texture

• To report any bleeding, white spots, ulcerations in mouth to prescriber; tell patient to examine mouth qd

• That urine and other body fluids may be red-orange for 48 hr

• To avoid crowds and persons with infections when granulocyte count is low

• That contraceptive measures are recommended during therapy and 4 mo after

• To avoid vaccinations; reactions may occur

doxycycline (℞)

(dox-i-sye'kleen)

Apo-Doxy✤, Atridox, Doryx, Doxy, Doxycin✤, doxycycline, Monodox, Novodoxyclin✤, Periostat, Vibramycin, Vibra-Tabs

Func. class.: Antiinfective

Chem. class.: Tetracycline

Action: Inhibits protein synthesis, prosphorylation in microorganisms by binding to 30S ribosomal subunits, reversibly binding to 50S ribosomal subunits; bacteriostatic

Uses: Syphilis, *Chlamydia trachomatis,* gonorrhea, *Rickettsia,* lymphogranuloma venereum, uncommon gram-negative/positive organisms, malaria prophylaxis, chronic periodontitis, acne, anthrax

Investigational uses: Traveler's diarrhea, Lyme disease, prevention of chronic bronchitis

Dosage and routes:

• *Adult:* **PO/IV** 100 mg q12h on day 1, then 100 mg/day; **IV** 200 mg in 1-2 inf on day 1, then 100-200 mg/day; delivery syst: 10% for cont rel

• *Child >8 yr:* **PO/IV** 2.2-4.4 mg/kg/day in divided doses q12h

Gonorrhea (uncomplicated) in patients allergic to penicillin

• *Adult:* **PO** 200 mg, then 100 mg hs and 100 mg bid × 3 days or 300 mg, then 300 mg in 1 hr; disseminated; 100 mg **PO** bid × at least 7 days

Malaria prophylaxis
• *Adult:* 100 mg qd 1-2 days prior to travel and daily during travel
C. trachomatis
• *Adult:* **PO** 100 mg bid × 7 days
Syphilis
• *Adult:* **PO** 300 mg/day in divided doses × 10 days
Periodontitis
• *Adult:* 20 mg bid after scaling and root planing for ≤9 mo; give ≥1 hr prior to meal AM or PM

Available forms: Tabs 50, 75, 100 mg; caps 50, 100 mg; cap, coated pellets 75, 100 mg; syr 50 mg/5 ml; powder for inj 100, 200 mg; powder for oral susp 25 mg/5 ml; inj 42.5 mg

Side effects/adverse reactions:
CNS: Fever
HEMA: ***Eosinophilia, neutropenia, thrombocytopenia, hemolytic anemia***
EENT: Dysphagia, glossitis, decreased calcification of deciduous teeth, oral candidiasis
GI: Nausea, abdominal pain, vomiting, diarrhea, anorexia, enterocolitis, ***hepatotoxicity,*** flatulence, abdominal cramps, gastric burning, stomatitis
CV: Pericarditis
GU: Increased BUN
INTEG: Rash, urticaria, photosensitivity, increased pigmentation, ***exfoliative dermatitis,*** pruritus, ***angioedema***

Contraindications: Hypersensitivity to tetracyclines, children <8 yr, pregnancy (D)

Precautions: Hepatic disease, lactation

Do not confuse:
doxycycline/doxepin

Pharmacokinetics:
PO: Well absorbed, widely distributed peak 1½-4 hr, half-life 14-17 hr; excreted in urine, feces, bile, 90% protein bound, crosses placenta, enters breast milk

Interactions:
• ↓ doxycycline effect: antacids, $NaHCO_3$, dairy products, alkali products, iron, kaolin/pectin, barbiturates, carbamazepine, phenytoin, cimetidine sucralfate, cholestyramine, colestipol
• ↑ effect: warfarin
• ↓ effects: penicillins, oral contraceptives
↑ action: bromelain
Do not use acidophilus with anti-infectives

Lab test interferences:
False increase: Urinary catecholamines; ALT, AST

NURSING CONSIDERATIONS

Assess:
• I&O ratio
• Blood studies: PT, CBC, AST, ALT, BUN, creatinine
• Signs of infection
• Allergic reactions: rash, itching, pruritus, angioedema
• Nausea, vomiting, diarrhea; administer antiemetic, antacids as ordered
• Overgrowth of infection: fever, malaise, redness, pain, swelling, drainage, perineal itching, diarrhea, changes in cough or sputum
• IV site for phlebitis/thrombosis; drug is highly irritating

Administer:
• After C&S
• 2 hr before or after laxative or iron products; 3 hr after antacid or kaolin-pectin products

IV route
• After diluting 100 mg or less/10 ml of sterile H_2O or NS for inj; further dilute with 100-1000 ml of NaCl, D_5, Ringer's LR D_5LR, Normosol-M, Normosol-R in D_5W; run 100 mg or less over 1-4 hr; do not give IM/SC; inf must be com-

pleted in 6 hr, when diluted in LR sol, or 12 hr in other sol
Additive compatibilities: Ranitidine
Syringe compatibilities: Doxapram
Y-site compatibilities: Acyclovir, amifostine, amiodarone, aztreonam, cisatracurium, cyclophosphamide, diltiazem, filgrastim, fludarabine, granisetron, hydromorphone, magnesium sulfate, melphalan, meperidine, morphine, ondansetron, perphenazine, propofol, remifentanil, sargramostim, tacrolimus, teniposide, theophylline, thiotepa, vinorelbine
Perform/provide:
- Storage in tight, light-resistant container at room temperature; IV stable for 12 hr at room temperature, 72 hr refrigerated; discard if precipitate forms

Evaluate:
- Therapeutic response: decreased temp, absence of lesions, negative C&S

Teach patient/family:
- To avoid sun, since burns may occur; sunscreen does not seem to decrease photosensitivity
- That all prescribed medication must be taken to prevent superinfection
- ⃠ Not to break, crush, or chew caps
- To take with a full glass of water; may take with food

RARELY USED

D-penicillamine (℞)

(pen-i-sill'a-meen)
Cuprimine, Depen
Func. class.: Heavy metal antagonist

Uses: Wilson's disease, rheumatoid arthritis, cystinuria, heavy metal poisoning (lead, mercury, gold)
Dosage and routes:
Cystinuria
- *Adult:* **PO** 250 mg qid ac, not to exceed 5 g/day
- *Child:* **PO** 30 mg/kg/day in divided doses qid ac

Wilson's disease
- *Adult:* **PO** 250 mg qid ac
- *Child:* **PO** 20 mg/kg/day in divided doses ac

Rheumatoid arthritis
- *Adult:* **PO** 125-250 mg/day, then increase 250 mg q2-3mo if needed, not to exceed 1 g/day
- *Child:* **PO** 3 mg/kg/day × 3 mo, then 6 mg/kg/day in divided doses for 3 mo, then increase to max 10 mg/kg/day

Contraindications: Hypersensitivity to penicillins, anuria, agranulocytosis, severe renal disease, pregnancy (D), lactation

HIGH ALERT

droperidol (℞)

(droe-per'i-dole)
droperidol, Inapsine
Func. class.: Neuroleptic
Chem. class.: Butyrophenone

Action: Acts on CNS at subcortical levels, produces tranquilization, sleep; antiemetic; mild α-blockade
Uses: Premedication for surgery; induction, maintenance in general anesthesia; postoperatively for nausea, vomiting
Dosage and routes:
Induction
- *Adult:* **IV/IM** 0.22-0.275 mg/kg given with analgesic or general anesthetic; may give 1.25-2.5 mg additionally
- *Child 2-12 yr:* **IV** 88-165 mcg/kg, titrated to response needed

Premedication
• *Adult:* **IM** 2.5-10 mg ½-1 hr before surgery, may give 1.25-2.5 mg additionally
• *Child 2-12 yr:* **IM** 88-165 mcg/kg
Maintaining general anesthesia
• *Adult:* **IV** 1.25-2.5 mg
Regional anesthesia adjunct
• *Adult:* **IV/IM** 2.5-5 mg
Diagnostic procedures without general anesthesia
• *Adult:* **IM** 2.5-10 mg ½-1 hr prior to procedure; 1.25-2.5 mg may be needed
Antiemetic
• *Adult:* **IV** 0.5-1.25 mg q4h prn (unlabeled)
Available forms: Inj 2.5 mg/ml
Side effects/adverse reactions:
RESP: ***Laryngospasm, bronchospasm***
CNS: Dystonia, akathisia, flexion of arms, fine tremors, dizziness, anxiety, drowsiness, restlessness, hallucination, depression, ***seizures,*** extrapyramidal symptoms, ***neuroleptic malignant syndrome***
CV: Tachycardia, hypotension
EENT: Upward rotation of eyes, oculogyric crisis
INTEG: Chills, facial sweating, shivering
Contraindications: Hypersensitivity, child <2 yr, pregnancy (C), lactation
Precautions: Elderly, cardiovascular disease (hypotension, bradydysrhythmias), renal disease, liver disease, Parkinson's disease, pheochromocytoma
Pharmacokinetics:
IM/IV: Onset 3-10 min, peak ½ hr, duration 3-6 hr; metabolized in liver; excreted in urine as metabolites; crosses placenta, half-life 2-3 hr
Interactions:
• ↑ CNS depression: alcohol, opiates, barbiturates, antihistamines, antipsychotics, or other CNS depressants
• ↑ hypotension: nitrates, antihypertensives
• ↑ side effects of: lithium
↑ action: kava
NURSING CONSIDERATIONS
Assess:
• VS q10min during IV administration, q30min after IM dose
• EPS: dystonia, akathisia
For increasing heart rate or decreasing B/P, notify prescriber at once; do not place patient in Trendelenburg position, or sympathetic blockade may occur, causing respiratory arrest
Administer:
• Anticholinergics (benztropine, diphenhydramine) for EPS
• Only with crash cart, resuscitative equipment nearby
• IM deep in large muscle mass
IV direct route
• Undiluted; give through Y-tube at 10 mg or less/min; titrate to patient response
Intermittent INF route
• May be given as an infusion by adding dose to 250 ml LR, D_5W, 0.9% NaCl, give slowly, titrate to patient response
Syringe compatibilities: Atropine, bleomycin, butorphanol, chlorproMAZINE, cimetidine, cisplatin, cyclophosphamide, dimenhyDRINATE, diphenhydrAMINE, DOXOrubicin, fentanyl, glycopyrrolate, hydroxyzine, meperidine, metoclopramide, midazolam, mitomycin, morphine, nalbuphine, pentazocine, perphenazine, prochlorperazine, promazine, promethazine, scopolamine, vinBLAStine, vinCRIStine
Y-site compatibilities: Amifostine, aztreonam, bleomycin, cisatracurium, cisplatin, cladribine, cyclo-

phosphamide, cytarabine, DOXOrubicin, DOXOrubicin liposome, famotidine, filgrastim, fluconazole, fludarabine, granisetron, hydrocortisone, idarubicin, melphalan, meperidine, metoclopramide, mitomycin, ondansetron, paclitaxel, potassium chloride, propofol, remifentanil, sargramostim, teniposide, thiotepa, vinBLAStine, vinCRIStine, vinorelbine, vit B/C

Evaluate:

• Therapeutic response: decreased anxiety, absence of vomiting during and after surgery

Teach patient/family:

• To rise slowly from sitting or standing to minimize orthostatic hypotension

• To avoid ambulation without assistance

drotrecogin alfa (℞)

(droh'treh-koh-jin al'fah)

Xigris

Func. class.: Thrombolytic agent

Chem. class.: Recombinant human activated protein C

Action: Activated protein C exerts an antithrombotic effect by inhibiting factor Va/VIIIa

Uses: Severe sepsis associated with organ dysfunction

Dosage and routes:

• *Adult:* IV INF 24 mcg/kg/hr × 96 hr

Available forms: Powder for inj, lyophilized, 5, 20 mg

Side effects/adverse reactions:

HEMA: Decreased Hct, ***bleeding***

SYST: ***GI, GU, intracranial, intraabdominal, intrathoracic, retroperitoneal bleeding; surface bleeding***

Contraindications: Hypersensitivity, internal active bleeding, intraspinal surgery, CNS neoplasms, ulcerative colitis, enteritis, hepatic disease, hypocoagulation, hemorrhagic stroke, epidural catheter in place, cerebral embolism/thrombosis/hemorrhage, recent major surgery, trauma

Precautions: Recent GI bleeding, prothrombin time – INR >3, pregnancy (C), lactation, children, use >96 hr

Pharmacokinetics: Inactivated by endogenous plasma protease inhibitors

Interactions:

• Bleeding potential: aspirin, indomethacin, phenylbutazone, anticoagulants, thrombolytics, glycoprotein IIb/IIIa inhibitors

NURSING CONSIDERATIONS

Assess:

➧ For bleeding during treatment; hematuria, hematemesis, bleeding from mucous membranes, epistaxis, ecchymosis; may require transfusion (rare), continue to assess for bleeding

• Blood studies (Hct, platelets, PTT, PT, TT, aPTT) before starting therapy; PT or aPTT must be less than 2× control before starting therapy; PTT or PT q3-4h during treatment

• VS, B/P, pulse, respirations, neurologic signs, temp at least q4h; temp >104° F (40° C) indicates internal bleeding; systolic pressure increase >25 mm Hg should be reported to prescriber

➧ For neurologic changes that may indicate intracranial bleeding

➧ Retroperitoneal bleeding: back pain, leg weakness, diminished pulses

Administer:

IV route

• Reconstitute 5 mg vial/2.5 ml; 20 mg vial/10 ml sterile water for inj to a concentration of 2 mg/ml; slowly add sterile water for inj, do not shake or invert, gently swirl until dissolved

- Further dilute with 0.9% NaCl, slowly withdraw prescribed amount and add to bag of 0.9% NaCl, direct stream to side of bag, gently invert bag; do not transport infusion bag between locations using mechanical delivery systems
- Use immediately after reconstituting, may be held for only 3 hr at controlled room temperature 59°-86° F; must complete infusion within 12 hr after preparation
- Do not use if discolored or if particulate is present
- If using an infusion pump, usual concentration is 100-200 mcg/ml; if using a syringe pump, usual concentration is 100-1000 mcg/ml
- Use a dedicated IV line, or dedicated lumen of central venous catheter; may use only 0.9% NaCl, LR, dextrose, or dextrose/saline mixtures through same line
- Do not expose to heat or direct sunlight
- Discontinue 2 hr prior to invasive surgery or procedures introducing risk of bleeding

Perform/provide:

- Refrigerated storage at 2° to 8° C (36° to 46° F); do not freeze
- Protect unreconstituted vials from light; keep in carton until time of use

Evaluate:

- Therapeutic response: Decreasing symptoms of sepsis, lack of mortality

dutasteride (℞)

(doo-tass'ter-ide)

Duagen

Func. class.: Sex hormone 5α-reductase inhibitor

Chem. class.: Synthetic 4-azasteroid compound

Action: Inhibits both types 1 and 2 forms of a steroid enzyme that converts testosterone to 5α-dihydrotestosterone (DHT), which is responsible for the initial growth of prostatic tissue

Uses: Treatment of benign prostatic hyperplasia (BPH) in men with an enlarged prostate gland

Dosage and routes:

- *Adult:* **PO** 0.5 mg qd

Available form: Caps 0.5 mg

Side effects/adverse reactions:

GU: Decreased libido, impotence, gynecomastia, ejaculation disorders (rare)

Contraindications: Hypersensitivity, pregnancy (X), lactation, women, children, lactation

Precautions: Hepatic disease

Pharmacokinetics: Peak 2-3 hr, protein binding 99%; metabolized in liver by CYP3A4, excreted in feces; half-life 5 wk at steady state

Interactions:

- ↑ dutasteride concentrations: ritonavir, ketoconazole, verapamil, diltiazem, cimetidine, ciprofloxacin, or other drugs metabolized by the CYP3A4 pathway

Lab test interferences:

Increase: TSH

Decrease: PSA

NURSING CONSIDERATIONS

Assess:

- For decreasing symptoms in BPH: decreasing urinary retention, frequency, urgency, nocturia

• PSA levels, digital rectal, urinary obstruction; determine the absence of urinary cancer before starting treatment
• Hepatic studies: ALT, AST, bilirubin

Administer:
• Without regard to meals
• ⃠ Caps whole; do not break, open, or chew

Evaluate:
• Therapeutic response: Decreasing symptoms of BPH—decreased urinary frequency, retention, urgency, nocturia

Teach patient/family:
• To read patient information leaflet before starting therapy and reread it upon prescription renewal
• To notify prescriber if therapeutic response decreases; if edema occurs
• Not to discontinue drug abruptly
• About changes in sex characteristics
• That men taking dutasteride should not donate blood for at least 6 mo after last dose, to prevent blood administration to pregnant female
• That caps should not be handled by a pregnant woman because this drug can be absorbed through the skin
• That ejaculate volume may decrease during treatment; that drug rarely interferes with sexual function

dyphylline (℞)

(dye'fi-lin)
Dilor, Dyflex-200, Dylline, dyphylline, Lufyllin, Neothylline
Func. class.: Bronchodilator
Chem. class.: Xanthine, theophylline derivative

Action: Relaxes smooth muscle of respiratory system by blocking phosphodiesterase, which increases cyclic AMP; cyclic AMP results in positive inotropic, chronotropic effects, bronchodilation, stimulation of CNS

Uses: Bronchial asthma, bronchospasm in chronic bronchitis and emphysema, COPD

Dosage and routes:
• *Adult:* **PO** 200-800 mg q6h; **IM** 250-500 mg q6h injected slowly, max 15 mg/kg q6h
• *Child>6 yr:* **PO** 4-7 mg/kg/day in 4 divided doses

Available forms: Tabs 200, 400 mg; elix 33.3, 53.3 mg/5 ml; inj 250 mg/ml

Side effects/adverse reactions:
CNS: Anxiety, restlessness, insomnia, dizziness, ***convulsions,*** headache, light-headedness, muscle twitching
CV: Palpitations, ***circulatory failure,*** *sinus tachycardia,* hypotension, flushing, ***dysrhythmias***
GI: Nausea, diarrhea, *vomiting, anorexia,* dyspepsia, epigastric pain, rectal irritation, bleeding
INTEG: Flushing, urticaria
RESP: Tachypnea, ***respiratory arrest***
OTHER: Fever, dehydration, ***albuminuria,*** hyperglycemia, increased diuresis

Contraindications: Hypersensitivity to xanthines, seizure disorder, peptic ulcer

Precautions: Elderly, CHF, cor pulmonale, hepatic disease, diabetes mellitus, hypertension, children, renal disease, pregnancy (B), lactation, glaucoma, hyperthyroidism

Pharmacokinetics: Well absorbed, peak 1 hr, duration 6 hr, half-life 2 hr, excreted in urine (85%) unchanged, and in breast milk

Interactions:
- ↑ action of dyphylline: cimetidine, propranolol, erythromycin, probenecid
- Cardiotoxicity: β-blockers
- ↑ dyphylline metabolism: barbiturates, phenytoin
- ↓ dyphylline elimination: uricosurics
- ↓ phenytoin levels

NURSING CONSIDERATIONS
Assess:
- Dyphylline blood levels; toxicity may occur with small increase above 20 mcg/ml; assess for drug toxicity: nausea, vomiting, anorexia, cramping, diarrhea, confusion, dysrhythmias, seizures, diuresis, flushing, headache
- Monitor I&O; diuresis occurs; dehydration may be the result in elderly or children
- Whether theophylline was given recently
- Auscultate lung fields bilaterally; notify prescriber of abnormalities, monitor pulmonary function studies baseline and periodically
- Allergic reactions: rash, urticaria; drug should be discontinued

Administer:
- Give around the clock to maintain blood levels, give qd dose each AM
- PO after meals to decrease GI symptoms; absorption may be affected
- Avoid IM inj, do not give IV; pain occurs, do not use if precipitate occurs

Perform/provide:
- Storage protected from light, at room temperature

Evaluate:
- Therapeutic response: decreased dyspnea, respiratory rate, rhythm

Teach patient/family:
- To check OTC medications, current prescription medications for epHEDrine; will increase stimulation; not to drink alcohol, caffeine, or other xanthine products; not to change brands
- To avoid hazardous activities; dizziness, drowsiness, blurred vision may occur
- For GI upset, to take drug with 8 oz water and food
- To avoid smoking, condition may worsen
- To obtain blood levels 6-12 mo

econazole topical

See appendix c

ecothiophate ophthalmic

See appendix c

RARELY USED

edetate calcium disodium (℞)

(ee'de-tate)

calcium disodium versenate, calcium EDTA, edathamil calcium disodium, sodium calcium edetate

Func. class.: Heavy metal antagonist (antidote)

Uses: Lead poisoning, acute lead encephalopathy

Dosage and routes:

Acute lead encephalopathy
- *Adult and child:* 1.5 g/m^2/day × 3-5 days in 2-3 divided doses **IM** or slow **IV** with dimercaprol; may be given again after 4 days off drug

Lead poisoning
- *Adult:* **IV** 1 g/250-500 ml D_5W or 0.9% NaCl over 1-2 hr or q12h × 3-5 days; may repeat after 2 days; not to exceed 50 mg/kg/day;

may be given as **CONT INF** over 8-24 hr

- *Adult:* **IM** 35 mg/kg bid
- *Child:* **IM** 35 mg/kg/day in divided doses q8-12h, not to exceed 50 mg/kg/day; may give for 3-5 days, off 4 days before next course

Contraindications: Hypersensitivity, anuria, poisoning of other metals, severe renal disease, child <3 yr

RARELY USED

edetate disodium (℞)

(ee'de-tate)

Chealamide, Disodium EDTA, Disotate, Endrate

Func. class.: Metal antagonist

Uses: Hypercalcemic crisis, control of ventricular dysrhythmias associated with digitalis toxicity

Dosage and routes: *Adult and child:* **IV INF** 15-50 mg/kg/day in 2 divided doses, diluted in 500 ml D_5W or 0.9% NaCl, given over 3-4 hr, not to exceed 3 g/day (adult) or 70 mg/kg/day (child); allow 5 days between courses (child), 2 days (adult)

Contraindications: Hypersensitivity, anuria, hepatic insufficiency, poisoning of other metals, severe renal disease, child <3 yr, seizure disorders, active/inactive TB

edrophonium (℞)

(ed-roh-fone'ee-um)

Enlon, Reversol, Tensilon

Func. class.: Cholinergics, anticholinesterase

Chem. class.: Quaternary ammonium compound

Action: Inhibits destruction of acetylcholine, which increases concentration at sites where acetylcholine is released; this facilitates transmission of impulses across myoneural junction

Uses: To diagnose myasthenia gravis; curare antagonist; differentiation of myasthenic crisis from cholinergic crisis

Dosage and routes:

Tensilon test (myasthenia gravis diagnosis)

- *Adult:* **IV** 1-2 mg over 15-30 sec, then 8 mg if no response; **IM** 10 mg; if cholinergic reaction occurs, retest after ½ hr with 2 mg **IM**
- *Child >34 kg:* **IV** 2 mg; if no response in 45 sec, then 1 mg q45sec, not to exceed 10 mg; **IM** 5 mg
- *Child <34 kg:* **IV** 1 mg; if no response in 45 sec, then 1 mg q45sec, not to exceed 5 mg; **IM** 2 mg
- *Infant:* **IV** 0.5 mg

Reversal of nondepolarizing neuromuscular blockers

- *Adult:* **IV** 10 mg over 30-45 sec, may repeat, not to exceed 40 mg

Differentiation of myasthenic crisis from cholinergic crisis

- *Adult:* **IV** 1 mg, if no response in 1 min, may repeat

Available forms: Inj 10 mg/ml

Side effects/adverse reactions:

INTEG: Rash, urticaria

CNS: Dizziness, headache, sweating, weakness, ***convulsions,*** incoordination, ***paralysis,*** drowsiness, ***loss of consciousness***

GI: Nausea, diarrhea, vomiting, cramps, increased salivary and gastric secretions, dysphagia, increased peristalsis

CV: Dysrhythmias, bradycardia, hypotension, ***AV block***, ECG changes, ***cardiac arrest,*** syncope

GU: Urinary frequency, incontinence, urgency

RESP: ***Respiratory depression, bronchospasm, constriction, laryngo-***

spasm, respiratory arrest, dyspnea, increased bronchial secretions

EENT: Miosis, blurred vision, lacrimation, visual changes

Contraindications: Obstruction of intestine, renal system, hypersensitivity

Precautions: Seizure disorders, bronchial asthma, coronary occlusion, hyperthyroidism, dysrhythmias, peptic ulcer, megacolon, poor GI motility, pregnancy (C), bradycardia, hypotension

Pharmacokinetics:

IV: Onset 30-60 sec, duration 6-15 min

IM: Onset 2-10 min, duration 12-45 min

Interactions:

- ↓ action of edrophonium: procainamide, quinidine, atropine, anesthetics, phenothiazines, antihistamines, haloperidol, magnesium, corticosteroids, antidysrhythmics
- Bradycardia: digitalis
- Prolonged action of: depolarizing muscle relaxants

NURSING CONSIDERATIONS

Assess:

- VS, respiration during test; muscle strength
- Diabetic patient carefully, since this drug lowers blood glucose

Administer:

- Only with atropine sulfate available for cholinergic crisis
- Only after all other cholinergics have been discontinued

IV direct route

- 2 mg or less over 15-30 sec; as a curare antagonist, over 30-45 sec; or given as continuous infusion in myasthenic crisis

Y-site compatibilities: Heparin, hydrocortisone, potassium chloride, vit B/C

Perform/provide:

- Storage at room temperature

Evaluate:

- Therapeutic response: increased muscle strength, hand grasp; improved gait; absence of labored breathing (if severe)

Teach patient/family:

- To wear emergency ID specifying myasthenia gravis, drugs taken

Treatment of overdose: Respiratory support, atropine 1-4 mg (IV)

efalizumab

See appendix a—selected new drugs

efavirenz (℞)

(ef-ah-veer′enz)

Sustiva

Func. class.: Antiretroviral

Chem. class.: Nonnucleoside reverse transcriptase inhibitor (NNRTI)

Action: Binds directly to reverse transcriptase and blocks RNA, DNA causing a disruption of the enzyme's site

Uses: HIV-1 in combination with other antivirals

Dosage and routes:

Given in combination with protease inhibitor or nucleoside analog reverse transcriptase inhibitors (NARTIs)

- *Adult and child >40 kg:* **PO** 600 mg qd hs
- *Child: 10-15 kg:* **PO** 200 mg qd hs
- *Child: 15-20 kg:* **PO** 250 mg qd hs
- *Child: 20-25 kg:* **PO** 300 mg qd hs
- *Child: 25-32.5 kg:* **PO** 350 mg qd hs
- *Child: 32.5-40 kg:* **PO** 400 mg qd hs

Available forms: Caps 50, 100, 200 mg; 600 mg tabs

Side effects/adverse reactions:

GU: Hematuria, kidney stones

CNS: Fatigue, impaired concentration, insomnia, abnormal dreams, depression, headache, dizziness
GI: Diarrhea, abdominal pain, *nausea,* hyperlipidemia
INTEG: Rash, ***erythema multiforme, Stevens-Johnson syndrome, toxic epidermal necrolysis***
Contraindication: Hypersensitivity
Precautions: Hepatic disease, pregnancy (C), lactation, children <3 yr, renal disease, myelosuppression
Pharmacokinetics: Well absorbed, metabolized by liver, terminal half-life 52-76 hr, >99% protein binding, metabolized by liver
Interactions:
• ↑ CNS depression: alcohol, antidepressants, antihistamines, opioids
• ↓ efavirenz levels: rifamycins
• Do not give together with benzodiazepines, ergots, midazolam, triazolam, cisapride
• ↓ levels of: indinavir, saquinavir, clarithromycin
• ↑ levels of both drugs: ritonavir, estrogens
• ↑ levels of: warfarin, ergots, midazolam, triazolam
• Drug/food: ↑ absorption: high-fat foods
↓ efavirenz level: St. John's wort, do not use together
Lab interferences:
Increase: ALT
False-positive: cannibinoids
NURSING CONSIDERATIONS
Assess:
• Signs of infection, anemia
• Hepatic studies: ALT, AST: renal studies
• Bowel pattern before, during treatment; if severe abdominal pain with bleeding occurs, drug should be discontinued; monitor hydration
• Skin eruptions; rash, urticaria, itching
• Allergies before treatment, reaction to each medication
• CBC, blood chemistry, plasma HIV RNA, absolute CD4+/CD8+ cell counts/%, serum β_2 microglobulin, serum ICD+24 antigen levels, cholesterol, hepatic enzymes
• Signs of toxicity: severe nausea/vomiting, maculopapular rash
Administer:
• Give on empty stomach; hs to decrease CNS side effects
Evaluate:
• Therapeutic response: increased CD4 cell counts; decreased viral load; slowing progression of HIV
Teach patient/family:
• To take as prescribed; if dose is missed, take as soon as remembered; do not double dose; take with water, juice; taken on empty stomach hs
• To make sure health-care provider knows all the medications, supplements, or OTC drugs taken
• That if severe rash occurs, to notify health care provider; that adverse reactions (rash, dizziness, abnormal dreams, insomnia) lessen after a month
• Not to breastfeed or become pregnant if taking this drug, use nonhormonal contraception
• To avoid hazardous activities if dizziness/drowsiness occur
• That drug does not cure disease, but controls symptoms, HIV can be transmitted to others even while taking this drug, to continue with safe-sex practices

eletriptan (℞)

(el-ee-trip'tan)
Relpax
Func. class.: Antimigraine agent
Chem. class.: 5-HT_1-Receptor agonist

Action: Binds selectively to the vas-

cular 5-HT_1-receptor subtype, exerts antimigraine effect; causes vasoconstriction in cranial arteries
Uses: Acute treatment of migraine with or without aura
Dosage and routes:
• *Adult:* **PO** 20 mg, may increase if needed, max 40 mg (single dose); may repeat in 2 hr if headache improves but returns, max 80 mg/day
Available forms: Tabs 20, 40 mg
Side effects/adverse reactions:
GI: Nausea, dry mouth
MS: Weakness
CNS: Dizziness, headache, anxiety, paresthesia, asthenia, somnolence, flushing, fatigue, hot/cold sensation
RESP: Chest tightness, pressure
CV: Chest pain, palpitations, hypertension
Contraindications: Concurrent use of ergotamine-containing preparations, uncontrolled hypertension, hypersensitivity, basilar or hemiplegic migraine; ischemic bowel disease; severe hepatic disease
Precautions: Postmenopausal women, men >40 yr, risk factors of CAD, MI, or other cardiac disease, hypercholesterolemia, obesity, diabetes, impaired hepatic or renal function, pregnancy (C), lactation, children, elderly
Pharmacokinetics: Onset of pain relief 2 hr; metabolized in the liver; excreted in urine, feces
Interactions:
• ↑ plasma concentration of eletriptan: CYP3A4 inhibitors (clarithromycin, ketoconazole, or propranolol)
↑ effect: butterbur
NURSING CONSIDERATIONS
Assess:
• B/P; signs/symptoms of coronary vasospasms
• Tingling, hot sensation, burning, feeling of pressure, numbness, flushing
• For stress level, activity, recreation, coping mechanisms
• Neurologic status: LOC, blurring vision, nausea, vomiting, tingling in extremities preceding headache
• Ingestion of tyramine foods (pickled products, beer, wine, aged cheese), food additives, preservatives, colorings, artificial sweeteners, chocolate, caffeine, which may precipitate these types of headaches
Administer:
PO, swallow whole
Perform/provide:
• Quiet, calm environment with decreased stimulation from noise, bright light, excessive talking
Evaluate:
• Therapeutic response: decrease in severity of migraine
Teach patient/family:
• To report any side effects to prescriber
• To use contraception while taking drug
• To provide dark, quiet environment
• That drug does not prevent or reduce number of migraine attacks

emedastine ophthalmic

See appendix c

enalapril/ enalaprilat (℞)

(e-nal′a-pril)/(e-nal′a-pril-at)
Vasotec, Vasotec IV
Func. class.: Antihypertensive
Chem. class.: Angiotensin-converting enzyme (ACE) inhibitor

Action: Selectively suppresses renin-angiotensin-aldosterone system; inhibits ACE; prevents conversion of angiotensin I to angiotensin II, dilation of arterial, venous vessels

Uses: Hypertension, CHF, left ventricular dysfunction

Dosage and routes:

Hypertension

• *Adult:* **PO** 5 mg/day, may increase or decrease to desired response, range 10-40 mg/day; **IV** 1.25 mg q6h over 5 min

• *Child:* **PO** 0.08 mg/kg/day in 1-2 divided doses, max 0.58 mg/kg/day

• *Child:* **IV** 5-10 mcg/kg/dose q8-24h

Patients on diuretics

• *Adult:* **IV** 0.625 mg over 5 min, may give additional doses of 1.25 mg q6h

Renal impairment

• *Adult:* **PO** 2.5 mg qd (CCr <30 ml/min) increase gradually; **IV** CCr >30 ml/min 1.25 mg q6h; CCr <30 ml/min 0.625 mg as one-time dose, increase as per B/P

CHF

• *Adult:* **PO** 2.5-20 mg/day in 2 divided doses, max 40 mg qd in divided doses

Available forms: enalapril: tabs 2.5, 5, 10, 20 mg; enalaprilat: inj 1.25 mg/ml

Side effects/adverse reactions:

CV: Hypotension, chest pain, tachycardia, ***dysrhythmias,*** syncope, angina, ***MI,*** orthostatic hypotension

CNS: Insomnia, dizziness, paresthesias, headache, fatigue, anxiety

GI: Nausea, vomiting, colitis, cramps, diarrhea, constipation, flatulence, dry mouth, loss of taste

INTEG: Rash, purpura, alopecia, hyperhidrosis, photosensitivity

HEMA: ***Agranulocytosis, neutropenia***

EENT: Tinnitus, visual changes, sore throat, double vision, dry burning eyes

GU: ***Proteinuria, renal failure,*** increased frequency of polyuria or oliguria

RESP: Dyspnea, dry cough, rales, angioedema

META: Hyperkalemia

Contraindications: Hypersensitivity, history of angioedema, pregnancy (D) 2nd/3rd trimester

Precautions: Renal disease, hyperkalemia, pregnancy (C) 1st trimester, lactation, hepatic failure, dehydration, bilateral renal artery stenosis

Do not confuse:

enalapril/ramipril/Anafranil

enalapril/Eldepryl

Pharmacokinetics:

PO: Peak 4-6 hr; half-life 1½ hr; metabolized by liver to active metabolite, excreted in urine

IV: Onset 5-15 min, peak up to 4 hr

Interactions:

• Hypersensitivity: allopurinol

• ↑ hypotension: diuretics, other antihypertensives, phenothiazines, nitrates, acute alcohol ingestion, general anesthesia

• ↓ effects of enalapril: antacids, rifampin

• ↑ potassium levels: salt substitutes, potassium-sparing diuretics, potassium supplements, cycloSPORINE, indomethacin

• ↑ levels of lithium, digoxin

Fatal hypokalemia: arginine

↓ effect: pineapple, yohimbe

↑ effect: pill-bearing spurge

severe photosensitivity: St. John's wort

Lab test interferences:

False positive: ANA titer

Increase: ALT, AST, bilirubin, alk phosphatase, glucose, uric acid

NURSING CONSIDERATIONS

Assess:

• Blood studies: neutrophils, decreased platelets; WBC with diff baseline and q3mo, if neutrophils <1000/mm^3, discontinue treatment

• B/P, peak/trough level, orthostatic hypotension, syncope when used with diuretic, pulse q4h; note rate, rhythm, quality
• Electrolytes: K, Na, Cl during 1st 2 wk of therapy
• Baselines in renal, liver studies before therapy begins and 1 wk into therapy
• Edema in feet, legs daily
• Skin turgor, dryness of mucous membranes for hydration status
• Symptoms of CHF: edema, dyspnea, wet rales

Administer:

IV direct/Intermittent INF route

• Undiluted over 5 min, use diluent provided or 50 ml D_5W, 0.9% NaCl, 0.9% NaCl in D_5W or LR, Isolyte E, give through Y-tube of free-flowing inf of 0.9% NaCl, D_5W, LR, Isolyte E

Additive compatibilities: DOBUTamine, DOPamine, heparin, meropenem, nitroglycerin, nitroprusside, potassium chloride

Y-site compatibilities: Allopurinol, amifostine, amikacin, aminophylline, ampicillin, ampicillin/sulbactam, aztreonam, butorphanol, calcium gluconate, cefazolin, cefoperazone, ceftazidime, ceftizoxime, chloramphenicol, cimetidine, cisatracurium, cladribine, clindamycin, dextran 40, DOBUTamine, DOPamine, doxorubicin liposome, erythromycin, esmolol, famotidine, fentanyl, filgrastim, ganciclovir, gentamicin, granisetron, heparin, hetastarch, hydrocortisone, labetalol, lidocaine, magnesium sulfate, melphalan, meropenem, methylPREDNISolone, metronidazole, morphine, nafcillin, niCARdipine, nitroprusside, penicillin G potassium, phenobarbital, piperacillin, piperacillin/tazobactam, potassium chloride, potassium phosphate, propofol, ranitidine, remifentanil, teniposide, thiotepa, tobramycin, trimethoprim-sulfamethoxazole, vancomycin, vinorelbine

Evaluate:

• Therapeutic response: decreased B/P

Teach patient/family:

• Not to use OTC (cough, cold, or allergy) products unless directed by prescriber; to avoid potassium, salt substitutes
• To avoid sunlight or wear sunscreen for photosensitivity
• To comply with dosage schedule, even if feeling better
• To notify prescriber of mouth sores, sore throat, fever, swelling of hands or feet, irregular heartbeat, chest pain, signs of angioedema
• That excessive perspiration, dehydration, vomiting, diarrhea may lead to fall in blood pressure; consult prescriber if these occur
• That drug may cause dizziness, fainting; light-headedness may occur during 1st few days of therapy
• That drug may cause skin rash or impaired perspiration; angioedema may occur and to D/C if it occurs
• Not to discontinue drug abruptly
• That CV adverse reactions may reoccur
• To rise slowly to sitting or standing position to minimize orthostatic hypotension

Treatment of overdose: Lavage, IV atropine for bradycardia, IV theophylline for bronchospasm, digitalis, O_2, diuretic for cardiac failure

enoxacin (℞)

(e-nox′a-sin)
Penetrex
Func. class.: Antiinfective
Chem. class.: Fluoroquinolone

Action: Inhibits the enzyme that repairs bacterial DNA, thereby preventing bacterial replication; DNA-gyrase inhibitor

Uses: Uncomplicated urethral or cervical gonorrhea, uncomplicated and complicated UTI; effective against staphylococci, *Aeromonas* sp., *Citrobacter* sp., *Enterobacter* sp., *Escherichia coli, Haemophilus ducreyi, Klebsiella* sp., *Morganella morganii, Neisseria gonorrheae, Proteus vulgaris, Proteus mirabilis, Providencia* sp., *Pseudomonas aeruginosa, Serratia*

Dosage and routes:

Gonorrhea
• *Adult:* **PO** 400 mg as a single dose

Uncomplicated UTI
• *Adult:* **PO** 200 mg q12h × 7 days

Complicated UTI
• *Adult:* **PO** 400 mg q12h × 14 days

Renal disease
• CCr <30 ml/min give initial dose, then give 50% of dose q12h

Available forms: Tabs 200, 400 mg

Side effects/adverse reactions:

SYST: ***Anaphylaxis, Stevens-Johnson syndrome***

CNS: Dizziness, headache, fatigue, somnolence, depression, insomnia, anxiety, ***seizures***

GI: Diarrhea, nausea, vomiting, anorexia, flatulence, heartburn, abdominal pain, dry mouth, increased AST, ALT, ***pseudomembranous colitis***

INTEG: Rash, pruritus, photosensitivity

EENT: Visual disturbances, dizziness

Contraindications: Hypersensitivity to quinolones

Precautions: Pregnancy (C), lactation, children, elderly, renal disease, seizure disorders

Do not confuse:
enoxacin/enoxaparin

Pharmacokinetics:
PO: Peak 1 hr, half-life 3-6 hr, steady state 2 days; excreted in urine as unchanged drug, metabolites

Interactions:
• ↑ levels of: aminophylline, cimetidine, cycloSPORINE, oral anticoagulants, use cautiously
• ↑ levels toxicity: theophylline; do not use together
• ↓ absorption of enoxacin: antacids with magnesium, aluminum; iron salts, sucralfate, bismuth subsalicylate
• ↑ digoxin levels: digoxin, monitor for toxicity
• Drug/food: ↓ absorption with food, dairy products
• Do not use acidophilus with antiinfectives

NURSING CONSIDERATIONS

Assess:
• Renal, hepatic studies: BUN, creatinine, AST, ALT, alk phosphatase
• I&O ratio, urine pH; <5.5 is ideal
• CNS symptoms: insomnia, vertigo, headache, agitation, confusion
• Allergic reactions and anaphylaxis: rash, flushing, urticaria, pruritus; may occur a few days after therapy begins, emergency equipment should be available

Administer:
• After clean-catch urine for C&S
• 2 hr before or 2 hr after antacids, zinc, iron, calcium

Perform/provide:
• Limited intake of alkaline foods, drugs; milk, dairy products, peanuts, vegetables, alkaline actacids, sodium bicarbonate

Evaluate:

• Therapeutic response: negative C&S, absence of symptoms of infection

Teach patient/family:

• That fluids must be increased to 2 L/day to avoid crystallization in kidneys

• If dizziness occurs, to ambulate, perform activities with assistance, do not perform hazardous activities

• Not to take within 2 hr of antacids, calcium, iron, milk, sucralfate; not to double or miss doses

• To use sunscreen, protective clothing for photosensitivity

• To complete full course of drug therapy, take 1 hr ac or 2 hr pc

• To contact prescriber if adverse reactions occur or if inflammation or pain of tendon occurs

• To avoid use with OTC medications unless approved by prescriber

---

HIGH ALERT

enoxaparin (℞)

(ee-nox'a-par-in)

Lovenox

Func. class.: Anticoagulant, antithrombotic

Chem. class.: Unfractionated porcine heparin

Action: Prevents conversion of fibrinogen to fibrin and prothrombin to thrombin by enhancing inhibitory effects of antithrombin III; produces higher ratio of anti–factor Xa to IIa

Uses: Prevention of deep-vein thrombosis, pulmonary emboli in hip and knee replacement, abdominal surgery at risk for thrombosis; unstable angina/non–Q wave MI

Dosage and routes:

Hip/knee replacement

• *Adult:* **SC** 30 mg bid given 12-24 hr postop for 7-10 days, provided that hemostasis has been established

Abdominal surgery

• *Adult:* **SC** 40 mg qd × 7-10 days to prevent thromboembolic complications, start 2 hr before surgery

DVT/PE

• *Adult:* **SC** (Outpatient) (without PE) 1 mg/kg q12h or 1.5 mg/kg qd (Outpatient and inpatient)

• *Adult:* initiate with warfarin therapy usually within 72 hr of enoxaparin, continue enoxaparin for ≥5 days until INR is 2-3

Prevention of ischemic complications in unstable angina/non-Q-wave MI with aspirin

• *Adult:* SC 1 mg/kg q12h until stable with aspirin 100-325 mg qd

Available forms: Inj 30 mg/0.3 ml, 40 mg/0.4 ml, 60 mg/0.6 ml, 80 mg/0.8 ml, 100 mg/1 ml, 120 mg/0.8 ml, 150 mg/ml, 300 mg/3 ml

Side effects/adverse reactions:

CNS: Fever, confusion

GI: Nausea

SYST: Edema, peripheral edema

HEMA: ***Hemorrhage, hypochromic anemia, thrombocytopenia,*** bleeding

INTEG: Ecchymosis, inj site hematoma

Contraindications: Hypersensitivity to this drug, heparin, or pork; hemophilia, leukemia with bleeding, peptic ulcer disease, thrombocytopenic purpura, heparin-induced thrombocytopenia

Precautions: Alcoholism, elderly, pregnancy (B), hepatic disease (severe), renal disease (severe), blood dyscrasias, severe hypertension, subacute bacterial endocarditis, acute nephritis, lactation, children, recent burn, spinal surgery

Do not confuse:
enoxaparin/enoxacin
Lovenox/Lotronex

Pharmacokinetics:
SC: 90% absorbed, maximum antithrombin activity (3-5 hr), elimination half-life 4½ hr, excreted in urine

Interactions:
• ↑ enoxaparin action: anticoagulants, salicylates, NSAIDs, antiplatelets, thrombolytics
• ↑ hypoprothrombinemia: plicamycin, valproic acid
• Do not mix with other drugs or infusion fluids
↑ risk of bleeding: agrimony, alfalfa, angelica, anise, basil, bay, bilberry, black haw, bogbean, bromelain, buchu, chondroitin, cinchona bark, dong quai, fenugreek, feverfew, garlic, ginger, ginkgo, ginseng, horse chestnut, Irish moss, kelp, kelpware, khella, lovage, lungwort, meadowsweet, motherwort, mugwort, nettle, papaya, parsley (large amts), Pau D'arco, pineapple, poplar, prickly ash, safflower, saw palmetto, tonka bean, turmeric, wintergreen, yarrow
↓ anticoagulant effect: chamomile, coenzyme Q10, flax, glucomannan, goldenseal, guar gum

Lab test interferences:
Decrease: Platelet count
Increase: AST, ALT

NURSING CONSIDERATIONS

Assess:
• Blood studies (Hct, CBC, coagulation studies, platelets, occult blood in stools), anti–factor Xa; thrombocytopenia may occur
• For bleeding: gums, petechiae, ecchymosis, black tarry stools, hematuria; notify prescriber
• For neurologic symptoms in patients who have received spinal anesthesia

Administer:
• Only after screening patient for bleeding disorders
• SC only; do not give IM, begin 2 hr prior to surgery, do not aspirate, rotate sites, do not expel bubble from syringe before administration
• To recumbent patient; give SC; rotate inj sites (left/right anterolateral, left/right posterolateral abdominal wall)
• Insert whole length of needle into skin fold held with thumb and forefinger
Only this drug when ordered; not interchangeable with heparin or LMWHs
• At same time each day to maintain steady blood levels
• Leave vascular access sheath in place for 6 hr after dose, then give next dose 6 hr after sheath removal
• Avoiding all IM inj that may cause bleeding

Perform/provide:
• Storage at 77° F (25° C); do not freeze

Evaluate:
• Therapeutic response: prevention of deep vein thrombosis

Teach patient/family:
• To use soft-bristle toothbrush to avoid bleeding gums, to use electric razor
• To report any signs of bleeding: gums, under skin, urine, stools
• To avoid OTC drugs containing aspirin

Treatment of overdose: Protamine SO_4 1% sol; dose should equal dose of enoxaparin

entacapone (℞)

(en'ta-kah-pone)
Comtan
Func. class.: Antiparkinson agent
Chem. class.: COMT inhibitor

Action: Inhibits COMT (catechol *O*-methyltransferase) and alters the plasma pharmacokinetics of levodopa. Given with levodopa/carbidopa

Uses: Parkinsonism in those experiencing end of dose, decreased effect as adjunct to levodopa/carbidopa

Research note: Motor impairment was improved in patients with severe Parkinson's disease when entacapone was given to patients taking levodopa[10]

Dosage and routes:

• *Adult:* **PO** 200 mg given with carbidopa/levodopa, max 1600 mg/day

Available forms: Tabs 200 mg film coated

Side effects/adverse reactions:

CNS: Involuntary choreiform movements, hand tremors, fatigue, headache, anxiety, twitching, numbness, dyskinesia, hypokinesia, hyperkinesia, weakness, confusion, agitation, nightmares, psychosis, hallucination, hypomania, severe depression, dizziness, ***neuroleptic malignant syndrome***

GI: Nausea, vomiting, anorexia, abdominal distress, dry mouth, flatulence, bitter taste, diarrhea, constipation, dyspepsia, gastritis, GI disorder

INTEG: Rash, sweating, alopecia

CV: Orthostatic hypotension

MISC: Dark urine, back pain, dyspnea, purpura, fatigue, asthenia, infection-bacterial, ***rhabdomyolysis***

Contraindications: Hypersensitivity

Precautions: Renal disease, hepatic disease, pregnancy (C), affective disorders, psychosis, lactation, children

Pharmacokinetics: Duration up to 8 hr; excreted in urine, feces; well absorbed, protein binding 98%, metabolized liver extensively, enters breast milk; half-life of levodopa is extended, half-life 0.5 hr initial, 2.5 hr second

Interactions:

• ↑ B/P, tachycardia, dysrhythmias, avoid use: bitolterol, apomorphine, DOPamine, DOBUTamine, epINEPHrine, methyldopa, isoetharine, norepinephrine

• ↓ excretion of entacapone: ampicillin, chloramphenicol, probenecid, erythromycin, rifampin

• Prevents catecholamine metabolism, do not use together: MAOIs

↓ effect: kava

NURSING CONSIDERATIONS

Assess:

Neuroleptic malignant syndrome: high temp, increased CPK, rigidity, change in consciousness

• Involuntary movements in parkinsonism: akinesia, tremors, staggering gait, muscle rigidity, drooling when given with levodopa/carbidopa

• B/P, respiration during initial treatment

• Mental status: affect, mood, behavioral changes, depression; complete suicide assessment

Administer:

• Only after MAOIs have been discontinued for 2 wk

Perform/provide:

• Assistance with ambulation during beginning therapy

Evaluate:

• Therapeutic response: decrease in akathisia, increased mood when given with levodopa/carbidopa

Teach patient/family:

- That hallucinations, mental changes, nausea, dyskinesia can occur
- To change positions slowly to prevent orthostatic hypotension; not to drive or operate machinery until stabilized on medication and mental performance is not affected
- To use drug exactly as prescribed
- That urine, sweat may darken
- To notify prescriber if pregnancy is suspected; or if lactating, drug is excreted in breast milk

---

HIGH ALERT

✤ epHEDrine (℞)

(e-fed′rin)

epHEDrine sulfate

Func. class.: Bronchodilator, nonselective adrenergic, mixed direct and indirect effects

Chem. class.: Phenylisopropylamine

Action: Causes increased contractility and heart rate by acting on β-receptors in the heart; also acts on α-receptors, causing vasoconstriction in blood vessels

Uses: Shock; increased perfusion; hypotension, bronchodilation

Dosage and routes:

Vasopressor

- *Adult:* **IM/SC** 25-50 mg, not to exceed 150 mg/24 hr; **IV** 10-25 mg, not to exceed 150 mg/24 hr
- *Child:* **SC/IV** 3 mg/kg/day or 25-100 mg/m^2/day in divided doses q4-6h or 16.7 mg/m^2 q4-6h

Bronchodilator

- *Adult and child ≥12 yr:* **PO** 25-50 mg bid-qid, not to exceed 400 mg/day; **IM/SC** 12.5-25 mg
- *Child 6-12 yr:* 6.25-12.5 mg q4h, max 75 mg/24 hr
- *Child >2 yr:* **PO** 2-3 mg/kg/day or 100 mg/m^2/day in 4-6 divided doses

Orthostatic hypotension

- *Adult:* **PO** 25 mg qd-qid
- *Child:* **PO** 3 mg/kg/day in 4-6 divided doses

Stimulation

- *Adult:* **PO** 25-50 mg q3-4h prn
- *Child:* **PO** 3 mg/kg/day or 100 mg/m^2/day in divided doses

Labor

- *Adult:* Administer **IV** dose to maintain B/P at or <130/80 mm Hg

Available forms: Inj 25, 30, 50 mg/ml; caps 25, 50 mg

Side effects/adverse reactions:

CNS: Tremors, anxiety, insomnia, sweating, headache, dizziness, confusion, hallucinations, ***convulsions, CNS depression, cerebral hemorrhage***

GU: Dysuria, urinary retention

CV: Palpitations, tachycardia, hypertension, chest pain, ***dysrhythmias***

GI: Anorexia, nausea, vomiting

RESP: ***Dyspnea***

Contraindications: Hypersensitivity to sympathomimetics, narrow-angle glaucoma, nonanaphylactic shock during general anesthesia

Precautions: Pregnancy (C), lactation, cardiac disorders, hyperthyroidism, diabetes mellitus, prostatic hypertrophy, hypertension

Do not confuse:

epHEDrine/epINEPHrine

Pharmacokinetics:

PO: Onset 15-60 min, duration 2-4 hr

IM: Onset 10-20 min, duration 1 hr

IV: Onset 5 min, duration 2 hr

Metabolized in liver; excreted in urine (unchanged), breast milk; crosses blood-brain barrier, placenta

Interactions:

- Severe hypertension: oxytocics
- Do not use with MAOIs; hypertensive crisis may occur

• ↓ effect of epHEDrine: methyldopa, urinary acidifiers, rauwolfia alkaloids, α-adrenergic blockers, diuretics, tricyclics
• ↑ effect of epHEDrine: urinary alkalizers
• Dysrhythmia: halothane anesthetics, cardiac glycosides, levodopa
• ↓ effect of guanethidine

NURSING CONSIDERATIONS
Assess:
• I&O ratio
• ECG continuously during administration; if B/P increases, drug is decreased; B/P and pulse q5min after parenteral route; CVP or PWP during infusion if possible
• For paresthesias and coldness of extremities; peripheral blood flow may decrease; long-term use may produce a pseudoanxiety state requiring sedative; increased lactic acid with severe metabolic acidosis can occur
• Injection site: tissue sloughing; if this occurs, administer phentolamine mixed with 0.9% NaCl

Administer:
IV direct route
• Through Y-tube or 3-way stopcock; give 10-25 mg slowly; may repeat in 5-10 min, protect from light
• Plasma expanders for hypovolemia

Additive compatibilities: Chloramphenicol, lidocaine, metaraminol, nafcillin, penicillin G potassium
Solution compatibilities: D_5W, $D_{10}W$, LR, 0.9% NaCl, 0.45% NaCl, Ringer's
Syringe compatibilities: Pentobarbital
Y-site compatibilities: Etomidate, propofol

Perform/provide:
• Storage of reconstituted sol refrigerated no longer than 24 hr
• Do not use discolored sol

Evaluate:
• Therapeutic response: increased B/P with stabilization

Teach patient/family:
• The reason for drug administration

*epHEDrine nasal agent

See appendix c

HIGH ALERT

*epINEPHrine (℞)

(ep-i-nef′rin)

Adrenalin Ana-Guard, AsthmaHaler Mist, AsthmaNefrin (racepinephrine), Bronitin Mist, Bronkaid Mist, Epinal, epINEPHrine, EpINEPHrine Pediatric, EpiPen, EpiPen Jr., Epitrate, Eppy/N, Medihaler microNefrin, Nephron, Primatene Mist, S-2, Sus-Phrine, Vaponefrin (racepinephrine)

Func. class.: Bronchodilator nonselective adrenergic agonist, vasopressor
Chem. class.: Catecholamine

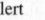

Action: β_1- and β_2-agonist causing increased levels of cAMP producing bronchodilation, cardiac, and CNS stimulation; large doses cause vasoconstriction via α-receptors; small doses can cause vasodilation via β_2-vascular receptors
Uses: Acute asthmatic attacks, hemostasis, bronchospasm, anaphylaxis, allergic reactions, cardiac arrest, adjunct in anesthesia, shock

Dosage and routes:

Asthma

• *Adult and child:* **INH** 1-2 puffs of 1:100 or 2.25% racemic q15min

Bronchodilator

• *Adult:* **SC** 0.2-0.5 mg q20min-4h, max 1 mg/dose

Anaphylactic shock/vasopressor

• *Adult:* **SC/IM** 0.1-0.5 mg, repeat q5min if needed, then **IV; IV** 0.1-0.25 mg, repeat q5-15min or inf 1 mcg/min, increase to 4 mcg/min if needed

• *Child <30 kg:* **SC/IM/IV** 10 mcg/kg, repeat q5-15min up to 0.3 mg

Anaphylactic reaction/asthma

• *Adult:* **SC/IM** 0.1-0.5 mg, repeat q10-15min, do not exceed 1 mg/dose; epINEPHrine susp 0.5 mg **SC,** may repeat 0.5-1.5 mg q6h

• *Child:* **SC** 0.01 mg/kg, repeat q15min, × 2 doses, then q4h, max 0.5 mg/dose; epINEPHrine susp 0.025 mg/kg **SC,** may repeat q6h, max 0.75 mg in child ≤30 kg

Cardiac arrest

• *Adult:* **IC, IV, ENDOTRACH** 0.1-1 mg, repeat q5min prn

• *Child:* **IC, IV, ENDOTRACH** 5-10 mcg q5min, may use 0.1 mcg/kg/min **IV INF** after initial dose

Available forms: Aerosol 0.16 mg/spray, 0.2 mg/spray, 0.25 mg/spray; inj 1:1000 (1 mg/ml), 1:200 (5 mg/ml), 0.01 mg/ml (1:100,000), 0.1 mg/ml (1:10,000), 0.5 mg/ml (1:2000); sol for nebulization 1:100, 1.25%, 2.25% (base)

Side effects/adverse reactions:

CNS: Tremors, anxiety, insomnia, headache, *dizziness,* confusion, hallucinations, ***cerebral hemorrhage***, weakness, drowsiness, headache

CV: Palpitations, tachycardia, hypertension, *dysrhythmias,* increased T wave

GI: Anorexia, nausea, vomiting

RESP: Dyspnea

Contraindications: Hypersensitivity to sympathomimetics, narrow-angle glaucoma, nonanaphylactic shock during general anesthesia, organic brain syndrome, local anesthesia of certain areas, labor, cardiac dilation, coronary insufficiency, cerebral arteriosclerosis, organic heart disease

Precautions: Pregnancy (C), lactation, cardiac disorders, hyperthyroidism, diabetes mellitus, prostatic hypertrophy, hypertension

Do not confuse:

epINEPHrine/epHEDrine

Pharmacokinetics:

SC: Onset 3-5 min, duration 20 min

PO, INH: Onset 1 min

Crosses placenta; metabolized in liver

Interactions:

• Do not use with MAOIs or tricyclics; hypertensive crisis may occur

• Toxicity: other sympathomimetics

• ↓ hypertensive effects: α-adrenergic blockers

• Dysrhythmias: bretylium, cardiac glycosides, halothane anesthetics

• ↓ vascular response: diuretics, ergot alkaloids, phenothiazines

• ↑ pressor response: guanethidine, antihistamines, levothyroxine

• Severe hypertension: oxytocics

NURSING CONSIDERATIONS

Assess:

• ECG during administration continuously; if B/P increases, drug is decreased; B/P and pulse q5min after parenteral route; CVP, ISVR, PCWP during infusion if possible; inadvertent high arterial B/P can result in angina, aortic rupture, cerebral hemorrhage

• Injection site: tissue sloughing; administer phentolamine with NS

• Sulfite sensitivity, which may be life-threatening

Administer:
• Increased dose of insulin in diabetic patients
• Check for correct concentration, route, dosage before administering
IM/SC route
• Rotate inj sites, massage after inj, shake before using
IV route
• Parenteral dose slowly, after reconstituting 1 mg (1:1000 sol)/10 ml or more 0.9% NaCl; to prepare a 1:10,000 sol for maintenance, may be further diluted in 500 ml D_5W; give 1 mg or less over 1 min or more through Y-tube or 3-way stopcock; 1 mg = 1 ml of 1:1000 or 10 ml of 1:10,000; protect from light
Additive compatibilities: Amikacin, cimetidine, DOBUTamine, floxacillin, furosemide, metaraminol, ranitidine, verapamil
Syringe compatibilities: Doxapram, heparin, milrinone
Y-site compatibilities: Amrinone, atracurium, calcium chloride, calcium gluconate, cisatracurium, diltiazem, DOBUTamine, DOPamine, famotidine, fentanyl, furosemide, heparin, hydrocortisone sodium succinate, hydromorphone, labetalol, lorazepam, midazolam, milrinone, morphine, niCARdipine, nitroglycerin, norepinephrine, pancuronium, phytonadione, potassium chloride, propofol, ranitidine, remifentanil, vecuronium, vit B/C, warfarin
Endotracheal route
• Give directly via endrotracheal tube
Inhalation route
• Place in nebulizer (10 gtts of a 1% base sol)
• Dilute racepinephrine 2.25% sol
Perform/provide:
• Storage of reconstituted sol refrigerated no longer than 24 hr
• Do not use discolored sol

Evaluate:
• Therapeutic response: increased B/P with stabilization or ease of breathing
Teach patient/family:
• The reason for drug administration
• To rinse mouth after use to prevent dryness after inhalation
• Not to take OTC preparations
Treatment of overdose: Administer an α-blocker and a β-blocker

*epINEPHrine bitartrate/ epINEPHrine HCl/ epinephryl borate ophthalmic

See appendix c

*epINEPHrine nasal agent

See appendix c

HIGH ALERT

epirubicin (℞)

(ep-ih-roo′bi-sin)
Ellence
Func. class.: Antineoplastic, antibiotic
Chem. class.: Anthracycline

Action: Inhibits DNA synthesis primarily; replication is decreased by binding to DNA, which causes strand splitting; maximum cytotoxic effects at Sand G_2 phases, a vesicant
Uses: Breast cancer as an adjuvant therapy, with axillary node involvement following resection
Research note: One study has concluded that epirubicin produces mild

subclinical myocardial damage with a decline in LVEF[11]

Dosage and routes:

• *Adult:* **IV Inf** 100-120 mg/m^2 initially, given with other antineoplastics; given in repeated cycles; 3-4 wk cycles

Hepatic dose

• *Adult:* **IV** bilirubin 1.2-3 mg/dl or AST 2-4 × normal upper limit 50% of starting dose; bilirubin >3 mg/dl or AST >4 × normal upper limit 25% of starting dose

Available forms: Inj 2 mg/ml

Side effects/adverse reactions:

HEMA: ***Thrombocytopenia, leukopenia, anemia, neutropenia, secondary AML***

GI: Nausea, vomiting, anorexia, mucositis, diarrhea

GU: Amenorrhea, hot flashes, hyperuricemia

INTEG: Rash, necrosis at inj site, reversible alopecia

MISC: Infection, febrile neutropenia, lethargy, fever, conjunctivitis

CV: Increased B/P, ***sinus tachycardia, PVCs,*** chest pain, ***bradycardia, extrasystoles, CHF***

Contraindications: Hypersensitivity to this drug, anthracyclines, anthracenediones, severe hepatic disease, baseline neutrophil count <1500 cell/mm^3, severe myocardial insufficiency, recent MI, pregnancy (D), lactation, systemic infections

Precautions: Renal, hepatic, cardiac disease; gout, bone marrow depression (severe), elderly, children

Pharmacokinetics: Triphasic pattern of elimination; half-life 3 min, 2.5 hr, 33 hr; metabolized by liver; crosses placenta; excreted in urine, bile, breast milk

Interactions:

• ↑ toxicity: other antineoplastics or radiation, cimetidine

• ↓ antibody response: live virus vaccine

NURSING CONSIDERATIONS

Assess:

• Bone marrow depression, infection: increased temp

• CBC, differential, platelet count weekly; withhold drug if baseline neutrophil ≤1500/mm^3; leukocyte nadir occurs 10-14 days after administration, recovery by 21st day; notify prescriber of these results

• Blood, urine uric acid levels; swelling, joint pain primarily in extremities, patient should be well hydrated to prevent urate deposits

• Renal studies: BUN, serum uric acid, urine CCr, electrolytes before, during therapy; I&O ratio; report fall in urine output to <30 ml/hr; dosage adjustment is needed if serum creatinine >5 mg/dl

• Hepatic studies before, during therapy: bilirubin, AST, ALT, alk phosphatase as needed or monthly

• Cardiac status: B/P, pulse, character, rhythm, rate, ABGs, ECG, LVEF, MUGA scan, or ECHO; watch for ST-T wave changes, low QRS and T, possible dysrhythmias (sinus tachycardia, heart block, PVCs)

• Bleeding: hematuria, guaiac, bruising, or petechiae, mucosa or orifices q8h

• Effects of alopecia on body image; discuss feelings about body changes

• Alkalosis if severe vomiting is present

• Local irritation, pain, burning at inj site

• GI symptoms: frequency of stools, cramping

• Acidosis, signs of dehydration: rapid respirations, poor skin turgor, decreased urine output, dry skin, restlessness, weakness

Administer:

⊘ Do not break, crush, or chew;

only chewable tabs should be chewed
• Antiemetic 30-60 min before giving drug to prevent vomiting
• Allopurinol or sodium bicarbonate to maintain uric acid levels, alkalinization of urine
IV route
• Hydrocortisone, dexamethasone, or sodium bicarbonate (1 mEq/1 ml) for extravasation; apply ice compresses
• Given into tubing of free-flowing IV infusion (0.9% NaCl or D_5) give over 3-5 min; do not mix with other drugs in syringe
Perform/provide:
• Strict hand-washing technique, gloves, protective clothing
• Liquid diet: carbonated beverages, gelatin may be added if patient is not nauseated or vomiting
• Increased fluid intake to 2-3 L/day to prevent urate, calculi formation
Evaluate:
• Therapeutic response: decreased tumor size, spread of malignancy
Teach patient/family:
• To report any complaints, side effects to nurse or prescriber
• That hair may be lost during treatment and wig or hairpiece may make patient feel better; tell patient that new hair may be different in color, texture
• To avoid crowds and persons with infections when granulocyte count is low
• That contraceptive measures are recommended during therapy and 4 mo thereafter
• To avoid vaccinations, reactions may occur; to avoid cimetidine during therapy
• That urine may appear red for 2 days
• To avoid crowds, persons with known infections
• To avoid OTC medications, supplements unless approved by prescriber

eplerenone (℞)

(ep-ler-ee'known)
Inspra
Func. class.: Antihypertensive
Chem. class.: Selective aldosterone receptor antagonist

Action: Binds to mineralocorticoid receptor and blocks the binding of aldosterone, a component of the renin-angiotensin aldosterone system (RAAS)
Uses: Hypertension, alone or in combination with thiazide diuretics
Dosage and routes:
• *Adult:* **PO** 50 mg qd, initially, may increase to 50 mg bid after 4 wk; start dose at 25 mg qd if patient is taking CYP 3A4 inhibitors
Available forms: Tabs 25, 50, 100 mg
Side effects/adverse reactions:
CV: angina, ***MI***
GU: Increased BUN, creatinine, gynecomastia, mastodynia (males), abnormal vaginal bleeding
RESP: Cough
META: Hyperkalemia, hyponatremia, hypercholesteremia, hypertriglyceridemia, increased uric acid
GI: Increased GGT diarrhea, abdominal pain, increased ALT
CNS: Headache, dizziness, fatigue
Contraindications: Hypersensitivity, lactation, children, increased serum creatinine >2 mg/dl (male), >1.8 mg/dl (female), potassium >5.5 mEq/L, type 2 diabetes with microalbuminuria, hepatic disease, creatinine clearance >50 ml/min
Precautions: Impaired renal, liver function, elderly, pregnancy (B), hyperkalemia, lactation

Pharmacokinetics:
PO: Peak 1½ hr, serum protein binding 50%, half-life 4-6 hr, metabolized by liver (CYP 3A4 inhibitor), excreted in urine
Interactions:
• ↑ hyperkalemia: ACE inhibitors, angiotensin II antagonists, NSAIDs, potassium supplements
• ↑ serum levels of lithium
• ↑ levels of eplerenone: CYP 3A4 inhibitors (ketoconazole, itraconazole, saquinavir, erythromycin, verapamil, fluconazole), reduce dose of eplerenone
• ↓ antihypertensive effect: NSAIDs
• Drug/food: Grapefruit juice ↑ drug level by 25%
↓ levels of eplerenone: St. John's wort
↑ toxicity, death: aconite
↑ or ↓ antihypertensive effect: astragalus, cola tree
↑ antihypertensive effect: barberry, betony, black catechu, black cohosh, bloodroot, broom, burdock, cat's claw, dandelion, goldenseal, Irish moss, Jamaican dogwood, kelp, khella, mistletoe, parsley
↓ antihypertensive effect: coltsfoot, guarana, khat, licorice
NURSING CONSIDERATIONS
Assess:
• B/P at peak/trough level of drug, orthostatic hypotension, syncope when used with diuretic
• Renal studies: Protein, BUN, creatinine; increased LFTs, uric acid may be increased
• Potassium levels, hyperkalemia may occur
Perform/provide:
• Storage in tight container at 86° F (30° C) or less
Evaluate:
• Therapeutic response: decrease in B/P
Teach patient/family:
• Not to discontinue drug abruptly
• Not to use OTC products (cough, cold, allergy) unless directed by prescriber; do not use salt substitutes containing potassium without consulting prescriber
• Important to comply with dosage schedule, even if feeling better
• That drug may cause dizziness, fainting, light-headedness; may occur during first few days of therapy
• How to take B/P, and normal readings for age-group

epoetin (℞)
(ee-poe'e-tin)
EPO, Epogen, Eprex ♣, Procrit
Func. class.: Antianemic, biologic modifier, hormone
Chem. class.: Amino acid polypeptide

Action: Erythropoietin is one factor controlling rate of red cell production; drug is developed by recombinant DNA technology
Uses: Anemia caused by reduced endogenous erythropoietin production, primarily end-stage renal disease; to correct hemostatic defect in uremia; anemia due to AZT treatment in HIV patients or chemotherapy; reduction of allogenic blood transfusion in surgery patients
Investigational uses:
Pruritus; anemia in: premature preterm infants, myelodysplastic syndrome, chronic inflammatory disorders
Dosage and routes:
Anemia related to chemotherapy
• *Adult:* **SC** 150 units/kg 3 ×/wk, may increase after 2 mo up to 300 units/kg 3 ×/wk
Anemia in chronic renal failure not on dialysis
• *Adult:* **SC/IV** 75-150 units/kg q wk to maintain Hct

• *Child:* **IV/SC** 50 units/kg 3 ×/wk

Anemia secondary to zidovudine treatment

• *Adult:* **SC/IV** 100 units/kg 3 ×/wk × 2 mo, may increase by 50-100 units/kg q1-2mo, up to 300 units/kg 3 ×/wk

Surgery

• *Adult:* **SC** 300 units/kg/day × 10 days prior to surgery, the day of surgery, and for 4 days postsurgery or 600 units/kg at 3 wk, 2 wk, 1 wk, prior to and on day of surgery

Available forms: Inj 2000, 3000, 4000, 10,000, 20,000, 40,000 units/ml

Side effects/adverse reactions:

CV: Hypertension, ***hypertensive encephalopathy***

CNS: ***Seizures,*** coldness, sweating, headache

MS: Bone pain

Contraindications: Hypersensitivity to mammalian cell–derived products, or human albumin, uncontrolled hypertension

Precautions: Seizure disorder, porphyria, pregnancy (C), children <1 mo, lactation, multidose preserved formulation contains benzyl alcohol and should not be used in premature infants

Pharmacokinetics:

IV: Metabolized in body; extent of metabolism unknown; onset of increased reticulocyte count 1-6 wk; peak, immediate

Interactions:

• Need for ↑ anticoagulant during hemodialysis

NURSING CONSIDERATIONS

Assess:

• Renal studies: urinalysis, protein, blood, BUN, creatinine; I&O, report drop in output <50 ml/hr

• Blood studies: ferritin, transferrin monthly; transferrin sat ≥20%, ferritin ≥100 ng/ml; Hct 2 ×/wk until stabilized in target range (30%-36%) then at regular intervals; those with endogenous erythropoietin levels of <500 units/L respond to this agent; monitor HCT 2×/wk in chronic renal failure; patients treated w/zidovudine or cancer patients should be monitored wk, then periodically after stabilization

• B/P; check for rising B/P as Hct rises, antihypertensives may be needed; hypertension may occur rapidly leading to hypertensive encephalopathy

• CNS symptoms: coldness, sweating, pain in long bones; for seizures if Hct is increased within 2 wk by 4 pts

• For hypersensitivity reactions: skin rashes, urticaria (rare), antibody development does not occur

For pure cell aplasia (PRCA) in CRF patients: any loss of response to epoetin should be evaluated

• Dialysis patients: thrill, bruit of shunts, monitor for circulation impairment

Administer:

• Do not shake vial

IV route

• Additional heparin to lower chance of clots

• By direct inj or bolus into IV tubing or venous line at end of dialysis

• Decrease dose by 25 units/kg, if Hct increases by 4% in 2 wk; increase dose if Hct does not increase by 5-6 pts after 8 wk of therapy, suggested target Hct range 30%–50%

Solution compatibilities: NaCl 0.9%, $D_{10}W$, $D_{10}W$/albumin, sterile water for inj, TPN

SC route

• Used for patients not on dialysis; admix before giving, using 0.9% NaCl with benzyl alcohol 0.9% 1 : 1

Evaluate:

• Therapeutic response: increase in reticulocyte count in 1-6 wk, Hgb/

Hct; increased appetite, enhanced sense of well-being

Teach patient/family:

- To avoid driving or hazardous activity during beginning of treatment
- To monitor B/P
- To take iron supplements, vitamin B_{12}, folic acid as directed

eprosartan (℞)

(ep-roh-sar'tan)

Teveten HCT

Func. class.: Antihypertensive

Chem. class.: Angiotensin II–receptor antagonist (Subtype AT_1)

Action: Blocks the vasoconstrictor and aldosterone-secreting effects of angiotensin II; selectively blocks the binding of angiotensin II to the AT_1 receptor found in tissues

Uses: Hypertension, alone or with other antihypertensives

Dosage and routes:

- *Adult:* **PO** 600 mg qd; dose may be divided and given bid with total daily doses ranging from 400-800 mg

Available forms: Tabs 600 mg/12.5, 600 mg/25

Side effects/adverse reactions:

CNS: Dizziness, depression, fatigue, headache

CV: Chest pain

EENT: Sinusitis

GI: Diarrhea, dyspepsia, abdominal pain

GU: UTI

META: Hypertriglyceridemia

MS: Myalgia, arthralgia

RESP: Cough, upper respiratory infection, rhinitis, pharyngitis, viral infection

Contraindications: Hypersensitivity, pregnancy (D) 2nd/3rd trimesters

Precautions: Hypersensitivity to ACE inhibitors; pregnancy (C) 1st trimester, lactation, children, elderly; renal, hepatic disease

Pharmacokinetics: Peak 1-2 hr, food delays absorption, protein binding 98%, moderate renal impairment increases drug levels by 30%, hepatic impairment increases levels by 40%, excreted in urine and feces

Interactions:

↑ toxicity, death: aconite

↑ or ↓ antihypertensive effect: astragalus, cola tree

↑ antihypertensive effect: barberry, betony, black catechu, black cohosh, bloodroot, broom, burdock, cat's claw, dandelion, goldenseal, Irish moss, Jamaican dogwood, kelp, khella, mistletoe, parsley

↓ antihypertensive effect: coltsfoot, guarana, khat, licorice

Lab test interferences:

Decrease: Hgb

Increase: ALT, AST, alk phosphatase

NURSING CONSIDERATIONS

Assess:

- B/P with position changes, pulse q4h; note rate, rhythm, quality
- Electrolytes (K, Na, Cl)
- Baselines in renal, hepatic studies before therapy begins
- Edema in feet, legs qd
- Skin turgor, dryness of mucous membranes for hydration status

Administer:

- Without regard to meals

Evaluate:

- Therapeutic response: decreased B/P

Teach patient/family:

- To comply with dosage schedule, even if feeling better
- To notify prescriber of fever, swelling of hands or feet, chest pain
- That excessive perspiration, dehydration, diarrhea may lead to fall in blood pressure; consult prescriber if these occur

• That drug may cause dizziness, avoid hazardous activities until effect is known
• Not to take this medication if pregnant or breastfeeding, or have had an allergic reaction to this drug
• To take missed dose as soon as possible, unless within 1 hr before next dose

HIGH ALERT

eptifibatide (℞)

(ep-tih-fib'ah-tide)
Integrilin
Func. class.: Antiplatelet agent
Chem. class.: Glycoprotein IIb/IIIa inhibitor

Action: Platelet glycoprotein antagonist. this agent reversibly prevents fibrinogen, von Willebrand's factor from binding to the glycoprotein IIb/IIIa receptor, inhibiting platelet aggregation
Uses: Acute coronary syndrome including those with PCI (percutaneous coronary intervention)
Dosage and routes:
Acute coronary syndrome
• *Adult:* **IV BOL** 180 mcg/kg as soon as diagnosed, then **IV CONT** 2 mcg/kg/min until discharge or CABG up to 72 hr; may decrease inf rate to 0.5 mcg/kg/min if undergoing PCI; continue inf for 20-24 hr postprocedure, allowing up to 96 hr of treatment
PCI in patients without acute coronary syndrome
• *Adult:* **IV BOL** 135 mcg/kg given immediately before PCI; then 0.5 mcg/kg/min × 20-24 hr
Available forms: Sol for inj 2 mg/ml (10 ml), 0.75 mg/ml (100 ml)
Side effects/adverse reactions:
CV: ***Stroke,*** hypotension
SYST: ***Bleeding, anaphylaxis***
GU: Hematuria
HEMA: ***Thrombocytopenia***
Contraindications: Hypersensitivity, active internal bleeding; history of bleeding, stroke within 1 mo; major surgery with severe trauma, severe hypotension, history of intracranial bleeding, intracranial neoplasm, arteriovenous malformation/aneurysm, aortic dissection, dependence on renal dialysis, platelets <100,000/mm^3
Precautions: Bleeding, pregnancy (B), lactation, children, elderly, renal function impairment
Interactions:
• ↑ bleeding: aspirin, heparin, NSAIDs, anticoagulants, ticlopidine, clopidogrel, dipyridamole, thrombolytics, plicamycin, valproate, abciximab
• Do not give with glycoprotein inhibitors IIb, IIIa
Pharmacokinetics: half-life 2.5 hr, steady state 4-6 hr, metabolism limited, excretion via kidneys
NURSING CONSIDERATIONS
Assess:
◆ Platelets, Hgb, Hct, creatinine, PT/APTT baseline INR within 6 hr of loading dose and qd therafter, patients undergoing PCI should have ACT monitored; maintain APTT 50-70 sec unless PCI is to be performed; during PCI, ACT should be 300-350 sec; if platelets drop <100,000/mm^3, obtain additional platelet counts; if thrombocytopenia is confirmed, discontinue drug; also, draw Hct, Hgb, serum creatinine
◆ For bleeding: gums, bruising, ecchymosis, petechiae; from GI, GU tract, cardiac cath sites, IM inj sites

Administer:
- Aspirin and heparin may be given with this drug
- D/C heparin before removing femoral artery sheath, after PCI

IV route
- After withdrawing bolus dose from 10 ml vial, give IV push over 1-2 min; follow bolus dose with continuous inf using pump, give drug undiluted directly from 100 ml vial, spike 100 ml vial with vented infusion set, use caution when centering spike on circle of stopper top

Y-site compatabilities: alteplase, atropine, DOBUTamine, heparin, lidocaine, meperidine, metoprolol, midazolam, morphine, nitroglycerin, verapamil

Solution compatibilities: 0.9% NaCl, D_5/0.9% NaCl

Perform/provide:
- Do not give discolored solutions or those with particulates, discard unused amount
- Discontinuing drug prior to CABG
- All medications PO if possible, avoid IM inj and all catheters

Teach patient/family:
- Reason for medication and expected results
- To report bruising, bleeding, chest pain immediately

ergonovine (℞)

(er-goe-noe′veen)
ergonovine, Ergotrate
Func. class.: Oxytocic
Chem. class.: Ergot alkaloid

Action: Stimulates uterine contractions and vascular smooth muscle, decreases bleeding

Uses: Postpartum or postabortion hemorrhage

Investigational uses: To induce a coronary artery spasm for diagnostic purposes

Dosage and routes:

Oxytocic
- *Adult:* **PO/SL** 0.2-0.4 mg q6-12h; **IM** 0.2 mg q2-4h, not to exceed 5 doses; **IV** 0.2 mg given over 1 min

Induced coronary artery spasm
- *Adult:* **IV** 50 mcg q5min up to 400 mcg or when chest pain occurs

Available forms: Inj 0.2, 0.25 mg/ml; tab 0.2 mg

Side effects/adverse reactions:
CNS: Headache, dizziness, fainting
CV: Hypertension, chest pain
GI: Nausea, vomiting, diarrhea
INTEG: Sweating
RESP: Dyspnea
EENT: Tinnitus
GU: Cramping

Contraindications: Hypersensitivity to ergot medication, augmentation of labor, before delivery of placenta, spontaneous abortion (threatened), pelvic inflammatory disease

Precautions: Hepatic disease, renal disease, cardiac disease, asthma, anemia, convulsive disorders, hypertension, glaucoma, obliterative vascular disease

Pharmacokinetics:
IM: Onset 2-5 min, duration 3 hr
IV: Onset immediate, duration 45 min
Metabolized in liver, excreted in urine

Interactions:
- Hypertension: sympathomimetics, ergots
- ↑ serotonin effect: horehound

NURSING CONSIDERATIONS

Assess:
- Ergotism: nausea, vomiting, weakness, muscular pain, insensitivity to cold, paresthesias of extremities; drug should be discontinued
- B/P, pulse; watch for change that may indicate hemorrhage

E

• Respiratory rate, rhythm, depth; notify prescriber of abnormalities
• Fundal tone, nonphasic contractions; check for relaxation

Administer:

• IM inj deep in large muscle mass; rotate inj sites if additional doses are given
• With emergency equipment available

IV direct route

• Dilute with 5 ml 0.9% NaCl, give through Y-tube or 3-way stopcock over 1 min

Additive compatibilities: Amikacin, cephapirin, sodium bicarbonate

Evaluate:

• Therapeutic response: decreased blood loss, severe cramping

Teach patient/family:

• To report increased blood loss, increased temp, or foul-smelling lochia; that cramping is normal
• The importance of pad count
• To avoid nicotine products

Treatment of overdose: Stop drug, give vasodilators, heparin, dextran

ergotamine (℞)

(er-got'a-meen)

Ergomar♣, Ergostat, Gynergen♣

dihydroergotamine

(dye-hye-droe-er-got'a-meen)

DHE45, Dihydroergotamine-Sandoz♣, Migranal

Func. class.: α-Adrenergic blocker, vascular headache suppressant

Chem. class.: Ergot alkaloid—amino acid

Action: Constricts smooth muscle in peripheral, cranial blood vessels, relaxes uterine muscle; blocks serotonin release

Uses: Vascular headache (migraine, cluster histamine)

Dosage and routes:

ergotamine

• *Adult:* **SL** 1 tab, may use q30min, max 3 tabs/24 hr

dihydroergotamine

• *Adults:* **SC/IM** 1 mg, may repeat in 1 hr to 3 mg, max 3 mg/day or 6 mg/wk; **IV** 0.5 mg, may repeat in 1 hr, max 2 mg/day or 6 mg/wk
• *Child ≥6 yr:* **SC/IM** 0.5 mg, may repeat in 1 hr; **IV:** 0.25 mg, may repeat in 1 hr

Severe acute migraine

• *Child 12-16 yr:* **IV** 0.25-0.5 mg, may repeat q20min for 1-2 doses

Available forms: ergotamine: SL tabs 2 mg; dihydroergotamine: inj 1 mg/ml; nasal spray 4 mg/ml

Side effects/adverse reactions:

CNS: Numbness in fingers, toes, headache, weakness

CV: Transient tachycardia, chest pain, bradycardia, edema, claudication, increase or decrease in B/P, ***MI***

GI: Nausea, vomiting, diarrhea, abdominal cramps

MS: Muscle pain

Contraindications: Hypersensitivity to ergot preparations, occlusion (peripheral, vascular), CAD, hepatic disease, renal disease, peptic ulcer, hypertension, pregnancy (X), Raynaud's disease, peripheral vascular disease, intermittent claudication

Precautions: Lactation, children, anemia, elderly

Pharmacokinetics:

IM/SC: Duration 8 hr

IV: Peak ¼-2 hr, duration 8 hr

PO: Peak 30 min-3 hr; metabolized in liver; excreted as metabolites in feces; crosses blood-brain barrier; excreted in breast milk

Interactions:

• ↑ ergot toxicity: macrolides
• ↑ vasoconstriction: β-blockers
• ↑ serotonin effect: horehound

NURSING CONSIDERATIONS

Assess:

• Ergotism: nausea, vomiting, weakness, muscular pain, insensitivity to cold, paresthesia of extremities; drug should be discontinued
• Weight daily, check for peripheral edema in feet, legs
• For stress level, activity, recreation, coping mechanisms
• Neurologic status: LOC, blurring vision, nausea, vomiting, tingling in extremities that occurs preceding the headache
• Ingestion of tyramine foods (pickled products, beer, wine, aged cheese), food additives, preservatives, colorings, artificial sweeteners, chocolate, caffeine; may precipitate headaches
• Toxicity: dyspnea, hypotension or hypertension, rapid, weak pulse, delirium, nausea, vomiting

Administer:

• At beginning of headache; dose must be titrated to patient response
• Not to pregnant women; harm to fetus may occur

IV route

• Give dihydroergotamine undiluted over 1 min

Perform/provide:

• Quiet, calm environment with decreased stimulation for noise, bright light, or excessive talking

Evaluate:

• Therapeutic response: decrease in frequency, severity of headache

Teach patient/family:

• Not to use OTC medications; serious drug interactions may occur
• To maintain dose at approved level; not to increase even if drug does not relieve headache
• To report side effects including increased vasoconstriction starting with cold extremities, then paresthesia, weakness
• That an increase in headaches may occur when this drug is discontinued after long-term use
• To keep drug out of reach of children; death may occur

Treatment of overdose: Induce emesis or gastric lavage if orally ingested; administer saline cathartic; keep warm

E

ertapenem (℞)

(er-tah-pen′em)
Invanz
Func. class.: Antiinfective-misc.
Chem. class.: Carbapenem

Action: Interferes with cell wall replication of susceptible organisms; osmotically unstable cell wall swells, bursts from osmotic pressure

Uses: Adult patients with moderate to severe infections caused by the following organisms: intraabdominal infections—*Escherichia coli, Clostridium clostridioforme, Eubacterium lentum, Peptostreptococcus* sp., *Bacteroides fragilis, Bacteroides distasonis, Bacteroides ovatus, Bacteroides thetaiotaomicron, Bacteroides uniformis;* complicated skin/skin structure infections—*Staphylococcus aureus* (methicillin-susceptible), *Streptococcus pyogenes, E. coli, Peptostreptococcus* sp.; community-acquired pneumonia—*Streptococcus pneumoniae* (penicillin-susceptible), *Haemophilus influenzae* (β-lactamase–negative), *Moraxella catarrhalis;* complicated UTI—*E. coli, Klebsiella pneumoniae;* acute pelvic infections—*Streptococcus agalactiae, E. coli, B. fragilis, Porphyromonas asaccharolytica, Peptostreptococcus* sp., *Prevotella bivia*

Dosage and routes:

Complicated intraabdominal infections

• *Adult:* **IV/IM** 1 g qd × 5-14 days

Complicated skin/skin structure infections

• *Adult:* **IV/IM** 1 g qd × 7-14 days

Community-acquired pneumonia

• *Adult:* **IV/IM** 1 g qd × 10-14 days

Complicated UTI

• *Adult:* **IV/IM** 1 g qd × 10-14 days

Acute pelvic infections

• *Adult:* **IV/IM** 1 g qd × 3-10 days

Available form: Powder, lyophilized, 1 g

Side effects/adverse reactions:

CNS: Insomnia, ***seizures***, dizziness, *headache*

GI: Diarrhea, nausea, vomiting, ***pseudomembranous colitis***

GU: Vaginitis

INTEG: Rash, urticaria, *pruritus,* pain at inj site, *infused vein complication, phlebitis/thrombophlebitis*, erythema at inj site

RESP: Dyspnea, cough, pharyngitis, rales, respiratory distress

SYST: ***Anaphylaxis***

Contraindications: Hypersensitivity to this drug or its components, to amide-type local anesthetics (IM only); anaphylactic reactions to β-lactams

Precautions: Pregnancy (B), lactation, elderly, children, renal disease

Do not confuse:

Invanz/Avinza

Pharmacokinetics:

IV: Onset immediate, peak dose dependent, half-life 4 hr, metabolized by liver, excreted in urine, feces, breast milk

Interactions:

• ↑ ertapenem levels: probenecid; do not coadminister

Do not use acidophilus with anti-infectives

NURSING CONSIDERATIONS

Assess:

• Sensitivity to carbapenem antibiotics, other β-lactam antibiotics, penicillins

• Renal disease: lower dose may be required

• Bowel pattern qd: if severe diarrhea occurs, drug should be discontinued; may indicate pseudomembranous colitis

• For infection: temp, sputum, characteristics of wound before, during, after treatment

Allergic reactions, anaphylaxis; rash, urticaria, pruritus; may occur a few days after therapy begins

• Overgrowth of infection: perineal itching, fever, malaise, redness, pain, swelling, drainage, rash, diarrhea, change in cough or sputum

Administer:

• By IV or IM

• After C&S is taken

IM route

• Reconstitute 1 g vial of ertapenem with 3.2 ml of 1% lidocaine HCl without epINEPHrine, shake well

• Withdraw contents, administer deep IM in large muscle mass, use within 1 hr

IV route

• Do not coinfuse or mix with other medications; do not use diluents containing dextrose

• Reconstitute 1 g vial of ertapenem with either 10 ml of water for inj, 0.9% NaCl, or bacteriostatic water for inj

• Shake well to dissolve, transfer contents of reconstituted vial to 50 ml 0.9% NaCl inj

• Complete inf within 6 hr

Evaluate:

• Therapeutic response: negative C&S, absence of signs and symptoms of infection

Teach patient/family:
- To report severe diarrhea; may indicate pseudomembranous colitis
- To report overgrowth of infection: black, furry tongue, vaginal itching, foul-smelling stools
- To avoid breastfeeding; drug is excreted in breast milk

Treatment of overdose: EpINEPHrine, antihistamines; resuscitate if needed (anaphylaxis)

erythromycin base (℞)

(eh-rith-roh-my′sin)
Apo-Erythro♣, E-Mycin, Eramycin, Erybid♣, Eryc, Ery-Tab, E-Base, Erythromid♣, Erythromycin Base Filmtab, Erythromycin Delayed-Release, Novo-Rythro Encap♣, PCE

erythromycin estolate (℞)

Ilosone, Novo-Rythro♣

erythromycin ethylsuccinate (℞)

Apo-Erythro-Es♣, E.E.S., Ery Ped, Novo-Rythro♣

erythromycin gluceptate

erythromycin lactobionate (℞)

Erythrocin

erythromycin stearate (℞)

Apo-Erythro-S♣, Novo-Rythro♣

Func. class.: Antiinfective
Chem. class.: Macrolide

Action: Binds to 50S ribosomal subunits of susceptible bacteria and suppresses protein synthesis

Uses: Infections caused by *Neisseria gonorrhoeae;* mild to moderate respiratory tract, skin, soft tissue infections caused by *Bordetella pertussis, Borrelia burgdorferi, Chlamydia trachomatis; Corynebacterium diphtheriae, Haemophilus influenzae* (when used with sulfonamides); *Legionella pneumophila,* Legionnaire's disease, *Listeria monocytogenes; Mycoplasma pneumoniae, Streptococcus pneumoniae,* syphilis: *Treponema pallidum*

Research note: Grapefruit juice increased erythromycin concentrations in a study of 6 people[12]

Dosage and routes:

Soft tissue infections
- *Adult:* **PO** 250-500 mg q6h (base, estolate, stearate); **PO** 400-800 mg q6h (ethylsuccinate); **IV INF** 15-20 mg/kg/day (lactobionate) divided q6h
- *Child:* **PO** 30-50 mg/kg/day in divided doses q6h (salts); **IV** 20-40 mg/kg/day in divided doses q6h (lactobionate)

Neisseria gonorrhoeae/PID
- *Adult:* **IV** 500 mg q6h × 3 days (gluceptate, lactobionate), then **PO** 250 mg (base, estolate, stearate) or 400 mg (ethylsuccinate) q6h × 1 wk

Syphilis
- *Adult:* **PO** 30 g in divided doses over 15 days (base, estolate, stearate)

Chlamydia
- *Adult:* **PO** 500 mg q6h × 1 wk or 250 mg qid × 2 wk
- *Infant:* **PO** 50 mg/kg/day in 4 divided doses × 3 wk or more
- *Newborn:* **PO** 50 mg/kg/day in 4 divided doses × 2 wk or more

Intestinal amebiasis
- *Adult:* **PO** 250 mg q6h × 10-14 days (base, estolate, stearate)
- *Child:* **PO** 30-50 mg/kg/day in divided doses q6h × 10-14 days (base, estolate, stearate)

Available forms: Base: tabs, enteric-coated 250, 333 mg; tabs, film-coated 250, 500 mg; caps, enteric-coated 125, 250 mg; estolate: tabs, chewable 125, 250 mg; tabs 500 mg; caps 125, 250 mg; drops 100 mg/ml; susp 125, 250 mg/5 ml; stearate: tabs, film-coated 250, 500 mg; ethylsuccinate: tabs, chewable 200, 400 mg; 100 mg/2.5 ml, 200, 400 mg/5 ml; susp 200, 400 mg; powder for suspension: 100 mg/2.5 ml, 200 and 400 mg/5 ml; powder for inj: 500 mg and 1 g (lactobionate), 250 mg, 500 mg, 1 g (as gluceptate)

Side effects/adverse reactions:
CV: ***Dysrhythmias***
INTEG: Rash, urticaria, pruritus, thrombophlebitis (IV site)
GI: Nausea, vomiting, diarrhea, ***hepatotoxicity,*** abdominal pain, stomatitis, heartburn, anorexia, pruritus ani
GU: Vaginitis, moniliasis
EENT: Hearing loss, tinnitus
SYST: ***Anaphylaxis***

Contraindications: Hypersensitivity, preexisting hepatic disease (estolate), hepatic disease

Precautions: Pregnancy (B), hepatic disease, lactation

Do not confuse:
erythromycin/azithromycin

Pharmacokinetics: Peak 4 hr (base): ½–2½ hr (ethylsuccinate), duration 6 hr, half-life 1-2 hr; metabolized in liver; excreted in bile, feces, protein binding 75%-90%

Interactions:
- ↑ action, toxicity of: bromocriptine, calcium antagonists, clindamycin, cycloSPORINE, digoxin, dihydropyridine, disopyramide, ergots, lovastatin, methylPREDNISolone, midazolam, oral anticoagulants, simvastatin, theophylline, triazolam

Serious dysrhythmias: pimozide, sparfloxacin; do not use together

Do not use acidophilus with anti-infectives

Lab test interferences:
False increase: 17-OHCS/17-KS
Increase: AST/ALT
Decrease: Folate assay

NURSING CONSIDERATIONS

Assess:
- For infection: temp, characteristics of wounds, urine, stools, sputum, WBCs, baseline and periodically
- I&O ratio; report hematuria, oliguria in renal disease
- Hepatic studies: AST, ALT, if patient is on long-term therapy
- Renal studies: urinalysis, protein, blood
- C&S before drug therapy; drug may be given as soon as culture is taken; C&S may be repeated after treatment
- Bowel pattern before, during treatment
- Skin eruptions, itching
- Respiratory status: rate, character, wheezing, tightness in chest; discontinue drug if these occur
- Allergies before treatment, reaction of each medication

Administer:
- Do not give by IM or IV push
- Enteric-coated tablets may be given with food

Do not break, crush, or chew; only chewable tabs should be chewed

IV route
- After diluting 500 mg or less/10 ml sterile H_2O without preservatives; dilute further in 80-250 ml of 0.9% NaCl, LR, Normosol-R; may be further diluted to 1 mg/ml and given as cont inf; run 1 g or less/100 ml over ½-1 hr; cont inf over 6 hr, may require buffers to neutralize pH if dilution is <250 ml, use inf pump

Additive compatibilities: *Gluceptate:* Calcium gluconate, hydrocortisone, methicillin, penicillin G

potassium, potassium chloride, sodium bicarbonate
Lactobionate: Aminophylline, ampicillin, cimetidine, diphenhydrAMINE, hydrocortisone, lidocaine, methicillin, penicillin G potassium or sodium, pentobarbital, polymyxin B, potassium chloride, prednisoLONE, prochlorperazine, promazine, ranitidine, sodium bicarbonate, verapamil
Syringe compatibilities: *Lactobionate:* Methicillin
Y-site compatibilities: Acyclovir, amiodarone, cyclophosphamide, diltiazem, enalaprilat, esmolol, famotidine, foscarnet, heparin, hydromorphone, idarubicin, labetalol, lorazepam, magnesium sulfate, meperidine, midazolam, morphine, multivitamins, perphenazine, tacrolimus, theophylline, vit B/C, zidovudine
Perform/provide:
- Storage at room temperature; store susp in refrigerator
- Adequate intake of fluids (2 L) during diarrhea episodes

Evaluate:
- Therapeutic response: decreased symptoms of infection

Teach patient/family:
- To take oral drug with full glass of water; with food for GI symptoms
- Not to take with fruit juice
- To report sore throat, fever, fatigue (could indicate superinfection)
- To notify nurse of diarrhea stools, dark urine, pale stools, jaundice of eyes or skin, and severe abdominal pain
- To take at evenly spaced intervals; complete dosage regimen

Treatment of hypersensitivity: Withdraw drug; maintain airway; administer epINEPHrine, aminophylline, O_2, IV corticosteroids

erythromycin ophthalmic
See appendix c

erythromycin topical
See appendix c

escitalopram (℞)
(es-sit-tal'oh-pram)
Lexapro
Func. class.: Antidepressant, SSRI (selective serotonin reuptake inhibitor)

Action: Inhibits CNS neuron uptake of serotonin but not of norepinephrine
Uses: Major depressive disorder
Dosage and routes:
- *Adult:* **PO** 10 mg qd in AM or PM; after 1 wk if no clinical improvement is noted, dose may be increased to 20 mg qd PM; maintenance 10-20 mg/day, reassess to determine need for treatment
- *Geriatric/hepatic dose:* **PO** 10 mg/day

Available forms: Tabs 10, 20 mg; oral sol 5 mg (as base)/5 ml
Side effects/adverse reactions:
CNS: Headache, nervousness, insomnia, drowsiness, anxiety, tremor, dizziness, fatigue, sedation, poor concentration, abnormal dreams, agitation, ***seizures,*** apathy, euphoria, hallucinations, delusions, psychosis
GI: Nausea, diarrhea, dry mouth, anorexia, dyspepsia, constipation, cramps, vomiting, taste changes, flatulence, decreased appetite
INTEG: Sweating, rash, pruritus, acne, alopecia, urticaria, photosensitivity
RESP: Infection, pharyngitis, nasal

congestion, sinus headache, sinusitis, cough, dyspnea, bronchitis, asthma, hyperventilation, pneumonia
CV: Hot flashes, palpitations, angina pectoris, ***hemorrhage,*** hypertension, ***tachycardia,*** 1st-degree AV block, ***bradycardia, MI, thrombophlebitis,*** postural hypotension
MS: Pain, arthritis, twitching
GU: Dysmenorrhea, decreased libido, urinary frequency, UTI, amenorrhea, cystitis, impotence, urine retention
EENT: Visual changes, ear/eye pain, photophobia, tinnitus
SYST: Asthenia, viral infection, fever, allergy, chills

Contraindications: Hypersensitivity

Precautions: Pregnancy (C), lactation, children, elderly, renal disease, history of seizures

Pharmacokinetics:
PO: Metabolized in liver; excreted in urine

Interactions:
- Do not use MAOIs with or 14 days before escitalopram
- ↑ side effects of escitalopram: highly protein-bound drugs
- ↑ effect: haloperidol
- ↓ escitalopram effect: cyproheptadine
- ↑ half-life of: diazepam
- ↑ levels or toxicity of: carbamazepine, lithium, warfarin, phenytoin
- ↑ levels of: tricyclics, phenothiazines
- Paradoxical worsening of OCD: busPIRone
- ↑ CNS depression: alcohol, antidepressants, opioids, sedatives
- Serotonin syndrome: tryptophan, amphetamines, antidepressants, busPIRone, lithium, amantadine, bromocriptine
- SAM-e, St. John's wort: do not use together

↑ anticholinergic effect: corkwood, jimsonweed
↑ CNS effect: hops, kava, lavender
↑ hypertension: yohimbe

Lab test interferences:
Increase: Serum bilirubin, blood glucose, alk phosphatase
Decrease: VMA, 5-HIAA
False increase: Urinary catecholamines

NURSING CONSIDERATIONS

Assess:
- Mental status: mood, sensorium, affect, suicidal tendencies, increase in psychiatric symptoms, depression, panic
- Appetite in bulemia nervosa, weight qd, increase nutritious foods in diet, watch for binging and vomiting
- Allergic reactions: itching, rash urticaria, drug should be discontinued, may need to give antihistamine
- B/P (lying/standing), pulse q4h; if systolic B/P drops 20 mm Hg, hold drug, notify prescriber; take VS q4h in patients with cardiovascular disease
- Blood studies: CBC, leukocytes, differential, cardiac enzymes if patient is receiving long-term therapy; check platelets; bleeding can occur
- Hepatic studies: AST, ALT, bilirubin, creatinine
- Weight qwk; appetite may decrease with drug
- ECG for flattening of T wave, bundle branch, AV block, dysrhythmias in cardiac patients
- Alcohol consumption; if alcohol is consumed, hold dose until AM

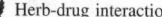

Administer:
- With food or milk for GI symptoms
- Crushed if patient is unable to swallow medication whole

• Dosage hs if oversedation occurs during the day
• Gum, hard candy, frequent sips of water for dry mouth

Perform/provide:
• Storage at room temperature; do not freeze
• Assistance with ambulation during therapy, since drowsiness, dizziness occur
• Safety measures primarily in elderly
• Checking to see if PO medication swallowed

Evaluate:
• Therapeutic response: decreased depression

Teach patient/family:
• That therapeutic effect may take 1-4 wk
• To use caution in driving, other activities requiring alertness because of drowsiness, dizziness, blurred vision
• To use sunscreen to prevent photosensitivity
• To avoid alcohol ingestion, other CNS depressants
• To notify prescriber if pregnant or plan to become pregnant or breastfeed
• To change positions slowly, orthostatic hypotension may occur
• To avoid all OTC drugs unless approved by prescriber
• To report immediately signs of urinary retention

esmolol (℞)
(ez'moe-lole)
Brevibloc
Func. class.: β-Adrenergic blocker (antidysrhythmic II)

Action: Competitively blocks stimulation of β_1-adrenergic receptors in the myocardium; produces negative chronotropic, inotropic activity (decreases rate of SA node discharge, increases recovery time), slows conduction of AV node, decreases heart rate, decreases O_2 consumption in myocardium; also decreases renin-aldosterone-angiotensin system at high doses; inhibits β_2-receptors in bronchial system at higher doses

Uses: Supraventricular tachycardia, noncompensatory sinus tachycardia, hypertensive crisis, intraoperative and postoperative tachycardia and hypertension

Dosage and routes:
• *Adult:* **IV** loading dose 500 mcg/kg/min over 1 min; maintenance 50 mcg/kg/min for 4 min; if no response in 5 min, give 2nd loading dose; then increase inf to 100 mcg/kg/min for 4 min; if no response, repeat loading dose, then increase maintenance inf by 50 mcg/kg/min (max of 200 mcg/kg/min), titrate to patient response
• *Child:* **IV** 50 mcg/kg/min, may increase q10min (max 300 mcg/kg/min)

Available forms: Inj 10 mg, 250 mg/ml

Side effects/adverse reactions:
INTEG: Induration, inflammation at site, discoloration, edema, erythema, burning pallor, flushing, rash, pruritus, dry skin, alopecia
CNS: Confusion, light-headedness, paresthesia, somnolence, fever, dizziness, fatigue, headache, depression, anxiety, ***seizures***
GI: Nausea, vomiting, anorexia, gastric pain, flatulence, constipation, heartburn, bloating
CV: Hypotension, bradycardia, chest pain, peripheral ischemia, shortness of breath, ***CHF,*** conduction disturbances, 1st, 2nd, 3rd degree heart block
GU: Urinary retention, impotence, dysuria

RESP: ***Bronchospasm,*** dyspnea, cough, wheeziness, nasal stuffiness

Contraindications: 2nd- or 3rd-degree heart block, cardiogenic shock, CHF, cardiac failure, hypersensitivity

Precautions: Hypotension, pregnancy (C), peripheral vascular disease, diabetes, hypoglycemia, thyrotoxicosis, renal disease, lactation

Do not confuse:

Brevibloc/Brevital

esmolol/Osmitrol

Pharmacokinetics:

Onset very rapid, duration short, half-life 9 min; metabolized by hydrolysis of the ester linkage; excreted via kidneys

Interactions:

- ↑ digoxin levels: digoxin
- ↑ α-adrenergic stimulation: epHEDrine, epINEPHrine, amphetamine, norepinephrine, phenylephrine, pseudoephedrine
- ↓ action of: thyroid hormones
- ↓ action of esmolol: thyroid hormone
- Avoid use with MAOIs

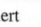

Potassium deficiency: aloe, buckthorn, cascara sagrada, senna

↑ β-blocking effect: betel palm, butterbur, cola tree, figwort, fumitory, guarana, hawthorn, lily of the valley, motherwort, plantain

↓ β-blocking effect: coenzyme Q10, yohimbe

↑ CV reactions: jaborandi tree

Lab test interferences:

Interference: Glucose/insulin tolerance test

NURSING CONSIDERATIONS

Assess:

- I&O ratio, weight daily, watch for signs of CHF (jugular vein distention, weight gain, rales or crackles, edema)
- B/P, pulse q4h; note rate, rhythm, quality; rapid changes can cause shock; if systolic <100 or diastolic <60, notify prescriber before giving drug
- ECG continuously during inf, hypotension is common
- Baselines in renal, hepatic studies before therapy begins
- Breath sounds and respiratory pattern: wheezing from bronchospasm

Administer:

- Reduced dosage in cool environment

IV route

- IV diluted 5 g/20 ml of D_5W, D_5R, D_5 0.9% NaCl, 0.45% NaCl, LR, D_5 0.45% NaCl, 0.9% NaCl further dilute in the remaining 480 ml (10 mg/ml) and give as infusion; give loading dose over 1 min, then maintenance over 4 min; may repeat loading dose q5min with increased maintenance dose; maintenance dose should not be >200 mcg/kg/min and be given up to 48 hr; dose should be tapered at 25 mcg/kg/min; use infusion pump

Additive compatibilities: Aminophylline, atracurium, bretylium, heparin

Y-site compatibilities: Amikacin, aminophylline, amiodarone, ampicillin, atracurium, butorphanol, calcium chloride, cefazolin, cefmetazole, cefoperazone, ceftazidime, ceftizoxime, chloramphenicol, cimetidine, cisatracurium, clindamycin, diltiazem, DOPamine, enalaprilat, erythromycin, famotidine, fentanyl, gentamicin, heparin, hydrocortisone, insulin (regular), labetalol, magnesium sulfate, methyldopate, metronidazole, midazolam, morphine, nafcillin, nitroglycerin, nitroprusside, norepinephrine, pancuronium, penicillin G potassium, phenytoin, piperacillin, polymyxin B, potassium chloride, potassium phosphate, propofol, ranitidine, remifentanil, streptomycin, tacrolimus, tobramycin, trimethoprim-sulfamethoxazole, vancomycin, vecuronium

Perform/provide:

• Storage protected from light, moisture; in cool environment

Evaluate:

• Therapeutic response: lower B/P immediately, lower heart rate

Teach patient/family:

• To notify prescriber if pain, swelling occurs at IV site

Treatment of overdose: Discontinue drug

esomeprazole (℞)

(es′oh-mep′rah-zohl)

Nexium

Func. class.: Antiulcer, proton pump inhibitor

Chem. class.: Benzimidazole

Action: Suppresses gastric secretion by inhibiting hydrogen/potassium ATPase enzyme system in gastric parietal cell; characterized as gastric acid pump inhibitor, because it blocks final step of acid production

Uses: Gastroesophageal reflux disease (GERD), severe erosive esophagitis; treatment of active duodenal ulcers in combination with antiinfectives for *Helicobacter pylori* infection

Dosage and routes:

***Active duodenal ulcers associated with* H. pylori**

• *Adult:* **PO** 40 mg qd × 10 days in combination with clarithromycin 500 mg bid × 10 days and amoxicillin 1000 mg bid × 10 days

GERD

• *Adult:* **PO** 20 or 40 mg qd × 4-8 wk

Available forms: Caps 20, 40 mg

Side effects/adverse reactions:

CNS: Headache, dizziness

GI: Diarrhea, flatulence, anorexia, dry mouth

RESP: Cough

INTEG: Rash, dry skin

GU: UTI, urinary frequency

MISC: Fatigue

Contraindications: Hypersensitivity

Precautions: Pregnancy (B), lactation, children, elderly

Pharmacokinetics: Eliminated in urine as metabolites and in feces; in elderly, elimination rate decreased, bioavailability increased

Interactions:

• ↑ esomeprazole serum levels: flurazepam, triazolam

• ↑ bleeding: warfarin

• ↓ diazepam clearance resulting in ↑ diazepam serum concentrations

NURSING CONSIDERATIONS

Assess:

• GI system: bowel sounds q8h, abdomen for pain, swelling, anorexia

• Hepatic enzymes: AST, ALT, alk phosphatase during treatment

Administer:

• At least 1 hr before eating

⃠ Capsule swallowed whole; do not break, crush, or chew

Evaluate:

• Therapeutic response: absence of epigastric pain, swelling, fullness

Teach patient/family:

• To report severe diarrhea; drug may have to be discontinued

• That diabetic patient should know hypoglycemia may occur

• To avoid hazardous activities; dizziness may occur

• To avoid alcohol, salicylates, ibuprofen; may cause GI irritation

estradiol
(es-tra-dye'ole)
Estrace

estradiol cypionate
depGynogen, Depo-Estradiol, Depogen, Dura-Estrin, E-Cypionate, Estragyn LA5, Estro-Cyp, Estrofem, Estroject-LA, Estrol-L.A.

estradiol valerate
Clinigen LA, Delestrogen, Dioval, Duragen, Estra-L, Estro-span, Femogex✱, Gynogen LA, Menaval, Valergen

estradiol transdermal system
Alora, ClimAra, Esclim, Estraderm, FemPatch, Vivelle

estradiol vaginal tablet
Vagifem

estradiol vaginal ring
Estring
Func. class.: Estrogen, progestins

Action: Needed for adequate functioning of female reproductive system; affects release of pituitary gonadotropins, inhibits ovulation, adequate calcium use in bone

Uses: Symptoms associated with menopause, inoperable breast cancer (selected cases), prostatic cancer, atrophic vaginitis, kraurosis vulvae, hypogonadism, primary ovarian failure, prevention of osteoporosis

Dosage and routes:

Hormone replacement

• *Adult:* **TD** 0.05-0.1 mg/24 hr, apply 2 ×/wk

Menopause/hypogonadism/castration/ovarian failure

• *Adult:* **PO** 1-2 mg qd 3 wk on, 1 wk off or 5 days on, 2 days off **IM** 1-5 mg q3-4wk (cypionate); 10-20 mg q4wk (valerate)

• *Adult:* **TOP** Estraderm 0.05 mg/24 hr applied 2 ×/wk ClimAra 0.05 mg/hr applied 1 ×/wk in a cyclic regimen; women with hysterectomy may use continuously

Prostatic cancer

• *Adult:* **IM** 30 mg q1-2wk (valerate); **PO** 1-2 mg tid (oral estradiol)

Breast cancer

• *Adult:* **PO** 10 mg tid × 3 mo or longer

Atropic vaginitis/kraurosis vulvae

• *Adult:* **VAG CREAM** 2-4 g qd × 1-2 wk, then 1 g 1-3 ×/wk cycled; vag tab 1 qd × 2 wk, maintenance 1 tab 2 ×/wk; **VAG RING** inserted and left in place continuously for 3 mo

Available forms: Estradiol tabs 0.5, 1, 2 mg; valerate inj 10, 20, 40 mg/ml; transderm 0.025, 0.0375, 0.05, 0.075, 0.1 mg/24 hr release rate; vag cream 100 mcg/g; vag tab 25 mcg; vag ring 2 mg/90 days

Side effects/adverse reactions:

CNS: Dizziness, headache, migraines, depression, ***seizures***

CV: Hypotension, thrombophlebitis, edema, ***thromboembolism, stroke, pulmonary embolism, myocardial infarction***

GI: Nausea, vomiting, diarrhea, anorexia, pancreatitis, cramps, constipation, increased appetite, increased weight, ***cholestatic jaundice, hepatic adenoma***

EENT: Contact lens intolerance, increased myopia, astigmatism

GU: Amenorrhea, cervical erosion, breakthrough bleeding, dysmenorrhea, vaginal candidiasis, breast changes, *gynecomastia, testicular atrophy, impotence,* ***increased risk of breast cancer, endometrial cancer,*** changes in libido

INTEG: Rash, urticaria, acne, hirsutism, alopecia, oily skin, seborrhea, purpura, melasma

META: Folic acid deficiency, hypercalcemia, hyperglycemia

Contraindications: Breast cancer, thromboembolic disorders, reproductive cancer, genital bleeding (abnormal, undiagnosed), pregnancy (X), lactation

Precautions: Hypertension, asthma, blood dyscrasias, gallbladder disease, CHF, diabetes mellitus, bone disease, depression, migraine headache, seizure disorders, hepatic disease, renal disease, family history of cancer of breast or reproductive tract, smoking

Pharmacokinetics:

PO/INJ/TD: Degraded in liver; excreted in urine; crosses placenta; excreted in breast milk

Interactions:

• ↓ action of anticoagulants, oral hypoglycemics, tamoxifen

• ↓ estradiol action: anticonvulsants, barbiturates, phenylbutazone, rifampin, calcium

• ↑ action of: corticosteroids

• ↑ toxicity: cycloSPORINE, dantrolene

• Drug/food: ↑ estrogen level: grapefruit juice

↑ estrogen effect: alfalfa, hops

↓ estrogen effect: saw palmetto

Altered estrogen effect: black cohosh, DHEA

Lab test interferences:

Increase: BSP retention test, PBI, T_4, serum sodium, platelet aggregation, thyroxine-binding globulin (TBG), prothrombin, factors VII, VIII, IX, X, triglycerides

Decrease: Serum folate, serum triglyceride, T_3 resin uptake test, glucose tolerance test, antithrombin III, pregnanediol, metyrapone test

False positive: LE prep, antinuclear antibodies

NURSING CONSIDERATIONS

Assess:

• Blood glucose of diabetic patient, hyperglycemia may occur

• Weight daily, notify prescriber of weekly weight gain >5 lb; if increase, diuretic may be ordered

• B/P q4h, watch for increase caused by H_2O and sodium retention

• I&O ratio; decreasing urinary output, increasing edema, report changes

• Hepatic studies, including AST, ALT, bilirubin, alk phosphatase baseline, periodically

• Hypertension, cardiac symptoms, jaundice, hypercalcemia

• Mental status: affect, mood, behavioral changes, aggression

• Female patient for intact uterus, if so, progesterone should be added to estrogen therapy to decrease risk of endometrial cancer

Administer:

• Titrated dose; use lowest effective dose

• IM inj deeply in large muscle mass

PO route

• With food or milk to decrease GI symptoms

Transdermal route

• Apply to trunk of body 2 ×/wk; press firmly and hold in place for 10 sec to ensure good contact

• On intermittent cycle schedule: 3 wk on, then 1 wk off; if patch falls off, reapply

Vaginal route

• Use applicator provided

Evaluate:

• Therapeutic response: reversal of menopause symptoms or decrease in tumor size in prostatic, breast cancer

Teach patient/family:

• To weigh weekly, report gain >5 lb

To report breast lumps, vaginal bleeding, edema, jaundice, dark urine, clay-colored stools, dyspnea, headache, blurred vision, abdominal pain, numbness or stiffness in legs, chest pain, tenderness, redness, and swelling in extremities; male to report impotence or gynecomastia

RARELY USED

estramustine
(ess-tra-muss'teen)
Emcyt
Func. class.: Antineoplastic

Uses: Metastatic prostate cancer
Dosage and routes:
• *Adult:* **PO** 10-16 mg/kg in 3-4 divided doses/day; treatment may continue for ≥3 mo or 600 mg/m^2/day in 3 divided doses
Contraindications: Hypersensitivity to estradiol, thromboembolic disorders, pregnancy (D)

estrogens, conjugated
Cenestin, C.E.S.✤, Congest, Premarin
estrogens, conjugated synthetic A
Cenestin
Func. class.: Estrogen, hormone

Action: Needed for adequate functioning of female reproductive system; affects release of pituitary gonadotropins, inhibits ovulation, adequate calcium use in bone
Uses: Symptoms associated with menopause, inoperable breast cancer, prostatic cancer, abnormal uterine bleeding, hypogonadism, primary ovarian failure, prevention of osteoporosis
Research notes: Women who take thyroxine and estrogen concurrently may need to have their thyroxine dose increased.[13]
When thyroid replacement is used with estrogens, a dosage adjustment increase may be required in the thyroid agent.[14]
Dosage and routes:
Menopause
• *Adult:* **PO** 0.3-1.25 mg qd 3 wk on, 1 wk off
Prevention of osteoporosis
• *Adult:* **PO** 0.625 mg qd or in cycle
Atrophic vaginitis
• *Adult:* **VAG CREAM** 2-4 g ml qd × 21 days, off 7 days, repeat
Prostatic cancer
• *Adult:* **PO** 1.25-2.5 mg tid
Breast cancer
• *Adult:* **PO** 10 mg tid × 3 mo or longer
Abnormal uterine bleeding
• *Adult:* **IV/IM** 25 mg, repeat in 6-12 hr
Castration/primary ovarian failure
• *Adult:* **PO** 1.25 mg qd 3 wk on, 1 wk off
Hypogonadism
• *Adult:* **PO** 2.5 mg bid-tid × 20 days/mo
Available forms: Tabs 0.3, 0.625, 0.9, 1.25, 2.5 mg; inj 25 mg/vial; vag cream 0.625 mg/g; synthetic A tabs 0.625, 0.9 mg
Side effects/adverse reactions:
CNS: Dizziness, headache, migraine, depression, ***seizures***
CV: Hypotension, thrombophlebitis, edema, ***thromboembolism, stroke, pulmonary embolism, myocardial infarction***
GI: Nausea, vomiting, diarrhea, anorexia, pancreatitis, cramps, constipation, increased appetite, increased weight, ***cholestatic jaundice, hepatic adenoma***
EENT: Contact lens intolerance, increased myopia, astigmatism
GU: Amenorrhea, cervical erosion,

breakthrough bleeding, dysmenorrhea, vaginal candidiasis, breast changes, *gynecomastia, testicular atrophy, impotence,* ***increased risk of breast cancer, endometrial cancer,*** libido changes
INTEG: Rash, urticaria, acne, hirsutism, alopecia, oily skin, seborrhea, purpura, melasma
META: Folic acid deficiency, hypercalcemia, hyperglycemia
Contraindications: Breast cancer, thromboembolic disorders, reproductive cancer, genital bleeding (abnormal, undiagnosed), pregnancy (X), lactation
Precautions: Hypertension, asthma, blood dyscrasias, gallbladder disease, CHF, diabetes mellitus, bone disease, depression, migraine headache, convulsive disorders, hepatic disease, renal disease, family history of cancer of breast or reproductive tract, smoking
Do not confuse:
Premarin/Provera
Pharmacokinetics:
PO/IV/IM: Degraded in liver, excreted in urine, crosses placenta, excreted in breast milk
Interactions:
- ↑ toxicity: cycloSPORINE, dantrolene
- ↓ action of anticoagulants, oral hypoglycemics, tamoxifen
- ↓ action of estrogens: anticonvulsants, barbiturates, phenylbutazone, rifampin
- ↑ action of corticosteroids
- Drug/food: ↑ estrogen level: grapefruit juice

↑ estrogen effect: alfalfa, hops
↓ estrogen effect: saw palmetto
Altered estrogen effect: black cohosh, DHEA
Lab test interferences:
Increase: BSP retention test, PBI, T_4, serum sodium, platelet aggregation, thyroxine-binding globulin (TBG), prothrombin, factors VII, VIII, IX, X, triglycerides
Decrease: Serum folate, serum triglyceride, T_3 resin uptake test, glucose tolerance test, antithrombin III, pregnanediol, metyrapone test
False positive: LE prep, antinuclear antibodies

NURSING CONSIDERATIONS
Assess:
- Blood glucose if diabetic patient, hyperglycemia may occur
- Weight daily; notify prescriber of weekly weight gain >5 lb; if increase, diuretic may be ordered
- B/P q4h; watch for increase caused by H_2O and Na retention
- I&O ratio; be alert for decreasing urinary output, increasing edema
- Hepatic studies: AST, ALT, bilirubin, alk phosphatase
- Hypertension, cardiac symptoms, jaundice, hypercalcemia
- Mental status: affect, mood, behavioral changes, aggression
- Female patient for intact uterus, if so, progesterone should be added to estrogen therapy to decrease risk of endometrial cancer

Administer:
- Titrated dose, use lowest effective dose

IM route
- IM reconstitute after withdrawing >5 ml of air from container and inject sterile diluent on vial side, rotate to dissolve; give inj deep in large muscle mass
- With food or milk to decrease GI symptoms (PO)

IV direct route
- IV, after reconstituting as for IM, inject into distal port of running IV line of D_5W, 0.9% NaCl, LR at 5 mg/min or less

Y-site compatibilities: Heparin/hydrocortisone, potassium chloride, vit B/C

Vaginal route
- Use applicator provided

Evaluate:
- Therapeutic response: absence of breast engorgement, reversal of menopause symptoms, or decrease in tumor size in prostatic cancer

Teach patient/family:
- To avoid breastfeeding, since drug is excreted in breast milk
- To weigh weekly, report gain >5 lb
- To report breast lumps, vaginal bleeding, edema, jaundice, dark urine, clay-colored stools, dyspnea, headache, blurred vision, abdominal pain, leg pain and redness, numbness or stiffness in legs, chest pain; male to report impotence or gynecomastia
- To avoid sunlight or wear sunscreen; burns may occur
- To notify prescriber if pregnancy is suspected

etanercept (℞)
(eh-tan′er-sept)
Enbrel
Func. class.: Antirheumatic agent (disease modifying)

Action: Binds tumor necrosis factor (TNF), which is involved in immune and inflammatory reactions
Uses: Acute, chronic rheumatoid arthritis that has not responded to other disease-modifying agents, polyarticular course juvenile rheumatoid arthritis (JRA)
Investigational uses: CHF, psoriasis/psoriatic arthritis
Dosage and routes:
Osteoarthritis
- *Adult:* **SC** 25 mg 2×/wk, may be given with other drugs for rheumatoid arthritis
- *Child 4-17 yr:* **SC** 0.4 mg/kg 2×/wk, max 25 mg 1 dose

CHF
- *Adult:* **SC** 5-12 mg/m^2 2×/wk × 3 mo

Psoriasis/psoriatic arthritis
- *Adult:* **SC** 25 mg 2×/wk × 12 wk

Available forms: Powder for inj: 25 mg
Side effects/adverse reactions:
GI: Abdominal pain, dyspepsia
CNS: Headache, asthenia, dizziness
INTEG: Rash, *inj site reaction*
RESP: Pharyngitis, cough, URI, non-URI, sinusitis, *rhinitis*
Contraindications: Hypersensitivity, sepsis
Precautions: Pregnancy (B), lactation, children <4 yr, elderly
Pharmacokinetics: Elimination half-life 115 hr, 60% absorbed SC
Interactions:
- Do not give concurrently with vaccines, immunizations should be brought up to date before treatment

NURSING CONSIDERATIONS
Assess:
- Pain, stiffness, ROM, swelling of joints during treatment
- For injection site pain, swelling, usually occur after 2 inj (4-5 days)

Administer:
- After reconstituting 1 ml of supplied diluent, slowly inject diluent into vial, swirl contents, do not shake, sol should be clear/colorless, do not use if cloudy or discolored
- Do not admix with other sol or medications, do not use filter
- May be injected SC into upper arm, abdomen, or thigh, rotate injection sites

Evaluate:
- Therapeutic response: decreased inflammation, pain in joints

Teach patient/family:
- That drug must be continued for prescribed time to be effective

• To use caution when driving; dizziness may occur
• About self-administration if appropriate: inj should be made in thigh, abdomen, upper arm; rotate sites at least 1 in from old site

ethambutol (℞)

(e-tham′byoo-tole)
Etibi♣, Myambutol
Func. class.: Antitubercular
Chem. class.: Diisopropylethylene diamide derivative

Action: Inhibits RNA synthesis, decreases tubercle bacilli replication
Uses: Pulmonary tuberculosis, as an adjunct, other mycobacterial infections
Dosage and routes:
• *Adult and child >13 yr:* **PO** 15-25 mg/kg/day as a single dose or 50 mg/kg 2×/wk or 25-30 mg/kg 3 ×/wk
Renal disease
• CCr 10-50 ml/min dose q24-36h; CCr <10 ml/min dose q48h
Retreatment
• *Adult:* **PO** 25 mg/kg/day as single dose × 2 mo with at least 1 other drug, then decrease to 15 mg/kg/day as single dose, max 2.5 g/day
• *Child:* 15 mg/kg/day
Available forms: Tabs 100, 400 mg
Side effects/adverse reactions:
GI: Abdominal distress, anorexia, nausea, vomiting
INTEG: Dermatitis, pruritus, ***toxic epidermal necrolysis***
CNS: Headache, confusion, fever, malaise, dizziness, *disorientation,* hallucinations
EENT: Blurred vision, optic neuritis, photophobia, decreased visual acuity
META: Elevated uric acid, acute gout, liver function impairment
MISC: ***Thrombocytopenia,*** joint pain, bloody sputum, ***anaphylaxis***
Contraindications: Hypersensitivity, optic neuritis, child <13 yr
Precautions: Pregnancy (B), lactation, renal disease, diabetic retinopathy, cataracts, ocular defects, hepatic and hematopoietic disorders
Do not confuse:
ethambutol/Ethmozine
Pharmacokinetics:
PO: Peak 2-4 hr, half-life 3 hr; metabolized in liver; excreted in urine (unchanged drug/inactive metabolites, unchanged drug in feces)
Interactions:
• Delayed absorption of ethambutol: aluminum salts
• Neurotoxicity: other neurotoxics

NURSING CONSIDERATIONS
Assess:
• Hepatic studies qwk × 2 wk, then q2mo: ALT, AST, bilirubin
• Signs of anemia: Hct, Hgb, fatigue
• Mental status often: affect, mood, behavioral changes; psychosis may occur
• Hepatic status: decreased appetite, jaundice, dark urine, fatigue
• C&S, including sputum, before treatment
• Visual status: decreased activity, altered color perception
Administer:
PO route
• With meals to decrease GI symptoms
• Antiemetic if vomiting occurs
• After C&S is completed; qmo to detect resistance
• 2 hr before antacids

Evaluate:

- Therapeutic response: decreased symptoms of TB, decrease in acid-fast bacteria

Teach patient/family:

- To avoid alcohol products
- That compliance with dosage schedule, duration is necessary
- That scheduled appointments must be kept or relapse may occur
- To report any visual changes, rash, hot, swollen, painful joints, numbness or tingling of extremities to prescriber

RARELY USED

ethosuximide (℞)

(eth-oh-sux′i-mide)

Zarontin

Func. class.: Anticonvulsant

Uses: Absence seizures, partial seizures, tonic-clonic seizures

Dosage and routes:

- *Adult and child >6 yr:* **PO** 250 mg bid initially; may increase by 250 mg q4-7d
- *Child 3-6 yr:* **PO** 250 mg/day or 125 mg bid; may increase by 250 mg q4-7d

Contraindications: Hypersensitivity to succinimide derivatives

etidronate (℞)

(eh-tih-droe′nate)

Didronel, Didronel IV

Func. class.: Bone resorption inhibitor

Chem. class.: Biphosphonate

Action: Decreases bone resorption and new bone development (accretion)

Uses: Paget's disease, heterotopic ossification, hypercalcemia of malignancy

Dosage and routes:

Paget's disease

- *Adult:* **PO** 5-10 mg/kg/day, 2 hr ac with H_2O, not to exceed 20 mg/kg/day, max 6 mo or 11-20 mg/kg/day for max of 3 mo

Heterotopic ossification

- *Adult:* **PO** 20 mg/kg qd × 2 wk, then 10 mg/kg/day for 10 wk, total 12 wk

Hypercalcemia

- *Adult:* **IV** 7.5 mg/kg/day × 3 days, then **PO** 20 mg/kg/day

Heterotopic ossification/hip replacement

- *Adult:* **PO** 20 mg/kg/day × 4 wk before and 3 mo after surgery

Available forms: Tabs 200, 400 mg; inj 50 mg/ml

Side effects/adverse reactions:

GI: Nausea, constipation; metallic taste (IV)

MS: Bone pain, hypocalcemia, decreased mineralization of nonaffected bones

GU: ***Nephrotoxicity***

MISC: Dyspnea, low magnesium, phosphorus

Contraindications: Pathologic fractures, clinically overt osteomalacia, severe renal disease with creatinine >5 mg/dl

Precautions: Pregnancy (C), renal disease, lactation, restricted vit D, calcium for children

Do not confuse:

etidronate/etretinate

etidronate/etomidate

Pharmacokinetics: Absorbed poorly (PO), not metabolized; excreted in urine/feces; therapeutic response: 1-3 mo

Interactions:

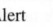

- ↓ absorption: calcium, aluminum, magnesium antacids/supplements, iron products

• ↑ protime: warfarin
• Drug/food: dairy products: ↓ absorption

NURSING CONSIDERATIONS

Assess:

• I&O ratio; check for decreased output in renal patients
• BUN, creatinine, uric acid, phosphate chloride, albumin, pH, urine calcium, magnesium, alk phosphatase, urinalysis; calcium should be kept at 9-10 mg/dl, vit D 50-135 international units/dl
• Muscle spasm, laryngospasm, paresthesias, facial twitching, colic; may indicate hypocalcemia
• Nutritional status, diet for sources of vit D (milk, some seafood), calcium (dairy products, dark green vegetables), phosphates—adequate intake is necessary
• Persistent nausea or diarrhea

Administer:

PO route

• Drug therapy should not last longer than 6 mo
• On empty stomach with H_2O 2 hr ac

IV route

• IV after diluting in 250 ml or more 0.9% NaCl; give over 2 hr or longer
• Food, especially high in calcium; vitamins with mineral supplements or antacids high in metals should not be given within 2 hr of dose

Evaluate:

• Therapeutic response: management of bone deficiencies, Paget's disease

Teach patient/family:

• To avoid OTC products
• That therapeutic response may take 1-3 mo; effects persist for months after drug is discontinued
• That adequate intake of calcium, vit D is necessary
• To report sudden onset of unexplained pain, restricted mobility, heat over bone; hypercalcemic relapse

etodolac (℞)

(ee-toe'doe-lak)

Lodine, Lodine XL

Func. class.: Nonsteroidal antiinflammatory/nonopioid analgesic

Action: Inhibits prostaglandin synthesis by decreasing an enzyme needed for biosynthesis; analgesic, antiinflammatory, antipyretic

Uses: Mild to moderate pain, osteoarthritis

Dosage and routes:

Osteoarthritis

• *Adult:* **PO** 800-1200 mg/day in divided doses q6-8h initially, then adjust dose to 600-1200 mg/day in divided doses; do not exceed 1200 mg/day; patients <60 kg not to exceed 20 mg/kg

Analgesia

• *Adult:* **PO** 200-400 mg q6-8h prn for acute pain; do not exceed 1200 mg/day; patients <60 kg, not to exceed 20 mg/kg

Available forms: Caps 200, 300 mg; tabs 400, 500 mg; ext rel 400, 600 mg

Side effects/adverse reactions:

CV: Tachycardia, peripheral edema, fluid retention, palpitations, dysrhythmias, CHF

GU: ***Nephrotoxicity:*** *dysuria,* ***hematuria,*** *oliguria, azotemia,* cystitis, urinary tract infection

HEMA: ***Blood dyscrasias***

INTEG: Erythema, urticaria, purpura, rash, pruritus, sweating, ***Stevens-Johnson syndrome***

GI: Nausea, anorexia, vomiting, diarrhea, jaundice, ***cholestatic hepatitis,*** constipation, flatulence, cramps, dry mouth, peptic ulcer, dyspepsia, ***GI bleeding***

CNS: Dizziness, headache, drowsiness, fatigue, tremors, confusion, insomnia, anxiety, depression, lightheadedness, vertigo

EENT: Tinnitus, hearing loss, blurred vision, photophobia

SYST: ***Angioedema, anaphylaxis***

Contraindications: Hypersensitivity; patients in whom aspirin, iodides, or other nonsteroidal antiinflammatories have produced asthma; rhinitis, urticaria, nasal polyps, angioedema, bronchospasm

Precautions: Pregnancy (C), avoid in 2nd half of pregnancy, lactation; children; bleeding; GI, cardiac disorders; elderly; renal, hepatic disorders

Do not confuse:

Lodine/codeine/iodine

Pharmacokinetics:

PO: Peak 1-2 hr, serum protein binding >90%, half-life 7 hr; metabolized by liver (metabolites excreted in urine)

Interactions:

- ↑ toxicity: cycloSPORINE, digoxin, lithium, methotrexate, phenytoin
- ↑ GI toxicity: aspirin
- ↓ effect of etodolac: antacids
- ↓ effect of: β-blockers, diuretics

↑ gastric irritation: arginine, gossypol

↑ NSAIDs effect: bearberry, bilberry

↑ bleeding risk: bogbean, chondroitin, saw palmetto, turmeric

Severe photosensitivity: St. John's wort

NURSING CONSIDERATIONS

Assess:

- Pain: location, frequency, characteristics; relief after med
- Blood, renal, hepatic studies: BUN, creatinine, AST, ALT, Hgb, before treatment, periodically thereafter
- For GI bleeding: black stools, hematemesis
- Audiometric, ophthalmic examination before, during, after treatment
- For eye, ear problems: blurred vision, tinnitus; may indicate toxicity
- For asthma, aspirin hypersensitivity, nasal polyps that may be hypersensitive to etodolac

Administer:

PO route

- With food to decrease GI symptoms, since extent of absorption is not affected by food

Perform/provide:

- Storage at room temperature

Evaluate:

- Therapeutic response: decreased pain, stiffness, swelling in joints, ability to move more easily

Teach patient/family:

- To report blurred vision or ringing, roaring in ears; may indicate toxicity

Not to break, crush, or chew ext rel tabs

- To avoid driving, other hazardous activities if dizziness or drowsiness occurs

To report change in urine pattern, weight increase, edema, pain increase in joints, fever, blood in urine; indicates nephrotoxicity

- That therapeutic effects may take up to 1 mo
- To avoid aspirin, NSAIDs, acetaminophen, alcoholic beverages while taking this medication

RARELY USED

etomidate (℞)

(e-tom'i-date)

Amidate

Func. class.: General anesthetic

Uses: Induction of general anesthesia

Dosage and routes:

• *Adult and child >10 yr:* **IV** 0.2-0.6 mg/kg over ½-1 min

Contraindications: Hypersensitivity, labor/delivery

HIGH ALERT

etoposide (℞)

(e-toe-poe'side)

Etopophos, VePesid, VP-16

Func. class.: Antineoplastic-misc.

Chem. class.: Semisynthetic podophyllotoxin

Action: Inhibits mitotic activity through metaphase to mitosis; also inhibits cells from entering mitosis, depresses DNA, RNA synthesis, cell cycle specific S and G_2

Uses: Leukemias, lung, testicular cancer, lymphomas, neuroblastoma, melanoma, ovarian cancer

Research note: A study showed an increase in etoposide when combined with atovaquone[14]

Dosage and routes:

Testicular cancer

• *Adult:* **IV** 50-100 mg/m²/day × 3-5 days given q3-5wk or 200-250 mg/m²/wk, or 125-140 mg/m²/day 3 × wk, q5wk

Lung cancer

• *Adult:* **PO** 35 mg/m²/day × 4 days, given q3-4wk, **IV** 35 mg/m²/day × 4 days

Available forms: Inj 20 mg/ml; caps 50, 100 mg; 113.6 etoposide phosphate = 100 etoposide

Side effects/adverse reactions:

HEMA: ***Thrombocytopenia, leukopenia, myelosuppression, anemia***

GI: Nausea, vomiting, anorexia, ***hepatotoxicity,*** dyspepsia, diarrhea, constipation

INTEG: Rash, alopecia, phlebitis at IV site, radiation recall

RESP: ***Bronchospasm,*** pleural effusion

CV: Hypotension, ***MI, dysrhythmias***

CNS: Headache, *fever,* peripheral neuropathy, paresthesias, confusion

GU: ***Nephrotoxicity***

SYST: ***Anaphylaxis***

Contraindications: Hypersensitivity, bone marrow depression, severe hepatic disease, severe renal disease, bacterial infection, pregnancy (D), viral infection

Precautions: Renal disease, hepatic disease, lactation, children, gout

Pharmacokinetics: Half-life 3 hr, terminal 15 hr; metabolized in liver; excreted in urine; crosses placental barrier

Do not confuse:

VePesid/Versed

Interactions:

• ↑ PT: warfarin

NURSING CONSIDERATIONS

Assess:

• CBC, differential, platelet count weekly; withhold drug if WBC is <1000 or platelet count is <50,000; notify prescriber

• Renal studies: BUN, serum uric acid, urine CCr, electrolytes before, during therapy

• I&O ratio; report fall in urine output to <30 ml/hr; check blood pressure bid and report any significant decrease

• Monitor temp q4h; may indicate beginning infection
• Hepatic studies before, during therapy (bilirubin, AST, ALT, LDH) as needed or monthly
• RBC, Hct, Hgb; may be decreased
• Bleeding: hematuria, guaiac stools, bruising or petechiae, mucosa or orifices q8h
• Effects of alopecia on body image; discuss feelings about body changes
• Jaundice of skin and sclera, dark urine, clay-colored stools, itchy skin, abdominal pain, fever, diarrhea
• B/P q15 min during inf, if systolic reading <90 mm Hg, discontinue inf and notify prescriber
• Buccal cavity q8h for dryness, sores or ulceration, white patches, oral pain, bleeding, dysphagia
• Local irritation, pain, burning, discoloration at inj site
Symptoms indicating severe allergic reaction: rash, pruritus, urticaria, purpuric skin lesions, itching, flushing
Symptoms of anaphylaxis: flushing, restlessness, coughing, difficulty breathing
• Frequency of stools, characteristics: cramping, acidosis; signs of dehydration: rapid respirations, poor skin turgor, decreased urine output, dry skin, restlessness, weakness

Administer:
• Antiemetic 30-60 min before giving drug and prn to prevent vomiting
• Allopurinol or sodium bicarbonate to maintain uric acid levels, alkalinization of urine
• Hyaluronidase 150 units/ml to 1 ml NaCl to infiltration area, ice compress for vesicant activity
• Antispasmodic, epINEPHrine, corticosteroids, antihistamines for reactions

IV route (VePesid)
• After diluting 100 mg/250 ml or more D_5W or NaCl to 0.2-0.4 mg/ml, infuse over 30-60 min; phosphate may be given over 5 min-3½ hr; may dilute further to 0.1 mg/ml in 0.9% NaCl, D_5W

Additive compatibilities: Carboplatin, cisplatin, cytarabine, floxuridine, fluorouracil, hydrOXYzine, ifosfamide, ondansetron

Y-site compatibilities: Allopurinol, amifostine, aztreonam, cladribine, DOXOrubicin liposome, fludarabine, granisetron, melphalan, ondansetron, paclitaxel, piperacillin/tazobactam, sargramostim, sodium bicarbonate, teniposide, thiotepa, vinorelbine

Perform/provide:
• Liquid diet: carbonated beverages, Jell-O; dry toast or crackers may be added if patient is not nauseated or vomiting
• Increase fluid intake to 2-3 L/day to prevent urate deposits, calculi formation
• Diet low in purines: organ meats (kidney, liver), dried beans, peas to maintain alkaline urine
• Nutritious diet with iron, vitamin supplements

Evaluate:
• Therapeutic response: decreased tumor size, spread of malignancy

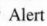

Teach patient/family:
• To report any complaints or side effects to nurse or prescriber
• To report any changes in breathing or coughing
• That hair may be lost during treatment; a wig or hairpiece may make patient feel better; tell patient that new hair may be different in color, texture

exemestane (℞)

(ex-em'eh-stane)
Aromasin
Func. class.: Antineoplastic
Chem. class.: Aromatase inhibitor

Action: Lowers serum estradiol concentrations; many breast cancers have strong estrogen receptors
Uses: Advanced breast carcinoma not responsive to other therapy in estrogen-receptor-positive patients (postmenopausal)
Research note: One study showed that this drug produced no change in parturition and was not teratogenic in rats and rabbits[15]
Dosage and routes:
- *Adult:* **PO** 25 mg qd pc

Available forms: Tabs 25 mg
Side effects/adverse reactions:
GI: Nausea, vomiting, diarrhea, constipation, abdominal pain, increased appetite
CV: Hypertension
CNS: Hot flashes, headache, depression, insomnia, anxiety, fatigue
RESP: Cough, dyspnea
Contraindications: Hypersensitivity, pregnancy (D), premenopausal women
Precautions: Lactation, children, elderly, liver disease, renal disease
Pharmacokinetics: Half-life 24 hr, excreted in feces, urine
NURSING CONSIDERATIONS
Assess:
- B/P, hypertension may occur

Perform/provide:
- Liquid diet, if needed including cola, gelatin; dry toast or crackers may be added if patient is not nauseated or vomiting
- Increase fluid intake to 2-3 L/day to prevent dehydration
- Nutritious diet with iron, vitamin supplements as ordered
- Storage in light-resistant container at room temperature

Evaluate:
- Therapeutic response: decreased tumor size, spread of malignancy

Teach patient/family:
- To report any complaints, side effects to prescriber
- That hot flashes are reversible after discontinuing treatment

ezetimibe (℞)

(ehz-eh-tim'bee)
Zetia
Func. class.: Antilipemic

Action: Inhibits absorption of cholesterol by the small intestine
Uses: Hypercholesterolemia, homozygous familial hypercholesterolemia (HoFH), homozygous sitosterolemia
Dosage and routes:
- *Adult:* **PO** 10 mg qd; may be given with HMG-CoA reductase inhibitor at same time; may be given with bile acid sequestrant; give ezetimibe 2 hr before or 4 hr after the bile acid sequestrant

Available forms: Tabs 10 mg
Side effects/adverse reactions:
CNS: Fatigue, dizziness, headache
GI: Diarrhea, abdominal pain
MISC: Chest pain
MS: Myalgias, arthralgias, back pain
RESP: Pharyngitis, sinusitis, cough, URI
Contraindications: Hypersensitivity, severe hepatic disease
Precautions: Pregnancy (C), lactation, children, hepatic disease
Pharmacokinetics: Metabolized in

E

small intestine, liver, excreted in feces 78%, urine 11%

Interactions:

- ↓ action of ezetimibe: antacids, cholestyramine
- ↑ action of ezetimibe: fibric acid derivatives, cycloSPORINE
- ↑ effect: glucomannan
- ↓ effect: gotu kola

NURSING CONSIDERATIONS

Assess:

- Lipid levels, LFTs baseline and periodically during treatment

Administer:

- Without regard to meals

Evaluate:

- Therapeutic response: decreased cholesterol

Teach patient/family:

- That compliance is needed
- That risk factors should be decreased: high-fat diet, smoking, alcohol consumption, absence of exercise
- To notify prescriber if pregnancy is suspected or planned

HIGH ALERT

factor IX complex (human)/factor IV (℞)

Alpha-Nine SD, Benefix, Konyne 80, Mononine, Profilnine/Alpha Nine, Proplex SX-T, Proplex T

Func. class.: Hemostatic

Chem. class.: Factors II, VII, IX, X

Action: Causes an increase in blood levels of clotting factors II, VII, IX, X; factor IX (human) has IX activity

Uses: Hemophilia B (Christmas disease), factor IX deficiency, anticoagulant reversal, control of bleeding in patients with factor VIII inhibitors, reversal of overdose of anticoagulants in emergencies

Dosage and routes:

Factor IX complex (human) bleeding in hemophilia B

- *Adult and child:* **IV** establish 25% of normal factor IX or 60-75 units/kg, then 10-20 units/kg/day 1-2 ×/wk

Prophylaxis for bleeding in hemophilia B

- *Adult and child:* **IV** 10-20 units/kg 1-2 ×/wk

Bleeding in hemophilia A/inhibitors of factor VIII (Proplex T, Konyne 80)

- *Adult and child:* **IV** 75 units/kg, repeat in 12 hr

Oral anticoagulant reversal

- *Adult and child:* **IV** 15 units/kg

Factor VII deficiency (use Proplex T only)

- *Adult and child:* **IV** 0.5 units/kg × weight (kg) × desired factor IX increase (% of normal); repeat q4-6h if needed

Factor IX (human) minor-moderate hemorrhage

Use only Alpha Nine, Alpha-Nine SD

- *Adult and child:* **IV** dose to increase factor IX level to 20%-30% in one dose

Serious hemorrhage

- *Adult and child:* **IV** dose to increase factor IX to 30%-50% as daily inf

Minor hemorrhage (mononine only)

- *Adult and child:* **IV** dose to increase factor IX to 15%-25% (20-30 units/kg), repeat in 24 hr if needed

Major hemorrhage

- *Adult and child:* **IV** dose to increase factor IX to 25%-50% (75 units/kg) q18-30h × 10 days or less

Available forms: Inj (number of units noted on label)

Side effects/adverse reactions:
GI: Nausea, vomiting, abdominal cramps, jaundice, ***viral hepatitis***
INTEG: Rash, flushing, *urticaria*
CNS: Headache, dizziness, malaise, paresthesia, *lethargy, chills, fever, flushing*
HEMA: ***Thrombosis, hemolysis, AIDS, DIC***
CV: Hypotension, tachycardia, *MI,* ***venous thrombosis, pulmonary embolism***
RESP: ***Bronchospasm***
Contraindications: Hypersensitivity to mouse protein, hepatic disease, DIC, elective surgery, mild factor IX deficiency
Precautions: Neonates/infants, pregnancy (C)
Pharmacokinetics:
IV: Half-life factor VII–3-6 hr, factor IX–24-36 hr; rapidly cleared from plasma
Interactions:
• Incompatible with protein products
⬌ ↑ thrombosis risk: aminocaproic acid; do not administer

NURSING CONSIDERATIONS
Assess:
• Blood studies (coagulation factors assays by % normal: 5% prevents spontaneous hemorrhage, 30%-50% for surgery, 80%-100% for severe hemorrhage)
• Increased B/P, pulse
• For bleeding q15-30min, immobilize and apply ice to affected joints
• I&O; if urine becomes orange or red, notify prescriber
• Allergic or pyrogenic reaction: fever, chills, rash, itching, slow inf rate if not severe
⬌ DIC: bleeding, ecchymosis, hypersensitivity, changes in coagulation tests
Administer:
• Hepatitis B vaccine before administration
• IV after warming to room temperature 3 ml/min or less, with plastic syringe only; do not admix
• After dilution with provided diluent, 50 units/ml or 25 units/ml; do not exceed 10 ml/min; decrease rate if fever, headache, flushing, tingling occur
• After crossmatch if patient has blood type A, B, AB, to determine incompatibility with factor
Perform/provide:
• Storage of reconstituted sol for 3 hr at room temperature or up to 2 yr refrigeration (powder); check expiration date
Evaluate:
• Therapeutic response: prevention of hemorrhage
Teach patient/family:
• To report any signs of bleeding: gums, under skin, urine, stools, emesis
• The risk of viral hepatitis, AIDS; to be tested q2-3mo for HIV, even though risk is low
• That immunization for hepatitis B may be given first
• To carry emergency ID identifying disease; avoid salicylates, NSAIDs; inform other health professionals of condition

famciclovir (℞)
(fam-cy′clo-veer)
Famvir
Func. class.: Antiviral
Chem. class.: Guanosine nucleoside

Action: Inhibits DNA polymerase and viral DNA synthesis by conversion of this guanosine nucleoside to penciclovir
Uses: Treatment of acute herpes

zoster (shingles), genital herpes; recurrent mucocutaneous herpes simplex virus (HSV) in HIV patients
Investigational uses: Initial episodes of herpes genitalis
Dosage and routes:
Herpes zoster
• *Adult:* **PO** 500 mg q8h
Renal dose: CCr ≥60 ml/min, 500 mg q8h; 40-59 ml/min, 500 mg q12h; 20-39 ml/min, 500 mg q24h
Recurrent mucocutaneous herpes simplex
• *Adult:* **PO** 500 mg q12h × 1 wk
Recurrent herpes simplex virus
• *Adult:* **PO** 125 mg q12h × 5 days
Suppression of recurrent herpes simplex virus
• *Adult:* **PO** 250 mg q12h up to 1 yr
Genital herpes (recurrent)
• *Adult:* **PO** 125 mg bid × 5 day; begin treatment at first sign of recurrence
Suppression of recurrent genital herpes
• *Adult:* **PO** 250 mg bid for up to a year
Herpes genitalis initial episodes (off-label)
• *Adult:* **PO** 25 mg tid × 7-10 days
Available forms: Tabs 125, 250, 500 mg
Side effects/adverse reactions:
MS: Back pain, arthralgia
GU: Decreased sperm count
CNS: Headache, fatigue, dizziness, paresthesia, somnolence, fever
RESP: Pharyngitis, sinusitis
GI: Nausea, vomiting, diarrhea, constipation, abdominal pain, anorexia
INTEG: Pruritus
Contraindications: Hypersensitivity to this drug, penciclovir
Precautions: Renal disease, pregnancy (B), hypersensitivity to acyclovir, ganciclovir, lactation
Pharmacokinetics: Unknown
Interactions:
• ↓ renal excretion: theophylline, probenecid, digoxin
• ↓ metabolism: cimetidine

NURSING CONSIDERATIONS
Assess:
• For number, distribution of lesions; burning, itching, pain, which are early symptoms of herpes infection
• Renal studies: urine CCr, BUN before and during treatment if decreased renal function; dose may have to be lowered
• Bowel pattern before, during treatment; diarrhea may occur
• Posttherapeutic neuralgia during and after treatment
Administer:
• With or without meals; absorption does not appear to be lowered when taken with food
• Within 72 hr of the appearance of rash in herpes zoster
Evaluate:
• Therapeutic response: decreased size, spread of lesions
Teach patient/family:
• How to recognize beginning infection
• How to prevent spread of infection; that this medication does not prevent the spread to others, that condoms should be used
• The reason for medication, expected results
• That women with genital herpes should have yearly Pap smears, cervical cancer is more likely

famotidine (OTC, ℞)
(fa-moe'ti-deen)
Mylanta AR, Pepcid, Pepcid AC, Pepcid IV, Pepcid RPD✦
Func. class.: H_2-histamine receptor antagonist

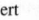

Action: Competitively inhibits

histamine at histamine H_2-receptor site, decreasing gastric secretion while pepsin remains at a stable level

Uses: Short-term treatment of active duodenal ulcer, maintenance therapy for duodenal ulcer, Zollinger-Ellison syndrome, multiple endocrine adenomas, gastric ulcers; gastroesophageal reflux disease, heartburn

Investigational uses: GI disorders in those taking NSAIDs; urticaria; prevention of stress ulcers, aspiration pneumonitis, inactivation of oral pancreatic enzymes in pancreatic disorders, prevention of paclitaxel hypersensitivity reactions

Dosage and routes:

Active ulcer

• *Adult:* **PO** 40 mg qd hs × 4-8 wk, then 20 mg qd hs if needed (maintenance); **IV** 20 mg q12h if unable to take **PO**

• *Child 1-16 yr:* 0.5 mg/kg/day hs or divided bid, max 40 mg qd

Hypersecretory conditions

• *Adult:* **PO** 20 mg q6h; may give 160 mg q6h if needed; **IV** 20 mg q12h if unable to take **PO**

• *Child* 1-16 yr: 1 mg/kg/day divide bid, max 40 mg bid

Heartburn relief/prevention

• *Adult:* **PO** 10 mg with water or 1 hr before eating

Paclitaxel hypersensitivity reactions

• *Adult:* **IV** 20 mg ½ hr prior to infusion

Renal disease

• CCr <10 ml/min 20 mg hs or dose q36-48h

Available forms: Tabs 10, 20, 40 mg; powder for oral susp 40 mg/5 ml; inj 10 mg/ml, 20 mg/50 ml 0.9% NaCl; orally disintegrating tabs (RPD) 20, 40 mg; chew tabs 10 mg

Side effects/adverse reactions:

HEMA: ***Thrombocytopenia, aplastic anemia***

CNS: Headache, dizziness, paresthesia, depression, anxiety, somnolence, insomnia, fever

EENT: Taste change, tinnitus, orbital edema

GI: Constipation, nausea, vomiting, anorexia, cramps, abnormal liver enzymes, diarrhea

INTEG: Rash

MS: Myalgia, arthralgia

CV: ***Dysrhythmias***

Contraindications: Hypersensitivity

Precautions: Pregnancy (B), lactation, children <12 yr, severe renal disease, severe hepatic disease, elderly

Pharmacokinetics: Absorption 50% (PO)

PO: Onset 30-60 min, duration 6-12 hr, peak 1-3 hr

IV: Onset immediate, peak 30-60 min, duration 8-15 hr, plasma protein-binding 15%-20%; metabolized in liver 30% (active metabolites), 70% excreted by kidneys, half-life 2½-3½ hr

Interactions:

• ↓ absorption: ketoconazole

• ↓ famotidine absorption: antacids

NURSING CONSIDERATIONS

Assess:

• For epigastric pain, adominal pain, frank or occult blood in emesis, stools

• Blood counts during therapy; watch for decreasing platelets; if low, therapy may have to be discontinued and restarted after hematologic recovery

• For bleeding, hematuria, hematuresis, occult blood in stools; abdominal pain

• Blood dyscrasias (thrombocytopenia): bruising, fatigue, bleeding, poor healing

Administer:
• Antacids 1 hr before or 2 hr after famotidine; may be given with foods or liquids
• After shaking oral suspension

IV direct route
• After diluting 2 ml of drug (10 mg/ml) in 0.9% NaCl to total volume of 5-10 ml; inject over 2 min to prevent hypotension

IV Intermittent INF route
• After diluting 20 mg (2 ml) of drug in 100 ml of LR, 0.9% NaCl, D_5W, $D_{10}W$; run over 15-30 min

Additive compatibilities: Cefazolin, cefmetazole, flumazenil, vancomycin

Y-site compatibilities: Acyclovir, allopurinol, amifostine, aminophylline, amphotericin, ampicillin, ampicillin/sulbactam, amrinone, amsacrine, atropine, aztreonam, bretylium, calcium gluconate, cefazolin, cefoperazone, cefotaxime, cefotetan, cefoxitin, ceftazidime, ceftizoxime, ceftriaxone, cefuroxime, cephalothin, cephapirin, chlorproMAZINE, cisatracurium, cisplatin, cladribine, cyclophosphamide, cytarabine, dexamethasone, dextran 40, digoxin, diphenhydrAMINE, DOBUTamine, DOPamine, DOXOrubicin, DOXOrubicin liposome, droperidol, enalaprilat, epINEPHrine, erythromycin, esmolol, filgrastim, fluconazole, fludarabine, folic acid, gentamicin, granisetron, haloperidol, heparin, hydrocortisone, hydromorphone, hydrOXYzine, imipenem/cilastatin, insulin (regular), isoproterenol, labetalol, lidocaine, lorazepam, magnesium sulfate, melphalan, meperidine, methotrexate, methylPREDNISolone, metoclopramide, mezlocillin, midazolam, morphine, nafcillin, nitroglycerin, nitroprusside, norepinephrine, ondansetron, oxacillin, paclitaxel, perphenazine, phenylephrine, phenytoin, phytonadione, piperacillin, potassium chloride/phosphate, procainamide, propofol, remifentanil, sargramostim, sodium bicarbonate, teniposide, theophylline, thiamine, thiotepa, ticarcillin, ticarcillin/clavulanate, verapamil, vinorelbine

Perform/provide:
• Storage in cool environment (oral); IV sol is stable for 48 hr at room temperature; do not use discolored sol; discard unused oral sol after 1 mo

Evaluate:
• Therapeutic response: decreased abdominal pain

Teach patient/family:
• That drug must be continued for prescribed time in prescribed method to be effective; do not double dose
• To report bleeding, bruising, fatigue, malaise, since blood dyscrasias occur
• About possibility of decreased libido, reversible after discontinuing therapy
• To avoid irritating foods, alcohol, aspirin, and extreme temperature of foods that may irritate GI system
• That smoking should be avoided; diminishes effectiveness of drug
• To avoid tasks requiring alertness; dizziness, drowsiness may occur
• To increase bulk and fluids in the diet to prevent constipation

fat emulsions (℞)

Intralipid 10%, Intralipid 20%, Liposyn II 10%, Liposyn II 20%, Liposyn III 10%, Liposyn III 20%, Soyacal 20%

Func. class.: Caloric

Chem. class.: Fatty acid, long chain

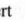

Action: Needed for energy, heat production; consist of neutral triglycerides, primarily unsaturated fatty acids

Uses: Increase calorie intake, fatty acid deficiency, prevention

Dosage and routes:

Deficiency

• *Adult and child:* **IV** 8%-10% of required calorie intake (intralipid)

Adjunct to TPN

• *Adult:* **IV** 1 ml/min over 15-30 min (10%) or 0.5 ml/min over 15-30 min (20%); may increase to 500 ml over 4-8 hr if no adverse reactions occur; not to exceed 2.5 g/kg

• *Child:* **IV** 0.1 ml/min over 10-15 min (10%) or 0.05 ml/min over 10-15 min (20%); may increase to 1 g/kg over 4 hr if no adverse reactions occur; not to exceed 4 g/kg

Prevention of deficiency

• *Adult:* **IV** 500 ml 2 ×/wk (10%), given 1 ml/min for 30 min, not to exceed 500 ml over 6 hr

• *Child:* **IV** 5-10 ml/kg/day (10%), given 0.1 ml/min for 30 min, not to exceed 100 ml/hr

Available forms: Inj 10% (50, 100, 200, 250, 500 ml), 20% (50, 100, 200, 250, 500 ml)

Side effects/adverse reactions:

CNS: Dizziness, headache, drowsiness, ***focal seizures***

CV: ***Shock***

GI: Nausea, vomiting, ***hepatomegaly***

RESP: Dyspnea, ***fat in lung tissue***

HEMA: ***Hyperlipemia, hypercoagulation, thrombocytopenia, leukopenia, leukocytosis***

Contraindications: Hypersensitivity, hyperlipemia, lipid necrosis, acute pancreatitis accompanied by hyperlipemia, hyperbilirubinemia of the newborn

Precautions: Severe hepatic disease, diabetes mellitus, thrombocytopenia, gastric ulcers, premature/term newborns, pregnancy (C), sepsis

NURSING CONSIDERATIONS

Assess:

• Triglycerides, free fatty acid levels, platelet counts daily to prevent fat overload, thrombocytopenia

• Hepatic studies: AST, ALT, Hct, Hgb; notify prescriber if abnormal

• Nutritional status: calorie count by dietitian; monitor weight daily

Administer:

IV Intermittent INF route

• At 10% (1 ml/min); 20% (0.5 ml/min) initially × 15-30 min, may increase 10% (120 ml/hr); 20% (62.5 ml/hr) if no adverse reaction; do not give more than 500 ml on first day

• After changing IV tubing at each infusion: infection may occur with old tubing

• With inf pump at prescribed rate; do not use in-line filter sized for lipid emulsion; clogging will occur

Additive compatibilities: Cefamandole, chloramphenicol, cimetidine, cycloSPORINE, diphenhydrAMINE, famotidine, heparin, hydrocortisone, multivitamins, nizatidine, penicillin G potassium

Y-site compatibilities: Ampicillin, cefamandole, cefazolin, cefoxitin, cephapirin, clindamycin, digoxin, DOPamine, erythromycin, furosemide, gentamicin, IL-2, isoproterenol, kanamycin, lidocaine, norepinephrine, oxacillin, penicillin G potassium, ticarcillin, tobramycin

Perform/provide:

• Do not use mixed sol if separated or oily looking

Evaluate:

• Therapeutic response: increased weight

Teach patient/family:

• The reason for use of lipids

RARELY USED

felbamate (℞)

(fell'ba-mate)
Felbatol
Func. class.: Anticonvulsant

Uses: Partial seizures, with or without generalization in adults; partial and generalized seizures in children with Lennox-Gastaut syndrome

Dosage and routes:

Adjunctive therapy

• *Adult or child >14 yr:* **PO** add 1.2 g/day in 3-4 divided doses; reduce other anticonvulsants (valproic acid, phenytoin, carbamazepine and derivatives) by 20% to control plasma concentrations; may increase felbamate 1.2 g/day increments qwk, up to 3.6 g/day

Monotherapy

• *Adult:* **PO** 1.2 g/day in 3-4 divided doses; titrate with close supervision; increase dose by 600-mg increments q2wk to 3.6 g/day if needed

Lennox-Gastaut syndrome adjunctive therapy

• *Child 2-14 yr:* **PO** add 15 mg/kg/day in 3-4 divided doses; reduce other anticonvulsants (valproic acid, phenytoin, carbamazepine and derivatives) by 20% to control plasma concentrations; may increase felbamate 15 mg/kg/day qwk up to 45 mg/day

Contraindications: Hypersensitivity to this drug, other carbamates, history of blood dyscrasia, aplastic anemia, hepatic disease

felodipine (℞)

(fe-loe'-di-peen)
Plendil, Renedil✱
Func. class.: Antihypertensive, calcium channel blocker, antianginal
Chem. class.: Dihydropyridine

Action: Inhibits calcium ion influx across cell membrane, resulting in inhibition of excitation/contraction

Uses: Essential hypertension, alone or with other antihypertensives, angina pectoris, Prinzmetal's angina (vasospastic)

Dosage and routes:

• *Adult:* **PO** 5 mg qd initially, usual range 5-10 mg qd; max 10 mg qd; do not adjust dosage at intervals of <2 wk

• *Geriatric:* **PO** 2.5 mg qd

Hepatic disease

• **PO** 2.5-5 mg, max 10 mg/day

Available forms: Ext rel tabs 2.5, 5, 10 mg

Side effects/adverse reactions:

CV: ***Dysrhythmia,*** edema, ***CHF,*** hypotension, palpitations, ***MI, pulmonary edema,*** tachycardia, syncope, AV block, angina

GI: Nausea, vomiting, diarrhea, gastric upset, constipation, increased liver function studies, dry mouth

GU: Nocturia, polyuria

INTEG: Rash, pruritus

MISC: Flushing, sexual difficulties, cough, nasal congestion, shortness of breath, wheezing, epistaxis, respiratory infection, chest pain, ***Stevens-Johnson syndrome,*** gingival hyperplasia

CNS: Headache, fatigue, drowsiness, dizziness, anxiety, depression, nervousness, insomnia, lightheadedness, paresthesia, tinnitus, psychosis, somnolence

HEMA: Anemia

Contraindications: Hypersensitivity, sick sinus syndrome, 2nd- or 3rd-degree heart block

Precautions: CHF, hypotension <90 mm Hg systolic, hepatic injury, pregnancy (C), lactation, children, renal disease, elderly

Do not confuse:
Plendil/pindolol/Pletal/Prilosec
Plendil/Prinivil

Pharmacokinetics: Peak plasma levels 2.5-5 hr; highly protein bound, >99% metabolized in liver, 0.5% excreted unchanged in urine; elimination half-life 11-16 hr

Interactions:

- ↑ toxicity: ketoconazole, erythromycin, itraconazole, propranolol
- Bradycardia, CHF: β-blockers, digoxin, phenytoin, disopyramide
- ↑ hypotension: fentanyl, nitrates, alcohol, quinidine
- ↓ antihypertensive effects: NSAIDs
- Drug/food: ↑ felodipine level: grapefruit juice

↑ toxicity, death: aconite

↑ or ↓ antihypertensive effect: astragalus, cola tree

↑ antihypertensive effect: barberry, betony, black catechu, black cohosh, bloodroot, broom, burdock, cat's claw, dandelion, goldenseal, Irish moss, Jamaican dogwood, kelp, khella, mistletoe, parsley

↓ antihypertensive effect: coltsfoot, guarana, khat, licorice

NURSING CONSIDERATIONS

Assess:

- I&O, weight daily; for CHF: weight gain, rales, crackles, dyspnea, edema, jugular venous distention
- Renal, hepatic studies
- Cardiac status: B/P, pulse, respiration; ECG periodically
- For angina pain: location, duration, intensity; ameliorating, aggravating factors

Administer:

- Once daily without regard to meals

Evaluate:

- Therapeutic response: decreased B/P, decreased anginal attacks, increase in activity tolerance

Teach patient/family:

To swallow whole; do not break, crush, or chew sus rel products

- To avoid hazardous activities until stabilized on drug, dizziness is no longer a problem
- To avoid OTC drugs, alcohol, unless directed by a prescriber, to limit caffeine consumption
- The importance of complying with all areas of medical regimen: diet, exercise, stress reduction, drug therapy
- That tablets may appear in stools, but are insignificant
- To report dyspnea, palpitations, irregular heart beat, swelling of extremities, nausea, vomiting, severe dizziness, severe headache
- To change positions slowly to prevent orthostatic hypotension
- To obtain correct pulse, to contact prescriber if pulse is <50 bpm
- To use protective clothing, sunscreen to prevent photosensitivity

Treatment of overdose: Atropine for AV block, vasopressor for hypotension

fenofibrate (℞)

(fen-oh-fee'brate)

Tricor

Func. class.: Antilipemic

Chem. class.: Fibric acid derivative

Action: Increases lipolysis and elimination of triglyceride rich particles from plasma by activating lipoprotein lipase, resulting in triglyceride change in size and composition of

LDL leading to rapid breakdown of LDL; mobilizes triglycerides from tissue; increases excretion of neutral sterols

Uses: Hypercholesterolemia, types IV, V hyperlipidemia that do not respond to other treatment and are at risk for pancreatitis, Fredrickson type IIa, IIb, hypertriglyceridemia

Investigational uses: Polymetabolic syndrome X

Dosage and routes:

Hypertriglyceridemia

• *Adult:* **PO** 54-160 mg/day, may increase q4-8wk, max 160 mg/day

Primary hypercholesterolemia/ mixed hyperlipidemia

• *Adult:* **PO** 160 mg/day

Renal dose

• *Adult:* **PO** 54 mg/day (CCr <50 ml/min)

Available forms: Tabs 54, 160 mg

Side effects/adverse reactions:

CNS: Fatigue, weakness, drowsiness, dizziness, insomnia, depression, vertigo

CV: Angina, ***dysrhythmias,*** hypertension

GI: Nausea, vomiting, dyspepsia, increased liver enzymes, flatulence, hepatomegaly, gastritis

GU: Dysuria, proteinuria, oliguria, urinary frequency

INTEG: Rash, urticaria, pruritus

MISC: Polyphagia, weight gain

MS: Myalgias, arthralgias, myopathy

HEMA: Anemia, leukopenia, ecchymosis

RESP: Pharyngitis, bronchitis, cough

Contraindications: Hypertensivity, severe hepatic disease, severe renal disease, primary biliary cirrhosis, preexisting gallbladder disease

Precautions: Peptic ulcer, pregnancy (C), lactation, pancreatitis, renal, hepatic disease, elderly

Pharmacokinetics: Peak 6-8h; protein binding 99%, converted to fenofibric acid, metabolized in liver, excreted in urine (60%), half-life 20 hr

Interactions:

• Nephrotoxicity: cycloSPORINE

• ↓ absorption of fenofibrate: bile acid sequestrants

• Avoid use with HMG-CoA reductase inhibitors, rhabdomyolysis may occur

↑ effect: glucomannan

↓ effect: gotu kola

• ↑ anticoagulant effects: oral anticoagulants

• Drug/food: ↑ absorption

NURSING CONSIDERATIONS

Assess:

• Lipid levels, LFTs baseline and periodically during treatment, CPK if muscle pain occurs, CBC, Hct, Hgb; PT with anticoagulant therapy

• Pancreatitis, cholelithiasis renal failure, rhabdomyolyis (when combined with HMG Co-A reductase inhibitors), myositis, drug should be discontinued

Administer:

• Drug with meals; may increase q4-8wk

Evaluate:

• Therapeutic response: decreased triglycerides

Teach patient/family:

• That compliance is needed

• That risk factors should be decreased: high-fat diet, smoking, alcohol consumption, absence of exercise

• To notify prescriber if pregnancy is suspected or planned

• To report GU symptoms: decreased

libido, impotence, dysuria, proteinuria, oliguria, hematuria
• To notify prescriber of muscle pain, weakness, fever, fatigue; epigastric pain

fenoldopam (℞)

(feh-nahl'doh-pam)
Corlopam
Func. class.: Antihypertensive, vasodilator

Action: Agonist at D_1-like dopamine receptors; binds to α_2-adrenoceptors; increases renal blood flow
Uses: Hypertensive crisis, malignant hypertension
Dosage and routes:
• *Adult:* **IV** 0.01-1.6 mcg/kg/min
Available forms: Inj conc 10 mg/ml in single use ampules
Side effects/adverse reactions:
CNS: Headache, anxiety, dizziness
CV: ***Hypotension,*** ST-T-wave changes, angina pectoris, palpitations, ***MI, ischemic heart disease, flushing***
GI: Nausea, vomiting, constipation, diarrhea
HEMA: ***Leukocytosis,*** bleeding
META: Increased BUN, glucose, LDH, creatinine, hypokalemia
Contraindications: Hypersensitivity, sulfite sensitivity
Precautions: Tachycardia, pregnancy (B), lactation, children, intraocular pressure, hypokalemia
Pharmacokinetics: Elimination half-life 5 min, steady state 20 min
Interactions:
• ↑ hypotension: avoid use with β-blockers
↑ toxicity, death: aconite
↑ or ↓ antihypertensive effect: astragalus, cola tree
↑ antihypertensive effect: barberry, betony, black catechu, black cohosh, bloodroot, broom, burdock, cat's claw, dandelion, goldenseal, Irish moss, Jamaican dogwood, kelp, khella, mistletoe, parsley
↓ antihypertensive effect: coltsfoot, guarana, khat, licorice

NURSING CONSIDERATIONS
Assess:
• B/P q5min until stabilized, then q1h × 2 hr, then q4h; pulse, jugular venous distention q4h
• Electrolytes, blood studies: K, Na, C1, CO_2, CBC, serum glucose
• Skin turgor, dryness of mucous membranes for hydration status
• IV site for extravasation, rate
Administer:
IV route
• After diluting contents of ampules in 0.9% NaCl, or 5% dextrose inj (40 mcg/ml); then add 4 ml of conc (40 mg of drug/1000 ml); 2 ml of conc (20 mg of drug/500 ml); 1 ml of conc (10 mg of drug/250 ml); do not admix
• To patient in recumbent position; keep in that position for 1 hr after administration
Perform/provide:
• Diluted sol is stable in normal light/temperature for 24 hr
Evaluate:
• Therapeutic response: decreased B/P
Teach patient/family:
• To report dyspnea, chest pain, bleeding
• Reason for medication and expected results

F

RARELY USED

fenoprofen (℞)

(fen-oh-proe′fen)

Fenoprofen, Nalfon

Func. class.: Nonsteroidal antiinflammatory/nonopioid analgesic

Uses: Mild to moderate pain, osteoarthritis, rheumatoid arthritis, acute gout, arthritis, ankylosing spondylitis, inflammation, dysmenorrhea

Dosage and routes:

Pain

• *Adult:* **PO** 200 mg q4-6h prn

Arthritis

• *Adult:* **PO** 300-600 mg qid, not to exceed 3.2 g/day

Contraindications: Hypersensitivity, asthma, severe renal disease, severe hepatic disease

HIGH ALERT

fentanyl (℞)

(fen′ta-nill)

Actiq, Fentanyl, Fentanyl Oralet, Sublimaze

Func. class.: Opioid analgesic

Chem. class.: Synthetic phenylpiperidine

Controlled Substance Schedule II

Action: Inhibits ascending pain pathways in CNS, increases pain threshold, alters pain perception by binding to opiate receptors

Uses: Preoperatively, postoperatively; adjunct to general anesthetic, adjunct to regional anesthesia; Fentanyl Oralet—anesthesia as premedication, conscious sedation; Actiq—breakthrough cancer pain

Dosage and routes:

Anesthetic

• *Adult:* **IV** 25-100 mcg (0.7-2 mcg/kg) q2-3 min prn

Anesthesia supplement

• *Adult:* **IV** 2-20 mcg/kg **IV INF** 0.025-0.25 mcg/kg/min

Induction and maintenance

• *Adult:* **IV BOL** 5-40 mcg/kg

• *Child 2-12 yr:* **IV** 2-3 mcg/kg

Preoperatively

• *Adult:* **IM** 0.05-0.1 mg q30-60 min before surgery

Postoperatively

• *Adult:* **IM** 0.05-0.1 mg q1-2h prn

Fentanyl Oralet

• *Adult:* Transmucosal 5 mcg/kg = fentanyl IM 0.75-1.25 mcg/kg, do not exceed 5 mcg/kg

• *Child:* Transmucosal may need doses of 5-15 mcg/kg; must be watched continuously for hypoventilation

Actiq

• *Adult:* Transmucosal 200 mcg, redose if needed 15 min after completion of 1st dose, do not give more than 2 doses during titration period

Available forms: Inj 0.05 mg/ml; lozenges 100, 200, 300, 400 mcg; lozenges on a stick 200, 400, 600, 800, 1200, 1600 mcg

Side effects/adverse reactions:

CNS: Dizziness, delirium, euphoria

GI: Nausea, vomiting

MS: Muscle rigidity

EENT: Blurred vision, miosis

CV: ***Bradycardia, arrest,*** hypotension or hypertension

RESP: ***Respiratory depression, arrest, laryngospasm***

GU: Urinary retention

INTEG: Rash, diaphoresis

Contraindications: Hypersensitivity to opiates, myasthenia gravis

Precautions: Elderly, respiratory depression, increased intracranial pressure, seizure disorders, severe respiratory disorders, cardiac dysrhythmias, pregnancy (C), lactation

Do not confuse:
fentanyl/Sufenta

Pharmacokinetics:
IM: Onset 7-8 min, peak 30 min, duration 1-2 hr
IV: Onset 1 min, peak 3-5 min, duration ½-1 hr; metabolized by liver; excreted by kidneys; crosses placenta; excreted in breast milk; half-life 1½-6 hr; 80% bound to plasma proteins

Interactions:
• ↑ with other CNS depressants: alcohol, opioids, sedative/hypnotics, antipsychotics, skeletal muscle relaxants
• ↑ anticholinergic effect: corkwood
• ↑ action: Jamaican dogwood, kava, lavender, mistletoe, nettle, pokeweed, poppy, senega, valerian

NURSING CONSIDERATIONS

Assess:
• VS after parenteral route; note muscle rigidity, drug history, liver, kidney function test
• CNS changes: dizziness, drowsiness, hallucinations, euphoria, LOC, pupil reaction
• Allergic reactions: rash, urticaria
• Respiratory dysfunction: respiratory depression, character, rate, rhythm; notify prescriber if respirations are <10/min

Administer:
• By injection (IM, IV); give slowly to prevent rigidity
• Only with resuscitative equipment available

IV route
• IV undiluted by anesthesiologist or diluted with 5 ml or more sterile H_2O or 0.9% NaCl given through Y-tube or 3-way stopcock at 0.1 mg or less/1-2 min

Additive compatibilities: Bupivacaine

Solution compatibilities: D_5W, 0.9% NaCl

Syringe compatibilities: Atracurium, atropine, bupivacaine/ketamine, butorphanol, chlorproMAZINE, cimetidine, clonidine/lidocaine, diphenhydrinate, diphenhydrAMINE, droperidol, heparin, hydromorphone, hydrOXYzine, meperidine, metoclopramide, midazolam, morphine, pentazocine, perphenazine, prochlorperazine, promazine, promethazine, ranitidine, scopolamine

Y-site compatibilities: Amphotericin B cholesteryl, atracurium, cisatracurium, diltiazem, DOBUTamine, DOPamine, enalaprilat, epINEPHrine, esmolol, etomidate, furosemide, heparin, hydrocortisone, hydromorphone, labetalol, lorazepam, midazolam, milrinone, morphine, nafcillin, niCARdipine, nitroglycerin, norepinephrine, pancuronium, potassium chloride, propofol, ranitidine, remifentanil, sargramostim, thiopental, vecuronium, vit B/C

Transmucosal
• Remove foil just before administration, instruct patient to place under tongue and suck, not chew (Oralet); place between cheek and lower gum, moving it back and forth and suck, not chew (Actiq); all products not used or partially used should be flushed down the toilet

Perform/provide:
• Storage in light-resistant area at room temperature

Teach patient/family:
• Coughing, turning, deep breathing for postoperative patients

• Safety measures: side rails, nightlight, call bell within reach

Evaluate:

• Therapeutic response: induction of anesthesia, breakthrough cancer pain

HIGH ALERT

fentanyl/droperidol combination (℞)

(fen'ta-nil)/(droe-per'i-dole)

Innovar

Func. class.: General anesthetic, opioid analgesic

Chem. class.: Phenylpiperone derivative

Controlled Substance Schedule II

Action: Action at subcortical levels to reduce motor activity, produces analgesia

Uses: Premedication, adjunct to general anesthesia, maintenance of anesthesia

Dosage and routes:

Induction

• *Adult:* **IV** 1 ml/20-25 lb

• *Child:* **IV** 0.5 ml/20 lb

Premedication

• *Adult:* **IM** 0.5-2 ml 45-60 min before surgery or procedure

• *Child:* **IM** 0.25 ml/20 lb 45-60 min before surgery or procedure

Available forms: Inj 0.05 mg fentanyl, 2.5 mg droperidol/ml

Side effects/adverse reactions:

RESP: ***Laryngospasm, bronchospasm, respiratory arrest***

CNS: Dystonia, akathisia, flexion of arms, fine tremors, dizziness, anxiety, drowsiness, restlessness, hallucination, depression, muscular rigidity, EPS

CV: Tachycardia, hypotension, circulatory depression

EENT: Upward rotation of eyes, oculogyric crisis, blurred vision

INTEG: Chills, facial sweating, shivering, diaphoresis

GI: Nausea, vomiting

Contraindications: Hypersensitivity, child <2 yr, myasthenia gravis

Precautions: Elderly, increased intracranial pressure, cardiovascular disease (bradydysrhythmias), renal disease, liver disease, Parkinson's disease, COPD, pregnancy (C)

Pharmacokinetics:

IV: Onset 20 sec, peak 2-10 min, duration ½-2 hr; tranquilizing effect may last up to 12 hr

IM: Onset 7 min, duration 1-2 hr; metabolized in liver; excreted in urine metabolites (90%)

Interactions:

• ↑ CNS depression: alcohol, opioids, barbiturates, antipsychotics, other CNS depressants

• ↓ effects of amphetamines, anticonvulsants, anticoagulants

• ↑ intraocular pressure: anticholinergics, antiparkinson drugs

• ↑ side effects of lithium

↑ anticholinergic effect: corkwood

↑ action: Jamaican dogwood, kava, lavender, mistletoe, nettle, pokeweed, poppy, senega, valerian

NURSING CONSIDERATIONS

Assess:

• VS q10min during IV administration, q30min after IM dose

• LFTs and BUN, creatinine, $Paco_2$

• Rigidity of skeletal muscles

• EPS: dystonia, akathisia

• Increasing heart rate or decreasing B/P by >10% from baseline; notify prescriber at once; do not place patient in Trendelenburg position or sympathetic blockade may occur, causing respiratory arrest

Administer:

• Anticholinergics (benztropine, diphenhydrAMINE) for EPS

• Only with crash cart, resuscitative equipment nearby; opioid antagonist for severe respiratory depression, cardiac monitor

IV route

• IV direct undiluted through Y-tube or 3-way stopcock; give each 1 ml undiluted drug/1min or more; 0.1 ml/kg may be diluted in 250 ml D_5W and given as IV INF over 5-10 min; titrate to response

Additive compatibilities: Sodium bicarbonate

Syringe compatibilities: Benzquinamide, glycopyrrolate

Y-site compatibilities: Hydrocortisone, potassium chloride, vit B/C

Perform/provide:

• Slow movement of patient to avoid orthostatic hypotension

Evaluate:

• Therapeutic response: decreased anxiety, absence of vomiting, maintenance of anesthesia

Teach patient/family:

• To use deep breathing, turning, coughing after surgery to prevent increased secretions in lungs

fentanyl transdermal (℞)

Duragesic

Func. class.: Opioid analgesic

Chem. class.: Synthetic phenylpiperidine

Controlled Substance Schedule II

Action: Inhibits ascending pain pathways in CNS, increases pain threshold, alters pain perception by binding to opiate receptors

Uses: Management of chronic pain for those requiring opioid analgesia

Dosage and routes:

• *Adult:* 25 mcg/hr; may increase until pain relief occurs; apply patch to flat surface on upper torso and wear for 72 hr; apply new patch on different site for continued relief

Available forms: Patch 25, 50, 75, 100 mcg/hr

Side effects/adverse reactions:

MS: Asthenia

GU: Urinary retention, urgency, dysuria, frequency, oliguria

INTEG: Sweating, pruritus, rash, erythema, papules

CNS: Dizziness, delirium, euphoria, light-headedness, sedation, dysphoria, agitation, anxiety, confusion, headache, depression

GI: Nausea, vomiting, diarrhea, cramps, anorexia, constipation, dyspepsia

EENT: Blurred vision, miosis

CV: Bradycardia, ***cardiac arrest,*** hypotension or hypertension, facial flushing, chills, chest pain, dysrhythmias

RESP: ***Respiratory depression, laryngospasm, bronchospasm,*** depresses cough, hypoventilation, dyspnea, hiccups, apnea

Contraindications: Hypersensitivity to opiates, myasthenia gravis, children <12 yr, patient <18 yr with weight <110 lb

Precautions: Elderly, respiratory depression, increased intracranial pressure, seizure disorders, severe respiratory disorders, cardiac dysrhythmias, pregnancy (C), fever

Interactions:

• ↑ with other CNS depressants: alcohol, opioids, sedative/hypnotics, antipsychotics, skeletal muscle relaxants

• ↑ anticholinergic effect: corkwood

• ↑ action: Jamaican dogwood, kava, lavender, mistletoe, nettle, pokeweed, poppy, senega, valerian

NURSING CONSIDERATIONS

Assess:

- Pain control; check for duration, site, character of pain, fever; use pain and sedation scoring
- CNS changes: dizziness, drowsiness, hallucinations, euphoria, LOC, pupil reaction
- Allergic reactions: rash, urticaria
- Respiratory dysfunction: respiratory depression, character, rate, rhythm; notify prescriber if respirations are <10/min

Administer:

- q72h for continuous pain relief; dosage is adjusted after at least two applications, apply to clean, dry skin, press firmly
- Give short-acting analgesics until patch takes effect (24 hr); when reducing dosage or switching to alternate treatment, withdraw gradually; serum levels drop gradually, give ½ the equianalgesic dose of new analgesic 12-18 hr after removal as ordered

Perform/provide:

- Safety measures: side rails, nightlight, call bell within reach

Evaluate:

- Therapeutic response: decreased pain

Teach patient/family:

- To avoid activities that require alertness
- That excessive heat may increase absorption
- That excessive perspiration may alter adhesiveness
- To dispose of patch by placing sticky sides together and flushing in toilet
- That patient may need to clip hair before applying to ensure adhesion

ferrous fumarate (℞)

Femiron, Feostat, Feostat Drops, Hemocyte, Ircon, Nephro-Fer, Novofumar♣, Palafer♣, Span-FF

ferrous gluconate (℞)

Fergon, Fertinic♣, Novoferrogluc♣

ferrous sulfate (℞)

Apo-Ferrous Sulfate♣, ED-IN-SOL, Feosol, Fer-gen-sol, Fer-Iron Drops, Fero-Grad, Mol-Iron

ferrous sulfate, dried (℞)

Fe^{50}, Feosol, Feratab, Novoferrosulfa♣, PMS-Ferrous Sulfate, Slow Fe

ferric gluconate complex (℞)

Ferrlecit

carbonyl iron

(kar′bo-nil)

Feosol

iron polysaccharide

Hytinic, Niferex, Nu-Iron, Nu-Iron 150

Func. class.: Hematinic

Chem. class.: Iron preparation

Action: Replaces iron stores needed for red blood cell development, energy and O_2 transport, utilization; fumarate contains 33% elemental iron; gluconate, 12%; sulfate, 20%; iron, 30%; ferrous sulfate exsiccated

Uses: Iron deficiency anemia, prophylaxis for iron deficiency in pregnancy

Dosage and routes:

Fumarate

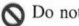

- *Adult:* **PO** 200 mg tid-qid
- *Child 2-12 yr:* **PO** 3 mg/kg/day (elemental iron) tid-qid
- *Child 6 mo-2 yr:* **PO** up to 6 mg/kg/day (elemental iron) tid-qid

• *Infant:* **PO** 10-25 mg/day (elemental iron) in 3-4 divided doses, max 15 mg/day

Gluconate

• *Adult:* **PO** 200-600 mg tid

• *Child 6-12 yr:* **PO** 300-900 mg qd

• *Child <6 yr:* **PO** 100-300 mg qd

Sulfate

• *Adult:* **PO** 0.75-1.5 g/day in divided doses tid

• *Child 6-12 yr:* **PO** 600 mg/day in divided doses

Pregnancy

• *Adult:* **PO** 300-600 mg/day in divided doses

Complex

Adult IV Inf (125 mg) 10 ml/100 ml of NaCl for inj given over 1 hr

Iron polysaccaride

• *Adult:* **PO** 100-200 mg tid

• *Child:* **PO** 4-6 mg/kg/day in 3 divided doses

Available forms:

Fumarate

Tabs 63, 195, 200, 324, 325 mg; tabs chewable 100 mg; tabs cont rel 300 mg; oral susp 100 mg/5 ml, 45 mg/0.6 ml

Gluconate

Tabs 300, 320, 325 mg; caps 86, 325, 435 mg; tabs film-coated 300 mg; elix 300 mg/5 ml

Sulfate

Tabs, 195, 300, 325 mg; tabs enteric-coated 325 mg; tabs ext rel, time-rel caps, 525 mg

Dried

Tabs, 200 mg; tabs ext rel 160 mg; caplets ext rel 160 mg

Complex

Inj. 62.5 mg/5 ml (12.5 mg/ml)

Iron polysaccharide

Tabs 50 mg, caps 150 mg, sol 100 mg/5 ml

Side effects/adverse reactions:

GI: Nausea, constipation, epigastric pain, black and red tarry stools, vomiting, diarrhea

INTEG: Temporarily discolored tooth enamel and eyes

Contraindications: Hypersensitivity, ulcerative colitis/regional enteritis, hemosiderosis/hemochromatosis, peptic ulcer disease, hemolytic anemia, cirrhosis

Precautions: Anemia (long-term), pregnancy (B) (ferric gluconate complex), (C) (iron dextran, oral products)

Pharmacokinetics:

PO: Excreted in feces, urine, skin, breast milk; enters bloodstream; bound to transferrin; crosses placenta

Interactions:

• ↓ absorption of: penicillamine, levodopa, methyldopa, fluoroquinolones, L-thyroxine, tetracycline

• ↓ absorption of iron preparations: antacids, cimetidine, cholestyramine, vit E

• ↑ action of iron preparation: ascorbic acid, chloramphenicol

• Drug/food: ↓ absorption: dairy products, caffeine, eggs

↓ iron absorption: allspice, bilberry, condurango, elderberry, eyebright (PO), gentian, ground ivy, hawthorn, horse chestnut, lady mantle, lemon balm, marshmallow, meadowsweet, mistletoe, motherwort, nettle, oak bark, plantain, poplar, prickly ash, raspberry, sage, tea made with artichoke, valerian

↑ iron effect: anise

Forms insoluble complex: black catechu

Lab test interferences:

False positive: Occult blood

NURSING CONSIDERATIONS

Assess:

• Blood studies: Hct, Hgb, reticulocytes, bilirubin before treatment, at least monthly

Toxicity: nausea, vomiting, diarrhea (green, then tarry stools), he-

matemesis, pallor, cyanosis, shock, coma
• Elimination; if constipation occurs, increase water, bulk, activity
• Nutrition: amount of iron in diet (meat, dark green leafy vegetables, dried beans, dried fruits, eggs)
• Cause of iron loss or anemia, including salicylates, sulfonamides, antimalarials, quinidine

Administer:
• Between meals for best absorption; may give with juice; do not give with antacids or milk, delay at least 1 hr; if GI symptoms occur, give pc even if absorption is decreased; eggs, milk products, chocolate, caffeine interfere with absorption
• Liquid through plastic straw to avoid discoloration of tooth enamel; dilute thoroughly
• At least 1 hr before hs, since corrosion may occur in stomach; ferrous gluconate is less GI irritating than ferrous sulfate
• For <6 mo for anemia

Perform/provide:
• Storage in tight, light-resistant container

Evaluate:
• Therapeutic response: improvement in Hct, Hgb, reticulocytes; decreased fatigue, weakness

Teach patient/family:
• That iron will change stools black or dark green
• That iron poisoning may occur if increased beyond recommended level
⊘ To swallow tab whole; not to break, crush, or chew unless labeled as chewable
• To keep out of reach of children
• Not to substitute one iron salt for another; elemental iron content differs (e.g., 300 mg ferrous fumarate contains about 100 mg elemental iron; 300 mg ferrous gluconate contains only about 30 mg elemental iron)
• To avoid reclining position for 15-30 min after taking drug to avoid esophageal corrosion
• To follow diet high in iron

Treatment of overdose: Induce vomiting; give eggs, milk until lavage can be done

fexofenadine (℞)

(fex-oh-fi′na-deen)

Allegra

Func. class.: Antihistamine

Chem. class.: Piperidine, peripherally selective

Action: Acts on blood vessels, GI, respiratory system by competing with histamine for H_1-receptor site; decreases allergic response by blocking pharmacologic effects of histamine

Uses: Rhinitis, allergy symptoms, chronic idiopathic urticaria

Dosage and routes:
• *Adult and child >12 yr:* 60 mg bid
• *Child 6-11 yr:* **PO** 30 mg bid

Renal dose:
• CCr <80 ml/min 60 mg qd

Available forms: Caps 60 mg; ext rel tab 180 mg; tab 30 mg

Side effects/adverse reactions:

GU: Frequency, dysuria, urinary retention, impotence

HEMA: ***Hemolytic anemia, thrombocytopenia, leukopenia, agranulocytosis, pancytopenia***

RESP: Thickening of bronchial secretions, dry nose, throat

GI: Nausea, diarrhea, abdominal pain, vomiting, constipation

CNS: Headache, stimulation, drowsiness, sedation, fatigue, confusion, blurred vision, tinnitus, restlessness, tremors, paradoxical excitation in children or elderly

INTEG: Rash, eczema, photosensitivity, urticaria
CV: Hypotension, palpitations, bradycardia, tachycardia, ***dysrhythmias*** (rare)
Contraindications: Hypersensitivity, newborn or premature infants, lactation, severe hepatic disease
Precautions: Pregnancy (C), elderly, children, respiratory disease, narrow-angle glaucoma, prostatic hypertrophy, bladder neck obstruction, asthma
Do not confuse:
Allegra/Viagra
Pharmacokinetics: Well absorbed; onset 3-5 min, peak 1-2 hr, duration 8-12 hr
Interactions:
- ↑ sedation: alcohol, other CNS depressants
- ↑ sedation: hops, Jamaican dogwood, khat, senega
- ↑ anticholinergic effect: corkwood, henbane leaf

Lab test interferences:
False negative: Skin allergy tests
NURSING CONSIDERATIONS
Assess:
- I&O ratio: be alert for urinary retention, frequency, dysuria, especially elderly; drug should be discontinued if these occur
- Respiratory status: rate, rhythm, increase in bronchial secretions, wheezing, chest tightness

Administer:
- On empty stomach 1 hr before or 2 hr after meals

Perform/provide:
- Hard candy, gum, frequent rinsing of mouth for dryness
- Storage in tight, light-resistant container

Evaluate:
- Therapeutic response: absence of running or congested nose or rashes

Teach patient/family:
- All aspects of drug use; to notify prescriber if confusion, sedation, hypotension occur
- To avoid driving, other hazardous activity if drowsiness occurs
- To avoid alcohol, other CNS depressants
- Not to exceed recommended dose; dysrhythmias may occur
- Not to break, crush, or chew caps, ext rel tabs

Treatment of overdose: Lavage, diazepam, vasopressors, barbiturates (short-acting)

fibrinolysin/ desoxyribonuclease (℞)

(fye-brin-oh-lye'sin)/(dez-ox-ee-rye-boo-nuke'lee-ase)
Elase
Func. class.: Enzyme
Chem. class.: Proteolytic, bovine

Action: Dissolves fibrin in clots and fibrinous exudates; attacks DNA in areas of disintegrating cells
Uses: Debridement of wounds, vaginitis, cervicitis, ulcerative colitis; 2nd-, 3rd-degree burns; irrigating wounds, topically
Dosage and routes:
Debridement/intravaginally
- *Adult:* **OINT** 5 g × 5 applications

Irrigating
- *Adult:* **IRIG** dilution depends on type of wound

Available forms: Fibrinolysin with desoxyribonuclease 666.6 units/g; powder for reconstitution fibrinolysin 25 units/desoxyribonuclease 15,000 units
Side effects/adverse reactions:
INTEG: Hyperemia
Contraindications: Hypersensitivity to bovine or mercury products, hematoma

Precautions: Pregnancy (C)

NURSING CONSIDERATIONS

Assess:

- For signs of irritation and inflammation; drug should be discontinued
- Wound: drainage, color, odor, size, depth

Administer:

- After reconstituting with 10 ml sterile NaCl sol; use only fresh sol
- After removing necrotic debris, dry eschar
- Wet dressing by mixing 1 vial Elase/10-50 ml NS; saturate gauze with sol; pack area; remove in 6-8 hr; repeat tid-qid

Perform/provide:

- Cleansing of wound using aseptic technique; cover with drug, then dressing; change at least qid

Evaluate:

- Therapeutic response: decrease in wound scarring, tissue necrosis

filgrastim (℞)

(fill-grass'stim)

G-CSF, granulocyte colony stimulator, Neupogen

Func. class.: Biologic modifier

Chem. class.: Granulocyte colony-stimulating factor

Action: Stimulates proliferation and differentiation of neutrophils

Uses: To decrease infection in patients receiving antineoplastics that are myelosuppressive; to increase WBC in patients with drug-induced neutropenia; bone marrow transplantation

Investigational uses: Neutropenia in HIV infection

Dosage and routes:

After myelosuppressive chemotherapy

- *Adult and child:* **IV/SC** 5 mcg/kg/day in a single dose × 14 days; may increase by 5 mcg/kg in each cycle; give qd for up to 2 wk until the absolute neutrophil count (ANC) is 10,000/mm^3; response to G-CSF is much greater with **SC** than **IV** therapy

After bone marrow transplantation

- **IV/SC** 10 mcg/kg/day as an **INF (IV)** over 4 hr or 24 hr, begin 24 hr after chemotherapy and 24 hr after bone marrow transplantation

Peripheral blood progenitor cell collection/therapy

- 10 mcg/kg/day as a bolus or **CONT INF** × 4 days or more before leukapheresis, continue to last leukapheresis; may alter dose if WBC >100,000 cells/mm^3

Severe neutropenia (chronic)

- *Adult:* **SC** 5 mcg/kg qd-bid

Available forms: Inj 300 mcg/ml

Side effects/adverse reactions:

RESP: Respiratory distress syndrome

CNS: Fever

HEMA: ***Thrombocytopenia***

INTEG: Alopecia, exacerbation of skin conditions

MS: Osteoporosis, skeletal pain

GI: Nausea, vomiting, diarrhea, mucositis, anorexia

Contraindications: Hypersensitivity to proteins of *E. coli*

Precautions: Pregnancy (C), lactation, cardiac conditions, children, myeloid malignancies

Pharmacokinetics:

IV: Onset 5-60 min, peak 24 hr, duration up to a week

SC: Onset 5-60 min, peak 2-8 hr, duration up to a week

Interactions:

- Do not use this drug concomitantly with antineoplastics

Lab test interferences:

Increase: Uric acid, lactate dehydrogenase, alk phosphatase

NURSING CONSIDERATIONS

Assess:

• Blood studies: CBC, platelet count before treatment and twice weekly; neutrophil counts may be increased for 2 days after therapy

• B/P, respirations, pulse before and during therapy

• Bone pain, give mild analgesics

Administer:

• Using single-use vials; after dose is withdrawn, do not reenter vial

• For 2 wk or until ANC is 10,000/mm^3 after the expected chemotherapy neutrophil nadir

CONT IV INF route

• Dilute in D_5W to a conc of >15 mcg/ml, vial is for one-time use; give over 15-30 min (chemotherapy); over 4-24 hr (bone marrow transplantation); do not use 0.9% NaCl to dilute drug

Y-site compatibilities: Acyclovir, allopurinol, amikacin, aminophylline, ampicillin, ampicillin/sulbactam, aztreonam, bleomycin, bumetanide, buprenorphine, butorphanol, calcium gluconate, carboplatin, carmustine, cefazolin, cefotetan, ceftazidime, chlorproMAZINE, cimetidine, cisplatin, cyclophosphamide, cytarabine, dacarbazine, DAUNOrubicin, dexamethasone, diphenhydrAMINE, DOXOrubicin, doxycycline, droperidol, enalaprilat, famotidine, floxuridine, fluconazole, fludarabine, gallium, ganciclovir, granisetron, haloperidol, hydrocortisone, hydromorphone, hydrOXYzine, idarubicin, ifosfamide, leucovorin, lorazepam, mechlorethamine, melphalan, meperidine, mesna, methotrexate, metoclopramide, miconazole, minocycline, mitoxantrone, morphine, nalbuphine, netilmicin, ondansetron, plicamycin, potassium chloride, promethazine, ranitidine, sodium bicarbonate, streptozocin, ticarcillin, ticarcillin/clavulanate, tobramycin, trimethoprim-sulfamethoxazole, vancomycin, vinBLAStine, vinCRIStine, vinorelbine, zidovudine

Perform/provide:

• Storage in refrigerator; do not freeze; may store at room temperature up to 6 hr

• Avoid shaking

Evaluate:

• Therapeutic response: absence of infection

Teach patient/family:

• The technique for self-administration: dose, side effects, disposal of containers and needles; provide instruction sheet

F

finasteride (℞)

(fin-ass'te-ride)

Propecia, Proscar

Func. class.: Hormone, androgen inhibitor, hair stimulant

Chem. class.: 5-α-Reductase inhibitor

Action: Inhibits 5-α-reductase and reduction in DHT; DHT induces androgenic effects by binding to androgen receptors in the cell nuclei of the prostate gland, liver, skin; prevents development of BHP

Uses: Symptomatic benign prostatic hyperplasia (Proscar); male-pattern baldness (Propecia)

Dosage and routes:

BPH

• *Adult:* **PO** 5 mg qd × 6-12 mo

Male pattern baldness

• *Adult:* **PO** 1 mg qd

Available forms: Tabs 1, 5 mg

Side effects/adverse reactions:

GU: Impotence, decreased libido, decreased volume of ejaculate

Contraindications: Hypersensitivity, children, women who are pregnant or may become pregnant should not handle tabs, pregnancy (X)

Precautions: Large residual urinary volume, severely diminished urinary flow, hepatic function abnormalities

Do not confuse:
Proscar/Prosom
Proscar/Prozac

Pharmacokinetics: Bioavailability 63%, readily absorbed from GI tract, plasma protein binding 90%; metabolized in the liver; excreted in urine (metabolites) 39%, feces (57%); crosses blood-brain barrier; peak 1-2 hr, duration 24 hr

Interactions:
- ↓ finasteride effect: theophylline, adrenergic bronchodilators, anticholinergics

NURSING CONSIDERATIONS

Assess:
- Urinary patterns, residual urinary volume, severely diminished urinary flow
- PSA levels and digital rectal exam prior to initiating therapy and periodically thereafter
- Hepatic studies prior to treatment; extensively metabolized in liver

Administer:
- Without regard to meals
- For a minimum of 6 mo; not all patients will respond

Perform/provide:
- Storage <86° F (30° C); protect from light; keep container tightly closed

Evaluate:
- Therapeutic response: increased urinary flow, decreased postvoiding dribbling, frequency, nocturia or hair growth within 3-6 mo

Teach patient/family:
- Pregnant women or women who may become pregnant should not touch crushed tabs or come into contact with semen of a patient taking this drug; may adversely affect developing male fetus
- That volume of ejaculate may be decreased during treatment; impotence and decreased libido may also occur
- Propecia results may not occur for 3 mo
- Proscar results may not occur for 6-12 mo

RARELY USED

flavoxate (℞)

(fla-vox'ate)

Func. class.: Spasmolytic

Uses: Relief of nocturia, incontinence, suprapubic pain, dysuria, frequency associated with urologic conditions (symptomatic only)

Dosage and routes:
- *Adult and child >12 yr:* **PO** 100-200 mg tid-qid

Contraindications: Hypersensitivity, GI obstruction, GI hemorrhage, GU obstruction

flecainide (℞)

(flek-ay'nide)

Tambocor

Func. class.: Antidysrhythmic (Class IC)

Action: Decreases conduction in all parts of the heart, with greatest effect on His-Purkinje system, which stabilizes cardiac membrane

Uses: Life-threatening ventricular dysrhythmias, sustained ventricular tachycardia, supraventricular tachydysrhythmias, paroxysmal atrial fibrillation/flutter associated with disabling symptoms

Dosage and routes:
- *Adult:* **PO** 50-100 mg q12h; may

increase q4d by 50 mg q12h to desired response, not to exceed 400 mg/day

Renal disease

• CCr <35 ml/min dose 50%-75%

Available forms: Tabs 50, 100, 150 mg

Side effects/adverse reactions:

CNS: Headache, dizziness, involuntary movement, confusion, psychosis, restlessness, irritability, paresthesias, ataxia, flushing, somnolence, depression, anxiety, malaise, fatigue, asthenia, tremors

EENT: Tinnitus, *blurred vision,* hearing loss

GI: Nausea, vomiting, anorexia, constipation, abdominal pain, flatulence, change in taste

CV: Hypotension, bradycardia, angina, PVCs, ***heart block, cardiovascular collapse, arrest,*** dysrhythmias, ***CHF, fatal ventricular tachycardia***

RESP: Dyspnea, ***respiratory depression***

INTEG: Rash, urticaria, edema, swelling

HEMA: Leukopenia, thrombocytopenia

GU: Impotence, decreased libido, polyuria, urinary retention

Contraindications: Hypersensitivity, severe heart block, cardiogenic shock, nonsustained ventricular dysrhythmias, frequent PVCs, non–life-threatening dysrhythmias

Precautions: Pregnancy (C), lactation, children, renal disease, liver disease, CHF, respiratory depression, myasthenia gravis

Pharmacokinetics:

PO: Peak 3 hr; half-life 12-27 hr; metabolized by liver; excreted unchanged by kidneys (10%); excreted in breast milk

Interactions:

• ↑ CV depressant action: β-blockers, disopyramide, verapamil

• ↑ flecainide level: amiodarone, cimetidine

• ↑ digoxin level: digoxin

• ↑ or ↓ effect: alkalinizing agents, acidifying agents

↑ toxicity, death: aconite

↑ effect: aloe, broom, chronic buckthorn use, cascara sagrada (chronic use), Chinese rhubarb, figwort, fumitory, goldenseal, kudzu, licorice

↓ effect: coltsfoot

↑ serotonin effect: horehound

Lab test interferences:

Increase: CPK

NURSING CONSIDERATIONS

Assess:

• I&O, daily weight; CHF: edema, weight gain, dyspnea, jugular vein distention, rales, crackles

• For hypokalemia, hyperkalemia before administration; correct electrolytes

• Blood levels: trough (0.2-1 mcg/ml)

• B/P, ECG continuously for fluctuations, watch for QRS widening, prolongation of QT and PR

• CNS effects: dizziness, confusion, psychosis, paresthesias, convulsions; drug should be discontinued

• Increased respiration, increased pulse; drug should be discontinued

Administer:

• Reduced dosage as soon as dysrhythmia is controlled

• May give with meals for GI upset

Evaluate:

• Therapeutic response: decreased dysrhythmias

Teach patient/family:

• To change position slowly from lying or sitting to standing to minimize orthostatic hypotension

• To take as prescribed, not to skip or double dose

• To avoid hazardous activities that

require alertness until response is known

- To carry emergency ID with disorder, medications taken
- To notify all health care providers of treatment

Treatment of overdose: O_2, artificial ventilation, ECG, DOPamine for circulatory depression, diazepam or thiopental for convulsions, treat ventricular dysrhythmias

---

RARELY USED

floxuridine (℞)

(flox-yoor′i-deen)

Floxuridine, FUDR

Func. class.: Antineoplastic, antimetabolite

Uses: GI adenocarcinoma metastatic to liver; cancer of breast, head, neck, liver, brain, gallbladder, bile duct

Dosage and routes:

- *Adult:* **INTRAARTERIAL** by cont inf 0.1-0.6 mg/kg/day × 1-6 wk; **HEPATIC ARTERY INJ** 0.4-0.6 mg/kg/day × 1-6 wk

Contraindications: Hypersensitivity, myelosuppression, pregnancy (D), poor nutritional status, serious infections

fluconazole (℞)

(floo-kon′a-zole)

Diflucan

Func. class.: Antifungal

Action: Inhibits ergosterol biosynthesis, causes direct damage to membrane phospholipids

Uses: Oropharyngeal candidiasis in AIDS patients, chronic mucocutaneous candidiasis, urinary candidiasis, cryptococcal meningitis

Dosage and routes:

Renal disease

- CCr 11-50 ml/min dose 50%

Vaginal candidiasis

- *Adult:* **PO** 150 mg as a single dose

Serious fungal infections

- *Adult:* **PO/IV** 50-400 mg initially, then 200 mg qd for 4 wk
- *Child:* 6-12 mg/kg/day

Oropharyngeal candidiasis

- *Adult:* **PO/IV** 200 mg initially, then 100 mg qd for at least 2 wk
- *Child:* 3 mg/kg/day

Available forms: Tabs 50, 100, 150, 200 mg; inj 2 mg/ml; powder for oral susp 50, 200 mg/ml

Side effects/adverse reactions:

GI: Nausea, vomiting, diarrhea, cramping, flatus, increased AST, ALT, ***hepatotoxicity***

CNS: Headache

INTEG: ***Stevens-Johnson syndrome***

Contraindications: Hypersensitivity

Precautions: Renal disease, pregnancy (C), lactation

Do not confuse:

Diflucan/Diprivan

Pharmacokinetics: Peak 2-4 hr, bioavailability (PO) 90%, excreted unchanged in urine 80%

Interactions:

- ↑ anticoagulation: warfarin
- ↑ plasma concentrations: cycloSPORINE, phenytoin, theophylline, rifabutin, tacrolimus
- Hypoglycemia: oral antidiabetics
- ↑ effect of zidovudine
- ↑ nephrotoxicity: gossypol

NURSING CONSIDERATIONS

Assess:

- For infection: clearing of CSF culture during treatment, obtain C&S baseline and throughout, drug may be started as soon as culture is taken
- For hepatotoxicity: increasing AST, ALT, periodically alk phosphatase, bilirubin

Administer:

PO route

• Shake oral susp before each use

IV route

• After diluting according to package directions; run at 200 mg/hr or less; do not use plastic containers in connections; check for bag leaks

• Using an infusion pump check for extravasation and necrosis q2h

Additive compatibilities: Acyclovir, amikacin, amphotericin B, cefazolin, ceftazidime, clindamycin, gentamicin, heparin, meropenem, metronidazole, morphine, piperacillin, potassium chloride, theophylline

Y-site compatibilities: Acyclovir, aldesleukin, allopurinol, amifostine, amikacin, aminophylline, ampicillin/sulbactam, aztreonam, benztropine, cefazolin, cefepime, cefotetan, cefoxitin, chlorproMAZINE, cimetidine, cisatracurium, dexamethasone, diphenhydrAMINE, DOBUTamine, DOPamine, DOXOrubicin liposome, droperidol, famotidine, filgrastim, fludarabine, foscarnet, gallium, ganciclovir, gentamicin, granisetron, heparin, hydrocortisone, immune globulin, leucovorin, lorazepam, melphalan, meperidine, meropenem, metoclopramide, metronidazole, midazolam, morphine, nafcillin, nitroglycerin, ondansetron, oxacillin, paclitaxel, pancuronium, penicillin G potassium, phenytoin, piperacillin/tazobactam, prochlorperazine, promethazine, propofol, ranitidine, remifentanil, sargramostim, tacrolimus, teniposide, theophylline, thiotepa, ticarcillin/clavulanate, tobramycin, vancomycin, vecuronium, vinorelbine, zidovudine

Perform/provide:

• Storage protected from moisture and light, diluted sol is stable 24 hr

Evaluate:

• Therapeutic response: decreasing oral candidiasis, fever, malaise, rash; negative C&S for infection organism

Teach patient/family:

• That long-term therapy may be needed to clear infection

• That medication may be taken with food to reduce GI effects

• To notify prescriber of nausea, vomiting, diarrhea, jaundice, anorexia, clay-colored stools, dark urine

F

RAREY USED

fludarabine (℞)

(floo-dar′a-been)

Fludara

Func. class.: Antineoplastic, antimetabolite

Uses: Chronic lymphocytic leukemia, non-Hodgkin's lymphoma

Dosage and routes:

• *Adult:* **IV** 25 mg/m^2 over 30 min qd × 5 days, may repeat q28d; reconstitute with 2 ml of sterile water for inj; dissolution should occur in <15 sec

Contraindications: Hypersensitivity, pregnancy (D), lactation

fludrocortisone (℞)

(floo-droe-kor′ti-sone)

Florinef

Func. class.: Corticosteroid

Chem. class.: Mineralocorticoid

Action: Promotes increased reabsorption of sodium and loss of potassium, water, hydrogen from distal renal tubules

Uses: Adrenal insufficiency, salt-losing adrenogenital syndrome

Investigational uses: Renal tubular acidosis (type IV) idiopathic orthostatic hypotension

Dosage and routes:

- *Adult:* **PO** 0.1-0.2 mg qd
- *Child:* **PO** 0.05-0.1 mg/day

Available forms: Tabs 0.1 mg

Side effects/adverse reactions:

CNS: Flushing, sweating, headache, paralysis, dizziness

CV: Hypertension, ***circulatory collapse, thrombophlebitis, embolism,*** tachycardia, ***CHF,*** edema

MS: Fractures, osteoporosis, weakness

ENDO: Weight gain, adrenal suppression

MISC: Hypersensitivity

META: Hypokalemia

Contraindications: Hypersensitivity, acute glomerulonephritis, amebiasis, psychoses, Cushing's syndrome, fungal infections, child <2 yr

Precautions: Pregnancy (C), osteoporosis, CHF, lactation, child >2 yr, hypertension, diabetes

Pharmacokinetics:

PO: Half-life 3.5 hr, metabolized by liver, excreted in urine

Interactions:

- ↓ fludrocortisone action: barbiturates, rifampin, phenytoin
- ↓ potassium levels: thiazides, potassium-wasting drugs, loop diuretics, amphotericin B, piperacillin, mezlocillin
- ↑ B/P: sodium-containing food or medication

↑ Hypokalemia: aloe, buckthorn, cascara sagrada, Chinese rhubarb, senna

↑ corticosteroid effect: aloe, licorice, perilla

Lab test interferences:

Increase: Potassium, sodium

Decrease: Hct

NURSING CONSIDERATIONS

Assess:

- Weight daily; notify prescriber of weekly gain >5 lb; I&O ratio; be alert for decreasing urinary output, increasing edema
- B/P q4h, pulse; notify prescriber if chest pain occurs
- Potassium depletion: paresthesias, fatigue, nausea, vomiting, depression, polyuria, dysrhythmias, weakness
- Electrolytes: sodium, potassium, chloride, hypokalemia is common

Administer:

- Titrated dose; use lowest effective dose
- With food or milk to decrease GI symptoms

Perform/provide:

- Assistance with ambulation in patient with bone tissue disease to prevent fractures

Evaluate:

- Therapeutic response: correction of adrenal insufficiency

Teach patient/family:

- That emergency ID as steroid user should be carried
- Not to discontinue this medication abruptly
- To notify health care provider of muscle cramps, weight gain, edema, nausea, infection, trauma, stress
- Not to breastfeed while taking this medication

flumazenil (℞)

(flu-maz′e-nill)

Anexate✱, Romazicon

Func. class.: Antidote: Benzodiazepine receptor antagonist

Chem. class.: Imidazobenzodiazepine derivative

Action: Antagonizes actions of benzodiazepines on CNS, competitively inhibits activity at benzodiazepine recognition site on GABA/benzodiazepine receptor complex

Uses: Reversal of sedative effects of benzodiazepines

Dosage and routes:

Reversal of conscious sedation or in general anesthesia

• *Adult:* **IV** 0.2 mg given over 15 sec; wait 45 sec, then give 0.2 mg if consciousness does not occur; may be repeated at 60-sec intervals prn (max 3 mg/hr)

• *Child:* **IV** 10 mcg (0.01 mg)/kg; cumulative dose of 1 mg or less

Management of suspected benzodiazepine overdose

• *Adult:* **IV** 0.2 mg given over 30 sec; wait 30 sec, then give 0.3 mg over 30 sec if consciousness does not occur; further doses of 0.5 mg can be given over 30 sec at intervals of 1 min up to cumulative dose of 3 mg

• *Child:* **IV** 100 mcg (0.1 mg)/kg; cumulative dose of 1 mg or less

Available forms: Inj 0.1 mg/ml

Side effects/adverse reactions:

EENT: Abnormal vision, blurred vision, tinnitus

CV: Hypertension, palpitations, cutaneous vasodilation, ***dysrhythmias,*** bradycardia, tachycardia, chest pain

GI: Nausea, vomiting, hiccups

CNS: Dizziness, agitation, emotional lability, confusion, ***seizures,*** somnolence

SYST: Headache, injection site pain, increased sweating, fatigue, rigors

Contraindications: Hypersensitivity to this drug or benzodiazepines, serious cyclic antidepressant overdose, patients given benzodiazepine for control of life-threatening condition

Precautions: Pregnancy (C), lactation, children, elderly, renal disease, seizure disorders, head injury, labor/delivery, hepatic disease, hypoventilation, panic disorder, drug and alcohol dependency, ambulatory patients

Do not confuse:

Mazicon/Mivacron

Pharmacokinetics: Terminal half-life 41-79 min; metabolized in liver

Interactions:

• Toxicity: mixed drug overdosage

NURSING CONSIDERATIONS

Assess:

• Cardiac status using continuous monitoring

• For seizures; protect patient from injury; most likely those that have withdrawals from sedatives

• GI symptoms: nausea, vomiting; place in side-lying position to prevent aspiration

• Allergic reactions: flushing, rash, urticaria, pruritus

Administer:

• Check airway and IV access before administration

IV direct route

• Give undiluted or diluted with 0.9% NaCl, D_5W, LR, give over 15 sec into running IV

Additive compatibilities: Aminophylline, cimetidine, DOBUTamine, DOPamine, famotidine, heparin, lidocaine, procainamide, ranitidine

Solution compatibilities: D_5W

Evaluate:

• Therapeutic response: decreased sedation, respiratory depression, toxicity

Teach patient/family:

• That amnesia may continue

• Not to engage in hazardous activities for 18-24 hr after discharge

• Not to take any alcohol or nonprescription drugs for 18-24 hr

fluocinolone topical

See appendix c

fluoride (PO) (℞)

(floor'ide)

Fluor-A-Day🍁, Fluoride Loz, Fluoritab, Flura-Loz, Karidium, Luride, Pediaflor, Pharmaflur, Phos-Flur, Solu-Flur🍁

fluoride (top) (℞)

ACT, Fluorigard, Fluorinse, Gel Kam, Gel-Tin, Karigel, MouthKote, Stop, Thera-Flur

Func. class.: Trace elements

Chem. class.: Fluoride ion

Action: Needed for hard tooth enamel and for resistance to periodontal disease; reduces acid production by dental bacteria

Uses: Prevention of dental caries, osteoporosis

Dosage and routes:

Prevention of dental caries

- *Adult and child >12 yr:* **Top** 10 ml 0.2% sol qd after brushing teeth, rinse mouth for >1 min with sol
- *Child 6-12 yr:* **Top** 5 ml 0.2% sol
- *Child >3 yr:* **PO** 1 mg qd
- *Child <3 yr:* **PO** 0.5 mg qd

Mild-moderate osteoporosis

- *Adult:* **PO** slow rel fluoride 25 mg, given as calcium citrate 400 mg bid

Available forms: Tabs chewable 0.5, 1 mg; tabs 1 mg, tabs effervescent 10 mg; drops 0.125, 0.25, 0.5 mg/drop; rinse supplements 0.2 mg/ml, rinse 0.01%, 0.02%, 0.04%, 0.09%; gel 0.1%, 0.5%; lozenges 1 mg; sol 0.2 mg/ml; honey-wax, slow rel sodium fluoride tab

Side effects/adverse reactions:

ACUTE OVERDOSE: ***Black tarry stools, bloody vomit, diarrhea, decreased respiration, increased salivation, watery eyes***

CHRONIC OVERDOSE: ***Hypocalcemia and tetany, respiratory arrest, sores in mouth, constipation, loss of appetite, nausea, vomiting, weight loss, discoloration of teeth*** (white, black, brown)

Contraindications: Hypersensitivity, pregnancy (NR)

Precautions: Child <6 yr

Pharmacokinetics:

PO: Excreted in urine and feces; crosses placenta, breast milk

Interactions:

- Drug/food: avoid use with dairy products

NURSING CONSIDERATIONS

Assess:

- For mottling of teeth, during treatment

Administer:

- Drops after meals with fluids or undiluted tabs; may be chewed; do not swallow whole; may be given with water or juice; avoid milk

Evaluate:

- Therapeutic response: absence of dental caries

Teach patient/family:

- To monitor children using gel or rinse; not to be swallowed
- Not to drink, eat, or rinse mouth for at least ½ hr
- Not to use during pregnancy
- To apply after brushing and flossing hs
- To store out of children's reach

fluorometholone ophthalmic

See appendix c

HIGH ALERT

fluorouracil (℞)

(flure-oh-yoor′a-sil)

Adrucil, Efudex, 5-FU

Func. class.: Antineoplastic, antimetabolite

Chem. class.: Pyrimidine antagonist

Action: Inhibits DNA, RNA synthesis; interferes with cell replication by competitively inhibiting thymidylate synthesis, S phase of cell cycle–specific, a vesicant

Uses:
Systemic: Cancer of breast, colon, rectum, stomach, pancreas; Topical: Multiple actinic keratoses, superficial basal cell carcinomas

Dosage and routes:
• *Adult:* **IV** 12 mg/kg/day × 4 days, not to exceed 800 mg/day; may repeat with 6 mg/kg on day 6, 8, 10, 12; maintenance is 10-15 mg/kg/wk as a single dose, not to exceed 1 g/wk

Actinic/solar keratoses
• *Adult:* **Top** 1% cream/sol 1-2 ×/day

Superficial basal cell carcinoma
• *Adult:* **Top** 5% sol 2 ×/day × 3-12 wk

Available forms: Inj 50 mg/ml; cream 1%, 5%; sol 1%, 2%, 5%

Side effects/adverse reactions:

Systemic use

CV: Myocardial ischemia, angina

HEMA: ***Thrombocytopenia, leukopenia, myelosuppression, anemia, agranulocytosis***

GI: Anorexia, stomatitis, diarrhea, nausea, vomiting, ***hemorrhage,*** enteritis glossitis

EENT: Epistaxis

INTEG: Rash, fever, photosensitivity

CNS: Lethargy, malaise, weakness, acute cerebellar dysfunction

Contraindications: Hypersensitivity, myelosuppression, pregnancy (D), poor nutritional status, serious infections, major surgery within 1 month

Precautions: Renal disease, hepatic disease, bone marrow depression, angina, lactation, children

Do not confuse:
fluorouracil/flucytosine

Pharmacokinetics: Half-life 20 hr terminal; metabolized in the liver; excreted in the urine; crosses blood-brain barrier

Interactions:
• ↑ toxicity, bone marrow depression: radiation or other antineoplastics
• ↓ antibody response: live virus vaccines

Lab test interferences:
Increase: LFTs, 6-HIAA
Decrease: Albumin

NURSING CONSIDERATIONS

Assess:
• CBC, differential, platelet count qd (IV); withhold drug if WBC is <3500/mm^3 or platelet count is <100,000/mm^3; notify prescriber of these results; drug should be discontinued; nadir of leukopenia within 2 wk, recovery 1 mo
• Renal studies: BUN, serum uric acid, urine CCr, electrolytes before, during therapy
• Temp q4h; fever may indicate beginning infection
• Hepatic studies before, during therapy: bilirubin, alk phosphatase, AST, ALT, LDH; before and during therapy
• Bleeding: hematuria, guaiac, bruising or petechiae, mucosa or orifices q8h
• Inflammation of mucosa, breaks in skin; buccal cavity q8h for dry-

F

ness, sores or ulceration, white patches, oral pain, bleeding, dysphagia
• GI symptoms: frequency of stools, cramping, intractable vomiting, stomatitis

Administer:
• Antiemetic 30-60 min before giving drug to prevent vomiting and for several days thereafter

IV route
• Prepared in biologic cabinet using gloves, gown, mask
• Undiluted; may inject through Y-tube or 3-way stopcock; give over 1-3 min; may be diluted in NS, D_5W, given over 2-8 hr as IV INF

Additive compatibilities: Bleomycin, cephalothin, cyclophosphamide, etoposide, floxuridine, hydromorphone, ifosfamide, methotrexate, mitoxantrone, prednisoLONE, vinCRIStine

Solution compatibilities: Amino acids 4.25%/D_{25}, D_5/LR, $D_{3.3}$/0.3 NaCl, D_5W, 0.9% NaCl, TPN #23

Syringe compatibilities: Bleomycin, cisplatin, cyclophosphamide, furosemide, heparin, leucovorin, methotrexate, metoclopramide, mitomycin, vinBLAStine, vinCRIStine

Y-site compatibilities: Allopurinol, amifostine, aztreonam, bleomycin, cefepime, cisplatin, cyclophosphamide, DOXOrubicin, DOXOrubicin liposome, fludarabine, furosemide, granisetron, heparin, hydrocortisone, leucovorin, mannitol, melphalan, methotrexate, metoclopramide, mitomycin, paclitaxel, piperacillin/tazobactam, potassium chloride, propofol, sargramostim, teniposide, thiotepa, vinBLAStine, vinCRIStine, vit B/C

Topical
• Wear gloves when applying; may use with a loose dressing; use a plastic or wooden applicator

Perform/provide:
• Strict asepsis, protective isolation if WBC levels are low
• Changing of IV site q48h
• Rinsing of mouth tid-qid with water, club soda; brushing of teeth bid-tid with soft brush or cotton-tipped applicator for stomatitis; use unwaxed dental floss
• Nutritious diet with iron, vitamin supplements, low fiber, few dairy products, especially when combined with radiotherapy as ordered

Evaluate:
• Therapeutic response: decreased tumor size, spread of malignancy

Teach patient/family:
• To avoid crowds, persons with known infections
• To avoid foods with citric acid, hot or rough texture if stomatitis is present; to drink adequate fluids
• To report stomatitis: any bleeding, white spots, ulcerations in mouth; tell patient to examine mouth qd, report symptoms; viscous lidocaine may be used
• To report signs of infection: fever, sore throat, flulike symptoms
• To report signs of anemia: fatigue, headache, faintness, shortness of breath, irritability
• To report bleeding: avoid use of razors, commercial mouthwash
• To avoid use of aspirin products, or NSAIDs
• To use contraception during therapy (men and women)
• Not to receive vaccinations during therapy
• To use sunscreen or stay out of the sun to prevent photosensitivity
• About hair loss, explore use of wigs or other products until hair regrowth occurs

fluoxetine (℞)

(floo-ox′eh-teen)

Prozac, Prozac Weekly, Sarafem

Func. class.: Antidepressant, SSRI (selective serotonin reuptake inhibitor)

Action: Inhibits CNS neuron uptake of serotonin but not of norepinephrine

Uses: Major depressive disorder, obsessive-compulsive disorder (OCD), bulimia nervosa; Sarafem: premenstrual dysphoric disorder (PMDD)

Investigational uses: Alcoholism, anorexia nervosa, ADHD, bipolar II affective disorder, borderline personality disorder, cataplexy, narcolepsy, kleptomania, migraine, obesity, posttraumatic stress disorder, schizophrenia, Tourette's syndrome, trichotillomania, levodopa-induced dyskinesia, social phobia, premenstrual dysphoric disorder

Dosage and routes:

ADHD (unlabeled)

• *Adult:* **PO** 20-60 mg/day

Alcoholism (unlabeled)

• *Adult:* **PO** 20-80 mg/day

Anorexia nervosa (unlabeled)

• *Adult:* **PO** 10 mg qod-20 mg/day

Bipolar II affective disorder (unlabeled)

• *Adult:* **PO** 10 mg qod-20 mg/day

Borderline personality disorder (unlabeled)

• *Adult:* **PO** 20 mg/day

Bulimia nervosa

• *Adult:* **PO** 60 mg/day in AM

Depression/obsessive-compulsive disorder

• *Adult:* **PO** 20 mg qd in AM; after 4 wk if no clinical improvement is noted, dose may be increased to 20 mg bid in AM, PM, not to exceed 80 mg/day; **PO** weekly

• *Geriatric:* **PO** 5-10 mg/day, increase as needed

• *Child 5-18 yr:* **PO** 5-10 mg/day, max 20 mg/day

Kleptomania (unlabeled)

• *Adult:* **PO** 60-80 mg/day

Migraine, chronic daily headaches (unlabeled)

• *Adult:* **PO** 10-80 mg/day

Narcolepsy (unlabeled)

• *Adult:* **PO** 20-40 mg/day

Posttraumatic stress disorder (unlabeled)

• *Adult:* **PO** 10-80 mg/day

Premenstrual dysphoric disorder (Sarafem)

• *Adult:* **PO** 20 mg qd, may be taken qd week before menses

Schizophrenia (unlabeled)

• *Adult:* **PO** 20-60 mg/day

Available forms: Caps 10, 20, 40 mg; tabs 10, 20 mg; oral sol 20 mg/5 ml; caps, del rel 90 mg

Side effects/adverse reactions:

CNS: Headache, nervousness, insomnia, drowsiness, anxiety, tremor, dizziness, fatigue, sedation, poor concentration, abnormal dreams, agitation, ***seizures,*** apathy, euphoria, hallucinations, delusions, psychosis

GI: Nausea, diarrhea, dry mouth, anorexia, dyspepsia, constipation, cramps, vomiting, taste changes, flatulence, decreased appetite

INTEG: Sweating, rash, pruritus, acne, alopecia, urticaria

RESP: Infection, pharyngitis, nasal congestion, sinus headache, sinusitis, cough, dyspnea, bronchitis, asthma, hyperventilation, pneumonia

CV: Hot flashes, palpitations, angina pectoris, ***hemorrhage,*** hypertension, ***tachycardia,*** first-degree AV block, ***bradycardia, MI, thrombophlebitis***

MS: Pain, arthritis, twitching
GU: Dysmenorrhea, decreased libido, urinary frequency, UTI, amenorrhea, cystitis, impotence, urine retention
EENT: Visual changes, ear/eye pain, photophobia, tinnitus
SYST: Asthenia, viral infection, fever, allergy, chills

Contraindications: Hypersensitivity

Precautions: Pregnancy (B), lactation, children, elderly, diabetes mellitus

Do not confuse:
Prozac/Proscar/Prosom
Sarafem/Serophene
Prozac/Prilosec

Pharmacokinetics:
PO: Peak 6-8 hr; metabolized in liver; excreted in urine; terminal half-life 2-3 days; steady state 28-35 days, protein binding 94%

Interactions:
Do not use MAOIs with or 14 days prior to fluoxetine
• Do not use with thioridazine, or within 5 wk of discontinuing fluoxetine
• ↑ side effects: highly protein-bound drugs
• ↑ effect: haloperidol
• ↓ fluoxetine effect: cyproheptadine
• ↑ half-life of: diazepam
• ↑ levels or toxicity of: carbamazepine, lithium, digoxin, warfarin, phenytoin
• ↑ levels of: tricyclics, phenothiazines
• Paradoxical worsening of OCD: busPIRone
• ↑ CNS depression: alcohol, antidepressants, opioids, sedatives
↑ anticholinergic effect: corkwood, jimsonweed
↑ CNS effect: hops, kava, lavender
Do not use together; ↑ risk of serotonin syndrome: St. John's wort, SAM-e

Lab test interferences:
Increase: Serum bilirubin, blood glucose, alk phosphatase
Decrease: VMA, 5-HIAA
False increase: Urinary catecholamines

NURSING CONSIDERATIONS

Assess:
• Mental status: mood, sensorium, affect, suicidal tendencies, increase in psychiatric symptoms, depression, panic
• Appetite in bulemia nervosa, weight qd, increase nutritious foods in diet, watch for binging and vomiting
• Allergic reactions: itching, rash urticaria, drug should be discontinued, may need to give antihistamine
• B/P (lying/standing), pulse q4h; if systolic B/P drops 20 mm Hg, hold drug, notify prescriber; take vital signs q4h in patients with cardiovascular disease
• Blood studies: CBC, leukocytes, differential, cardiac enzymes if patient is receiving long-term therapy; check platelets; bleeding can occur
• Hepatic studies: AST, ALT, bilirubin, creatinine
• Weight qwk; appetite may decrease with drug
• ECG for flattening of T wave, bundle branch, AV block, dysrhythmias in cardiac patients
• Alcohol consumption; if alcohol is consumed, hold dose until AM

Administer:
• With food or milk for GI symptoms
• Crushed if patient is unable to swallow medication whole (tab only)
• Dosage hs if oversedation occurs during the day; may take entire dose hs; elderly may not tolerate once/day dosing

• Gum, hard candy, frequent sips of water for dry mouth
• Prozac weekly on the same day each week

Perform/provide:
• Storage at room temperature; do not freeze
• Assistance with ambulation during therapy, since drowsiness, dizziness occur
• Safety measures primarily in elderly
• Checking to see if PO medication swallowed

Evaluate:
• Therapeutic response: decreased depression, symptoms of OCD

Teach patient/family:
• That therapeutic effect may take 1-4 wk
• To use caution in driving, other activities requiring alertness because of drowsiness, dizziness, blurred vision
• To use sunscreen to prevent photosensitivity
• To avoid alcohol ingestion, other CNS depressants
• To notify prescriber if pregnant or plan to become pregnant or breastfeed
• To change positions slowly, orthostatic hypotension may occur
• To avoid all OTC drugs unless approved by prescriber

fluphenazine decanoate (℞)

(floo-fen'a-zeen)
Modecate✤, Modecate Concentrate✤, Prolixin Decanoate

fluphenazine enanthate (℞)

Moditen Enanthate✤, Prolixin Enanthate

fluphenazine hydrochloride (℞)

Apo-Fluphenazine✤, Moditen HCL✤, Moditen HCl-H.P.✤, Permitil✤, Prolixin
Func. class.: Antipsychotic
Chem. class.: Phenothiazine, piperazine

Action: Depresses cerebral cortex, hypothalamus, limbic system, which control activity and aggression; blocks neurotransmission produced by dopamine at synapse; exhibits strong α-adrenergic and anticholinergic blocking action; mechanism for antipsychotic effects is unclear

Uses: Psychotic disorders, schizophrenia

Dosage and routes:

decanoate
• *Adult and child >16 yr:* **SC/IM** 12.5-25 mg q1-3wk, may increase slowly
• *Child 12-16 yr:* **IM/SC** 6.25-18.75 mg, then repeat q1-3wk, then increase slowly, max 25 mg
• *Child 5-12 yr:* **IM/SC** 3.125-12.5 mg, then repeat q1-3wk, increase slowly

HCl
• *Adult:* **PO** 2.5-10 mg, in divided doses q6-8h, not to exceed 20 mg qd; **IM** initially 1.25 mg then 2.5-10 mg in divided doses q6-8h

• *Child:* **PO** 0.25-3.5 mg qd in divided doses q4-6h, max 10 mg/qd
enanthate
• *Adult:* **IM/SC** 25 mg q1-3wk, may increase slowly, max 100 mg/dose
Available forms: HCl tabs 1, 2.5, 5, 10 mg; elix 2.5 mg/5 ml; conc 5 mg/ml; inj 2.5, 10 mg/ml; enanthate, decanoate inj 25 mg/ml

Side effects/adverse reactions:
RESP: ***Laryngospasm,*** dyspnea, ***respiratory depression***
CNS: EPS: pseudoparkinsonism, akathisia, dystonia, tardive dyskinesia, drowsiness, headache, ***seizures, neuroleptic malignant syndrome***
HEMA: Anemia, ***leukopenia, leukocytosis, agranulocytosis, aplastic anemia, thrombocytopenia***
INTEG: Rash, photosensitivity, dermatitis
EENT: Blurred vision, glaucoma, dry eyes
GI: Dry mouth, nausea, vomiting, anorexia, constipation, diarrhea, jaundice, weight gain, ***paralytic ileus, hepatitis***
GU: Urinary retention, urinary frequency, enuresis, impotence, amenorrhea, gynecomastia
CV: Orthostatic hypotension, hypertension, ***cardiac arrest,*** ECG changes, ***tachycardia***

Contraindications: Hypersensitivity, circulatory collapse, liver damage, cerebral arteriosclerosis, coronary disease, severe hypertension/hypotension, blood dyscrasias, coma, brain damage, narrow-angle glaucoma, bone marrow depression, alcohol and barbiturate withdrawal

Precautions: Pregnancy (C), lactation, seizure disorders, hypertension, hepatic disease, cardiac disease, elderly, child <12 yr

Do not confuse:
Prolixin/Proloid

Pharmacokinetics:
PO/IM (HCl): Onset 1 hr, peak 2-4 hr, duration 6-8 hr
SC (enanthate): Onset 1-2 days, peak 2-3 days, duration 1-3 wk, half-life 3.5-4 days; decanoate: onset 1-3 days, peak 1-2 days, duration over 4 wk, single-dose half-life 6.8-9.6 days; multiple dose, 14.3 days; metabolized by liver; excreted in urine (metabolites); crosses placenta; enters breast milk

Interactions:
• Oversedation: other CNS depressants, alcohol, barbiturate anesthetics
• Toxicity: epINEPHrine
• ↓ effects of levodopa, lithium
• ↓ fluphenazine effects: smoking, barbiturates
• ↑ anticholinergic effects: anticholinergics
↑ EPS: betel palm, kava
↑ anticholinergic effect: henbane leaf
↑ action: cola tree, hops, kava, nettle, nutmeg

Lab test interferences:
Increase: LFTs, cardiac enzymes, cholesterol, blood glucose, prolactin, bilirubin, PBI, cholinesterase
Decrease: Hormones (blood and urine)
False positive: Pregnancy tests, PKU urinary steroids, 17-OHCS

NURSING CONSIDERATIONS
Assess:
• Swallowing of PO medication; check for hoarding, giving of medication to other patients
• I&O ratio; palpate bladder if low urinary output occurs, urinary retention may be the cause
• Bilirubin, CBC, LFTs monthly
• Urinalysis is recommended before and during prolonged therapy
• Affect, orientation, LOC, reflexes, gait, coordination, sleep pattern disturbances

• B/P standing and lying; take pulse and respirations q4h during initial treatment; establish baseline before starting treatment; report drops of 30 mm Hg
• Dizziness, faintness, palpitations, tachycardia on rising
• EPS including akathisia (inability to sit still, no pattern to movements), tardive dyskinesia (bizarre movements of jaw, mouth, tongue, extremities), pseudoparkinsonism (rigidity, tremors, pill rolling, shuffling gait)
• Skin turgor qd
• Constipation, urinary retention qd; if these occur, increase bulk, H_2O in diet

Administer:
• Concentrate with juice, milk, or uncaffeinated drinks
• Antiparkinsonian agent if EPS occur
• IM inj into large muscle mass; to minimize postural hypotension, give inj and have patient remain seated or recumbent for ½ hr
• Use dry needle, or solution will become cloudy; use 21G or larger due to viscosity

Syringe compatibilities: Benztropine, diphenhydrAMINE, hydrOXYzine

Perform/provide:
• Decreased sensory input by dimming lights, avoiding loud noises
• Supervised ambulation until stabilized on medication; do not involve in strenuous exercise; fainting is possible; patient should not stand still for long periods
• Increased fluids to prevent constipation
• Sips of water, candy, gum for dry mouth
• Storage in tight, light-resistant container in cool environment

Evaluate:
• Therapeutic response: decrease in emotional excitement, hallucinations, delusions, paranoia, reorganization of patterns of thought, speech

Teach patient/family:
• That orthostatic hypotension occurs often; to rise from sitting or lying position gradually; avoid hazardous activities until stabilized on medication
• To avoid hot tubs, hot showers, tub baths, since hypotension may occur; that in hot weather, heat stroke may occur; take extra precautions to stay cool
◆ To avoid abrupt withdrawal of this drug, or EPS may result; drug should be withdrawn slowly
• To avoid OTC preparations (cough, hay fever, cold) unless approved by prescriber; serious drug interactions may occur; avoid use with alcohol, CNS depressants; increased drowsiness may occur
• To use a sunscreen to prevent burns
• About importance of compliance with drug regimen
• About EPS and necessity for meticulous oral hygiene, since oral candidiasis may occur
• To report sore throat, malaise, fever, bleeding, mouth sores; if these occur, CBC should be drawn and drug discontinued
• That urine may turn pink to reddish-brown

Treatment of overdose: Lavage; if orally ingested, provide an airway; *do not induce vomiting*

flurandrenolide topical

See appendix c

flurazepam (℞)

(flure-az′e-pam)

Apo-Flurazepam✦, Dalmane, flurazepam, Novoflupam✦, Somnol✦

Func. class.: Sedative/hypnotic

Chem. class.: Benzodiazepine derivative

Controlled Substance Schedule IV (USA), Schedule F (Canada)

Action: Produces CNS depression at the limbic, thalamic, hypothalamic levels of CNS; may be mediated by neurotransmitter γ-aminobutyric acid (GABA); results are sedation, hypnosis, skeletal muscle relaxation, anticonvulsant activity, anxiolytic action

Uses: Insomnia

Dosage and routes:

• *Adult:* **PO** 15-30 mg hs; may repeat dose once if needed

• *Elderly:* **PO** 15 mg hs; may increase if needed

Available forms: Caps 15, 30 mg

Side effects/adverse reactions:

HEMA: ***Leukopenia, granulocytopenia*** (rare)

CNS: Lethargy, drowsiness, daytime sedation, dizziness, confusion, lightheadedness, headache, anxiety, irritability

GI: Nausea, vomiting, diarrhea, heartburn, abdominal pain, constipation

CV: Chest pain, pulse changes, palpitations

MISC: Physical, psychological dependence

Contraindications: Hypersensitivity to benzodiazepines, lactation, intermittent porphyria, uncontrolled pain, pregnancy (UK)

Precautions: Anemia, hepatic disease, renal disease, suicidal individuals, drug abuse, elderly, psychosis, child <15 yr

Do not confuse:

flurazepam/temazepam

Pharmacokinetics:

PO: Onset 15-45 min, duration 7-8 hr; metabolized by liver; excreted by kidneys (inactive/active metabolites); crosses placenta; excreted in breast milk; half-life 47-100 hr

Interactions:

• ↑ flurazepam effects: cimetidine, disulfiram, probenicid, isoniazid, oral contraceptives, fluoxetine, ketoconazole, propranolol, valproic acid

• ↑ CNS depression: alcohol, CNS depressants

• ↓ flurazepam effect: rifampin, barbiturates, theophylline

↑ sedative effect: catnip, chamomile, clary, cowslip, kava, lavender, mistletoe, nettle, pokeweed, poppy, Queen Anne's lace, senega, valerian

↑ hypotension: black cohosh

Lab test interferences:

Increase: AST, ALT, serum bilirubin

False increase: Urinary 17-OHCS

Decrease: RAI uptake

NURSING CONSIDERATIONS

Assess:

• Blood studies: Hct, Hgb, RBC (if on long-term therapy)

• Hepatic studies: AST, ALT, bilirubin

• Mental status: mood, sensorium, affect, memory (long, short), physical, psychological dependence or tolerance

• Type of sleep problem: falling asleep, staying asleep

Administer:

• After removal of cigarettes to prevent fires

• After trying conservative measures for insomnia
• ½-1 hr before hs for sleeplessness
• Caps may be opened and mixed with food

Perform/provide:
• Assistance with ambulation after receiving dose
• Safety measures: night-light, call bell within easy reach
• Checking to see if PO medication has been swallowed
• Storage in tight container in cool environment

Evaluate:
• Therapeutic response: ability to sleep at night, decreased amount of early morning awakening if taking drug for insomnia

Teach patient/family:
• To avoid driving or other activities requiring alertness until drug is stabilized
• To avoid alcohol ingestion or CNS depressants; serious CNS depression may result
• That effects may take 2 nights for benefits to be noticed
• Alternative measures to improve sleep: reading, exercise several hr before hs, warm bath, warm milk, TV, self-hypnosis, deep breathing
• That hangover is common in elderly

Treatment of overdose: Lavage, activated charcoal; monitor electrolytes, vital signs

flurbiprofen ophthalmic
See appendix c

flutamide (℞)
(floo′-ta-mide)
Eulexin
Func. class.: Antineoplastic, hormone
Chem. class.: Antiandrogen

Action: Interferes with testosterone uptake in the nucleus or testosterone activity in target tissues; arrests tumor growth in androgen-sensitive tissue (i.e., prostate gland)

Uses: Metastatic prostatic carcinoma, stage D_2 in combination with LHRH agonistic analogs (leuprolide)

Dosage and routes:
• *Adult:* **PO** 250 mg q8h tid, for a daily dosage of 750 mg

Stage B_2-C prostatic carcinoma
• *Adult:* Start 8 wk prior to radiation therapy and continue during radiation therapy; give with goserelin

Stage D_2 metastatic carcinoma
• *Adult:* Give with LHRH agonist and continue until progression

Available forms: Caps 125 mg

Side effects/adverse reactions:
CNS: Hot flashes, drowsiness, confusion, depression, anxiety, paresthesia
GU: Decreased libido, impotence, gynecomastia
GI: Diarrhea, nausea, vomiting, increased levels in hepatic studies, ***hepatitis,*** anorexia
HEMA: ***Leukopenia, thrombocytopenia, hemolytic anemia***
INTEG: Irritation at site, rash, photosensitivity
MISC: Edema, neuromuscular and pulmonary symptoms, hypertension

Contraindications: Hypersensitivity, pregnancy (D)

Pharmacokinetics: Rapidly and completely absorbed; excreted in urine and feces as metabolites; half-life 6 hr, geriatric half-life 8 hr; 94% bound to plasma proteins

NURSING CONSIDERATIONS

Assess:

- Hepatic studies: AST, ALT, alk phosphatase, which may be elevated; if LFTs are elevated, drug may need to be discontinued; monitor CBC, bilirubin, creatinine
- For CNS symptoms including: drowsiness, confusion, depression, anxiety

Evaluate:

- Therapeutic response: decrease in prostatic tumor size, decrease in spread of cancer

Teach patient/family:

- Not to break, crush, or chew caps
- That flutamide must be taken with leuprolide, do not change dosing
- To report side effects: decreased libido, impotence, breast enlargement, hot flashes, diarrhea
- To report nausea, vomiting, yellow eyes or skin, dark urine, clay-colored stools, hepatotoxicity may be the cause

fluticasone topical

See appendix c

fluvastatin (℞)

(flu′vah-stay-tin)

Lescol

Func. class.: Antilipidemic

Chem. class.: HMG-CoA reductase inhibitor

Action: Inhibits HMG-CoA reductase enzyme, which reduces cholesterol synthesis

Uses: As an adjunct in primary hypercholesterolemia (types Ia, Ib), coronary atherosclerosis in CAD

Dosage and routes:

- *Adult:* **PO** 20-40 mg qd in PM initially, usual range 20-80 mg, not to exceed 80 mg; may be given in 2 doses (40 mg AM, 40 mg PM); dosage adjustments may be made in 4 wk intervals or more

Available forms: Caps 20, 40 mg; 80 mg ext rel tab

Side effects/adverse reactions:

INTEG: Rash, pruritus

GI: Abdominal pain, cramps, nausea, constipation, diarrhea, dyspepsia, flatus, ***liver dysfunction,*** pancreatitis

EENT: Lens opacities

MS: Myalgia, ***myositis, rhabdomyolysis,*** *arthritis, arthralgia*

CNS: Headache, dizziness, insomnia

MISC: Fatigue, influenza, photosensitivity

HEMA: ***Thrombocytopenia, hemolytic anemia, leukopenia***

RESP: Upper respiratory infection, rhinitis, cough, pharyngitis, sinusitis

Contraindications: Hypersensitivity, pregnancy (X), lactation, active liver disease

Precautions: Past hepatic disease, alcoholism, severe acute infections, trauma, hypotension, uncontrolled seizure disorders, severe metabolic disorders, electrolyte imbalance

Pharmacokinetics: Metabolized in liver, highly protein bound, excreted primarily in feces, half-life <1 hr

Interactions:

- ↓ fluvastatin effect: rifampin
- ↑ effects of warfarin, digoxin
- ↑ myalgia, myositis: cycloSPORINE, gemfibrozil, niacin, erythromycin, clofibrate; azole antiinfectives
- ↑ effects of fluvastatin: alcohol, cimetidine, ranitidine, omeprazole, saquinavir

• Drug/food: Grapefruit juice: possible ↑ toxicity

↑ effect: glucomannan

↓ effect: gotu kola

NURSING CONSIDERATIONS

Assess:

• Fasting lipid profile (cholesterol, LDL, HDL, TG) q8wk, then q3-6 mo when stable

• Hepatic studies q1-2mo during the first 1½ yr of treatment; AST, ALT, LFTs may be increased

• Renal studies in patients with compromised renal system: BUN, I&O ratio, creatinine

• Ophthalmic exam before, 1 mo after treatment begins, annually; lens opacities may occur

Perform/provide:

• Storage in cool environment in tight container protected from light

Evaluate:

• Therapeutic response: decrease in LDL, VLDL, total cholesterol; increased HDL, decreased triglycerides

Teach patient/family:

• That blood work will be necessary during treatment, to take as prescribed

• To report severe GI symptoms, headache, muscle pain, weakness, tenderness

• That previously prescribed regimen will continue: low-cholesterol diet, exercise program, smoking cessation

Not to break, crush, or chew caps

• To report suspected pregnancy, not to use during pregnancy

• To use sunscreen or stay out of sun to prevent photosensitivity

• To notify all health care providers of drugs taken

fluvoxamine (℞)

(flu-vox'a-meen)

Luvox

Func. class.: Antidepressant SSRI (selective serotonin reuptake inhibitor)

Action: Inhibits CNS neuron uptake of serotonin but not of norepinephrine

Uses: Obsessive-compulsive disorder

Investigational uses: Depression

Dosage and routes:

• *Adult:* **PO** 50 mg hs, increase by 50 mg at 4-7 day intervals, max 300 mg, doses over 100 mg should be divided

• *Child 8-17 yr:* **PO** 25 mg hs, increase by 25 mg/day q4-7 days, max 200 mg/day, doses over 50 mg should be divided

Available forms: Tabs 25, 50, 100 mg

Side effects/adverse reactions:

CNS: Headache, drowsiness, dizziness, convulsions, sleep disorders, insomnia

*GI: Nausea, anorexia, constipation, **hepatotoxicity,** vomiting, diarrhea,* dry mouth

INTEG: Rash, sweating

GU: Decreased libido

Contraindications: Hypersensitivity

Precautions: Pregnancy (C), lactation, children, elderly

Do not confuse:

Luvox/Levoxyl

Pharmacokinetics: Crosses blood-brain barrier, 77% protein binding, metabolism by the liver, terminal half-life 16.9 hr, peak 2-8 hr

Interactions:

• ↓ metabolism, ↑ action of: propranolol, diazepam, lithium, theophylline, carbamazepine, warfarin

• ↑ CNS depression: alcohol, barbiturates, benzodiazepines
• ↑ fluvoxamine, toxicity levels: tricyclics, clozapine
Fatal reaction: MAO inhibitors
• Drug/smoking: ↑ metabolism, ↓ effects
↑ effect, possible fatal reaction: St. John's wort
↑ anticholinergic effect: corkwood, jimsonweed
↑ CNS effect: hops, kava, lavender

NURSING CONSIDERATIONS

Assess:
• Hepatic studies: AST, ALT, bilirubin
• Mental status: mood, sensorium, affect, suicidal tendencies; increase in psychiatric symptoms: depression, panic, obsessive-compulsive symptoms
• Constipation; most likely in elderly
For toxicity: nausea, vomiting, diarrhea, syncope, increased pulse, seizures

Administer:
• With food, milk for GI symptoms

Perform/provide:
• Storage at room temperature; do not freeze

Evaluate:
• Therapeutic response: decrease in depression

Teach patient/family:
• That therapeutic effects may take 2-3 wk
• To use caution in driving, other activities requiring alertness because of drowsiness, dizziness that may occur
• Not to use other CNS depressants, alcohol, barbiturates, benzodiazepines, St. John's wort, kava
• To notify prescriber if pregnancy is suspected or planned
• To notify prescriber of allergic reaction
• To increase bulk in diet if constipation occurs, especially elderly

folic acid (vit B_9) (OTC)

(foe'lik a'sid)
Apo-Folic♣, Folate, Folvite, Novofolacid♣, Vitamin B_9
Func. class.: Vit B complex group

Action: Needed for erythropoiesis; increases RBC, WBC, platelet formation in megaloblastic anemias

Uses: Megaloblastic or macrocytic anemia caused by folic acid deficiency; hepatic disease, alcoholism, hemolysis, intestinal obstruction, pregnancy

Dosage and routes:

Therapeutic dose
• *Adult and child:* **PO/IM/SC/IV** up to 1 mg qd

Maintenance dose
• *Adult and child >4 yr:* **PO/IM/IV/SC** 0.4 mg/day
• *Pregnant and lactating:* **PO/IM/IV/SC** 0.8 mg/day
• *Child <4 yr:* **PO/IM/IV/SC** up to 0.3 mg/day
• *Infants:* **PO/IM/IV/SC** up to 0.1 mg/day

Available forms: Tabs 0.1, 0.4, 0.8, 1, 5 mg; inj 5, 10 mg/ml

Side effects/adverse reactions:
RESP: ***Bronchospasm***
INTEG: Flushing

Contraindications: Hypersensitivity, anemias other than megaloblastic/macrocytic anemia, vit B_{12} deficiency anemia, uncorrected pernicious anemia

Precautions: Pregnancy (A)

Pharmacokinetics:
PO: Peak ½-1 hr; bound to plasma proteins; excreted in breast milk;

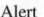

metabolized by liver; excreted in urine (small amounts)

Interactions:

- ↓ folate levels: methotrexate, sulfonamides, sulfasalazine
- ↑ need for folic acid: estrogen, hydantoins, carbamazepine, glucocorticoids
- ↓ phenytoin levels, fosphenytoin, may ↑ seizures

NURSING CONSIDERATIONS

Assess:

- For fatigue, dyspnea, weakness, dyspnea that are signs of megaloblastic anemia
- Folate levels: 6-15 mcg/ml, Hgb, Hct, and reticulocyte count
- Nutritional status: bran, yeast, dried beans, nuts, fruits, fresh vegetables, asparagus
- Drugs currently taken: estrogen, carbamazepine, glucocorticoids, hydantoins; these drugs may cause increased folic acid use by body and contribute to a deficiency

Administer:

IV route

- Direct undiluted 5 mg or less/1 min or more; or may be added to most IV sol or TPN

Solution compatibilities: $D_{20}W$

Y-site compatibilities: Famotidine

Perform/provide:

- Storage in light-resistant container

Evaluate:

- Therapeutic response: increased weight, oriented, well-being; absence of fatigue; increase in reticulocyte count within 5 days of beginning treatment

Teach patient/family:

- To take drug exactly as prescribed; periodic lab work is required
- To alter nutrition to include high-folic-acid foods: organ meats, vegetables, fruit
- That urine will turn bright yellow
- To notify prescriber of allergic reaction

fondaparinux (℞)

(fon-dah-pair'ih-nux)

Arixtra

Func. class.: Anticoagulant, antithrombotic

Chem. class.: Synthetic, selective factor Xa inhibitor

Action: Acts by antithrombin III (ATIII)-mediated selective inhibition of factor Xa; neutralization of factor Xa interrupts blood coagulation and inhibits thrombin formation; does not inactivate thrombin (activated factor II) or affect platelets

Uses: Prevention of deep-vein thrombosis, pulmonary emboli in hip and knee replacement, hip fracture surgery

Dosage and routes:

- *Adult:* **SC** 2.5 mg qd; after hemostasis established, initial dose is given 6-8 hr after surgery, usual duration 5-9 days

Available forms: Inj 2.5 mg/0.5 ml single-dose syringe

Side effects/adverse reactions:

CNS: Fever, confusion, headache, dizziness, *insomnia*

GI: Nausea, vomiting, diarrhea, dyspepsia, *constipation,* increased AST, ALT

GU: UTI, urinary retention

HEMA: Anemia, minor bleeding, purpura, hematoma, ***thrombocytopenia, major bleeding (intracranial, cerebral, retroperitoneal hemorrhage), postoperative hemorrhage***

INTEG: Increased wound drainage, bullous eruption, local reaction—*rash,* pruritus, inj site bleeding

META: Hypokalemia

OTHER: Hypotension, pain, *edema*

Contraindications: Hypersensitivity to this drug; hemophilia, leukemia with bleeding, peptic ulcer dis-

F

ease, hemorrhagic stroke, surgery, thrombocytopenic purpura, weight <50 kg, severe renal disease (CCr <30 ml/min)

Precautions: Alcoholism, hepatic disease (severe), blood dyscrasias, heparin-induced thrombocytopenia, uncontrolled, severe hypertension, subacute bacterial endocarditis, acute nephritis, lactation, pregnancy (B), elderly, children, mild to moderate renal disease

Do not confuse:
Arixtra/Anti-Xa

Pharmacokinetics: Rapidly, completely absorbed; peak steady state 3 hr; distributed primarily in blood, does not bind to plasma proteins except 94% to ATIII; metabolism unknown; eliminated unchanged in urine in 72 hr in normal renal function

Interactions:

• Do not mix with other drugs or infusion fluids

• Discontinue use of other drugs that may ↑ the risk of hemorrhage before starting fondaparinux; monitor closely if coadministration is essential

↑ risk of bleeding: agrimony, alfalfa, angelica, anise, basil, bay, bilberry, black haw, bogbean, bromelain, buchu, chondroitin, cinchona bark, dong quai, fenugreek, feverfew, garlic, ginger, ginkgo, ginseng, horse chestnut, Irish moss, kelp, kelpware, khella, lovage, lungwort, meadowsweet, motherwort, mugwort, nettle, papaya, parsley (large amts), pau d'arco, pineapple, poplar, prickly ash, safflower, saw palmetto, tonka bean, turmeric, wintergreen, yarrow

↓ anticoagulant effect: chamomile, coenzyme Q10, flax, glucomannan, goldenseal, guar gum

NURSING CONSIDERATIONS

Assess:

• Blood studies (Hct, CBC, coagulation studies, platelets, occult blood in stools), anti-Xa; thrombocytopenia may occur

• For bleeding: gums, petechiae, ecchymosis, black tarry stools, hematuria; notify prescriber

• For neurologic symptoms in patients who have received spinal anesthesia

Administer:

• Alone; do not mix with other drugs or solutions; cannot be used interchangeably (unit to unit) with other anticoagulants

• For 5-9 days

• Only after screening patient for bleeding disorders

• SC only; do not give IM

SC route

• Check for discolored sol or sol with particulate; if present, do not give

• Administer 6-8 hr after surgery

• Administer to recumbent patient, rotate inj sites (left/right anterolateral, left/right posterolateral abdominal wall)

• Wipe surface of inj site with alcohol swab, twist plunger cap and remove, remove rigid needle guard by pulling straight off needle, do not aspirate, do not expel air bubble from surface

• Insert whole length of needle into skinfold held with thumb and forefinger

• When drug is injected, a soft click may be felt or heard

• Give at same time each day to maintain steady blood levels

• Avoid all IM injections that may cause bleeding

Administer only this drug when ordered; not interchangeable with heparin

Perform/provide:
• Storage at 25° C (77° F); do not freeze

Evaluate:
• Therapeutic response: Prevention of deep vein thrombosis

Teach patient/family:
• To use soft-bristle toothbrush to avoid bleeding gums, to use electric razor
• To report any signs of bleeding: gums, under skin, urine, stools
• To avoid OTC drugs containing aspirin

formoterol fumarate (℞)

(for-moh′ter-ahl fyoo′mah-rayt)

Foradil Aerolizer

Func. class.: β-Adrenergic agonist

Chem. class.: Sympathomimetic catecholamine

Action: Has β_1 and β_2 action; relaxes bronchial smooth muscle and dilates the trachea and main bronchi by increasing levels of cAMP, which relaxes smooth muscles; causes increased contractility and heart rate by acting on β-receptors in heart

Uses: Maintenance, treatment of asthma, COPD, prevention of exercise-induced bronchospasm

Dosage and routes:

Maintenance, treatment of asthma
• *Adult/child ≥5 yr:* INH AM and PM long term 1 cap q12h using aerolizer inhaler

Maintenance of COPD
• *Adult:* **INH** 12 mcg q12h

Prevention of exercise-induced bronchospasm
• *Adult/child ≥12 yr:* prn occasionally 1 cap at least 15 min before exercise

Available form: INH powder in cap 12 mcg

Side effects/adverse reactions:

CNS: Tremors, anxiety, insomnia, headache, dizziness, stimulation

CV: Palpitations, tachycardia, hypertension

GI: Nausea, vomiting

RESP: Bronchial irritation, dryness of oropharynx, ***bronchospasms*** (overuse)

Contraindications: Hypersensitivity to sympathomimetics, narrow-angle glaucoma

Precautions: Pregnancy (C), cardiac disorders, hyperthyroidism, diabetes mellitus, prostatic hypertrophy, elderly

Do not confuse:
Foradil/Toradol

Pharmacokinetics:
INH: Onset 15 min
Metabolized in liver, lungs, GI tract

Interactions:
• ↑ effects of both drugs: other sympathomimetics
• ↓ action when used with β-blockers

NURSING CONSIDERATIONS

Assess:
• Respiratory function: B/P, pulse, lung sounds
• I&O ratio; check for urinary retention, frequency, hesitancy
• For paresthesias and coldness of extremities; peripheral blood flow may decrease

Perform/provide:
• Storage at room temperature, protection from heat, moisture; do not use discolored solution

Evaluate:
• Therapeutic response: ease of breathing

Teach patient/family:
• To rinse mouth after use
• Correct use of inhaler; review package insert with patient; to avoid

getting aerosol in eyes; to wash inhaler in warm water and dry qd
• Use of spacer device in elderly or children
• About all aspects of drug; to avoid smoking, smoke-filled rooms, persons with respiratory infections
Treatment of overdose: Administration of a β-blocker

foscarnet (℞)

(foss-kar′net)
Foscavir
Func. class.: Antiviral
Chem. class.: Inorganic pyrophosphate organic analog

Action: Antiviral activity is produced by selective inhibition at the pyrophosphate binding site on virus-specific DNA polymerases and reverse transcriptases at concentrations that do not affect cellular DNA polymerases
Uses: Treatment of CMV retinitis, HSV infections, used with ganciclovir for relapsing patients
Dosage and routes:
CMV retinitis
• *Adult:* **IV INF** 60 mg/kg given over at least 1 hr, q8h × 2-3 wk initially, then 90-120 mg/kg/day over 2 hr, usually give with at least 750-1000 ml **NS** qd
HSV
• *Adult:* **IV** 40 mg/kg q8-12h × 2-3 wk
In renal abnormalities:
• *Adult:* **IV**
Male:

$$\frac{140 - \text{age}}{\text{serum creatinine} \times 72} = \text{CCr}$$

Female: 0.85 × above value
Dose based on table provided in package insert
Available forms: Inj 24 mg/ml

Side effects/adverse reactions:
CNS: Fever, dizziness, *headache*, ***seizures,*** *fatigue*, neuropathy, tremor, ataxia, dementia, stupor, EEG abnormalities, vertigo, ***coma,*** abnormal gait, hypertonia, EPS, hemiparesis, ***paralysis,*** hyperreflexia, paraplegia, ***tetany,*** hyporeflexia, neuralgia, neuritis, ***cerebral edema,*** *paresthesia*, depression, *confusion*, *anxiety*, insomnia, somnolence, amnesia, hallucinations, agitation
GI: Nausea, vomiting, diarrhea, anorexia, abdominal pain, constipation, dysphagia, rectal hemorrhage, dry mouth, melena, flatulence, ulcerative stomatitis, pancreatitis, enteritis, enterocolitis, glossitis, proctitis, stomatitis, increased amylases, gastroenteritis, ***pseudomembranous colitis,*** duodenal ulcer, ***paralytic ileus, esophageal ulceration,*** abnormal A-G ratio, increased AST, ALT, cholecystitis, ***hepatitis,*** dyspepsia, tenesmus, hepatosplenomegaly, jaundice
INTEG: Rash, sweating, pruritus, skin ulceration, seborrhea, skin discoloration, alopecia, acne, dermatitis, pain/inflammation at injection site, facial edema, dry skin, urticaria
HEMA: Anemia, ***granulocytopenia, leukopenia, thrombocytopenia,*** platelet abnormalities, ***thrombosis, pulmonary embolism, coagulation disorders, decreased prothrombin, hypochromic anemia, pancytopenia, hemolysis, leukocytosis,*** lymphadenopathy, epistaxis, lymphopenia
SYST: Hypokalemia, hypocalcemia, hypomagnesemia; increased alk phosphatase, LDH, BUN; acidosis, hypophosphatemia, hyperphosphatemia, dehydration, glycosuria, increased CPK, hypervolemia, infection, ***sepsis, death, ascites,*** hyponatremia, hypochloremia, hypercalcemia

GU: ***Acute renal failure,*** decreased CCr and increased serum creatinine, ***glomerulonephritis, toxic nephropathy, nephrosis, renal tubular disorders, pyelonephritis, uremia, hematuria, albuminuria,*** dysuria, polyuria

RESP: Coughing, dyspnea, pneumonia, sinusitis, pharyngitis, ***pulmonary infiltration,*** stridor, ***pneumothorax, hemoptysis, bronchospasm,*** bronchitis, ***respiratory depression, pleural effusion, pulmonary hemorrhage,*** rhinitis

EENT: Visual field defects, vocal cord paralysis, speech disorders, taste perversion, eye pain, conjunctivitis, tinnitus, otitis

CV: Hypertension, palpitations, ECG abnormalities, 1st-degree AV block, nonspecific ST-T segment changes, hypotension, cerebrovascular disorder, cardiomyopathy, ***cardiac arrest,*** bradycardia, dysrhythmias

MS: Arthralgia, myalgia

Contraindications: Hypersensitivity, CCr <0.4 ml/min/kg

Precautions: Pregnancy (C), lactation, children, elderly, renal disease, seizure disorders, electrolyte/mineral imbalances, severe anemia

Pharmacokinetics: 14%-17% plasma protein bound, half-life 2-8 hr in normal renal function

Interactions:

- Nephrotoxicity: aminoglycosides, amphotericin B
- Hypocalcemia: pentamidine

NURSING CONSIDERATIONS

Assess:

General

- Renal, hepatic studies: BUN, creatinine, AST, ALT
- I&O ratio, urine pH, serum creatinine baseline, 3×/wk during initial therapy, then 2×/wk thereafter; CCr baseline, throughout treatment; if CCr <0.4 ml/min/kg, discontinue
- Blood counts q2wk; watch for decreasing granulocytes, Hgb; if low, therapy may have to be discontinued and restarted after hematologic recovery; blood transfusions may be required
- Electrolytes and minerals (Ca, P, Mg, Na, K); watch closely for tetany during first administration
- GI symptoms: nausea, vomiting, diarrhea; severe symptoms may necessitate discontinuing drug

◆ Blood dyscrasias (anemia, granulocytopenia); bruising, fatigue, bleeding, poor healing

- Allergic reactions: flushing, rash, urticaria, pruritus

CMV retinitis

- Culture should be done prior to treatment (blood, urine, throat)
- Ophthalmic exam should confirm diagnosis

Administer:

- Increased fluids before and during drug administration to induce diuresis and minimize renal toxicity

IV Intermittent INF route

- Using inf device, at no more than 1 mg/kg/min; do not give by rapid or bolus IV; give by CVP or peripheral vein; standard 24 mg/ml sol may be used without dilution if using by CVP; dilute the 24 mg/ml sol to 12 mg/ml with D_5W or NS if using peripheral vein

Y-site compatibilities: Aldesleukin, amikacin, aminophylline, ampicillin, aztreonam, benzquinamide, cefazolin, cefoperazone, cefoxitin, ceftazidime, ceftizoxime, ceftriaxone, cefuroxime, chloramphenicol, cimetidine, clindamycin, dexamethasone, DOPamine, erythromycin, fluconazole, flucytosine, furosemide, gentamicin, heparin, hydrocortisone, hydromorphone, hydrOXYzine, imipenem-cilastatin, metoclopramide, metronidazole, miconazole, morphine, nafcillin, oxacillin, penicillin G potassium, phenytoin, piperacillin, ranitidine, ticarcillin/clavulanate, tobramycin

Perform/provide:

- Regular ophthalmologic exams
- Close monitoring during therapy for tingling, numbness, paresthesias; if these occur, stop infusion, obtain lab sample for electrolytes

Evaluate:

- Therapeutic response: improvement in CMV retinitis

Teach patient/family:

- To call prescriber if sore throat, swollen lymph nodes, malaise, fever occur, since other infections may occur
- To report perioral tingling, numbness in extremities, and paresthesias
- That serious drug interactions may occur if OTC products are ingested; check first with prescriber
- That drug is not a cure but will control symptoms

fosinopril (℞)

(foss'in-oh-pril)

Monopril

Func. class.: Antihypertensive

Chem. class.: Angiotensin-converting enzyme (ACE) inhibitor

Action: Selectively suppresses renin-angiotensin-aldosterone system; inhibits ACE; prevents conversion of angiotensin I to angiotensin II; results in dilation of arterial, venous vessels

Uses: Hypertension, alone or in combination with thiazide diuretics, systolic CHF

Dosage and routes:

CHF

- *Adult:* **PO** 10 mg qd, then up to 40 mg/day increased over several wk; use lower dose in those diuresed before fosinopril

Hypertension

- *Adult:* **PO** 10 mg qd initially, then 20-40 mg/day divided bid or qd, max 80 mg/day

Available forms: Tabs 10, 20, 40 mg

Side effects/adverse reactions:

CV: *Hypotension,* chest pain, palpitations, angina, orthostatic hypotension, dysrhythmias, tachycardia

GU: ***Proteinuria,*** increased BUN, creatinine, decreased libido

HEMA: Decreased Hct, Hgb; ***eosinophilia, leukopenia, neutropenia***

INTEG: ***Angioedema,*** rash, flushing, sweating, photosensitivity, pruritus

RESP: Cough, sinusitis, dyspnea, ***bronchospasm***

META: Hyperkalemia

GI: *Nausea,* constipation, vomiting, diarrhea

CNS: *Insomnia, paresthesia, headache, dizziness,* fatigue, memory disturbance, tremor, mood change

MS: Arthralgia, myalgia

Contraindications: Hypersensitivity to ACE inhibitors, pregnancy (D) 2nd/3rd trimester, lactation, children

Precautions: Impaired hepatic function, hypovolemia, blood dyscrasias, CHF, COPD, asthma, elderly

Do not confuse:

Monopril/minoxidil/Accupril/Monoket

Pharmacokinetics:

PO: Peak 2-6 hr; serum protein binding 97%; half-life 12 hr; metabolized by liver (metabolites excreted in urine, feces)

Interactions:

- ↑ hypotension: diuretics, other antihypertensives, ganglionic blockers, adrenergic blockers, phenothiazines, nitrates, acute alcohol ingestion

• ↑ toxicity: vasodilators, hydrALAZINE, prazosin, potassium-sparing diuretics, sympathomimetics, digoxin, lithium
• ↓ absorption: antacids
• ↓ antihypertensive effect: indomethacin
• Hypersensitivity reactions: allopurinol
Fatal hypokalemia: arginine
↑ antihypertensive effect: pill-bearing spurge
↓ antihypertensive effect: pineapple, yohimbe
Severe photosensitivity: St. John's wort

Lab test interferences:
False-positive: Urine acetone
Positive: ANA titer
Increase: AST, ALT, alk phosphatase, glucose, bilirubin, uric acid

NURSING CONSIDERATIONS

Assess:
• Blood studies: neutrophils, decreased platelets; obtain WBC with diff baseline and qmo × 6 mo, then q2-3 mo × 1 yr; if neutrophils <1000/mm^3, discontinue
• B/P, orthostatic hypotension, syncope
• Renal studies: protein, BUN, creatinine; increased levels may indicate nephrotic syndrome
• Baselines in renal, hepatic studies before therapy begins
• Potassium levels, although hyperkalemia rarely occurs
• Edema in feet, legs daily, weigh daily in CHF
• Allergic reactions: rash, fever, pruritus, urticaria; drug should be discontinued if antihistamines fail to help

Administer:
• IV infusion of 0.9% NaCl (as ordered) to expand fluid volume if severe hypotension occurs

Perform/provide:
• Storage in tight container at 86° F (30° C) or less
• Supine position for severe hypotension

Evaluate:
• Therapeutic response: decrease in B/P

Teach patient/family:
• Not to discontinue drug abruptly
• Not to use OTC products (cough, cold, allergy) unless directed by prescriber; not to use salt substitutes containing potassium without consulting prescriber
• The importance of complying with dosage schedule, even if feeling better
• To rise slowly to sitting or standing position to minimize orthostatic hypotension
• To notify prescriber of mouth sores, sore throat, fever, swelling of hands or feet, irregular heartbeat, chest pain
• To report excessive perspiration, dehydration, vomiting, diarrhea; may lead to fall in B/P
• That drug may cause dizziness, fainting, light-headedness during first few days of therapy
• That drug may cause skin rash or impaired perspiration
• How to take B/P; normal readings for age-group
• To notify prescriber if pregnancy is planned or suspected

Treatment of overdose: 0.9% NaCl IV inf, hemodialysis

fosphenytoin (℞)

(foss-fen'i-toy-in)
Cerebyx
Func. class.: Anticonvulsant
Chem. class.: Hydantoin

Action: Inhibits spread of seizure activity in motor cortex by altering ion transport; increases AV conduction

Uses: Generalized tonic-clonic seizures; status epilepticus

Dosage and routes:

Status epilepticus

• *Adult and child:* **IV** loading dose 15-20 mg PE/kg given at 100-150 mg PE/min (PE = phenytoin equivalent)

Nonemergent/maintenance dosing

• *Adult and child:* **IV** loading dose 10-20 mg PE/kg; maintenance dosing 4-6 mg PE/kg/day given at a rate of <150 mg PE/min

Available forms: Inj 150 mg (100 mg phenytoin equiv), 750 mg (500 mg phenytoin equiv)

Side effects/adverse reactions:

CNS: Drowsiness, dizziness, insomnia, paresthesias, depression, suicidal tendencies, aggression, headache, confusion

CV: Hypotension, ***ventricular fibrillation***

EENT: Nystagmus, diplopia, blurred vision

GI: Nausea, vomiting, diarrhea, constipation, anorexia, weight loss, hepatitis, jaundice, gingival hyperplasia

HEMA: ***Agranulocytosis, leukopenia, aplastic anemia, thrombocytopenia, megaloblastic anemia***

INTEG: Rash, lupus erythematosus, ***Stevens-Johnson syndrome,*** hirsutism

SYST: Hyperglycemia

Contraindications: Hypersensitivity, psychiatric conditions, pregnancy (D), bradycardia, SA and AV block, Stokes-Adams syndrome

Precautions: Allergies, hepatic disease, renal disease, lactation, myocardial insufficiency

Pharmacokinetics: Metabolized by liver, excreted by kidneys

Interactions:

• ↓ fosphenytoin effects: alcohol (chronic use), antihistamines, antacids, antineoplastics, rifampin, folic acid, carbamazepine, theophylline

• ↑ fosphenytoin level: cimetidine, amiodarone, chloramphenicol, estrogens, H_2 antagonists, phenothiazines, salicylates, sulfonamides, tricyclics

↓ anticonvulsant effect: ginseng, santonica, valerian

↑ anticonvulsant effect: ginkgo

Lab test interferences:

Decrease: Dexamethasone, metyrapone test serum, PBI, urinary steroids

Increase: Glucose, alk phosphatase

NURSING CONSIDERATIONS

Assess:

• Drug level: toxic level 30-50 mcg/ml

• Blood studies: CBC, platelets q2 wk until stabilized, then qmo × 12 mo, then q3mo; discontinue drug if neutrophils <1600/mm^3

• Mental status: mood, sensorium, affect, memory (long, short)

• Seizure activity including type, location, duration, and character; provide seizure precaution

• Renal studies; urinalysis, BUN, urine creatine

• Hepatic studies: ALT, AST, bilirubin, creatinine

• Allergic reaction: red raised rash; if this occurs, drug should be discontinued

• For toxicity: bone marrow depression, nausea, vomiting, ataxia, diplopia, cardiovascular collapse, slurred speech, confusion

- Respiratory depression; rate, depth, character of respirations
- Blood dyscrasias: fever, sore throat, bruising, rash, jaundice
- Continuous monitoring of ECG, B/P, respiratory function
- Rash, discontinue as soon as rash develops, serious adverse reactions such as Stevens-Johnson syndrome can occur

Administer:

IV route

- Dilute in D_5 or 0.9% NaCl to 1.5-25 mg PE/ml, give <150 mg PE/min

Y-site compatibilities: Esmolol, famotidine, foscarnet

Additive compatibilities: Potassium chloride

Solution compatibilities: D_5W, $D_{10}W$, amino acid inj 10%, D_5LR, D_5/0.9% NaCl, Plasmalyte A, LR, sterile water for inj

Evaluate:

- Therapeutic response: decrease in severity of seizures

Teach patient/family:

- The reason for and expected outcome of treatment
- Not to use machinery or engage in hazardous activity, as drowsiness, dizziness may occur
- To carry emergency ID denoting drug use, name of prescriber
- To notify prescriber of rash, bleeding, bruising, slurred speech, jaundice of skin or eyes, joint pain, nausea, vomiting, severe headaches
- To keep all medical appointments, including lab work, physical assessment
- To notify prescriber if pregnancy is planned, suspected
- To use contraception while using this product

frovatriptan (℞)

(froh-vah-trip'tan)

Frova

Func. class.: Antimigraine agent

Chem. class.: 5-HT_1-Receptor agonist

Action: Binds selectively to the vascular 5-HT_{1B}, 5-HT_{1D} receptor subtypes, exerts antimigraine effect; binds to benzodiazepine receptor sites

Uses: Acute treatment of migraine with or without aura

Dosage and routes:

- *Adult:* **PO** 2.5 mg, a 2nd dose may be taken after ≥2 hr; max 3 tabs (7.5 mg/day)

Available form: Tabs 2.5 mg

Side effects/adverse reactions:

CNS: Hot sensation, paresthesia, *dizziness,* headache, fatigue, cold sensation

CV: Flushing, ***MI,*** chest pain

GI: Dry mouth, dyspepsia

INTEG: Photosensitivity

MS: Skeletal pain

Contraindications: Angina pectoris, history of MI, documented silent ischemia, Prinzmetal's angina, ischemic heart disease; concurrent ergotamine-containing preparations; uncontrolled hypertension; hypersensitivity; basilar or hemiplegic migraine; ischemic bowel disease; peripheral vascular disease

Precautions: Postmenopausal women, men >40 yr, risk factors for CAD, hypercholesterolemia, obesity, diabetes, impaired hepatic function, pregnancy (C), lactation, children, elderly

Pharmacokinetics: Onset of pain relief 10 min–2 hr, terminal half-life 25-29 hr, protein binding 15%

Interactions:

- ↑ vasospastic effects: ergot, ergot derivatives, other 5-HT_1 agonists
- ↑ frovatriptan effect: oral contraceptives, propranolol
- Weakness, incoordination, hyperreflexia: SSRIs

↑ effect: butterbur

NURSING CONSIDERATIONS

Assess:

- B/P; signs/symptoms of coronary vasospasms
- For stress level, activity, recreation, coping mechanisms
- Neurologic status: LOC, paresthesia, hot/cold sensations, dizziness, headache, fatigue
- Ingestion of tyramine-containing foods (pickled products, beer, wine, aged cheese), food additives, preservatives, colorings, artificial sweeteners, chocolate, caffeine, which may precipitate these types of headaches

Administer:

PO, swallow whole

Perform/provide:

- Quiet, calm environment with decreased stimulation from noise, bright light, excessive talking

Evaluate:

- Therapeutic response: decrease in frequency, severity of migraine

Teach patient/family:

- To report any side effects to prescriber
- To use sunscreen, wear protective clothing because of increased photosensitivity
- To use contraception while taking drug
- To have dark, quiet environment available

fulvestrant (℞)

(full-vess′trant)

Faslodex

Func. class.: Antineoplastic

Chem. class.: Antiestrogen hormone

Action: Inhibits cell division by binding to cytoplasmic estrogen receptors; resembles normal cell complex but inhibits DNA synthesis and estrogen response of target tissue

Uses: Advanced breast carcinoma in estrogen-receptor-positive patients (usually postmenopausal)

Dosage and routes:

- *Adult:* **IM** 250 mg qmo

Available forms: Inj 50 mg/ml

Side effects/adverse reactions:

GI: Nausea, vomiting, anorexia, constipation, diarrhea, abdominal pain

INTEG: Rash, sweating, hot flashes

CNS: Headache, depression, dizziness, insomnia, paresthesia, anxiety

RESP: Pharyngitis, dyspnea, cough

MS: Bone pain, arthritis, back pain

Contraindications: Hypersensitivity, pregnancy (D)

Precautions: Lactation, children, hepatic disease

Pharmacokinetics: Half-life 40 days, metabolized by CYP 3A4, excretion feces 90%

NURSING CONSIDERATIONS

Assess:

- For side effects, report to prescriber

Administer:

IM route

- IM 5 ml as a single inj or 2, 2.5 ml inj; give slowly in buttock
- Antacid before oral agent; give drug after evening meal, before bedtime
- Antiemetic 30-60 min before giving drug to prevent vomiting

Perform/provide:
- Liquid diet, if needed, including cola, Jell-O; dry toast or crackers may be added if patient is not nauseated or vomiting
- Nutritious diet with iron, vitamin supplements as ordered
- Store in refrigerator

Evaluate:
- Therapeutic response: decreased tumor size, spread of malignancy

Teach patient/family:
- To report any complaints, side effects to prescriber
- To increase fluids to 2 L/day unless contraindicated
- To report vaginal bleeding immediately
- That tumor flare—increase in size of tumor, increased bone pain—may occur and will subside rapidly; may take analgesics for pain
- That premenopausal women must use mechanical birth control because ovulation may be induced

furosemide (℞)

(fur-oh'se-mide)
Apo-Furosemide✤, Furoside✤, Lasix, Lasix Special✤, Myrosemide✤, Novosemide✤, Uritol✤

Func. class.: Loop diuretic
Chem. class.: Sulfonamide derivative

Action: Inhibits reabsorption of sodium and chloride at proximal and distal tubule and in the loop of Henle

Uses: Pulmonary edema; edema in CHF, hepatic disease, nephrotic syndrome, ascites, hypertension

Investigational uses: Hypercalcemia in malignancy

Dosage and routes:
- *Adult:* **PO** 20-80 mg/day in AM; may give another dose in 6 hr up to 600 mg/day; **IM/IV** 20-40 mg, increased by 20 mg q2h until desired response
- *Child:* **PO/IM/IV** 2 mg/kg; may increase by 1-2 mg/kg/q6-8h up to 6 mg/kg

Pulmonary edema
- *Adult:* **IV** 40 mg given over several min, repeated in 1 hr; increase to 80 mg if needed

Hypertensive crisis/acute renal failure
- *Adult:* **IV** 100-200 mg over 1-2 min

Antihypercalcemia
- *Adult:* **IM/IV** 80-100 mg q1-4h or **PO** 120 mg qd or divided bid
- *Child:* **IM/IV** 25-50 mg, repeat q4h if needed

Available forms: Tabs 20, 40, 80 mg; oral sol 10 mg/ml, 40 mg/5 ml; inj 10 mg/ml

Side effects/adverse reactions:
CNS: Headache, fatigue, weakness, vertigo, paresthesias
CV: Orthostatic hypotension, chest pain, ECG changes, ***circulatory collapse***
EENT: ***Loss of hearing,*** ear pain, tinnitus, blurred vision
ELECT: *Hypokalemia, hypochloremic alkalosis, hypomagnesemia, hyperuricemia, hypocalcemia, hyponatremia,* metabolic alkalosis
ENDO: *Hyperglycemia*
GI: *Nausea,* diarrhea, dry mouth, vomiting, anorexia, cramps, oral, gastric irritations, pancreatitis
GU: *Polyuria,* ***renal failure,*** glycosuria
HEMA: ***Thrombocytopenia, agranulocytosis, leukopenia, neutropenia, anemia***
INTEG: *Rash, pruritus,* purpura, ***Stevens-Johnson syndrome,*** sweating, photosensitivity, urticaria
MS: Cramps, stiffness

Contraindications: Hypersensitivity to sulfonamides, anuria, hypovolemia, infants, lactation, electrolyte depletion

Precautions: Diabetes mellitus, dehydration, severe renal disease, pregnancy (C), cirrhosis, ascites

Do not confuse:
furosemide/torsemide
Lasix/Luvox/Lomotil
Lasix/Lanoxin

Pharmacokinetics:
PO: Onset 1 hr, peak 1-2 hr, duration 6-8 hr; absorbed 70%
IV: Onset 5 min, peak ½ hr, duration 2 hr (metabolized by the liver 30%)
Excreted in urine, some as unchanged drug, feces; crosses placenta; excreted in breast milk; half-life ½-1 hr

Interactions:
- ↑ toxicity: lithium, nondepolarizing skeletal muscle relaxants, digitalis
- ↑ hypotensive action of antihypertensives, nitrates
- ↑ ototoxicity: aminoglycosides, cisplatin, vancomycin

↑ diuretic effect: aloe, cucumber, dandelion, khella, horsetail, pumpkin, Queen Anne's lace

Severe photosensitivity: St. John's wort

Lab test interferences:
Interference: GTT

NURSING CONSIDERATIONS

Assess:
- Signs of metabolic alkalosis: drowsiness, restlessness
- Signs of hypokalemia: postural hypotension, malaise, fatigue, tachycardia, leg cramps, weakness
- Rashes, temp elevation qd
- Confusion, especially in elderly; take safety precautions if needed
- Hearing, including tinnitus and hearing loss, when giving high doses for extended periods
- Weight, I&O qd to determine fluid loss; effect of drug may be decreased if used qd
- Rate, depth, rhythm of respiration, effect of exertion, lung sounds
- B/P lying, standing; postural hypotension may occur
- Electrolytes (K, Na, Cl); include BUN, blood glucose, CBC, serum creatinine, blood pH, ABGs, uric acid, calcium, magnesium
- Skin turgor, edema, condition of mucous membranes in mouth and nose
- Glucose in urine if patient is diabetic
- Allergies to sulfonamides, thiazides

Administer:
- In AM to avoid interference with sleep if using drug as a diuretic
- Potassium replacement if potassium <3 mg/dl
- PO with food if nausea occurs; absorption may be decreased slightly; tabs may be crushed

IV route
- Undiluted; may be given through Y-tube or 3-way stopcock; give 20 mg or less/min; may be added to NS or D_5W if large doses are required and given as IV inf, not to exceed 4 mg/min; use infusion pump

Additive compatibilities: Amikacin, aminophylline, ampicillin, atropine, bumetanide, calcium gluconate, cefamandole, cefoperazone, cefuroxime, cimetidine, cloxacillin, dexamethasone, diamorphine, digoxin, epINEPHrine, heparin, isosorbide, kanamycin, lidocaine, meropenem, morphine, nitroglycerin, penicillin G, potassium chloride, ranitidine, scopolamine, sodium bicarbonate, theophylline, tobramycin, verapamil

Syringe compatibilities: Bleomycin, cisplatin, cyclophosphamide, fluorouracil, heparin, leucovorin, methotrexate, mitomycin

Y-site compatibilities: Allopurinol, amifostine, amikacin, amphotericin B cholesteryl, aztreonam, bleomycin, cefepime, cefmetazole, cisplatin, cladribine, cyclophosphamide, cytarabine, DOXOrubicin liposome, epINEPHrine, fentanyl, fludarabine, fluorouracil, foscarnet, gallium, granisetron, heparin, hydrocortisone, hydromorphone, indomethacin, kanamycin, leucovorin, lorazepam, melphalan, meropenem, methotrexate, mitomycin, nitroglycerin, norepinephrine, paclitaxel, piperacillin/tazobactam, potassium chloride, propofol, ranitidine, remifentanil, sargramostim, tacrolimus, teniposide, thiotepa, tobramycin, tolazoline, vit B/C

Evaluate:

• Therapeutic response: improvement in edema of feet, legs, sacral area daily if medication is being used for CHF

Teach patient/family:

• To discuss the need for a high-potassium diet or potassium replacement with prescriber

• To increase fluid intake 2-3 L/day unless contraindicated

• To rise slowly from lying or sitting position; orthostatic hypotension may occur

• To recognize adverse reactions that may occur: muscle cramps, weakness, nausea, dizziness

• Regarding entire regimen, including exercise, diet, stress relief for hypertension

• To take with food or milk for GI symptoms

• To use sunscreen or protective clothing to prevent photosensitivity

• To take early in day to prevent sleeplessness

• To avoid OTC medication unless directed by prescriber

Treatment of overdose: Lavage if taken orally; monitor electrolytes; administer dextrose in saline; monitor hydration, CV, renal status

gabapentin (℞)

(gab'a-pen-tin)

Neurontin

Func. class.: Anticonvulsant

Action: Mechanism unknown; may increase seizure threshold; structurally similar to GABA; gabapentin binding sites in neocortex, hippocampus

Uses: Adjunct treatment of partial seizures, with or without generalization in patients >12 yr; adjunct in partial seizures in children 3-12 yr, postherpetic neuralgia

Investigational uses: Tremors in multiple sclerosis, neuropathic pain, bipolar disorder, migraine prophylaxis, diabetic neuropathy

Dosage and routes:

• *Adult and child >12 yr:* **PO** 900-1800 mg/day in 3 divided doses; may titrate by giving 300 mg on first day, 300 mg bid on second day, 300 mg tid on third day; may increase to 1800 mg/day by adding 300 mg on subsequent days

• *Child 5-12 yr:* **PO** 10-15 mg/kg/day in 3 divided doses, initially titrate dose upward over approximately 3 days; 25-35 mg/kg/day; all given in 3 divided doses; rect 200 mg as single dose

• *Child 3-4 yr:* **PO** 10-15 mg/kg/day in 3 divided doses, initially titrate dose upward over approximately 3 days; 40 mg/kg/day; all given in 3 divided doses; rect 200 mg as single dose

Postherpetic neuralgia

• *Adult:* **PO** 300 mg on day 1, 600 mg/day divided bid on day 2, 900 mg/day divided tid, may titrate to 1800 mg divided tid if needed

Renal dose

• *Adult and child >12 yr:* CCr 30-60 ml/min 300 mg bid, CCr 15-30 ml/

G

min 300 mg qd, CCr <15 ml/min 125 mg qd
Available forms: Caps 100, 300, 400 mg; tabs 600, 800 mg; oral sol 250 mg/5 ml
Side effects/adverse reactions:
CNS: Dizziness, fatigue, anxiety, somnolence, ataxia, amnesia, abnormal thinking, unsteady gait, depression; 3-12 yr old, emotional lability, aggression, thought disorder, hyperkinesia
CV: Vasodilation, peripheral edema
EENT: Dry mouth, blurred vision, *diplopia,* nystagmus
GI: Constipation, increased appetite, dental abnormalities, nausea, vomiting
GU: Impotence, bleeding, *UTI*
HEMA: ***Leukopenia,*** decreased WBC
INTEG: Pruritus, abrasion
MS: Myalgia
RESP: Rhinitis, pharyngitis, cough
Contraindications: Hypersensitivity to this drug
Precautions: Renal disease, pregnancy (C), lactation, children <12 yr, elderly, hemodialysis
Do not confuse:
Neurontin/Noroxin/Neoral
Pharmacokinetics: Largely unbound to plasma proteins; not metabolized; excreted in urine (unchanged); elimination half-life 5-7 hr
Interactions:
- ↑ CNS depression: alcohol, sedatives, antihistamines, all other CNS depressants
- ↓ gabapentin levels: antacids

↑ CNS depression: chamomile, hops, kava, skullcap, valerian
Lab test interferences:
False-positive: Urinary protein using Ames N-multistix SG
NURSING CONSIDERATIONS
Assess:
- Seizures: aura, location, duration, activity at onset
- Pain: location, duration, characteristics if using for chronic pain
- Renal studies: urinalysis, BUN, urine creatinine q3mo
- Description of seizures; location, duration, characteristics
- Mental status: mood, sensorium, affect, behavioral changes; if mental status changes, notify prescriber
- Eye problems, need for ophthalmic exam before, during, after treatment (slit lamp, fundoscopy, tonometry)

Administer:
- 2 hr apart when giving antacids
- Caps may be opened and contents put in applesauce or dissolved in juice
- Give without regard to meals
- Gradually withdraw over 7 days, abrupt withdrawal may precipitate seizures

Perform/provide:
- Storage at room temperature away from heat and light
- Hard candy, frequent rinsing of mouth, gum for dry mouth
- Assistance with ambulation during early part of treatment; dizziness occurs
- Seizure precautions: padded side rails; move objects that may harm patient
- Increased fluids, bulk in diet for constipation

Evaluate:
- Therapeutic response: decreased seizure activity; decrease in chronic pain

Teach patient/family:
- To carry emergency ID stating patient's name, drugs taken, condition, prescriber's name and phone number
- To avoid driving, other activities that require alertness: dizziness, drowsiness may occur
- Not to discontinue medication quickly after long-term use, taper

over ≥1 wk; withdrawal-precipitated seizures may occur, not to double doses if dose is missed, take if 2 hr or more before next dose

🚫 Not to crush or chew caps

• To notify prescriber if pregnancy planned or suspected, avoid breastfeeding

Treatment of overdose: Lavage, VS

galantamine (℞)

(gah-lan'tah-meen)

Reminyl

Func. class.: Anti-Alzheimer agent, cholinesterase inhibitor

Action: May enhance cholinergic functioning by increasing acetylcholine

Uses: Alzheimer's dementia

Dosage and routes:

• *Adult:* **PO** 4 mg bid; after 4 wk or more may increase to 8 mg bid; may increase to 12 mg bid after another 4 wk

Available forms: Tabs 4, 8, 12 mg; oral sol 4 mg/ml

Side effects/adverse reactions:

CNS: Tremors, insomnia, depression, dizziness, headache, somnolence, fatigue

CV: Bradycardia, anemia, hematuria, chest pain

GI: Nausea, vomiting, anorexia, abdominal distress, flatulence, diarrhea

GU: Urinary incontinence, bladder outflow obstruction, hematuria

META: Weight decrease

MS: Asthenia, anemia

RESP: URI, rhinitis

Contraindications: Hypersensitivity to this drug

Precautions: Renal disease, hepatic disease, respiratory disease, seizure disorder, peptic ulcer, pregnancy (B), asthma, lactation, children

Pharmacokinetics: Rapidly and completely absorbed, metabolized by CYP450 enzyme, excreted via kidneys; clearance is lower in the elderly, hepatic disease; clearance is 20% lower in females

Interactions:

• Synergistic effect: cholinomimetics, other cholinesterase inhibitors

• ↑ galantamine bioavailability: cimetidine, paroxetine, ketoconazole, erythromycin, quinidine, amitriptyline, fluvoxamine

Cholinergic antagonism: jimsonweed, scopolia

↑ effect: pill-bearing spurge

NURSING CONSIDERATIONS

Assess:

• Hepatic studies: AST, ALT, alk phosphatase, LDH, bilirubin, CBC

• For severe GI effects: nausea, vomiting, anorexia, weight loss

• B/P, respiration during initial treatment

• Mental status: affect, mood, behavioral changes, depression

Administer:

• With meals; take with morning and evening meal

Perform/provide:

• Assistance with ambulation during beginning therapy

• Complete suicide assessment

Evaluate:

• Therapeutic response: decreased confusion

Teach patient/family:

• Correct procedure for giving oral solution, using instruction sheet provided

• To notify prescriber of severe GI effects

• To report hypo/hypertension

HIGH ALERT/RARELY USED

gallamine (℞)

(gal'a-meen)

Flaxedil

Func. class.: Neuromuscular blocker (nondepolarizing)

Uses: Facilitation of endotracheal intubation, skeletal muscle relaxation during mechanical ventilation, surgery, general anesthesia

Dosage and routes:

• *Adult and child >1 mo:* **IV** 1 mg/kg, not to exceed 100 mg, then 0.5-1 mg/kg q30-40min

• *Child <1 mo, >5 kg:* **IV** 0.25-0.75 mg/kg, then 0.01-0.05 mg/kg q30-40min

Contraindications: Hypersensitivity to iodides

gallium (℞)

(gal'ee-um)

Ganite

Func. class.: Electrolyte modifier

Chem. class.: Hypocalcemic drug

Action: Lowers serum calcium levels by inhibiting calcium resorption from bone

Uses: Cancer-related hypercalcemia

Dosage and routes:

• *Adult:* **IV** 100-200 mg/m^2 qd × 5 days; infuse over 24 hr, rest period of 2-4 wk between courses

Available forms: 25 mg/ml inj

Side effects/adverse reactions:

HEMA: ***Anemia, leukopenia, thrombocytopenia***

CV: Tachycardia, hypotension

EENT: Blurred vision, optic neuritis, hearing loss

GU: ***Nephrotoxicity,*** increased BUN, creatinine

GI: Nausea, vomiting, diarrhea, constipation, mucositis, metallic taste

META: Hypophosphatemia, hypocalcemia, decreased serum bicarbonate

Contraindications: Hypersensitivity, severe renal disease

Precautions: Pregnancy (C), lactation, children, mild renal disease

Pharmacokinetics:

IV: Onset 12-48 hr, peak 5 days, duration 4-14 days, excreted by kidneys

Interactions:

• ↑ nephrotoxicity: aminoglycosides, amphotericin B

NURSING CONSIDERATIONS

Assess:

• Renal status: BUN, creatinine, urine output; if creatinine level is 2.5 mg/dl or more, drug should be discontinued

• Monitor calcium, phosphate, bicarbonate, since all levels may be decreased and supplements of phosphate may be needed

• For hypercalcemia: nausea, vomiting, fatigue, weakness, thirst, dehydration, dysrhythmias, change in mental status

• For hypocalcemia: dysrhythmias; paresthesia; twitching; colic; laryngospasm; Trousseau's, Chvostek's sign; tremors

• For hypophosphatemia: confusion, decreased reflexes, joint stiffness and pain, portal hypotension

Administer:

IV route

• Adequate hydration with IV saline, 2 L/day during treatment

• After dilution of dose/1 L 0.9% NaCl or D_5W, run over 24 hr, use infusion pump

Y-site compatibilities: Acyclovir, allopurinol, amifostine, aminophylline, ampicillin/sulbactam, aztreonam, cefazolin, ceftazidime, ceftriaxone, cimetidine, ciprofloxacin, cladribine, cyclophosphamide, dexamethasone, diphenhydrAMINE, filgrastim, fluconazole, furosemide, granisetron, heparin, hydrocortisone, ifosfamide, magnesium sulfate, mannitol, melphalan, meperidine, mesna, methotrexate, metoclopramide, ondansetron, piperacillin, piperacillin/tazobactam, potassium chloride, ranitidine, sodium bicarbonate, teniposide, thiotepa, ticarcillin/clavulanate, trimethoprim-sulfamethoxazole, vancomycin, vinorelbine

Perform/provide:

- Storage of solution 48 hr at room temperature, 1 wk in refrigerator

Evaluate:

- Therapeutic response: decreased serum calcium levels

Teach patient/family:

- To follow dietary guidelines given by prescriber, including avoiding calcium (dairy products, broccoli) and vit D (fortified milk, grain products, fish oil)

ganciclovir (℞)

(gan-sye'kloe-vir)

Cytovene, Vitrasert

Func. class.: Antiviral

Chem. class.: Synthetic nucleoside analog

Action: Inhibits replication of herpesviruses in vitro, in vivo by selective inhibition of the human CMV DNA polymerase and by direct incorporation into viral DNA

Uses: Cytomegalovirus (CMV) retinitis in immunocompromised persons, including those with AIDS, after indirect ophthalmoscopy confirms diagnosis

Investigational uses: CMV pneumonia in organ transplant patients, CMV gastroenteritis in patients with IBS, CMV pneumonitis

Dosage and routes:

- Reduce dose in renal disease CCr <70 ml/min

Prevention of CMV

- *Adult:* **IV** 5 mg/kg q12h × 1-2 wk, then 5 mg/kg/day 7 day/wk, then 5 mg/kg/day or 6 mg/kg × 5 days/wk; **PO** 1000 mg tid

Induction treatment

- *Adult:* **IV** 5 mg/kg given over 1 hr, q12h × 2-3 wk

Maintenance treatment

- *Adult:* **IV INF** 5 mg/kg given over 1 hr, qd × 7 days/wk; or 6 mg/kg qd × 5 days/wk; **PO** 1000 mg tid with food or 500 mg q3h while awake; **INTRAVITREAL:** 4.5 mg implant

Available forms: Powder for inj 500 mg/vial; caps 250, 500 mg; implant, intraviteral 4.5 mg

Side effects/adverse reactions:

HEMA: ***Granulocytopenia, thrombocytopenia, irreversible neutropenia, anemia, eosinophilia***

GI: Abnormal LFTs, nausea, vomiting, anorexia, diarrhea, abdominal pain, ***hemorrhage***

INTEG: Rash, alopecia, *pruritus,* urticaria, pain at site, phlebitis

CNS: Fever, chills, ***coma,*** *confusion,* abnormal thoughts, dizziness, bizarre dreams, *headache,* psychosis, tremors, somnolence, *paresthesia, weakness,* ***seizures***

CV: Dysrhythmia, hyper/hypotension

RESP: Dyspnea

EENT: Retinal detachment in CMV retinitis

GU: ***Hematuria,*** increased creatinine, BUN

Contraindications: Hypersensitivity to acyclovir or ganciclovir, absolute neutrophil count <500, platelet count <25,000

Precautions: Preexisting cytopenias, renal function impairment, pregnancy (C), lactation, children <6 mo, elderly

Do not confuse:

Cytovene/Cytosar

Pharmacokinetics: Half-life 3-4½ hr; excreted by kidneys (unchanged); crosses blood-brain barrier, CSF

Interactions:

• ↓ ganciclovir renal clearance: probenecid

• ↑ toxicity: adriamycin, amphotericin B, cycloSPORINE, dapsone, DOXOrubicin, flucytosine, pentamidine, probenecid, trimethoprim-sulfa combinations, vinBLAStine, vinCRIStine, or other nucleoside analogs

◆ Severe granulocytopenia: zidovudine, antineoplastics, radiation; do not give together

• ↑ seizures: imipenem/cilastatin

NURSING CONSIDERATIONS

Assess:

• For leukopenia/neutropenia/thrombocytopenia: WBCs, platelets q2d during 2×/day dosing and then q1wk

• For leukopenia with qd WBC count in patients with prior leukopenia with other nucleoside analogs or for whom leukopenia counts are <1000 cells/mm^3 at start of treatment

• Serum creatinine or CCr ≥q2wk

Administer:

PO route

• With food

IV route

• Mixed in biologic cabinet, using gown, gloves, mask

Intermittent INF route

• IV after diluting 500 mg/10 ml sterile H_2O for inj (50 mg/ml); shake; further dilute in 100 ml D_5W, 0.9% NaCl, LR, Ringer's and run over 1 hr; use infusion pump, in-line filter

• Slowly; do not give by bolus IV, IM, SC inj

• Using diluted sol within 12 hr; do not refrigerate or freeze

Y-site compatibilities: Allopurinol, amphotericin B cholesteryl, cisplatin, cyclophosphamide, DOXOrubicin liposome, enalaprilat, filgrastim, fluconazole, granisetron, melphalan, methotrexate, paclitaxel, propofol, remifentanil, tacrolimus, teniposide, thiotepa

Evaluate:

• Therapeutic response: decreased symptoms of CMV

Teach patient/family:

• That drug does not cure condition, that regular ophthalmologic exams are necessary

• That major toxicities may necessitate discontinuing drug

• To use contraception during treatment and that infertility may occur; men should use barrier contraception for 90 days after treatment

• To take PO with food

◆ To report infection: fever, chills, sore throat; blood dyscrasias: bruising, bleeding, petechiae

• To avoid crowds, persons with respiratory infections

• To use sunscreen to prevent burns

ganirelix (℞)

Antagon

Func. class.: Gonadotropin-releasing hormone antagonist

Chem. class.: Synthetic decapeptide

Action: Inhibitor of pituitary gonadotropin secretion; initially increases LH and FSH, induces a rapid suppression of gonadotropin secretion

Uses: For inhibition of premature LH surges in women undergoing controlled ovarian hyperstimulation

Dosage and routes:

• *Adult:* **SC** 250 mcg qd during early to mid follicular phase, continue until the day of hCG administration

Available forms: Inj 250 mcg/0.5 ml

Side effects/adverse reactions:

CNS: Headache

ENDO: Ovarian hyperstimulation syndrome, abdominal pain (gyn)

GI: Nausea

GU: Spotting, breakthrough bleeding

INTEG: Pain on inj

SYST: ***Fetal death***

Contraindications: Hypersensitivity, pregnancy (X), latex allergy, lactation

Pharmacokinetics: Excreted in feces/urine, half-life 13-16 hr, metabolized to metabolites, protein binding 82%

NURSING CONSIDERATIONS

Assess:

• For suspected pregnancy, drug should not be used

• For latex allergy, drug should not be used

Administer:

• SC using abdomen, around navel or upper thigh, swab inj area with disinfectant, clean a 2 in circle and allow to dry, pinch up area between thumb and finger, insert needle at 45°-90° to surface, if positioned correctly, no blood will be drawn back into syringe, if blood is drawn into syringe, reposition needle without removing it

Perform/provide:

• Protection from light

Evaluate:

• Therapeutic response: pregnancy

Teach patient/family:

• To report abdominal pain, vaginal bleeding

gatifloxacin (℞)

(gat-ih-floks′ah-sin)

Tequin

Func. class.: Broad-spectrum antiinfective

Chem. class.: Fluoroquinolone

Action: Interferes with conversion of intermediate DNA fragments into high–molecular weight DNA in bacteria; DNA gyrase inhibitor

Uses: Infection caused by susceptible *Escherichia coli, Staphylococcus aureus, Haemophilus influenzae, Haemophilus parainfluenzae, Klebsiella pneumoniae, Moraxella catarrhalis, Neisseria gonorrhoeae, Proteus mirabilis,* and other microorganisms: *Chlamydia pneumoniae, Legionella pneumophila, Mycoplasma pneumoniae,* acute bacterial exacerbation of chronic bronchitis, acute sinusitis, community-acquired respiratory tract infections, gonorrhea

Investigational uses: Multidrug-resistant *Streptococcus pneumoniae* in children with acute otitis media, sinusitis; *Mycobacterium leprae,* atypical pneumonia, uncomplicated skin, soft tissue infections, chronic prostatitis

Dosage and routes:

Renal dose

• CCr ≥40 ml/min 400 mg qd; <40 ml/min 200 mg qd after 400 mg initially; hemodialysis 200 mg qd after 400 mg initially

Uncomplicated urinary tract infections

• *Adult:* **PO/IV** 400 mg single dose

Complicated/severe urinary tract infections

• *Adult:* **PO/IV** 400 mg × 7-10 days

Chronic bronchitis

• *Adult:* **PO/IV** 400 mg × 7-10 days

Acute sinusitis
• *Adult:* **PO/IV** 400 mg × 10 days
Community-acquired pneumonia
• *Adult:* **PO/IV** 400 mg × 7-14 days
Gonorrhea
• *Adult:* **PO/IV** 400 mg single dose

Available forms: Tabs 200, 400 mg; inj 20 ml (200 mg), 40 ml (400 mg); inj premix 200, 400 mg

Side effects/adverse reactions:
CNS: Headache, dizziness, insomnia, paresthesia, tremor, vasodilation
GI: Nausea, diarrhea, increased ALT, AST, ***pseudomembranous colitis***
INTEG: Rash, pruritus, urticaria, photosensitivity, flushing, fever, chills
RESP: Dyspnea, pharyngitis
SYST: ***Anaphylaxis, Stevens-Johnson syndrome***
ENDO: Increased blood glucose

Contraindications: Hypersensitivity to quinolones

Precautions: Pregnancy (C), lactation, children, renal disease

Pharmacokinetics: Half-life 6½-14 hr; excreted in urine unchanged, protein binding 20%, peak 1-2 hr (PO) depending on dose, duration 24 hr

Interactions:
• ↓ gatifloxacin absorption: magnesium antacids, aluminum hydroxide, sucralfate, calcium
• ↑ gatifloxacin serum levels: probenecid, cimetidine
• ↑ warfarin level
• ↑ nephrotoxicity risk: cycloSPORINE

NURSING CONSIDERATIONS

Assess:
• CNS symptoms: headache, dizziness, insomnia
• Renal, hepatic studies, blood glucose: BUN, creatinine, AST, ALT
• I&O ratio, urine pH <5.5 is ideal
• Allergic reactions and anaphylaxis: fever, flushing, rash, urticaria, pruritus, emergency equipment should be nearby

Administer:

PO route
• 2 hr before or 2 hr after antacids, zinc, iron, calcium

IV route
• Do not use flexible containers in series connections, air embolism may occur
• Do not use if particulate matter is present
• Do not admix with other drugs
• Dilute with compatible sol to 2 mg/ml before administration, give over 1 hr; do not give by bolus or rapid IV

Solution compatibilities: D_5, 0.9% NaCl, D_5/0.9% NaCl, LR/D_5, water for inj

Perform/provide:
• Limited intake of alkaline foods, drugs: milk, dairy products, alkaline antacids, sodium bicarbonate

Evaluate:
• Therapeutic response: decreased pain, frequency, urgency, C&S; absence of infection

Teach patient/family:
• Not to take any products containing magnesium or calcium (such as antacids), iron, or aluminum with this drug or within 4 hr of drug; to increase fluid intake to 2 L/day to prevent crystalluria
• That photosensitivity may occur; patient should avoid sunlight or use sunscreen to prevent burns
• If dizziness occurs, to ambulate, perform activities with assistance
• To contact prescriber if adverse reaction occurs or if inflammation or pain in tendon occurs
• To use frequent rinsing of mouth, sugarless candy, or gum for dry mouth
• To avoid other medications unless approved by prescriber

• Not to use theophylline with this product, will cause toxicity; contact prescriber if taking theophylline
• To take as prescribed, not to double or miss doses, to take all medications

gemcitabine (℞)

(jem-sit'a-been)
Gemzar
Func. class.: Misc. antineoplastic
Chem. class.: Nucleoside analog

Action: Exhibits antitumor activity by killing cells undergoing DNA synthesis (S-phase) and blocking G1/S-phase boundary
Uses: Adenocarcinoma of the pancreas (nonresectable stage II, III, or metastatic stage IV); non–small cell lung cancer (stage IIIA or B, IV); in combination with cisplatin for inoperable, advanced, or metastatic non–small cell lung cancer
Dosage and routes:
Pancreatic carcinoma
• *Adult:* **IV** 1000 mg/m^2 given over ½ hr qwk × 7 wk, then 1 wk rest period; subsequent cycles should be infused once qwk × 3 wk out of every 4 wk
Non–small cell lung cancer
4-wk schedule:
• *Adult:* **IV** 1000 mg/m^2 given over ½ hr on days 1, 8, 15, of each 28-day cycle. Give cisplatin **IV** 100 mg/m^2 on day 1 after gemcitabine
3-wk schedule:
• *Adult:* **IV** 1250 mg/m^2 given over ½ hr on days 1, 8 of each 21-day cycle. Give cisplatin 100 mg/m^2 after the inf of gemcitabine on day 1
Available forms: Lyophilized powder for inj 20 mg/ml
Side effects/adverse reactions:
GI: Diarrhea, nausea, vomiting, anorexia, constipation, stomatitis
INTEG: Irritation at site, rash, alopecia
HEMA: ***Leukopenia, anemia, neutropenia, thrombocytopenia***
GU: Proteinuria, hematuria
OTHER: Dyspnea, fever, ***hemorrhage,*** infection, flulike symptoms, paresthesia
Contraindications: Hypersensitivity, pregnancy (D)
Precautions: Lactation, children, elderly, myelosuppression, irradiation
Do not confuse:
Gemzar/Zinecard
Pharmacokinetics: Half-life 42-79 min, crosses placenta
Interactions:
• ↑ bleeding: NSAIDs, alcohol, salicylates
• ↑ myelosuppression, diarrhea: other antineoplastics, radiation
• ↓ antibody response: live virus vaccines

NURSING CONSIDERATIONS

Assess:
• CBC, differential, platelet count before each dose; absolute granulocyte count >1000, platelets >100,000, give complete dose; absolute granulocyte count 500-1000, platelets 50,000-100,000, give 75%; absolute granulocyte count <500, platelets <50,000, do not give
• Blood dyscrasias: bruising, bleeding, petechiae
• I&O, nutritional intake; food preferences: list likes, dislikes
• Renal, hepatic studies before and during treatment; may increase AST, ALT, alk phosphatase, bilirubin, BUN, creatinine

• Buccal cavity q8h for dryness, sores/ulceration, white patches, oral pain, bleeding, dysphagia
• GI symptoms: frequency of stools; cramping
• Signs of dehydration: rapid respirations, poor skin turgor, decreased urine output, dry skin, restlessness, weakness

Administer:

IV route

• Prepare in biologic cabinet using gown, mask, gloves
• After reconstituting with 0.9% NaCl 5 ml/200 mg vial of drug or 25 ml/1 g of drug, shake = 40 mg/ml may be further diluted with 0.9% NaCl to conc as low as 0.1 mg/ml; discard unused portions, give over ½ hr, do not admix

Perform/provide:

• Increased fluid intake to 2-3 L/day to prevent dehydration, unless contraindicated
• Changing of IV site q48h
• Rinsing of mouth tid-qid with water, club soda; brushing of teeth bid-tid with soft brush or cotton-tipped applicator for stomatitis; use unwaxed dental floss
• Nutritious diet with iron, vitamin supplement, low fiber, few dairy products

Evaluate:

• Therapeutic response: decrease in tumor size, decrease in spread of cancer

Teach patient/family:

• To avoid foods with citric acid or hot or rough texture if stomatitis is present; to drink adequate fluids
• To avoid use with NSAIDs, alcohol, salicylates
• To report stomatitis; any bleeding, white spots, ulcerations in mouth; tell patient to examine mouth qd, report symptoms
• To report signs of anemia: fatigue, headache, faintness, shortness of breath, irritability; hematuria, dysuria
• To use contraception during therapy
• Not to receive vaccinations during treatment

gemfibrozil (℞)

(jem-fi'broe-zil)

gemfibrozil, Lopid

Func. class.: Antilipemic

Chem. class.: Fibric acid derivative

Action: Inhibits biosynthesis of VLDL, decreases triglycerides, increases HDL

Uses: Type IIb, IV, V hyperlipidemia as adjunct with diet therapy

Dosage and routes:

• *Adult:* **PO** 1200 mg in divided doses bid 30 min before AM, PM meal

Available forms: Tabs 600 mg

Side effects/adverse reactions:

GI: Dyspepsia, diarrhea, abdominal pain, nausea, vomiting

INTEG: Rash, urticaria, pruritus

HEMA: ***Leukopenia, anemia, eosinophilia, thrombocytopenia***

CNS: Fatigue, vertigo, headache, paresthesia, dizziness, somnolence

MISC: Taste perversion

Contraindications: Severe hepatic disease, preexisting gallbladder disease, severe renal disease, primary biliary cirrhosis, hypersensitivity

Precautions: Monitor hematologic and hepatic function, pregnancy (C), lactation

Do not confuse:

Lopid/Levbid/Slo-bid

Pharmacokinetics:

PO: Peak 1-2 hr; plasma protein binding >90%; half-life 1½ hr; 70% excreted in urine as conjugate; <2%

excreted unchanged; metabolized in liver (minimal)

Interactions:

• ↑ hypoglycemic effect: sulfonylureas

• ↑ anticoagulant properties: oral anticoagulants

• ↑ risk of myositis, myalgia: HMG-CoA reductase inhibitors

• ↓ effect of: cycloSPORINE

↑ effect: glucomannan

↓ effect: gotu kola

Lab test interferences:

Increase: LFTs, CPK, BSP, thymol turbidity, glucose

Decrease: Hgb, Hct, WBC

NURSING CONSIDERATIONS

Assess:

• Triglycerides, cholesterol; if lipids increase, drug should be discontinued; LDL, VLDL baseline and periodically

• Renal, hepatic studies, CBC, blood glucose if patient is on long-term therapy; if LFTs increase, therapy should be discontinued

• Bowel pattern daily; watch for increasing diarrhea (common)

Administer:

PO route

• 30 min before morning and evening meals

Evaluate:

• Therapeutic response: decreased cholesterol, triglyceride levels, HDL, cholesterol ratios improved

Teach patient/family:

• That compliance is needed for positive results; do not double or skip dose

• That risk factors should be decreased: high-fat diet, smoking, alcohol consumption, absence of exercise

• To notify prescriber of diarrhea, nausea, vomiting, chills, fever, sore throat, muscle cramps, abdominal cramps, severe flatulence

• That drug may be discontinued, if no improvement in 3 mo

HIGH ALERT

gemtuzumab (℞)

(gem-tue-zue′mab)

Mylotarg

Func. class.: Misc. antineoplastic

Chem. class.: Monoclonal antibody

Action: Composed of recombinant humanized IgG_4 kappa antibody, binds to CD33 antigen that is released in myeloid cells

Uses: Acute myeloid leukemia (AML)

Dosage and routes:

• *Adult:* **IV** 9 mg/m^2 as a 2 hr inf; before giving inf, give diphenhydrAMINE 50 mg **PO,** acetaminophen 650-1000 mg **PO** 1 hr prior to inf; then use acetaminophen 650-1000 mg q1-4h prn

Available forms: Powder for inj, lyophilized 5 mg

Side effects/adverse reactions:

CNS: Dizziness, insomnia, depression

CV: Hypertension, hemorrhage, tachycardia, hypotension

INTEG: Rash, herpes simplex, local reaction, petechiae

GI: Anorexia, diarrhea, constipation, nausea, stomatitis, vomiting

GU: Hematuria, vaginal hemorrhage

MISC: Fever, myalgias, headache, chills

RESP: Cough, pneumonia, epistaxis, rhinitis

META: Hypokalemia, hypomagnesemia

Contraindications: Hypersensitivity, pregnancy (D), severe myelosuppression

Precautions: Lactation, children, severe renal or hepatic disease

Pharmacokinetics: Half-life 45 and 100 hr, respectively

NURSING CONSIDERATIONS

Assess:

- For symptoms of infection; chills, fever, headache, may be masked by drug fever
- CNS reaction: LOC, mental status, dizziness, confusion
- Cardiac status: Lung sounds; ECG before and during treatment, especially in those with cardiac disease
- Bone marrow depression: bruising, bleeding, blood in stools, urine, sputum, emesis

Administer:

- Do not give IV push or bolus
- Protect from light, use biologic safety hood, allow to come to room temp
- Reconstitute each vial with 5 ml sterile water for inj using sterile syringes, swirl each vial, check for discoloration or particulate matter, give over 2 hr, use a separate line with 1.2 micron terminal filter

Perform/provide:

- Storage of reconstituted sol for ≤8 hr in refrigerator

Evaluate:

- Therapeutic response: decrease in size, number of lesions

Teach patient/family:

- To take acetaminophen for fever
- To avoid hazardous tasks, since confusion, dizziness may occur; avoid prolonged sunlight, use sunscreen
- To report signs of infection: sore throat, fever, diarrhea, vomiting

gentamicin (℞)

(jen-ta-mye'sin)

Cidomycin✱, Garamycin, gentamicin sulfate, G-Mycin, Jenamicin

Func. class.: Antiinfective

Chem. class.: Aminoglycoside

Action: Interferes with protein synthesis in bacterial cell by binding to ribosomal subunit, causing misreading of genetic code; inaccurate peptide sequence forms in protein chain, causing bacterial death

Uses: Severe systemic infections of CNS, respiratory, GI, urinary tract, bone, skin, soft tissues caused by susceptible strains of *Pseudomonas aeruginosa, Proteus, Klebsiella, Serratia, Escherichia coli, Enterobacter, Citrobacter, Staphylococcus, Shigella, Salmonella, Acinetobacter*, acute PID

Dosage and routes:

Severe systemic infections

- *Adult:* **IV INF** 3-5 mg/kg/day in 3 divided doses q8h; dilute in 50-200 ml 0.9% NaCl or D_5W given over 30 min-1 hr; **IM** 3 mg/kg/day in divided doses q8h
- *Child:* **IV/IM** 2-2.5 mg/kg q8h
- *Neonate and infant:* **IV/IM** 2.5 mg/kg q8-12h
- *Neonate <1 wk:* 2.5 mg/kg q12-24h

Once daily dosing/extended interval dosing (unlabeled)

- *Adult:* **IV** 4-7 mg/kg/q24h, adjust according to levels

Renal dose

- *Adult:* **IV/IM** 1-1.7 mg/kg initially, then adjust according to levels

Available forms: Inj 10, 40 mg/ml; premixed inj 40, 60, 70, 80, 100 mg/50 ml; 40, 60, 80, 90, 100, 120, 160, 180 mg/ml

Side effects/adverse reactions:
GU: ***Oliguria, hematuria, renal damage, azotemia, renal failure, nephrotoxicity***
CNS: Confusion, depression, numbness, tremors, ***convulsions,*** muscle twitching, ***neurotoxicity,*** dizziness, vertigo
EENT: ***Ototoxicity,*** *deafness,* visual disturbances, tinnitus
HEMA: ***Agranulocytosis, thrombocytopenia, leukopenia, eosinophilia,*** anemia
GI: Nausea, vomiting, anorexia; increased ALT, AST, bilirubin; hepatomegaly, ***hepatic necrosis,*** splenomegaly
CV: Hypotension, hypertension, palpitations
INTEG: Rash, burning, urticaria, dermatitis, alopecia
Contraindications: Severe renal disease, hypersensitivity
Precautions: Neonates, mild renal disease, pregnancy (C), hearing deficits, myasthenia gravis, lactation, elderly, Parkinson's disease
Do not confuse:
Geramycin/kanamycin
Pharmacokinetics:
IM: Onset rapid, peak 1-2 hr
IV: Onset immediate, peak 1-2 hr; plasma half-life 1-2 hr, infants 6-7 hr; duration 6-8 hr; not metabolized; excreted unchanged in urine; crosses placental barrier; poor penetration into CSF
Interactions:
- ↑ ototoxicity, neurotoxicity, nephrotoxicity: other aminoglycosides, amphotericin B, polymyxin, vancomycin, ethacrynic acid, furosemide, mannitol, methoxyflurane, cisplatin, cephalosporins, penicillins
- ↑ effects: nondepolarizing neuromuscular blockers

NURSING CONSIDERATIONS
Assess:
- Weight before treatment; calculation of dosage is usually based on ideal body weight, but may be calculated on actual body weight
- I&O ratio, urinalysis daily for proteinuria, cells, casts; report sudden change in urine output; toxicity is increased in patients with decreased renal function if high doses are given
- VS during infusion; watch for hypotension, change in pulse
- IV site for thrombophlebitis, including pain, redness, swelling, q30min, change site if needed; discontinue, apply warm compresses to site
- Serum peak, drawn at 30-60 min after IV inf or 60 min after IM inj, and trough level drawn just before next dose; blood level should be 2-4 times bacteriostatic level; peak = 4-12 mcg/ml, trough = 1-2 mcg/ml
- Urine pH if drug is used for UTI; urine should be kept alkaline
- Renal impairment by securing urine for CCr testing, BUN, serum creatinine; lower dosage should be given in renal impairment (CCr <80 ml/min)
- Deafness by audiometric testing, ringing, roaring in ears, vertigo; assess hearing before, during, after treatment
- Dehydration: high specific gravity, decrease in skin turgor, dry mucous membranes, dark urine
- Overgrowth of infection including fever, malaise, redness, pain, swelling, perineal itching, diarrhea, stomatitis, change in cough or sputum
- C&S before starting treatment to identify infecting organism
- Vestibular dysfunction: nausea, vomiting, dizziness, headache; drug should be discontinued if severe
- Injection sites for redness, swelling, abscesses; use warm compresses at site

Administer:
- IM inj in large muscle mass; rotate inj sites
- Drug in evenly spaced doses to maintain blood level
- Bicarbonate to alkalinize urine if ordered for UTI, as drug is most active in alkaline environment

IV route
- After diluting in 50-200 ml NS or D_5W; sol concentration should be 1 mg/ml or less; decrease vol of diluent in child; maintain 0.1% sol run over ½-1 hr (adults) or up to 2 hr (children); flush IV line with NS or D_5W after administration

Additive compatibilities: Atracurium, aztreonam, bleomycin, cefoxitin, cimetidine, ciprofloxacin, fluconazole, meropenem, methicillin, metronidazole, ofloxacin, penicillin G sodium, ranitidine, verapamil

Syringe compatibilities: Clindamycin, methicillin, penicillin G sodium

Y-site compatibilities: Acyclovir, amifostine, amiodarone, amsacrine, atracurium, aztreonam, cefpirome, ciprofloxacin, cyclophosphamide, cytarabine, diltiazem, enalaprilat, esmolol, famotidine, filgrastim, fluconazole, fludarabine, foscarnet, granisetron, hydromorphone, IL-2, insulin, labetalol, lorazepam, magnesium sulfate, melphalan, meperidine, meropenem, midazolam, morphine, multivitamins, ondansetron, paclitaxel, pancuronium, perphenazine, sargramostim, tacrolimus, teniposide, theophylline, thiotepa, tolazine, vecuronium, vinorelbine, vit B/C, zidovudine

Perform/provide:
- Adequate fluids of 2-3 L/day, unless contraindicated, to prevent irritation of tubules
- Supervised ambulation, other safety measures with vestibular dysfunction

Evaluate:
- Therapeutic response: absence of fever, draining wounds, negative C&S after treatment

Teach patient/family:
- To report headache, dizziness, symptoms of overgrowth of infection, renal impairment
- To report loss of hearing, ringing, roaring in ears, or feeling of fullness in head

gentamicin ophthalmic

See appendix c

gentamicin topical

See appendix c

glatiramer (℞)

(glah-tear′a-meer)

Copaxone

Func. class.: Multiple sclerosis agent

Action: Unknown, may modify the immune responses responsible for multiple sclerosis (MS)

Uses: Reduction of the frequency of relapses in patients with relapsing-remitting MS

Dosage and routes:
- *Adult:* **SC** 20 mg/day

Available forms: Inj 20 mg/ml

Side effects/adverse reactions:

CV: Migraine, palpitations, syncope, tachycardia, vasodilation

GI: Nausea, vomiting, diarrhea, anorexia, gastroenteritis

HEMA: Ecchymosis, lymphadenopathy

META: Edema, weight gain

MS: Arthralgia

CNS: Anxiety, hypertonia, tremor,

vertigo, speech disorder, agitation, confusion
RESP: Bronchitis, dyspnea
INTEG: Pruritus, rash, sweating, urticaria, erythema
EENT: Ear pain
GU: Urinary urgency, dysmenorrhea, vaginal moniliasis
Contraindications: Hypersensitivity to this drug or mannitol
Precautions: Immune disorders, renal disease, pregnancy (B), lactation
Pharmacokinetics: Unknown

NURSING CONSIDERATIONS

Assess:
• Blood, renal, hepatic studies: prior to treatment
• For CNS symptoms: anxiety, confusion, vertigo
• GI status: diarrhea, vomiting, abdominal pain, gastroenteritis
• Cardiac status: tachycardia, palpitations, vasodilation, chest pain

Administer:
• SC route
• Using a sterile syringe/needle to transfer the supplied diluent into the vial, rotate vial gently, do not shake; withdraw medication using a syringe with 27G needle; administer SC into hip, thigh, arm; discard unused portion
• Use SC route only; do not give IM or IV
• Do not use sol that contains precipitate or is discolored
• Use immediately

Evaluate:
• Therapeutic response: decreased symptoms of MS

Teach patient/family:
• Give written, detailed instructions about the drug; provide initial and return demonstrations on inj procedure; give information on use and disposal of drug
• That blurred vision, sweating may occur
• That irregular menses, dysmenorrhea, or metrorrhagia as well as breast pain may occur; use contraception during treatment
• That if pregnancy is suspected, or if nursing, notify prescriber
• Not to change dosing or to stop taking drug without advice of prescriber

* glipiZIDE (℞)
(glip-i′zide)
Glucotrol, Glucotrol XL

glimepiride
(glye-me′pi-ride)
Amaryl

Func. class.: Antidiabetic
Chem. class.: Sulfonylurea (2nd generation)

Action: Causes functioning β-cells in pancreas to release insulin, leading to drop in blood glucose levels; may improve insulin binding to insulin receptors or increase the number of insulin receptors with prolonged administration; may also reduce basal hepatic glucose secretion; not effective if patient lacks functioning β-cells
Uses: Stable adult-onset diabetes mellitus (type 2)
Dosage and routes:
GlipiZIDE
• *Adult:* **PO** 5 mg initially, then increase to desired response; max 40 mg/day in divided doses or 15 mg/dose
• *Elderly/hepatic disease:* **PO** 2.5 mg initially, then increase to desired response; max 40 mg/day in divided doses or 15 mg/dose
Glimepiride
• *Adult:* **PO** 1-2 mg qd, then increase q1-2wk up to 8 mg/day
Renal dose
Adult: **PO** CCr <20 ml/min, 1 mg

qd with breakfast, may titrate upward as needed

Available forms: *glipiZIDE:* tabs 5, 10 mg scored; ext rel tab 5, 10 mg; *glimepiride:* tabs 1, 2, 4 mg

Side effects/adverse reactions:

CNS: Headache, weakness, dizziness, drowsiness, tinnitus, fatigue, vertigo

GI: ***Hepatotoxicity, cholestatic jaundice,*** nausea, vomiting, diarrhea, heartburn

HEMA: ***Leukopenia, thrombocytopenia, agranulocytosis, aplastic anemia;*** increased AST, ALT, alk phosphatase; ***pancytopenia, hemolytic anemia***

INTEG: Rash, allergic reactions, pruritus, urticaria, eczema, photosensitivity, erythema

ENDO: ***Hypoglycemia***

Contraindications: Hypersensitivity to sulfonylureas, juvenile or type 1 diabetes, diabetic ketoacidosis

Precautions: Pregnancy (C), elderly, cardiac disease, severe renal disease, severe hepatic disease, thyroid disease

Do not confuse:

glipiZIDE/Glucotrol/glyBURIDE

Pharmacokinetics:

PO: Completely absorbed by GI route, onset 1-1½ hr, peak 1-3 hr, duration 10-24 hr, half-life 2-4 hr; metabolized in liver; excreted in urine; 90%-95% is plasma protein bound

Interactions:

• ↑ action of: digitalis, glycosides

• ↑ hypoglycemic effects: insulin, MAOIs, cimetidine, chloramphenicol, guanethidine, methyldopa, nonsteroidal antiinflammatories, salicylates, probenecid, androgens, anticoagulants, clofibrate, fenfluramine, fluconazole, gemfibrozil, histamine H_2 antagonists, magnesium salts, phenylbutazone, sulfinpyrazone, sulfonamides, tricyclics, urinary acidifiers

• Effect may be ↓: thiazide diuretics, rifampin, isoniazid, cholestyramine, diazoxide, hydantoins, urinary alkalinizers, charcoal

• May mask symptoms of hypoglycemia: β-blockers

↓ hypoglycemic effect: broom, buchu, dandelion, glucosamine, juniper

↑ or ↓ hypoglycemic effect: chromium, fenugreek, ginseng, coenzyme Q-10

↑ glucose tolerance: karela

↓ antidiabetic effect: bee pollen, blue cohosh, broom, chromium, elecampane, eucalyptus, gotu kola

↑ antidiabetic effect: alfalfa, aloe, basil, bay, bilberry, bitter melon, black catechu, buchu, burdock, coriander, dandelion, eyebright (po), fenugreek, garlic, ginseng, glucomannan, glucosamine, goat's rue, gymnema, horehound, horse chestnut, jambul, myrrh, myrtle

NURSING CONSIDERATIONS

Assess:

• Blood, urine glucose, glycosylated Hgb levels during treatment to determine diabetes control

• CBC baseline and throughout treatment

• Hypo/hyperglycemic reaction that can occur soon after meals; for severe hypoglycemia give IV $D_{50}W$, then IV dextrose solution

Administer:

• Drug 30 min before meals; if patient is NPO, may need to hold dose to prevent hypoglycemia

• May crush tabs and mix with fluids, if unable to swallow whole

Do not crush, break, or chew ext rel tabs

Perform/provide:
• Storage in tight, light-resistant container at room temperature

Evaluate:
• Therapeutic response: decrease in polyuria, polydipsia, polyphagia, clear sensorium, absence of dizziness, stable gait

Teach patient/family:
• Not to drink alcohol; explain disulfiram reaction (nausea, headache, cramps, flushing, hypoglycemia)
• To check for symptoms of cholestatic jaundice: dark urine, pruritus, yellow sclera; prescriber should be notified
• The symptoms of hypo/hyperglycemia, what to do about each; to have glucagon emergency kit available, carry sugar packets
• That drug must be continued on daily basis; explain consequence of discontinuing drug abruptly
• To take drug in morning to prevent hypoglycemic reactions at night
• To use sunscreen or stay out of the sun to prevent photosensitivity
• To avoid OTC medications unless ordered by prescriber
• That diabetes is a lifelong illness; drug will not cure disease
• That all food in diet plan must be eaten to prevent hypoglycemia
• To carry emergency ID with prescriber and medications
• To test urine for glucose/ketones tid if this drug is replacing insulin; to use a capillary blood glucose test while on this drug
• To continue weight control, dietary restrictions, exercise, hygiene
• Ext rel tab may appear in stool

Treatment of overdose: Glucose 25 g IV via dextrose 50% solution 50 ml or 1 mg glucagon

*glyBURIDE (℞)

(glye'byoor-ide)

Apo-Glyburide✤, DiaBeta✤, Euglucon✤, Gen-Glybe✤, Glynase PresTab, Micronase, Novo-Glyburide✤, Nu-Glyburide✤

Func. class.: Antidiabetic

Chem. class.: Sulfonylurea (2nd generation)

Action: Causes functioning β-cells in pancreas to release insulin, leading to drop in blood glucose levels; may improve insulin binding to insulin receptors and increase number of insulin receptors with prolonged administration; may also reduce basal hepatic glucose secretion; not effective if patient lacks functioning β-cells

Uses: Stable adult-onset diabetes mellitus (type 2)

Dosage and routes:

DiaBeta/Micronase
• *Adult:* **PO** 1.25-5 mg initially, then increased to desired response at weekly intervals up to 20 mg/day
• *Elderly:* **PO** 1.25 mg initially, then increased to desired response; max 20 mg/day, maintenance 1.25-20 mg/qd

Glynase PresTab (micronized)
• *Adult:* **PO** 1.5-3 mg/day initially, may increase by 1.5 mg/wk, max 12 mg/day
• *Elderly:* **PO** 0.75-3 mg/day, may increase by 1.5 mg/wk

Available forms: (Diabeta) Tabs 1.25, 2.5, 5 mg; (Glynase PresTab) 1.5, 3, 6 mg

Side effects/adverse reactions:

CNS: Headache, weakness, paresthesia, tinnitus, fatigue, vertigo

GI: Nausea, fullness, heartburn, ***hepatotoxicity, cholestatic jaundice,*** vomiting, diarrhea

HEMA: ***Leukopenia, thrombocytopenia, agranulocytosis, aplastic anemia,*** increased AST, ALT, alk phosphatase
INTEG: Rash, allergic reactions, pruritus, urticaria, eczema, photosensitivity, erythema
ENDO: ***Hypoglycemia***
MS: Joint pain

Contraindications: Hypersensitivity to sulfonylureas, juvenile or type 1 diabetes, diabetic ketoacidosis

Precautions: Pregnancy (B), elderly, cardiac disease, severe renal disease, severe hepatic disease, thyroid disease, severe hypoglycemic reactions

Do not confuse:
glyBURIDE/Glucotrol/glipiZIDE
DiaBeta/Zebeta

Pharmacokinetics:
PO: Completely absorbed by GI route; onset 2-4 hr, peak 4 hr, duration 24 hr; half-life 10 hr; metabolized in liver; excreted in urine, feces (metabolites); crosses placenta; 99% is plasma protein bound

Interactions:
- Both drugs' effects may be ↓: diazoxide
- ↑ level: digoxin
- ↑ hypoglycemic effects: insulin, MAOIs, oral anticoagulants, chloramphenicol, guanethidine, methyldopa, NSAIDs, salicylates, probenecid, androgens, fenfluramine, fluconazole, gemfibrozil, histamine H_2 antagonists, magnesium salts, phenylbutazone, sulfinpyrazone, sulfonamides, tricyclics, urinary acidifiers
- ↓ glyBURIDE action: thiazide diuretics, rifampin, isoniazid, cholestyramine, diazoxide, hydantoins, urinary alkalinizers, charcoal
- Mask symptoms of hypoglycemia: β-blockers

↓ antidiabetic effect: bee pollen, blue cohosh, broom, chromium, elecampane, eucalyptus, gotu kola

↑ antidiabetic effect: alfalfa, aloe, basil, bay, bilberry, bitter melon, black catechu, buchu, burdock, coriander, dandelion, eyebright (po), fenugreek, garlic, ginseng, glucomannan, glucosamine, goat's rue, gymnema, horehound, horse chestnut, jambul, myrrh, myrtle

↓ hypoglycemic effect: broom, buchu, dandelion, glucosamine, juniper

↑ or ↓ hypoglycemic effect: chromium, coenzyme Q-10, fenugreek, ginseng

↑ glucose tolerance: karela

NURSING CONSIDERATIONS

Assess:
- Hypo/hyperglycemic reaction that can occur soon after meals; for severe hypoglycemia, give IV $D_{50}W$, then IV dextrose sol
- Blood, urine glucose; glycosylated Hgb levels during treatment
- CBC baseline and throughout treatment

Administer:
- With breakfast, hold dose if NPO to avoid hypoglycemia

Perform/provide:
- Storage in tight container in cool environment

Evaluate:
- Therapeutic response: decrease in polyuria, polydipsia, polyphagia, clear sensorium, absence of dizziness, stable gait

Teach patient/family:
- To check for symptoms of cholestatic jaundice: dark urine, pruritus, jaundiced sclera; if these occur, notify prescriber
- To use a capillary blood glucose test while on this drug
- The symptoms of hypo/hyperglycemia, what to do about each
- That drug must be continued on

daily basis; explain consequence of discontinuing drug abruptly
• To take drug in morning to prevent hypoglycemic reactions at night
• To avoid OTC medications unless ordered by prescriber
• That diabetes is a lifelong illness; drug will not cure disease
• That all food included in diet plan must be eaten to prevent hypoglycemia; to have glucagon emergency kit, sugar packets available
• To use sunscreen or stay out of the sun to prevent photosensitivity
• To carry an emergency ID with prescriber and medications

Treatment of overdose: Glucose 25 g IV via dextrose 50% sol, 50 ml or 1 mg glucagon

RARELY USED

glycerin (OTC)

(gli'ser-in)
Fleet Babylax, Glycerin USP, Glycerol, Osmoglyn, Sani-Supp
Func. class.: Laxative, hyperosmotic

Uses: Constipation, intraocular pressure reduction
Dosage and routes:
Laxative
• *Adult and child >6 yr:* **RECT SUPP** 3 g; **ENEMA** 5-15 ml
• *Child <6 yr:* **RECT SUPP** 1-1.5 g; **ENEMA** 2-5 ml
Intraocular pressure reduction
• *Adult:* **PO** 1-1.5 g/kg once, then may be given 500 mg/kg q6h
• *Child:* **PO** 1-1.5 g/kg once, then 500 mg/kg 4-8 hr after first dose
Contraindications: Hypersensitivity

glycopyrrolate (℞)

(glye-koe-pye'roe-late)
glycopyrrolate, Robinul, Robinul-Forte
Func. class.: Cholinergic blocker
Chem. class.: Quaternary ammonium compound

Action: Inhibits the action of acetylcholine at receptor sites in autonomic nervous system, which controls secretions, free acids in stomach
Uses: Decreased secretions before surgery, reversal of neuromuscular blockade, peptic ulcer disease, irritable bowel syndrome
Investigational uses: Drooling
Dosage and routes:
Preoperatively
• *Adult:* **IM** 4.4 mcg/kg ½-1 hr before surgery, max 0.1 mg
• *Child:* **IM** 4.4-8.8 mcg/kg
Reversal of neuromuscular blockade
• *Adult and child:* **IV** 200 mcg for each 1 mg of neostigmine or 5 mg **IV** of pyridostigmine simultaneously
GI disorders
• *Adult:* **PO** 1-2 mg bid-tid; **IM/IV** 100-200 mcg tid-qid, titrated to patient response
Antidysrhythmic
• *Adult:* **IV** 100 mcg, may repeat q2min
• *Child:* **IV** 4.4 mcg/kg, may repeat q2min, max 100 mcg
Drooling
• *Adult:* **PO** doses vary widely
Available forms: Tabs 1, 2 mg; inj 200 mcg (0.2 mg)/ml
Side effects/adverse reactions:
INTEG: Urticaria, allergic reactions
MISC: Suppression of lactation, nasal congestion, decreased sweating
CNS: Confusion, anxiety, restless-

ness, irritability, delusions, hallucinations, headache, sedation, depression, incoherence, dizziness, lethargy, flushing, weakness
EENT: Blurred vision, photophobia, dilated pupils, difficulty swallowing, increased intraocular pressure, mydriasis, cycloplegia
CV: Palpitations, tachycardia, postural hypotension, paradoxical bradycardia
GI: Dryness of mouth, constipation, nausea, vomiting, abdominal distress, paralytic ileus, altered taste perception
SYST: ***Anaphylaxis***
GU: Urinary hesitancy, retention, impotence

Contraindications: Hypersensitivity, narrow-angle glaucoma, myasthenia gravis, GI/GU obstruction, child <3 yr, tachycardia, myocardial ischemia, hepatic disease, ulcerative colitis, toxic megacolon

Precautions: Pregnancy (B), elderly, lactation, prostatic hypertrophy, renal disease, CHF, pulmonary disease, hyperthyroidism

Pharmacokinetics:
PO: Peak 1 hr, duration 8-12 hr
IM: Peak 30-45 min, duration 2-7 hr
IV: Peak 10-15 min, duration 2-7 hr; excreted in urine (50%) (unchanged); half-life 1-2 hr

Interactions:
- ↑ anticholinergic effect: alcohol, antihistamines, phenothiazines, amantadine, tricyclics
- ↓ glycopyrrolate absorption: antacids, antidiarrheals

NURSING CONSIDERATIONS
Assess:
- I&O ratio; retention commonly causes decreased urinary output
- Urinary hesitancy, retention: palpate bladder if retention occurs
- Constipation; increase fluids, bulk, exercise if this occurs
- Mental status: affect, mood, CNS depression, worsening of mental symptoms during early therapy

Administer:
- Parenteral dose with patient recumbent to prevent postural hypotension
- Parenteral dose slowly; keep in bed for at least 1 hr after dose; monitor VS
- After checking dose carefully; even slight overdose may lead to toxicity
- With or after meals to prevent GI upset; may give with fluids other than water

IV route
- Undiluted, give through a Y-tube or 3-way stopcock; give 0.2 mg or less over 1-2 min

Syringe compatibilities: Atropine, benzquinamide, chlorproMAZINE, cimetidine, codeine, diphenhydrAMINE, droperidol, droperidol/fentanyl, hydromorphone, hydrOXYzine, levorphanol, lidocaine, meperidine, meperidine/promethazine, midazolam, morphine, nalbuphine, neostigmine, oxymorphone, procaine, prochlorperazine, promazine, promethazine, pyridostigmine, ranitidine, scopolamine, triflupromazine, trimethobenzamide

Solution compatibilities: D_5W, 0.9% NaCl, Ringer's, D_5/0.45% NaCl

Perform/provide:
- Storage at room temperature

Evaluate:
- Therapeutic response: decreased secretions; decreased pain in GI disorders; reversal of neuromuscular blockers

Teach patient/family:
- Hard candy, frequent drinks, sugarless gum to relieve dry mouth
- Not to discontinue this drug abruptly; to taper off over 1 wk; to take PO ½-1 hr ac

• To avoid driving, other hazardous activities; drowsiness, blurred vision may occur
• To avoid OTC medication: cough, cold preparations with alcohol, antihistamines unless directed by prescriber
• To avoid hot temperatures, since sweating is decreased, heat stroke is possible
• To change positions slowly to prevent orthostatic hypotension
• To notify prescriber of eye pain, blurred vision, light sensitivity

goserelin (℞)

(goe'se-rel-lin)
Zoladex

Func. class.: Gonadotropin-releasing hormone, antineoplastic (hormone)

Chem. class.: Synthetic decapeptide analog of LHRH

Action: Inhibitor of pituitary gonadotropin secretion; initially increases LH and FSH, with increases in testosterone, reduction in sex steroid levels (substitute serum testosterone levels)

Uses: Advanced prostate cancer (10.8 mg), endometriosis, advanced breast cancer, endometrial thinning (3.6 mg)

Dosage and routes:
• *Adult:* **SC** 3.6 mg q4wk or 10.8 mg q12wk

Endometrial thinning
• *Adult:* **SC** 1-2 depot inj, usually 1 depot, surgery performed at 4 wk, if 2 depots, surgery performed 2-4 wk after 2nd depot

Available forms: Depot inj 3.6, 10.8 mg

Side effects/adverse reactions:
CNS: Headaches, ***spinal cord compression,*** anxiety, depression
CV: ***Dysrhythmia, cerebrovascular accident,*** hypertension, ***MI,*** chest pain
ENDO: Gynecomastia, breast tenderness, hot flashes
GI: Nausea, vomiting, constipation, diarrhea, ulcer
GU: Spotting, breakthrough bleeding, decreased libido, renal insufficiency, urinary obstruction, urinary tract infection, impotence
INTEG: Rash, pain on inj
MS: Osteoneuralgia

Contraindications: Hypersensitivity to LHRH, LHRH-agonist analogs, pregnancy (D) (breast cancer), (X)—endometriosis, lactation, nondiagnosed vaginal bleeding

Pharmacokinetics: Peak serum concentrations in 14-28 days; half-life 4½ hr

Lab test interferences:
Increase: Alk phosphatase, estradiol, FSH, LH, testosterone levels
Decrease: Testosterone levels, progesterone

NURSING CONSIDERATIONS

Assess:
• I&O ratios; palpate bladder for distention in urinary obstruction
• For relief of bone pain (back pain), change in motor function
• Acid phosphatase PSA baseline and periodically

Administer:

Depot
• SC using implant, inserted by qualified person into upper subcutaneous tissue in abdominal wall q28d or q12wk (10.8 mg)

Evaluate:
• Therapeutic response: more normal levels of prostate-specific antigen, acid phosphatase, alk phosphatase; testosterone level of <25 ng/dl

Teach patient/family:
• That gynecomastia and postmeno-

pausal symptoms may occur but will decrease after treatment is discontinued
• That bone pain may increase, then decrease
• To notify prescriber of difficulty urinating, hot flashes
• To keep appointments
• Not to breastfeed while taking drug

granisetron (℞)

(grane-iss'e-tron)

Kytril

Func. class.: Antiemetic

Chem. class.: 5-HT_3 receptor antagonist

Action: Prevents nausea, vomiting by blocking serotonin peripherally, centrally, and in the small intestine

Uses: Prevention of nausea, vomiting associated with cancer chemotherapy including high-dose cisplatin

Investigational uses: Acute nausea, vomiting following surgery

Dosage and routes:

Nausea, vomiting in chemotherapy

• *Adult and child:* **IV** 10 mcg/kg over 5 min, 30 min before the start of cancer chemotherapy
• *Adult:* **PO** 1 mg bid, give first dose 1 hr before chemotherapy and next dose 12 hr after first

Nausea, vomiting in radiation therapy

• *Adult:* **PO** 2 mg qd 1 hr prior to radiation

Available forms: Inj 1 mg/ml; tab 1 mg

Side effects/adverse reactions:

CNS: Headache, asthenia, anxiety, dizziness

CV: Hypertension

GI: Diarrhea, *constipation,* increased AST, ALT, *nausea*

HEMA: ***Leukopenia,*** anemia, ***thrombocytopenia***

MISC: Rash, ***bronchospasm***

Contraindications: Hypersensitivity

Precautions: Pregnancy (B), lactation, children, elderly

Pharmacokinetics: Metabolized in liver to an active metabolite, half-life 10-12 hr

NURSING CONSIDERATIONS

Assess:

• For absence of nausea, vomiting during chemotherapy
• Hypersensitive reaction: rash, bronchospasm

Administer:

IV direct route

• Dilute in 0.9% NaCl for inj or D_5W (20-50 ml); give over 5-15 min; ½ hr before chemotherapy

Additive compatibilities: Dexamethasone, methylPREDNISolone

Solution compatibilities: D_5W, 0.9% NaCl

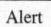

Y-site compatibilities: Acyclovir, allopurinol, amifostine, amikacin, aminophylline, amphotericin B cholesteryl, ampicillin, ampicillin/sulbactam, amsacrine, aztreonam, bleomycin, bumetanide, buprenorphine, butorphanol, calcium gluconate, carboplatin, carmustine, cefazolin, cefepime, cefonicid, cefoperazone, cefotaxime, cefotetan, cefoxitin, ceftazidime, ceftizoxime, ceftriaxone, cefuroxime, chlorproMAZINE, cimetidine, ciprofloxacin, cisplatin, cladribine, clindamycin, cyclophosphamide, cytarabine, dacarbazine, dactinomycin, DAUNOrubicin, dexamethasone, diphenhydrAMINE, DOBUTamine, DOPamine, DOXOrubicin, DOXOrubicin liposome, doxycycline, droperidol, enalaprilat, etoposide, famotidine, filgrastim, fluconazole, fluorouracil, floxuridine, fludarabine, furosemide, gallium, ganciclovir, gentamicin, haloperidol, heparin hydrocortisone, hydromorphone, hydrOXYzine, idarubicin, ifosfamide, imipenem-cilastatin, leucovorin, lorazepam, magnesium sulfate, melphalan, meperidine, mesna, methotrexate, methylPREDNISolone, metoclopramide, metronidazole, mezlocillin, miconazole, minocycline, mitomycin, mitoxantrone, morphine, nalbuphine, netilmicin, ofloxacin, paclitaxel, piperacillin, piperacillin/tazobactam, plicamycin, potassium chloride, prochlorperazine, promethazine, propofol, ranitidine, sargramostim, sodium bicarbonate, streptozocin, teniposide, thiotepa, ticarcillin, ticarcillin/clavulanate, tobramycin, trimethoprim - sulfamethoxazole, vancomycin, vinBLAStine, vinCRIStine, vinorelbine, zidovudine

Perform/provide:

• Storage at room temperature for 24 hr after dilution

Evaluate:

• Therapeutic response: absence of nausea, vomiting during cancer chemotherapy

Teach patient/family:

• To report diarrhea, constipation, rash, changes in respirations

RARELY USED

griseofulvin microsize (℞)

(gris-ee-oh-ful'vin)

Fulvicin-U/F, Grifulvin V, Grisactin, Grisovin-FP✤

griseofulvin ultramicrosize (℞)

Fulvicin P/G, Grisactin Ultra, Gris-PEG

Func. class.: Antifungal

Uses: Mycotic infections: tinea corporis, tinea pedis, tinea cruris, tinea barbae, tinea capitis, tinea unguium if caused by *Epidermophyton, Microsporum, Trichophyton*

Dosage and routes:

• *Adult:* **PO** 500-1000 mg qd in single or divided doses (microsize), 125-165 mg bid (ultramicrosize) or 250-330 mg qd; may need 500-660 mg in divided doses for severe infections

• *Child:* **PO** 10 mg/kg/day or 30 mg/m^2/day (microsize) or 5 mg/kg/day (ultramicrosize)

Contraindications: Hypersensitivity, porphyria, hepatic disease, lupus erythematosus

G

guaifenesin (OTC, ℞)

(gwye-fen'e-sin)

Anti-Tuss, Benylin-E♣, Breonesin, Calmylin Expectorant♣, Diabetic Tussin Ex, Duratuss-G, Fenesin, Gee-Gee, Genatuss, GG-Cen, Glyate, Glycotuss, Glytuss, guaifenesin, Guaifenex LA, Guiatuss, Halotussin, Humibid, Humibid L.A., Hytuss, Hytuss 2X, Liquibid, Monafed, Muco-Fen-LA, Mytussin, Naldecon Senior EX, Organidin NR, Pneumomist, Respa-GF, Resyl♣, Robitussin, Scot-Tussin Expectorant, Sinumist-SR, Unitussin

Func. class.: Expectorant

Action: Acts as an expectorant by stimulating a gastric mucosal reflex to increase the production of lung mucus

Uses: Dry, nonproductive cough

Dosage and routes:

• *Adult:* **PO** 200-400 mg q4-6h, not to exceed 1.2 g/day; **EXT REL** 600-1200 mg q12h, not to exceed 2.4 g/day

• *Child 6-12 yr:* **PO** 100-200 mg q4h; 600 mg q12h **(EXT REL)** not to exceed 1.2 g/day

• *Child 2-6 yr:* **PO** 50-100 mg q4h; not to exceed 600 mg/day

Available forms: Tabs 100, 200 mg; tabs, ext rel 600, 1200 mg; caps 200 mg; caps, ext rel 300 mg; syr 100, 200 mg/5 ml

Side effects/adverse reactions:

CNS: Drowsiness

GI: Nausea, anorexia, vomiting

Contraindications: Hypersensitivity, persistent cough

Precautions: Pregnancy (C)

NURSING CONSIDERATIONS

Assess:

• Cough: type, frequency, character, including sputum; fluids should be increased to 2 L/day

Perform/provide:

• Storage at room temperature

• Increased fluids, room humidification to liquefy secretions

Evaluate:

• Therapeutic response: absence of cough

Teach patient/family:

• To avoid driving, other hazardous activities if drowsiness occurs (rare)

• To avoid smoking, smoke-filled room, perfumes, dust, environmental pollutants, cleansers

---

RARELY USED

guanfacine (℞)

(gwahn'fa-seen)

Func. class.: Antihypertensive

Uses: Hypertension in individual using a thiazide diuretic or other antihypertensive

Investigational uses: Heroin withdrawal

Dosage and routes:

• *Adult:* **PO** 1 mg/day hs; may increase dose in 3-4 wk to 2 mg/day

Contraindications: Hypersensitivity

RARELY USED

halcinonide (℞)

(hal-sin'oh-nide)

Func. class.: Corticosteroid, synthetic

Uses: Inflammation of corticosteroid-responsive dermatoses

Dosage and routes:
• *Adult:* **TOP** apply to affected area bid-tid (not around eyes)
Contraindications: Hypersensitivity, viral infections, fungal infections

halcinonide topical

See appendix c

halobetasol topical

See appendix c

haloperidol (℞)

(hal-oh-pehr'ih-dol)
Apo-Haloperidol✤, Haldol, Novo-Peridol✤, Peridol✤

haloperidol decanoate (℞)

Haldol Decanoate, Haldol LA✤

haloperidol lactate (℞)

Haldol, Haloperidol Injection, Haloperidol Intensol
Func. class.: Antipsychotic, neuroleptic
Chem. class.: Butyrophenone

Action: Depresses cerebral cortex, hypothalamus, limbic system, which control activity and aggression; blocks neurotransmission produced by dopamine at synapse; exhibits strong α-adrenergic, anticholinergic blocking action; mechanism for antipsychotic effects unclear
Uses: Psychotic disorders, control of tics, vocal utterances in Gilles de la Tourette's syndrome, short-term treatment of hyperactive children showing excessive motor activity, prolonged parenteral therapy in chronic schizophrenia, control of severe nausea and vomiting in chemotherapy, organic mental syndrome with psychotic features, hiccups (short-term), emergency sedation of severely agitated or delirious patients
Investigational uses: Nausea, vomiting in chemotherapy, surgery
Dosage and routes:
Psychosis
• *Adult:* **PO** 0.5-5 mg bid or tid initially depending on severity of condition; dose is increased to desired dose, max 100 mg/day; **IM** 2-5 mg q4-8h or bid-tid
• *Geriatric:* 0.25-0.5 mg qd-bid, titrate q3-4 days by 0.25-0.5 mg/dose
• *Child 3-12 yr:* **PO/IM** 0.05-0.15 mg/kg/day
• *Decanoate:* Initial dose **IM** is 10-15 mg × daily oral dose at 4 wk interval; do not administer **IV**; not to exceed 100 mg
Chronic schizophrenia
• *Adult:* **IM** 50-100 mg q4wk (decanoate)
• *Child 3-12 yr:* **PO/IM** 0.05-0.15 mg/kg/day
Tics/vocal utterances
• *Adult:* **PO** 0.5-5 mg bid or tid, increased until desired response occurs
• *Child 3-12 yr:* **PO** 0.05-0.075 mg/kg/day
Hyperactive children
• *Child 3-12 yr:* **PO** 0.05-0.075 mg/kg/day
Available forms: Tabs 0.5, 1, 2, 5, 10, 20 mg; lactate conc 2 mg/ml; inj 5 mg/ml, decanoate 50 mg base/ml, 100 mg base/ml
Side effects/adverse reactions:
RESP: ***Laryngospasm,*** dyspnea, ***respiratory depression***
CNS: EPS: pseudoparkinsonism, akathisia, dystonia, tardive dyskinesia, drowsiness, headache, ***seizures, neuroleptic malignant syndrome,*** confusion

INTEG: Rash, photosensitivity, dermatitis
EENT: Blurred vision, glaucoma, dry eyes
GI: Dry mouth, nausea, vomiting, anorexia, constipation, diarrhea, jaundice, weight gain, ***ileus, hepatitis***
GU: Urinary retention, dysuria, urinary frequency, enuresis, impotence, amenorrhea, gynecomastia
CV: Orthostatic hypotension, hypertension, ***cardiac arrest,*** ECG changes, ***tachycardia***

Contraindications: Hypersensitivity, blood dyscrasias, coma, child <3 yr, brain damage, bone marrow depression, alcohol and barbiturate withdrawal states, Parkinson's disease, angina, epilepsy, urinary retention, narrow-angle glaucoma

Precautions: Pregnancy (C), lactation, seizure disorders, hypertension, hepatic disease, cardiac disease, elderly

Do not confuse:
haloperidol/Halotestin
Haldol/Stadol

Pharmacokinetics:
PO: Onset erratic, peak 2-6 hr, half-life 24 hr
IM: Onset 15-30 min, peak 15-20 min, half-life 21 hr
IM (Decanoate): Peak 4-11 days, half-life 3 wk
Metabolized by liver; excreted in urine, bile; crosses placenta; enters breast milk

Interactions:
• Oversedation: other CNS depressants, alcohol, barbiturate anesthetics
• Toxicity: epinephrine, lithium
• ↓ effects: lithium, levodopa
• ↑ both drugs effects: β-adrenergic blockers, alcohol
• ↑ anticholinergic effects: anticholinergics
• ↓ haloperidol effects: phenobarbital, carbamazepine
↑ action: chamomile, cola tree, hops, kava, nettle, nutmeg, skullcap, valerian
Antagonist action: jimsonweed, scopolia
↑ EPS: betel palm, kava

Lab test interferences:
Increase: LFTs, cardiac enzymes, cholesterol, blood glucose, prolactin, bilirubin, PBI, cholinesterase, alk phosphatase
Decrease: Hormones (blood, urine), PT
False positive: Pregnancy tests, PKU
False negative: Urinary steroids

NURSING CONSIDERATIONS

Assess:
• Swallowing of PO medication; check for hoarding or giving of medication to other patients
• I&O ratio; palpate bladder if low urinary output occurs
• Bilirubin, CBC, LFTs monthly
• Urinalysis is recommended before and during prolonged therapy
• Affect, orientation, LOC, reflexes, gait, coordination, sleep pattern disturbances
• B/P standing and lying; take pulse and respirations q4h during initial treatment; establish baseline before starting treatment; report drops of 30 mm Hg
• Dizziness, faintness, palpitations, tachycardia on rising
• EPS including akathisia (inability to sit still, no pattern to movements), tardive dyskinesia (bizarre movements of jaw, mouth, tongue, extremities), pseudoparkinsonism (rigidity, tremors, pill rolling, shuffling gait)
• Skin turgor daily
For neuroleptic malignant syndrome: hyperthermia, muscle rigidity, altered mental status, increased CPK, seizures, hyper/hypotension,

tachycardia, notify prescriber immediately
• Constipation, urinary retention daily; if these occur, increase bulk, water in diet

Administer:
• Reduced dose to elderly
• Antiparkinsonian agent, to be used if EPS occur

IM route
• IM inj into large muscle mass, use 21G, 2-in needle; give no more than 3 ml/inj site; patient should remain recumbent for ½ hr

PO route
• Oral liquid: use calibrated dropper; do not mix in coffee or tea
• PO with food or milk

IV route
• Give undiluted for psychotic episode at 5 mg/min
• Give by intermittent inf after dilution in 30-50 ml of D_5W, run over ½ hr

Solution compatibilities: D_5W

Syringe compatibilities: Hydromorphone, sufentanil

Y-site compatibilities: Amifostine, amsacrine, aztreonam, cimetidine, cisatracurium, cladribine, DOBUTamine, DOPamine, DOXOrubicin liposome, famotidine, filgrastim, fludarabine, granisetron, lidocaine, lorazepam, melphalan, midazolam, nitroglycerin, norepinephrine, ondansetron, paclitaxel, phenylephrine, propofol, remifentanil, sufentanil, tacrolimus, teniposide, theophylline, thiotepa, vinorelbine

Perform/provide:
• Decreased sensory input by dimming lights, avoiding loud noises
• Supervised ambulation until stabilized on medication; do not involve in strenuous exercise program because fainting is possible; patient should not stand still for long periods
• Increased fluids, roughage to prevent constipation
• Sips of water, sugarless candy, gum for dry mouth
• Storage in tight, light-resistant container

Evaluate:
• Therapeutic response: decrease in emotional excitement, hallucinations, delusions, paranoia, reorganization of patterns of thought, speech, improvement in specific behaviors

Teach patient/family:
• That orthostatic hypotension occurs often and to rise from sitting or lying position gradually
• To avoid hazardous activities until stabilized on medication
• To remain lying down after IM inj for at least 30 min
• To avoid hot tubs, hot showers, tub baths, since hypotension may occur
• To avoid abrupt withdrawal of this drug, or EPS may result; drug should be withdrawn slowly
• To avoid OTC preparations (cough, hay fever, cold) unless approved by prescriber, since serious drug interactions may occur; avoid use with alcohol, CNS depressants; increased drowsiness may occur
• To use a sunscreen to prevent burns
• Regarding compliance with drug regimen
• About EPS and necessity for meticulous oral hygiene, since oral candidiasis may occur
• To report impaired vision, jaundice, tremors, muscle twitching
• That in hot weather, heat stroke may occur; take extra precautions to stay cool

Treatment of overdose: Activated charcoal, lavage if orally ingested; provide an airway; do not induce vomiting

haloprogin topical

See appendix c

HIGH ALERT

heparin (℞)

(hep'a-rin)

Calcilean✤, Calciparine✤, Hepalean✤, Heparin Leo✤, heparin sodium, Hep-Lock, Hep-Lock U/P

Func. class.: Anticoagulant, antithrombotic

Action: Prevents conversion of fibrinogen to fibrin and prothrombin to thrombin by enhancing inhibitory effects of antithrombin III

Uses: Prevention of deep-vein thrombosis, pulmonary emboli, myocardial infarction, open heart surgery, disseminated intravascular clotting syndrome, atrial fibrillation with embolization, as an anticoagulant in transfusion and dialysis procedures, prevention of DVT/PE, to maintain patency of indwelling venipuncture devices, diagnosis, treatment of disseminated intravascular coagulation (DIC)

Dosage and routes:

Deep-vein thrombosis/MI

• *Adult:* **IV PUSH** 5000-7000 units q4h then titrated to PTT or ACT level; **IV BOL** 5000-7500 units, then **IV INF; IV INF** after bolus dose, then 1000 units/hr titrated to PTT or ACT level

• *Child:* **IV INF** 50 units/kg, maintenance 100 units/kg q4h or 20,000 units/m^2 qd

Pulmonary embolism

• *Adult:* **IV PUSH** 7500-10,000 units q4h then titrated to PTT or ACT level; **IV BOL** 7500-10,000, then **IV INF; IV INF** after bolus dose, then 1000 units/hr titrated to PTT or ACT level

• *Child:* **IV INF** 50 units/kg, maintenance 100 units/kg q4h or 20,000 units/m^2 qd

Cardiovascular surgery

• *Adult:* **IV INF** 150-300 units/kg

Prophylaxis for DVT/PE

• *Adult:* **SC** 5000 units q8-12h

Heparin flush

• *Adult and child:* **IV** 10-100 units

Available forms:

Sodium carpaject: 5000 units/ml; disposable inj: 1000, 2500, 5000, 7500, 10,000, 15,000, 20,000, 40,000 units/ml; unit dose: 1000, 5000, 10,000, 20,000, 40,000 units/ml; vials: 1000, 2000, 2500, 5000, 7500, 10,000, 20,000, 40,000 units/ml; disposable syringes flush: 10 units/ml; vials: 100 units/ml; Ca inj: 5000 units/0.2 ml; ampules: 12,500 units/0.5 ml; 20,000 units/0.8 ml

Side effects/adverse reactions:

CNS: Fever, chills

GU: ***Hematuria***

HEMA: ***Hemorrhage, thrombocytopenia, anemia***

SYST: ***Anaphylaxis***

INTEG: Rash, dermatitis, urticaria, pruritus, delayed transient alopecia, hematoma, cutaneous necrosis (SC)

Contraindications: Hypersensitivity, hemophilia, leukemia with bleeding, peptic ulcer disease, severe thrombocytopenic purpura, hepatic disease (severe), renal disease (severe), blood dyscrasias, severe hypertension, subacute bacterial endocarditis, acute nephritis

Precautions: Alcoholism, elderly, pregnancy (C), children, hyperlipidemia, diabetes, renal disease

Do not confuse:

heparin/Hespan

Pharmacokinetics: Well absorbed (SC)

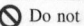

IV: Peak 5 min, duration 2-6 hr

SC: Onset 20-60 min, duration 8-12 hr
Half-life 1½ hr, excreted in urine, 95% bound to plasma proteins, does not cross placenta or alter breast milk; removed from the system via the lymph and spleen, partially metabolized in kidney, liver, excreted in urine (<50% unchanged)

Interactions:

- ↓ corticosteroids action
- Resistance to heparin: streptokinase
- ↑ diazepam action
- ↓ heparin action: digitalis, tetracyclines, antihistamines
- ↑ heparin action: oral anticoagulants, salicylates, dextran, nonsteroidal antiinflammatories, platelet inhibitors, cephalosporins, penicillins, ticlopidine, dipyridamole

↑ risk of bleeding: agrimony, alfalfa, angelica, anise, basil, bay, bilberry, black haw, bogbean, bromelain, buchu, chondroitin, cinchona bark, dong quai, fenugreek, feverfew, garlic, ginger, ginkgo, ginseng, horse chestnut, Irish moss, kelp, kelpware, khella, lovage, lungwort, meadowsweet, motherwort, mugwort, nettle, papaya, parsley (large amts), pau d'arco, pineapple, poplar, prickly ash, safflower, saw palmetto, tonka bean, turmeric, wintergreen, yarrow

↓ anticoagulant effect: chamomile, coenzyme Q10, flax, glucomannan, goldenseal, guar gum

Lab test interferences:
Increase: ALT, AST, INR, PT, PTT
Decrease: Platelets

NURSING CONSIDERATIONS

Assess:

- Blood studies (Hct, occult blood in stools) q3mo
- Partial prothrombin time, which should be 1.5-2 × control, PTT often done qd, also APTT, ACT
- Platelet count q2-3d; thrombocytopenia may occur on 4th day of treatment

Bleeding gums, petechiae, ecchymosis, black tarry stools, hematuria, epistaxis, decrease in Hct, B/P; may indicate bleeding, hemorrhage

- Fever, skin rash, urticaria
- Needed dosage change q1-2wk

Administer:

- Cannot be used interchangeably (unit for unit) with LMWHS or heparinoids
- At same time each day to maintain steady blood levels
- SC deep with 25G ⅜-in needle; do not massage area or aspirate when giving SC inj; give in abdomen between pelvic bones, rotate sites; do not pull back on plunger, leave in for 10 sec; apply gentle pressure for 1 min
- Changing needles is not recommended
- Avoiding all IM inj that may cause bleeding, hematoma

IV route

- Diluted in 0.9% NaCl, dextrose, Ringer's sol and given by direct, intermittent, or continuous infusion; give 1000 units or less over 1 min; then 5000 units or less over 1 min; infusion may run from 4-24 hr; use infusion pump
- When drug is added to inf sol for cont IV, invert container at least 6 times to ensure adequate mixing
- Blood after adding 7500 units/100 ml NaCl inj, add 6-8 ml of this sol/100 ml of whole blood

Additive compatibilities: Aminophylline, amphotericin, ascorbic acid, bleomycin, calcium gluconate, cefepime, cephapirin, chloramphenicol, clindamycin, cloxacillin, colistimethate, dimenhyDRINATE, DOPamine, enalaprilat, erythromycin gluceptate, esmolol, floxacillin, fluconazole, flumazenil, furosemide, hydrocortisone, isoproterenol, lidocaine, lincomycin, magnesium sulfate, meropenem, methyldopate, methylPREDNISolone, metronidazole/sodium bicarbonate, nafcillin, norepinephrine, octreotide, penicillin G, potassium chloride, prednisoLONE, promazine, ranitidine, sodium bicarbonate, verapamil, vit B, vit B/C

Syringe compatibilities: Aminophylline, amphotericin B, ampicillin, atropine, azlocillin, bleomycin, cefamandole, cefazolin, cefoperazone, cefotaxime, cefoxitin, chloramphenicol, cimetidine, cisplatin, clindamycin, cyclophosphamide, diazoxide, digoxin, dimenhyDRINATE, DOBUTamine, DOPamine, epinephrine, fentanyl, fluorouracil, furosemide, leucovorin, lidocaine, lincomycin, methotrexate, metoclopramide, mezlocillin, mitomycin, moxalactam, nafcillin, naloxone, neostigmine, nitroglycerin, norepinephrine, pancuronium, penicillin G, phenobarbital, piperacillin, sodium nitroprusside, succinylcholine, trimethoprim-sulfamethoxazole, verapamil

Y-site compatibilities: Acyclovir, aldesleukin, allopurinol, amifostine, aminophylline, ampicillin, ampicillin/sulbactam, atracurium, atropine, aztreonam, betamethasone, bleomycin, calcium gluconate, cefazolin, cefotetan, cefotiam, ceftazidime, ceftriaxone, cephalothin, cephapirin, chlordiazepoxide, chlorproMAZINE, cimetidine, cisplatin, cladribine, clindamycin, conjugated estrogens, cyanocobalamin, cyclophosphamide, cytarabine, dexamethasone, digoxin, diphenhydrAMINE, DOPamine, DOXOrubicin liposome, edrophonium, enalaprilat, epINEPHrine, erythromycin, esmolol, ethacrynate, famotidine, fentanyl, fluconazole, fludarabine, fluorouracil, foscarnet, furosemide, gallium, granisetron, hydrALAZINE, hydrocortisone, hydromorphone, insulin (regular), isoproterenol, kanamycin, leucovorin, lidocaine, lorazepam, magnesium sulfate, melphalan, menadiol, meperidine, meropenem, methicillin, methotrexate, methoxamine, methyldopate, methylergonovine, metoclopramide, metronidazole, midazolam, milrinone, minocycline, mitomycin, morphine, nafcillin, neostigmine, nitroglycerin, nitroprusside, norepinephrine, ondansetron, oxacillin, oxytocin, paclitaxel, pancuronium, penicillin G potassium, pentazocine, phytonadione, piperacillin, piperacillin/tazobactam, potassium chloride, prednisoLONE, procainamide, prochlorperazine, propofol, propranolol, pyridostigmine, ranitidine, remifentanil, sargramostim, scopolamine, sodium bicarbonate, streptokinase, succinylcholine, tacrolimus, teniposide, theophylline, thiopental, thiotepa, ticarcillin, ticarcillin/clavulanate, trimethobenzamide, vecuronium, vinBLAStine, vinorelbine, warfarin, zidovudine

Perform/provide:

- Storage in tight container

Evaluate:

- Therapeutic response: decrease of deep-vein thrombosis, PTT 1.5-2.5 × control, free flowing IV

Teach patient/family:

- To avoid OTC preparations that may cause serious drug interactions unless directed by prescriber
- That drug may be held during active bleeding (menstruation), depending on condition
- To use soft-bristle toothbrush to avoid bleeding gums, avoid contact sports, use electric razor, avoid IM inj
- To carry emergency ID identifying drug taken

• To report any signs of bleeding: gums, under skin, urine, stools

Treatment of overdose: Withdraw drug, protamine 1 mg protamine/ 100 units heparin

hepatitis B immune globulin (℞)

Bay Hep B, Nabi-HB

Func. class.: Immune globulin

Action: Provides passive immunity to hepatitis B

Uses: Prevention of hepatitis B virus in exposed patients, including passive immunity in neonates born to HBsAg-positive mother

Dosage and routes:

Acute exposure to blood with HBsAg

• *Adult:* 2 doses, given after exposure and 1 mo later

Perinatal exposure of infants born to HBsAg-positive mothers

• *Infant:* 1 dose at birth, then start hepatitis B vaccine series soon after birth

Sexual exposure to HBsAg

• *Adult:* Administer 1 dose within 2 wk of exposure

Available forms:

Bay Hep B: Sol for inj 15%-18% protein

Nabi-HB: Sol for inj 5% ± 1% protein

Side effects/adverse reactions:

INTEG: Soreness at inj site, urticaria, erythema, swelling

SYST: Induration, ***anaphylaxis, angioedema***

CNS: Headache, dizziness, fever

GI: Nausea, vomiting

Contraindications: Hypersensitivity to immune globulins, coagulation disorders

Precautions: Pregnancy (C), elderly, lactation, children; active infection, IgA deficiency

NURSING CONSIDERATIONS

Assess:

• For history of allergies, skin conditions (eczema, psoriasis, dermatitis), reactions to vaccinations

• For skin reactions: rash, induration, urticaria

◆ For anaphylaxis: inability to breathe, bronchospasm, hypotension, wheezing, diaphoresis, fever, flushing

Administer:

• After rotating vial; do not shake

• Only with epinephrine 1:1000 on unit to treat laryngospasm

• In deltoid for better absorption (adult)

Perform/provide:

• Written record of immunization

• Comfort measures

Evaluate:

• Prevention of hepatitis B

Teach patient/family:

• That discomfort may occur at site

• To report any rash, wheezing, inability to breathe immediately

hetastarch (℞)

(het′a-starch)

Hespan

Func. class.: Plasma expander

Chem. class.: Synthetic polymer

Action: Similar to human albumin, which expands plasma volume by colloidal osmotic pressure

Uses: Plasma volume expander, leukapheresis

Dosage and routes:

• *Adult:* **IV INF** 500-1000 ml (30-60 g), total dose not to exceed 1500 ml/day, not to exceed 20 ml/kg/hr (hemorrhagic shock)

Leukapheresis
• *Adult:* **IV INF** 250-700 ml infused at 1:8 ratio with whole blood, may be repeated 2/wk up to 10 treatments

Available forms: 6% hetastarch/0.9% NaCl inj

Side effects/adverse reactions:
HEMA: Decreased Hct, platelet function, increased bleeding/coagulation times, increased sed rate
INTEG: Rash, urticaria, pruritus, angioedema, chills, fever, flushing, peripheral edema
RESP: Wheezing, dyspnea, ***bronchospasm, pulmonary edema***
GI: Nausea, vomiting
EENT: Periorbital edema
SYST: ***Anaphylaxis***
CNS: Headache

Contraindications: Hypersensitivity, severe bleeding disorders, renal failure, CHF (severe)

Precautions: Pregnancy (C), hepatic disease, pulmonary edema

Do not confuse:
Hespan/heparin

Pharmacokinetics:
IV: Expands blood volume 1-2 × amount infused, excreted in urine

Lab test interferences:
False increase: Bilirubin

NURSING CONSIDERATIONS

Assess:
• VS q5min × 30 min; CVP during infusion (5-10 cm H_2O normal range), PCWP
• Monitor CBC with differential, Hgb, Hct, PT, PTT, platelet count, clotting time during treatment; Hct may drop; do not allow to drop >30% by vol
• Urine output q1h, watch for increase in urinary output (common); if output does not increase, decrease or discontinue infusion
• I&O ratio and specific gravity, urine osmolarity; if specific gravity is very low, renal clearance is low; drug should be discontinued
• Allergy: rash, urticaria, pruritus, wheezing, dyspnea, bronchospasm; drug should be discontinued immediately
◆ For circulatory overload: increased pulse, respirations, dyspnea, wheezing, chest tightness, chest pain
• For dehydration after infusion: decreased output, fever, poor skin turgor, increased specific gravity, dry skin

Administer:

IV route
• INF undiluted, run at 20 ml/kg/hr (1.2 g/kg); reduced rate in septic shock, burns

Additive compatibilities: Cloxacillin, fosphenytoin

Y-site compatibilities: Cimetidine, diltiazem, enalaprilat
• Storage at room temperature; discard unused portion, do not freeze, do not use if turbid or deep brown or if precipitate forms

Evaluate:
• Therapeutic response: increased plasma volume

Teach patient/family:
• When to notify prescriber

homatropine ophthalmic

See appendix c

RARELY USED

hyaluronidase (℞)

(hye-al-yoor-on'i-dase)
Wydase
Func. class.: Enzyme

Uses: Hypodermoclysis, subcutane-

ous urography; adjunct to dispersion of other drugs
Dosage and routes:
Adjunct
• *Adult and child:* **INJ** 150 units with other drug
Urography
• *Adult and child:* **SC** 75 units over scapula, then contrast medium injected at same site
Hypodermoclysis
• *Adult and child >3 yr:* **SC** 150 units/L of lysis sol
Contraindications: Hypersensitivity to bovine products, CHF, hypoproteinemia, around infected/inflamed or cancerous area

*hydrALAZINE (℞)

(hye-dral'a-zeen)
Alazine, Apresoline, hydrALAZINE HCl, Novo-Hylazin✤, Pralzine, Rolzine, Supres✤
Func. class.: Antihypertensive, direct-acting peripheral vasodilator
Chem. class.: Phthalazine

Action: Vasodilates arteriolar smooth muscle by direct relaxation; reduction in blood pressure with reflex increases in heart rate, stroke volume, cardiac output
Uses: Essential hypertension; severe essential hypertension
Investigational uses: CHF
Dosage and routes:
• *Adult:* **PO** 10 mg qid 2-4 days, then 25 mg for rest of first wk, then 50 mg qid individualized to desired response, not to exceed 300 mg qd; **IV/IM BOL** 20-40 mg q4-6h, administer **PO** as soon as possible; **IM** 20-40 mg q4-6h
• *Child:* **PO** 0.75-3 mg/kg/day in 4 divided doses, max 7.5 mg/kg/24 hr; **IV BOL** 0.1-0.2 mg/kg q4-6h; **IM** 0.1-0.2 mg/kg q4-6h
Available forms: Inj 20 mg/ml; tabs 10, 25, 50, 100 mg
Side effects/adverse reactions:
MISC: Nasal congestion, muscle cramps, *lupuslike symptoms,* flushing, edema, dyspnea
CV: Palpitations, reflex tachycardia, angina, ***shock,*** rebound hypertension
CNS: Headache, tremors, dizziness, anxiety, peripheral neuritis, depression, fever, chills
GI: Nausea, vomiting, anorexia, diarrhea, constipation, paralytic ileus
INTEG: Rash, pruritus, urticaria
HEMA: ***Leukopenia, agranulocytosis,*** anemia, ***thrombocytopenia***
GU: Urinary retention
Contraindications: Hypersensitivity to hydrALAZINEs, coronary artery disease, mitral valvular rheumatic heart disease
Precautions: Pregnancy (C), CVA, advanced renal disease, elderly, coronary artery disease, lactation
Do not confuse:
Apresoline/allopurinol
hydrALAZINE/hydrOXYzine
Pharmacokinetics:
PO: Onset 20-30 min, peak 1-2 hr, duration 6-12 hr
IM: Onset 5-10 min, peak 1 hr, duration 2-4 hr
IV: Onset 5-20 min, peak 10-80 min, duration 2-6 hr
Half-life 2-8 hr; metabolized by liver; 12%-14% excreted in urine
Interactions:
• ↓ hydrALAZINE effects: indomethacin
• ↑ tachycardia, angina: sympathomimetics (epINEPHrine, norepinephrine)
• ↑ effects of: β-blockers
• Severe hypotension: MAOIs
↑ toxicity, death: aconite

↑ or ↓ antihypertensive effect: astragalus, cola tree

↑ antihypertensive effect: barberry, betony, black catechu, black cohosh, bloodroot, broom, burdock, cat's claw, dandelion, goldenseal, Irish moss, Jamaican dogwood, kelp, khella, mistletoe, parsley

↓ antihypertensive effect: coltsfoot, guarana, khat, licorice

NURSING CONSIDERATIONS

Assess:

- B/P q5min × 2 hr, then q1h × 2 hr, then q4h
- Pulse, jugular venous distention q4h
- Electrolytes, blood studies: K, Na, Cl, CO_2, CBC, serum glucose
- Weight daily, I&O
- LE prep, ANA titer before starting therapy and during treatment; assess for fever, joint pain, rash, sore throat (lupuslike symptoms); notify prescriber
- Edema in feet, legs daily
- Skin turgor, dryness of mucous membranes for hydration status
- Rales, dyspnea, orthopnea
- IV site for extravasation, rate
- Fever, joint pain, tachycardia, palpitations, headache, nausea
- Mental status: affect, mood, behavior, anxiety; check for personality changes

Administer:

- Give with meals (PO) to enhance absorption
- To recumbent patient, keep for 1 hr after administration

IV route

- IV undiluted; give through Y-tube or 3-way stopcock, give each 10 mg ≤min

Additive compatibilities: DOBUTamine

Y-site compatibilities: Heparin, hydrocortisone, potassium chloride, verapamil, vit B/C

Evaluate:

- Therapeutic response: decreased B/P

Teach patient/family:

- To take with food to increase bioavailability (PO)
- To avoid OTC preparations unless directed by prescriber
- To notify prescriber if chest pain, severe fatigue, fever, muscle or joint pain occurs
- To rise slowly to prevent orthostatic hypotension
- To notify prescriber if pregnancy is suspected

Treatment of overdose: Administer vasopressors, volume expanders for shock; if PO, lavage or give activated charcoal, digitalization

hydrochlorothiazide (℞)

(hye-droe-klor-oh-thye'a-zide)

Apo-Hydrol✤, Esidrix, HCTZ, Hydro-Chlor, hydrochlorothiazide, HydroDIURIL, Microzide, Neo-Codema✤, Novohydrazide✤, Oretic, Urozide✤

Func. class.: Thiazide diuretic, antihypertensive

Chem. class.: Sulfonamide derivative

Action: Acts on distal tubule and ascending limb of loop of Henle by increasing excretion of water, sodium, chloride, potassium

Uses: Edema, hypertension, diuresis, CHF; edema in corticosteroid, estrogen, NSAIDs, idiopathic lower extremity edema therapy

Dosage and routes:

- *Adult:* **PO** 25-100 mg/day
- *Geriatric:* **PO** 12.5 mg/day, initially

• *Child >6 mo:* **PO** 2 mg/kg/day in divided doses
• *Child <6 mo:* **PO** up to 4 mg/kg/day in divided doses

Available forms: Tabs 25, 50, 100 mg; caps 12.5 mg; oral sol 10 mg/5 ml, 100 mg/ml

Side effects/adverse reactions:
GU: Urinary frequency, polyuria, ***uremia, glucosuria,*** hyperuricemia
CNS: Drowsiness, paresthesia, depression, headache, *dizziness, fatigue, weakness,* fever
GI: Nausea, vomiting, anorexia, constipation, diarrhea, cramps, pancreatitis, GI irritation, ***hepatitis***
EENT: Blurred vision
INTEG: Rash, urticaria, purpura, photosensitivity, alopecia, erythema multiforme
META: Hyperglycemia, hyperuricemia, increased creatinine, BUN
HEMA: ***Aplastic anemia, hemolytic anemia, leukopenia, agranulocytosis, thrombocytopenia, neutropenia***
CV: Irregular pulse, orthostatic hypotension, palpitations, volume depletion, allergic myocarditis
ELECT: Hypokalemia, hypercalcemia, hyponatremia, hypochloremia, hypomagnesemia

Contraindications: Hypersensitivity to thiazides or sulfonamides, anuria, renal decompensation, hypomagnesemia

Precautions: Hypokalemia, renal disease, pregnancy (B), lactation, hepatic disease, gout, COPD, LE, diabetes mellitus, hyperlipidemia, CCr <25 ml/min

Pharmacokinetics:
PO: Onset 2 hr, peak 4 hr, duration 6-12 hr, half-life 6-15 hr; excreted unchanged by kidneys; crosses placenta; enters breast milk

Interactions:
• ↑ toxicity, lithium, nondepolarizing skeletal muscle relaxants, cardiac glycosides
• ↓ antidiabetics effects
• ↓ thiazides absorption: cholestyramine, colestipol
• ↑ renal failure risk: NSAIDs
• Hyperglycemia, hyperuricemia, ↑ antihypertensives: diazoxide
• Hypokalemia: glucocorticoids, amphotericin B
• ↑ effects: loop diuretics
↑ hypokalemia: aloe, buckthorn, cascara sagrada, Chinese rhubarb, gossypol, licorice, nettle, senna
↑ diuretic effect: cucumber, dandelion, ginkgo, horsetail, khella, licorice, nettle, pumpkin, Queen Anne's lace
Severe photosensitivity: St. John's wort

Lab test interferences:
Increase: BSP retention, amylase, parathyroid test
Decrease: PBI, PSP

NURSING CONSIDERATIONS

Assess:
• Weight, I&O daily to determine fluid loss; effect of drug may be decreased if used qd
• Rate, depth, rhythm of respiration, effect of exertion
• B/P lying, standing; postural hypotension may occur
• Electrolytes: K, Mg, Na, Cl; include BUN, blood glucose, CBC, serum creatinine, blood pH, ABGs, uric acid, Ca; renal function
• Glucose in urine if patient is diabetic
• Signs of metabolic alkalosis: drowsiness, restlessness
• Signs of hypokalemia: postural hypotension, malaise, fatigue, tachycardia, leg cramps, weakness, dehydration
• Rashes, temp qd

H

• Confusion, especially in elderly; take safety precautions if needed

Administer:

• In AM to avoid interference with sleep if using drug as a diuretic

• Potassium replacement if potassium <3 mg/dl

• With food; if nausea occurs, absorption may be decreased slightly

Evaluate:

• Therapeutic response: improvement in edema of feet, legs, sacral area qd, decreased B/P

Teach patient/family:

• To increase fluid intake to 2-3 L/day unless contraindicated; to rise slowly from lying or sitting position

• To notify prescriber of muscle weakness, cramps, nausea, dizziness

• That drug may be taken with food or milk

• To use sunscreen for photosensitivity

• That blood glucose may be increased in diabetics

• To take early in day to avoid nocturia

Treatment of overdose: Lavage if taken orally; monitor electrolytes; administer dextrose in saline; monitor hydration, CV, renal status

hydrocodone (℞)

(hye-droe-koe′done)

Hycodan, Robidone✱, Tussigon

hydrocodone/ acetaminophen

Allay, Anexsia, Anolor DH, Bancap HC, Co-Gesic, Dolacet, Dolagesic, Duocet, Hycomed, Hyco-Pap, Hydrocet, Hydrogesic, Lorcet, Lortab, Onset, Pancet, Panlor, Polygesic, Stagesic, T-Gesic, Ugesic, Vanacet, Vandone, Vicodin, Zydone

hydrocodone/aspirin

Azdone, Damason-P, Lortab ASA, Panasal

hydrocodone/ ibuprofen

Vicoprofen

Func. class.: Antitussive opioid analgesic, nonopioid analgesic

Controlled Substance Schedule III

Action: Acts directly on cough center in medulla to suppress cough; binds to opiate receptors in CNS to reduce pain

Uses: Hyperactive and nonproductive cough, mild pain

Dosage and routes:

• *Adult:* **PO** 5-10 mg q4h prn

• *Child:* **PO** 1.25-5 mg q4h prn or 0.2 mg/kg q3-4h

Available forms: Syr 5 mg/5 ml; tabs 5 mg (long-acting)

Side effects/adverse reactions:

CNS: Drowsiness, dizziness, lightheadedness, confusion, headache, sedation, euphoria, dysphoria, weakness, hallucinations, disorientation, mood changes, dependence, ***convulsions***

GI: Nausea, vomiting, anorexia, constipation, cramps, dry mouth

GU: Increased urinary output, dysuria, urinary retention
INTEG: Rash, urticaria, flushing, pruritus
EENT: Tinnitus, blurred vision, miosis, diplopia
CV: Palpitations, tachycardia, bradycardia, change in B/P, ***circulatory depression,*** syncope
RESP: ***Respiratory depression***

Contraindications: Hypersensitivity, addiction (opioid)

Precautions: Addictive personality, pregnancy (C), lactation, increased intracranial pressure, MI (acute), severe heart disease, respiratory depression, hepatic disease, renal disease

Do not confuse:
hydrocodone/hydrocortisone
Hycodan/Vicodan

Pharmacokinetics: Onset 10-20 min, duration 4-6 hr, half-life 3½-4½ hr; metabolized in liver; excreted in urine; crosses placenta

Interactions:
• ↑ CNS depression: alcohol, opioids, sedative/hypnotics, phenothiazines, skeletal muscle relaxants, general anesthetics, tricyclics
↑ CNS depression: Jamaican dogwood, lavender, mistletoe, nettle, pokeweed, poppy, senega, valerian
↑ anticholinergic effect: corkwood

Lab test interferences:
Increase: Amylase, lipase

NURSING CONSIDERATIONS

Assess:
• Pain: intensity, type, location, and other characteristics
• CNS changes: dizziness, drowsiness, hallucinations, euphoria, LOC, pupil reaction
• Allergic reactions: rash, urticaria
• Cough and respiratory dysfunction: respiratory depression, character, rate, rhythm; notify prescriber if respirations are <10/min
• Need for pain medication, physical dependence

Administer:
• With antiemetic after meals if nausea or vomiting occurs

Perform/provide:
• Storage in light-resistant area at room temperature
• Assistance with ambulation
• Safety measures: night-light, call bell within easy reach

Evaluate:
• Therapeutic response: decrease in pain or cough

Teach patient/family:
• To report any symptoms of CNS changes, allergic reactions
• That physical dependency may result when used for extended periods
• That withdrawal symptoms may occur: nausea, vomiting, cramps, fever, faintness, anorexia
Not to break, crush, or chew tabs
• To avoid driving, other hazardous activities, drowsiness occurs
• To avoid other CNS depressants, will enhance sedating properties of this drug

Treatment of overdose: Naloxone HCl (Narcan) 0.2-0.8 mg IV, O_2, IV fluids, vasopressors

hydrocortisone (℞)

(hy-dro-kor′tih-sone)

Cortef, Cortenema, Hydrocortone

hydrocortisone acetate (℞)

Cortifoam, Hydrocortone Acetate

hydrocortisone cypionate (℞)

Cortef

hydrocortisone sodium phosphate (℞)

Hydrocortone Phosphate

hydrocortisone sodium succinate (℞)

A-hydroCort, Solu-Cortef

Func. class.: Corticosteroid

Chem. class.: Short-acting glucocorticoid

Action: Decreases inflammation by suppression of migration of polymorphonuclear leukocytes, fibroblasts, reversal of increased capillary permeability and lysosomal stabilization

Uses: Severe inflammation, septic shock, adrenal insufficiency, ulcerative colitis, collagen disorders

Dosage and routes:

Adrenal insufficiency/inflammation

• *Adult:* **PO** 5-30 mg bid-qid; **IM/IV** 100-250 mg (succinate), then 50-100 mg **IM** as needed; **IM/IV** 15-240 mg q12h (phosphate)

Shock

• *Adult:* 500 mg-2 g q2-6h (succinate)

• *Child:* **IM/IV** 0.186-1 mg/kg bid-tid (succinate)

Colitis

• *Adult:* **ENEMA** 100 mg nightly for 21 days

Available forms: Tabs 5, 10, 20 mg; inj 25, 50 mg/ml; enema 100 mg/60 ml; acetate—inj 25✤, 50 mg/ml✤, enema 10% aerosol foam; supp 25 mg; cypionate—oral susp 10 mg/5 ml; phosphate—inj 50 mg/ml; succinate inj 100 mg✤, 250 mg✤, 500 mg✤, 1000 mg/vial✤

Side effects/adverse reactions:

CNS: Depression, flushing, sweating, headache, mood changes

CV: Hypertension, ***circulatory collapse, thrombophlebitis, embolism,*** tachycardia, edema

EENT: Fungal infections, increased intraocular pressure, blurred vision

GI: Diarrhea, nausea, abdominal distention, ***GI hemorrhage,*** increased appetite, ***pancreatitis***

HEMA: ***Thrombocytopenia***

INTEG: Acne, poor wound healing, ecchymosis, petechiae

MS: Fractures, osteoporosis, weakness

Contraindications: Psychosis, hypersensitivity, idiopathic thrombocytopenia (IM), acute glomerulonephritis, amebiasis, fungal infections, non-asthmatic bronchial disease, child <2 yr, AIDS, TB

Precautions: Pregnancy (C), lactation, diabetes mellitus, glaucoma, osteoporosis, seizure disorders, ulcerative colitis, CHF, myasthenia gravis, renal disease, esophagitis, peptic ulcer

Do not confuse:

hydrocortisone/hydrocodone

Pharmacokinetics:

PO: Onset 1-2 hr, peak 1 hr, duration 1-1½ days

IM/IV: Onset 20 min, peak 4-8 hr, duration 1-1½ days

RECT: Onset 3-5 days

Metabolized by liver, excreted in urine (17-OHCS, 17-KS), crosses placenta

Interactions:

• ↓ hydrocortisone action: cholestyramine, colestipol, barbiturates, rifampin, epHEDrine, phenytoin, theophylline

• ↓ anticoagulants effects, anticonvulsants, antidiabetics, toxoids, vaccines
• ↑ side effects: alcohol, amphotericin B, digitalis, cycloSPORINE, diuretics
• Risk of GI bleeding: salicylates, NSAIDs
↑ hypokalemia: aloe, buckthorn, cascara sagrada, Chinese rhubarb, senna
↑ corticosteroid effect: aloe, licorice, perilla

Lab test interferences:
Increase: Cholesterol, sodium, blood glucose, uric acid, calcium, urine glucose
Decrease: Ca, K, T_4, T_3, thyroid ^{131}I uptake test, urine 17-OHCS, 17-KS
False negative: Skin allergy tests

NURSING CONSIDERATIONS

Assess:
• Potassium, blood glucose, urine glucose while on long-term therapy; hypokalemia and hyperglycemia
• Weight daily, notify prescriber of weekly gain >5 lb
• B/P q4h, pulse; notify prescriber of chest pain
• I&O ratio; be alert for decreasing urinary output, increasing edema
• Plasma cortisol levels during long-term therapy (normal level: 138-635 nmol/L SI units when drawn at 8 AM)
• Infection: increased temp, WBC, even after withdrawal of medication; drug masks infection
• Potassium depletion: paresthesias, fatigue, nausea, vomiting, depression, polyuria, dysrhythmias, weakness
• Edema, hypertension, cardiac symptoms
• Mental status: affect, mood, behavioral changes, aggression

Administer:
• Daily dose in AM for better results
• IM inj deep in large muscle mass; rotate sites; avoid deltoid; use 21G needle
• In one dose in AM to prevent adrenal suppression; avoid SC administration; may damage tissue
• With food or milk for GI symptoms (PO)
• Rectal: telling patient to retain for 20 min if possible

IV route
• Phosphate: IV undiluted or added to dextrose or saline inj and given by inf; give 25 mg or less/min
• Succinate: IV in mix-o-vial, or reconstitute 250 mg or less/2 ml bacteriostatic H_2O for inj; mix gently; give direct IV over 1 min or more; may be further diluted in 100, 250, 500, or 1000 ml of D_5W, D_5 0.9%, NaCl 0.9% given over ordered rate

Sodium phosphate preparations
Additive compatibilities: Amikacin, amphotericin B, bleomycin, cephapirin, metaraminol, sodium bicarbonate, verapamil
Syringe compatibilities: Metoclopramide
Y-site compatibilities: Allpurinol, amifostine, aztreonam, cefepime, cladribine, famotidine, filgrastim, fluconazole, fludarabine, granisetron, melphalan, ondansetron, paclitaxel, piperacillin/tazobactam, teniposide, thiotepa, vinorelbine

Sodium succinate preparations
Additive compatibilities: Amikacin, aminophylline, amphotericin B, calcium chloride, calcium gluconate, cephalothin, cephapirin, chloramphenicol, clindamycin, cloxacillin, corticotropin, DAUNOrubicin, diphenhydrAMINE, DOPamine, erythromycin, floxacillin, lidocaine, magnesium sulfate, mephentermine, metronidazole/sodium bicarbonate, mitomycin, mitoxantrone,

H

netilmicin, netilmicin/potassium chloride, norepinephrine, penicillin G potassium/sodium, piperacillin, polymyxin B, potassium chloride, sodium bicarbonate, theophylline, thiopental, vancomycin, verapamil, vit B/C

Syringe compatibilities: Metoclopramide, thiopental

Y-site compatibilities: Acyclovir, allopurinol, amifostine, aminophylline, amphotericin B cholesteryl, ampicillin, amrinone, amsacrine, atracurium, atropine, aztreonam, betamethasone, calcium gluconate, cefepime, cefmetazole, cephalothin, cephapirin, chlordiazepoxide, chlorproMAZINE, cisatracurium, cladribine, cyanocobalamin, cytarabine, dexamethasone, digoxin, diphenhydrAMINE, DOPamine, DOXOrubicin liposome, droperidol, edrophonium, enalaprilat, epINEPHrine, esmolol, estrogens conjugated, ethacrynate, famotidine, fentanyl, fentanyl/droperidol, filgrastim, fludarabine, fluorouracil, foscarnet, furosemide, gallium, granisetron, heparin, hydrALAZINE, insulin (regular), isoproterenol, kanamycin, lidocaine, lorazepam, magnesium sulfate, melphalan, menadiol, meperidine, methicillin, methoxamine, methylergonovine, minocycline, morphine, neostigmine, norepinephrine, ondansetron, oxacillin, oxytocin, paclitaxel, pancuronium, penicillin G potassium, pentazocine, phytonadione, piperacillin/tazobactam, prednisolone, procainamide, prochlorperazine, propofol, propranolol, pyridostigmine, remifentanil, scopolamine, sodium bicarbonate, succinylcholine, tacrolimus, teniposide, theophylline, thiotepa, trimethaphan, trimethobenzamide, vecuronium, vinorelbine

Perform/provide:

- Assistance with ambulation in patient with bone tissue disease to prevent fractures

Evaluate:

- Therapeutic response: ease of respirations, decreased inflammation

Teach patient/family:

- That emergency ID as steroid user should be carried
- To notify prescriber if therapeutic response decreases; dosage adjustment may be needed; of signs of infection
- Not to discontinue abruptly, or adrenal crisis can result; drug should be tapered off
- To avoid OTC products: salicylates, alcohol in cough products, cold preparations unless directed by prescriber
- About cushingoid symptoms of adrenal insufficiency: nausea, anorexia, fatigue, dizziness, dyspnea, weakness, joint pain

hydrocortisone otic

See appendix c

hydrocortisone topical

See appendix c

HIGH ALERT

hydromorphone (℞)

(hye-droe-mor'fone)

Dilaudid, Dilaudid HP, hydromorphone HCl, Hydrostat IR, PMS-Hydromorphone

Func. class.: Opiate analgesic

Chem. class.: Semisynthetic phenanthrene

Controlled Substance Schedule II
Action: Inhibits ascending pain pathways in CNS, increases pain threshold, alters pain perception
Uses: Moderate to severe pain, nonproductive cough
Dosage and routes:
• *Adult:* **PO** 1-6 mg q4-6h prn; **IM/SC/IV** 2-4 mg q4-6h; **RECT** 3 mg q4-6h prn
• *Geriatric:* **PO** 1-2 mg q4-6h
• *Child:* 0.03-0.08 mg/kg q4-6h, max 5 mg/dose
Antitussive
• *Adult:* **PO** 1 mg q3-4h prn
Available forms: Inj 1, 2, 3, 4, 10 mg/ml; tabs 1, 2, 3, 4, 8 mg; supp 3 mg; oral sol 5 mg/5 ml; syrup 1 mg/5 ml
Side effects/adverse reactions:
CNS: Drowsiness, dizziness, confusion, headache, sedation, euphoria, mood changes, ***seizures***
GI: Nausea, vomiting, anorexia, constipation, cramps, dry mouth
GU: Increased urinary output, dysuria, urinary retention
INTEG: Rash, urticaria, bruising, flushing, diaphoresis, pruritus
EENT: Tinnitus, blurred vision, miosis, diplopia
CV: Palpitations, bradycardia, change in B/P, hypotension, tachycardia
RESP: ***Respiratory depression***
Contraindications: Hypersensitivity, addiction (opiate)
Precautions: Addictive personality, pregnancy (C), lactation, increased intracranial pressure, MI (acute), severe heart disease, respiratory depression, hepatic disease, renal disease, child <18 yr
Do not confuse:
Dilaudid/Demerol
hydromorphone/meperidine
hydromorphone/morphine
Pharmacokinetics: Onset 15-30 min, peak ½-1 hr, duration 4-5 hr; metabolized by liver; excreted by kidneys; crosses placenta; excreted in breast milk, half-life 2-3 hr
Interactions:
• ↑ with other CNS depressants: alcohol, opiates, sedative/hypnotics, antipsychotics, skeletal muscle relaxants
↑ action: chamomile, hops, Jamaican dogwood, kava, lavender, mistletoe, nettle, pokeweed, poppy, senega, skullcap, valerian
↑ anticholinergic effect: corkwood
Lab test interferences:
Increase: Amylase

NURSING CONSIDERATIONS
Assess:
• I&O ratio; check for decreasing output; may indicate urinary retention
• CNS changes: dizziness, drowsiness, hallucinations, euphoria, LOC, pupil reaction
• Bowel function, constipation
• Allergic reactions: rash, urticaria
• Respiratory dysfunction: respiratory depression, character, rate, rhythm; notify prescriber if respirations are <10/min
• Need for pain medication, physical dependence
• Pain control, sedation by scoring on 0-10 scale, ATC dosing is best for pain control
Administer:
• With antiemetic if nausea, vomiting occur
• When pain is beginning to return; determine interval by response
• Rotate inj sites when giving SC
IV route
• Direct, diluted with 5 ml sterile H_2O or NS; give through Y-connector or 3-way stopcock; give 2 mg or less/3-5 min
• IV INF: Dilute each 0.1-1 mg/ml NS (0.1-1 mg/ml), deliver by opioid syringe infusor; may be diluted in

H

D_5W, D_5/NaCl, 0.45% NaCl, or NS for larger amounts and delivery through an infusion pump
Additive compatibilities: Bupivacaine, fluorouracil, midazolam, ondansetron, promethazine, verapamil
Solution compatibilities: D_5W, D_5/0.45% NaCl, D_5/0.9% NaCl, D_5/LR, D_5/Ringer's sol, 0.45% NaCl, 0.9% NaCl, Ringer's and lactated Ringer's sol
Syringe compatibilities: Atropine, bupivacaine, ceftazidime, chlorproMAZINE, cimetidine, dimenhyDRINATE, diphenhydrAMINE, fentanyl, glycopyrrolate, haloperidol, hydrOXYzine, lorazepam, midazolam, pentazocine, pentobarbital, prochlorperazine, promethazine, ranitidine, scopolamine, tetracaine, thiethylperazine, trimethobenzamide
Y-site compatibilities: Acyclovir, allopurinol, amifostine, amikacin, amsacrine, aztreonam, cefamandole, cefazolin, cefepime, cefmetazole, cefoperazone, cefotaxime, cefoxitin, ceftazidime, ceftizoxime, cefuroxime, cephalothin, cephapirin, chloramphenicol, cisatracurium, cisplatin, cladribine, clindamycin, cyclophosphamide, cytarabine, diltiazem, DOBUTamine, DOPamine, DOXOrubicin, DOXOrubicin liposome, doxycycline, epINEPHrine, erythromycin lactobionate, famotidine, fentanyl, filgrastim, fludarabine, foscarnet, furosemide, gentamicin, granisetron, heparin, kanamycin, labetalol, lorazepam, magnesium sulfate, melphalan, methotrexate, metronidazole, mezlocillin, midazolam, milrinone, morphine, moxalactam, nafcillin, niCARdipine, nitroglycerin, norepinephrine, ondansetron, oxacillin, paclitaxel, penicillin G potassium, piperacillin, piperacillin/tazobactam, propofol, ranitidine, remifentanil, teniposide, thiotepa, ticarcillin, tobramycin, trimethoprim-sulfamethoxazole, vancomycin, vecuronium, vinorelbine
Perform/provide:
- Storage in light-resistant area at room temperature
- Assistance with ambulation
- Safety measures: side rails, nightlight, call bell within easy reach

Evaluate:
- Therapeutic response: decrease in pain

Teach patient/family:
- To report any symptoms of CNS changes, allergic reactions
- That physical dependency may result when used for extended periods
- That withdrawal symptoms may occur: nausea, vomiting, cramps, fever, faintness, anorexia
- To avoid driving, other hazardous activities, drowsiness occurs

Treatment of overdose: Naloxone HCl (Narcan) 0.2-0.8 mg IV, O_2, IV fluids, vasopressors

hydromorphone/guaifenesin/alcohol (℞)

(hye-droe-mor′fone)
Dilaudid Cough Syrup
Func. class.: Antitussive, opioid
Chem. class.: Phenanthrene derivative

Controlled Substance Schedule II
Action: Increases respiratory tract fluid by decreasing surface tension, adhesiveness, which increases removal of mucus; analgesic, antitussive suppresses the cough reflex by a direct central action
Uses: Cough
Dosage and routes:
- *Adult:* **PO** 1 mg q3-4h prn

Available forms: Syr 1 mg/5 ml

Side effects/adverse reactions:
CNS: Dizziness, drowsiness
GI: Nausea, constipation, vomiting, anorexia
CV: Hypotension
INTEG: Urticaria, rash
RESP: ***Respiratory depression***
Contraindications: Hypersensitivity, increased intracranial pressure, status asthmaticus
Precautions: Hypothyroidism, Addison's disease, CNS depression, brain tumor, asthma, hepatic disease, renal disease, COPD, psychosis, alcoholism, convulsive disorders, pregnancy (C), lactation
Do not confuse:
hydromorphone/meperidine/morphine
Pharmacokinetics: Metabolized by liver; half-life 2-4 hr
Interactions:
• ↑ CNS depression: barbiturates, opioids, antipsychotics, antidepressants
• ↑ anticholinergic effect: corkwood
• ↑ sedative effect: chamomile, hops, Jamaican dogwood, lavender, mistletoe, nettle, pokeweed, poppy, senega, skullcap, valerian
NURSING CONSIDERATIONS
Assess:
• VS, cardiac status, including hypotension
• Respiratory rate, depth
• Cough: type, frequency, character, including sputum
Administer:
• Decreased dose to elderly patients; metabolism may be slowed
Perform/provide:
• Storage at room temperature
• Increased fluids, bulk, exercise to decrease constipation
Evaluate:
• Therapeutic response: absence of cough
Teach patient/family:
• To avoid driving, other hazardous activities until patient stabilized on medication if drowsiness occurs
• To avoid alcohol, other CNS depressants; will enhance sedating properties of this drug
• May be taken with food for GI upset
• Physical dependency may result when used for extended periods of time

hydroxocobalamin (vit B_{12}) (℞)

(hye-drox'-o-ko-bal'a-min)
Acti-B_{12} ✤, Alphamin, Hydrobexan, Hydro-Crysti 12, Hydroxo-12, hydroxycobalamin, LA-12
Func. class.: Vitamin
Chem. class.: B_{12}—water-soluble vitamin

Action: Needed for adequate nerve functioning, protein and carbohydrate metabolism, normal growth, RBC development
Uses: Vit B_{12} deficiency, pernicious anemia, vit B_{12} malabsorption syndrome, Schilling test
Dosage and routes:
Vitamin B_{12} deficiency
Adult: **IM** 30-100 mcg qd × 5-10 days, maintenance 100-200 mg **IM** qmo
Child: **IM** 1-30 mcg qd × 5-10 days, maintenance 60 mcg **IM** qmo or more often
Pernicious anemia/malabsorption syndrome
• *Adult:* **IM** 100-1000 mcg qd × 2 wk, then 100-1000 mcg **IM** qmo
• *Child:* **IM** 1000-5000 mcg × 2 wk or more given in 100-500 mcg doses, then 60 mcg **IM/SC** qmo

Schilling test
- *Adult and child:* **IM** 1000 mcg in 1 dose

Available forms: Inj 1000 mcg/ml
Side effects/adverse reactions:
CNS: Flushing, optic nerve atrophy
GI: Diarrhea
CV: ***CHF,*** peripheral vascular thrombosis, ***pulmonary edema***
INTEG: Itching, rash
MISC: Hypersensitivity reaction: ***anaphylaxis***
Contraindications: Hypersensitivity, optic nerve atrophy, cardiac disease
Precautions: Pregnancy (A), (C) if used above RDA level, lactation, children
Pharmacokinetics: Stored in liver, kidneys, stomach; 50%-90% excreted in urine; crosses placenta, breast milk
Interactions:
- ↓ hydroxocobalamin absorption: aminoglycosides, anticonvulsants, colchicine, chloramphenicol, antineoplastics, cimetidine, alcohol, vit C, K preparations

Lab test interferences:
False positive: Intrinsic factor
NURSING CONSIDERATIONS
Assess:
- For deficiency, red, beefy tongue, pale skin, neuropathy, psychotic episodes; before and after treatment
- Megaloblastic anemia: potassium levels during beginning treatment
- CBC for increased reticulocyte count during first week of therapy, followed by increase in RBC and hemoglobin; folic acid levels, vit B_{12} levels, before and during treatment
- For pulmonary edema or worsening of CHF in cardiac patients

Administer:
- By IM inj for pernicious anemia unless contraindicated

Evaluate:
- Therapeutic response: decreased anorexia, dyspnea on excretion, palpitations, paresthesias, psychosis, visual disturbances

Teach patient/family:
- That treatment must continue for life in pernicious anemia
- The importance of a well-balanced diet

hydroxychloroquine (℞)
(hye-drox-ee-klor′oh-kwin)
Plaquenil
Func. class.: Antimalarial, antirheumatic (DMARDs)
Chem. class.: 4-Aminoquinoline derivative

Action: Inhibits parasite replications, transcription of DNA to RNA by forming complexes with DNA in parasite
Uses: Malaria caused by *Plasmodium vivax, P. malariae, P. ovale, P. falciparum* (some strains): LE, rheumatoid arthritis
Dosage and routes:
Malaria
- *Adult:* **PO** suppression or prevention 200 mg qwk, begin 1-2 wk before travel, continue 4 wk after returning; treatment 400 mg, then 200 mg at 6, 24, 48 hr after 1st dose
- *Child:* **PO** suppression or prevention 5 mg/kg qwk, begin 1-2 wk before travel, continue 4 wk after returning; treatment 10 mg/kg, then 5 mg/kg at 6, 24, 48 hr after 1st dose

Lupus erythematosus
- *Adult:* **PO** 400 mg qd-bid; length depends on patient response; maintenance 200-400 mg qd

Rheumatoid arthritis
- *Adult:* **PO** 400-600 mg qd for 4-12

wk; then 200-300 mg qd after good response

• *Child:* **PO** 3-5 mg/kg/day max 400 mg/day

Available forms: Tabs 200 mg

Side effects/adverse reactions:

CV: Hypotension, heart block, ***asystole with syncope***

INTEG: Pruritus, pigmentation changes, skin eruptions, lichen planus–like eruptions, eczema, ***exfoliative dermatitis,*** alopecia

CNS: Headache, stimulation, fatigue, irritability, ***seizures,*** bad dreams, dizziness, confusion, psychosis, decreased reflexes

EENT: Blurred vision, corneal changes, retinal changes, difficulty focusing, tinnitus, vertigo, deafness, photophobia, corneal edema

GI: Nausea, vomiting, anorexia, diarrhea, cramps

HEMA: ***Thrombocytopenia, agranulocytosis, leukopenia, aplastic anemia***

Contraindications: Hypersensitivity, retinal field changes, children (long-term)

Precautions: Blood dyscrasias, severe GI disease, neurologic disease, alcoholism, hepatic disease, G6PD deficiency, psoriasis, eczema, pregnancy (C), lactation

Pharmacokinetics:

PO: Peak 1-2 hr, half-life 3-5 days; metabolized in liver; excreted in urine, feces, breast milk; crosses placenta

Interactions:

• ↓ hydroxychloroquine action: Mg or Al compounds

• ↑ digoxin levels

• ↑ antibody titer: rabies vaccine

NURSING CONSIDERATIONS

Assess:

• For lupus erythematosus, malaria symptoms

• For rheumatoid arthritis: pain, swelling, ROM, temperature of joints

• Ophthalmic exam baseline and q6mo if long-term treatment or drug dosage >150 mg/day

• Hepatic studies qwk: AST, ALT, bilirubin

• Blood studies: CBC, platelets; WBC, RBC, platelets may be decreased; if severe, drug should be discontinued

• For decreased reflexes: knee, ankle

• ECG during therapy

• Watch for depression of T waves, widening of QRS complex

• Allergic reactions: pruritus, rash, urticaria

• Blood dyscrasias: malaise, fever, bruising, bleeding (rare)

• For ototoxicity (tinnitus, vertigo, change in hearing); audiometric testing should be done before, after treatment

◆ For toxicity: blurring vision, difficulty focusing, headache, dizziness, knee, ankle reflexes; drug should be discontinued immediately

Administer:

PO route

• Before or after meals or with milk; at same time each day to maintain drug level

• Tabs may be crushed and mixed with food, fluids

• For malaria prophylaxis should be started 2 wk prior to exposure and 4-6 wk after leaving exposure area

Perform/provide:

• Storage in tight, light-resistant container at room temperature; keep inj in cool environment

Evaluate:

• Therapeutic response: decreased symptoms of malaria, LE, rheumatoid arthritis

Teach patient/family:

• To use sunglasses in bright sunlight to decrease photophobia
• That urine may turn rust or brown
• To report hearing, visual problems, fever, fatigue, bruising, bleeding, which may indicate blood dyscrasias

Treatment of overdose: Induce vomiting; gastric lavage; administer barbiturate (ultrashort-acting), vasopressor, ammonium chloride; tracheostomy may be necessary

hydroxyurea (℞)

(hye-drox'ee-yoo-ree-ah)
Droxia, Hydrea
Func. class.: Antineoplastic, antimetabolite
Chem. class.: Synthetic urea analog

Action: Acts by inhibiting DNA synthesis without interfering with RNA or protein synthesis; incorporates thymidine into DNA, causing direct damage to DNA strands; S phase specific of cell cycle

Uses: Melanoma, chronic myelocytic leukemia, recurrent or metastatic ovarian cancer, squamous cell carcinoma of the head and neck, sickle cell anemia, psoriasis

Dosage and routes:

Renal disease
• CCr 10-50 ml/min dose 50%; CCr <10 ml/min dose 20%

Solid tumors
• *Adult:* **PO** 80 mg/kg as a single dose q3d or 20-30 mg/kg as a single dose qd

In combination with radiation
• *Adult:* **PO** 80 mg/kg as a single dose q3d; should be started 7 days before irradiation

Resistant chronic myelocytic leukemia
• *Adult:* **PO** 20-30 mg/kg/day as a single daily dose

Sickle cell anemia
• *Adult:* **PO** 15 mg/kg/day, may increase by 5 mg/kg/day, max 35 mg/kg/day

Available forms: Caps 200, 300, 400, 500 mg

Side effects/adverse reactions:
HEMA: ***Leukopenia, anemia, thrombocytopenia, megalobastic erythropoiesis***
GI: Nausea, vomiting, anorexia, diarrhea, stomatitis, constipation
GU: Increased BUN, uric acid, creatinine, temporary renal function impairment
INTEG: *Rash,* urticaria, pruritus, dry skin, facial erythema
CV: Angina, ischemia
CNS: Headache, confusion, hallucinations, dizziness, ***convulsions***
MISC: Fever, chills, malaise

Contraindications: Hypersensitivity, leukopenia (<2500/mm^3), thrombocytopenia (<100,000/mm^3), anemia (severe), pregnancy (D), lactation

Precautions: Renal disease (severe)

Pharmacokinetics: Readily absorbed when taken orally, peak level in 2 hr; degraded in liver; excreted in urine, almost totally eliminated in 24 hr; readily crosses blood-brain barrier, eliminated as CO_2

Interactions:
• ↑ toxicity: radiation or other antineoplastics

Lab test interferences:
Increase: Renal studies

NURSING CONSIDERATIONS

Assess:
• CBC, differential, platelet count qwk; withhold drug if WBC is <2500/mm^3 or platelet count is <100,000/mm^3; notify prescriber; drug should be discontinued

• Renal studies: BUN, serum uric acid, urine CCr, electrolytes before, during therapy
• I&O ratio; report fall in urine output to <30 ml/hr
• Monitor temp q4h; fever may indicate beginning infection
• Hepatic studies before, during therapy: bilirubin, alk phosphatase, AST, ALT, LDH; prn or qmo
• B/P q3-4h; check for chest pain; angina, ischemia may occur
• Bleeding: hematuria, guaiac, bruising or petechiae, mucosa or orifices q8h
• Food preferences; list likes, dislikes
• Inflammation of mucosa, breaks in skin
• Buccal cavity q8h for dryness, sores or ulceration, white patches, oral pain, bleeding, dysphagia
• Symptoms indicating severe allergic reaction: rash, urticaria, itching, flushing
• Neurotoxicity: headaches, hallucinations, convulsions, dizziness

Administer:
• Allopurinol or $NaHCO_3$ concurrently to prevent high uric acid levels; extra fluids
• Antiemetic 30-60 min before giving drug and prn
• Antibiotics for prophylaxis of infection
• Transfusion for anemia

Perform/provide:
• Rinsing of mouth tid-qid with water, club soda; brushing of teeth bid-tid with soft brush or cotton-tipped applicators for stomatitis; use unwaxed dental floss
• Nutritious diet with iron, vitamin supplements as ordered

Evaluate:
• Therapeutic response: decreased tumor size, spread of malignancy

Teach patient/family:
⊘ Not to break, crush, or chew caps
• To report signs of infection: elevated temp, sore throat, flulike symptoms
• To report signs of anemia: fatigue, headache, faintness, shortness of breath, irritability
• To report bleeding: avoid use of razors, commercial mouthwash
• To avoid use of aspirin products, ibuprofen
• To avoid foods with citric acid, hot or rough texture if stomatitis is present
• To report stomatitis: any bleeding, white spots, ulcerations in the mouth; tell patient to examine mouth qd, report symptoms
• That contraceptive measures are recommended during therapy
• To notify prescriber of fever, chills, sore throat, nausea, vomiting, anorexia, diarrhea, bleeding, bruising; may indicate blood dyscrasias

* hydrOXYzine (℞)

(hye-drox'i-zeen)
Apo-Hydroxyzine♣, Atarax, hydroxyzine, Multi-pax♣, Novohydroxyzine♣, Vistaril
Func. class.: Antianxiety/antihistamine/sedative-hypnotic, antiemetic
Chem. class.: Piperazine derivative

Action: Depresses subcortical levels of CNS, including limbic system, reticular formation; competes with H_1-receptor sites
Uses: Anxiety preoperatively, postoperatively to prevent nausea, vomiting, to potentiate opioid analgesics; sedation; pruritus

Dosage and routes:

• *Adult:* **PO** 25-100 mg tid-qid, max 600 mg/day

• *Geriatric:* **PO** 10 mg tid-qid (pruritus)

• *Child >6 yr:* 50-100 mg/day in divided doses

• *Child <6 yr:* 50 mg/day in divided doses

Preoperatively/postoperatively

• *Adult:* **IM** 25-100 mg q4-6h

• *Child:* **IM** 0.5-1.1 mg/kg q4-6h

Pruritus

• *Adult:* **PO** 25 mg tid-qid

Antiemetic

• *Adult:* **IM** 25-100 mg/dose q4-6h prn

Available forms: Tabs 10, 25, 50, 100 mg; caps 10, 25, 50, 100 mg; oral susp 25 mg/5 ml; inj 25, 50 mg/ml

Side effects/adverse reactions:

CV: Hypotension

CNS: Dizziness, drowsiness, confusion, headache, tremors, fatigue, depression, ***seizures***

GI: Dry mouth, increased appetite, nausea, diarrhea, weight gain

Contraindications: Hypersensitivity to this drug or cetirizine, pregnancy (1st trimester), lactation, acute asthma

Precautions: Elderly, debilitated, hepatic disease, renal disease, narrow-angle glaucoma, COPD, prostatic hypertrophy, pregnancy (2nd/3rd trimester) (C)

Do not confuse:

Atarax/amoxicillin/Ativan

Vistaril/Versed

hydrOXYzine/hydrALAZINE

Pharmacokinetics:

PO: Onset 15-30 min, duration 4-6 hr, half-life 3 hr, metabolized by liver, excreted by kidneys

Interactions:

• ↑ CNS depressant effect: barbiturates, opioids, analgesics, alcohol

• ↑ anticholinergic effects: phenothiazines, quinidine, disopyramide, antihistamines, antidepressants, atropine, haloperidol

↑ anticholinergic effect: corkwood, henbane leaf, jimsonweed, scopolia

↑ sedative action: chamomile, cowslip, hops, Jamaican dogwood, kava, khat, Queen Anne's lace, senega, skullcap, valerian

NURSING CONSIDERATIONS

Assess:

• B/P (lying, standing), pulse; if systolic B/P drops 20 mm Hg, hold drug, notify prescriber

• Mental status: mood, sensorium, affect, anxiety, behavior, increased sedation

Administer:

PO route

• With food or milk for GI symptoms (PO)

• Crushed if patient is unable to swallow medication whole

• Gum, hard candy, frequent sips of water for dry mouth

IM route

• By Z-track inj in large muscle for IM to decrease pain, chance of necrosis, never give IV/SC

Additive compatibilities: Cisplatin, cyclophosphamide, cytarabine, dimenhyDRINATE, etoposide, lidocaine, mesna, methotrexate, nafcillin

Syringe compatibilities: Atropine, atropine/meperidine, benzquinamide, bupivacaine, butorphanol, chlorproMAZINE, cimetidine, codeine, diphenhydrAMINE, doxapram, droperidol, fentanyl, fluphenazine, glycopyrrolate, hydromorphone, lidocaine, meperidine, meperidine/atropine, methotrimeprazine, metoclopramide, midazolam, morphine, nalbuphine, oxymorphone, pentazocine, perphenazine, procaine, prochlorperazine, promazine, promethazine, scopolamine, sufentanil, thiothixene

Perform/provide:

- Assistance with ambulation during beginning therapy, since drowsiness/dizziness occurs
- Safety measures, including side rails
- Checking to see if PO medication has been swallowed

Evaluate:

- Therapeutic response: decreased anxiety

Teach patient/family:

- That medication is not to be used for everyday stress or used longer than 4 mo
- To avoid OTC preparations (cold, cough, hay fever) unless approved by prescriber
- To avoid driving, activities that require alertness
- To avoid alcohol ingestion, psychotropic medications
- Not to discontinue medication quickly after long-term use
- To rise slowly or fainting may occur

Treatment of overdose: Lavage if orally ingested; VS, supportive care; IV norepinephrine for hypotension

hyoscyamine (℞)

(hye-oh-sye'a-meen)

Anaspaz, A-Spas S/L, Cystospaz, Cystospaz-M, Donnamar, ED-SPAZ, Gastrosed, Levsin, Levsinex, NuLev Timecaps

Func. class.: Anticholinergic

Chem. class.: Belladonna alkaloid

Action: Inhibits muscarinic actions of acetylcholine at postganglionic parasympathetic neuroeffector sites, reduces rigidity, tremors, hyperhidrosis of Parkinsonism

Uses: Treatment of peptic ulcer disease in combination with other drugs; other GI disorders, other spastic disorders, urinary incontinence

Dosage and routes:

- *Adult:* **PO/SL** 0.125-0.25 mg tid-qid ac, hs; **TIME REL** 0.375 q12h; **IM/SC/IV** 0.25-0.5 mg q6h
- *Child 2-10 yr:* ½ adult dose
- *Child <2 yr:* ¼ adult dose

Available forms: Tabs 0.125, 0.13, 0.15 mg; caps time rel 0.375 mg; sol 0.125 mg/ml; elix 0.125 mg/5 ml; inj 0.5 mg/ml

Side effects/adverse reactions:

CNS: Confusion, stimulation in elderly, headache, insomnia, dizziness, drowsiness, anxiety, weakness, hallucination

GI: Dry mouth, constipation, paralytic ileus, heartburn, nausea, vomiting, dysphagia, absence of taste

GU: Urinary hesitancy, retention, impotence

CV: Palpitations, tachycardia

EENT: Blurred vision, photophobia, mydriasis, cycloplegia, increased ocular tension

INTEG: Urticaria, rash, pruritus, anhidrosis, fever, allergic reactions

Contraindications: Hypersensitivity to anticholinergics, narrow-angle glaucoma, GI obstruction, myasthenia gravis, paralytic ileus, GI atony, toxic megacolon, prostatic hypertrophy

Precautions: Hyperthyroidism, coronary artery disease, dysrhythmias, CHF, ulcerative colitis, hypertension, hiatal hernia, hepatic disease, renal disease, pregnancy (C), urinary retention, elderly

Pharmacokinetics:

PO: Duration 4-6 hr; metabolized by liver; excreted in urine; half-life 3.5 hr

Interactions:
- ↓ hyoscyamine effect: antacids
- ↑ anticholinergic effect: amantadine, tricyclics, MAOIs, H_1-antihistamines
- ↓ effect of phenothiazines, levodopa, ketoconazole

↑ constipation: black catechu

↑ anticholinergic effect: butterbur, jimsonweed

↓ anticholinergic effect: jaborandi tree, pill-bearing spurge

NURSING CONSIDERATIONS

Assess:
- VS, cardiac status: checking for dysrhythmias, increased rate, palpitations
- I&O ratio; check for urinary retention or hesitancy
- GI complaints: pain, bleeding (frank or occult), nausea, vomiting, anorexia

Administer:
- ½ hr ac for better absorption
- Decreased dose to elderly patients; metabolism may be slowed
- Gum, hard candy, frequent rinsing of mouth for dryness of oral cavity

Perform/provide:
- Storage in tight container protected from light
- Increased fluids, bulk, exercise to decrease constipation

Evaluate:
- Therapeutic response: absence of epigastric pain, bleeding, nausea, vomiting

Teach patient/family:
- To avoid driving, other hazardous activities until stabilized on medication
- To avoid alcohol or other CNS depressants; will enhance sedating properties of this drug
- To avoid hot environments; heat stroke may occur; drug suppresses perspiration
- To use sunglasses when outside to prevent photophobia; may cause blurred vision

Not to break, crush, or chew time rel caps

ibandonate

See appendix a—selected new drugs

ibritumomab tiuxetan (℞)

(ee-brit-u-moe′mab)

Zevalin

Func. class.: Misc. antineoplastic

Chem. class.: Monoclonal antibody

Action: High affinity for indium-111, yttrium-90; induces CD20 + B-cell lines

Uses: Non-Hodgkin's lymphoma, B-cell NHL

Dosage and routes:
- *Adult:* **IV INF** 250 mg/m^2 at a rate of 50 mg/hr; if hypersensitivity does not occur, increase rate by 50 mg/hr $q^1/_2h$, max 400 mg/hr; slow/interrupt inf if hypersensitivity occurs

Available forms: Inj 3.2 mg/2 ml

Side effects/adverse reactions:

CV: ***Cardiac dysrhythmias***

GU: ***Renal failure***

SYST: ***Stevens-Johnson syndrome***

GI: Nausea, vomiting, anorexia, abdominal pain, diarrhea

INTEG: Irritation at site, rash, ***fatal mucocutaneous infections (rare)***

HEMA: ***Leukopenia, neutropenia, thrombocytopenia,*** anemia

OTHER: Fever, chills, asthenia, headache, angioedema, hypotension, myalgia, ***bronchospasm, hemorrhage,*** infections, cough, dyspnea, dizziness, anxiety

Contraindications: Hypersensitiv-

ity to this agent or murine proteins, pregnancy (D)
Precautions: Lactation, children, elderly, cardiac conditions, immunizations after therapy
Pharmacokinetics: Half-life 30 hr
NURSING CONSIDERATIONS
Assess:
- For signs of fatal infusion reaction: hypoxia, pulmonary infiltrates, ARDS, MI, ventricular fibrillation, cardiogenic shock; most fatal infusion reactions occur with first infusion; potentially fatal
- Biodistribution: 1st image 2-24 hr, 2nd image 48-72 hr, 3rd image 90-120 hr (optimal)
- For signs of severe mucocutaneous reactions: Stevens-Johnson syndrome, lichenoid dermatitis, toxic epidermal lysis; occur 1-13 wk after drug was given
- Tumor lysis syndrome: acute renal failure requiring hemodialysis, hyperkalemia, hypocalcemia, hyperuricemia, hyperphosphatemia
- CBC, differential, platelet count weekly; withhold drug if WBC is <3500/mm^3, or platelet count <100,000/mm^3; notify prescriber of these results; drug should be discontinued
- GI symptoms: frequency of stools
- Signs of dehydration: rapid respirations, poor skin turgor, decreased urine output, dry skin, restlessness, weakness

Administer:
- Do not use as bolus or IV direct

IV INF route
- See manufacturer's product labeling for preparation

Perform/provide:
- Increased fluid intake to 2-3 L/day to prevent dehydration, unless contraindicated
- Emergency equipment nearby with epINEPHrine, antihistamines, corticosteroids
- Changing of IV site q48h
- Nutritious diet with iron, vitamin supplement, low fiber, few dairy products
- Storage of vials at 36°-46° F, do not freeze

Evaluate:
- Therapeutic response: decrease in tumor size, decrease in spread of cancer

Teach patient/family:
- To report adverse reactions

ibuprofen (OTC, ℞)

(eye-byoo-proe'fen)
Actiprofen ✦, Advil, Advil Migraine, Apo-Ibuprofen ✦, Bayer Select Ibuprofen Pain Relief, Children's Advil, Children's Motrin, Excedrin IB, Genpril, Haltran, ibuprofen, Medipren, Menadol, Midol Maximum Strength Cramp Formula, Motrin, Motrin IB, Motrin Junior Strength, Motrin Migraine Pain, Novoprofen ✦, Nuprin, Nu-Ibuprofen, PediaCare Children's Fever

Func. class.: Nonsteroidal anti-inflammatory, antipyretic, nonopioid analgesics
Chem. class.: Propionic acid derivative

Action: Inhibits prostaglandin synthesis by decreasing enzyme needed for biosynthesis; analgesic, antiinflammatory, antipyretic
Uses: Rheumatoid arthritis, osteoarthritis, primary dysmenorrhea, gout, dental pain, musculoskeletal disorders, fever
Dosage and routes:
Analgesic
- *Adult:* **PO** 200-400 mg q4-6h, not to exceed 3.2 g/day

• *Child:* **PO** 4-10 mg/kg/dose q6-8h

Antipyretic

• *Child 6 mo-12 yr:* **PO** 5 mg/kg (temp <102.5° F or 39.2° C), 10 mg/kg, (temp >102.5° F), may repeat q4-6h, max 40 mg/kg/day

Antiinflammatory

• *Adult:* **PO** 300-800 mg tid-qid, max 3.2 g/day

• *Child:* **PO** 30-40 mg/kg/day in 3-4 divided doses, max 50 mg/kg/day

Available forms: Tabs 100, 200, 300, 400, 600, 800 mg; cap, liq gels 200 mg; oral susp 100 mg/2.5 ml, 100 mg/5 ml; liq 100 mg/5 ml; tabs, chew 50, 100 mg; drops 50 mg/1.25 ml

Side effects/adverse reactions:

CV: Tachycardia, peripheral edema, palpitations, dysrhythmias

CNS: Headache, dizziness, drowsiness, fatigue, tremors, confusion, insomnia, anxiety, depression

EENT: Tinnitus, hearing loss, blurred vision

GI: Nausea, anorexia, vomiting, diarrhea, jaundice, ***hepatitis,*** constipation, flatulence, cramps, dry mouth, peptic ulcer, ***GI bleeding***

GU: ***Nephrotoxicity:*** dysuria, hematuria, oliguria, azotemia

HEMA: ***Blood dyscrasias,*** increased bleeding time

INTEG: Purpura, rash, pruritus, sweating

SYST: ***Anaphylaxis***

Contraindications: Hypersensitivity, asthma, severe renal disease, severe hepatic disease, avoid in 2nd/3rd trimester of pregnancy

Precautions: Pregnancy (B) 1st trimester, lactation, children, bleeding disorders, GI disorders, cardiac disorders, hypersensitivity to other antiinflammatory agents, elderly, CHF, CCr <25 ml/min

Do not confuse:

Nuprin/Lupron

Pharmacokinetics: Well absorbed (PO)

PO: Onset ½ hr; peak 1-2 hr, half-life 2-4 hr, metabolized in liver (inactive metabolites), excreted in urine (inactive metabolites), 90%-99% plasma protein binding, does not enter breast milk

Interactions:

• ↓ effect of: antihypertensives, thiazides, furosemide

• ↓ ibuprofen action: aspirin

• ↑ bleeding risk: cefamandole, cefotetan, cefoperazone, valproic acid, thrombolytics, antiplatelets, warfarin

• ↑ blood dyscrasias possibility: antineoplastics, radiation

• ↑ toxicity: digoxin, lithium, oral anticoagulants, cyclosporine, probenecid

• ↑ GI reactions: aspirin, corticosteroids, NSAIDs, alcohol

• ↑ hypoglycemia: oral antidiabetics, insulin

↑ bleeding risk: arnica, chamomile, clove, dong quai, fenugreek, feverfew, garlic, ginger, ginkgo, ginseng *(Panax)*

↑ gastric irritation: arginine, gossypol

↑ NSAIDs effect: bearberry, bilberry

↑ bleeding risk: bogbean, chondroitin

NURSING CONSIDERATIONS

Assess:

• Renal, hepatic, blood studies: BUN, creatinine, AST, ALT, Hgb, before treatment, periodically thereafter

• Pain: note type, duration, location and intensity with ROM 1 hr after administration

• Audiometric, ophthalmic exam be-

fore, during, after treatment; for eye, ear problems: blurred vision, tinnitus; may indicate toxicity
• Fever: temp before and 1 hr after administration
• Cardiac status: edema (peripheral), tachycardia, palpitations; monitor B/P, pulse for character, quality, rhythm especially in patients with cardiac disease/elderly
• For history of peptic ulcer disorder; asthma, aspirin, hypersensitivity, check closely for hypersensitivity reactions

Administer:
• With food, milk, or antacid to decrease GI symptoms; however, taking on empty stomach best facilitates absorption; if nausea and vomiting occur/persist, notify prescriber

Perform/provide:
• Storage at room temperature

Evaluate:
• Therapeutic response: decreased pain, stiffness in joints; decreased swelling in joints; ability to move more easily; reduction in fever or menstrual cramping

Teach patient/family:
• To report blurred vision, ringing, roaring in ears; may indicate toxicity; eye and hearing tests should be done during long-term therapy
• To avoid driving, other hazardous activities if dizziness or drowsiness occurs
⬥ To report change in urinary pattern, increased weight, edema, increased pain in joints, fever, blood in urine; indicate nephrotoxicity
• That therapeutic inflammatory effects may take up to 1 mo
⬥ To avoid alcohol, NSAIDs, salicylates; bleeding may occur
• To use sunscreen to prevent photosensitivity

HIGH ALERT

ibutilide (℞)

(eye-byoo′tih-lide)

Corvert

Func. class.: Antidysrhythmic (Class III)

Action: Prolongs duration of action potential and effective refractory period

Uses: For rapid conversion of atrial fibrillation/flutter occurring within 1 wk of coronary artery bypass or valve surgery

Dosage and routes:
• *Adult:* **IV INF** (≥60 kg) 1 vial (1 mg) given over 10 min, may repeat same dose in 10 min; **IV INF** (<60 kg) 0.01 mg/kg given over 10 min, may repeat same dose in 10 min

Available forms: Inj 0.1 mg/ml

Side effects/adverse reactions:

CNS: Headache

GI: Nausea

CV: Hypotension, bradycardia, ***sinus arrest, CHF, dysrhythmias,*** hypertension, extrasystoles, ventricular tachycardia, bundle branch block, AV block, palpitations, supraventricular extrasystoles, syncope

Contraindications: Hypersensitivity

Precautions: Sinus node dysfunction, 2nd- or 3rd-degree AV block, electrolyte imbalances, pregnancy (C), bradycardia, lactation, children <18 yr, renal/hepatic disease, elderly

Pharmacokinetics: Elimination half-life in 6 hr; metabolized by liver, excreted by kidneys

Interactions:
• Prodysrhythmia: phenothiazines, tricyclics, tetracyclics, antidepressants, H_1-receptor antagonists, antihistamines
• Masking of cardiotoxicity: digoxin

• Do not use within 4 hr of ibutilide: Class Ia antidysrhythmics (disopyramide, quinidine, procainamide), Class III agents (amiodarone, sotalol)
↑ toxicity, death: aconite
↑ effect: aloe, broom, chronic buckthorn use, cascara sagrada (chronic use), Chinese rhubarb, figwort, fumitory, goldenseal, kudzu, licorice
↓ effect: coltsfoot
↑ serotonin effect: horehound

NURSING CONSIDERATIONS

Assess:

• I&O ratio; electrolytes: K, Na, Cl
• Hepatic studies: AST, ALT, bilirubin, alk phosphatase
• ECG continuously to determine drug effectiveness, measure PR, QRS, QT intervals, check for PVCs, other dysrhythmias, discontinue if atrial fibrillation/flutter ceases
• For dehydration or hypovolemia
• For rebound hypertension after 1-2 hr
• Cardiac rate, respiration: rate, rhythm, character, chest pain

Administer:

IV route

• Undiluted or diluted in 50 ml 0.9% NaCl, or D_5W (0.017 mg/ml) give over 10 min
• Solution is stable for 48 hr refrigerated or 24 hr, room temperature
• Do not admix with other solution, drugs
• Reduce dosage slowly with ECG monitoring

Evaluate:

• Therapeutic response: decrease in atrial fibrillation/flutter

Teach patient/family:

• To report side effects immediately
• Reason for medication

HIGH ALERT

idarubicin (℞)

(eye-dah-roob'ih-sin)

Idamycin, Idamycin PFS

Func. class.: Antineoplastic, antibiotic

Chem. class.: Anthracycline glycoside

Action: Inhibits DNA synthesis by binding to DNA, a vesicant derived from daunorubicin by binding to DNA, which causes strand splitting; cell cycle specific (S phase)

Uses: Used in combination with other antineoplastics for acute myelocytic leukemia in adults

Investigational uses: Breast cancer, solid tumors

Dosage and routes:

• *Adult:* **IV** 12 mg/m^2/day × 3 days in combination with cytosine (induction)

Available forms: Inj 1 mg/ml; powder for inj, lyophilized 5, 10, 20 mg

Side effects/adverse reactions:

HEMA: ***Thrombocytopenia, leukopenia, anemia***

GI: Nausea, vomiting, abdominal pain, mucositis, diarrhea, ***hepatotoxicity***

INTEG: Rash, extravasation, dermatitis, reversible alopecia, urticaria, thrombophlebitis and tissue necrosis at inj site

CV: ***Dysrhythmias, CHF, pericarditis, myocarditis,*** peripheral edema, angina, ***MI***

CNS: Fever, chills, headache

GU: ***Nephrotoxicity***

Contraindications: Hypersensitivity, pregnancy (D), lactation, myelosuppression

Precautions: Renal and hepatic disease, gout, bone marrow depression, children

Do not confuse:
Idamycin/Adriamycin
idarubicin/DOXOrubicin

Pharmacokinetics: Half-life 22 hr; metabolized by liver; crosses placenta; excreted in bile, urine (primarily as metabolites)

Interactions:

- ↑ toxicity: other antineoplastics or radiation
- ↓ antibody response: live virus vaccines

Lab test interferences:
Increase: Uric acid

NURSING CONSIDERATIONS

Assess:

- CBC, differential, platelet count weekly; withhold drug if WBC is <4000/mm^3 or platelet count is <75,000/mm^3; notify prescriber of these results
- Blood, urine, uric acid levels
- Renal studies: BUN, serum uric acid, urine CCr, electrolytes before, during therapy
- I&O ratio; report fall in urine output to <30 ml/hr
- Monitor temp q4h; fever may indicate beginning infection
- Hepatic studies before, during therapy: bilirubin, AST, ALT, alk phosphatase prn or qmo; check for jaundice of skin, sclera, dark urine, clay-colored stools, itchy skin, abdominal pain, fever, diarrhea
- Cardiac toxicity: CHF, dysrythmias, cardiomyopathy; cardiac studies should be done before and periodically during treatment: ECG, chest x-ray
- ECG: watch for ST-T wave changes, low QRS and T, possible dysrhythmias (sinus tachycardia, heart block, PVCs)
- Bleeding: hematuria, guaiac stools, bruising or petechiae, mucosa or orifices q8h
- Effects of alopecia on body image; discuss feelings about body changes
- Inflammation of mucosa, breaks in skin
- Buccal cavity q8h for dryness, sores, ulceration, white patches, oral pain, bleeding, dysphagia
- Local irritation, pain, burning at inj site
- GI symptoms: frequency of stools, cramping
- Acidosis, signs of dehydration: rapid respirations, poor skin turgor, decreased urine output, dry skin, restlessness, weakness

Administer:

- Allopurinol or sodium bicarbonate to reduce uric acid levels, alkalinization of urine
- Transfusion for anemia
- Hydrocortisone for extravasation; apply ice compress after stopping infusion

IV direct route

- After preparing in biologic cabinet wearing gown, gloves, mask
- Antiemetic 30-60 min before giving drug and 6-10 hr after treatment to prevent vomiting
- After reconstituting 5 mg vial with 5 ml 0.9% NaCl (1 mg/1 ml); give over 10-15 min through Y-tube or 3-way stopcock of inf of D_5 or NS; discard unused portion

Solution compatibilities: $D_{3.3}$/0.3% NaCl, D_5/0.9% NaCl, D_5W, LR, 0.9% NaCl

Y-site compatibilities: Amifostine, amikacin, aztreonam, cimetidine, cladribine, cyclophosphamide, cytarabine, diphenhydrAMINE, droperidol, erythromycin, filgrastim, granisetron, imipenem/cisplatin, magnesium sulfate, mannitol, melphalan, metoclopramide, potassium chloride, ranitidine, sargramostim, thiotepa, vinorelbine

Perform/provide:

- Strict hand-washing technique, gloves, protective clothing
- Liquid diet: carbonated beverages, gelatin may be added if patient is not nauseated or vomiting
- Increase fluid intake to 2-3 L/day to prevent urate and calculi formation
- Diet low in purines: absence of organ meats (kidney, liver), dried beans, peas to reduce uric acid level
- Rinsing of mouth tid-qid with water, club soda; brushing of teeth tid-qid with soft brush or cotton-tipped applicators for stomatitis; use unwaxed dental floss
- Storage at room temperature for 3 days after reconstituting or 7 days refrigerated

Evaluate:

- Therapeutic response: decreased tumor size, spread of malignancy

Teach patient/family:

- To report any complaints, side effects to nurse or prescriber
- That hair may be lost during treatment and wig or hairpiece may make patient feel better; tell patient that new hair may be different in color, texture
- To avoid foods with citric acid, hot or rough texture
- To report any bleeding, white spots, ulcerations in mouth; tell patient to examine mouth qd
- That urine may be red-orange for 48 hr
- To use contraception during treatment with this drug and for ≥4 mo after treatment

idoxuridine-IDU ophthalmic

See appendix c

HIGH ALERT

ifosfamide (℞)

(i-foss′fa-mide)

Ifex

Func. class.: Antineoplastic alkylating agent

Chem. class.: Nitrogen mustard

Action: Alkylates DNA, RNA, inhibits enzymes that allow synthesis of amino acids in proteins; also responsible for cross-linking DNA strands; activity is not cell cycle stage specific

Uses: Testicular cancer, soft tissue sarcoma, Ewing's sarcoma, non-Hodgkin's lymphoma, lung, pancreatic sarcoma

Dosage and routes:

- *Adult:* **IV** 1.2 g/m^2/day × 5 days, repeat course q3wk, given with mesna

Available forms: Inj 1, 3 g

Side effects/adverse reactions:

CNS: Facial paresthesia, fever, malaise, somnolence, confusion, depression, hallucinations, dizziness, disorientation, ***seizures, coma,*** cranial nerve dysfunction

GI: Nausea, vomiting, anorexia, ***hepatotoxicity,*** stomatitis, constipation, diarrhea

INTEG: Dermatitis, alopecia, pain at injection site

GU: ***Hematuria, nephrotoxicity, hemorrhagic cystitis,*** dysuria, urinary frequency

HEMA: ***Thrombocytopenia, leukopenia, anemia***

Contraindications: Hypersensitivity, bone marrow suppression, pregnancy (D)

Precautions: Renal disease, lactation, children

Pharmacokinetics: Metabolized by liver; saturation occurs at high doses; excreted in urine; half-life 7-15 hr

Interactions:

- ↑ myelosuppression: other antineoplastics, radiation
- ↓ antibody response: live virus vaccines
- ↑ toxicity: barbiturates, allopurinol

NURSING CONSIDERATIONS

Assess:

- Hepatic studies before, during therapy (bilirubin, AST, ALT, LDH) as needed or monthly
- CBC, differential, platelet count weekly; withhold drug if WBC <2000 or platelet count <50,000; notify prescriber
- Monitor temp q4h (may indicate beginning infection)
- Blood dyscrasias (anemia, granulocytopenia); bruising, fatigue, bleeding, poor healing
- Allergic reactions: dermatitis, exfoliative dermatitis, pruritus, urticaria
- I&O ratio; monitor for hematuria; hemorrhagic cystitis can occur; increase fluids to 3 L/day
- Neurologic symptoms: hallucinations, confusion, disorientation, drug should be discontinued
- Bleeding: hematuria, guaiac, bruising or petechiae, mucosa or orifices q8h
- Jaundice of skin, sclera, dark urine, clay-colored stools, itchy skin, abdominal pain, fever, diarrhea

Administer:

- Antiemetic 30-60 min before giving drug to prevent vomiting
- Antibiotics for prophylaxis of infection
- Always give with mesna to prevent ifosfamide-induced hemorrhagic cystitis

IV route

- After diluting 1 g/20 ml sterile or bacteriostatic H_2O for inj with parabens or benzyl only; shake; may be diluted further with D_5W, LR, NS, sterile H_2O for inj; 1 g/20 ml = 50 mg/ml; 1 g/50 ml = 20 mg/ml; 1 g/200 ml = 5 mg/ml; give over ≥30 min; may also give as cont inf over 72 hr

Additive compatibilities: Carboplatin, cisplatin, etoposide, fluorouracil, mesna

Syringe compatibilities: Mesna

Y-site compatibilities: Allopurinol, amifostine, amphotericin B cholesteryl, aztreonam, DOXOrubicin liposome, filgrastim, fludarabine, gallium, granisetron, melphalan, ondansetron, paclitaxel, piperacillin/tazobactam, propofol, sargramostim, sodium bicarbonate, teniposide, thiotepa, vinorelbine

Perform/provide:

- Storage of powder at room temperature
- Increase fluid intake to 3 L/day to prevent hemorrhagic cystitis
- Warm compresses at inj site for inflammation

Evaluate:

- Therapeutic response: decrease in size and spread of tumor

Teach patient/family:

- To notify prescriber of sore throat, swollen lymph nodes, malaise, fever; other infections may occur
- Not to have vaccinations during treatment
- That hair may be lost during treatment; a wig or hairpiece may make the patient feel better; new hair may be different in color, texture
- To report signs of anemia: fatigue, headache, faintness, shortness of breath, irritability
- To report bleeding; avoid use of razors, commercial mouthwash
- To avoid use of aspirin products, NSAIDs, ibuprofen, hemorrhage can occur

• To use contraceptive measures during therapy
• To avoid crowds, those with infections

imatinib (℞)

(im-ah-tin′ib)

Gleevec

Func. class.: Antineoplastic, misc.

Chem. class.: Protein-tyrosine kinase inhibitor

Action: Inhibits Bcr-Abl tyrosine kinase created in chronic myeloid leukemia (CML)

Uses: Treatment of chronic myeloid leukemia (CML) in blast cell crisis or chronic failure after treatment failure with interferon alfa; gastrointestinal stromal tumors (GIST)

Investigational uses: Polycythemia vera, medullary thyroid carcinoma, recurrent extraabdominal desmoid tumors

Dosage and routes:

• *Adult:* **PO** 400-600 mg/day, may increase to 800 mg qd give in 2 divided doses; give with meal or large glass of water, continue as long as response is good, may increase by 200 mg/day as needed

Available form: Cap 100 mg

Side effects/adverse reactions:

CV: Hemorrhage

CNS: ***CNS hemorrhage,*** headache, dizziness, insomnia

GI: Nausea, ***hepatotoxicity, vomiting, dyspepsia,*** GI hemorrhage, *anorexia, abdominal pain*

HEMA: ***Neutropenia, thrombocytopenia, bleeding***

INTEG: Rash, pruritus

META: Fluid retention, hypokalemia, edema

MISC: Fatigue, epistaxis, pyrexia, night sweats, increased weight

MS: Cramps, pain, arthralgia, myalgia

RESP: Cough, dyspnea, nasopharyngitis, pneumonia, URI

Contraindications: Hypersensitivity, pregnancy (D)

Precautions: Lactation, children, elderly

Pharmacokinetics: Well absorbed (98%) (PO), protein binding 95%, metabolized by CYP3A4, excreted in feces, small amount in urine; peak 2-4 hr, duration 24 hr (imatinib), 40 hr (metabolite), half-life 18 hr

Interactions:

• ↑ hepatotoxicity: acetaminophen
• ↑ imatinib concentrations: ketoconazole, itraconazole, erythromycin, clarithromycin
• ↓ imatinib concentrations: dexamethasone, phenytoin, carbamazepine, rifampin, phenobarbital
• ↑ plasma concentrations of simvastatin, calcium channel blockers
• ↑ plasma concentration of warfarin; avoid use with warfarin, use low-molecular-weight anticoagulants instead

↓ imatinib concentration: St. John's wort

NURSING CONSIDERATIONS

Assess:

• ANC and platelets; in chronic phase if ANC <1 $\times 10^9$/L and/or platelets <50 $\times 10^9$/L, stop until ANC >1.5 $\times 10^9$/L and platelets >75 $\times 10^9$/L; in accelerated phase/blast crisis if ANC <0.5 $\times 10^9$/L and/or platelets <10 $\times 10^9$/L, determine whether cytopenia is related to biopsy/aspirate, if not, reduce dose by 200 mg, if cytopenia continues, reduce dose by another 100 mg; if cytopenia continues for 4 wk, stop drug until ANC ≥1 $\times 10^9$/L
• For hepatotoxicity: monitor LFTs, before treatment and qmo

- CBC, differential, platelet count weekly; withhold drug if WBC is <3500/mm³, or platelet count <100,000/mm³; notify prescriber of these results; drug should be discontinued
- Signs of fluid retention, edema: weigh, monitor lung sounds, assess for edema, some fluid retention is dose dependent

Administer:
- With meal and large glass of water, to decrease GI symptoms

Perform/provide:
- Nutritious diet with iron, vitamin supplement, low fiber, few dairy products
- Storage at 25° C (77° F)

Evaluate:
- Therapeutic response: decrease in leukemic cells or size of tumor

Teach patient/family:
- To report adverse reactions immediately: SOB, swelling of extremities, bleeding
- Reason for treatment, expected result

imipenem/cilastatin (℞)

(i-me-pen'em sye-la-stat'in)
Primaxin IM, Primaxin IV
Func. class.: Antiinfective, misc.
Chem. class.: Carbapenem

Action: Interferes with cell wall replication of susceptible organisms; osmotically unstable cell wall swells, bursts from osmotic pressure; addition of cilastatin prevents renal inactivation that occurs with high urinary concentrations of imipenem

Uses: Serious infections caused by gram-positive: *Streptococcus pneumoniae,* group A β-hemolytic streptococci, *Staphylococcus aureus,* enterococcus; gram-negative: *Klebsiella, Proteus, Escherichia coli, Acinetobacter, Serratia, Pseudomonas aeruginosa, Salmonella, Shigella*

Dosage and routes:
- *Adult:* **IV** 250-500 mg q8h; severe infections may require 1 g q8h; may give **IM** q12h (total daily **IM** dosage >1500 mg not recommended); mild to moderate infections
- *Child:* **IV** 60-100 mg/kg/day in divided doses, max 4 g/day

Renal dose
- *Adult:* **IV** CCr 30-70 ml/min give 50% dose q6-8h; CCr 20-30 ml/min give 40% dose q8-12h; CCr 5-20 ml/min give 25% dose q12h

Available forms: Inj 250, 500 mg (IV); inj 500, 750 mg (IM)

Side effects/adverse reactions:
CNS: Fever, somnolence, ***seizures,*** confusion, dizziness, weakness, myoclonia
GI: Diarrhea, nausea, vomiting, ***pseudomembranous colitis, hepatitis,*** glossitis
CV: Hypotension, palpitations
HEMA: ***Eosinophilia, neutropenia,*** decreased Hgb, Hct
INTEG: Rash, urticaria, pruritus, pain at injection site, phlebitis, erythema at injection site
SYST: ***Anaphylaxis***
RESP: Chest discomfort, dyspnea, hyperventilation

Contraindications: Hypersensitivity, IM hypersensitivity to local anesthetics of the amide type

Precautions: Pregnancy (C), lactation, elderly, hypersensitivity to penicillins, seizure disorders, renal disease, children

Do not confuse:
imipenem/Omnipen
Primaxin/Premarin

Pharmacokinetics:
IV: Onset immediate, peak ½-1 hr, half-life 1 hr; 70%-80% excreted unchanged in urine

Interactions:
• ↑ imipenem plasma levels: probenecid
• ↑ toxicity: β-lactam antibiotics
• ↑ seizures risk: ganciclovir, cyclosporine

Lab test interferences:
Increase: AST, ALT, LDH, BUN, alk phosphatase, bilirubin, creatinine
False-positive: Direct Coombs' test

NURSING CONSIDERATIONS
Assess:
• For infection: increased temp, WBC, characteristics of wounds, sputum, urine culture or stool culture
• Sensitivity to penicillin—may have sensitivity to this drug
• Renal disease: lower dose may be required
• Bowel pattern qd; if severe diarrhea occurs, drug should be discontinued; may indicate pseudomembranous colitis
Allergic reactions, anaphylaxis: rash, urticaria, pruritus, wheezing, laryngeal edema; may occur few days after therapy begins; have epINEPHrine, antihistamine, emergency equipment available
• Overgrowth of infection: perineal itching, fever, malaise, redness, pain, swelling, drainage, rash, diarrhea, change in cough, sputum

Administer:
• After C&S is taken

IV route
• After reconstitution of 250 or 500 mg with 10 ml of diluent and shake; add to at least 100 ml of same inf sol
• 250-500 mg over 20-30 min; 1 g over 40-60 min; give through Y-tube or 3-way stopcock; do not give by IV bolus or if cloudy

Y-site compatibilities: Acyclovir, amifostine, aztreonam, cefepime, cisatracurium, diltiazem, famotidine, fludarabine, foscarnet, granisetron, idarubicin, insulin (regular), melphalan, methotrexate, ondansetron, propofol, remifentanil, tacrolimus, teniposide, thiotepa, vinorelbine, zidovudine

Evaluate:
• Therapeutic response: negative C&S; absence of signs and symptoms of infection

Teach patient/family:
To report severe diarrhea; may indicate pseudomembranous colitis
To report sore throat, bruising, bleeding, joint pain; may indicate blood dyscrasias (rare)

Treatment of anaphylaxis: EpINEPHrine, antihistamines; resuscitate if needed

imipramine (℞)

(im-ip′ra-meen)
Apo-Imipramine♣, imipramine HCl♣, Impril♣, Norfranil, Novo Pramine♣, Tipramine, Tofranil, Tofranil PM

Func. class.: Antidepressant, tricyclic
Chem. class.: Dibenzazepine, tertiary amine

Action: Blocks reuptake of norepinephrine, serotonin into nerve endings, increasing action of norepinephrine, serotonin in nerve cells

Uses: Depression, enuresis in children

Investigational uses: Chronic pain, migraine headaches, cluster headaches as adjunct, incontinence

Dosage and routes:
• *Adult:* **PO/IM** 75-100 mg/day in divided doses, may increase by 25-50 mg to 200 mg, not to exceed 300 mg/day; may give daily dose hs
• *Geriatric:* **PO** 25 mg hs, may in-

crease to 100 mg/day in divided doses
• *Child:* **PO** 25-75 mg/day
Enuresis
• *Child 6-12 yr:* **PO** 10 mg at hs, max 50 mg
Available forms: Tabs 10, 25, 50, 75 mg; inj 25 mg/2 ml; caps 75, 100, 125, 150 mg
Side effects/adverse reactions:
HEMA: ***Agranulocytosis, thrombocytopenia, eosinophilia, leukopenia***
CNS: Dizziness, drowsiness, confusion, ***seizures,*** headache, anxiety, tremors, stimulation, weakness, insomnia, nightmares, EPS (elderly), increased psychiatric symptoms, paresthesia
GI: Diarrhea, dry mouth, nausea, vomiting, ***paralytic ileus;*** increased appetite; cramps, epigastric distress, jaundice, ***hepatitis,*** stomatitis, constipation, taste change
GU: Retention, ***acute renal failure***
INTEG: Rash, urticaria, sweating, pruritus, photosensitivity
CV: Orthostatic hypotension, ECG changes, tachycardia, hypertension, palpitations, ***dysrhythmias***
EENT: Blurred vision, tinnitus, mydriasis
Contraindications: Hypersensitivity to tricyclics, recovery phase of MI, convulsive disorders, prostatic hypertrophy
Precautions: Suicidal patients, severe depression, increased intraocular pressure, narrow-angle glaucoma, urinary retention, cardiac disease, hepatic disease, hyperthyroidism, electroshock therapy, elective surgery, elderly, pregnancy (C), lactation
Do not confuse:
imipramine/desipramine
Pharmacokinetics:
PO: Steady state 2-5 days; metabolized by liver; excreted in urine, breast milk, feces; crosses placenta; half-life 6-20 hr
Interactions:
• ↓ effects of guanethidine, clonidine, indirect-acting sympathomimetics (ephedrine)
• ↑ effects of direct-acting sympathomimetics (epINEPHrine), alcohol, barbiturates, benzodiazepines, CNS depressants
↑ toxicity: SSRIs, avoid concurrent use
Hyperpyretic crisis, convulsions, hypertensive episode: MAOIs, clonidine
↑ anticholinergic effect: belladonna, corkwood, henbane, jimsonweed, scopolia
↑ imipramine action: chamomile, hops, kava, lavender, skullcap, valerian
Serotonin syndrome: SAM-e, St. John's wort
↑ hypertension: yohimbe
Lab test interferences:
Increase: Serum bilirubin, alk phosphatase, blood glucose
Decrease: 5-HIAA, VMA, urinary catecholamines
NURSING CONSIDERATIONS
Assess:
• B/P (lying, standing), pulse q4h; if systolic B/P drops 20 mm Hg, hold drug, notify prescriber; take vital signs q4h in patients with cardiovascular disease
• Blood studies: CBC, leukocytes, differential, cardiac enzymes if patient is receiving long-term therapy
• Hepatic studies: AST, ALT, bilirubin
• Weight qwk; appetite may increase with drug
ECG for flattening of T wave, bundle branch block, AV block, dysrhythmias in cardiac patients
• EPS primarily in elderly: rigidity, dystonia, akathisia
• Mental status: mood, sensorium,

affect, suicidal tendencies, increase in psychiatric symptoms: depression, panic
• Urinary retention, constipation; constipation is more likely to occur in children, elderly
Withdrawal symptoms: headache, nausea, vomiting, muscle pain, weakness, diarrhea, insomnia, restlessness; not usual unless drug discontinued abruptly
• Alcohol consumption; if alcohol is consumed, hold dose until morning

Administer:
• Increased fluids, bulk in diet for constipation, urinary retention
• With food or milk for GI symptoms
• Dosage hs if oversedation occurs during day; may take entire dose hs; elderly may not tolerate once/day dosing
• Sugarless gum, hard candy, or frequent sips of water for dry mouth
• In IM route after running warm water over ampule to dissolve crystals

Syringe compatibilities: Doxapram
Y-site compatibilities: Cladribine

Perform/provide:
• Storage in tight container at room temperature; do not freeze
• Assistance with ambulation during beginning therapy, since drowsiness/dizziness, orthostatic hypotension occurs
• Safety measures, primarily in elderly

Evaluate:
• Therapeutic response: decreased depression, enuresis, pain

Teach patient/family:
• That therapeutic effects may take 2-3 wk
• That drug is dispensed in small amounts because of suicide potential, especially in beginning of therapy
• To use caution in driving, other activities requiring alertness because of drowsiness, dizziness, blurred vision
• To report urinary retention immediately
• To avoid alcohol ingestion, other CNS depressants during treatment
• Not to discontinue medication quickly after long-term use; may cause nausea, headache, malaise
• To wear sunscreen or large hat, since photosensitivity occurs
Not to break, crush, or chew caps
• To rise slowly, orthostatic hypotension may occur

Treatment of overdose: ECG monitoring; induce emesis; lavage, activated charcoal; administer anticonvulsant

immune globulin (℞)

Gamimune N, Gammagard S/D, gamma globulin, Gammar–P IV, Iveegam, Polygam, Polygam S/D, Sandoglobulin, Venoglobulin-I, Venoglobulin-S

Func. class.: Immune serum
Chem. class.: IgG

Action: Provides passive immunity to hepatitis A, measles, varicella, rubella, immune globulin deficiency; contains gamma globulin antibodies (IgG)

Uses: Immunodeficiency syndrome, B-cell chronic lymphocytic leukemia, Kawasaki syndrome, bone marrow transplantation, pediatric HIV infection, agammaglobulinemia, hepatitis A, B exposure, measles exposure, measles vaccine complications, purpura, rubella exposure, chickenpox exposure

Dosage and routes:
• *Adult:* **IM** 30-50 ml qmo; **IV** 100

mg/kg qmo, 0.01-0.02 ml/kg/min × ½ hr (Gamimune N); **IV** 200 mg/kg qmo, 0.05-1 ml/min × 15-30 min, then increase to 1.5-2.5 ml/min (Sandoglobulin)

• *Child:* **IM** 20-40 ml qmo

Hepatitis A exposure

• *Adult and child:* **IM** 0.02-0.04 ml/kg or 0.1 mg/kg if treatment is delayed

Hepatitis B exposure

• *Adult and child:* **IM** 0.06 ml/kg within 1 wk, qmo

Measles (postexposure)

• *Child:* **IM** 0.25 ml/kg within 6 days

Immunoglobulin deficiency

• *Adult and child:* **IM** 1.3 ml/kg, then 0.66 ml/kg after 2-4 wk and q2-4wk thereafter

Idiopathic thrombocytopenia, purpura

• *Adult and child:* **IV** 0.4 g/kg × 5 days or 1 g/kg/day × 1-2 days

Kawasaki syndrome

• *Child:* **PO** 2 g/kg as a single dose

Available forms: Inj 2, 10 ml/vial; 5% sol, 0.5, 1, 2.5, 3, 6, 10 g vials

Side effects/adverse reactions:

INTEG: Pain at inj site, rash, pruritus, chills

MS: Arthralgia, chest pain

SYST: Lymphadenopathy, ***anaphylaxis***

CNS: Headache, fatigue, malaise

GI: Abdominal pain

Contraindications: Hypersensitivity

Precautions: Pregnancy (C)

Interactions:

• Do not administer live virus vaccines within 3 mo of this drug

NURSING CONSIDERATIONS

Assess:

• For exposure date: this drug should be given within 6 days of measles, 7 days of hepatitis B, 14 days of hepatitis A

• For anaphylaxis: diaphoresis, wheezing, chest tightness, hypotension

Administer:

• IM ≤3 ml in one site, use large muscle mass

• Only with epINEPHrine 1:1000, resuscitative equipment available

• Only within 2 wk of exposure to hepatitis A

IV route

• Gamimune N: IV undiluted or dilute with D_5; give 0.01 ml/kg/min; may increase to 0.02-0.04 ml/kg/min

• Sandoglobulin: IV diluted with provided diluent; give 0.5-1 ml/min × 15-30 min; may increase to 1.5-2.5 ml/min

• Venoglobulin-I: (50 mg/ml sol) give 0.01-0.02 ml/kg/min; if no adverse reaction in ½ hr, increase to 0.04 ml/kg/min, store at room temperature

• Gammagard: reconstitute with sterile H_2O for inj (50 mg protein/ml); give 0.5 ml/kg/hr, may increase to 4 ml/kg/hr, use infusion set provided

• Gammar-IV: give 0.01 ml/kg/min (50 mg/ml sol) × 15-30 min, may increase to 0.02 ml/kg/min, may increase to 0.03-0.06 ml/kg/min

Y-site compatibilities: Fluconazole, sargramostim

Perform/provide:

• Storage at 36°-46° F (2°-8° C)

Evaluate:

• Prevention of infection, increased platelets

Teach patient/family:

• That passive immunity is temporary

• The treatment of anaphylaxis: epINEPHrine, diphenhydrAMINE, O_2, vasopressors, corticosteroids

HIGH ALERT

inamrinone (℞)

(in-am′rih-nohn)

Inocor

Func. class.: Inotropic

Chem. class.: Bipyrimidine derivative

Action: Positive inotropic agent with vasodilator properties; reduces preload and afterload by direct relaxation of vascular smooth muscle, increases cardiac output

Uses: Short-term management of CHF that has not responded to other medication; can be used with digitalis

Dosage and routes:

- *Adult and child:* **IV BOL** 0.75 mg/kg given over 2-3 min; start inf of 5-10 mcg/kg/min; may give another bol 30 min after start of therapy, max 10 mg/kg total daily dose
- *Infant:* **IV** 3-4.5 mg/kg in divided doses, then give by inf 10 mcg/kg/min
- *Neonate:* **IV** 3-4.5 mg/kg in divided doses, then give by inf 3-5 mcg/kg/min

Available forms: Inj 5 mg/ml

Side effects/adverse reactions:

CV: ***Dysrhythmias,*** *hypotension,* chest pain

GI: Nausea, vomiting, anorexia, abdominal pain, ***hepatotoxicity (rare), ascites,*** jaundice, hiccups

INTEG: Allergic reactions, burning at inj site

HEMA: ***Thrombocytopenia***

RESP: Pleuritis, ***pulmonary densities, hypoxemia***

Contraindications: Hypersensitivity to this drug or bisulfites, severe aortic disease, severe pulmonic valvular disease, acute MI

Precautions: Lactation, pregnancy (C), children, renal disease, hepatic disease, atrial flutter/fibrillation, elderly, asthma

Do not confuse:

inamrinone/amiodarone

Pharmacokinetics:

IV: Onset 2-5 min, peak 10 min, duration variable; half-life 4-6 hr, metabolized in liver, excreted in urine as drug and metabolites 60%-90%

Interactions:

- Excessive hypotension: antihypertensives, disopyramide
- Additive effect: cardiac glycosides

↑ amrinone action: aloe, buckthorn, cascara sagrada, senna

Lab test interferences:

Decrease: Serum K

Increase: Hepatic enzymes

NURSING CONSIDERATIONS

Assess:

- B/P and pulse q5min during infusion; if B/P drops 30 mm Hg, stop infusion and call prescriber
- Electrolytes: K, S, Cl, Ca; renal studies: BUN, creatinine; blood studies: platelet count; monitor fluid status (CVP) in elderly
- ALT, AST, bilirubin daily
- I&O ratio and weight qd; diuresis should increase with continuing therapy

If platelets are <150,000/mm^3, drug is usually discontinued and another drug started

- Extravasation; change site q48h

Administer:

IV route

- Do not mix directly with dextrose solutions; chemical reaction occurs over 24 hr; precipitate forms if inamrinone and furosemide come in contact
- May inject into running dextrose infusion through Y-connector or directly into tubing; may give undi-

luted over 2-3 min or dilute with 0.9%, 0.45% NaCl to 1-3 mg/ml, run at prescribed rate by continuous infusion

- By infusion pump for doses other than bolus
- Potassium supplements if ordered for potassium levels <3.0, correct before using amrinone

Syringe compatibilities: Propranolol, verapamil

Y-site compatibilities: Aminophylline, atropine, bretylium, calcium chloride, cimetidine, cisatracurium, digoxin, DOBUTamine, DOPamine, epINEPHrine, famotidine, hydrocortisone, isoproterenol, lidocaine, metaraminol, methylPREDNISolone, nitroglycerin, nitroprusside, norepinephrine, phenylephrine, potassium chloride, propofol, propranolol, remifentanil, verapamil

Evaluate:

- Therapeutic response: increased cardiac output, decreased PCWP, adequate CVP, decreased dyspnea, fatigue, edema, ECG

Teach patient/family:

- That burning may occur at IV site
- To report adverse reactions promptly

Treatment of overdose: Discontinue drug, support circulation

indapamide (℞)

(in-dap'a-mide)

indapamide, Lozide✤, Lozol

Func. class.: Diuretic—thiazide-like, antihypertensive

Chem. class.: Indoline

Action: Acts on proximal section of distal renal tubule and thick ascending loop of Henle by inhibiting reabsorption of sodium; may act by direct vasodilation caused by blocking of calcium channel

Uses: Edema of CHF, hypertension, diuresis

Dosage and routes:

Edema

- *Adult:* **PO** 2.5 mg qd in AM; may be increased to 5 mg qd if needed

Antihypertensive

- *Adult:* 1.25-5 mg qd; may increase to 5 mg/day over 8 wk

Available forms: Tabs 1.25, 2.5 mg

Side effects/adverse reactions:

GU: Polyuria, nocturia, urinary frequency, impotence

ELECT: Hypochloremic alkalosis, hypomagnesemia, hyperuricemia, hypercalcemia, hyponatremia, hypokalemia, hyperglycemia

CNS: Headache, dizziness, fatigue, weakness, nervousness, agitation, extremity numbness, depression

GI: Nausea, diarrhea, dry mouth, vomiting, anorexia, cramps, constipation, abdominal pain

EENT: Blurred vision, nasal congestion, increased intraocular pressure

INTEG: Rash, pruritus

MS: Cramps

CV: Orthostatic hypotension, volume depletion, palpitations, dysrhythmias, PVCs

Contraindications: Hypersensitivity, anuria, hepatic coma

Precautions: Hypokalemia, dehydration, ascites, hepatic disease, severe renal disease, pregnancy (B), lactation, CCr <25 ml/min (not effective)

Pharmacokinetics: Well absorbed (PO), widely distributed, metabolized by liver, excreted by kidney (small amounts); onset 1-2 hr, peak 2 hr, duration up to 36 hr; excreted in urine, feces; half-life 14-18 hr

Interactions:

- Hyperglycemia: diazoxide
- ↑ toxicity of: muscle relaxants, steroids, lithium, digitalis

• ↓ hypokalemia: steroids, amphotericin B, other diuretics
• ↓ effects: antidiabetics, antigout agents, anticoagulants
• ↓ absorption: cholestyramine, colestipol
• ↓ hypotensive effect: indomethacin, NSAIDs
↑ hypokalemia: aloe, buckthorn, cascara sagrada, Chinese cucumber, licorice, senna
Severe photosensitivity: St. John's wort
↑ diuretic effect: aloe, cucumber, dandelion, horsetail, pumpkin, Queen Anne's lace

Lab test interferences:
Increase: Calcium, parathyroid test glucose, uric acid

NURSING CONSIDERATIONS

Assess:
• Weight daily, I&O daily to determine fluid loss; effect of drug may be decreased if used qd
• Rate, depth, rhythm of respiration, effect of exertion
• B/P lying, standing; postural hypotension may occur
• Electrolytes: K, Mg, Na, Cl: include BUN, CBC, serum creatinine, blood pH, ABGs, uric acid, Ca, glucose
• Signs of metabolic alkalosis, hypokalemia
• Rashes, fever qd
• Confusion, especially in elderly; take safety precautions if needed
• Hydration: skin turgor, thirst, dry mucous membranes

Administer:
• In AM to avoid interference with sleep
• With food; if nausea occurs, absorption may be decreased slightly

Evaluate:
• Therapeutic response: improvement in edema of feet, legs, sacral area daily, decreased B/P

Teach patient/family:
• Diet high in potassium; to rise slowly from lying or sitting position
• To recognize adverse reactions: muscle cramps, weakness, nausea, dizziness
• To take with food or milk for GI symptoms
• To use sunscreen for photosensitivity
• To take early in day to prevent nocturia

Treatment of overdose: Lavage if taken orally; monitor electrolytes, administer IV fluids; monitor hydration, CV, renal status

indinavir (℞)

(en-den′a-veer)
Crixivan
Func. class.: Antiretroviral
Chem. class.: Protease inhibitor

Action: Inhibits human immunodeficiency virus (HIV) protease; this prevents maturation of virus

Uses: HIV in combination with other antiretrovirals

Investigational uses: Prevention of HIV after exposure

Dosage and routes:
• Reduce dose in mild/moderate hepatic impairment and ketoconazole coadministration
• *Adult:* **PO** 800 mg q8h; if given with ddI, give 1 hr apart on empty stomach

Available forms: Caps 200, 400 mg

Side effects/adverse reactions:
GU: Nephrolithiasis
GI: Diarrhea, abdominal pain, nausea, vomiting, anorexia, dry mouth
CNS: Headache, insomnia, dizziness, somnolence
INTEG: Rash
MS: Pain
OTHER: Asthenia, ***insulin-resistant***

hyperglycemia, hyperlipidemia, ***ketoacidosis***
Contraindications: Hypersensitivity
Precautions: Hepatic disease, pregnancy (C), lactation, children, renal disease, history of renal stones
Do not confuse:
indinavir/Denavir
Pharmacokinetics: Terminal half-life 1-2 hr
Interactions:
• ↑ myopathy: lovastatin, simvastatin
• ↑ indinavir levels: ketoconazole, delavirdine, itraconazole
• ↓ indinavir levels: rifamycins, fluconazole, nevirapine, efavirenz
• ↑ levels of both drugs: clarithromycin, zidovudine
• ↑ levels of isoniazid, oral contraceptives
Life-threatening dysrhythmias: ergots, midazolam, rifampin, triazolam
• Drug/food: ↓ indinavir absorption: grapefruit juice, high-fat, high-protein foods
↓ indinavir levels: St. John's wort; avoid concurrent use
NURSING CONSIDERATIONS
Assess:
• For complaints of lower back, flank pain, indicates kidney stones
• Signs of infection, anemia, the presence of other sexually transmitted diseases
• Hepatic studies: ALT, AST; total bilirubin, amylase, all may be elevated
• Viral load, CD4 during treatment
• Bowel pattern before, during treatment; if severe abdominal pain with bleeding occurs, drug should be discontinued; monitor hydration
• Skin eruptions; rash, urticaria, itching
• Allergies before treatment, reaction of each medication; place allergies on chart
Administer:
• With water, 1 hr ac or 2 hr pc; may be given with other liquids or small meal; do not give with high-fat, high-protein meals
• Dosage adjustment will need to be considered when given with efavirenz
• Water to 1.5 L/day minimum to prevent nephrolithiasis
Teach patient/family:
• To take as prescribed; if dose is missed, take as soon as remembered up to 1 hr before next dose; do not double dose
Not to break, crush, or chew caps
• That drug must be taken in equal intervals around the clock to maintain blood levels for duration of therapy
That hyperglycemia may occur; watch for increased thirst, weight loss, hunger, dry, itchy skin; notify prescriber
• To increase fluids to prevent kidney stones, if stone formation occurs, treatment may need to be interrupted
• That drug does not cure AIDS, only controls symptoms; not to donate blood

I

indomethacin (℞)

(in-doe-meth'a-sin)

Apo-Indomethacin ♣, Indameth ♣, Indocid ♣, Indocin, Indocin IV, Indocin PDA ♣, Indocin SR, indomethacin, Indochron E-R, Novomethacin ♣, Nu-Indo ♣

Func. class.: Nonsteroidal antiinflammatory (NSAID), antirheumatic

Chem. class.: Propionic acid derivative

Action: Inhibits prostaglandin synthesis by decreasing enzyme needed for biosynthesis; analgesic, antiinflammatory, antipyretic

Uses: Rheumatoid arthritis, ankylosing rheumatoid spondylitis, acute gouty arthritis, closure of patent ductus arteriosus in premature infants

Research note: Indomethacin reduces the antihypertensive effects of captopril and losartan; monitor carefully[17]

Dosage and routes:

Arthritis/antiinflammatory

• *Adult:* **PO/RECT** 25-50 mg bid; may increase by 25 mg/day qwk, not to exceed 200 mg/day; **SUS REL** 75 mg qd, may increase to 75 mg bid

Acute arthritis

• *Adult:* **PO/RECT** 50 mg tid; use only for acute attack, then reduce dose

Patent ductus arteriosus

Longer or repeated treatment courses may be necessary for very premature infants

• *Infant <2 days:* **IV** 0.2 mg/kg, then 0.1 mg/kg × 2 doses after 12, 24 hr

• *Infant 2-7 days:* **IV** 0.2 mg/kg, then 0.2 mg/kg × 2 doses after 12, 24 hr

• *Infant >7 days:* **IV** 0.2 mg/kg, then 0.25 mg/kg × 2 doses after 12, 24 hr

Available forms: Caps 25, 50 mg; caps sus rel 75 mg; susp 25 mg/5 ml; rec supp 50, 100 mg; inj 1 mg vial

Side effects/adverse reactions:

GI: Nausea, anorexia, *vomiting,* diarrhea, jaundice, ***cholestatic hepatitis,*** *constipation,* flatulence, cramps, dry mouth, peptic ulcer, ***ulceration, perforation, GI bleeding***

CNS: Dizziness, drowsiness, fatigue, tremors, confusion, insomnia, anxiety, depression, headache

CV: Tachycardia, peripheral edema, palpitations, dysrhythmias, hypertension

INTEG: Purpura, rash, pruritus, sweating

GU: ***Nephrotoxicity: dysuria, hematuria, oliguria, azotemia***

HEMA: ***Blood dyscrasias,*** prolonged bleeding

EENT: Tinnitus, hearing loss, blurred vision

Contraindications: Hypersensitivity, asthma, severe renal disease, severe hepatic disease, ulcer disease, avoid in 2nd/3rd trimester of pregnancy

Precautions: Lactation, children, bleeding disorders, GI disorders, cardiac disorders, hypersensitivity to other antiinflammatory agents, pregnancy (B) 1st trimester, depression

Pharmacokinetics:

PO: Onset 1-2 hr, peak 3 hr, duration 4-6 hr; metabolized in liver, kidneys; excreted in urine, bile, feces; crosses placenta; excreted in breast milk; 99% plasma protein binding

Interactions:

• ↑ effect of: digoxin, penicillamine, phenytoin, aminoglycosides

• ↓ effect of antihypertensives

• Hyperkalemia: potassium-sparing diuretics

• Toxicity: lithium, methotrexate, cycloSPORINE, zidovudine
• ↑ bleeding risk: anticoagulants, abciximab, cefamandole, cefoperazone, cefotetan, clopidogrel, eptifibatide, plicamycin, ticlopidine, tirofiban, valproic acid, thrombolytics, aspirin
↑ bleeding risk: anise, arnica, chamomile, clove, dong quai, feverfew, garlic, ginger, ginkgo, ginseng (Panax)
↑ gastric irritation: arginine, gossypol
↑ NSAIDs effect: bearberry, bilberry
↑ bleeding risk: bogbean, chondroitin

NURSING CONSIDERATIONS

Assess:
• Arthritis symptoms: ROM, pain, swelling before and 2 hr after treatment
• Patent ductus arteriosus: respiratory rate, character, heart sounds
• Renal, hepatic, blood studies: BUN, creatinine, AST, ALT, Hgb, before treatment, periodically thereafter; if renal function has decreased, do not give subsequent doses
• For eye, ear problems: blurred vision, tinnitus; may indicate toxicity; audiometric, ophthalmic exam before, during, after treatment if on long-term therapy
• For confusion, mood changes, hallucinations, especially in elderly
• For asthma, nasal polyps, aspirin sensitivity, may develop hypersensitivity to indomethacin

Administer:

PO route
• With food to decrease GI symptoms and prevent ulcerations
⊘ Do not crush, chew, or break sus rel cap
• Shake susp, do not mix with other liquids

Rectal route
• Have patient retain for 1 hr

IV route
• After diluting 1-2 mg/ml or more NS or sterile H_2O for inj without preservative; 5-10 sec to avoid dramatic shift in cerebral blood flow

Y-site compatibilities: Furosemide, insulin (regular), potassium chloride, sodium bicarbonate, sodium nitroprusside

Perform/provide:
• Storage at room temperature

Evaluate:
• Therapeutic response: decreased pain, stiffness in joints, decreased swelling in joints, ability to move more easily

Teach patient/family:
• To report blurred vision, ringing, roaring in ears; may indicate toxicity
• To avoid driving, other hazardous activities if dizziness, drowsiness occurs
• To report change in urine pattern, increased weight, edema, increased pain in joints, fever, blood in urine; indicate nephrotoxicity; to report mood changes: anxiety, depression
• That therapeutic antiinflammatory effects may take up to 1 mo
• To avoid alcohol, NSAIDs, salicylates; bleeding may occur
⊘ Not to break, crush, or chew sus rel or reg caps

infliximab

(in-fliks'ih-mab)

Remicade

Func. class.: Monoclonal antibody

Action: Monoclonal antibody that neutralizes the activity of tumor necrosis factor alpha (TNF α) found in Crohn's disease; decreased infiltration of inflammatory cells

Uses: Crohn's disease, fistulizing (moderate-severe); rheumatoid arthritis given with methotrexate

Investigational uses: Plaque psoriasis, ankylosing spondylitis, ulcerative colitis, psoriatic arthritis, psoriasis, Behçet's syndrome, uveitis, juvenile arthritis

Dosage and routes:

Crohn's disease (moderate-severe)

• *Adult:* **IV INF** 5 mg/kg × 1

Crohn's disease (fistulizing)

• *Adult:* **IV INF** 5 mg/kg initially, then repeat dose 2 wk, 6 wk after 1st dose

Rheumatoid arthritis

• *Adult:* **IV** 3 mg/kg initially and q2, 6, 8 wk thereafter given with methotrexate

Available forms: Powder for inj 100 mg

Side effects/adverse reactions:

SYST: ***Anaphylaxis, fatal infections, sepsis, malignancies, immunogenicity***

GI: Nausea, vomiting, abdominal pain, stomatitis, constipation, dyspepsia, flatulence

CNS: Headache, dizziness, depression, vertigo, fatigue, anxiety, fever, ***seizures***

HEMA: ***Anemia***

INTEG: Rash, dermatitis, urticaria, dry skin, sweating, flushing, hematoma, pruritus

RESP: URI, pharyngitis, bronchitis, cough, dyspnea, sinusitis

MS: Myalgia, back pain, arthralgia

GU: Dysuria, urinary frequency

CV: Chest pain, hyper/hypotension, ***tachycardia***

Contraindications: Hypersensitivity to murines, moderate to severe CHF (NYHA Class III/IV)

Precautions: Pregnancy (B), lactation, children, elderly

Pharmacokinetics: Distributed to vascular compartment, half-life 9.5 days

Interactions:

• Do not administer live vaccines concurrently

NURSING CONSIDERATIONS

Assess:

• GI symptoms: nausea, vomiting, abdominal pain

• Periodic blood counts (CBC)

• CV status: B/P, pulse, chest pain

◆ Allergic reaction, anaphylaxis: rash, dermatitis, urticaria, dyspnea, hypotension, fever, chills; discontinue if severe, administer epINEPHrine, corticosteroids, antihistamines; assess for allergies to murine proteins before starting therapy

◆ Fatal infections: discontinue if infection occurs, do not administer to patients with active infections

• Identify TB before beginning treatment, a TB test should be obtained, if present, TB should be treated prior to receiving infliximab

Administer:

IV INF route

• Give immediately after reconstitution; reconstitute each vial with 10 ml of sterile water for inj, further dilute total dose/250 ml of 0.9% NaCl inj to a total conc of 0.4-4 mg/ml; use 21G or smaller needle for reconstitution, direct sterile water at glass wall of vial, gently swirl

• Give over ≥2 hr, use polyethylene-lined infusion with in-line, sterile, low-protein-bind filter

• Do not admix

Perform/provide:

• Refrigerated storage, do not freeze

Evaluate:

• Therapeutic response: absence of fever, mucus in stools

Teach patient/family:

• Not to breastfeed while taking this drug

• To notify prescriber of GI symptoms, hypersensitivity reactions

• Not to operate machinery, drive if dizziness, vertigo occur

HIGH ALERT

insulin aspart
Novolog
insulin lispro (℞)
Humalog
insulin glargine
Lantus
insulin, isophane suspension (NPH) (℞)
Humulin N, Iletin NPH♣, Iletin II NPH♣, Novolin N
insulin, isophane suspension and regular insulin (℞)
Humulin 70/30, Humalin 30/70♣, Novolin 70/30, Novolin 70/30 PenFill, Novolin 70/30 Prefilled, Novolin ge 30/70♣
insulin, regular (℞)
Humulin R♣, Novolin ge Toronto♣, Iletin II Regular, Novolin R, Velosulin BR
insulin, regular concentrated
regular (concentrated), Iletin II U-500
insulin, zinc suspension (Lente) (℞)
Humulin L, Lente Iletin II, Lente L, Novolin ge Lente♣, Novolin L
insulin, zinc suspension extended (Ultralente) (℞)
Humulin U Ultralente, Novolin ge Ultralente♣, Novolin U, Ultralente U
isophane insulin suspension (NPH) and insulin mixtures (℞)
Humalin 50/50, Novolin 50/50

Func. class.: Antidiabetic, pancreatic hormone
Chem. class.: Exogenous unmodified insulin

Action: Decreases blood glucose; by transport of glucose into cells and the conversion of glucose to glycogen, indirectly increases blood pyruvate and lactate, decreases phosphate and potassium; insulin may be beef, pork, human (processed by recombinant DNA technologies)

Uses: Adult-onset diabetes, juvenile diabetes, ketoacidosis types I and II, type II (non–insulin-dependent) diabetes mellitus, type I (insulin-dependent) diabetes mellitus; insulin lispro may be used in combination with sulfonylureas in children >3 yr

Dosage and routes:

Insulin, isophane, suspension
- *Adult:* **SC** dosage individualized by blood, urine glucose; usual dose 7-26 units; may increase by 2-10 units/day if needed

Regular insulin (ketoacidosis)
- *Adult:* **IV** 5-10 units, then 5-10 units/hr until desired response, then switch to **SC** dose; **IV**/inf 2-12 units (50 units/500 ml of normal saline)
- *Child:* **IV** 0.1 units/kg

Replacement
- *Adult and child:* **SC** 0.5-1 units/kg/day qid given 30 min ac
- *Adolescent:* **SC** 0.8-1.2 mg/kg/day; this dosage is used during rapid growth

Available forms: NPH Inj 100 units/ml; regular inj 100 units/ml; zinc susp 100 units/ml; insulin analog inj 100 units/ml; insulin zinc susp, ext (Ultralente) 100 units/ml; isophane insulin/insulin inj 100 units/ml; insulin lispro 100 units/ml 1.5 ml cartridges

Side effects/adverse reactions:
EENT: Blurred vision, dry mouth
INTEG: Flushing, rash, urticaria,

warmth, *lipodystrophy,* lipohypertrophy, swelling, redness
META: Hypoglycemia, rebound hyperglycemia (Somogyi effect 12-72 hr or longer)
SYST: ***Anaphylaxis***
Contraindications: Hypersensitivity to protamine
Precautions: Pregnancy (C) glargine, (B) all others
Do not confuse:
Lantus/lente
Novolin 70/30 Penfill/Novolin 70/30 Prefilled
Pharmacokinetics:
SC (aspart): Onset 15 min, peak 1-3 hr, duration 3-5 hr
SC (glargine): Onset 1.1 hr, no pronounced peak, duration 24 hr
SC (lispro): Onset rapid, peak ½-1 hr, duration 3-4 hr
SC (NPH): Onset 1-2 hr, peak 4-12 hr, duration 18-24 hr
SC (regular susp): Onset ½ hr, peak 4-8 hr, duration 12-24 hr
SC (regular): Onset ½-1 hr, peak 2-4 hr, duration 5-7 hr
IV (regular): Onset 10-30 min, peak 10-30 min, duration ½-1 hr
SC (regular conc): Onset ½-1 hr, peak 2-5 hr, duration 5-7 hr
SC (zinc susp): Onset 1-2 ½ hr, peak 7-15 hr, duration 12-24 hr
SC (zinc susp conc): Onset 4-8 hr, peak 10-30 hr, duration 7-36 hr
SC (zinc susp prompt): Onset 1-1 ½ hr, peak 5-10 hr, duration 12-16 hr
Metabolized by liver, muscle, kidneys; excreted in urine
Interactions:
• ↑ hypoglycemia: salicylate, alcohol, β-blockers, anabolic steroids, fenfluramine, phenylbutazone, sulfinpyrazone, guanethidine, oral hypoglycemics, MAOIs, tetracycline
• ↓ hypoglycemia: thiazides, thyroid hormones, oral contraceptives, corticosteroids, estrogens, DOBUTamine, epINEPHrine
↓ hypoglycemic effect: annato, cocoa seeds, coffee seeds, cola seeds, guarana, ma huang, maté, rosemary
↓ antidiabetic effect: bee pollen, blue cohosh, broom, chromium, elecampane, eucalyptus, gotu kola
↑ antidiabetic effect: alfalfa, aloe, basil, bay, bilberry, bitter melon, black catechu, buchu, burdock, coriander, dandelion, eyebright (po), fenugreek, garlic, ginseng, glucomannan, glucosamine, goat's rue, gymnema, horehound, horse chestnut, jambul, myrrh, myrtle
↓ or ↑ hypoglycemic effect: chromium
↑ glucose tolerance: karela
↑ hypoglycemics: aceitilla, adiantum agrimony, aloe gel, banana flowers/roots, banyan stembark, bilberry, bitter melon, broom, bugleweed, burdock, carob, cumin, damiana, dandelion, eucalyptus, fenugreek, fo-ti, garlic, goat's rue, guar gum, horse chestnut, jambue, juniper, konjac, maitake, onion, psyllium, reishi
Lab test interferences:
Increase: VMA
Decrease: Potassium, calcium
Interference: LFTs, thyroid function studies

NURSING CONSIDERATIONS
Assess:
• Fasting blood glucose, 2 hr PP (80-150 mg/dl, normal fasting level; 70-130 mg/dl, normal 2 hr level); also glycosylated Hgb may be drawn to identify treatment effectiveness
• Urine ketones during illness; insulin requirements may increase during stress, illness, surgery
• For hypoglycemic reaction that can occur during peak time (sweating, weakness, dizziness, chills, confusion, headache, nausea, rapid weak pulse, fatigue, tachycardia,

NURSING CONSIDERATIONS
Assess:
• For symptoms of infection; chills, fever, headache; may be masked by drug fever
• CNS reaction: LOC, mental status, dizziness, confusion, paresthesia, slurred speech
• Cardiac status: Lung sounds; ECG before and during treatment, especially in those with cardiac disease
• Bone marrow depression: bruising, bleeding, blood in stools, urine, sputum, emesis
• Mental status: depression, suicidal thoughts, hallucinations, amnesia
Administer:
alfa-2a
• SC/IM after reconstituting 18 million units/3 ml of diluent provided (6 million units/ml)
• 36 million units/ml is used for Kaposi's sarcoma only
alfa-2b
• IM/SC after reconstituting 3-5 million international units/1 ml, 10 million international units/2 ml, 25 million international units/5 ml, of diluent provided, mix gently
• Intralesional after reconstituting 10 million international units/1 ml bacteriostatic water for inj; no more than 5 lesions can safely be treated at a time
• At hs to minimize side effects
• Acetaminophen as ordered to alleviate fever and headache
Perform/provide:
• Reconstituted sol must be used within 30 days
• Increased fluid intake to 2-3 L/day
Evaluate:
• Therapeutic response: decrease in size, number of lesions
Teach patient/family:
• To take acetaminophen for fever
• To avoid hazardous tasks, since confusion, dizziness may occur; avoid prolonged sunlight, use sunscreen
• That brands of this drug should not be changed; each form is different, with different doses
• That fatigue is common; activity may have to be altered to take hs to minimize flulike symptoms
• Not to become pregnant while taking drug; possible mutagenic effects
• To report signs of infection: sore throat, fever, diarrhea, vomiting, sore or white patches in mouth
• That impotence may occur during treatment but is temporary
• That emotional lability is common; notify prescriber if severe or incapacitating

interferon alfacon-1 (℞)

(in-ter-feer'on al'fa-kon)
Infergen
Func. class.: Recombinant type 1 interferon

Action: Induces biologic responses and has antiviral, antiproliferative and immunomodulatory effects
Uses: Chronic hepatitis C infections
Investigational uses:
Hairy cell leukemia when used with G-CSF
Dosage and routes:
• *Adult:* **SC** 9 mcg as a single inj 3×/wk × 24 wk
Available forms: Inj 9 mcg/0.3 ml, 15 mcg/0.5 ml
Side effects/adverse reactions:
CNS: Headache, fatigue, fever, rigors, insomnia, dizziness
GI: Abdominal pain, nausea, diarrhea, anorexia, dyspepsia, vomiting, constipation, flatulence, hemorrhoids, decreased salivation

MS: Back, limb, neck skeletal pain
GU: Dysmenorrhea, vaginitis, menstrual disorders
INTEG: Alopecia, pruritus, rash, erythema, dry skin
EENT: Tinnitus, earache, conjunctivitis, eye pain
HEMA: ***Granulocytopenia, thrombocytopenia, leukopenia,*** ecchymosis
CV: Hypertension, palpitation
PSYCH: Nervousness, depression, anxiety, lability, abnormal thinking
RESP: Pharyngitis, upper respiratory infection, cough, sinusitis, rhinitis, respiratory tract congestion, epistaxis, dyspnea, bronchitis

Contraindications: Hypersensitivity to alpha interferons, or products from *Escherichia coli*

Precautions: Thyroid disorders, myelosuppression, hepatic, cardiac disease, lactation, children <18 yr

Pharmacokinetics: Peak 24-36 hr

Interactions:

- None known

NURSING CONSIDERATIONS

Assess:

- Platelet counts, heme concentration, ANC, serum creatinine concentration, albumin, bilirubin, TSH, T_4
- For myelosuppression: hold dose if neutrophil count is $<500 \times 10^6$/L or if platelets are $<50 \times 10^9$/L
- For hypersensitivity: discontinue immediately if hypersensitivity occurs

Evaluate:

- Therapeutic response: decreased chronic hepatitis C signs/symptoms

Teach patient/family:

- Provide patient or family member with written, detailed information about drug

interferon alfa-n1 lymphoblastoid (℞)

(in-ter-feer′on al′fa n one lim-foh-blast′oid)

Wellferon

Func. class.: Recombinant type 1 interferon

Action: Induces biologic responses and has antiviral, antiproliferative and immunomodulatory effects; mixture of alpha interferons isolated from human cells after induction with parainfluenza virus

Uses: Chronic hepatitis C infections

Dosage and routes:

- *Adult:* **SC/IM** 3 MU × 3×/wk × 6-12 mo

Available forms: Solution 3 MU/ml

Side effects/adverse reactions:

CNS: Headache, fever, insomnia, dizziness, anxiety, hostility, lability, nervousness, depression, confusion, abnormal thinking, amnesia
GI: Abdominal pain, nausea, diarrhea, anorexia, vomiting
MS: Back pain
INTEG: Alopecia, pruritus, rash, erythema, dry skin
HEMA: ***Granulocytopenia, thrombocytopenia, leukopenia,*** ecchymosis
RESP: Pharyngitis, upper respiratory infection, cough, epistaxis, *dyspnea, bronchitis*

Contraindications: Hypersensitivity to alpha interferons, history of anaphylaxis to bovine or ovine immunoglobulins, egg protein, polymyxin B, neomycin sulfate

Precautions: Thyroid disorders, myelosuppression, hepatic, cardiac disease, lactation, children <18 yr, depression/suicide

Pharmacokinetics: Peak 24-36 hr

Interactions:

• Use caution when giving with theophylline, myelosuppressive agents

NURSING CONSIDERATIONS

Assess:

• ALT, HCV viral load; patients that show no reduction in ALT, HCV are unlikely to show benefit of treatment after 6 mo

• Platelet counts, heme concentration, ANC, serum creatinine concentration, albumin, bilirubin, TSH, T_4, AFP

• For myelosuppression, hold dose if neutrophil count is $<500 \times 10^6$/L or if platelets are $<50 \times 10^9$/L

• For hypersensitivity: discontinue immediately if hypersensitivity occurs

Administer:

• Same brand of product during course of treatment

Evaluate:

• Therapeutic response: decreased chronic hepatitis C signs/symptoms, undetectable viral load

Teach patient/family:

• Provide patient or family member with written, detailed information about drug

• Instructions for home use if appropriate

• Take in evening to reduce discomfort, sleep through some side effects

interferon alfa-n 3 (℞)

(in-ter-feer'on)

Alferon N

Func. class.: Antineoplastic

Chem. class.: Human interferon α-protein

Action: Binds interferon to membrane receptors on cell surface with high specificity; this produces protein synthesis, inhibition of virus replication, suppression of cell proliferation, increased phagocytosis

Uses: Condylomata acuminata (venereal/genital warts)

Dosage and routes:

• *Adult:* 0.05 ml (250,000 international units) per wart, given 2×/wk × 8 wk; not to exceed 0.5 ml (2.5 million international units); inject into base of wart

Available forms: Inj 5 m international units/L ml vial with 3.3 mg/ml phenol and 1 mg/ml human albumin

Side effects/adverse reactions:

CNS: Fever, headache, sweating, vasovagal reaction, chills, fatigue, dizziness, insomnia, sleepiness, depression

GI: Nausea, vomiting, heartburn, diarrhea, constipation, anorexia, stomatitis, dry mouth

MS: Myalgias, arthralgia, back pain, flulike symptoms

INTEG: Pain at inj site, pruritus

CV: Chest pain, hypotension

Contraindications: Hypersensitivity to this product, egg protein, IgG, neomycin

Precautions: Pregnancy (C), lactation, children, CHF, angina (unstable), COPD, diabetes mellitus with ketoacidosis, hemophilia, pulmonary embolism, thrombophlebitis, bone marrow depression, convulsive disorder

Pharmacokinetics: Unable to detect

Lab test interferences:

Interference: AST, ALT, LDH, alk phosphatase, WBC, platelets, granulocytes, creatinine

NURSING CONSIDERATIONS

Assess:

• For symptoms of infection; may be masked by drug fever

• CNS reaction: LOC, mental status, dizziness, confusion

• For body image disturbance

Administer:
- Acetaminophen to alleviate fever and headache

Perform/provide:
- Storage of reconstituted sol for 1 mo in refrigerator
- Increased fluid intake to 2-3 L/day

Evaluate:
- Therapeutic response: decrease in wart size

Teach patient/family:
- To avoid hazardous tasks, since confusion, dizziness may occur
- That brands of this drug should not be changed; each form is different, with different doses
- That fatigue is common; activity may have to be altered
- Not to become pregnant while taking drug; possible mutagenic effects
- To report signs of infection: sore throat, fever, diarrhea, vomiting
- To recognize the signs of hypersensitivity: liver, urticaria, wheezing, dyspnea; notify prescriber immediately

interferon beta-1a
(in-ter-feer′on)
Avonex
interferon beta-1b (℞)
Betaseron
Func. class.: Multiple sclerosis agent, immune modifier
Chem. class.: Interferon, *Escherichia coli* derivative

Action: Antiviral, immunoregulatory; action not clearly understood; biologic response modifying properties mediated through specific receptors on cells, inducing expression of interferon-induced gene products

Uses: Ambulatory patients with relapsing-remitting multiple sclerosis

Investigational uses: May be useful in treatment of AIDS, AIDS-related Kaposi's sarcoma, malignant melanoma, metastatic renal cell carcinoma, cutaneous T cell lymphoma, acute non-A, non-B hepatitis

Dosage and routes:

interferon beta-1a
- *Adult:* **IM** 30 mcg qwk

interferon beta-1b

Relapsing-remitting multiple sclerosis
- *Adult:* **SC** 0.25 mg (8 international units) qod

Available forms: beta-1a 33 mcg (6.6 million international units/ vial); beta-1b powder for inj 0.3 mg (9.6 m international units)

Side effects/adverse reactions:

CNS: Headache, fever, pain, chills, mental changes, hypertonia, ***suicide attempts, seizures***

CV: Migraine, palpitations, hypertension, tachycardia, peripheral vascular disorders

EENT: Conjunctivitis, blurred vision

GI: Diarrhea, constipation, vomiting, abdominal pain

GU: Dysmenorrhea, irregular menses, metrorrhagia, cystitis, breast pain

HEMA: ***Decreased lymphocytes, ANC, WBC;*** *lymphadenopathy*

INTEG: Sweating, inj site reaction

MS: Myalgia, **myasthenia**

RESP: Sinusitis, dyspnea

Contraindications: Hypersensitivity to natural or recombinant interferon-β or human albumin

Precautions: Pregnancy (C), lactation, child <18 yr, chronic progressive MS, depression, mental disorders

Pharmacokinetics:

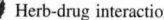

beta-1a: Onset up to 12 hr, peak 48 hr, duration 4 days, half-life 8-6 hr
beta-1b: Onset rapid, peak 2-8 hr,

duration unknown, half-life 8 min-4.3 hr

NURSING CONSIDERATIONS

Assess:

- Blood, renal, hepatic studies: CBC, differential, platelet counts, BUN, creatinine ALT, urinalysis; if absolute neutrophil count < 750/mm^3, or if AST/ALT is 10 × normal, drug is discontinued
- CNS symptoms: headache, fatigue, depression
- GI status: diarrhea or constipation, vomiting, abdominal pain
- Cardiac status: increased B/P, tachycardia
- Mental status: depression, depersonalization, suicidal thoughts, insomnia
- For multiple sclerosis symptoms

Administer:

- Acetaminophen for fever, headache
- SC only; products are not interchangeable

Interferon beta-1a

- Reconstitute with 1.1 ml diluent, swirl, give within 6 hr

Interferon beta-1b

- Reconstitute by injecting diluent provided (1.2 ml) into vial, swirl (8 m international units/ml), use 27G needle for inj

Perform/provide:

- Storage in refrigerator; do not freeze

Evaluate:

- Therapeutic response: decreased symptoms of multiple sclerosis

Teach patient/family:

- To provide patient or family member with written, detailed information about the drug
- That blurred vision, sweating may occur
- That female patients may experience irregular menses, dysmenorrhea, or metrorrhagia as well as breast pain
- To use sunscreen to prevent photosensitivity
- To notify prescriber if pregnancy is suspected
- Inj technique and care of equipment
- To notify prescriber of increased temp, chills, muscle soreness, fatigue

interferon gamma-1b (℞)

(in-ter-feer′on)

Actimmune

Func. class.: Biologic response modifier

Chem. class.: Lymphokine, interleukin type

Action: Species-specific protein synthesized in response to viruses, effects; can mediate killing of *Staphylococcus aureus, Toxoplasma gondii, Leishmania donovani, Listeria monocytogenes, Mycobacterium avium-intracellulare;* enhances oxidative metabolism of macrophages, enhances antibody-dependent cellular cytotoxicity

Uses: Serious infections associated with chronic granulomatous disease, osteoporosis

Dosage and routes:

- *Adult:* **SC** 50 mcg/m^2 (1.5 million units/m^2) for patients with surface area >0.5 m^2; 1.5 mcg/kg/dose for patient with surface area <0.5 m^2; give Monday, Wednesday, Friday for 3×/wk dosing

Available forms: Inj 100 mcg (3 million units)/single-dose vial

Side effects/adverse reactions:

GI: Nausea, anorexia, abdominal pain, weight loss, diarrhea, vomiting

CNS: Headache, fatigue, depression, fever, chills

INTEG: Rash, pain at inj site
MS: Myalgia, arthralgia
Contraindications: Hypersensitivity to interferon-γ, *Escherichia coli*-derived products
Precautions: Pregnancy (C), cardiac disease, seizure disorders, CNS disorders, myelosuppression, lactation, children
Pharmacokinetics:
SC: Dose absorbed 89%, elimination half-life 5.9 hr, peak 7 hr
Interactions:
- ↑ myelosuppression: other myelosuppressive agents

NURSING CONSIDERATIONS
Assess:
- Blood, renal, hepatic studies: CBC, differential, platelet counts, BUN, creatinine, ALT, urinalysis
- CNS symptoms: headache, fatigue, depression

Administer:
- At hs to minimize adverse reactions; administer acetaminophen for fever, headache
- 50% of dose if severe reactions occur or discontinue treatment until reactions subside
- In right and left deltoid and anterior thigh
- Warm to room temperature before use; do not leave at room temperature over 12 hr (unopened vial)

Perform/provide:
- Storage in refrigerator upon receipt; do not freeze; do not shake

Evaluate:
- Therapeutic response: decreased serious infections, improvement in existing infections and inflammatory conditions

Teach patient/family:
- The method of administration if family members will be giving medication
- Provide patient or family member with written, detailed information about drug

ipecac syrup (℞, OTC)
(ip′e-kak)
Func. class.: Emetic
Chem. class.: Cephaelis ipecacuanha derivative

Action: Acts on chemoreceptor trigger zone to induce vomiting; irritates gastric mucosa
Uses: In poisoning to induce vomiting
Dosage and routes:
- *Adult:* **PO** 15-30 ml, then 200-300 ml water; repeat 1×, if vomiting does not occur within 20 min
- *Child >1 yr:* **PO** 15 ml, then 200-300 ml water
- *Child 6-12 mo:* **PO** 5-10 ml, then 100-200 ml water; may repeat dose if needed

Available forms: Syr
Side effects/adverse reactions:
CNS: ***Depression, convulsions, coma***
GI: Nausea, vomiting, bloody diarrhea
CV: ***Circulatory failure, atrial fibrillation, fatal myocarditis, dysrhythmias***
Contraindications: Hypersensitivity, unconscious/semiconscious, depressed gag reflex, poisoning with petroleum products or caustic substances, convulsions
Precautions: Lactation, pregnancy (C)
Pharmacokinetics:
PO: Onset 15-30 min
Interactions:
- Do not administer with activated charcoal, other antiemetics; effect will be decreased
- Drug/food: ↓ effect: dairy products
- ↑ abdominal distention: carbonated drinks

NURSING CONSIDERATIONS

Assess:

• VS, B/P; check patients with cardiac disease more often

• Type of poisoning; do not administer if petroleum products or caustic substances have been ingested: kerosene, gasoline, lye, Draño

• Respiratory status before, during, after administration; check rate, rhythm, character; respiratory depression can occur rapidly with elderly or debilitated patients

Administer:

◆ Ipecac syrup, not ipecac fluid, which is 14 times stronger; death may occur

• Activated charcoal after vomiting completed; may begin lavage after 10-15 min after 2 doses of ipecac syrup with no result

Evaluate:

• Therapeutic response: vomiting

ipratropium (℞)

(i-pra-troe'pee-um)

Atrovent

Func. class.: Anticholinergic, bronchodilator

Chem. class.: Synthetic quaternary ammonium compound

Action: Inhibits interaction of acetylcholine at receptor sites on the bronchial smooth muscle, resulting in decreased cGMP and bronchodilation

Uses: Bronchodilation during bronchospasm in those with COPD; rhinorrhea in children 6-11 yr (nasal spray)

Dosage and routes:

• *Adult:* 2 **INH** 4 × day, not to exceed 12 **INH**/24 hr; sol 500 mcg (1 unit dose) given 3-4 ×/day

• *Child 6-11 yr:* **NASAL** 1 spray in each nostril

Available forms: Aerosol 18 mcg/actuation; nasal spray 0.03%, 0.06%; sol for inh 0.02%

Side effects/adverse reactions:

GI: Nausea, vomiting, cramps

EENT: Dry mouth, blurred vision

CNS: Anxiety, dizziness, headache, nervousness

*RESP: Cough, worsening of symptoms, **bronchospasms***

INTEG: Rash

CV: Palpitation

Contraindications: Hypersensitivity to this drug, atropine, soya lecithin

Precautions: Pregnancy (B), lactation, children <12 yr, narrow-angle glaucoma, prostatic hypertrophy, bladder neck obstruction

Do not confuse:

Atrovent/Alupent

Pharmacokinetics: Half-life 2 hr; does not cross blood-brain barrier

Interactions:

↑ constipation: black catechu

↓ anticholinergic effect: jaborandi tree, pill-bearing spurge

↑ anticholinergic effect: butterbur, jimsonweed

↑ bronchodilator effect: green tea (large amts), guarana

NURSING CONSIDERATIONS

Assess:

• For palpitations; if severe, drug may have to be changed

• For tolerance over long-term therapy; dose may have to be increased or changed

Administer:

Nebulizer

• Use sol in nebulizer with a mouthpiece rather than a face mask

Nasal spray

• Priming pump initially requires 7 actuations of the pump, priming again is not necessary if used regularly

Perform/provide:
- Storage at room temperature
- Hard candy, frequent drinks, sugarless gum to relieve dry mouth

Evaluate:
- Therapeutic response: ability to breathe adequately

Teach patient/family:
- That compliance is necessary with number of inhalations/24 hr, or overdose may occur; spacer device in the elderly
- To shake before using
- The correct method of inhalation and cleaning of equipment daily

irbesartan (℞)

(er-be-sar′tan)

Avapro

Func. class.: Antihypertensive

Chem. class.: Angiotensin II receptor blocker (Type AT_1)

Action: Blocks the vasoconstrictor and aldosterone-secreting effects of angiotensin II; selectively blocks the binding of angiotensin II to the AT_1 receptor found in tissues

Uses: Hypertension, alone or in combination; nephropathy in type 2 diabetic patients

Investigational uses: Heart failure

Dosages and routes:

Hypertension
- *Adult:* **PO** 150 mg qd; may be increased to 300 mg qd

Neuropathy in type 2 diabetic patients
- *Adult:* **PO** maintenance dose 300 mg qd
- *Child 13-16 yr:* **PO** 150 mg qd, may increase to 300 mg qd
- *Child 6-12 yr:* **PO** 75 mg qd, may increase to 150 mg qd

Volume- and salt-depleted patients
- *Adult:* **PO** 75 mg qd

Available forms: 75, 150, 300 mg

Side effects/adverse reactions:

CNS: Dizziness, anxiety, headache, fatigue

GI: Diarrhea, dyspepsia

MISC: Edema, chest pain, rash, tachycardia, UTI

RESP: Cough, upper respiratory infection, sinus disorder, pharyngitis, rhinitis

Contraindications: Hypersensitivity, pregnancy (D) 2nd/3rd trimester

Precautions: Hypersensitivity to ACE inhibitors; pregnancy (C) 1st trimester, lactation, children, elderly, renal disease

Do not confuse:
Avapro/Anaprox

Pharmacokinetics: Extensively metabolized, half-life 11-15 hr, highly bound to plasma proteins, excreted in urine and feces

Interactions:

↑ toxicity, death: aconite

↑ or ↓ antihypertensive effect: astragalus, cola tree

↑ antihypertensive effect: barberry, betony, black catechu, black cohosh, bloodroot, broom, burdock, cat's claw, dandelion, goldenseal, Irish moss, Jamaican dogwood, kelp, khella, mistletoe, parsley

↓ antihypertensive effect: coltsfoot, guarana, khat, licorice

NURSING CONSIDERATIONS

Assess:
- B/P, pulse q4h; note rate, rhythm, quality
- Electrolytes: K, Na, Cl
- Baselines in renal, hepatic studies before therapy begins
- Edema in feet, legs qd
- Skin turgor, dryness of mucous membranes for hydration status

Administer:
- Without regard to meals

Evaluate:
- Therapeutic response: decreased B/P

Teach patient/family:
- To comply with dosage schedule, even if feeling better
- That drug may cause dizziness, fainting; light-headedness may occur
- To rise slowly to sitting or standing position to minimize orthostatic hypotension
- To notify prescriber if pregnancy is suspected

HIGH ALERT

irinotecan (℞)

(ear-een-oh-tee'kan)

Camptosar

Func. class.: Antineoplastic hormone

Chem. class.: Topoisomerase inhibitor

Action: Cytotoxic by producing damage to double-strand DNA during DNA synthesis

Uses: Metastatic carcinoma of the colon or rectum, or 1st-line treatment in combination with 5-FU and leucovorin for metastatic colon or rectal carcinomas

Dosage and routes:

Single agent
- *Adult:* **IV** 125 mg/m^2 given over 1½ hr qwk × 4 wk, then 2 wk rest period, may be repeated; 4 wk or 2 wk off; dosage adjustments may be made to 150 mg/m^2 (high) or 50 mg/m^2 (low); adjustments should be made in increments of 25-50 mg/m^2 depending on patient's tolerance

Combination dosage schedules
- *Regimen 1:* irinotecan 75-125 mg/m^2, leucovorin 20 mg/m^2, 5-FU 300-500 mg/m^2 depending on dosing levels
- *Regimen 2:* irinotecan 120-180 mg/m^2, leucovorin 200 mg/m^2, 5-FU BOL 240-400 mg/m^2, 5-FU infusion 360-600 mg/m^2

Hepatic impairment
- *Adult:* **IV** 100 mg/m^2 qwk × 4 wk, then 2 wk rest, may repeat cycle or 300 mg/m^2 q3wk, dose may be adjusted up or down

Available forms: Inj 20 mg/ml

Side effects/adverse reactions:

CNS: Fever, headache, chills, dizziness

GI: ***Severe diarrhea,*** nausea, vomiting, anorexia, constipation, cramps, flatus, stomatitis, dyspepsia, ***hepatotoxicity***

INTEG: Irritation at site, rash, sweating, alopecia

HEMA: ***Leukopenia, anemia, neutropenia***

RESP: Dyspnea, increased cough, rhinitis

CV: Vasodilation

MISC: Edema, asthenia, weight loss

Contraindications: Hypersensitivity, pregnancy (D)

Precautions: Lactation, children, elderly, myelosuppression, irradiation

Pharmacokinetics: Rapidly and completely absorbed; excreted in urine and bile as metabolites; half-life 10 hr, bound to plasma proteins 30%-68%

Interactions:
- ↑ myelosuppression, diarrhea: other antineoplastics, radiation
- ↑ lymphocytopenia: dexamethasone
- ↑ akathisia: prochlorperazine
- ↑ dehydration: diuretics

NURSING CONSIDERATIONS

Assess:
- For CNS symptoms: fever, headache, chills, dizziness

• CBC, differential, platelet count weekly; withhold drug if WBC is <2000/mm^3, or platelet count <100,000/mm^3, Hgb ≤9 g/dl, neutrophil ≤1000/mm^3; notify prescriber of these results; drug should be discontinued, and colony-stimulating factor given
• Buccal cavity q8h for dryness, sores, or ulceration, white patches, oral pain, bleeding, dysphagia
◆GI symptoms: frequency of stools; cramping; severe life-threatening diarrhea may occur with fluid and electrolyte imbalances
• Signs of dehydration: rapid respirations, poor skin turgor, decreased urine output, dry skin, restlessness, weakness
• Bone marrow depression: bruising, bleeding, blood in stools, urine, sputum, emesis

Administer:
• Antiemetics and dexamethasone 10 mg at least ½ hr before antineoplastics
• After preparing in biologic cabinet using gloves, mask, gown
• Early diarrhea and other cholinergic symptoms can be treated with atropine
• Late diarrhea must be treated promptly with loperimide; late diarrhea can be life-threatening

IV route
• By intermittent inf after diluting with 0.9% NaCl or D_5 (0.12-1.1 mg/ml) give over 1½ hr
• Do not admix with other solutions or medications
• Stable for 24 hr at room temperature, 48 hr, refrigerated

Perform/provide:
• Increased fluid intake to 2-3 L/day to prevent dehydration, unless contraindicated
• Changing of IV site q48h
• Rinsing of mouth tid-qid with water, club soda; brushing of teeth bid-tid with soft brush or cotton-tipped applicator for stomatitis; use unwaxed dental floss
• Nutritious diet with iron, vitamin supplement, low fiber, few dairy products

Evaluate:
• Therapeutic response: decrease in tumor size, decrease in spread of cancer

Teach patient/family:
• To avoid foods with citric acid or hot or rough texture if stomatitis is present; to drink adequate fluids
• To report stomatitis; any bleeding, white spots, ulcerations in mouth; tell patient to examine mouth qd, report symptoms
• To report signs of anemia: fatigue, headache, faintness, shortness of breath, irritability
• To use contraception during therapy
• To avoid salicylates, NSAIDs, alcohol, bleeding may occur
• About alopecia, that when hair grows back, it will be different texture, thickness
• To avoid vaccinations while taking this drug
◆To report diarrhea that occurs 24 hr after administration, severe dehydration can occur rapidly

Treatment of overdose: Induce vomiting, provide supportive care, prevent dehydration

iron dextran (℞)

DexFerrum, Imferon, InFeD

Func. class.: Hematinic

Chem. class.: Ferric hydroxide complex with dextran

Action: Iron is carried by transferrin to the bone marrow, where it is incorporated into hemoglobin

Uses: Iron deficiency anemia

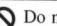

Dosage and routes:
• *Adult and child:* **IM** 0.5 ml as a test dose by Z-track, then no more than the following per day:
• *Adult <50 kg:* **IM** 100 mg
• *Adult >50 kg:* **IM** 250 mg
• *Infant <5 kg:* **IM** 25 mg
• *Child <5-9 kg:* **IM** 50 mg
• *Adult:* **IV** 0.5 ml (25 mg) test dose, then 100 mg qd after 2-3 days; give 25 mg test dose, wait 5 min, then infuse over 6-12 hr or use equation that follows:

$$\frac{0.3 \times \text{wt (lb)} \times 100\text{-Hgb (g/dl)} \times 100}{14.8} = \text{mg iron}$$

<30 lb (66 kg) should be given 80% of above formula dose
Available forms: Inj 50 mg/ml (2 ml, 10 ml vials)
Side effects/adverse reactions:
CNS: Headache, paresthesia, dizziness, shivering, weakness, ***seizures***
GI: Nausea, vomiting, metallic taste, abdominal pain
INTEG: Rash, pruritus, urticaria, fever, sweating, chills, brown skin discoloration, pain at inj site, necrosis, sterile abscesses, phlebitis
CV: Chest pain, ***shock,*** hypotension, tachycardia
RESP: Dyspnea
HEMA: ***Leukocytosis***
OTHER: ***Anaphylaxis***
Contraindications: Hypersensitivity, all anemias excluding iron deficiency anemia, hepatic disease
Precautions: Acute renal disease, children, asthma, lactation, rheumatoid arthritis (IV), infants <4 mo, pregnancy (C)
Do not confuse:
Imferon/Imuran
Imferon/Roferon-A
Pharmacokinetics:
IM: Excreted in feces, urine, bile, breast milk; crosses placenta; most absorbed through lymphatics; can be gradually absorbed over weeks/months from fixed locations
Interactions:
• ↓ reticulocyte response: chloramphenicol
• ↑ toxicity: oral iron—do not use
• ↓ absorption of fluoroquinolones, penicillamine
• Drug/food: iron absorption is ↓ by food
Lab test interferences:
False increase: Serum bilirubin
False decrease: Serum calcium
False positive: ^{99m}Tc diphosphate bone scan, iron test (large doses >2 ml)

NURSING CONSIDERATIONS
Assess:
• Blood studies: Hct, Hgb, reticulocytes, transferrin, plasma iron concentrations, ferritin, total iron-binding, bilirubin before treatment, at least monthly
• Allergy: anaphylaxis, rash, pruritus, fever, chills, wheezing; notify prescriber immediately, keep emergency equipment available
• Cardiac status: anginal pain, hypotension, tachycardia
• Nutrition: amount of iron in diet (meat, dark green leafy vegetables, dried beans, dried fruits, eggs)
• Cause of iron loss or anemia, including use of salicylates, sulfonamides
• Toxicity: nausea, vomiting, diarrhea, fever, abdominal pain (early symptoms), cyanotic-looking lips, nailbeds, seizures, CV collapse (late symptoms)
Administer:
• D/C oral iron before parenteral; give only after test dose of 25 mg by preferred route; wait at least 1 hr before giving remaining portion
• IM deeply in large muscle mass; use Z-track method and a 19-20G 2-3-in needle; ensure needle is long

enough to place drug deep in muscle, change needles after withdrawing drug and before injecting to prevent skin, tissue staining

 Only with epINEPHrine available in case of anaphylactic reaction during dose

IV route

• IV after flushing with 10 ml 0.9% NaCl; give undiluted; may be diluted in 50-250 ml NS for infusion; give 1 ml (50 mg) or less over 1 min or more; flush line after use with 10 ml 0.9% NaCl; patient should remain recumbent for ½-1 hr

• IV injection requires single-dose vial without preservative; verify on label IV use is approved

Additive compatibilities: Netilmicin

Solution compatibility: TPN #211

Perform/provide:

• Storage at room temperature in cool environment

• Recumbent position 30 min after IV inj to prevent orthostatic hypotension

• Therapeutic response: increased serum iron levels, Hct, Hgb

Teach patient/family:

• That iron poisoning may occur if increased beyond recommended level; not to take oral iron preparation

• That delayed reaction may occur 1-2 days after administration and last 3-4 days (IV), 3-7 days (IM); report fever, chills, malaise, muscle, joint aches, nausea, vomiting, backache

Treatment of overdose: Discontinue drug, treat allergic reaction, give diphenhydramine or epINEPHrine as needed, give iron-chelating drug in acute poisoning

iron sucrose (℞)

Venofer

Func. class.: Hematinic

Chem. class.: Ferric hydroxide complex with dextran

Action: Iron is carried by transferrin to the bone marrow, where it is incorporated into hemoglobin

Uses: Iron deficiency anemia

Investigational uses: Dystrophic epidermolysis bullosa (DEB)

Dosage and routes:

• *Adult:* **IV** 5 ml (100 mg of elemental iron) given during dialysis, most will need 1000 mg of elemental iron over 10 dialysis sessions

Available forms: Inj 20 mg/ml

Side effects/adverse reactions:

CNS: Headache, dizziness

GI: Nausea, vomiting, abdominal pain

INTEG: Rash, pruritus, urticaria, fever, sweating, chills

CV: Chest pain, hypotension, hypertension, hypervolemia

RESP: Dyspnea, pneumonia, cough

OTHER: ***Anaphylaxis***

Contraindications: Hypersensitivity, all anemias excluding iron deficiency anemia, iron overload

Precautions: Lactation, pregnancy (B), elderly, children

Pharmacokinetics: Excreted in urine, half-life 6 hr

Interactions:

• ↑ toxicity: oral iron—do not use

NURSING CONSIDERATIONS

Assess:

• Blood studies: Hct, Hgb, reticulocytes, transferrin, plasma iron concentrations, ferritin, total iron-binding, bilirubin before teratment, at least monthly

• Allergy: anaphylaxis, rash, pruritus, fever, chills, wheezing; notify prescriber immediately, keep emergency equipment available
• Cardiac status: hypotension, hypertension, hypervolemia
• Toxicity: nausea, vomiting, diarrhea, fever, abdominal pain (early symptoms), cyanotic-looking lips, nailbeds, seizures, CV collapse (late symptoms)

Administer:

◆ Only with epINEPHrine available in case of anaphylactic reaction during dose

IV route

• Give directly in dialysis line by slow inj or inf; give by slow inj at 1 ml/min (5 min/vial); inf dilute each vial exclusively in a maximum of 100 ml of 0.9% NaCl, give at rate of 100 mg of iron/15 min, discard unused portions

Perform/provide:

• Storage at room temperature in cool environment, do not freeze
• Therapeutic response: increased serum iron levels, Hct, Hgb

Teach patient/family:

• That iron poisoning may occur if increased beyond recommended level; not to take oral iron preparation

Treatment of overdose: Discontinue drug, treat allergic reaction, give diphenhydrAMINE or epINEPHrine as needed, give iron-chelating drug in acute poisoning

isoflurophate ophthalmic

See appendix c

isoniazid (℞)

(eye-soe-nye'a-zid)

INH, isoniazid, Isotamine♣, Laniazid, Nydrazid, PMS-Isoniazid♣

Func. class.: Antitubercular

Chem. class.: Isonicotinic acid hydrazide

Action: Bactericidal interference with lipid, nucleic acid biosynthesis

Uses: Treatment, prevention of TB

Dosage and routes:

Treatment

• *Adult:* **PO/IM** 300 mg/day or 15 mg/kg 2-3 ×/wk, max 900 mg 2-3 ×/wk
• *Child and infant:* **PO/IM** 10-20 mg/kg qd in 1-2 divided doses max 300 mg/day or 20-40 mg/kg, max 900 mg 2-3 ×/wk

Available forms: Tabs 50, 100, 300 mg; inj 100 mg/ml; powder, syr 50 mg/5 ml

Side effects/adverse reactions:

Hypersensitivity: fever, skin eruptions, lymphadenopathy, vasculitis

CNS: Peripheral neuropathy, dizziness, memory impairment, ***toxic encephalopathy, convulsions,*** psychosis, slurred speech

EENT: Blurred vision, optic neuritis

HEMA: ***Agranulocytosis, hemolytic, aplastic anemia, thrombocytopenia, eosinophilia, methemoglobinemia***

MISC: Dyspnea, B_6 deficiency, pellagra, hyperglycemia, metabolic acidosis, gynecomastia, rheumatic syndrome, SLE-like syndrome

GI: Nausea, vomiting, epigastric distress, ***jaundice, fatal hepatitis***

Contraindications: Hypersensitivity, acute liver disease

Precautions: Pregnancy (C), renal disease, diabetic retinopathy, cataracts, ocular defects, hepatic disease, child <13 yr

Pharmacokinetics:

PO: Peak 1-2 hr, duration 6-8 hr

IM: Peak 45-60 min

Metabolized in liver; excreted in urine (metabolites); crosses placenta; excreted in breast milk

Interactions:

- ↑ toxicity: tyramine foods, alcohol, cycloSERINE, ethionamide, rifampin, carbamazepine, warfarin, phenytoin, benzodiazepines, meperidine
- ↓ absorption: aluminum antacids
- ↓ effectiveness of BCG vaccine, ketoconazole
- Drug/food: do not give with high-tyramine foods

NURSING CONSIDERATIONS

Assess:

- Hepatic studies qwk: ALT, AST, bilirubin; increased test results may indicate hepatitis
- Mental status often: affect, mood, behavioral changes; psychosis may occur
- Hepatic status: decreased appetite, jaundice, dark urine, fatigue

Administer:

- PO with meals to decrease GI symptoms; better to take on empty stomach 1 hr ac or 2 hr pc
- Antiemetic if vomiting occurs
- After C&S is completed; qmo to detect resistance
- IM deep in large muscle mass, massage, rotate inj site, warm inj to room temperature to dissolve crystals

Evaluate:

- Therapeutic response: decreased symptoms of TB

Teach patient/family:

- That compliance with dosage schedule, duration is necessary, not to skip or double dose
- That scheduled appointments must be kept or relapse may occur
- To avoid alcohol while taking drug, may increase risk of hepatic injury
- That if diabetic, use blood glucose monitor to obtain correct result
- To report weakness, fatigue, loss of appetite, nausea, vomiting, jaundice of skin or eyes, tingling/numbness of hands/feet

Treatment of overdose: Pyridoxine

isoproterenol (℞)

(eye-soe-proe-ter′e-nole)

Aerolone, Dispos-a-Medisoproterenol HCl, Isoproterenol HCl, Isuprel, Isuprel Glossets, Isuprel Mistometer, Medihaler-Iso, Vapo-Iso

Func. class.: β-Adrenergic agonist

Chem. class.: Catecholamine

Action: Has β_1 and β_2 action; relaxes bronchial smooth muscle and dilates the trachea and main bronchi by increasing levels of cAMP, which relaxes smooth muscles; causes increased contractility and heart rate by acting on β-receptors in heart

Uses: Bronchospasm, asthma, heart block, ventricular dysrhythmias, shock

Dosage and routes:

Asthma, bronchospasm

- *Adult:* **SL** 10-20 mg q6-8h; **INH** 1 puff, may repeat in 2-5 min, maintenance 1-2 puffs 4-6×/day; **IV** 10-20 mcg during anesthesia
- *Child:* **SL** 5-10 mg q6-8h; **INH** 1 puff, may repeat in 2-5 min, maintenance 1-2 puffs 4-6×/day

Heart block/ventricular dysrhythmias

- *Adult:* **IV** 0.02-0.06, then 0.01-0.2 mg or 5 mcg/min HCl; 0.2 mg, then 0.02-1 mg as needed HCl

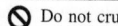

Shock

• *Adult:* **IV INF** 0.5-5 mcg/min 1 mg/500 ml D_5W, titrate to B/P, CVP, hourly urine output

Available forms: Sol for nebulization 1:400 (0.25%), 1:200 (0.5%), 1:100 (1%); aerosol 0.25%, 0.2%; pwd for inh 0.1 mg/cart; inj 1:5000 (0.2 mg/ml); glossets (SL) 10, 15 mg

Side effects/adverse reactions:

CNS: Tremors, anxiety, insomnia, headache, dizziness, stimulation

CV: Palpitations, tachycardia, hypertension, ***cardiac arrest***

GI: Nausea, vomiting

RESP: Bronchial irritation, edema, dryness of oropharynx, ***bronchospasms*** (overuse)

META: Hyperglycemia

Contraindications: Hypersensitivity to sympathomimetics, narrow-angle glaucoma, tachydysrhythmias

Precautions: Pregnancy (C), cardiac disorders, hyperthyroidism, diabetes mellitus, prostatic hypertrophy, elderly

Pharmacokinetics:

IV: Onset rapid, duration 10 min

INH/SL: Onset 1-2 hr

RECT: Onset 2-4 hr

Metabolized in liver, lungs, GI tract

Interactions:

• ↑ effects of both drugs: other sympathomimetics

• ↓ action when used with β-blockers

NURSING CONSIDERATIONS

Assess:

• Respiratory function: B/P, pulse, lung sounds

• Blood studies (CBC, WBC, differential), since blood dyscrasias may occur (rare)

• I&O ratio; check for urinary retention, frequency, hesitancy

• For paresthesias and coldness of extremities; peripheral blood flow may decrease

• Injection site: tissue sloughing; administer phentolamine mixed with 0.9% NaCl

Administer:

• With meals for GI symptoms

• SL ≤q3-4h or no more than tid

IV route

• Direct dilute 0.2 mg/10 ml 0.9% NaCl (1:50,000 sol); give over 1 min; IV INF 2 mg (1:5000 sol)/500 ml of D_5W; run each 1 ml (1:250,000) sol/min; may be increased; use infusion pump, intracardiac, 1:5000 sol undiluted

Additive compatibilities: Atracurium, calcium chloride, calcium gluceptate, cephalothin, cimetidine, DOBUTamine, floxacillin, heparin, magnesium sulfate, multivitamins, netilmicin, potassium chloride, ranitidine, succinylchloride, verapamil, vit B/C

Syringe compatibilities: Ranitidine

Y-site compatibilities: Amiodarone, amrinone, atracurium, bretylium, cisatracurium, famotidine, heparin, hydrocortisone, pancuronium, potassium chloride, propofol, remifentanil, tacrolimus, vecuronium, vit B/C

Perform/provide:

• Storage at room temperature; do not use discolored sol

Evaluate:

• Therapeutic response: increased B/P with stabilization, ease of breathing

Teach patient/family:

• To rinse mouth after use

• Use of inhaler; review package insert with patient; to avoid getting aerosol in eyes; to wash inhaler in warm water and dry qd

• Use of spacer device in elderly

• About all aspects of drug; avoid smoking, smoke-filled rooms, persons with respiratory infections

Treatment of overdose: Administer a β-blocker

isosorbide dinitrate (℞)

(eye-soe-sor′bide)

Apo-ISDN🍁, Cedocard-SR🍁, Coronex🍁, Dilatrate-SR, ISDN, Iso-Bid, Isonate, Isorbid, Isordil, Isosorbide dinitrate, Isotrate, Novasorbide🍁, Sorbitrate

isosorbide mononitrate

(eye-soe-sor′bide)

Imdur, Ismo, Isotrate ER, Monoket

Func. class.: Antianginal, vasodilator

Chem. class.: Nitrate

Action: Relaxation of vascular smooth muscle which leads to decreases preload, after-load, which is responsible for decreasing left ventricular end-diastolic pressure, systemic vascular resistance and reducing cardiac O_2 demand

Uses: Treatment, prevention of chronic stable angina pectoris

Dosage and routes:

Dinitrate

- *Adult:* **PO** 5-40 mg qid; **SL,** buccal 2.5-5 mg, may repeat q5-10 min × 3 doses; **CHEW TAB** 5-10 mg prn or q2-3h as prophylaxis; **SUS REL** 40-80 mg q8-12h

Mononitrate

- *Adult:* **PO** Ismo, Monoket: 10-20 mg bid, 7 hr apart; Imdur: initiate at 30-60 mg/day as a single dose, increase q3d as needed, may increase to 120 mg qd, max 240 mg/day

Available forms:

Dinitrate: Caps sus rel 40 mg; tabs 2.5, 5, 10, 20, 30, 40 mg; SL tabs 2.5, 5, 10 mg; sus rel tab 40 mg; chew tabs 5, 10 mg

Mononitrate: Tabs 10, 20 mg (Ismo, Monoket); ext rel (Imdur) 30, 60, 120 mg

Side effects/adverse reactions:

MISC: Twitching, hemolytic anemia, ***methemoglobinemia***

CV: Postural hypotension, tachycardia, ***collapse,*** syncope, palpitations

GI: Nausea, vomiting, diarrhea

INTEG: Pallor, sweating, rash

CNS: Vascular headache, flushing, dizziness, weakness, faintness

Contraindications: Hypersensitivity to this drug or nitrates, severe anemia, increased intracranial pressure, cerebral hemorrhage, acute MI

Precautions: Postural hypotension, pregnancy (C), lactation, children, MI, CHF, severe renal, hepatic disease

Do not confuse:

Monoket/Monopril

Imdur/Imuran/Inderal/K-Dur

Pharmacokinetics:

Mononitrate

Sus Rel: Duration 6-8 hr

Dinitrate

PO: Onset 15-30 min, duration 4-6 hr

SUS REL: Onset up to 4 hr, duration 6-8 hr

SL: Onset 2-5 min, duration 1-4 hr

CHEW TAB: Onset 3 min, duration ½-3 hr

Metabolized by liver, excreted in urine as metabolites (80%-100%)

Interactions:

- ↑ hypotension: β-blockers, diuretics, antihypertensives, alcohol, calcium channel blockers, phenothiazines

Fatal hypotension: sildenafil

↓ antianginal effect: blue cohosh

NURSING CONSIDERATIONS

Assess:

- Pain: duration, time started, activity being performed, character

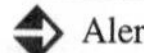

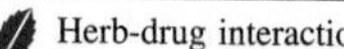
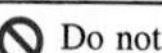

• B/P, pulse, respirations during beginning therapy
• Tolerance if taken over long period
• Headache, light-headedness, decreased B/P; may indicate a need for decreased dosage

Administer:
• After checking expiration date
⊘ Do not break, crush, or chew sus rel caps, SL tabs
• PO with 8 oz H_2O on empty stomach; do not crush SR or SL drug
• SL tabs should be placed under the tongue until dissolved

Evaluate:
• Therapeutic response: decrease or prevention of anginal pain

Teach patient/family:
• To leave tabs in original container
• To avoid alcohol products
• That drug may cause headache, but tolerance usually develops; taking with meals may reduce or eliminate headache
• That drug may be taken before stressful activity (exercise, sexual activity)
• That SL may sting when drug comes in contact with mucous membranes
• To avoid hazardous activities if dizziness occurs
• The importance of complying with complete medical regimen
• To make position changes slowly to prevent orthostatic hypotension
⊘ Not to crush, chew sus rel caps, SL tabs

RARELY USED

isotretinoin (℞)

(eye-soe-tret′i-noyn)

Func. class.: Antiacne agent

Uses: Severe recalcitrant cystic acne

Dosage and routes:
• *Adult:* **PO** 0.5-2 mg/kg/day in 2 divided doses × 15-20 wk; if relapse occurs, repeat after 2 mo off drug

Contraindications: Hypersensitivity, inflamed skin, pregnancy (X)

isradipine (℞)

(is-ra′di-peen)

DynaCirc, DynaCirc CR

Func. class.: Antihypertensive, antianginal (calcium channel blocker)

Chem. class.: Dihydropyridine

Action: Inhibits calcium ion influx across cell membrane during cardiac depolarization; produces relaxation of coronary vascular smooth muscle, peripheral vascular smooth muscle; dilates coronary vascular arteries

Uses: Essential hypertension, angina pectoris, vasospastic angina

Dosage and routes:
• *Adult:* **PO** 2.5 mg bid; increase at 2-4 wk intervals up to 10 mg bid or 5 mg qd; cont rel may be increased q2-4wk, max 20 mg/day

Available forms: Caps 2.5, 5 mg, cont rel tabs 5, 10 mg

Side effects/adverse reactions:
HEMA: ***Leukopenia***
CV: Peripheral edema, tachycardia, hypotension, chest pain, ***dysrhythmias,*** syncope
GI: Nausea, vomiting, diarrhea, gastric upset, constipation, ***hepatitis,*** abdominal pain, distention, dry mouth
GU: Nocturia, urinary frequency
INTEG: Rash, pruritus, urticaria
CNS: Headache, fatigue, dizziness, fainting, sleep disturbances, weakness, depression, drowsiness
MISC: Flushing

Contraindications: Sick sinus syndrome, 2nd- or 3rd-degree heart

block, hypotension less than 90 mm Hg systolic, hypersensitivity
Precautions: CHF, hypotension, hepatic disease, pregnancy (C), lactation, children, renal disease, elderly
Do not confuse:
DynaCirc/Dynabac/Dynacin
Pharmacokinetics: Metabolized in liver; metabolites excreted in urine, feces; secreted in breast milk, peak plasma levels at 1.5 hr immediate rel, 7-18 hr cont rel
Interactions:
• ↑ hypotension: nitrates, fentanyl, other antihypertensives
• Bradycardia, conduction defects: disopyramide
• Additive/synergistic effect: β-blockers
• ↑ serum conc of isradipine: cimetidine, ranitidine
• ↓ serum conc of isradipine: rifampin
• ↓ conc: fluvastatin
↑ toxicity, death: aconite
↑ or ↓ antihypertensive effect: astragalus, cola tree
↑ antihypertensive effect: barberry, betony, black catechu, black cohosh, bloodroot, broom, burdock, cat's claw, dandelion, goldenseal, Irish moss, Jamaican dogwood, kelp, khella, mistletoe, parsley
↓ antihypertensive effect: coltsfoot, guarana, khat, licorice

NURSING CONSIDERATIONS
Assess:
• I&O ratio, daily weight, watch for CHF: dyspnea, weight gain, rales, crackles, jugular vein distention
• Renal, hepatic studies, electrolytes prior to and during treatment
• Cardiac status: B/P, pulse, respiration, ECG; assess anginal pain, precipitating, ameliorating factors
Administer:
• Without regard to meals
Evaluate:
• Therapeutic response: decreased anginal pain, decreased B/P
Teach patient/family:
Not to break, crush, or chew cont rel tabs
• To avoid hazardous activities until stabilized on drug, dizziness is no longer a problem
• To limit caffeine consumption
• To avoid OTC drugs unless directed by prescriber
• The importance of compliance in all areas of regimen: diet, exercise, stress reduction, drug therapy
• To notify prescriber of irregular heartbeat, shortness of breath, swelling of feet and hands, pronounced dizziness, constipation, nausea, hypotension
Treatment of overdose: Defibrillation, β-agonists, IV calcium inotropic agents, diuretics, atropine for AV block, vasopressor for hypotension

itraconazole (℞)
(it-ra-con'a-zol)
Sporanox
Func. class.: Antifungal, systemic
Chem. class.: Triazole derivative

Action: Alters cell membranes and inhibits several fungal enzymes
Uses: Systemic candidiasis, chronic mucocandidiasis, oral thrush, candiduria, coccidioidomycosis, histoplasmosis, chromomycosis, paracoccidioidomycosis, blastomycosis (pulmonary and extrapulmonary), aspergillosis onychomycosis
Investigational uses: Dermatophytoses, pityriasis versicolor, sebopsoriasis, vaginal candidiasis, cryptococcus, subcutaneous my-

coses, dimorphic infections, leishmaniasis, fungal keratitis, alternariosis, zygomycosis

Dosage and routes:

Dose varies with type of infection

• *Adult:* **PO** 200 mg qd with food; may increase to 400 mg qd if needed; life-threatening infections may require a loading dose of 200 mg tid × 3 days; **IV** 200 mg bid × 4 doses, then 200 mg qd, give each dose over 1 hr; maintenance **PO** 100 mg/day

• *Child:* **PO** 3-5 mg/kg/day

Available forms: Caps 100 mg; oral sol 10 mg/ml; inj 10 mg/ml

Side effects/adverse reactions:

CV: Hypertension

GU: Gynecomastia, impotence, decreased libido

INTEG: Pruritus, fever, *rash,* ***toxic epidermal necrolysis***

CNS: Headache, dizziness, insomnia, somnolence, depression

GI: Nausea, vomiting, anorexia, diarrhea, cramps, abdominal pain, flatulence, ***GI bleeding, hepatotoxicity***

MISC: Edema, fatigue, malaise, hypokalemia, tinnitus, ***rhabdomyolysis***

Contraindications: Hypersensitivity, lactation, fungal meningitis, onychomycosis or dermatomycosis in cardiac dysfunction

Precautions: Hepatic disease, achlorhydria or hypochlorhydria (drug-induced), children, pregnancy (C)

Pharmacokinetics:

PO: Peak 3-5 hr, half-life 21 hr; metabolized in liver; excreted in bile, feces; requires acid pH for absorption; distributed poorly to CSF; highly protein bound; inhibits P4503A enzyme

Interactions:

• Edema: calcium channel blockers

• ↑ sedation: triazolam, oral midazolam

• Tinnitus, hearing loss: quinidine

• ↑ levels, toxicity: busPIRone, busulfan, clarithromycin, cycloSPORINE, diazepam, digoxin, felodipine, indinavir, isradipine, niCARdipine, niFEDipine, nimoldipine, phenytoin, quinidine, ritonavir, saquinavir, tacrolimus, warfarin

• Hepatotoxicity: other hepatotoxic drugs

• ↓ itraconazole action: antacids, H_2-receptor antagonists, rifamycins, didanosine

• Severe hypoglycemia: oral hypoglycemics

⬥ Life-threatening CV reactions: pimozide, quinidine, dofetilide

• Drug/food: food increases absorption

Nephrotoxicity: gossypol

NURSING CONSIDERATIONS

Assess:

• For type of infection, may begin treatment prior to obtaining results

• For infection: temp, WBC, sputum, baseline and periodically

• I&O ratio, potassium levels

• Hepatic studies (ALT, AST, bilirubin) if on long-term therapy

• For allergic reaction: rash, photosensitivity, urticaria, dermatitis

⬥ For hepatotoxicity: nausea, vomiting, jaundice, clay-colored stools, fatigue

Administer:

• In the presence of acid products only; do not use alkaline products or antacids within 2 hr of drug; may give coffee, tea, acidic fruit juices

• IV: after adding full contents 25-50 ml NaCl, mix gently, use flow control device, give over 1 hr; use separate line, flush after use

• Oral sol: patient should swish in mouth vigorously

• Oral sol and caps are not interchangeable on an mg/mg basis

• Give caps after full meal to ensure absorption, swallow whole

Perform/provide:
• Storage in tight container at room temperature

Evaluate:
• Therapeutic response: decreased fever, malaise, rash, negative C&S for infecting organism

Teach patient/family:
• That long-term therapy may be needed to clear infection (1 wk-6 mo depending on infection)
• To avoid hazardous activities if dizziness occurs
• To take 2 hr ac administration of other drugs that increase gastric pH (antacids, H_2-blockers, omeprazole, sucralfate, anticholinergics) to notify health-care provider of all medications taken; to take after a full meal (caps), on empty stomach (oral sol)
• The importance of compliance with drug regimen
• To notify prescriber of GI symptoms, signs of hepatic dysfunction (fatigue, nausea, anorexia, vomiting, dark urine, pale stools)
⃠ Not to break, crush, or chew caps; not to use oral sol, caps interchangeably

---

RARELY USED

kanamycin (℞)

(kan-a-mye'sin)
kanamycin sulfate, Kantrex
Func. class.: Antiinfective

Uses: Severe systemic infections of CNS, respiratory, GI, urinary tract, bone, skin, soft tissues caused by *Escherichia coli, Acinetobacter, Proteus, Klebsiella pneumoniae, Pseudomonas aeruginosa;* also used as adjunct in hepatic coma, peritonitis, preoperatively to sterilize bowel; decreases ammonia-producing bacteria in bowel and intraperitoneally after fecal spill during surgery

Dosage and routes:

Severe systemic infections
• *Adult and child:* **IV INF** 15 mg/kg/day in divided doses q8-12h; diluted 500 mg/200 ml of NS or D_5W given over 30-60 min, not to exceed 1.5 g/day; **IM** 15 mg/kg/day in divided doses q8-12h, not to exceed 1.5 g/day, irrigation not to exceed 1.5 g/day; **INH** 250 mg qid

Preoperative bowel sterilization
• *Adult:* **PO** 1 g qh × 4 doses, then q6h × 36-72 hr

Renal dose
• *Adult:* **IM/IV** 7.5 mg/kg, may increase or decrease dose based on renal status

Contraindications: Bowel obstruction, severe renal disease, hypersensitivity, pregnancy (D)

kaolin, pectin (OTC)

(kay'oh-lin, pek'tin)
Donnagel-MB🍁, Kao-Spen, Kapectolin, K-P
Func. class.: Antidiarrheal, adsorbent
Chem. class.: Hydrous magnesium aluminum silicate

Action: Decreases gastric motility, H_2O content of stool; adsorbent, demulcent

Uses: Diarrhea (cause undetermined)

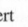

Dosage and routes:
• *Adult:* **PO** 60-120 ml (30 ml conc) after each loose BM
• *Child >12 yr:* **PO** 60 ml after each loose BM
• *Child 6-12 yr:* **PO** 30-60 ml (15 ml conc) after each loose BM
• *Child 3-6 yr:* **PO** 15-30 ml (7.5 ml conc) after each loose BM

Available forms: Susp kaolin 0.87 g/5 ml, pectin 43 mg/5 ml; kaolin 0.98 g/5 ml, pectin 21.7 mg/5 ml

Side effects/adverse reactions:

GI: Constipation (chronic use)

Precautions: Pregnancy (C)

Interactions:

- ↓ action of all other drugs
- ↑ antidiarrheal effect: nutmeg

NURSING CONSIDERATIONS

Assess:

- Bowel pattern before; for rebound constipation, after; bowel sounds
- For dehydration in children

Administer:

- After shaking suspension
- For 48 hr only

Evaluate:

- Therapeutic response: decreased diarrhea

Teach patient/family:

- Not to exceed recommended dose
- To shake well before administration
- To take all other medications ≥2 hr apart

ketoconazole (℞)

(kee-toe-koe′na-zole)

Nizoral

Func. class.: Antifungal

Chem. class.: Imidazole derivative

Action: Alters cell membranes and inhibits several fungal enzymes

Uses: Systemic candidiasis, chronic mucocandidiasis, oral thrush, candiduria, coccidioidomycosis, histoplasmosis, chromomycosis, paracoccidioidomycosis, blastomycosis; tinea cruris, tinea corporis, tinea versicolor, *Pityrosporum ovale*

Investigational uses: Cushing's syndrome, advanced prostatic cancer

Dosage and routes:

- *Adult:* **PO** 200-400 mg qd for 1-2 wk (candidiasis), 6 wk (other infections); 400 mg tid (prostate cancer—unlabeled)
- *Child >2 yr:* **PO:** 3.3-6.6 mg/kg/day as single daily dose

Available forms: Tabs 200 mg; oral susp 100 mg/5 ml✤

Side effects/adverse reactions:

GU: Gynecomastia, impotence

INTEG: Pruritus, fever, chills, photophobia, rash, dermatitis, purpura, urticaria

CNS: Headache, dizziness, somnolence

SYST: ***Anaphylaxis***

GI: Nausea, vomiting, anorexia, diarrhea, abdominal pain, ***hepatotoxicity***

HEMA: ***Thrombocytopenia, leukopenia, hemolytic anemia***

Contraindications: Hypersensitivity, lactation, fungal meningitis; coadministration with terfenadine

Precautions: Renal disease, hepatic disease, achlorhydria (drug-induced), pregnancy (C), children <2 yr, other hepatotoxic agents including terfenadine

Do not confuse:

Nizoral/Nasarel/Neoral

Pharmacokinetics:

PO: Peak 1-2 hr, half-life 2 hr, terminal 8 hr; metabolized in liver; excreted in bile, feces; requires acid pH for absorption; distributed poorly to CSF; highly protein bound

Interactions:

- Hepatotoxicity: other hepatotoxic drugs, alcohol
- Inhibition of CYP 450 3A4 pathway, toxicity: alfentanil, alprazolam, amprenavir, atorvastatin, calcium channel blockers, carbamazepine, cerivastatin, clarithromycin, corticosteroids, cyclophosphamide, cycloSPORINE, donepezil, erythro-

K

mycin, fentanyl, ifosfamide, indinavir, lovastatin, midazolam, nelfinavir, nisoldipine, quinidine, ritonavir, saquinavir, sildenafil, simvastatin, sufentanil, tamoxifen, triazolam, vinBLAStine, vinca alkaloids, vinCRIStine, zolpidem
• ↓ action of ketoconazole: antacids, H_2-receptor antagonists, anticholinergics, isoniazid, rifampin, ddI, gastric acid pump inhibitors
• ↑ anticoagulant effect: warfarin, anticoagulants
• ↓ effect of: oral contraceptives
• Ketoconazole may ↓ theophylline effect
• Inhibited metabolism: paclitaxel
↓ ketoconazole action: yew
Nephrotoxicity: gossypol

NURSING CONSIDERATIONS

Assess:
• For infection symptoms before and after treatment
• Hepatic studies (ALT, AST, bilirubin) if on long-term therapy
• For allergic reaction: rash, photosensitivity, urticaria, dermatitis
For hepatotoxicity: nausea, vomiting, jaundice, clay-colored stools, fatigue

Administer:
• In the presence of acid products only; do not use alkaline products, proton pump inhibitors, H_2-antagonists, antacids within 2 hr of drug; may give coffee, tea, acidic fruit juices, cola
• With food to decrease GI symptoms
• With HCl if achlorhydria is present; dissolve tab/4 ml of aqueous sol 0.2 NHCl, use straw to avoid contact, rinse with water afterward and swallow

Perform/provide:
• Storage in tight container at room temperature

Evaluate:
• Therapeutic response: decreased fever, malaise, rash, negative C&S for infecting organism, absence of scaling

Teach patient/family:
• That long-term therapy may be needed to clear infection (1 wk-6 mo depending on infection)
• To avoid hazardous activities if dizziness occurs
• To take 2 hr ac administration of other drugs that increase gastric pH (antacids, H_2-blockers, omeprazole, sucralfate, anticholinergics)
• The importance of compliance with drug regimen
To notify prescriber of GI symptoms, signs of hepatic dysfunction (fatigue, nausea, anorexia, vomiting, dark urine, pale stools)
• Use sunglasses to prevent photophobia

ketoconazole topical

See appendix c

ketoprofen (OTC, ℞)

(ke-toe-proe′fen)

Actron, Apo-Keto♣, Apo-Keto-E♣, ketoprofen, Orudis, Orudis-E♣, Orudis-KT, Orudis-SR♣, Oruvail, Rhodis♣

Func. class.: Nonsteroidal anti-inflammatory (NSAID), antirheumatic

Chem. class.: Propionic acid derivative

Action: Inhibits prostaglandin synthesis by decreasing enzyme needed for biosynthesis; analgesic, antiinflammatory, antipyretic

Uses: Mild to moderate pain, osteoarthritis, rheumatoid arthritis, dysmenorrhea

Dosage and routes:

Antiinflammatory

• *Adult:* **PO** 150-300 mg in divided doses tid-qid, not to exceed 300 mg/day or ext rel 150-200 mg qd

Analgesic

• *Adult:* **PO** 25-50 mg q6-8h

Available forms: Caps 25, 50, 75 mg; ext rel cap 100, 150, 200 mg; tabs 12.5 mg

Side effects/adverse reactions:

GI: Nausea, anorexia, vomiting, diarrhea, jaundice, ***hepatitis,*** constipation, flatulence, cramps, dry mouth, peptic ulcer, ***GI bleeding***

CNS: Dizziness, drowsiness, fatigue, tremors, confusion, insomnia, anxiety, depression, headache

CV: Tachycardia, peripheral edema, palpitations, dysrhythmias, hypertension

INTEG: Purpura, rash, pruritus, sweating

GU: ***Nephrotoxicity: dysuria, hematuria, oliguria, azotemia***

HEMA: ***Blood dyscrasias***

EENT: Tinnitus, hearing loss, blurred vision

SYST: ***Anaphylaxis***

Contraindications: Hypersensitivity, asthma, severe renal disease, severe hepatic disease, ulcer disease; avoid in 2nd/3rd trimester

Precautions: Pregnancy (B) 1st trimester, lactation, children, bleeding disorders, GI disorders, cardiac disorders, hypersensitivity to other antiinflammatory agents, elderly

Do not confuse:

Oruvail/Clinoril

Oruvail/Elavil

Pharmacokinetics:

PO: Peak 2 hr, half-life 2-4 hr; metabolized in liver; excreted in urine (metabolites); excreted in breast milk; 99% plasma protein binding

Interactions:

• ↑ hypoglycemia: insulin, sulfonylureas

• ↑ toxicity: cycloSPORINE, lithium, methotrexate, phenytoin, alcohol

• ↑ bleeding risk: cefamandole, cefoperazone, cefotetan, clopidogrel, eptifibatide, plicamycin, thrombolytics, ticlopidine, tirofiban, valproic acid, warfarin

• ↑ ketoprofen levels: aspirin, probenecid

• ↓ effect of: diuretics, antihypertensives

• ↑ adverse GI reactions: aspirin, corticosteroids, NSAIDs, alcohol

• ↑ hematologic toxicity: radiation

↑ bleeding risk: anise, arnica, chamomile, clove, dong quai, feverfew, garlic, ginger, ginkgo, ginseng *(Panax)*

↑ gastric irritation: arginine, gossypol

↑ NSAIDs effect: bearberry, bilberry

↑ bleeding risk: bogbean, chondroitin

Lab test interferences:

Increase: Potassium, BUN, alk phosphatase, AST, ALT, LDH, creatinine, bleeding time

Decrease: Blood glucose, HCT, Hgb, platelets, CCr, leukocyte

Interfere: Urine albumin, 17 KS, 17-Hydroxycorticosteroid, bilirubin

NURSING CONSIDERATIONS

Assess:

• For pain: type, location, intensity, ROM before and 1-2 hr after treatment

• Renal, hepatic, blood studies: BUN, creatinine, AST, ALT, Hgb,

K

before treatment, periodically thereafter

◆ For aspirin sensitivity, asthma; these patients may be more likely to develop hypersensitivity to NSAIDs

- Audiometric, ophthalmic exam before, during, after treatment
- For eye, ear problems: blurred vision, tinnitus; may indicate toxicity
- For GI bleeding: blood in sputum, emesis, stools

Administer:

⊘ Whole; do not crush, break, or chew ext rel caps

- With food to decrease GI symptoms; however, taking on empty stomach best facilitates absorption

Perform/provide:

- Storage at room temperature

Evaluate:

- Therapeutic response: decreased pain, stiffness in joints, decreased swelling in joints, ability to move more easily; decreased fever

Teach patient/family:

- To report blurred vision, ringing, roaring in ears; may indicate toxicity
- To avoid driving, other hazardous activities if dizziness, drowsiness occurs, especially elderly
- To report change in urine pattern, increased weight, edema, increased pain in joints, fever, blood in urine; indicate nephrotoxicity; rash, itching, blurred vision, ringing in the ears, flulike symptoms
- That therapeutic effects may take up to 1 mo, to take with 8 oz of water and sit upright for ½ hr after administration to prevent GI irritation
- To avoid aspirin, alcohol, steroids, acetaminophen or other medications, supplements unless approved by prescriber
- To wear sunscreen to prevent photosensitivity

ketorolac (℞)

(kee-toe′role-ak)

Acular, Toradol

Func. class.: Nonsteroidal antiinflammatory/nonopioid analgesic

Chem. class.: Pyrrolo-pyrrole

Action: Inhibits prostaglandin synthesis by decreasing an enzyme needed for biosynthesis; analgesic, antiinflammatory, antipyretic effects

Uses: Mild to moderate pain; seasonal allergic conjunctivitis (ophth)

Dosage and routes:

- *Adult <65 yr:* **PO** 20 mg then 10 mg q4-6h prn, max 40 mg/day
- *Adult >65 yr, renal disease, <50 kg:* **PO** 10 mg q4-6h prn, max 40 mg/day
- *Adult <65 yr:* **IM** (single dose) 60 mg **IV** 30 mg; **IM** (multiple dosing) 15 mg q6h, max 60 mg/day × 5 day combined either **PO/IM/IV**
- *Adult >65 yr, renal disease, <50 kg:* **IM** single dose 30 mg; **IV** 15 mg **IM/IV** (multiple dosing) 15 mg q6h, max 60 mg/day × 5 days combined either **PO/IM/IV**
- *Adult:* **OPHTH** 1 gtt qid

Available forms: Inj 15, 30 mg/ml (prefilled syringes); ophth 0.5% sol; tab 10 mg

Side effects/adverse reactions:

CV: Hypertension, flushing, syncope, pallor, edema, vasodilation

CNS: Dizziness, *drowsiness,* tremors

EENT: Tinnitus, hearing loss, blurred vision

GI: Nausea, anorexia, vomiting, diarrhea, constipation, flatulence, cramps, dry mouth, peptic ulcer, ***GI bleeding, perforation***, taste change

GU: ***Nephrotoxicity: dysuria, hematuria, oliguria, azotemia***
HEMA: ***Blood dyscrasias,*** prolonged bleeding
INTEG: Purpura, rash, pruritus, sweating
Contraindications: Hypersensitivity, asthma, severe renal disease, severe hepatic disease, peptic ulcer disease, L&D, lactation, CV bleeding
Precautions: Pregnancy (C), children, bleeding disorders, GI disorders, cardiac disorders, hypersensitivity to other antiinflammatory agents, elderly, CCr <25 ml/min
Do not confuse:
Toradol/Tegretol/Foradil
Toradol/Inderal
Toradol/Torecan
Toradol/tramadol
Pharmacokinetics:
PO: Peak 2-3 hr, duration 4-6 hr
IM: Peak 50 min, half-life 6 hr, enters breast milk, <50% metabolized by liver, excreted by kidneys
Interactions:
• ↑ toxicity: methotrexate, lithium, cycloSPORINE
• ↑ bleeding risk: anticoagulants, cefamandole, cefoperazone, cefotetan, clopidogrel, eptifibatide, plicamycin, salicylates, ticlopidine, tirofiban, thrombolytics, valproic acid
• ↓ effects: antihypertensives, diuretics
• ↑ renal impairment: ACE inhibitors
• ↑ ketorolac levels: aspirin, probenecid
• ↑ GI effects: steroids, alcohol, aspirin, NSAIDs, potassium products
↑ gastric irritation: arginine, gossypol
↑ NSAIDs effect: bearberry, bilberry
↑ bleeding risk: bogbean, chondroitin
↑ bleeding risk: anise, arnica, chamomile, clove, dong quai, feverfew, garlic, ginger, ginkgo, ginseng *(Panax)*
Lab test interferences:
Increase: Hepatic studies, bleeding time, BUN, creatinine, potassium
NURSING CONSIDERATIONS
Assess:
• Patients with aspirin sensitivity, asthma; may be more likely to develop hypersensitivity to NSAIDs, monitor for hypersensitivity
• For pain: type, location, intensity, ROM before and 1 hr after treatment
• Eyes: redness, swelling, tearing, itching (ophth)
• Renal, hepatic, blood studies: BUN, creatinine, AST, ALT, Hgb before treatment, periodically thereafter; check for dehydration
• Bleeding times; check for bruising, bleeding; test for occult blood in urine
• For eye, ear problems: blurred vision, tinnitus (may indicate toxicity)
Hepatic dysfunction: jaundice, yellow sclera and skin, clay-colored stools
• Audiometric, ophthalmic exam before, during, after treatment
• GI bleeding: blood in sputum, emesis, stools
Administer:
• IM/IV for 5 days or less; continue therapy with PO
IV route
• Give undiluted over ≥15 sec
Solution compatibility: D_5W, 0.9% NaCl, LR, D_5, plasmalate
Syringe compatibilities: Sufentanil

Y-site compatibilities: Cisatracurium, remifentanil, sufentanil

Perform/provide:

• Storage at room temperature

Evaluate:

• Therapeutic response: decreased pain, stiffness, swelling in joints, ability to move more easily; decreased ocular itching (ophth)

Teach patient/family:

• To report blurred vision or ringing, roaring in ears (may indicate toxicity)

• To avoid driving, other hazardous activities if dizziness or drowsiness occurs

• To report change in urine pattern, weight increase, edema, pain increase in joints, fever, blood in urine (indicates nephrotoxicity)

• To avoid alcohol, salicylates, other NSAIDs, acetaminophen

• This drug may cause redness, burning if soft contact lenses are worn (ophth)

ketorolac ophthalmic

See appendix c

ketotifen ophthalmic

See appendix c

labetalol (℞)

(la-bet′a-lole)

Normodyne, Trandate

Func. class.: Antihypertensive, antianginal

Chem. class.: α/β-Blocker

Action: Produces decreases in B/P without reflex tachycardia or significant reduction in heart rate through mixture of α-blocking, β-blocking effects; elevated plasma renins are reduced

Uses: Mild to moderate hypertension; treatment of severe hypertension (IV)

Investigational uses: Hypertension in patients with pheochromocytoma, hypertension in clonidine withdrawal

Dosage and routes:

Hypertension

• *Adult:* **PO** 100 mg bid; may be given with a diuretic; may increase to 200 mg bid after 2 days; may continue to increase q1-3 days; max 400 mg bid

Hypertensive crisis

• *Adult:* **IV INF** 200 mg/160 ml D_5W, run at 2 ml/min; stop inf at desired response, repeat q6-8h as needed; **IV BOL** 20 mg over 2 min, may repeat 40-80 mg q10min, not to exceed 300 mg

Available forms: Tabs 100, 200, 300 mg; inj 5 mg/ml in 20 ml amps

Side effects/adverse reactions:

CV: Orthostatic hypotension, bradycardia, ***CHF,*** chest pain, ***ventricular dysrhythmias,*** AV block, scalp tingling

CNS: Dizziness, mental changes, drowsiness, fatigue, headache, catatonia, depression, anxiety, nightmares, paresthesias, lethargy

GI: Nausea, vomiting, diarrhea, dyspepsia, taste distortion
INTEG: Rash, alopecia, urticaria, pruritus, fever
HEMA: ***Agranulocytosis, thrombocytopenia, purpura*** (rare)
EENT: Tinnitus, visual changes, sore throat, double vision, dry, burning eyes
GU: Impotence, dysuria, ejaculatory failure
RESP: ***Bronchospasm,*** dyspnea, wheezing

Contraindications: Hypersensitivity to β-blockers, cardiogenic shock, heart block (2nd or 3rd degree), sinus bradycardia, CHF, bronchial asthma

Precautions: Major surgery, pregnancy (C), lactation, diabetes mellitus, renal disease, thyroid disease, COPD, well-compensated heart failure, CAD, nonallergic bronchospasm, elderly, hepatic disease

Do not confuse:
Trandate/Tridrate

Pharmacokinetics:
PO: Onset ½-2 hr, peak 2-4 hr, duration 8-12 hr
IV: Onset 5 min, peak 15 min, duration 2-4 hr
Half-life 6-8 hr; metabolized by liver (metabolites inactive); excreted in urine; crosses placenta; excreted in breast milk

Interactions:
- Do not use within 2 wk of MAOIs
- Myocardial depression: hydantoins, general anesthetics, verapamil
- ↑ hypotension: diuretics, other antihypertensives, cimetidine, nitroglycerin, alcohol
- ↓ effects: sympathomimetics, lidocaine, indomethacin, theophylline, β-blockers, bronchodilators, xanthines
- ↓ labetolol effect: glutethimide

↑ toxicity, death: aconite
↑ or ↓ antihypertensive effect: astragalus, cola tree
↑ antihypertensive effect: barberry, betony, black catechu, black cohosh, bloodroot, broom, burdock, cat's claw, dandelion, goldenseal, Irish moss, Jamaican dogwood, kelp, khella, mistletoe, parsley
↓ antihypertensive effect: coltsfoot, guarana, khat, licorice

Lab test interferences:
Increase: ANA titer, blood glucose, alk phosphatase, LDH, AST, ALT, BUN, potassium, triglyceride, uric acid
False increase: Urinary catecholamines

NURSING CONSIDERATIONS
Assess:
I&O, weight daily; fluid overload: weight gain, jugular venous distention, edema, rales in lungs
- B/P during beginning treatment, periodically thereafter, pulse q4h; note rate, rhythm, quality
- Apical/radial pulse before administration; notify prescriber of any significant changes
- Baselines in renal, hepatic studies before therapy begins
- Edema in feet, legs daily
- Skin turgor, dryness of mucous membranes for hydration status

Administer:
- PO ac, hs; tab may be crushed or swallowed whole, give with meals to increase absorption
- Reduced dosage in renal dysfunction

IV route
- Undiluted or diluted in LR, D_5W, D_5 in 0.2%, 0.9%, 0.33% NaCl or Ringer's inj, give undiluted 20 mg or less/2 min; inf is titrated to patient response; 200 mg of drug/160 ml sol = 1 mg/ml; 300 mg of drug/240 ml sol = 1 mg/ml; 200 mg of drug/250 ml sol = 2 mg/3 ml; use infusion pump

• Keeping patient recumbent during and for 3 hr after administration, monitor VS q5-15min

Solution compatibilities: D_5R, D_5LR, $D_{2\frac{1}{2}}$/0.45% NaCl, D_5/0.2% NaCl, D_5/0.33% NaCl, $D_5$0.9% NaCl, D_5W, Ringer's, LR

Y-site compatibilities: Amikacin, aminophylline, amiodarone, ampicillin, butorphanol, calcium gluconate, cefazolin, ceftazidime, ceftizoxime, chloramphenicol, cimetidine, clindamycin, diltiazem, DOBUTamine, DOPamine, enalaprilat, epINEPHrine, erythromycin, esmolol, famotidine, fentanyl, gentamicin, hydromorphone, lidocaine, lorazepam, magnesium sulfate, meperidine, metronidazole, midazolam, milrinone, morphine, niCARdipine, nitroglycerin, norepinephrine, nitroprusside, oxacillin, penicillin G potassium, piperacillin, potassium chloride, potassium phosphate, propofol, ranitidine, sodium acetate, tobramycin, trimethoprim-sulfamethoxazole, vancomycin, vecuronium

Perform/provide:

• Storage in dry area at room temperature; do not freeze

Evaluate:

• Therapeutic response: decreased B/P after 1-2 wk

Teach patient/family:

• Not to discontinue drug abruptly; taper over 2 wk; may cause precipitate angina

• Not to use OTC products containing α-adrenergic stimulants (nasal decongestants, OTC cold preparations) unless directed by prescriber

• To report bradycardia, dizziness, confusion, depression, fever

• To take pulse at home, advise when to notify prescriber

• To avoid alcohol, smoking, sodium intake

• To comply with weight control, dietary adjustments, modified exercise program

• To carry emergency ID to identify drug, allergies

• To avoid hazardous activities if dizziness is present

• To report symptoms of CHF: difficulty breathing, especially on exertion or when lying down, night cough, swelling of extremities

• To take medication at bedtime to prevent effect of orthostatic hypotension

• To wear support hose to minimize effects of orthostatic hypotension

Treatment of overdose: Lavage, IV atropine for bradycardia, IV theophylline for bronchospasm, digitalis, O_2, diuretic for cardiac failure; hemodialysis is useful for removal, hypotension; administer vasopressor (norepinephrine)

lactulose (℞)

(lak'tyoo-lose)

Cephulac, Cholac, Chronulac, Constilac, Constulose, Duphalac, Enulose, Evalose, Heptalac, Kristalose, Lactulax✦, Lactulose PSE, Portalac

Func. class.: Laxative; ammonia detoxicant (hyperosmotic)

Chem. class.: Lactose synthetic derivative

Action: Prevents absorption of ammonia in colon; increases water in stool

Uses: Chronic constipation, portal-systemic encephalopathy in patients with hepatic disease

Dosage and routes:

Constipation

• *Adult:* **PO** 15-60 ml qd

• *Child* (unlabeled): **PO** 7.5 ml qd

Encephalopathy
• *Adult:* **PO** 30-45 ml tid or qid until stools are soft; **RETENTION ENEMA** 300 ml diluted
• *Infant:* (unlabeled) **PO** 2.5-10 ml/day in divided doses (unlabeled)
• *Child:* (unlabeled) **PO** 40-90 ml/day in divided doses given 2-4×/day (unlabeled)
Available forms: Syr 10 g/15 ml; single-use packets (Kristalose) 10, 20 g
Side effects/adverse reactions:
GI: Nausea, vomiting, anorexia, abdominal cramps, diarrhea, flatulence, distention, belching
Contraindications: Hypersensitivity, low-galactose diet
Precautions: Pregnancy (B), lactation, diabetes mellitus, elderly, debilitated patients
Pharmacokinetics: Metabolized in intestine, excreted by kidneys; onset 1-2 days, peak unknown, duration unknown
Interactions:
• Do not use with laxatives
• ↓ lactulose effects: neomycin, other oral antiinfectives
↑ laxative action: flax, senna
NURSING CONSIDERATIONS
Assess:
• Stool: amount, color, consistency
• Blood ammonia level (30-70 mg/100 ml); may decrease ammonia level by 25%-50%
• Blood, urine electrolytes if drug is used often; may cause diarrhea, hypokalemia, hyponatremia
• I&O ratio to identify fluid loss
• Cause of constipation; determine whether fluids, bulk, or exercise is missing from lifestyle
• Cramping, rectal bleeding, nausea, vomiting; if these symptoms occur, drug should be discontinued
• Clearing of confusion, lethargy, restlessness, irritability if portal-systemic encephalopathy

Administer:
PO route
• With 8 oz fruit juice, water, milk to increase palatability of oral form
RECT route
• Retention enema by diluting 300 ml lactose/700 ml of water; administer by rectal balloon catheter
• Increased fluids to 2 L/day; do not give with other laxatives; if diarrhea occurs, reduce dosage
Evaluate:
• Therapeutic response: decreased constipation, decreased blood ammonia level, clearing of mental state
Teach patient/family:
• Not to use laxatives long-term
• To dilute with water or fruit juice to counteract sweet taste
• To store in cool environment; do not freeze
• To take on an empty stomach for rapid action
• To report diarrhea; may indicate overdose

lamivudine (℞)
(lam-i-voo'deen)
Epivir, Epivir-HBV, 3TC
Func. class.: Antiretroviral
Chem. class.: Nucleoside reverse transcriptase inhibitor

Action: Inhibits replication of HIV virus by incorporating into cellular DNA by viral reverse transcriptase, thereby terminating cellular DNA chain
Uses: HIV infection in combination with other antiretrovirals; chronic hepatitis B (Epivir-HBV)
Investigational uses: Prophylaxis of HIV—postexposure with indinavir and zidovudine

Dosage and routes:

HIV

• *Adult and child >16 yr:* **PO** 150 mg bid or 300 mg qd

• *Child 3 mo to 16 yr:* **PO** 4 mg/kg bid, max 150 mg bid

Renal dose

• *Adult:* **PO** CCr 30-49 ml/min 150 mg qd; CCr 15-29 ml/min 150 mg 1st dose, then 100 mg qd; CCr 5-14 ml/min 150 mg qd, then 50 mg qd; CCr <5 ml/min, 50 mg 1st dose, then 25 mg qd

Chronic hepatitis B

• *Adult:* **PO** 100 mg qd

Renal dose

• *Adult:* **PO** CCr 30-49 ml/min 100 mg 1st dose, then 50 mg qd; CCr 15-29 ml/min 100 mg 1st dose, then 25 mg qd; CCr 5-14 ml/min 35 mg 1st dose, then 15 mg qd CCr <5 ml/min 35 mg 1st dose, then 10 mg qd

Available forms: Tabs 100, 150, 300 mg; oral sol 10 mg/ml

Side effects/adverse reactions:

HEMA: ***Neutropenia, anemia, thrombocytopenia***

CNS: Fever, headache, malaise, dizziness, insomnia, depression, fatigue, chills, ***seizures***

GI: Nausea, vomiting, diarrhea, anorexia, cramps, dyspepsia, ***hepatomegaly with steatosis, pancreatitis (pediatrics)***

RESP: Cough

EENT: Taste change, hearing loss, photophobia

INTEG: Rash

MS: Myalgia, arthralgia, pain

SYST: ***Lactic acidosis, anaphylaxis, Stevens-Johnson syndrome***

Contraindications: Hypersensitivity

Precautions: Granulocyte count <1000/mm^3 or Hgb <9.5 g/dl, pregnancy (C), lactation, children, renal disease, severe hepatic dysfunction, pancreatitis, elderly

Do not confuse:

lamivudine/lamotrigine

Pharmacokinetics: Rapidly absorbed, distributed to extravascular space, excreted unchanged in urine

Interactions:

• ↑ lamivudine level: trimethoprim-sulfamethoxazole

NURSING CONSIDERATIONS

Assess:

• Blood counts q2wk; watch for neutropenia, thrombocytopenia, Hgb, CD4, viral load; if low, therapy may have to be discontinued and restarted after hematologic recovery; blood transfusions may be required

• Hepatic studies: AST, ALT, bilirubin; amylase, lipase, triglycerides, CD4, viral load periodically during treatment

• Children for pancreatitis: abdominal pain, nausea, vomiting

◆ Lactic acidosis, severe hepatomegaly with steatosis: obtain baseline LFTs, if elevated discontinue treatment; discontinue even if LFTs are normal if lactic acidosis, severe hepatomegaly develop

Administer:

• PO qd or bid, without regard to meals

Perform/provide:

• With other antiretrovirals only

• Storage in cool environment; protect from light

Evaluate:

• Blood dyscrasias: bruising, fatigue, bleeding, poor healing

Teach patient/family:

• That GI complaints, insomnia resolve after 3-4 wk of treatment

• That drug is not a cure for HIV, but will control symptoms

• To notify prescriber of sore throat, swollen lymph nodes, malaise, fever; other infections may occur

• That patient is still infective, may pass HIV virus on to others

• That follow-up visits must be con-

tinued since serious toxicity may occur; blood counts must be done q2wk
• That drug must be taken as prescribed, even if patient feels better
• That other drugs may be necessary to prevent other infections
• That drug may cause fainting or dizziness

lamotrigine (℞)

(la-mot'ri-geen)
Lamictal, Lamictal Chewable Dispersible
Func. class.: Anticonvulsant, misc.
Chem. class.: Phenyltriazine

Action: Unknown, may inhibit voltage-sensitive sodium channels
Uses: Adjunct in the treatment of partial seizures; children with Lennox-Gastaut syndrome
Investigational uses: Generalized tonic-clonic, absence, atypical absence and myoclonic seizures; refractory bipolar disorder
Dosage and routes:
Monotherapy
• *Adult:* 50 mg/day for wk 1-2, then increase to 100 mg divided bid for wk 3-4; maintenance, 300-500 mg/day
• *Child:* 2 mg/kg/day in 2 divided doses × 2 wk, then 10 mg/kg/day, max 15 mg/kg/day or 400 mg/day
Multiple therapy
• *Adult:* 25 mg qod wk 1-4, then 150 mg/day in divided doses
• *Child:* 0.1-0.2 mg/kg/day initially, then increase q2wk as needed to 2 mg/kg/day or 150 mg/day
Hepatic Dose (Child-Pugh Grade B)
• *Adult:* **PO** Reduce by 50%; ***(Child-Pugh Grade C)*** Reduce by 75%
Available forms: Tabs 25, 100, 150, 200 mg; chew dispersible tabs 2, 5, 25 mg
Side effects/adverse reactions:
CNS: Dizziness, ataxia, *headache,* fever, insomnia, tremor, depression, anxiety
EENT: Nystagmus, *diplopia, blurred vision*
GI: Nausea, vomiting, anorexia, abdominal pain, ***hepatotoxicity***
GU: Dysmenorrhea
INTEG: ***Rash (potentially life-threatening),*** alopecia, photosensitivity
SYST: ***Stevens-Johnson syndrome***
Contraindications: Hypersensitivity
Precautions: Pregnancy (C), lactation, child <16 yr, renal, hepatic disease, elderly, cardiac disease
Do not confuse:
Lamictal/Lomotil/Lamisil
lamotrigine/lamivudine
Pharmacokinetics: Half-life varies depending on dose
Interactions:
• ↑ metabolic clearance of lamotrigine: carbamazepine, phenobarbital, phenytoin, primidone ethosuximide, oxcarbazepine
• ↓ metabolic clearance of lamotrigine: valproic acid
• ↓ lamotrigine serum concentration: rifamycins, oral contraceptives, acetaminophen
↑ anticonvulsant effect: ginkgo
↓ anticonvulsant effect: ginseng, santonica

NURSING CONSIDERATIONS
Assess:
• For seizure activity: duration, type, intensity, halo before seizure
• For rash (Stevens-Johnson syndrome or toxic epidermal necrolysis) in pediatric patients, drug should be discontinued at first sign of rash
Administer:
• Chewable dispersible tabs; swallow whole, chew, or dispersed in

water or diluted fruit juice; if chewed, drink a small amount of water

Evaluate:

• Therapeutic response: decrease in severity of seizures

Teach patient/family:

• To take PO doses divided with or after meals to decrease adverse effects, not to discontinue drug abruptly; seizures may occur

• To avoid hazardous activities until stabilized on drug

• To carry emergency ID, to notify prescriber of skin rash or increased seizure activity, to use sunscreen and protective clothing if photosensitivity occurs

• To notify prescriber if pregnant or intend to become pregnant

lansoprazole (℞)

(lan-so-prey'zole)

Prevacid

Func. class.: Antiulcer, proton pump inhibitor

Chem. class.: Benzimidazole

Action: Suppresses gastric secretion by inhibiting hydrogen/potassium ATPase enzyme system in gastric parietal cell; characterized as gastric acid pump inhibitor, since it blocks final step of acid production

Uses: Gastroesophageal reflux disease (GERD), severe erosive esophagitis, poorly responsive systemic GERD, pathologic hypersecretory conditions (Zollinger-Ellison syndrome, systemic mastocytosis, multiple endocrine adenomas); possibly effective for treatment of duodenal, gastric ulcers, maintenance of healed duodenal ulcers

Dosage and routes:

NG tube

• *Adult:* Use intact granules mixed in 40 ml of apple juice and injected through **NG** tube, then flush with apple juice

Duodenal ulcer

• *Adult:* **PO** 15 mg qd before eating for 4 wk, then 15 mg qd to maintain healing of ulcers; associated with *Helicobacter pylori*—30 mg lansoprazole, 500 mg clarithromycin, 1 g amoxicillin bid × 14 days or 30 mg lansoprazole, 1 g amoxicillin tid × 14 days

Erosive esophagitis

• *Adult:* **PO** 30 mg qd before eating for up to 8 wk, may use another 8 wk course if needed

Pathologic hypersecretory conditions

• *Adult:* **PO** 60 mg qd, may give up to 90 mg bid

Available forms: Caps, del rel 15, 30 mg

Side effects/adverse reactions:

CNS: Headache, dizziness, confusion, agitation, amnesia, depression

GI: Diarrhea, abdominal pain, vomiting, nausea, constipation, flatulence, acid regurgitation, anorexia, irritable colon

RESP: Upper respiratory infections, cough, epistaxis, asthma, bronchitis, dyspnea

INTEG: Rash, urticaria, pruritus, alopecia

META: Weight gain/loss, gout

EENT: Tinnitus, taste perversion, deafness, eye pain, otitis media

CV: Chest pain, angina, tachycardia, bradycardia, palpitations, ***CVA,*** hypertension/hypotension, ***MI, shock,*** vasodilation

GU: ***Hematuria,*** glycosuria, impotence, kidney calculus, breast enlargement

HEMA: ***Hemolysis,*** anemia

Contraindications: Hypersensitivity

Precautions: Pregnancy (B), lactation, children

Do not confuse:

Prevacid/Pravachol/Prinivil

Pharmacokinetics: Absorption after granules leave stomach—rapid; plasma half-life 1½ hr, protein binding 97%, extensively metabolized in liver, excreted in urine, feces; clearance decreased in the elderly, renal and hepatic impairment

Interactions:

• Delayed lansoprazole absorption: sucralfate

• ↓ absorption of ketoconazole, itraconazole, ampicillin, iron, digoxin

NURSING CONSIDERATIONS

Assess:

• GI system: bowel sounds q8h, abdomen for pain, swelling, anorexia

• Hepatic studies: AST, ALT, alk phosphatase during treatment

Administer:

⃠ Before eating; swallow capsule whole; do not break, crush, or chew caps

Evaluate:

• Therapeutic response: absence of epigastric pain, swelling, fullness

Teach patient/family:

• To report severe diarrhea; drug may have to be discontinued

• That diabetic patient should know that hypoglycemia may occur

• To avoid hazardous activities; dizziness may occur

• To avoid alcohol, salicylates, ibuprofen; may cause GI irritation

latanoprost ophthalmic

See appendix c

leflunomide (℞)

(leh-floo′noh-mide)

Arava

Func. class.: Antirheumatic (DMARDs)

Chem. class.: Immune modulator, pyrimidine synthesis inhibitor

Action: Inhibits an enzyme involved in pyrimidine synthesis and has antiproliferative, antiinflammatory effect

Uses: Rheumatoid arthritis, to reduce disease process and symptoms

Dosage and routes:

• *Adult:* **PO** loading dose 100 mg/day × 3 days, maintenance 20 mg/day, may be decreased to 10 mg/day if not well tolerated

Available forms: Tabs 10, 20, 100 mg

Side effects/adverse reactions:

GI: Nausea, anorexia, vomiting, constipation, flatulence, diarrhea, elevated LFTs

CNS: Headache, dizziness, insomnia, depression, paresthesia, anxiety, migraine, neuralgia

CV: Palpitations, hypertension, chest pain, angina pectoris, peripheral edema

INTEG: Rash, pruritus, alopecia, acne, hematoma, herpes infections

RESP: Pharyngitis, rhinitis, bronchitis, cough, respiratory infection, pneumonia, sinusitis

EENT: Pharyngitis, oral candidiasis, stomatitis, dry mouth, blurred vision

HEMA: Anemia, ecchymosis, hyperlipidemia

Contraindications: Hypersensitivity, pregnancy (X), lactation

Precautions: Hepatic, renal disorders

Pharmacokinetics:
PO: metabolized in liver to metabolite, excreted in urine
Interactions:
• ↓ antibody response: live virus vaccines
• ↑ NSAIDs effect: NSAIDs
• ↑ leflunomide side effects: hepatotoxic agents, methotrexate
• ↑ rifampin levels: rifampin
• ↓ leflunomide effect: activated charcoal, cholestyramine
NURSING CONSIDERATIONS
Assess:
• Arthritic symptoms: ROM, mobility, swelling of joints baseline and during treatment
• Hepatic studies: if ALT elevations are > twofold ULN, reduce dose to 10 mg/day
Administer:
PO route
• With food for GI upset
• To eliminate drug: give cholestyramine 8 g tid × 11 days, check levels
Evaluate:
• Therapeutic response: decreased inflammation, pain in joints
Teach patient/family:
• That drug must be continued for prescribed time to be effective
• To take with food, milk, or antacids to avoid GI upset
• To use caution when driving; drowsiness, dizziness may occur
• To take with a full glass of water to enhance absorption
• To avoid pregnancy while taking this drug; not to breastfeed while taking this drug; men should also discontinue drug and begin leflunomide removal protocol if a pregnancy is planned
• That hair may be lost, review alternatives
• To avoid vaccinations during treatment (live virus)

HIGH ALERT

lepirudin (℞)
(lep-ih-roo'din)
Refludan
Func. class.: Anticoagulant
Chem. class.: Thrombin inhibitor, hirudin

Action: Direct inhibitor of thrombin that is highly specific
Uses: Heparin-induced thrombocytopenia and other thromboembolic conditions
Investigational uses: Adjunct therapy in unstable angina, acute MI without ST elevation, prevention of deep vein thrombosis, percutaneous coronary intervention
Dosage and routes:
• *Adult:* **IV** 0.4 mg/kg (≤110 kg) over 15-20 sec; then 0.15 mg/kg (≤110 kg/hr) as a cont inf for 2-10 days or longer
Renal dose
• *Adult:* **IV BOLUS** 0.2 mg/kg over 15-20 sec, then CCr 45-60 ml/min 0.075 mg/kg/hr, CCr 30-44 ml/min 0.045 mg/kg/hr, CCr 15-29 ml/min 0.0225 mg/kg/hr
Concomitant use with thrombolytic therapy
• *Adult:* **IV BOLUS** 0.2 mg/kg initially
• *Adult:* **CONT IV INF** 0.1 mg/kg/hr
Available forms: Powder for inj 50 mg
Side effects/adverse reactions:
CV: ***Heart failure, pericardial effusion, ventricular fibrillation***
SYST: ***Multiorgan failure, sepsis, anaphylaxis***
CNS: Fever, vaginal bleeding
GI: GI bleeding, abnormal LFTs
GU: ***Hematuria,*** abnormal kidney function, ***intracranial bleeding***

HEMA: ***Hemorrhage, thrombocytopenia***
RESP: Pneumonia
INTEG: Allergic skin reactions
Contraindications: Hypersensitivity to hirudins
Precautions: Intracranial bleeding, lactation, children, hepatic disease, pregnancy (B), recent major surgery, hemorrhagic diathesis bacterial endocarditis, severe uncontrolled hypertension, advanced renal disease, recent active peptic ulcer, recent CVA, stroke, intracerebral surgery, elderly, women
Pharmacokinetics: May be metabolized by the release of amino acids during catabolism; 50% unchanged in urine
Interactions:
• ↑ bleeding risk: warfarin derivatives, thrombolytics, NSAIDs, plicamycin, cefamandole, cefotetan, cefoperazone, aspirin, clopidogrel, dipyridamole, eptifibatide, ticlopidine, tirofiban, valproic acid
↑ risk of bleeding: agrimony, alfalfa, angelica, anise, basil, bay, bilberry, black haw, bogbean, bromelain, buchu, chondroitin, cinchona bark, Dong quai, fenugreek, feverfew, garlic, ginger, ginkgo, ginseng, horse chestnut, Irish moss, kelp, kelpware, khella, lovage, lungwort, meadowsweet, motherwort, mugwort, nettle, papaya, parsley (large amts), pau d'arco, pineapple, poplar, prickly ash, safflower, saw palmetto, tonka bean, turmeric, wintergreen, yarrow
↓ anticoagulant effect: chamomile, coenzyme Q10, flax, glucomannan, goldenseal, guar gum
NURSING CONSIDERATIONS
Assess:
• Obtain baseline in APTT before treatment; do not start treatment if APTT ratio ≥2.5, then APTT 4 hr after initiation of treatment and at least qd thereafter, if APTT above target, stop inf for 2 hr, then restart at 50%, take APTT in 4 hr; if below target, increase inf rate by 20%, take APTT in 4 hr, do not exceed inf rate of 0.21 mg/kg/hr without checking for coagulation abnormalities
• APTT, which should be 1.5-2.5 × control
Bleeding gums, petechiae, ecchymosis, black tarry stools, hematuria/epistaxis, B/P, vaginal bleeding and possible hemorrhage
• Fever, skin rash, urticaria
Administer:
• Avoiding all IM inj that may cause bleeding
• After reconstitution and further dilution under sterile conditions; use water for inj or 0.9% NaCl; for further dilution 0.9% NaCl or D_5; for rapid and complete reconstitution, inject 1 ml of diluent into vial and shake gently, use immediately, warm to room temp before use
IV BOL route
• Use sol with conc. of 5 mg/ml, reconstitute 5 mg (1 vial)/1 ml of water for inj or 0.9% NaCl, use body wt for correct calculation as to wt
IV INF route
• Use sol with a conc. of 0.2 or 0.4 mg/ml; reconstitute 100 mg (2 vials) with 1 ml each (2 ml) water for inj or 0.9% NaCl, transfer to inf bag with either 500 or 250 ml of 0.9% NaCl or D_5
Evaluate:
• Therapeutic response
Teach patient/family:
• To use soft-bristle toothbrush to avoid bleeding gums, avoid contact sports, use electric razor, avoid IM inj
• To report any signs of bleeding: gums, under skin, urine, stools

L

letrozole (℞)

(let'tro-zohl)

Femara

Func. class.: Antineoplastic, nonsteroidal aromatase inhibitor

Action: Binds to the heme group of aromatase. Inhibits conversion of androgens to estrogens to reduce plasma estrogen levels. 30% of breast cancers decrease in size when deprived of estrogen

Uses: Metastatic breast cancer in postmenopausal women

Dosage and routes:

- *Adult:* **PO** 2.5 mg qd

Available forms: Tabs 2.5 mg

Side effects/adverse reactions:

RESP: Dyspnea, cough

GI: Nausea, vomiting, anorexia, ***hepatotoxicity,*** constipation, heartburn, diarrhea

INTEG: Rash, pruritus, alopecia, sweating, hot flashes

CV: Hypertension

CNS: Headache, lethargy, somnolence, dizziness, depression, anxiety

Contraindications: Hypersensitivity, pregnancy (D)

Precautions: Hepatic disease, respiratory disease

Pharmacokinetics: Metabolized in liver, excreted in urine

Interactions: Unknown

NURSING CONSIDERATIONS

Assess:

- Monitor temp q4h; may indicate beginning infection
- Hepatic studies before, during therapy (bilirubin, AST, ALT, LDH) as needed or monthly
- Jaundiced skin, sclera, dark urine, clay-colored stools, itchy skin, abdominal pain, fever, diarrhea

Perform/provide:

- Liquid diet, including cola, Jell-O; dry toast or crackers as ordered may be added if patient is not nauseated or vomiting
- Nutritious diet with iron and vitamin supplements as ordered

Evaluate:

- Therapeutic response: decrease in size of tumor

Teach patient/family:

- To report any complaints, side effects to nurse or prescriber
- That drowsiness may occur and to avoid driving or operating heavy machinery
- May take without regard to meals

leucovorin (℞)

(loo-koe-vor'in)

citrovorum factor, folinic acid, leucovorin calcium, Wellcovorin

Func. class.: Vitamin, folic acid/methotrexate antagonist antidote

Chem. class.: Tetrahydrofolic acid derivative

Action: Needed for normal growth patterns; prevents toxicity during antineoplastic therapy by protecting normal cells

Uses: Megaloblastic or macrocytic anemia caused by folic acid deficiency, overdose of folic acid antagonist, methotrexate toxicity, toxicity caused by pyrimethamine or trimethoprim, pneumocystosis, toxoplasmosis

Dosage and routes:

Megaloblastic anemia caused by enzyme deficiency

- *Adult and child:* **PO/IV/IM** up to 6 mg/day

Megaloblastic anemia caused by deficiency of folate

- *Adult and child:* **IM** 1 mg or less qd until adequate response

Methotrexate toxicity

- *Adult and child:* **PO/IM/IV** normal elimination given 6 hr after dose of methotrexate (10 mg/m^2) until methotrexate is <10^{-8} M; CCr is >50% above prior level or methotrexate level is 5 × 10 at 24 hr, or at 48 hr level is >9 × 10 M, give leucovorin 100 mg/m^2 q3h until level drops to <10 M

Pyrimethamine toxicity

• *Adult and child:* **PO/IM** 5-15 mg qd

Trimethoprim toxicity

• *Adult and child:* **PO/IM** 400 mg qd

Advanced colorectal cancer

• *Adult:* **IV** 200 mg/m^2, then 5-FU 370 mg/m^2; or leucovorin 20 mg/m^2, then 5-FU 425 mg/m^2; give qd × 5 days q4-5wk

Available forms: Tabs 5, 10, 15, 25 mg; inj 3, 5 mg/ml; powder for inj 10 mg/ml

Side effects/adverse reactions:

RESP: Wheezing

INTEG: Rash, pruritus, erythema, urticaria

HEMA: Thrombocytosis (intraarterial)

Contraindications: Hypersensitivity, anemias other than megaloblastic not associated with vit B_{12} deficiency

Precautions: Pregnancy (C)

Do not confuse:

leucovorin/Leukeran

leucovorin/leukine

Interactions:

• ↓ folate levels: chloramphenicol

• ↑ metabolism of phenobarbital, hydantoins

NURSING CONSIDERATIONS

Assess:

• CCr, creatinine before leucovorin rescue and qd to detect nephrotoxicity; methotrexate level

• I&O; watch for nausea and vomiting

• Other drugs taken: alcohol, hydantoins, trimethoprim may cause increased folic acid use by body

Administer:

• Within 1 hr of folic acid antagonist

IM route

• No reconstitution needed

• Treatment of megaloblastic anemia uses IM dosing

IV route

For IV reconstitute 50 mg/5 ml bacteriostatic or sterile H_2O for inj (10 mg/ml) or (100 mg/10 ml); use immediately if sterile H_2O is used

Give by direct IV over 160 mg/min or less (16 ml of 10 mg/ml sol/min)

Give by intermittent inf after diluting in 100-500 ml of 0.9% NaCl, D_5W, $D_{10}W$, LR, Ringer's sol

Additive compatibilities: Cisplatin, cisplatin/floxuridine, floxuridine

Syringe compatibilities: Bleomycin, cisplatin, cyclophosphamide, DOXOrubicin, fluorouracil, furosemide, heparin, methotrexate, metoclopramide, mitomycin, vinBLAStine, vinCRIStine

Y-site compatibilities: Amifostine, aztreonam, bleomycin, cefepime, cisplatin, cladribine, cyclophosphamide, DOXOrubicin, DOXOrubicin liposome, filgrastim, fluconazole, fluorouracil, furosemide, granisetron, heparin, methotrexate, metoclopramide, mitomycin, piperacillin/tazobactam, tacrolimus, teniposide, thiotepa, vinBLAStine, vinCRIStine

Perform/provide:

• Increase fluid intake if used to treat folic acid inhibitor overdose

• Protection from light and heat

Evaluate:

• Therapeutic response: increased weight; improved orientation, well-being; absence of fatigue; reversal of toxicity (methotrexate, folic acid antagonist overdose)

Teach patient/family:

• For leucovorin rescue have patient drink 3 L fluid qd of rescue
• For folic acid deficiency eat folic acid rich foods: bran, yeast, dried beans, nuts, fresh, green leafy vegetables
• To take drug exactly as prescribed
• To notify prescriber of side effects
• To report signs of hyposensitivity reaction immediately

leuprolide (℞)

(loo-proe'lide)
Leupron Depo PED, Lupron, Lupron Depot, Lupron Depot-3 month, Viadur

Func. class.: Antineoplastic hormone

Chem. class.: Gonadotropin-releasing hormone

Action: Causes initial increase in circulating levels of LH, FSH; continuous administration results in decreased LH, FSH; in men, testosterone is reduced to castrate levels; in premenopausal women, estrogen is reduced to menopausal levels

Uses: Metastatic prostate cancer, management of endometriosis, central precocious puberty

Dosage and routes:

Prostate cancer

• *Adult:* **SC** 1 mg/day; **IM:** 7.5 mg/dose qmo; Viadur implant (72 mg) qyr; or **IM** 22.5 mg q3mo; or **IM** 30 mg q4mo

Endometriosis/fibroids

• *Adult:* **IM** 3.75 mg qmo or 11.25 q3mo or 30 mg q4mo

Central precocious puberty

• *Child:* **SC** 50 mcg/kg/day; may increase by 10 mcg/kg/day as needed
• *Child >37.5 kg:* **IM** 15 mg q4wk
• *Child 25-37.5 kg:* **IM** 11.25 mg q4wk
• *Child ≤25 kg:* 7.5 mg q4wk

Available forms: Inj (depot) 3.75 mg, 7.5 mg single dose, multiple-dose vials (5 mg/ml), single-use kit 11.25 mg vial, pediatric depot 7.5, 11.25, 15 mg; 3 mo depot 22.5 mg single use; Viadur once a yr implant

Side effects/adverse reactions:

GU: Edema, hot flashes, impotence, decreased libido, amenorrhea, vaginal dryness, gynecomastia

CV: ***MI, pulmonary emboli, dysrhythmias***

GI: Anorexia, diarrhea, ***GI bleeding***

Contraindications: Hypersensitivity to GnRH or analogs, thromboembolic disorders, pregnancy (X), lactation, undiagnosed vaginal bleeding

Precautions: Edema, hepatic disease, CVA, MI, seizures, hypertension, diabetes mellitus

Do not confuse:

Lupron/Nuprin
Lupron/Lopurin

Pharmacokinetics:

SC: Onset 1-2 wk, peak 2-4 wk; absorbed rapidly (SC), slowly (IM depot); half-life 3 hr

Interactions:

• ↑ antineoplastic action: flutamide megestrol

NURSING CONSIDERATIONS

Assess:

• For symptoms of endometriosis (lower abdominal pain)/fibroids (pelvic pain, excessive vaginal bleeding, bloating) before, during, and after treatment
• For central precocious puberty (CPP) if treatment is for this condition; secondary S_4 characteristics to child <9 yr, estradiol/testosterone levels, GnRH test, tomography of head, adrenal steroids, chorionic gonadotropin, wrist x-ray, height, weight

• Hepatic studies before, during therapy (bilirubin, AST, ALT, LDH) as needed or monthly, PSA in prostate cancer
• Pituitary gonadotropic and gonadal function during therapy and 4-8 wk after therapy is decreased
• Worsening of signs and symptoms; normal during beginning therapy
• Fatigue, increased pulse, pallor, lethargy; edema in feet, joints; stomach pain
◆ Symptoms indicating severe allergic reaction: rash, pruritus, urticaria, purpuric skin lesions, itching, flushing

Administer:
• IM/SC using syringe and drug packaged together, give deep in large muscle mass, rotate sites
• Use depot IM only
• Monthly: reconstitute single-use vial with 1 ml of diluent, if multiple vials used, withdraw 0.5 ml and inject into each vial (1 ml), withdraw all and inject
• 3-month: reconstitute microspheres using 1.5 ml of diluent, and inject in vial, shake, withdraw, and inject
• 12-month: insert into upper arm; at the end of 12 months, implant must be removed

Perform/provide:
• Nutritious diet with iron, vitamin supplements as ordered
• Storage in tight container at room temperature

Evaluate:
• Therapeutic response: decreased tumor size and spread of malignancy, decrease in lesions, pain in endometriosis, fibroids, correction of CCP

Teach patient/family:
• To notify prescriber if menstruation continues; menstruation should stop
• To use a nonhormonal method of contraception during therapy
• That bone pain will disappear after 1 wk
• To report any complaints, side effects to nurse or prescriber; hot flashes may occur; record weight, report gain of >2 lb/day
• How to prepare, give; to rotate sites for SC inj
• To keep accurate records of dose
• That tumor flare may occur: increase in size of tumor, increased bone pain, will subside rapidly; may take analgesics for pain; premenopausal women must use mechanical birth control; ovulation may be induced
• Do not breastfeed while taking this drug
• Voiding problems may increase in beginning of therapy, but will decrease in several weeks

levalbuterol (℞)

(lev-al-byoo'ter-ole)
Xopenex
Func. class.: Bronchodilator, adrenergic β_2-agonist

Action: Causes bronchodilation by action on β_2 (pulmonary) receptors by increasing levels of cAMP, which relaxes smooth muscle; produces bronchodilation, CNS, cardiac stimulation, as well as increased diuresis and gastric acid secretion; longer acting than isoproterenol

Uses: Treatment or prevention of bronchospasm (reversible obstructive airway disease)

Dosage and routes:
• *Adult and child ≥12 yr:* **INH** 0.63 mg tid, q6-8h by nebulization, may increase 1.25 mg q8h
• *Child 6-11 yr:* **INH** 0.31 mg tid via neb, max 0.63 mg tid

Available forms: Sol, inh 0.63 mg, 1.25 mg/3 ml

Side effects/adverse reactions:

CNS: Tremors, anxiety, insomnia, headache, dizziness, stimulation, *restlessness,* hallucinations, flushing, irritability

EENT: Dry nose, irritation of nose and throat

CV: Palpitations, tachycardia, hypertension, angina, hypotension, dysrhythmias

GI: Heartburn, nausea, vomiting

MS: Muscle cramps

Contraindications: Hypersensitivity to sympathomimetics, tachydysrhythmias, severe cardiac disease

Precautions: Lactation, pregnancy (C), cardiac disorders, hyperthyroidism, diabetes mellitus, hypertension, prostatic hypertrophy, narrow-angle glaucoma, seizures

Pharmacokinetics: Metabolized in the liver and tissues, crosses placenta, breast milk, blood-brain barrier

INH: Onset 5-15 min, peak 1-1½ hr, duration 6-8 hr

Interactions:

• ↑ action of aerosol bronchodilators

• ↑ levalbuterol action: tricyclics, MAOIs, other adrenergics

• ↓ levalbuterol action: other β-blockers

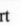

↑ stimulation: black/green tea, coffee, cola nut, guarana, yerba maté

NURSING CONSIDERATIONS

Assess:

• Respiratory function: vital capacity, forced expiratory volume, ABGs, lung sounds, heart rate and rhythm (baseline); character of sputum: color, consistency, amount

• That patient has not received theophylline therapy before giving dose

• For evidence of allergic reactions, paradoxical bronchospasm

Administer:

• By nebulization q6-8h; wait at least 1 min between inhalation of aerosols

Evaluate:

• Therapeutic response: absence of dyspnea, wheezing after 1 hr, improved airway exchange, improved ABGs

Teach patient/family:

• Not to use OTC medications; excess stimulation may occur

• To avoid getting aerosol in eyes; blurring may result

• To wash inhaler in warm water qd and dry

• To avoid smoking, smoke-filled rooms, persons with respiratory infections

That paradoxic bronchospasm may occur and to stop drug immediately, contact prescriber

• To limit caffeine products such as chocolate, coffee, tea, and colas or herbs such as cola nut, guarana, yerba maté

Treatment of overdose: Administer a β_1-adrenergic blocker

levetiracetam (℞)

(lev-eh-teer-ass'eh-tam)

Keppra

Func. class.: Anticonvulsant

Action: Unknown, may inhibit nerve impulses by limiting influx of sodium ions across cell membrane in motor cortex

Uses: Adjunctive therapy in partial onset seizures

Dosage and routes:

• *Adult:* **PO** 500 mg bid, may increase by 1000 mg/day q2wk max 3000 mg/day

Available forms: Tabs 250, 500, 750 mg

Side effects/adverse reactions:
HEMA: Lowered Hct, Hgb, RBC, infection
CNS: Dizziness, somnolence, asthenia
MISC: Infection, abdominal pain, pharyngitis
Contraindications: Hypersensitivity
Precautions: Renal disease, cardiac disease, psychosis, pregnancy (C), lactation, children
Pharmacokinetics: Rapidly absorbed, not protein bound, excreted via kidneys 66% unchanged; half-life 6-8 hr, longer in elderly

NURSING CONSIDERATIONS
Assess:
- Renal studies: urinalysis, BUN, urine creatinine q3mo
- Blood studies: RBC, Hct, Hgb
- Description of seizures
- Mental status: mood, sensorium, affect, behavioral changes; if mental status changes, notify prescriber

Administer:
- With food, milk to decrease GI symptoms (rare)

Perform/provide:
- Storage at room temperature
- Assistance with ambulation during early part of treatment; dizziness occurs

Evaluate:
- Therapeutic response: decreased seizure activity, document on patient's chart

Teach patient/family:
- To carry emergency ID stating patient's name, drugs taken, condition, prescriber's name, phone number
- To avoid driving, other activities that require alertness
- Not to discontinue medication quickly after long-term use

levobetaxolol ophthalmic
See appendix c

levobunolol ophthalmic
See appendix c

RARELY USED

levobupivacaine (℞)
(lee-voh-bu-piv′ah-kane)
Chirocaine
Func. class.: Local anesthetic

Uses: Local, regional anesthesia, surgical anesthesia, pain management, continuous epidural analgesia
Dosage and routes:
- Varies with route of anesthesia

Contraindications: Hypersensitivity, children <12 yr, elderly, severe hepatic disease

levocabastine ophthalmic
See appendix c

levodopa (℞)
(lee′voe-doe-pa)
Dopar, Larodopa, L-Dopa
Func. class.: Antiparkinson agent
Chem. class.: Dopamine agonist

Action: Decarboxylation to DOPamine, which increases DOPamine levels in brain
Uses: Parkinsonism
Research note: Levodopa may be

the cause of sleep attacks (daytime) in patients[19]

Dosage and routes:

• *Adult:* **PO** 0.5-1 g qd divided bid-qid with meals; may increase by up to 0.75 g q3-7d not to exceed 8 g/day unless closely supervised

Available forms: Caps 100, 250, 500 mg; tabs 100, 250, 500 mg

Side effects/adverse reactions:

HEMA: ***Hemolytic anemia, leukopenia, agranulocytosis***

CNS: Involuntary choreiform movements, hand tremors, fatigue, headache, anxiety, twitching, numbness, weakness, confusion, agitation, insomnia, nightmares, psychosis, hallucination, hypomania, severe depression, dizziness

GI: Nausea, vomiting, anorexia, abdominal distress, dry mouth, flatulence, dysphagia, bitter taste, diarrhea, constipation

INTEG: Rash, sweating, alopecia

CV: Orthostatic hypotension, tachycardia, hypertension, palpitation

EENT: Blurred vision, diplopia, dilated pupils

MISC: Urinary retention, incontinence, weight change, dark urine

Contraindications: Hypersensitivity, narrow-angle glaucoma, undiagnosed skin lesions

Precautions: Renal disease, cardiac disease, hepatic disease, respiratory disease, MI with dysrhythmias, convulsions, peptic ulcer, pregnancy (C), asthma, endocrine disease, affective disorders, psychosis, lactation, children <12 yr, peptic ulcer

Do not confuse:

L-dopa (levodopa)/methyldopa

Pharmacokinetics:

PO: Peak 1-3 hr, excreted in urine (metabolites)

Interactions:

Hypertensive crisis: MAOIs

• ↓ levodopa effects: anticholinergics, hydantoins, papaverine, pyridoxine

• ↑ levodopa effects: antacids

• Drug/food: ↓ levodopa absorption: high-protein foods

• ↑ pyridoxine will ↓ levodopa effect

↓ levodopa action, ↑ EPS: Indian snakeroot

↑ parkinsonian symptoms: kava

Lab test interferences:

False positive: Urine ketones, urine glucose, Coombs' test

False negative: Urine glucose (glucose oxidase)

False increase: Uric acid, urine protein

Decrease: VMA

NURSING CONSIDERATIONS

Assess:

• Renal, hepatic studies: AST, ALT, alk phosphatase, LDH, bilirubin, CBC, BUN, protein-bound iodine

• Involuntary movements in parkinsonism: akinesia, tremors, staggering gait, muscle rigidity, drooling

Levodopa toxicity: mental, personality changes, increased twitching, grimacing, tongue protrusion

• B/P, respiration during initial treatment; hypo/hypertension should be reported

• Mental status: affect, mood, behavioral changes, depression; complete suicide assessment

Administer:

• Drug until NPO before surgery

• Adjust dosage to patient response

• With meals; limit protein taken with drug

• Only after MAOIs have been discontinued for 2 wk

Perform/provide:

• Assistance with ambulation during beginning therapy

• Testing for diabetes mellitus, acromegaly if on long-term therapy

Evaluate:
- Therapeutic response: decrease in akathisia, increased mood

Teach patient/family:
- That therapeutic effects may take several wk to a few mo
- To change positions slowly to prevent orthostatic hypotension
- To report side effects: twitching, eye spasms; indicate overdose
- To use drug exactly as prescribed; if drug is discontinued abruptly, parkinsonian crisis may occur
- That urine, sweat may darken
- To avoid vit B_6 preparations, vitamin-fortified foods containing B_6; these foods can reverse effects of levodopa

levofloxacin (℞)

(lee-voh-floks'a-sin)
Levaquin
Func. class.: Antiinfective
Chem. class.: Fluoroquinolone

See Ophthalmic Appendix for Ophthalmic Product

Action: Interferes with conversion of intermediate DNA fragments into high-molecular-weight DNA in bacteria; DNA gyrase inhibitor

Uses: Acute sinusitis, acute chronic bronchitis, community-acquired pneumonia, uncomplicated skin infections, complicated UTI, acute pyelonephritis caused by *Streptococcus pneumoniae, Haemophilus influenzae, Haemophilis parainfluenzae, Moraxella catarrhalis*

Dosage and routes:
- *Adult:* **IV INF** 500 mg by slow inf over 1 hr q24h × 7-14 days depending on infection; **PO:** 500 mg q24h × 7-14 days depending on infection

Renal disease
- *Adult:* **PO/IV** CCr 20-49 ml/min initial 500 mg, then 250 mg, q24h; CCr 10-19 ml/min 250 or 500 mg, depending on condition; then 250 mg q48h

Available forms: Single-use vials (500 mg); 25 mg/ml 20 ml vials; premixed flexible containers; tabs 250, 500, 750 mg

Side effects/adverse reactions:
MISC: Hypoglycemia, hypersensitivity
CNS: Headache, dizziness, *insomnia,* anxiety, ***seizures,*** encephalopathy, paresthesia
CV: Chest pain, palpitations, vasodilation
EENT: Dry mouth
HEMA: Eosinophilia, ***hemolytic anemia,*** lymphopenia
RESP: Pneumonitis
GI: Nausea, flatulence, *vomiting,* diarrhea, abdominal pain, ***pseudomembranous colitis***
SYST: ***Anaphylaxis, multisystem organ failure, Stevens-Johnson syndrome***
GU: Vaginitis, crystalluria
INTEG: Rash, pruritus, *photosensitivity*

Contraindications: Hypersensitivity to quinolones, photosensitivity

Precautions: Pregnancy (C), lactation, children

Pharmacokinetics: Metabolized in liver, excreted in urine unchanged, half-life 6-8 hr

Interactions:
- Nephrotoxicity: cycloSPORINE
- ↓ levofloxacin absorption: antacids containing aluminum, magnesium; sucralfate, zinc, iron, calcium
- Altered blood glucose levels: antidiabetic agents
- ↑ CNS stimulation, seizures: NSAIDs, foscarnet
- ↓ clearance of: theophylline, toxicity may result

• ↑ bleeding risk: warfarin
• Do not use with magnesium in the same IV line
• ↑ toxicity/levels of digoxin, cimetidine
↑ antiinfective effect: cola tree

Lab test interferences:
Decrease: Glucose, lymphocytes

NURSING CONSIDERATIONS

Assess:
• For previous sensitivity reaction
• For signs and symptoms of infection: characteristics of sputum, WBC >10,000/mm^3, fever; obtain baseline information before and during treatment
• C&S before beginning drug therapy to identify if correct treatment has been initiated
For allergic reactions and anaphylaxis: rash, urticaria, pruritus, chills, fever, joint pain; may occur a few days after therapy begins; epINEPHrine and resuscitation equipment should be available for anaphylactic reaction
• Bowel pattern qd; if severe diarrhea occurs, drug should be discontinued
For overgrowth of infection: perineal itching, fever, malaise, redness, pain, swelling, drainage, rash, diarrhea, change in cough, sputum

Administer:
• PO 4 hr before or 2 hr after antacids, iron, calcium, zinc

IV route
• Only by slow IV infusion over 1 hr
• Discard any unused sol in the single-dose vial
• Using premix, tear outer wrap at notch and remove sol container, check for leaks, close control clamps; remove cover from port at bottom of container, insert pin into port with a twist; suspend container from hanger, squeeze and release drip chamber to proper fluid level, open flow control to expel air, close clamp; regulate rate with flow control clamps

Solution compatibilities: 0.9% NaCl, D_5W, D_5/0.9% NaCl, D_5LR, D_5/0.45% NaCl, sodium lactate

Evaluate:
• Therapeutic response: absence of signs/symptoms of infection (WBC <10,000/mm^3, temp WNL)

Teach patient/family:
• To contact prescriber if vaginal itching, loose, foul-smelling stools, furry tongue occur (may indicate superinfection); report itching, rash, pruritus, urticaria
• To notify prescriber of diarrhea with blood or pus
• To take 4 hr before or 2 hr after antacids, iron, calcium, zinc products
• To complete full course of therapy; to increase fluid intake to 2 L/day to prevent crystalluria
• To avoid hazardous activities until response is known
• To use frequent rinsing of mouth, sugarless candy or gum for dry mouth
• To avoid other medication unless approved by prescriber
• Not to use theophylline with this product, toxicity may result; contact prescriber if taking theophylline
• To prevent sun exposure or use sunscreen to prevent phototoxicity

levofloxacin ophthalmic

See appendix c

levonorgestrel implant (℞)

(lee-voe-nor-jess'trel)

Norplant, Mirena

Func. class.: Contraceptive system

Chem. class.: Synthetic progestin

Action: As a progestin, transforms proliferative endometrium into secretory endometrium; inhibits secretion of pituitary gonadotropins, which prevents follicular maturation and ovulation

Uses: Prevention of pregnancy for 5 yr

Dosage and routes:

• *Adult:* 6 caps subdermally implanted in the upper arm during first 7 days after onset of menses, replace q5yr

Available forms: Kit of 6 caps, 36 mg/cap

Side effects/adverse reactions:

CV: ***Cerebral hemorrhage, coronary thrombosis, pulmonary embolism, cerebral thrombosis***

CNS: Dizziness, headache, nervousness

GU: Amenorrhea, cervical erosion, breakthrough bleeding, dysmenorrhea, vaginal candidiasis, breast changes, vaginitis

GI: Nausea, abdominal discomfort

INTEG: Alopecia, dermatitis, hirsutism, acne, hypertrichosis, infection at site, pain/itching at site

OTHER: Change in appetite, weight gain

Contraindications: Hypersensitivity, pregnancy (X), thrombophlebitis, undiagnosed genital bleeding, liver tumors, breast carcinoma, liver disease

Precautions: Depression, psychosis, lactation, fluid retention, contact lens wearers

Pharmacokinetics: Onset 1 mo, peak 1 mo, duration 5 yr

Interactions:

• ↓ contraception: phenytoin, carbamazepine, penicillins, chloramphenicol, dihydroergotamine, mineral oil, corticosteroids, phenylbutazone, primadone, protease inhibitors, antiretrovirals, tetracyclines

↓ contraception: St. John's wort

• Possible toxicity: β-blockers, benzodiazepines, cycloSPORINE, corticosteroids, tricyclics, theophylline

NURSING CONSIDERATIONS

Assess:

• Blood studies: cholesterol, triglycerides; may be increased or decreased; sex hormone—binding globulin, thyroxine, T_3 uptake, LDL, HDL

• Menstrual irregularities: spotting, prolonged bleeding, amenorrhea; usually diminish

• For jaundice, thrombophlebitis; implants should be removed, hepatic studies

• For acne, dermatitis, hirsutism, alopecia

Administer:

• 8 cm (3 in) above the crease of the elbow; implantation should be during first 7 days after onset of menses; implantation should be fanlike, 15 degrees apart

Evaluate:

• Therapeutic response: absence of pregnancy

Teach patient/family:

• To notify prescriber if pregnancy is suspected

• To use sunscreen or stay out of the sun

• That this product only prevents pregnancy, does not protect against HIV or other STDs

L

• That if vision problems occur, an ophthalmologist should be seen
• That physical examinations are necessary
◆ To report fluid retention: weight gain, edema; hepatic symptoms: yellowing skin or eyes, clay-colored stools, dark urine; thrombosis: blurred vision, headache, tenderness in extremities

levothyroxine (T_4) (℞)

(lee-voe-thye-rox'een)
Eltroxin✱, Levo-T, Levothroid, levothyroxine sodium, Levoxyl, PMS-Levothyroxine Sodium✱, Synthroid, T_4
Func. class.: Thyroid hormone
Chem. class.: Levoisomer of thyroxine

Action: Increases metabolic rate, controls protein synthesis, increases cardiac output, renal blood flow, O_2 consumption, body temp, blood volume, growth, development at cellular level, exact mechanism unknown
Uses: Hypothyroidism, myxedema coma, thyroid hormone replacement, congenital hypothyroidism, thyrotoxicosis, congenital hypothyroidism, some types of thyroid cancer
Dosage and routes:
Severe hypothyroidism
• *Adult:* **PO** 50 mcg qd, increased by 50-100 mcg q1-4 wk until desired response, maintenance dose 75-125 mcg qd; **IM/IV** 50-100 mcg/day as a single dose or 50% of usual oral dosage
• *Child >12 yr:* **PO** 2-3 mcg/kg/day as a single dose AM
• *Child 6-12 yr:* **PO** 4-5 mcg/kg/day as a single dose AM
• *Child 1-5 yr:* **PO** 5-6 mcg/kg/day as a single dose AM
• *Child 6-12 mo:* **PO** 6-8 mcg/kg/day as a single dose AM
• *Child to 6 mo:* **PO** 8-10 mcg/kg/day as a single dose AM
Myxedema coma
• *Adult:* **IV** 200-500 mcg, may increase by 100-300 mcg after 24 hr; place on oral medication as soon as possible
Available forms: Powder for inj 50, 200, 500 mcg/vial; tabs 0.025, 0.05, 0.075, 0.088, 0.1, 0.112, 0.125, 0.137, 0.15, 0.175, 0.2, 0.3 mg
Side effects/adverse reactions:
CNS: Anxiety, insomnia, tremors, headache, ***thyroid storm***
CV: Tachycardia, palpitations, angina, dysrhythmias, hypertension, ***cardiac arrest***
GI: Nausea, diarrhea, increased or decreased appetite, cramps
MISC: Menstrual irregularities, weight loss, sweating, heat intolerance, fever, alopecia
Contraindications: Adrenal insufficiency, recent MI, thyrotoxicosis, hypersensitivity to beef, alcohol intolerance (inj only)
Precautions: Elderly, angina pectoris, hypertension, ischemia, cardiac disease, pregnancy (A), lactation, diabetes
Do not confuse:
Synthroid/Symmetrel
Pharmacokinetics:
PO: Onset 3-5 days, peak 1-3 wk, duration 1-3 wk
IV: Onset 6-8 hr, peak 24 hr, duration unknown
Half-life 6-7 days; distributed throughout body tissues
Interactions:
• ↑ cardiac insufficiency risk: epINEPHrine products
• ↓ levothyroxine absorption: cholestyramine, colestipol, ferrous sulfate

• ↑ effects of anticoagulants, sympathomimetics, tricyclics
• ↓ effects of digitalis drugs, insulin, hypoglycemics
• ↓ levothyroxine effects: estrogens
↓ thyroid hormone effect: agar, bugleweed carnitine, kelpware, soy, spirulina

Lab test interferences:
Increase: CPK, LDH, AST, PBI, blood glucose
Decrease: Thyroid function tests

NURSING CONSIDERATIONS

Assess:
• B/P, pulse periodically during treatment
• Weight qd in same clothing, using same scale, at same time of day
• Height, growth rate of a child
• T_3, T_4, FTIs, which are decreased; radioimmunoassay of TSH, which is increased; radio uptake, which is increased if patient is on too low a dose of medication
• PT may require decreased anticoagulant; check for bleeding, bruising
• Increased nervousness, excitability, irritability, which may indicate too high dose of medication, usually after 1-3 wk of treatment
• Cardiac status: angina, palpitation, chest pain, change in VS

Administer:
• IV after diluting with provided diluent 0.5 mg/5 ml; shake; give through Y-tube or 3-way stopcock; give 0.1 mg or less over 1 min; do not add to IV inf; 0.1 mg = 1 ml
• Considered to be incompatible in syringe with all other drugs
• In AM if possible as a single dose to decrease sleeplessness
• At same time each day to maintain drug level
• Only for hormone imbalances; not to be used for obesity, male infertility, menstrual conditions, lethargy
• Lowest dose that relieves symptoms; lower dose to the elderly and in cardiac diseases
• Crushed and mixed with water, nonsoy formula, or breast milk for infants/children

Perform/provide:
• Storage in tight, light-resistant container; sol should be discarded if not used immediately
• Withdrawal of medication 4 wk before RAIU test

Evaluate:
• Therapeutic response: absence of depression; increased weight loss, diuresis, pulse, appetite; absence of constipation, peripheral edema, cold intolerance; pale, cool, dry skin; brittle nails, alopecia, coarse hair, menorrhagia, night blindness, paresthesias, syncope, stupor, coma, rosy cheeks

Teach patient/family:
• That hair loss will occur in child, is temporary
• To report excitability, irritability, anxiety, which indicate overdose
• Not to switch brands unless approved by prescriber
• That drug may be discontinued after giving birth, thyroid panel evaluated after 1-2 mo
• That hypothyroid child will show almost immediate behavior/personality change
• That drug is not to be taken to reduce weight
• To avoid OTC preparations with iodine; read labels
• To avoid iodine food, iodized salt, soybeans, tofu, turnips, high-iodine seafood, some bread
• That drug is not a cure but controls symptoms and treatment is lifelong

L

HIGH ALERT

lidocaine (parenteral) (℞)

(lye'doe-kane)

LidoPen Auto-Injector, Xylocaine, Xylocard✱

Func. class.: Antidysrhythmic (Class Ib)

Chem. class.: Aminoacyl amide

Action: Increases electrical stimulation threshold of ventricle, His-Purkinje system, which stabilizes cardiac membrane, decreases automaticity

Uses: Ventricular tachycardia, ventricular dysrhythmias during cardiac surgery, myocardial infarction, digitalis toxicity, cardiac catheterization

Dosage and routes:

- *Adult:* **IV BOL** 50-100 mg (1 mg/kg) over 2-3 min, repeat q3-5min, not to exceed 300 mg in 1 hr; begin **IV INF; IV INF** 20-50 mcg/kg/min; **IM** 200-300 mg (4.3 mg/kg) in deltoid muscle, may repeat in 1-1½ hr if needed
- *Elderly, CHF, reduced hapatic function:* **IV BOL** give ½ adult dose
- *Child:* **IV BOL** 1 mg/kg, then **IV INF** 30 mcg/kg/min

Available forms: IV INF 0.2% (2 mg/ml), 0.4% (4 mg/ml), 0.8% (8 mg/ml); IV ad 4% (40 mg/ml), 10% (100 mg/ml), 20% (200 mg/ml); IV dir 1% (10 mg/ml), 2% (20 mg/ml); IM 10% 300 mg/ml

Side effects/adverse reactions:

CNS: Headache, dizziness, involuntary movement, confusion, tremor, drowsiness, euphoria, ***convulsions***

EENT: Tinnitus, blurred vision

GI: Nausea, vomiting, anorexia

CV: Hypotension, bradycardia, ***heart block, cardiovascular collapse, arrest***

RESP: Dyspnea, ***respiratory depression***

INTEG: Rash, urticaria, edema, swelling

MISC: Febrile response, phlebitis at injection site

Contraindications: Hypersensitivity to amides, severe heart block, supraventricular dysrhythmias, Adams-Stokes syndrome, Wolff-Parkinson-White syndrome

Precautions: Pregnancy (B), lactation, children, renal disease, hepatic disease, CHF, respiratory depression, malignant hyperthermia

Pharmacokinetics:

IV: Onset 2 min, duration 20 min

IM: Onset 5-15 min, duration 1½ hr; half-life 8 min, 1-2 hr (terminal); metabolized in liver; excreted in urine; crosses placenta

Interactions:

- ↑ neuromuscular blockade: neuromuscular blockers, tubocurarine
- ↑ lidocaine effects: cimetidine, phenytoin, propranolol, metoprolol
- ↓ lidocaine effects: barbiturates

↑ lidocaine action: aloe, buckthorn, cascara sagrada, senna

↑ toxicity, death: aconite

↑ effect: aloe, broom, chronic buckthorn use, cascara sagrada (chronic use), Chinese rhubarb, figwort, fumitory, goldenseal, kudzu, licorice

↓ effect: coltsfoot

↑ serotonin effect: horehound

Lab test interferences:

Increase: CPK

NURSING CONSIDERATIONS

Assess:

ECG continuously to determine increased PR or QRS segments; if these develop, discontinue or reduce rate; watch for increased ventricular ectopic beats; may have to rebolus, B/P

• IV infusion rate using infusion pump; run at less than 4 mg/min
• Blood levels (therapeutic level: 1.5-5 mcg/ml)
• I&O ratio, electrolytes (K, Na, Cl)
Malignant hyperthermia: tachypnea, tachycardia, changes in B/P, increased temp
• Respiratory status: rate, rhythm, lung fields for rales, watch for respiratory depression; lung fields, bilateral rales may occur in CHF patient; increased respiration, increased pulse; drug should be discontinued
• CNS effects: dizziness, confusion, psychosis, paresthesias, convulsions; drug should be discontinued

Administer:
• IM inj in deltoid; aspirate to avoid intravascular administration; check site daily for infiltration or extravasation

IV route
• Bolus undiluted (1%, 2% only) give 50 mg or less over 1 min or dilute 1 g/250-500 ml of D_5W; titrate to patient response; use infusion pump; pediatric inf is 120 mg of lidocaine/100 ml D_5W; 1-2.5 ml/kg/hr = 20-50 mcg/kg/min; use only 1%, 2% sol for IV bol

Additive compatibilities: Alteplase, aminophylline, amiodarone, atracurium, bretylium, calcium chloride, calcium gluceptate, calcium gluconate, chloramphenicol, chlorothiazide, cimetidine, dexamethasone, digoxin, diphenhydrAMINE, DOBUTamine, DOPamine, epHEDrine, erythromycin lactobionate, floxacillin, flumazenil, furosemide, heparin, hydrocortisone, hydrOXYzine, insulin (regular), mephentermine, metaraminol, nafcillin, nitroglycerin, penicillin G potassium, pentobarbital, phenylephrine, potassium chloride, procainamide, prochlorperazine, promazine, ranitidine, sodium bicarbonate, sodium lactate, theophylline, verapamil, vit B/C

Solution compatibilities: D_5W, D_5/0.9% NaCl, D_5/0.45% NaCl, D_5/LR, LR, 0.9% NaCl, 0.45% NaCl

Syringe compatibilities: Cloxacillin, glycopyrrolate, heparin, hydrOXYzine, methicillin, metoclopramide, milrinone, moxalactam, nalbuphine

Y-site compatibilities: Alteplase, amiodarone, amrinone, cefazolin, ciprofloxacin, cisatracurium, diltiazem, DOBUTamine, DOPamine, enalaprilat, etomidate, famotidine, haloperidol, heparin, heparin/hydrocortisone, labetalol, meperidine, morphine, nitroglycerin, nitroprusside, potassium chloride, propofol, remifentanil, streptokinase, theophylline, vit B/C, warfarin

Evaluate:
• Therapeutic response: decreased dysrhythmias

Teach patient/family:
• The use of automatic lidocaine injection device if ordered for personal use

Treatment of overdose: O_2, artificial ventilation, ECG; administer DOPamine for circulatory depression, diazepam or thiopental for convulsions; decrease drug if needed

lidocaine topical

See appendix c

lindane (℞)

(lin'dane)

GBH♣, G-Well, Hexit♣, Kwell, lindane, PMS-Lindane♣, Scabene

Func. class.: Scabicide, pediculicide

Chem. class.: Chlorinated hydrocarbon (synthetic)

Action: Stimulates nervous system of arthropods, resulting in seizures, death of organism

Uses: Scabies, lice (head/pubic/body), nits

Dosage and routes:

Lice

• *Adult and child:* **CREAM/LOTION** wash area with soap, water; remove visible crusts; apply to skin surfaces; remove with soap, water in 8-12 hr; may reapply in 1 wk if needed; shampoo using 30 ml: work into lather, rub for 5 min, rinse, dry with towel; comb with fine-toothed comb to remove nits

Scabies

• *Adult and child:* **TOP** apply 1% cream/lotion to skin, neck to bottom of feet, toes; repeat in 1 wk prn

Available forms: Lotion, shampoo, cream (1%)

Side effects/adverse reactions:

INTEG: Pruritus, rash, irritation, contact dermatitis

GI: Nausea, vomiting, diarrhea, liver damage (inhalation of vapors)

HEMA: ***Aplastic anemia*** (chronic inhalation of vapors)

CV: ***Ventricular fibrillation*** (chronic inhalation of vapors)

GU: ***Kidney damage*** (chronic inhalation of vapors)

CNS: Tremors, ***seizures, CNS toxicity,*** stimulation, dizziness (chronic inhalation of vapors)

Contraindications: Hypersensitivity; premature neonate; patients with known seizure disorders; inflammation of skin, abrasions, or skin breaks

Precautions: Pregnancy (B); avoid contact with eyes; children <10 yr, infants, lactation

Interactions:

• Oils may ↑ absorption; if an oil-based hair dressing is used, shampoo, rinse, dry hair before applying lindane shampoo

NURSING CONSIDERATIONS

Assess:

• Head, hair for lice and nits before and after treatment; if scabies are present check all skin surfaces

• Identify source of infection: school, family, sexual contacts

Administer:

• To body areas, scalp only; do not apply to face, lips, mouth, eyes, any mucous membrane, anus, or meatus

• Topical corticosteroids as ordered to decrease contact dermatitis

• Antihistamines

• Lotions of menthol or phenol to control itching

• Topical antibiotics for infection

Perform/provide:

• Isolation until areas on skin, scalp have cleared and treatment is completed

• Removal of nits by using a fine-toothed comb rinsed in vinegar after treatment; use gloves

Evaluate:

• Therapeutic response: decreased crusts, nits, brownish trails on skin, itching papules in skin folds, decreased itching after several wk

Teach patient/family:

• To wash all inhabitants' clothing, using insecticide; preventive treatment may be required of all persons living in same house, using lotion or shampoo to decrease spread of infection; use rubber gloves when applying drug

• That itching may continue for 4-6 wk
• That drug must be reapplied if accidently washed off, or treatment will be ineffective
• Not to apply to face; if accidental contact with eyes occurs, flush with water
• Instruct patient to remove after specified time to prevent toxicity
• To treat sexual contacts simultaneously
• To check for CNS toxicity: dizziness, cramps, anxiety, nausea, vomiting, seizures

Treatment of ingestion: Gastric lavage, saline laxatives, IV diazepam (Valium) for convulsions

linezolid (℞)

(line-zoe′lide)

Zyvox

Func. class.: Broad-spectrum antiinfective

Chem. class.: Oxazolidinone

Action: Binds to bacterial 235 ribosomal RNA of the 50S subunit preventing formation of the bacterial translation process

Uses: Vancomycin-resistant *Enterococcus faecium* infections, nosocomial pneumonia, uncomplicated or complicated skin and skin structure infections, community-acquired pneumonia

Research note: One case of myelosuppression occurring with linezolid led researchers to suggest monitoring of hematologic parameters[20]

Dosage and routes:

Vancomycin-resistant* Enterococcus faecium *infections
• *Adult:* **IV/PO** 600 mg q12h × 14-28 days

Nosocomial pneumonia/complicated skin infections/community-acquired pneumonia/concurrent bacterial infection
• *Adult:* **IV/PO** 600 mg q12h × 10-14 days

Uncomplicated skin infections
• *Adult:* **IV/PO** 400 mg q12h × 10-14 days

Available forms: Tab 400, 600 mg; oral sus 100 mg/5 ml; inj 2 mg/ml

Side effects/adverse reactions:

CNS: Headache, dizziness

GI: Nausea, diarrhea, increased ALT, AST, *vomiting,* taste change, tongue color change

MISC: Vaginal moniliasis, fungal infection, oral moniliasis

HEMA: ***Myelosuppression***

Contraindications: Hypersensitivity

Precautions: Pregnancy (C), lactation, children, thrombocytopenia

Do not confuse:

Zyvox/Vioxx

Pharmacokinetics: Rapidly and extensively absorbed, protein binding 31%, metabolized by oxidation of the morpholine ring

Interactions:

• ↓ MAOIs effects
• ↑ effects of adrenergic agents, serotonergic agents

NURSING CONSIDERATIONS

Assess:

• CBC weekly, assess for myelosuppression (anemias, leukopenia, pancytopenia, thrombocytopenia)
• CNS symptoms: headache, dizziness
• Hepatic studies: AST, ALT
• Allergic reactions: fever, flushing, rash, urticaria, pruritus
• For pseudomembranous colitis

Administer:

PO route

• Store reconstituted oral suspension at room temperature, use within 3 wk

IV route

• 30-120 min; do not use IV infusion bag in series connections, do not use with additives in sol, do not use with another drug, administer separately

Y-site compatibilities: acyclovir, alfentanil, amikacin, aminophylline, ampicillin, aztreonam, bretylium, buprenorphine, butorphanol, calcium gluconate, carboplatin, cefazolin, cefoperazone, cefotetan, cefoxitin, ceftazidine, ceftizoxime, ceftriaxone, cefuroxime, cimetidine, ciprofloxacin, cisatracurium, cisplatin, clindamycin, cyclophosphamide, cycloSPORINE, cytarabine, hydromorphone, ifosfamide, labetalol, leucovorin, levofloxacin, lidocaine, lorazepam, magnesium sulfate, mannitol, meperidine, meropenem, mesna, methotrexate, methylPREDNISolone, metoclopramide, metronidazole, midazolam, minocycline, mitoxantrone, morphine, nalbuphine, naloxone, nitroglycerin, ofloxacin, ondansetron, paclitaxel, pentobarbital, phenobarbital, piperacillin, potassium chloride, prochlorperazine, promethazine, propranolol, ranitidine, remifentanil, sufentanil, theophylline, ticarcillin, tobramycin, vancomycin, vecuronium, verapamil, vinCRIStine, zidovudine

Solution compatibilities: D_5, 0.9% NaCl, LR

Evaluate:

• Therapeutic response: decreased symptoms of infection, blood cultures negative

Teach patient/family:

• If dizziness occurs, to ambulate, perform activities with assistance

• To complete full course of drug therapy

• To contact prescriber if adverse reaction occurs

• To avoid large amounts of high-tyramine foods (provide list)

liothyronine (T_3) (℞)

(lye-oh-thye'roe-neen)

Cytomel, *l*-triiodothyronine, T_3, liothyronine sodium, Triostat

Func. class.: Thyroid hormone

Chem. class.: Synthetic T_3

Action: Increases metabolic rates, cardiac output, O_2 consumption, body temp, blood volume, growth, development at cellular level; exact mechanism unknown

Uses: Hypothyroidism, myxedema coma, thyroid hormone replacement, congenital hypothyroidism, nontoxic goiter, T_3 suppression test

Dosage and routes:

• *Adult:* **PO** 25 mcg qd, increased by 12.5-25 mcg q1-2wk until desired response, maintenance dose 25-75 mcg qd

• *Geriatric:* **PO** 5 mcg/day, increase by 5 mcg/day q1-2wk

Congenital hypothyroidism

• *Child >3 yr:* **PO** 50-100 mcg qd

• *Child <3 yr:* **PO** 5 mcg qd, increased by 5 mcg q3-4d titrated to response

Myxedema, severe hypothyroidism

• *Adult:* **PO** 25-50 mcg then may increase by 5-10 mcg q1-2wk; maintenance dose 50-100 mcg qd

Myxedema coma/precoma

• *Adult:* **IV** 25-50 mcg initially, 5 mcg in elderly, 10-20 mcg in cardiac disease; give doses q4-12h

Nontoxic goiter

• *Adult:* **PO** 5 mcg qd, increased by 12.5-25 mcg q1-2wk; maintenance dose 75 mcg qd

Suppression test

• *Adult:* **PO** 75-100 mcg qd × 1 wk;

radioactive ^{131}I is given before and after 1 wk dose
Available forms: Tabs 5, 25, 50 mcg; inj 10 mcg/ml
Side effects/adverse reactions:
CNS: Insomnia, tremors, headache, ***thyroid storm***
CV: Tachycardia, palpitations, angina, dysrhythmias, hypertension, ***cardiac arrest***
GI: Nausea, diarrhea, increased or decreased appetite, cramps
MISC: Menstrual irregularities, weight loss, sweating, heat intolerance, fever, alopecia
Contraindications: Adrenal insufficiency, myocardial infarction, thyrotoxicosis
Precautions: Elderly, angina pectoris, hypertension, ischemia, cardiac disease, pregnancy (A), lactation, diabetes
Pharmacokinetics:
PO/IV: Peak 12-48 hr, duration 72 hr, half-life 1-2 days
Interactions:
- ↓ absorption of liothyronine: cholestyramine, colestipol
- ↑ effects of anticoagulants, sympathomimetics, tricyclics, amphetamines, decongestants, vasopressors
- ↓ effects of digoxin, insulin, hypoglycemics
- ↓ effects of liothyronine: estrogens

↓ thyroid hormone effect: agar, bugleweed, carnitine, kelpware, soy, spirulina
Lab test interferences:
Increase: CPK, LDH, AST, PBI, blood glucose
Decrease: Thyroid function tests
NURSING CONSIDERATIONS
Assess:
- B/P, pulse, periodically during treatment
- Weight qd in same clothing, using same scale, at same time of day
- Height, growth rate of child
- T_3, T_4, which are decreased; radioimmunoassay of TSH, which is increased; radio uptake, which is increased if patient is on too low a dose of medication
- PT may require decreased anticoagulant; check for bleeding, bruising
- Increased nervousness, excitability, irritability, which may indicate too high dose of medication, usually after 1-3 wk of treatment
- Cardiac status: angina, palpitation, chest pain, change in VS

Administer:
- In AM if possible as a single dose to decrease sleeplessness
- At same time each day to maintain drug level
- Only for hormone imbalances; not to be used for obesity, male infertility, menstrual conditions, lethargy
- Lowest dose that relieves symptoms
- Liothyronine after discontinuing other thyroid preparation

Perform/provide:
- Removal of medication 4 wk before RAIU test

Evaluate:
- Therapeutic response: absence of depression; increased weight loss, diuresis, pulse, appetite; absence of constipation, peripheral edema, cold intolerance; pale, cool, dry skin; brittle nails, alopecia, coarse hair, menorrhagia, night blindness, paresthesia, syncope, stupor, coma, rosy cheeks

Teach patient/family:
- That hair loss will occur in child but is temporary
- To report excitability, irritability, anxiety, which indicates overdose
- Not to switch brands unless approved by prescriber
- That hypothyroid child will show

almost immediate behavior/personality change
• That drug is not to be taken to reduce weight
• To avoid OTC preparations with iodine; read labels
• To avoid iodine food, iodized salt, soybeans, tofu, turnips, high iodine seafood, some bread
• That drug controls symptoms but does not cure; treatment is lifelong

liotrix (℞)

(lye′oh-trix)
Thyrolar, T_3/T_4
Func. class.: Thyroid hormone
Chem. class.: Levothyroxine/liothyronine (synthetic T_4, T_3)

Action: Increases metabolic rates, cardiac output, O_2 consumption, body temp, blood volume, growth, development at cellular level, exact mechanism unknown

Uses: Hypothyroidism, thyroid hormone replacement

Dosage and routes:
• *Adult and child:* **PO** 50 mcg levothyroxine mg qd, increased by 12.5 mcg liothyronine mg q2-3wk until desired response
• *Elderly:* **PO** 12.5-25 mcg levothyroxine/3.1-6.2 mcg liothyronine, may increase by 12.5-25 mcg levothyroxine/3.1-6.2 mcg liothyronine q6-8wk until adequate response

Available forms: Tabs: 12.5 mcg levothyroxine/3.1 mcg liothyronine, 25 mcg levothyroxine/6.25 mcg liothyronine, 50 mcg levothyroxine/12.5 mcg liothyronine, 100 mcg levothyroxine/25 mcg liothyronine, 150 mcg levothyroxine/37.5 mcg liothyronine

Side effects/adverse reactions:
CNS: Insomnia, tremors, headache, ***thyroid storm***
CV: Tachycardia, palpitations, angina, dysrhythmias, hypertension, ***cardiac arrest***
GI: Nausea, diarrhea, increased or decreased appetite, cramps
MISC: Menstrual irregularities, weight loss, sweating, heat intolerance, fever

Contraindications: Adrenal insufficiency, myocardial infarction, thyrotoxicosis

Precautions: Elderly, angina pectoris, hypertension, ischemia, cardiac disease, pregnancy (A), lactation, diabetes

Do not confuse:
Thyrolar/Thyrar

Pharmacokinetics:
PO (T_4): Onset unknown, peak 1-3 wk, duration 1-3 wk
PO (T_3): Onset unknown, peak 24-72 hr, duration 72 hr, half-life 1 wk

Interactions:
• ↓ absorption of liotrix: cholestyramine, colestipol
• ↑ effects of amphetamines, decongestants, vasopressors, anticoagulants, sympathomimetics, tricyclics, catecholamines
• ↓ effects of digoxin, insulin, hypoglycemics
• ↓ effects of liotrix: estrogens
↓ thyroid hormone effect: agar, bugleweed, carnitine, kelpware, soy, spirulina

Lab test interferences:
Increase: CPK, LDH, AST, PBI, blood glucose
Decrease: Thyroid function tests

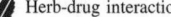

NURSING CONSIDERATIONS
Assess:
• B/P, pulse periodically during treatment
• Weight qd in same clothing, using same scale, at same time of day
• Height, growth rate of child
• T_3, T_4, FTIs, which are decreased; radioimmunoassay of TSH, which

is increased; radio uptake, which is increased if patient is on too low a dose of medication
• PT may require decreased anticoagulant; check for bleeding, bruising
• Increased nervousness, excitability, irritability, which may indicate too high dose of medication, usually after 1-3 wk of treatment
• Cardiac status: angina, palpitation, chest pain, change in VS

Administer:
• In AM if possible as a single dose to decrease sleeplessness
• At same time each day to maintain drug level
• Only for hormone imbalances; not to be used for obesity, male infertility, menstrual conditions, lethargy
• Lowest dose that relieves symptoms

Perform/provide:
• Withdrawal of medication 4 wk before RAIU test
• Storage in airtight, light-resistant container

Evaluate:
• Therapeutic response: absence of depression; increased weight loss, diuresis, pulse, appetite; absence of constipation, peripheral edema, cold intolerance; pale, cool, dry skin; brittle nails, coarse hair, menorrhagia, night blindness, paresthesias, syncope, stupor, coma, rosy cheeks

Teach patient/family:
• That hair loss will occur in child, is temporary
• To report excitability, irritability, chest pain, increased pulse rate, palpitations, excessive sweating, heat intolerance, nervousness, anxiety, which indicate overdose
• Not to switch brands unless approved by prescriber
• That hypothyroid child will show almost immediate behavior/personality change
• That drug is not to be taken to reduce weight
• To avoid OTC preparations with iodine; read labels
• To avoid iodine food, iodized salt, soybeans, tofu, turnips, high iodine seafood, some bread
• That drug does not cure, but controls symptoms, treatment is lifelong

lisinopril (℞)

(lyse-in′oh-pril)
Prinivil, Zestril
Func. class.: Antihypertensive, angiotensin converting enzyme inhibitor (ACE)
Chem. class.: Enalaprilat lysine analog

L

Action: Selectively suppresses renin-angiotensin-aldosterone system; inhibits ACE, preventing conversion of angiotensin I to angiotensin II

Uses: Mild to moderate hypertension, adjunctive therapy of systolic CHF, acute MI

Dosage and routes:

Hypertension
• *Adult:* **PO** 10-40 mg qd; may increase to 80 mg qd if required
• *Geriatric:* **PO** 2.5-5 mg/day, increase q7 days

CHF
• *Adult:* **PO** 5 mg initially with diuretics/digitalis, range 5-20 mg

Available forms: Tabs 2.5, 5, 10, 20, 40 mg

Side effects/adverse reactions:
GI: Nausea, vomiting, anorexia, constipation, flatulence, GI irritation, diarrhea

GU: ***Proteinuria, renal insufficiency,*** sexual dysfunction, impotence
INTEG: Rash, pruritus
CNS: *Vertigo,* depression, ***stroke,*** insomnia, paresthesias, headache, *fatigue,* asthenia, dizziness
EENT: Blurred vision, nasal congestion
SYST: ***Angioedema***
RESP: Dry cough, dyspnea
CV: Chest pain, hypotension
MISC: Muscle cramps

Contraindications: Hypersensitivity, pregnancy (D) 2nd/3rd trimesters

Precautions: Pregnancy (C) 1st trimester, lactation, renal disease, hyperkalemia, renal artery stenosis

Do not confuse:
lisinopril/Risperdal
Prinivil/Plendil/Proventil
Prinivil/Prilosec

Pharmacokinetics: Onset 1 hr, peak 6-8 hr, duration 24 hr; excreted unchanged in urine

Interactions:

- ↑ hypotensive effect: diuretics, other hypertensives, probenecid, phenothiazines, nitrates, acute alcohol ingestion
- ↓ lisinopril effects: aspirin, indomethacin, NSAIDs
- Hyperkalemia: potassium salt substitutes, potassium-sparing diuretics, potassium supplements, cycloSPORINE
- Possible toxicity: lithium, digoxin
- ↑ hypersensitivity: allopurinol
- Drug/food: high-potassium diet (bananas, orange juice, avocados, nuts, spinach) should be avoided; hyperkalemia may occur

↑ toxicity, death: aconite
↑ or ↓ antihypertensive effect: astragalus, cola tree
↑ antihypertensive effect: barberry, betony, black catechu, black cohosh, bloodroot, broom, burdock, cat's claw, dandelion, goldenseal, Irish moss, Jamaican dogwood, kelp, khella, mistletoe, parsley
↓ antihypertensive effect: coltsfoot, guarana, khat, licorice

Lab test interferences:
Interference: Glucose/insulin tolerance tests, ANA titer

NURSING CONSIDERATIONS

Assess:

Blood studies, platelets; WBC with diff baseline and periodically q3mo; if neutrophils <1000/mm^3, discontinue treatment

- B/P, pulse q4h; note rate, rhythm, quality
- Electrolytes: K, Na, Cl
- Apical/pedal pulse before administration; notify prescriber of any significant changes
- Baselines in renal, hepatic studies before therapy begins and periodically LFTs, uric acid and glucose may be increased
- Edema in feet, legs qd, weight qd in CHF
- Skin turgor, dryness of mucous membranes for hydration status
- Symptoms of CHF: edema, dyspnea, wet rales

Evaluate:

- Therapeutic response: decreased B/P, CHF symptoms

Teach patient/family:

- Not to discontinue drug abruptly
- To rise slowly to sitting or standing position to minimize orthostatic hypotension
- To avoid increasing potassium in the diet

Treatment of overdose: Lavage, IV atropine for bradycardia, IV theophylline for bronchospasm, digitalis, O_2, diuretic for cardiac failure

lithium (℞)

(li'thee-um)

Carbolith✱, Duralith✱, Eskalith, Eskalith-CR, lithium carbonate, Lithizine✱, Lithonate, Lithotabs

Func. class.: Antimanic, antipsychotic

Chem. class.: Alkali metal ion salt

Action: May alter sodium, potassium ion transport across cell membrane in nerve, muscle cells; may balance biogenic amines of norepinephrine, serotonin in CNS areas involved in emotional responses

Uses: Bipolar disorders (manic phase), prevention of bipolar manic-depressive psychosis

Dosage and routes:

• *Adult:* **PO** 300-600 mg tid, maintenance 300 mg tid or qid; slow rel tabs 300 mg bid; dose should be individualized to maintain blood levels at 0.5-1.5 mEq/L

• *Geriatric:* **PO** 300 mg bid, increase q7 days by 300 mg to desired dose

• *Child:* **PO** 15-20 mg (0.4-0.5 mEq/kg/day in 2-3 divided doses, ↑ as needed, do not exceed adult doses

Renal dose

• **PO** CCr 10-50 ml/min 50%-75% of dose; CCr <10 ml/min 25%-50% of dose

• *Child:* **PO** 15-20 mg (0.4-0.5 mEq)/kg/day in 2-3 divided doses, increase as needed, do not exceed adult doses

Available forms: Caps 150, 300, 600 mg; tabs 300 mg; tabs ext rel 300, 450 mg; syr 300 mg/5 ml (8 mEq/5 ml); cap slow rel 150, 300 mg✱

Side effects/adverse reactions:

CNS: Headache, drowsiness, dizziness, tremors, twitching, ataxia, ***seizure,*** slurred speech, restlessness, confusion, stupor, memory loss, clonic movements, fatigue

GI: Dry mouth, anorexia, nausea, vomiting, diarrhea, incontinence, abdominal pain, metallic taste

GU: ***Polyuria, glycosuria, proteinuria, albuminuria,*** urinary incontinence, polydipsia, edema

CV: Hypotension, ECG changes, ***dysrhythmias, circulatory collapse,*** edema

INTEG: Drying of hair, alopecia, rash, pruritus, hyperkeratosis, acneiform lesions, folliculitis

HEMA: ***Leukocytosis***

EENT: Tinnitus, blurred vision

ENDO: Hyponatremia, hypothyroidism, goiter, hyperglycemia, hyperthyroidism

MS: Muscle weakness

Contraindications: Hepatic disease, brain trauma, OBS, pregnancy (D), lactation, children <12 yr, schizophrenia, severe cardiac disease, severe renal disease, severe dehydration

Precautions: Elderly, thyroid disease, seizure disorders, diabetes mellitus, systemic infection, urinary retention

Pharmacokinetics:

PO: Onset rapid, peak ½-4 hr, half-life 18-36 hr depending on age; crosses blood-brain barrier; 80% of filtered lithium is reabsorbed by the renal tubules, excreted in urine; crosses placenta; enters breast milk; well absorbed by oral method

Interactions:

• ↑ hypothyroid effects: antithyroid agents, calcium iodide, potassium iodide, iodinated glycerol

• Neurotoxicity: haloperidol, thioridazine

• ↑ effects of neuromuscular blocking agents, phenothiazines

L

• ↑ renal clearance: sodium bicarbonate, acetaZOLAMIDE, mannitol, aminophylline
• ↑ toxicity: indomethacin, diuretics, nonsteroidal antiinflammatories, losartan
• ↓ lithium effects: theophyllines, urea, urinary alkalinizers
• ↑ lithium effect/toxicity: carbamazepine, fluoxetine, methyldopa, NSAIDs, thiazide diuretics, probenecid
• Drug/food: significant changes in sodium intake will alter lithium excretion
↑ lithium effects, ↑ toxicity: broom, buchu, dandelion, goldenrod, horsetail, juniper, nettle, parsley
↓ lithium levels: black/green tea, coffee, cola nut, guarana, plantain, yerba maté

Lab test interferences:
Increase: Potassium excretion, urine glucose, blood glucose, protein, BUN
Decrease: VMA, T_3, T_4, PBI, ^{131}I

NURSING CONSIDERATIONS

Assess:
• Weight qd; check for and report edema in legs, ankles, wrists
• Sodium intake; decreased sodium intake with decreased fluid intake may lead to lithium retention; increased sodium and fluids may decrease lithium retention
• Skin turgor at least qd
• Urine for albuminuria, glycosuria, uric acid during beginning treatment, q2mo thereafter
• Neurologic status: LOC, gait, motor reflexes, hand tremors
• Serum lithium levels qwk initially, then q2mo (therapeutic level: 0.5-1.5 mEq/L)

Administer:
• Reduced dose to elderly
• With meals to avoid GI upset
• Adequate fluids (2-3 L/day) to prevent dehydration during initial treatment, 1-2 L/day during maintenance

Evaluate:
• Therapeutic response: decrease in excitement, manic phase

Teach patient/family:
• The symptoms of minor toxicity: vomiting, diarrhea, poor coordination, fine motor tremors, weakness, lassitude; major toxicity: coarse tremors, severe thirst, tinnitus, diluted urine
• To monitor urine specific gravity, emphasize need for follow-up care to determine lithium levels
• That contraception is necessary, since lithium may harm fetus
• Not to operate machinery until lithium levels are stable
• That beneficial effects may take 1-3 wk
• About drugs that interact with lithium (provide list) and discuss need for adequate stable intake of salt and fluids
Not to break, crush, or chew caps, ext rel tabs

Treatment of overdose: Induce emesis or lavage, maintain airway, respiratory function; dialysis for severe intoxication

lodoxamide ophthalmic

See appendix c

lomefloxacin (℞)

(lo-meh-flox'a-sin)
Maxaquin
Func. class.: Antiinfective
Chem. class.: Fluoroquinolone

Action: Interferes with conversion of intermediate DNA fragments into

high-molecular-weight DNA in bacteria; DNA gyrase inhibitor
Uses: Treatment of lower respiratory tract infections (pneumonia, bronchitis), genitourinary infections (prostatitis, UTIs), preoperatively to reduce UTIs in transurethral surgical procedures; gram-negative bacteria: *Aeromonas, Citrobacter, Enterobacter, Escherichia coli, Haemophilus influenzae, Klebsiella, Legionella, Moraxella catarrhalis, Morganella morganii, Proteus vulgaris, Proteus mirabilis, Providencia alcalifaciens, Providencia rettgeri, Pseudomonas aeruginosa, Serratia;* gram-positive bacteria: *Staphylococcus aureus, Staphylococcus epidermidis, Staphylococcus saprophyticus*
Dosage and routes:
Lower respiratory tract infection/ uncomplicated cystitis
• *Adult:* **PO** 400 qd × 10 day
Complicated UTI
• *Adult:* **PO** 400 mg qd × 14 days depending on type of infection
Renal dose
• *Adult:* **PO** CCr ≤40 ml/min 400 mg, then 200 mg/day
Surgical prophylaxis
• *Adult:* **PO** 400 mg 2-6 hr before surgery
Available forms: Tabs 400 mg
Side effects/adverse reactions:
CNS: Dizziness, headache, somnolence, depression, insomnia, nervousness, confusion, agitation, ***seizures***
GI: Diarrhea, *nausea,* vomiting, anorexia, flatulence, heartburn, dry mouth; increased AST, ALT; constipation, abdominal pain, oral thrush, glossitis, stomatitis, ***pseudomembranous colitis***
INTEG: Rash, pruritus, urticaria, *photosensitivity*
EENT: Visual disturbances
SYST: ***Anaphylaxis, Stevens-Johnson syndrome***
Contraindications: Hypersensitivity to quinolones
Precautions: Pregnancy (C), lactation, children, elderly, renal disease, seizure disorders, excessive exposure to sunlight, psychosis, increased intracranial pressure
Pharmacokinetics:
PO: Peak 1-2 hr, half-life 6-8 hr; excreted in urine as active drug, metabolites
Interactions:
• ↓ absorption: antacids containing aluminum, magnesium, sucralfate, zinc, iron
• ↑ CNS stimulation, seizures: NSAIDs
• ↑ lomefloxacin toxicity: cimetidine, probenecid
• ↑ levels: cycloSPORINE, warfarin, watch for toxicity
• ↓ theophylline clearance, toxicity may result
↑ antiinfective effect: cola tree
NURSING CONSIDERATIONS
Assess:
• Renal, hepatic studies: BUN, creatinine, AST, ALT
• I&O ratio; urine pH, <5.5 is ideal
• CNS symptoms: insomnia, vertigo, headache, agitation, confusion
Allergic reactions and anaphylaxis: rash, flushing, urticaria, pruritus, chills, fever, joint pain; may occur a few days after therapy begins; epINEPHrine and resuscitation equipment should be available for anaphylactic reaction
• Bowel pattern qd, if severe diarrhea occurs, drug should be discontinued
• For overgrowth of infection: perineal itching, fever, malaise, redness, pain, swelling, drainage, rash, diarrhea, change in cough, sputum

L

Administer:
- After clean-catch urine for C&S
- 4 hr before or 2 hrs after antacids, iron, calcium, zinc products

Evaluate:
- Therapeutic response: negative C&S, absence of signs/symptoms of infection

Teach patient/family:
- That fluids must be increased to 2 L/day to avoid crystallization in kidneys
- That if dizziness or light-headedness occurs, to ambulate, perform activities with assistance
- To complete full course of drug therapy
- To contact prescriber if adverse reactions occur
- To avoid iron- or mineral-containing supplements or antacids within 4 hr before and after dosing
- That photosensitivity may occur and sunscreen should be used
- To use frequent rinsing of mouth, sugarless candy or gum for dry mouth
- To avoid other medication unless approved by prescriber
- Not to use theophylline with this product, toxicity may result; contact prescriber if taking theophylline

lomustine (℞)

(loe-mus'teen)

CCNU, CeeNU

Func. class.: Antineoplastic alkylating agent

Chem. class.: Nitrosourea

Action: Responsible for crosslinking DNA strands, which leads to cell death; activity is not cell cycle phase specific

Uses: Hodgkin's disease, lymphomas, melanomas, multiple myeloma; brain, lung, bladder, kidney, colon cancer

Investigational uses: Brain, breast, renal, GI tract, bronchogenic carcinoma; melanomas

Dosage and routes:
- *Adult:* **PO** 130 mg/m^2 as a single dose q6wk; titrate dose to WBC; do not give repeat dose unless WBC >4000/mm^3, platelet count >100,000/mm^3

Available forms: Caps 10, 40, 100 mg

Side effects/adverse reactions:

HEMA: ***Thrombocytopenia, leukopenia, myelosuppression, anemia***

GI: Nausea, vomiting, anorexia, stomatitis, ***hepatotoxicity***

GU: ***Azotemia, renal failure***

INTEG: Burning at inj site

RESP: ***Fibrosis, pulmonary infiltrate***

Contraindications: Hypersensitivity, leukopenia, thrombocytopenia, pregnancy (D), lactation, "blastic" phase of CML

Precautions: Radiation therapy

Pharmacokinetics: Metabolized in liver, excreted in urine; half-life 16-48 hr; 50% protein bound; crosses blood-brain barrier; appears in breast milk

Interactions:
- ↑ bleeding: aspirin, anticoagulants
- ↑ toxicity: barbiturates, phenytoin, chloral hydrate
- ↑ lomustine metabolism: phenobarbital
- Lomustine potentiation: succinylcholine
- ↑ bone marrow depression: allopurinol

Lab test interferences:

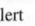

False positive: Cytology tests for breast, bladder, cervix, lung

NURSING CONSIDERATIONS
Assess:
- CBC, differential, platelet count qwk; withhold drug if WBC <4000/mm^3 or platelet count <100,000/mm^3; notify prescriber
- Pulmonary function tests, chest x-ray films before, during therapy; chest film should be obtained q2wk during treatment
- Renal studies: BUN, serum uric acid, urine CCr before, during therapy
- I&O ratio; report fall in urine output of 30 ml/hr
- Monitor temp q4h (may indicate beginning infection); no rectal temps
- Hepatic studies before, during therapy (bilirubin, AST, ALT, LDH) as needed or monthly
- Bleeding: hematuria, guaiac, bruising or petechiae, mucosa or orifices q8h
- Dyspnea, rales, unproductive cough, chest pain, tachypnea
- Food preferences; list likes, dislikes
- Jaundiced skin and sclera, dark urine, clay-colored stools, itchy skin, abdominal pain, fever, diarrhea
- Inflammation of mucosa, breaks in skin
- Buccal cavity q8h for dryness, sores or ulceration, white patches, oral pain, bleeding, dysphagia
- Local irritation, pain, burning, discoloration at inj site

⬥ Symptoms indicating severe allergic reaction: rash, pruritus, urticaria, purpuric skin lesions, itching, flushing

Administer:
- Antiemetic 30-60 min before giving drug to prevent vomiting
- Antibiotics for prophylaxis of infection

Perform/provide:
- Storage in tight container at room temperature
- Strict medical asepsis, protective isolation if WBC levels are low
- Deep-breathing exercises with patient tid-qid; place in semi-Fowler's position
- Increase fluid intake to 2-3 L/day to prevent urate deposits, calculi formation
- Rinsing of mouth tid-qid with water, club soda; brushing of teeth bid-tid with soft brush or cotton-tipped applicators for stomatitis; use unwaxed dental floss

Evaluate:
- Therapeutic response: decreased tumor size, spread of malignancy

Teach patient/family:
- About protective isolation
- To report any changes in breathing or coughing
- To avoid foods with citric acid, hot or rough texture if buccal inflammation is present
- To report any bleeding, white spots, or ulcerations in mouth to prescriber; tell patient to examine mouth qd
- To report signs of infection: fever, sore throat, flulike symptoms
- To report signs of anemia: fatigue, headache, faintness, shortness of breath, irritability
- To avoid use of razors, commercial mouthwash
- To avoid use of aspirin products or ibuprofen

loperamide (OTC, ℞)

(loe-per′a-mide)

loperamide solution, Imodium, Imodium A-D, Imodium A-D Caplet, loperamide, Kaopectate II Caplets, Maalox Antidiarrheal Caplets, Neo-Diaral, Pepto Diarrhea Control

Func. class.: Antidiarrheal

Chem. class.: Piperidine derivative

Action: Direct action on intestinal muscles to decrease GI peristalsis; reduces volume, increases bulk, electrolytes not lost

Uses: Diarrhea (cause undetermined), chronic diarrhea, to decrease amount of ileostomy discharge

Dosage and routes:

- *Adult:* **PO** 4 mg, then 2 mg after each loose stool, max 16 mg/day
- *Child 9-11 yr:* **PO** 2 mg, then 1 mg after each loose stool, max 6 mg/24 hr
- *Child 2-5 yr:* **PO** 1 mg then 0.1 mg/kg after each loose stool, max 4 mg/24 hr

Available forms: Caps 2 mg; liq 1 mg/5 ml; tabs 2 mg

Side effects/adverse reactions:

CNS: Dizziness, drowsiness, fatigue, fever

GI: Nausea, dry mouth, vomiting, constipation, abdominal pain, anorexia, ***toxic megacolon***

INTEG: Rash

Contraindications: Hypersensitivity, severe ulcerative colitis, pseudomembranous colitis, acute diarrhea associated with *Escherichia coli*

Precautions: Pregnancy (B), lactation, children <2 yr, liver disease, dehydration, bacterial disease

Pharmacokinetics:

PO: Onset ½-1 hr, duration 4-5 hr, half-life 7-14 hr; metabolized in liver; excreted in feces as unchanged drug; small amount in urine

Interactions:

- ↑ CNS depression: alcohol, antihistamines, analgesics, opioids, sedative/hypnotics
- Do not mix oral sol with other sols

↑ CNS depression: chamomile, hops, kava, skullcap, valerian

↑ antidiarrheal effect: nutmeg

NURSING CONSIDERATIONS

Assess:

- Stools: volume, color, characteristics
- Electrolytes (K, Na, Cl) if on long-term therapy
- Skin turgor q8h if dehydration is suspected
- Bowel pattern before; for rebound constipation
- Response after 48 hr; if no response, drug should be discontinued
- Dehydration, CNS problems in children
- Abdominal distention, toxic megacolon; may occur in ulcerative colitis

Administer:

- For 48 hr only

Perform/provide:

- Storage in tight container

Evaluate:

- Therapeutic response: decreased diarrhea

Teach patient/family:

- To avoid OTC products unless directed by prescriber
- That ileostomy patient may take this drug for extended time
- That if drowsiness occurs, not to operate machinery
- To use hard candy, sips of water for dry mouth

Not to break, crush, or chew caps

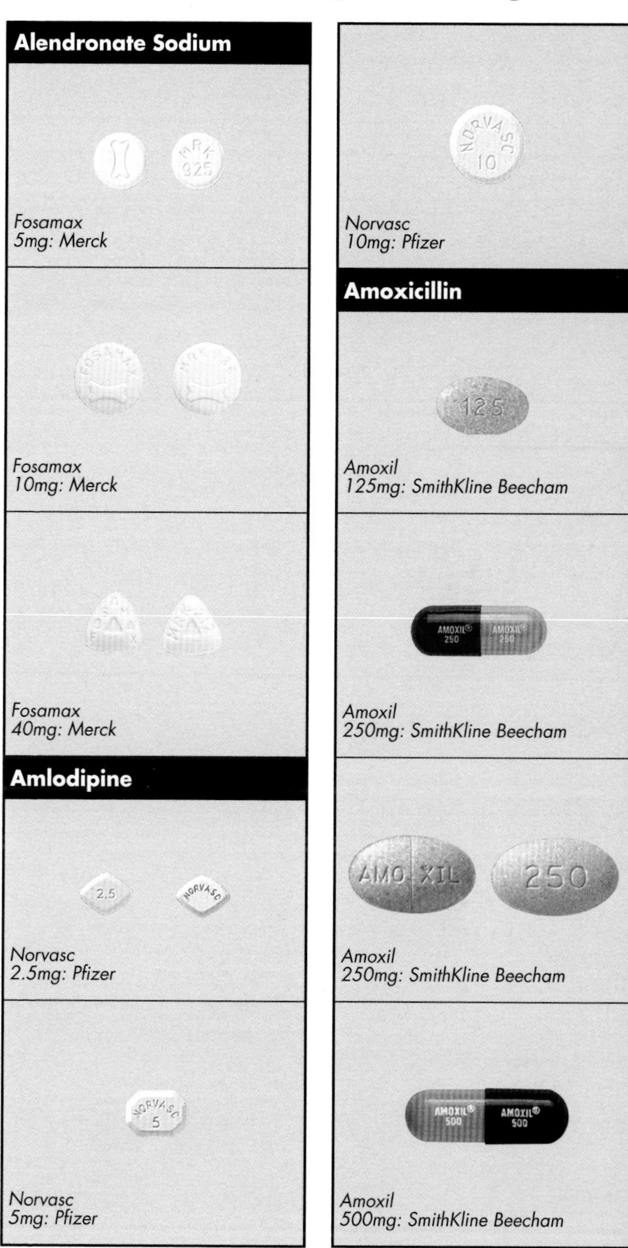
Alendronate Sodium
Fosamax
5mg: Merck
Fosamax
10mg: Merck
Fosamax
40mg: Merck
Amlodipine
Norvasc
2.5mg: Pfizer
Norvasc
5mg: Pfizer
Norvasc
10mg: Pfizer
Amoxicillin
Amoxil
125mg: SmithKline Beecham
Amoxil
250mg: SmithKline Beecham
Amoxil
250mg: SmithKline Beecham
Amoxil
500mg: SmithKline Beecham

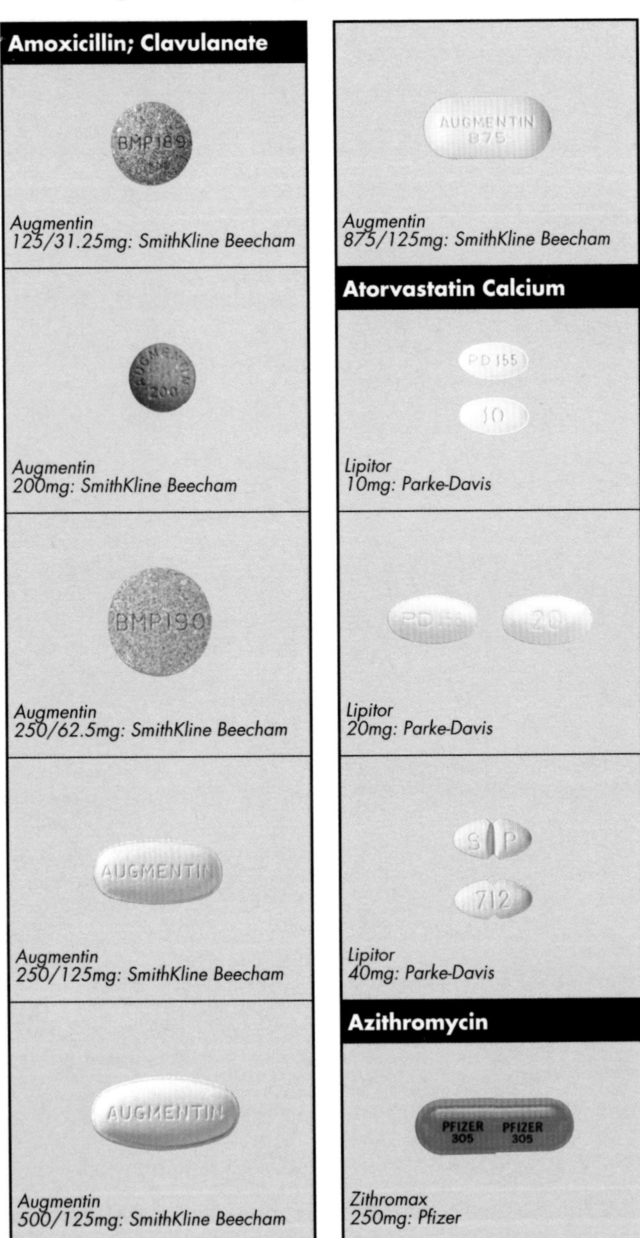

Amoxicillin; Clavulanate

Augmentin
125/31.25mg: SmithKline Beecham

Augmentin
200mg: SmithKline Beecham

Augmentin
250/62.5mg: SmithKline Beecham

Augmentin
250/125mg: SmithKline Beecham

Augmentin
500/125mg: SmithKline Beecham

Augmentin
875/125mg: SmithKline Beecham

Atorvastatin Calcium

Lipitor
10mg: Parke-Davis

Lipitor
20mg: Parke-Davis

Lipitor
40mg: Parke-Davis

Azithromycin

Zithromax
250mg: Pfizer

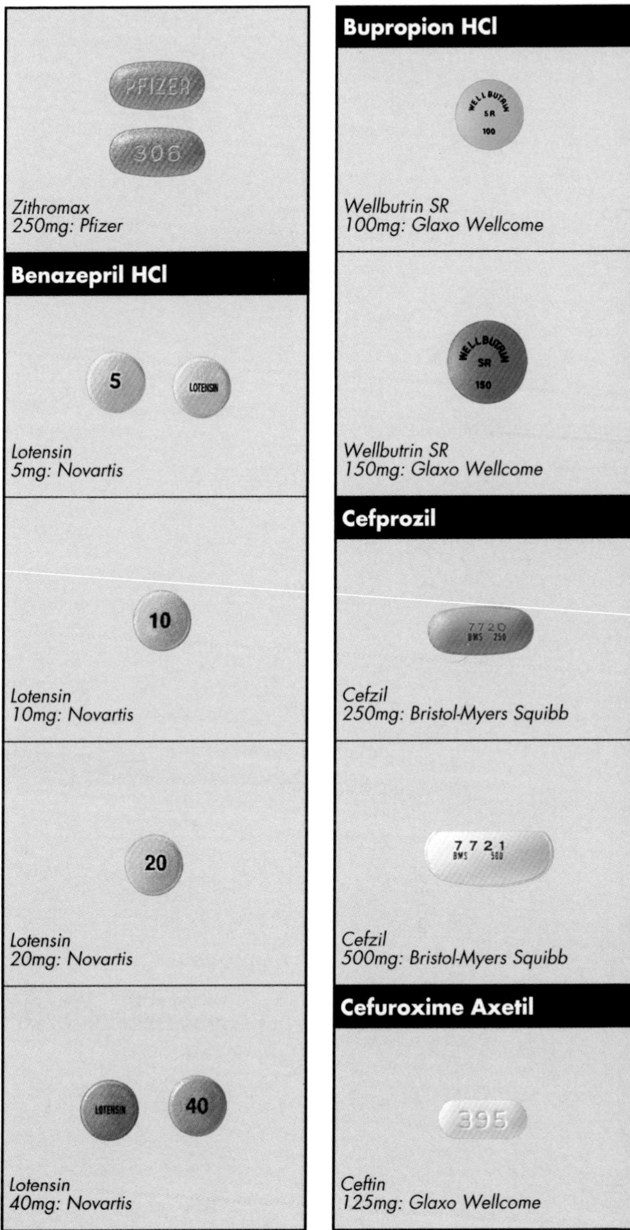

Zithromax
250mg: Pfizer

Benazepril HCl

Lotensin
5mg: Novartis

Lotensin
10mg: Novartis

Lotensin
20mg: Novartis

Lotensin
40mg: Novartis

Bupropion HCl

Wellbutrin SR
100mg: Glaxo Wellcome

Wellbutrin SR
150mg: Glaxo Wellcome

Cefprozil

Cefzil
250mg: Bristol-Myers Squibb

Cefzil
500mg: Bristol-Myers Squibb

Cefuroxime Axetil

Ceftin
125mg: Glaxo Wellcome

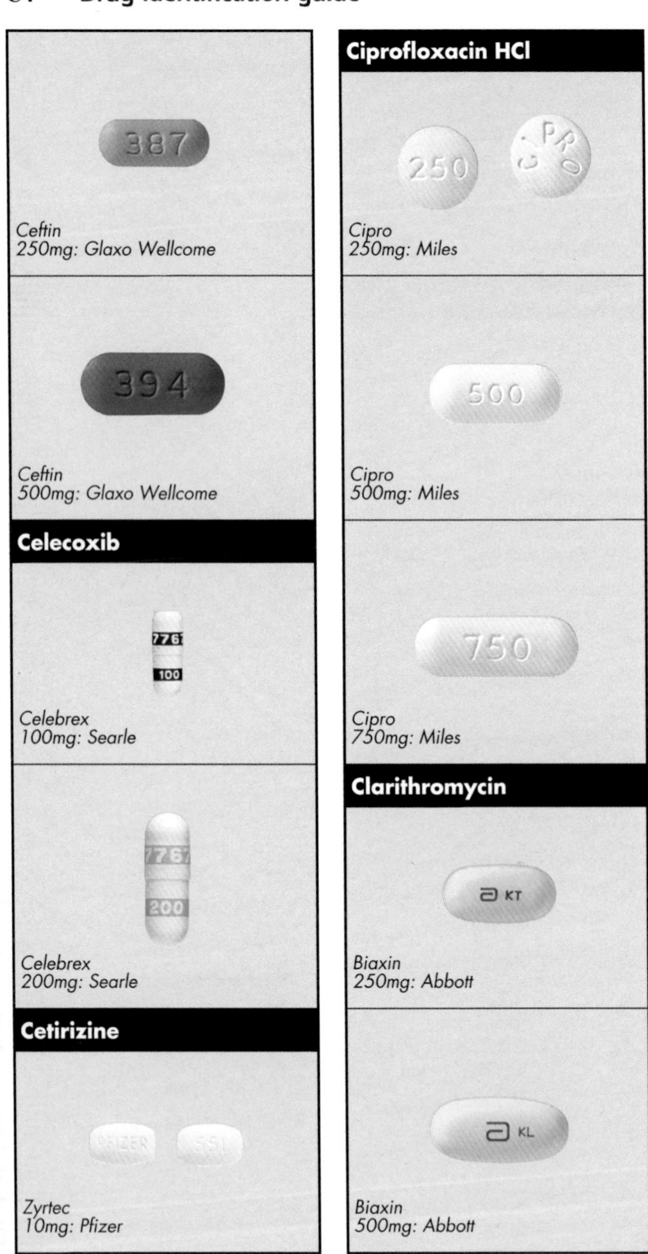

Ceftin
250mg: Glaxo Wellcome

Ceftin
500mg: Glaxo Wellcome

Celecoxib

Celebrex
100mg: Searle

Celebrex
200mg: Searle

Cetirizine

Zyrtec
10mg: Pfizer

Ciprofloxacin HCl

Cipro
250mg: Miles

Cipro
500mg: Miles

Cipro
750mg: Miles

Clarithromycin

Biaxin
250mg: Abbott

Biaxin
500mg: Abbott

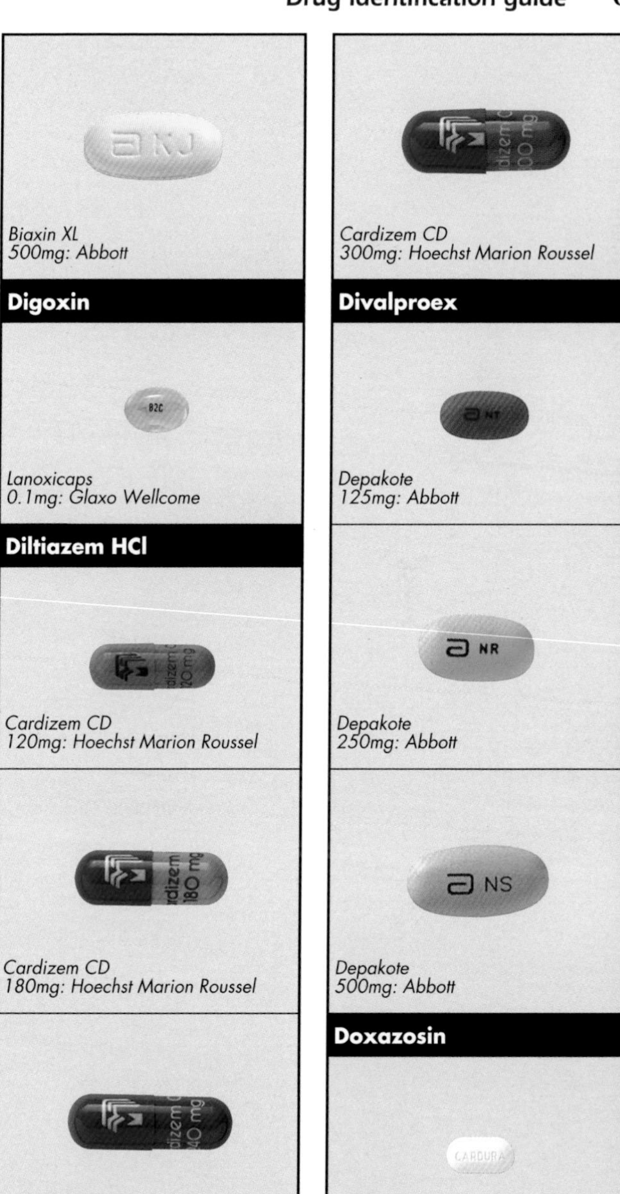

Biaxin XL
500mg: Abbott

Cardizem CD
300mg: Hoechst Marion Roussel

Digoxin

Lanoxicaps
0.1mg: Glaxo Wellcome

Diltiazem HCl

Cardizem CD
120mg: Hoechst Marion Roussel

Cardizem CD
180mg: Hoechst Marion Roussel

Cardizem CD
240mg: Hoechst Marion Roussel

Divalproex

Depakote
125mg: Abbott

Depakote
250mg: Abbott

Depakote
500mg: Abbott

Doxazosin

Cardura
1mg: Roerig

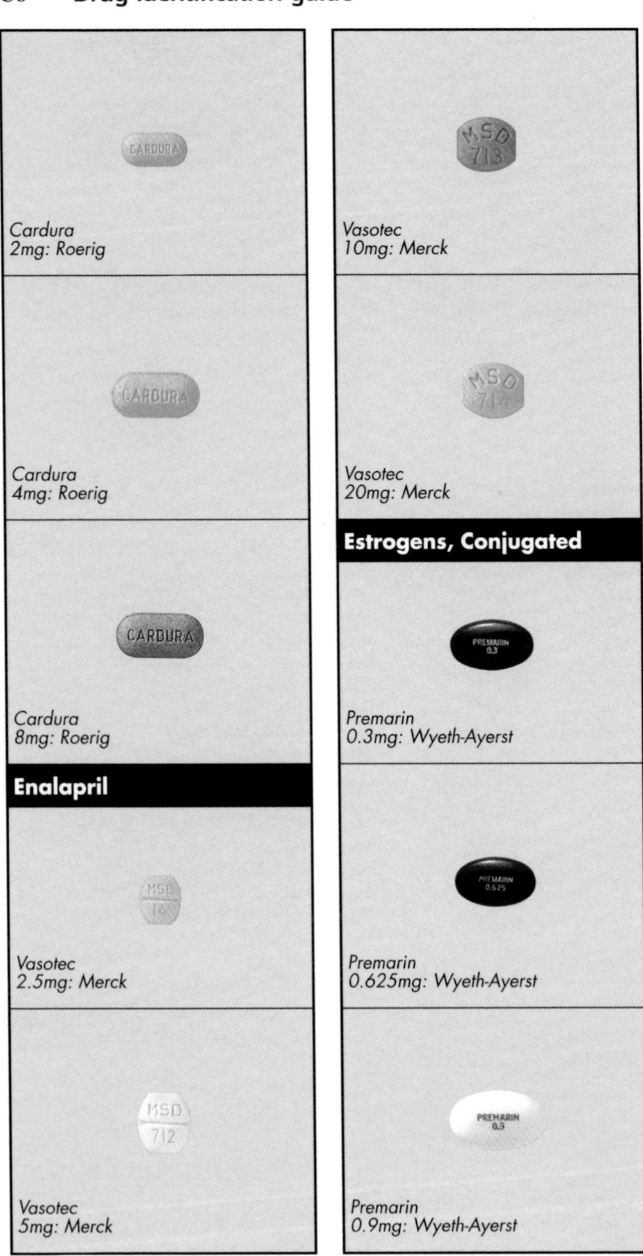

Cardura
2mg: Roerig

Cardura
4mg: Roerig

Cardura
8mg: Roerig

Enalapril

Vasotec
2.5mg: Merck

Vasotec
5mg: Merck

Vasotec
10mg: Merck

Vasotec
20mg: Merck

Estrogens, Conjugated

Premarin
0.3mg: Wyeth-Ayerst

Premarin
0.625mg: Wyeth-Ayerst

Premarin
0.9mg: Wyeth-Ayerst

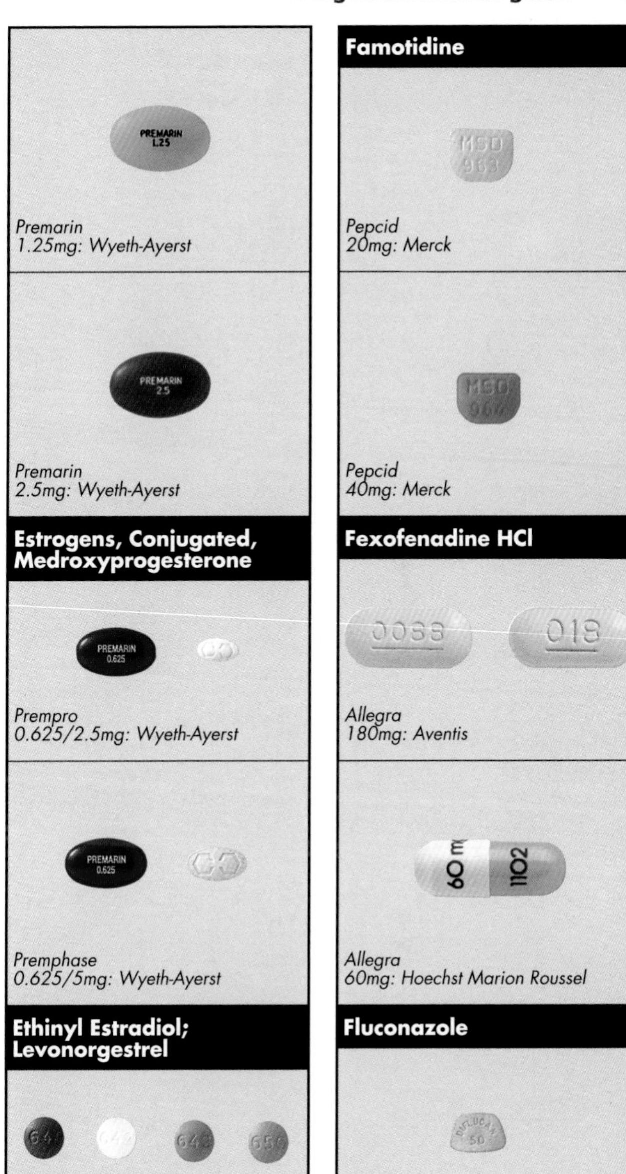

Premarin
1.25mg: Wyeth-Ayerst

Premarin
2.5mg: Wyeth-Ayerst

Estrogens, Conjugated, Medroxyprogesterone

Prempro
0.625/2.5mg: Wyeth-Ayerst

Premphase
0.625/5mg: Wyeth-Ayerst

Ethinyl Estradiol; Levonorgestrel

Triphasil Inert/ 0.03/0.125/0.03/ 0.05/0.04/0.075mg: Wyeth-Ayerst

Famotidine

Pepcid
20mg: Merck

Pepcid
40mg: Merck

Fexofenadine HCl

Allegra
180mg: Aventis

Allegra
60mg: Hoechst Marion Roussel

Fluconazole

Diflucan
50mg: Roerig

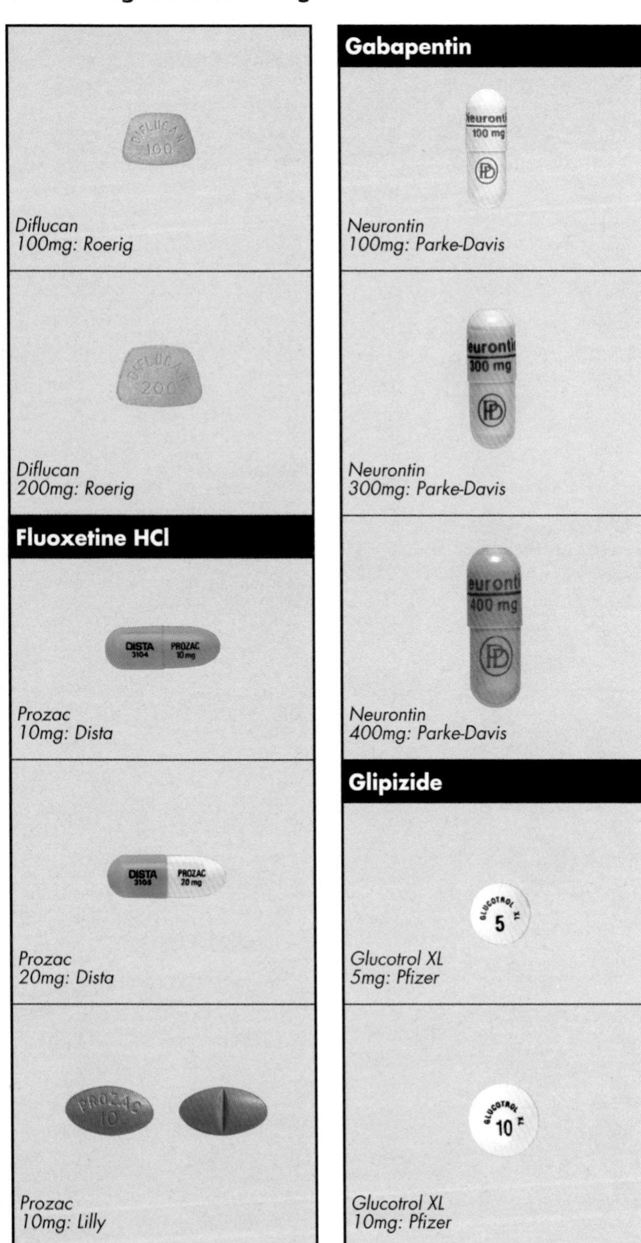

Diflucan
100mg: Roerig

Diflucan
200mg: Roerig

Fluoxetine HCl

Prozac
10mg: Dista

Prozac
20mg: Dista

Prozac
10mg: Lilly

Gabapentin

Neurontin
100mg: Parke-Davis

Neurontin
300mg: Parke-Davis

Neurontin
400mg: Parke-Davis

Glipizide

Glucotrol XL
5mg: Pfizer

Glucotrol XL
10mg: Pfizer

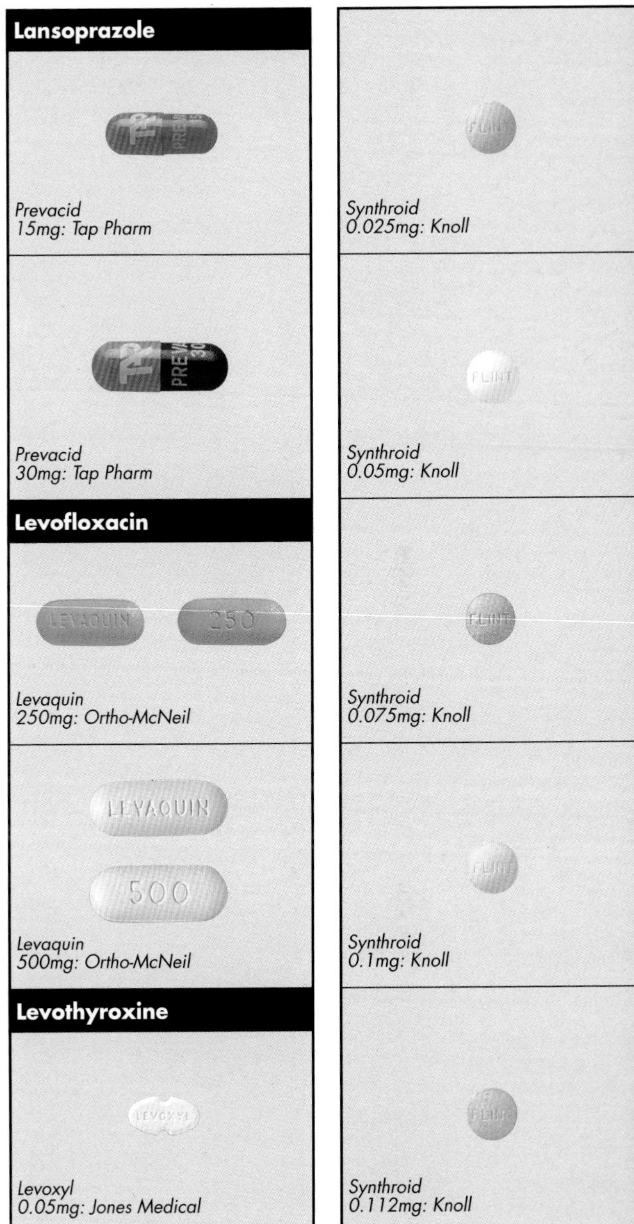

Lansoprazole

Prevacid
15mg: Tap Pharm

Prevacid
30mg: Tap Pharm

Levofloxacin

Levaquin
250mg: Ortho-McNeil

Levaquin
500mg: Ortho-McNeil

Levothyroxine

Levoxyl
0.05mg: Jones Medical

Synthroid
0.025mg: Knoll

Synthroid
0.05mg: Knoll

Synthroid
0.075mg: Knoll

Synthroid
0.1mg: Knoll

Synthroid
0.112mg: Knoll

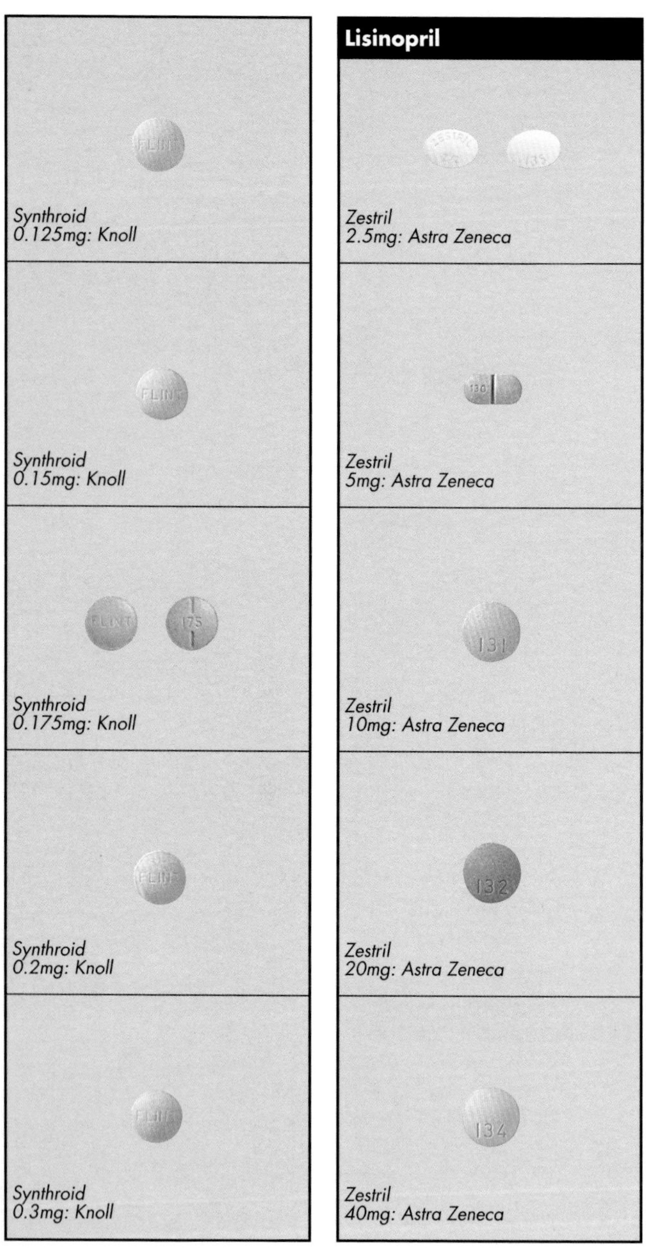

Synthroid
0.125mg: Knoll

Synthroid
0.15mg: Knoll

Synthroid
0.175mg: Knoll

Synthroid
0.2mg: Knoll

Synthroid
0.3mg: Knoll

Lisinopril

Zestril
2.5mg: Astra Zeneca

Zestril
5mg: Astra Zeneca

Zestril
10mg: Astra Zeneca

Zestril
20mg: Astra Zeneca

Zestril
40mg: Astra Zeneca

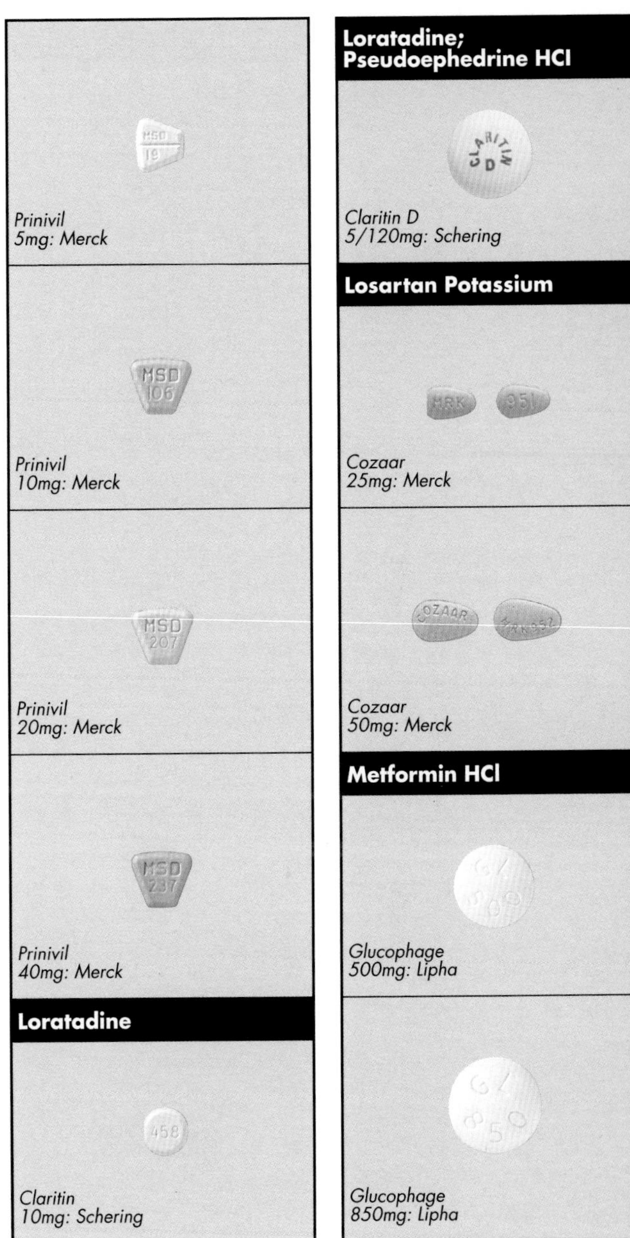

Prinivil
5mg: Merck

Prinivil
10mg: Merck

Prinivil
20mg: Merck

Prinivil
40mg: Merck

Loratadine

Claritin
10mg: Schering

Loratadine; Pseudoephedrine HCl

Claritin D
5/120mg: Schering

Losartan Potassium

Cozaar
25mg: Merck

Cozaar
50mg: Merck

Metformin HCl

Glucophage
500mg: Lipha

Glucophage
850mg: Lipha

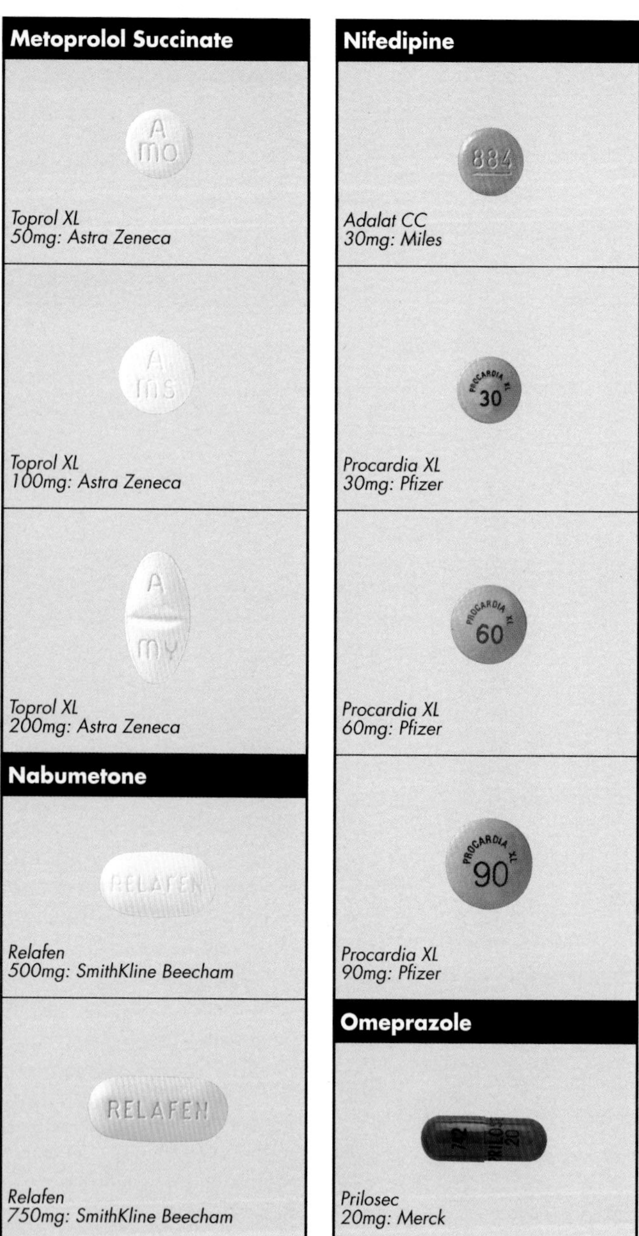
Metoprolol Succinate
A mo
Toprol XL
50mg: Astra Zeneca
A ms
Toprol XL
100mg: Astra Zeneca
A my
Toprol XL
200mg: Astra Zeneca
Nabumetone
RELAFEN
Relafen
500mg: SmithKline Beecham
RELAFEN
Relafen
750mg: SmithKline Beecham
Nifedipine
884
Adalat CC
30mg: Miles
PROCARDIA XL 30
Procardia XL
30mg: Pfizer
PROCARDIA XL 60
Procardia XL
60mg: Pfizer
PROCARDIA XL 90
Procardia XL
90mg: Pfizer
Omeprazole
742 PRILOSEC 20
Prilosec
20mg: Merck

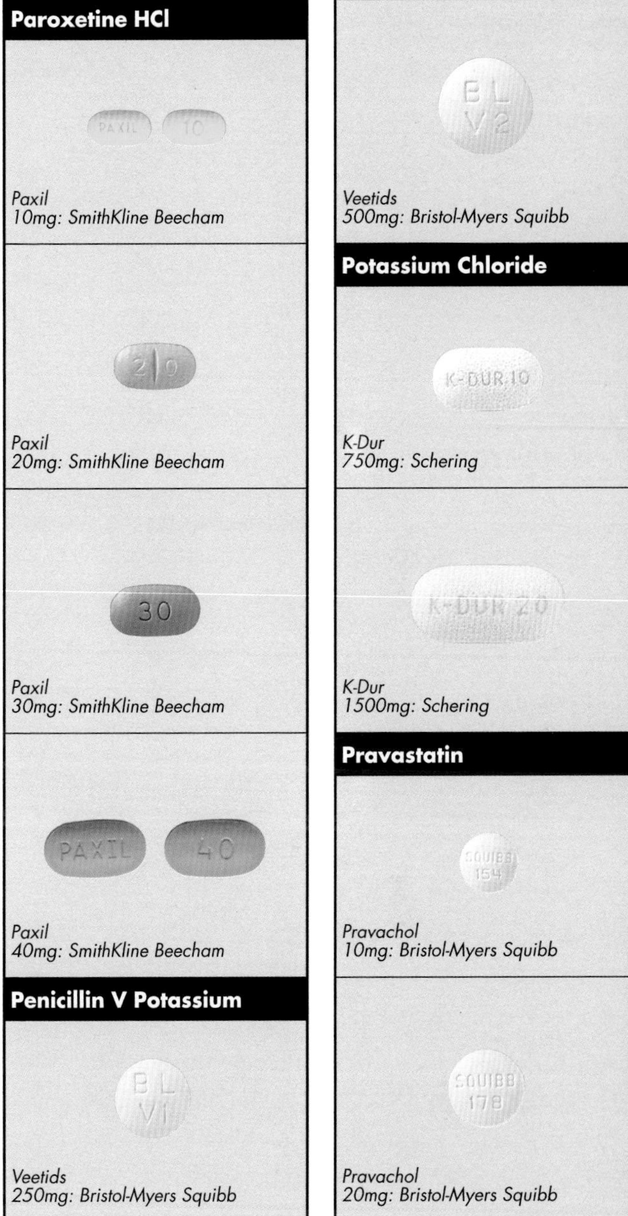

Paroxetine HCl

Paxil
10mg: SmithKline Beecham

Paxil
20mg: SmithKline Beecham

Paxil
30mg: SmithKline Beecham

Paxil
40mg: SmithKline Beecham

Penicillin V Potassium

Veetids
250mg: Bristol-Myers Squibb

Veetids
500mg: Bristol-Myers Squibb

Potassium Chloride

K-Dur
750mg: Schering

K-Dur
1500mg: Schering

Pravastatin

Pravachol
10mg: Bristol-Myers Squibb

Pravachol
20mg: Bristol-Myers Squibb

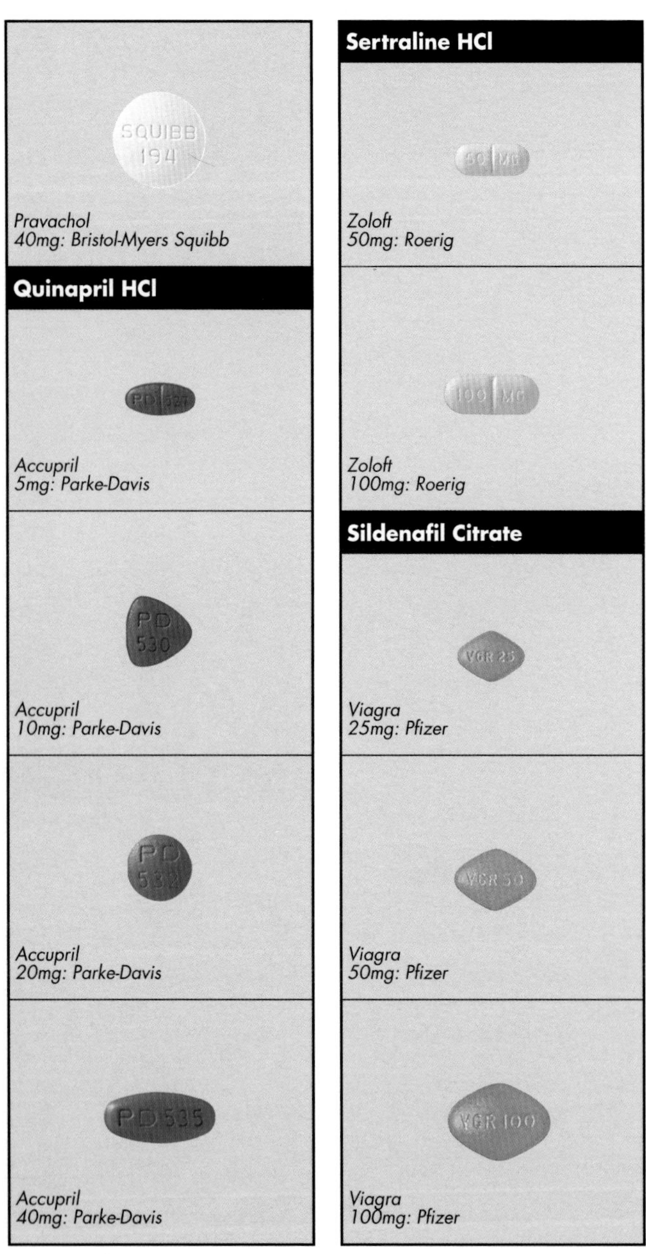

Pravachol
40mg: Bristol-Myers Squibb

Quinapril HCl

Accupril
5mg: Parke-Davis

Accupril
10mg: Parke-Davis

Accupril
20mg: Parke-Davis

Accupril
40mg: Parke-Davis

Sertraline HCl

Zoloft
50mg: Roerig

Zoloft
100mg: Roerig

Sildenafil Citrate

Viagra
25mg: Pfizer

Viagra
50mg: Pfizer

Viagra
100mg: Pfizer

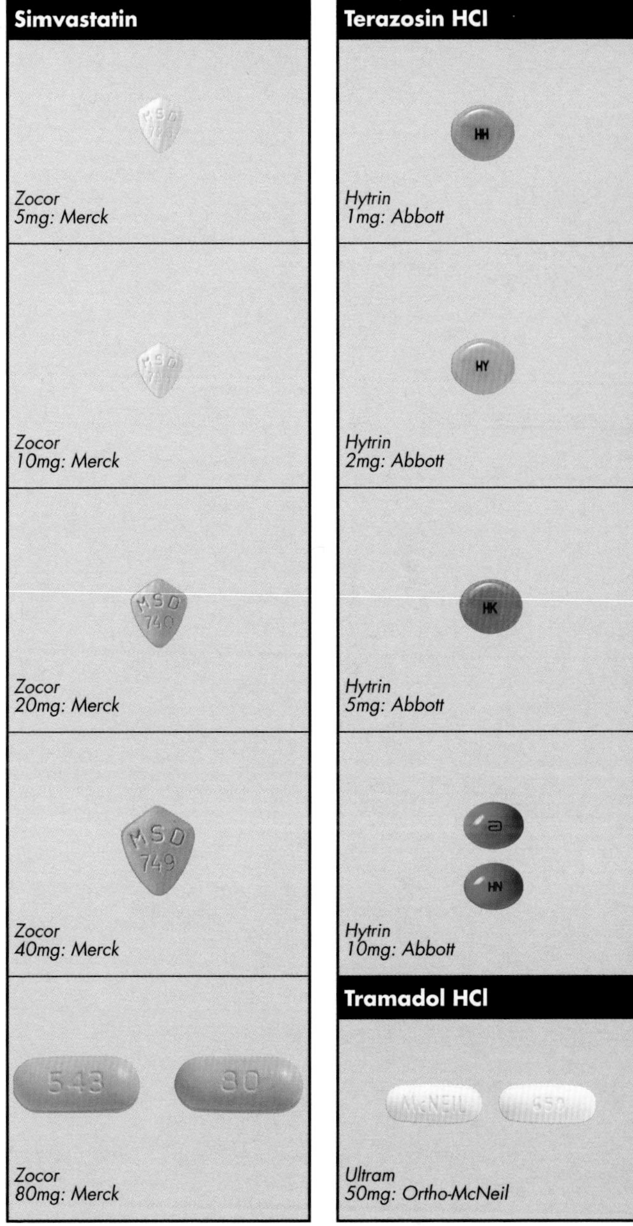

Simvastatin

Zocor
5mg: Merck

Zocor
10mg: Merck

Zocor
20mg: Merck

Zocor
40mg: Merck

Zocor
80mg: Merck

Terazosin HCl

Hytrin
1mg: Abbott

Hytrin
2mg: Abbott

Hytrin
5mg: Abbott

Hytrin
10mg: Abbott

Tramadol HCl

Ultram
50mg: Ortho-McNeil

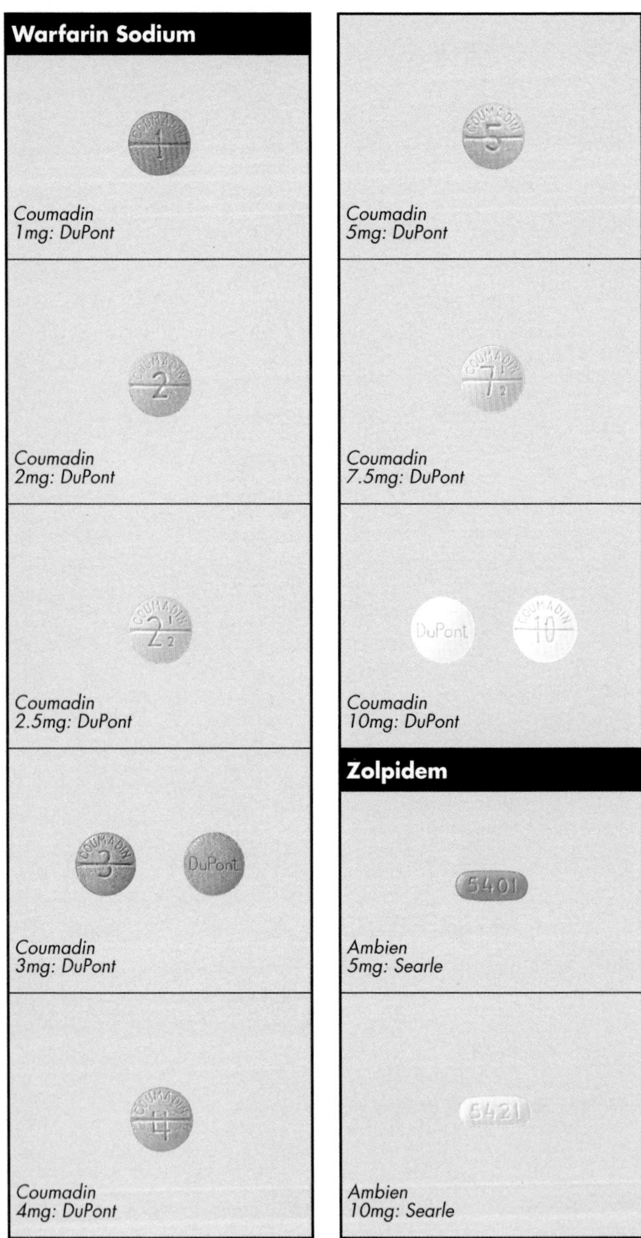

Warfarin Sodium

Coumadin
1mg: DuPont

Coumadin
2mg: DuPont

Coumadin
2.5mg: DuPont

Coumadin
3mg: DuPont

Coumadin
4mg: DuPont

Coumadin
5mg: DuPont

Coumadin
7.5mg: DuPont

Coumadin
10mg: DuPont

Zolpidem

Ambien
5mg: Searle

Ambien
10mg: Searle

loracarbef

See cephalosporins—2nd generation

loratadine (OTC, ℞)

(lor-a'ti-deen)

Alavert, Claritin, Claritin Non-Drowsy Allergy, Claritin Reditabs, Tavist ND

Func. class.: Antihistamine, 2nd generation

Chem. class.: Selective histamine (H_1)-receptor antagonist

Action: Binds to peripheral histamine receptors, providing antihistamine action without sedation

Uses: Seasonal rhinitis

Investigational uses: Chronic idiopathic urticaria for those ≥2 yr

Dosage and routes:

• *Adult and child ≥6 yr:* **PO** 10 mg qd

• *Child 2-5 yr:* **PO** 5 mg qd

Hepatic/renal dose

• *Adult/child ≥6 yr:* 10 mg qod

• *Child 2-5 yr:* 5 mg qod

• ***Available forms:*** Tabs 10 mg; tabs rapid-disintegrating 10 mg; tabs, orally disintegrating 10 mg; syr 1 mg/ml

Side effects/adverse reactions:

CNS: Sedation (more common with increased doses), headache

Contraindications: Hypersensitivity, acute asthma attacks, lower respiratory tract disease

Precautions: Pregnancy (B), increased intraocular pressure, bronchial asthma

Pharmacokinetics: Peak 1½ hr, elimination half-life 8½-28 hr; metabolized in liver to active metabolites, excreted in urine

Interactions:

• ↑ antihistamine effects: MAOIs

• ↑ CNS depressant effects: alcohol, antidepressants, other antihistamines, sedative/hypnotics

↑ CNS depression: chamomile, hops, Jamaican dogwood, kava, khat, senega, skullcap, valerian

↑ anticholinergic effect: corkwood, henbane leaf

NURSING CONSIDERATIONS

Assess:

• Allergy: hives, rash, rhinitis; monitor respiratory status

Administer:

• Rapid-disintegrating tabs by placing on tongue, then swallow after disintegrated with or without water

• On empty stomach qd

Perform/provide:

• Storage in tight container at room temperature

Evaluate:

• Therapeutic response: absence of running or congested nose, other allergy symptoms

Teach patient/family:

• To avoid driving, other hazardous activities if drowsiness occurs

• To use sunscreen or stay out of the sun to prevent photosensitivity

• To avoid use of other CNS depressants

lorazepam (℞)

(lor-a'ze-pam)

Apo-Lorazepam♣, Ativan, lorazepam, Novo-Lorazem♣, Nu-Loraz♣

Func. class.: Sedative, hypnotic; antianxiety

Chem. class.: Benzodiazepine

Controlled Substance Schedule IV

Action: Potentiates the actions of GABA, especially in system and reticular formation

Uses: Anxiety, irritability in psychiatric or organic disorders, preoperatively, insomnia, adjunct in endoscopic procedures

Investigational uses: Antiemetic prior to chemotherapy, status epilepticus, rectal use

Dosage and routes:

Anxiety

• *Adult:* **PO** 2-6 mg/day in divided doses, not to exceed 10 mg/day

• *Geriatric:* **PO** 0.5-1 mg/day in divided doses; or 0.5-1 mg hs

• *Child:* **PO** 0.05 mg/kg/dose, q4-8h

Insomnia

• *Adult:* **PO** 2-4 mg hs; only minimally effective after 2 wk continuous therapy

• *Elderly:* **PO** 1-2 mg initially

Preoperatively

• *Adult:* **IM** 50 mcg/kg 2 hr prior to surgery; **IV** 44 mcg/kg 15-20 min prior to surgery

• *Child:* **IV** 0.05 mg/kg

Status epilepticus

• *Neonate:* **IV** 0.05 mg/kg

• *Child:* **IV** 0.1 mg/kg up to 4 mg/dose; rectal (off label) 0.05-0.1 mg ×2; wait 7 min before giving 2nd dose

Available forms: Tabs 0.5, 1, 2 mg; inj 2, 4 mg/ml; conc sol 2 mg/ml

Side effects/adverse reactions:

CNS: Dizziness, drowsiness, confusion, headache, anxiety, tremors, stimulation, fatigue, depression, insomnia, hallucinations, weakness, unsteadiness

GI: Constipation, dry mouth, nausea, vomiting, anorexia, diarrhea

INTEG: Rash, dermatitis, itching

CV: Orthostatic hypotension, ***ECG changes, tachycardia,*** hypotension; ***apnea, cardiac arrest (IV, rapid)***

EENT: Blurred vision, tinnitus, mydriasis

Contraindications: Hypersensitivity to benzodiazepines, narrow-angle glaucoma, psychosis, pregnancy (D), lactation, child <12 yr, history of drug abuse, COPD

Precautions: Elderly, debilitated, hepatic disease, renal disease

Do not confuse:

lorazepam/alprazolam/clonazepam

Pharmacokinetics:

PO: Onset ½ hr, peak 1-6 hr, duration 24-48 hr

IM: Onset 15-30 min, peak 1-1½ hr, duration 24-48 hr

IV: Onset 5-15 min, peak unknown, duration 24-48 hr

Metabolized by liver; excreted by kidneys; crosses placenta, breast milk; half-life 14 hr

Interactions:

• ↓ lorazepam effects: valproic acid

• ↑ lorazepam effects: CNS depressants, alcohol, disulfiram, oral contraceptives

↑ hypotension: black cohosh

↑ CNS depression: catnip, chamomile, clary, cowslip, hops, kava, lavender, mistletoe, nettle, pokeweed, poppy, Queen Anne's lace, senega, skullcap, valerian

Lab test interferences:

Increase: AST, ALT, serum bilirubin

Decrease: RAIU

False increase: 17-OHCS

NURSING CONSIDERATIONS

Assess:

• B/P (lying, standing), pulse; if systolic B/P drops 20 mm Hg, hold drug, notify prescriber; respirations q5-15min if given IV

• Blood studies: CBC during long-term therapy; blood dyscrasias have occurred rarely

• Hepatic studies: AST, ALT, bilirubin, creatinine, LDH, alk phosphatase

• Mental status: mood, sensorium, affect, sleeping pattern, drowsiness, dizziness

• Physical dependency, withdrawal symptoms: headache, nausea, vomiting, muscle pain, weakness, tremors, convulsions, after long-term, excessive use

⬥ Suicidal tendencies

Administer:

• With food or milk for GI symptoms

• Crushed if patient is unable to swallow medication whole

• Sugarless gum, hard candy, frequent sips of water for dry mouth

• Deep into large muscle mass (IM inj)

IV route

• IV after diluting in equal vol sterile H_2O, 5% dextrose or 0.9% NaCl for inj; give through Y-tube or 3-way stopcock; give at 2 mg or less over 1 min

Syringe compatibilities: Cimetidine, hydromorphone

Y-site compatibilities: Acyclovir, albumin, allopurinol, amifostine, amikacin, amoxicillin, amoxicillin/clavulanate, amphotericin B cholesteryl, amsacrine, atracurium, bumetanide, cefepime, cefmetazole, cefotaxime, ciprofloxacin, cisatracurium, cisplatin, cladribine, clonidine, cyclophosphamide, cytarabine, dexamethasone, diltiazem, DOBUTamine, DOPamine, DOXOrubicin, DOXOrubicin liposome, epINEPHrine, erythromycin, etomidate, famotidine, fentanyl, filgrastim, fluconazole, fludarabine, furosemide, gentamicin, granisetron, haloperidol, heparin, hydrocortisone, hydromorphone, ketanserin, labetalol, melphalan, methotrexate, metronidazole, midazolam, milrinone, morphine, niCARdipine, nitroglycerin, norepinephrine, paclitaxel, pancuronium, piperacillin, piperacillin/tazobactam, potassium chloride, propofol, ranitidine, remifentanil, tacrolimus, teniposide, thiotepa, trimethoprim-sulfamethoxazole, vancomycin, vecuronium, vinorelbine, zidovudine

Perform/provide:

• Assistance with ambulation during beginning therapy, since drowsiness/dizziness occurs

• Check to see if PO medication has been swallowed

• Refrigerate parenteral form

Evaluate:

• Therapeutic response: decreased anxiety, restlessness, insomnia

Teach patient/family:

• That drug may be taken with food

• Not to use drug for everyday stress or used longer than 4 mo unless directed by prescriber

• Not to take more than prescribed amount; may be habit forming

• To avoid OTC preparations (cough, cold, hay fever) unless approved by prescriber

• To avoid driving, activities that require alertness, since drowsiness may occur

• To avoid alcohol ingestion, other psychotropic medications, unless directed by prescriber

• Not to discontinue medication abruptly after long-term use

• To rise slowly or fainting may occur, especially elderly

• That drowsiness may worsen at beginning of treatment

• To use birth control if child-bearing age

Treatment of overdose: Lavage, VS, supportive care, flumazenil

losartan (℞)

(lo-zar′tan)

Cozaar

Func. class.: Antihypertensive

Chem. class.: Angiotensin II receptor (type AT_1)

Action: Blocks the vasoconstrictor

and aldosterone-secreting effects of angiotensin II; selectively blocks the binding of angiotensin II to the AT_1 receptor found in tissues

Uses: Hypertension, alone or in combination, nephropathy in type 2 diabetes, hypertension with left ventricular hypertrophy

Dosage and routes:

Hypertension

• *Adult:* **PO** 50 mg qd alone or 25 mg qd when used in combination with diuretic

Hepatic dose

• *Adult:* **PO** 25 mg qd as starting dose

Hypertension with left ventricular hypertrophy

• *Adult:* **PO** 50 mg qd, add hydrochlorothiazide 12.5 mg/day and/or increase losartan to 100 mg qd, then increase hydrochlorothiazide to 25 mg qd

Nephropathy in type 2 diabetic patients

• *Adult:* **PO** 50 mg qd, may increase to 100 mg qd

Available forms: Tabs 25, 50, 100 mg

Side effects/adverse reactions:

CNS: Dizziness, insomnia, anxiety, confusion, abnormal dreams, migraine, tremor, vertigo, headache

CV: Angina pectoris, 2nd-degree AV block, ***cerebrovascular accident,*** hypotension, ***myocardial infarction,*** *dysrhythmias*

EENT: Blurred vision, burning eyes, conjunctivitis

GI: Diarrhea, dyspepsia, anorexia, constipation, dry mouth, flatulence, gastritis, vomiting

GU: Impotence, nocturia, urinary frequency, UTI, ***renal failure***

HEMA: Anemia

INTEG: Alopecia, dermatitis, dry skin, flushing, photosensitivity, rash, pruritus, sweating

META: Gout

MS: Cramps, myalgia, pain, stiffness

RESP: Cough, upper respiratory infection, congestion, dyspnea, bronchitis

Contraindications: Hypersensitivity, pregnancy (D) 2nd/3rd trimesters

Precautions: Hypersensitivity to ACE inhibitors; pregnancy (C) 1st trimester; lactation, children, elderly

Do not confuse:

Cozaar/Zocor

losartan/valsartan

Pharmacokinetics: Extensively metabolized, half-life 2 hr, metabolite 6-9 hr, highly bound to plasma proteins, excreted in urine and feces

Interactions:

• ↑ lithium toxicity: lithium

• ↓ antihypertensive effect: phenobarbital, rifamycin

• ↑ antihypertensive effect: fluconazole

↑ toxicity, death: aconite

↑ or ↓ antihypertensive effect: astragalus, cola tree

↑ antihypertensive effect: barberry, betony, black catechu, black cohosh, bloodroot, broom, burdock, cat's claw, dandelion, goldenseal, Irish moss, Jamaican dogwood, kelp, khella, mistletoe, parsley

↓ antihypertensive effect: coltsfoot, guarana, khat, licorice

NURSING CONSIDERATIONS

Assess:

• B/P with position changes, pulse q4h; note rate, rhythm, quality

• Electrolytes: K, Na, Cl

• Baselines in renal, hepatic studies before therapy begins

• Edema in feet, legs qd

• Skin turgor, dryness of mucous membranes for hydration status

Administer:

• Without regard to meals

Evaluate:

• Therapeutic response: decreased B/P

Teach patient/family:

• To avoid sunlight or wear sunscreen if in sunlight; photosensitivity may occur

• To comply with dosage schedule, even if feeling better

• To notify prescriber of mouth sores, fever, swelling of hands or feet, irregular heartbeat, chest pain

• That excessive perspiration, dehydration, vomiting, diarrhea may lead to fall in blood pressure; consult prescriber if these occur

• That drug may cause dizziness, fainting; light-headedness may occur

• To rise slowly to sitting or standing position to minimize orthostatic hypotension

• To use contraception while taking this product

lovastatin (℞)

(loh-vah-stat′in)

Altocor, Mevacor

Func. class.: Antilipemic

Chem. class.: HMG-CoA reductase inhibitor

Action: Inhibits HMG-CoA reductase enzyme, which reduces cholesterol synthesis

Uses: As an adjunct in primary hypercholesterolemia (types IIa, IIb), atherosclerosis, primary and secondary prevention of coronary events

Dosage and routes:

• *Adult:* **PO** 20 mg qd with evening meal; may increase to 20-80 mg/day in single or divided doses, not to exceed 80 mg/day; dosage adjustments should be made qmo, reduce dose in renal disease

Available forms: Tabs 10, 20, 40 mg; ext rel tab 10, 20, 40, 60 mg

Side effects/adverse reactions:

GI: Flatus, nausea, constipation, diarrhea, dyspepsia, abdominal pain, heartburn, ***hepatic dysfunction,*** vomiting, acid regurgitation, dry mouth, dysgeusia

MS: Muscle cramps, myalgia, ***myositis, rhabdomyolysis,*** leg, shoulder or localized pain

CNS: Dizziness, headache, tremor, insomnia, paresthesia

INTEG: Rash, pruritus, photosensitivity

HEMA: ***Thrombocytopenia, hemolytic anemia, leukopenia***

EENT: Blurred vision, lens opacities

Contraindications: Hypersensitivity, pregnancy (X), lactation, active liver disease

Precautions: Past hepatic disease, alcoholism, severe acute infections, trauma, hypotension, uncontrolled seizure disorders, severe metabolic disorders, electrolyte imbalances, visual disorder, children

Do not confuse:

lovastatin/Lotensin

Pharmacokinetics:

PO: Peak 2-4 hr, metabolized in liver (metabolites), highly protein bound; excreted in urine 10%, feces 83%; crosses placenta, excreted in breast milk; half-life 3-4 hr

Interactions:

• ↓ effects of lovastatin: bile acid sequestrants

• ↑ myalgia, myositis: cycloSPORINE, gemfibrozil, niacin, erythromycin, clofibrate, azole antifungals

• ↑ bleeding: warfarin

• ↑ effects of: digoxin

• Drug/food: ↑ levels of lovastatin with food, must be taken with food

• Possible toxicity: grapefruit juice

↑ effect: glucomannan

↓ effect: gotu kola

Lab test interferences:
Increase: CPK, LFTs

NURSING CONSIDERATIONS

Assess:

• Diet, obtain diet history including fat, cholesterol in diet
• Fasting cholesterol, LDL, HDL, triglycerides periodically during treatment
• Hepatic studies q1-2mo during the first 1½ yr of treatment; AST, ALT, LFTs may increase
• Renal function in patients with compromised renal system: BUN, creatinine, I&O ratio
• Ophthalmic exam before, 1 mo after treatment begins, annually; lens opacities may occur

For muscle pain, tenderness, obtain CPK; if these occur, drug may need to be discontinued

Administer:

• In evening with meal; if dose is increased, take with breakfast and evening meal

Perform/provide:

• Storage in cool environment in airtight, light-resistant container

Evaluate:

• Therapeutic response: cholesterol at desired level after 8 wk

Teach patient/family:

• To report suspected pregnancy
• That blood work and ophthalmic exam will be necessary during treatment
• To report blurred vision, severe GI symptoms, dizziness, headache, muscle pain, weakness
• To use sunscreen or stay out of the sun to prevent photosensitivity
• That previously prescribed regimen will continue: low-cholesterol diet, exercise program, smoking cessation

loxapine (℞)

(lox′a-peen)

Loxapac♣, loxapine succinate♣, Loxitane, Loxitane IM, Loxitane-C

Func. class.: Antipsychotic, neuroleptic

Chem. class.: Dibenzoxazepine

Action: Depresses cerebral cortex, hypothalamus, limbic system, which control activity and aggression; blocks neurotransmission produced by dopamine at synapse; exhibits strong α-adrenergic, anticholinergic blocking action; mechanism for antipsychotic effects is unclear

Uses: Psychotic disorders, nonpsychotic symptoms associated with dementia

Investigational uses: Depression, anxiety

Dosage and routes:

• *Adult:* **PO** 10 mg bid-qid initially, may be rapidly increased depending on severity of condition, maintenance 60-100 mg/day; **IM** 12.5-50 mg q4-6h or more until desired response, then start **PO** form
• *Geriatric:* **PO** 5-10 mg qd-bid, increase q4-7 days by 5-10 mg, max 125 mg

Available forms: Caps 5, 10, 25, 50 mg; tabs 5, 10, 25, 50 mg; conc 25 mg/ml; inj 50 mg/ml

Side effects/adverse reactions:

RESP: ***Laryngospasm,*** dyspnea, ***respiratory depression***

CNS: EPS: pseudoparkinsonism, akathisia, dystonia, tardive dyskinesia, drowsiness, headache, ***seizures,*** confusion, ***neuroleptic malignant syndrome***

HEMA: ***Anemia, leukopenia, leukocytosis, agranulocytosis***

INTEG: Rash, photosensitivity, dermatitis

EENT: Blurred vision, glaucoma
GI: Dry mouth, nausea, vomiting, anorexia, constipation, diarrhea, jaundice, weight gain
GU: Urinary retention, urinary frequency, enuresis, impotence, amenorrhea, gynecomastia
CV: Orthostatic hypotension, ***cardiac arrest,*** ECG changes, tachycardia

Contraindications: Hypersensitivity, blood dyscrasias, coma, brain damage, bone marrow depression, alcohol and barbiturate withdrawal states, severe CNS depression, narrow-angle glaucoma

Precautions: Pregnancy (C), lactation, seizure disorders, hepatic disease, cardiac disease, prostatic hypertrophy, cardiac conditions, child <16 yr, elderly

Do not confuse:
Loxitane/Soriatane

Pharmacokinetics:
PO: Onset 20-30 min, peak 2-4 hr, duration 12 hr
IM: Onset 15-30 min, peak 15-20 min, duration 12 hr
Metabolized by liver; excreted in urine; crosses placenta; enters breast milk; initial half-life 5 hr; terminal half-life 19 hr

Interactions:
- Toxicity: epINEPHrine
- ↑ EPS: other antipsychotics
- ↓ effects: guanadrel, guanethidine
- ↑ CNS depression: MAOIs, antidepressants, alcohol

↑ CNS depression: chamomile, cola tree, hops, kava, nettle, nutmeg, skullcap, valerian
↑ EPS: betel palm, kava

NURSING CONSIDERATIONS

Assess:
- Mental status before initial administration
- Swallowing of PO medication; check for hoarding or giving of medication to other patients
- I&O ratio; palpate bladder if low urinary output occurs, urinary retention may be the cause
- Bilirubin, CBC, LFTs qmo
- Urinalysis is recommended before and during prolonged therapy
- Affect, orientation, LOC, reflexes, gait, coordination, sleep pattern disturbances
- B/P standing and lying; take pulse and respirations q4h during initial treatment; establish baseline before starting treatment; report drops of 30 mm Hg
- Dizziness, faintness, palpitations, tachycardia on rising
- EPS including akathisia (inability to sit still, no pattern to movements), tardive dyskinesia (bizarre movements of the jaw, mouth, tongue, extremities), pseudoparkinsonism (rigidity, tremors, pill rolling, shuffling gait)

For neuroleptic malignant syndrome: muscle rigidity, increased CPK, altered mental status, hyperthermia

- Constipation, urinary retention qd; if these occur, increase bulk, water in diet

Administer:
- Reduced dose to elderly
- Antiparkinsonian agent if EPS symptoms occur

IM route
- IM inj into large muscle mass

PO route
- Concentrate mixed in orange or grapefruit juice

Perform/provide:
- Decreased sensory input by dimming lights, avoiding loud noises
- Supervised ambulation until stabilized on medication; do not involve in strenuous exercise program because fainting is possible; patient should not stand still for long periods

• Increased fluids to prevent constipation
• Sips of water, candy, gum for dry mouth
• Storage in airtight, light-resistant container

Evaluate:

• Therapeutic response: decrease in emotional excitement, hallucinations, delusions, paranoia; reorganization of patterns of thought, speech

Teach patient/family:

• That orthostatic hypotension may occur and to rise from sitting or lying position gradually
• To remain lying down after IM injection for at least 30 min
• To avoid hot tubs, hot showers, tub baths, as hypotension may occur; that in hot weather heat stroke may occur; take extra precautions to stay cool
• To avoid abrupt withdrawal of this drug, or EPS may result; drug should be withdrawn slowly
• To avoid OTC preparations (cough, hay fever, cold) unless approved by prescriber; serious drug interactions may occur; avoid use with alcohol, CNS depressants; increased drowsiness may occur
• To avoid hazardous activities until stabilized on medication
• To use a sunscreen during sun exposure to prevent burns
• About necessity for meticulous oral hygiene, since oral candidiasis may occur
• To report impaired vision, jaundice, tremors, muscle twitching

Treatment of overdose: Lavage if orally ingested; provide an airway

lymphocyte immune globulin (antithymocyte) (℞)

Atgam

Func. class.: Immune globulins—immunosuppressant

Action: Produces immunosuppression by inhibiting the function of lymphocytes (T)

Uses: Organ transplants to prevent rejection, aplastic anemia

Investigational uses: Multiple sclerosis; myasthenia gravis; immunosuppressant in liver, bone marrow, heart, and other organ transplants; pure red-cell aplasia; scleroderma

Dosage and routes:

Renal allograft

• *Adult:* **IV** 10-30 mg/kg/day
• *Child:* **IV** 5-25 mg/kg/day

Delay of renal allograft rejection

• *Adult:* **IV** 15 mg/kg/day × 14 days, then qod × 14 days for a total of 21 doses in 28 days

Aplastic anemia

• *Adult:* **IV** 10-20 mg/kg/day × 8-14 days

Available forms: Inj 50 mg horse gamma globulin/ml

Side effects/adverse reactions:

Renal transplant

CNS: Fever, chills, headache, dizziness, weakness, faintness, ***seizures***

INTEG: Rash, pruritus, urticaria, wheal

GI: Diarrhea, nausea, vomiting, epigastric pain

CV: Chest pain, hypertension, tachycardia

SYST: ***Anaphylaxis***

Aplastic anemia

CNS: Fever, chills, headache, ***seizures,*** lightheadedness, encephalitis, postviral encephalopathy

CV: Bradycardia, myocarditis, irregularity
GI: Nausea, LFTs abnormality
Contraindications: Hypersensitivity
Precautions: Severe renal disease, severe hepatic disease, pregnancy (C), lactation, children
Pharmacokinetics: Onset rapid, half-life 5.7 days
Interactions: None known

NURSING CONSIDERATIONS
Assess:
- For infection; if infection occurs, evaluation will be needed to continue therapy
- Renal studies: BUN, creatinine at least monthly during treatment, 3 mo after treatment
- Hepatic studies: alk phosphatase, AST, ALT, bilirubin

Administer:
- Do not infuse <4 hr

Aplastic anemia
- Skin testing must be completed prior to treatment; use intradermal inj of 0.1 ml of a 1:1000 dilution (5 mcg horse IgG) in 0.9% NaCl, if a wheal or rash >10 mm or both, use caution during inf
- Dilute in saline sol before inf, invert IV bag, so undiluted drug does not contact the air inside, concentration should not be >1 mg/ml
- Keep emergency equipment nearby for severe allergic reaction

Evaluate:
- Therapeutic response: absence of rejection; hematologic recovery (aplastic anemia)

Teach patient/family:
- To report fever, chills, sore throat, fatigue, since serious infections may occur
- To use contraceptive measures during treatment, for 12 wk after ending therapy

mafenide topical
See appendix c

magaldrate (OTC)
(mag′al-drate)
Losapan✦, Lowsium, Riopan, Riopan Extra Strength✦
Func. class.: Antacid
Chem. class.: Aluminum/magnesium hydroxide

Action: Neutralizes gastric acidity; drug is dissolved in gastric contents; combination of aluminum, magnesium
Uses: Antacid, peptic ulcer disease (adjunct), duodenal, gastric ulcers, reflux esophagitis, hyperacidity, indigestion, heartburn
Dosage and routes:
- *Adult:* **SUSP** 5-10 ml (400-800 mg) with H_2O between meals, hs, not to exceed 100 ml/day

Available forms: Susp 540 mg/5 ml, liquid 540 mg/5 ml
Side effects/adverse reactions:
GI: Constipation, diarrhea
META: Hypermagnesemia, hypophosphatemia
Contraindications: Hypersensitivity to this drug or aluminum
Precautions: Elderly, fluid restriction, decreased GI motility, GI obstruction, dehydration, renal disease, sodium-restricted diets, pregnancy (C)
Pharmacokinetics:
PO: Duration 60 min
Interactions:
- ↓ effectiveness of tetracyclines, ketoconazole
- ↓ absorption of anticholinergics, chlordiazepoxide, cimetidine, corticosteroids, iron salts, phenothiazines, phenytoin, salicylates

M

NURSING CONSIDERATIONS
Assess:
• GI status: location of pain, intensity, characteristics, heartburn, hematemesis
• Serum magnesium levels with impaired renal function; calcium, phosphate, potassium if using long term
• Constipation: increase bulk in diet if needed
Administer:
• Laxatives or stool softeners if constipation occurs
• After shaking; give between meals and hs
Evaluate:
• Therapeutic response: absence of pain, decreased acidity
Teach patient/family:
• To separate enteric-coated drugs and antacid by 2 hr
• To notify prescriber immediately of coffee-ground emesis, emesis with frank blood, black tarry stools

RARELY USED

magnesium salicylate (OTC, ℞)

Doan's Pills, Magan, Mobidin
Func. class.: Nonopioid analgesic, nonsteroidal antiinflammatory

Uses: Mild to moderate pain or fever including arthritis, juvenile rheumatoid arthritis
Dosage and routes:
Arthritis
• *Adult:* **PO** not to exceed 4.8 g/day in divided doses
Pain/fever
• *Adult:* **PO** 600 mg tid or qid
Available forms: Tabs 325, 500, 545, 600 mg
Contraindications: Hypersensitivity to salicylates, GI bleeding, bleeding disorders, children <12 yr, vit K deficiency, pregnancy (D) 1st trimester

magnesium salts

(mag-nee'zee-um)

magnesium chloride (℞)

Chloromag, Slo-Mag

magnesium citrate (OTC)

citrate of magnesia, Citroma, CitroMag♣, Evac-Q-Mag

magnesium gluconate
magtrate, mag-g
magnesium oxide (OTC)

Mag-Ox 400, Maox, Uro-Mag

magnesium hydroxide (OTC)

Phillips' Magnesium Tablets, Phillips' Milk of Magnesia, MOM

magnesium sulfate (OTC, ℞)

epsom salts
Func. class.: Electrolyte; anticonvulsant; saline laxative, antacid

Action: Increases osmotic pressure, draws fluid into colon, neutralizes HCl
Uses: Constipation, bowel preparation before surgery or exam, anticonvulsant in preeclampsia, eclampsia (magnesium sulfate), electrolyte
Dosage and routes:
Laxative
• *Adult:* **PO** 30-60 ml hs (Milk of Magnesia), 300 mg
• *Adult and child >6 yr:* **PO** 15 g in 8 oz H_2O (magnesium sulfate); **PO** 10-20 ml (Concentrated Milk of

Magnesia); **PO** 5-10 oz hs (magnesium citrate)
• *Child 2-6 yr:* 5-15 ml/day (Milk of Magnesia)
Prevention of magnesium deficiency
• *Adult and child ≥10 yr:* **PO** male: 350-400 mg/day; female: 280-300 mg/day; lactation: 335-350 mg/day; pregnancy 320 mg/day
• *Child 8-10 yr:* **PO** 170 mg/day
• *Child 4-7 yr:* **PO** 120 mg/day
• *Child infant to 4 yr:* 40-80 mg/day
Magnesium sulfate
Deficiency
• *Adult:* **PO** 200-400 mg in divided doses tid-qid; **IM** 1 g q6h × 4 doses; **IV** 5 g (severe)
• *Child 6-12 yr:* 3-6 mg/kg/day in divided doses tid-qid
Pre-eclampsia/eclampsia magnesium sulfate
• *Adult:* **IM/IV** 4-5 g **IV inf;** with 5 g **IM** in each gluteus, then 5 g q4h or 4 g **IV inf,** then 1-2 g/hr **cont inf**
Available forms:
• Chloride: sus rel tabs 535 mg (64 mg Mg) enteric tabs 833 mg (100 mg Mg)
• Hydroxide: Liq 400 mg/5 ml; conc liq 800 mg/5 ml; chew tabs 300, 600 mg
• Oxide: Tabs 200, 400 mg; caps 140 mg
• Sulfate: Powder for oral; bulk packages; epsom salts, bulk packages; inj 10%, 12.5%, 25%, 50%
Side effects/adverse reactions:
CNS: Muscle weakness, flushing, sweating, confusion, sedation, depressed reflexes, ***flaccid paralysis,*** hypothermia
GI: Nausea, vomiting, anorexia, cramps
CV: Hypotension, heart block, ***circulatory collapse***
RESP: Respiratory depression
META: Electrolyte, fluid imbalances
Contraindications: Hypersensitivity, abdominal pain, nausea/vomiting, obstruction, acute surgical abdomen, rectal bleeding
Precautions: Pregnancy (A); (B) magnesium sulfate, renal disease, cardiac disease
Pharmacokinetics:
PO: Onset 3-6 hr
IM: Onset 1 hr, duration 4 hr
IV: Duration ½ hr
Excreted by kidney, effective anticonvulsant serum levels 2.5-7.5 mEq/L
Interactions:
• ↑ effect of neuromuscular blockers
• ↓ absorption of tetracyclines, aminoquinolones, nitrofurantoin

NURSING CONSIDERATIONS
Assess:
• I&O ratio; check for decrease in urinary output
• Cause of constipation; lack of fluids, bulk, exercise
• Cramping, rectal bleeding, nausea, vomiting; drug should be discontinued
• Magnesium toxicity: thirst, confusion, decrease in reflexes
Administer:
• With 8 oz H_2O
• Refrigerate magnesium citrate before giving
• Shake susp before using as antacid at least 2 hr pc
IV route
• Only when calcium gluconate available for magnesium toxicity
• IV undiluted 1.5 ml of 10% sol over 1 min; may dilute to 20% sol, infuse over 3 hr
• IV at less than 150 mg/min; circulatory collapse may occur
Additive compatibilities: Cephalothin, chloramphenicol, cisplatin, heparin, hydrocortisone, isoproterenol, meropenem, methyldopate, norepinephrine, penicillin G potas-

M

sium, potassium phosphate, verapamil

Y-site compatibilities: Acyclovir, aldesleukin, amifostine, amikacin, ampicillin, aztreonam, cefamandole, cefazolin, cefmetazole, cefoperazone, cefotaxime, cefoxitin, cephalothin, cephapirin, chloramphenicol, cisatracurium, DOBUTamine, doxycycline, DOXOrubicin liposome, enalaprilat, erythromycin, esmolol, famotidine, fludarabine, gallium, gentamicin, granisetron, heparin, hydromorphone, idarubicin, insulin, kanamycin, labetalol, meperidine, metronidazole, minocycline, morphine, moxalactam, nafcillin, ondansetron, oxacillin, paclitaxel, penicillin G potassium, piperacillin, piperacillin/tazobactam, potassium chloride, propofol, remifentanil, sargramostim, thiotepa, ticarcillin, tobramycin, trimethoprim-sulfamethoxazole, vancomycin, vit B complex/C

Evaluate:
- Therapeutic response: decreased constipation

Teach patient/family:
- Not to use laxatives for long-term therapy; bowel tone will be lost
- That chilling helps the taste of magnesium citrate
- To shake suspension well
- To not give at hs as a laxative; may interfere with sleep
- To give citrus fruit after administering to counteract unpleasant taste

mannitol (℞)

(man′i-tole)

mannitol, Osmitrol, Resectisol

Func. class.: Diuretic, osmotic

Chem. class.: Hexahydric alcohol

Action: Acts by increasing osmolarity of glomerular filtrate, which raises osmotic pressure of fluid in renal tubules; decrease in reabsorption of water, electrolytes; increase in urinary output, sodium, chloride excretion

Uses: Edema, promote systemic diuresis in cerebral edema, decrease intraocular pressure, improve renal function in acute renal failure, chemical poisoning

Dosage and routes:

Oliguria, prevention
- *Adult:* **IV** 50-100 g 5%-25% sol, may use test dose 0.2 g/kg over 3-5 min

Oliguria, treatment
- *Adult:* **IV** 300-400 mg/kg 20%-25% sol up to 100 g 15%-20% sol, run over 30-60 min
- *Child:* **IV** 0.25-2 g/kg as 15%-20% sol run over 2-6 hr

Intraocular pressure/intracranial pressure
- *Adult:* **IV** 1½-2 g/kg 15%-25% sol over ½-1 hr
- *Child:* **IV** 1-2 g/kg (30-60 g/m^2) as 15%-20% sol run over ½-1 hr

Renal failure
- *Adult:* **IV** 50-200 g/24 hr, adjusted to maintain output of 30-50 mg/hr

Diuresis in drug intoxication
- *Adult and child >12 yr:* 5%-10% sol continuously up to 200 g **IV,** while maintaining 100-500 ml urine output/hr

Available forms: Inj 5%, 10%, 15%, 20%, 25%; GU irrigation: 5%

Side effects/adverse reactions:

GU: Marked diuresis, urinary retention, thirst

CNS: Dizziness, headache, ***convulsions, rebound increased ICP,*** confusion

GI: Nausea, vomiting, dry mouth, diarrhea

CV: Edema, thrombophlebitis, hypotension, hypertension, ***tachycar-***

dia, angina-like chest pains, fever, chills, ***CHF***
RESP: Pulmonary congestion
ELECT: Fluid, electrolyte imbalances, *acidosis,* electrolyte loss, dehydration
EENT: Loss of hearing, blurred vision, nasal congestion, decreased intraocular pressure
Contraindications: Active intracranial bleeding, hypersensitivity, anuria, severe pulmonary congestion, edema, severe dehydration, progressive heart, renal failure
Precautions: Dehydration, pregnancy (C), severe renal disease, CHF, lactation
Pharmacokinetics:
IV: Onset 30-60 min for diuresis, ½-1 hr for intraocular pressure, 25 min for cerebrospinal fluid; duration 4-6 hr for intraocular pressure, 3-8 hr for cerebrospinal fluid; excreted in urine, half-life 100 min
Interactions:
- ↓ effect: lithium
- Drug/food: potassium foods: ↑ hyperkalemia

Lab test interferences:
Interference: Inorganic phosphorus, ethylene glycol

NURSING CONSIDERATIONS
Assess:
- Weight, I&O qd to determine fluid loss; effect of drug may be decreased if used qd; output qh prn
- Rate, depth, rhythm of respiration, effect of exertion
- B/P lying, standing; postural hypotension may occur
- Electrolytes: K, Na, Cl; include BUN, CBC, serum creatinine, blood pH, ABGs, CVP, PAP
- Signs of metabolic acidosis: drowsiness, restlessness
- Signs of hypokalemia: postural hypotension, malaise, fatigue, tachycardia, leg cramps, weakness
- Rashes, temp qd
- Confusion, especially in elderly; take safety precautions if needed
- Hydration including skin turgor, thirst, dry mucous membranes
- For blurred vision, pain in eyes, before and during treatment (increased intraocular pressure); neurologic checks, intracranial pressure during treatment (increased intracranial pressure)

Administer:
IV route
- In 15%-25% sol with filter; give over ½-1½ hr; rapid infusion may worsen CHF; warm in hot water and shake to dissolve crystals
- Test dose in severe oliguria, 0.2 g/kg over 3-5 min; if no urine increase, give second test dose; if no response, reassess patient

Irrigation
- 100 ml of 25%/900 ml of sterile water for inj (2.5% sol)

Additive compatibilities: Amikacin, bretylium, cefamandole, cefoxitin, cimetidine, cisplatin, DOPamine, fosphenytoin, furosemide, gentamicin, metoclopramide, netilmicin, nizatidine, ofloxacin, ondansetron, sodium bicarbonate, tobramycin, verapamil
Y-site compatibilities: Allopurinol, amifostine, amphotericin B cholesteryl, aztreonam, cisatracurium, cladribine, fludarabine, fluorouracil, gallium, idarubicin, melphalan, ondansetron, paclitaxel, piperacillin, propofol, remifentanil, sargramostim, teniposide, thiotepa, vinorelbine
Evaluate:
- Therapeutic response: improvement in edema of feet, legs, sacral area daily if medication is being used in CHF; decreased intraocular pressure, prevention of hypokalemia, increased excretion of toxic substances; decreased ICP

M

Teach patient/family:
• To rise slowly from lying or sitting position
• The reason for and method of treatment

Treatment of overdose: Discontinue infusion; correct fluid, electrolyte imbalances; hemodialysis; monitor hydration, CV, renal function

mebendazole (℞)

(me-ben′da-zole)
Vermox
Func. class.: Anthelmintic
Chem. class.: Carbamate

Action: Inhibits glucose uptake, degeneration of cytoplasmic microtubules in the cell; interferes with absorption, secretory function

Uses: Pinworms, roundworms, hookworms, whipworms, threadworms, pork tapeworms, dwarf tapeworms, beef tapeworms, hydatid cyst

Dosage and routes:
• *Adult and child >2 yr:* **PO** 100 mg as a single dose (pinworms) or bid × 3 days (whipworms, roundworms, or hookworms); course may be repeated in 3 wk if needed

Available forms: Tabs, chew 100 mg

Side effects/adverse reactions:
CNS: Dizziness, fever, headache
GI: Transient diarrhea, abdominal pain, nausea, vomiting

Contraindications: Hypersensitivity

Precautions: Child <2 yr, lactation, pregnancy (C) (1st trimester)

Pharmacokinetics:
PO: Peak ½-7 hr; excreted in feces primarily (metabolites), small amount in urine (unchanged); highly bound to plasma proteins 95%

Interactions:
• ↓ mebendazole effect: carbamazepine, hydantoins
• Drug/food: ↑ absorption: high-fat meal

NURSING CONSIDERATIONS

Assess:
• Stools during entire treatment; specimens must be sent to lab while still warm, also 1-3 wk after treatment is completed
• For allergic reaction: rash (rare)
• For diarrhea during expulsion of worms; avoid self-contamination with patient's feces
• For infection in other family members, since infection from person to person is common
• Blood studies: AST, ALT, alk phosphatase, BUN, CBC during treatment

Administer:
• May be crushed, chewed, swallowed whole, mixed with food
• PO after meals to avoid GI symptoms, since absorption is not altered by food
• Second course after 3 wk if needed; usually recommended

Perform/provide:
• Storage in tight container

Evaluate:
• Therapeutic response: expulsion of worms and 3 negative stool cultures after completion of treatment

Teach patient/family:
• Proper hygiene after BM, including hand-washing technique; tell patient to avoid putting fingers in mouth; clean fingernails
• That infected person should sleep alone; do not shake bed linen, change bed linen qd, wash in hot water, change and wash undergarments daily
• To clean toilet qd with disinfectant (green soap solution)
• The need for compliance with dosage schedule, duration of treatment

• To wear shoes, wash all fruits and vegetables well before eating; use commercial fruit/vegetable cleaner
• That all members of the family should be treated (pinworms)

mechlorethamine (℞)

(me-klor-eth'a-meen)
Mustargen, nitrogen mustard
Func. class.: Antineoplastic alkylating agent
Chem. class.: Nitrogen mustard

Action: Responsible for cross-linking DNA strands leading to cell death; rapidly degraded, a vesicant; activity is not cell cycle phase-specific

Uses: Hodgkin's disease, leukemias, lymphomas, lymphosarcoma; ovarian, breast, lung carcinoma; neoplastic effusions

Dosage and routes:
• *Adult:* **IV** 0.4 mg/kg or 10 mg/m^2 as 1 dose or 2-4 divided doses over 2-4 days; second course after 3 wk depending on blood cell count

Neoplastic effusions
• *Adult:* **INTRACAVITARY** 0.4 mg/kg, may be 200-400 mcg/kg

Available forms: Inj 10 mg

Side effects/adverse reactions:
EENT: Tinnitus, hearing loss
HEMA: ***Thrombocytopenia, leukopenia, agranulocytosis,*** anemia
GI: Nausea, vomiting, diarrhea, stomatitis, weight loss, colitis, ***hepatotoxicity***
CNS: Headache, dizziness, drowsiness, paresthesia, peripheral neuropathy, ***coma***
INTEG: Alopecia, pruritus, herpes zoster, extravasation

Contraindications: Lactation, pregnancy (D), myelosuppression, acute herpes zoster

Precautions: Radiation therapy, chronic lymphocytic leukopenia

Pharmacokinetics: Metabolized in liver, excreted in urine

Interactions:
• ↑ bleeding: aspirin, anticoagulants
• ↑ toxicity: antineoplastics, radiation
• Blood dyscrasias: amphotericin B
• ↓ antibody reaction: live virus vaccines

NURSING CONSIDERATIONS

Assess:
• CBC, differential, platelet count qwk; withhold drug if WBC is <1000/mm^3 or platelet count is <75,000/mm^3; notify prescriber, recovery of WBCs, platelets within 20 days
• Renal function tests: BUN, serum uric acid, urine CCr before, during therapy
• I&O ratio; report fall in urine output of 30 ml/hr
• Monitor temp q4h (may indicate beginning infection); no rectal temps
• Hepatic studies before, during therapy (bilirubin, AST, ALT, LDH) as needed or monthly
• Bleeding: hematuria, guaiac, bruising or petechiae, mucosa or orifices q8h
• Jaundiced skin and sclera, dark urine, clay-colored stools, itchy skin, abdominal pain, fever, diarrhea
• Effects of alopecia on body image; discuss feelings about body changes
• Buccal cavity q8h for dryness, sores, ulceration, white patches, oral pain, bleeding, dysphagia
• Local irritation, pain, burning, discoloration at inj site
⬥ Symptoms indicating severe allergic reaction: rash, pruritus, urticaria, purpuric skin lesions, itching, flushing

Administer:
- After using guidelines for preparation of cytotoxic drugs
- Antiemetic 30-60 min before giving drug and prn
- IV after diluting 10 mg/10 ml sterile H_2O or NaCl; leave needle in vial, shake, withdraw dose, give through Y-tube or 3-way stopcock or directly over 3-5 min
- Watch for infiltration; infiltrate area with isotonic sodium thiosulfate or 1% lidocaine; apply ice for 6-12 hr
- Topical or systemic analgesics for pain
- Local or systemic drugs for infection

Y-site compatibilities: Amifostine, aztreonam, filgrastim, fludarabine, granisetron, melphalan, ondansetron, sargramostim, teniposide, vinorelbine

Perform/provide:
- Storage at room temperature in dry form
- Increase fluid intake to 2-3 L/day to prevent urate deposits, calculi formation
- Diet low in purines: organ meats (kidney, liver), dried beans, peas to maintain alkaline urine
- Preparation under hood using gloves and mask
- Rinsing of mouth tid-qid with water, club soda; brushing of teeth bid-tid with soft brush or cotton-tipped applicators for stomatitis; use unwaxed dental floss
- Warm compresses at inj site for inflammation

Evaluate:
- Therapeutic response: decreased tumor size, spread of malignancy

Teach patient/family:
- The rationale for and techniques of protective isolation
- That sterility, amenorrhea can occur; reversible after discontinuing treatment
- That hair may be lost during treatment; a wig or hairpiece may make patient feel better; new hair may be different in color, texture
- To avoid foods with citric acid, hot or rough texture
- To report any bleeding, white spots, or ulcerations in mouth to prescriber; tell patient to examine mouth qd
- To report signs of infection: fever, sore throat, flulike symptoms
- To report signs of anemia: fatigue, headache, faintness, shortness of breath, irritability
- To avoid use of razors, commercial mouthwash
- To avoid use of aspirin products, NSAIDs
- To notify prescriber if pregnancy is suspected; to use contraception during treatment

meclizine (OTC, ℞)

(mek'li-zeen)

Antivert, Antrizine, Bonamine✤, Bonine, Dramamine Less Drowsy Formula, meclizine HCl, Meni-D, Vergan

Func. class.: Antiemetic, antihistamine, anticholinergic

Chem. class.: H_1-Receptor antagonist, piperazine derivative

Action: Acts centrally by blocking chemoreceptor trigger zone, which in turn acts on vomiting center

Uses: Vertigo, motion sickness

Dosage and routes:
- *Adult:* **PO** 25-100 mg qd in divided doses or 1 hr before traveling

Available forms: Tabs 12.5, 25, 50 mg; chew tabs 25 mg; caps 15, 25, 30 mg

Side effects/adverse reactions:
CNS: Drowsiness, fatigue, restlessness, headache, insomnia
CV: Hypotension
GU: Urinary retention
GI: Nausea, anorexia
EENT: Dry mouth, blurred vision
Contraindications: Hypersensitivity to cyclizines, shock
Precautions: Children, narrow-angle glaucoma, glaucoma, urinary retention, lactation, prostatic hypertrophy, elderly, pregnancy (B), CV disease, hypertension, seizure disease
Pharmacokinetics:
PO: Duration 8-24 hr, half-life 6 hr
Interactions:
• ↑ effect of alcohol, opioids, other CNS depressants
↑ anticholinergic effect: corkwood, henbane leaf
↑ sedative effect: hops, Jamaican dogwood, khat, senega
Lab test interferences:
False negative: Allergy skin testing

NURSING CONSIDERATIONS

Assess:
• VS, B/P
Signs of toxicity of other drugs or masking of symptoms of disease: brain tumor, intestinal obstruction
• Observe for drowsiness, dizziness, level of consciousness

Administer:

PO route
• Tablets may be swallowed whole, chewed, or allowed to dissolve; give with food to decrease GI upset
• Lowest possible dose in elderly, anticholinergic effects

Evaluate:
• Therapeutic response: absence of dizziness, vomiting

Teach patient/family:
• That a false-negative result may occur with skin testing for allergies; these procedures should not be scheduled for 4 days after discontinuing use
• To avoid hazardous activities, activities requiring alertness; dizziness may occur; instruct patient to request assistance with ambulation
• To avoid alcohol, other depressants

*medroxyPROGESTERone (℞)

(me-drox'ee-proe-jess'te-rone)
Amen, Curretab, Cycrin, Depo-Provera, medroxyPROGESTERone, Provera
Func. class.: Antineoplastic, hormone, contraceptive
Chem. class.: Progesterone derivative

Action: Inhibits secretion of pituitary gonadotropins, which prevents follicular maturation and ovulation; stimulates growth of mammary tissue; antineoplastic action against endometrial cancer
Uses: Uterine bleeding (abnormal), secondary amenorrhea, endometrial cancer, renal cancer, contraceptive, prevent endometrial changes associated with estrogen replacement therapy (ERT)
Investigational uses: Pickwickian syndrome, sleep apnea, hypersomnolence
Dosage and routes:
Secondary amenorrhea
• *Adult:* **PO** 5-10 mg qd × 5-10 days
Endometrial/renal cancer
• *Adult:* **IM** 400-1000 mg/wk may repeat qwk, dose may be decreased after adequate response
Uterine bleeding
• *Adult:* **PO** 5-10 mg qd × 5-10 days starting on 16th or 21st day of menstrual cycle

Contraceptive
- *Adult:* **IM** 150 mg q3mo

With ERT
- *Adult:* **PO** monophasic 2.5 mg qd; Biphasic 5 mg days 15-28 of cycle

Available forms: Tabs 2.5, 5, 10 mg; inj susp 50, 100, 150, 400 mg/ml

Side effects/adverse reactions:
CNS: Dizziness, headache, migraines, depression, fatigue
CV: Hypotension, thrombophlebitis, edema, ***thromboembolism, stroke, pulmonary embolism, MI***
GI: Nausea, vomiting, anorexia, cramps, increased weight, ***cholestatic jaundice***
EENT: Diplopia
GU: Amenorrhea, cervical erosion, breakthrough bleeding, dysmenorrhea, vaginal candidiasis, breast changes, *gynecomastia, testicular atrophy, impotence,* endometriosis, ***spontaneous abortion***
INTEG: Rash, urticaria, acne, hirsutism, alopecia, oily skin, seborrhea, purpura, melasma, photosensitivity
META: Hyperglycemia
SYST: ***Angioedema, anaphylaxis***

Contraindications: Breast cancer, hypersensitivity, thromboembolic disorders, reproductive cancer, genital bleeding (abnormal, undiagnosed), pregnancy (X)

Precautions: Lactation, hypertension, asthma, blood dyscrasias, gallbladder disease, CHF, diabetes mellitus, bone disease, depression, migraine headache, convulsive disorders, hepatic disease, renal disease, family history of cancer of breast or reproductive tract

Do not confuse:
Amen/Ambien
medroxyPROGESTERone/methylPREDNISolone
Provera/Premarin

Pharmacokinetics:
PO: Duration 24 hr, excreted in urine and feces, metabolized in liver

Lab test interferences:
Increase: Alk phosphatase, sodium (urine), pregnanediol, amino acids
Decrease: GTT, HDL

NURSING CONSIDERATIONS

Assess:
- Symptoms indicating severe allergic reaction, angioedema, have epINEPHrine and rescusiative equipment available
- Weight qd; notify prescriber of weekly weight gain >5 lb
- B/P at beginning of treatment and periodically
- I&O ratio; be alert for decreasing urinary output, increasing edema
- Hepatic studies: ALT, AST, bilirubin, periodically during long-term therapy
- Edema, hypertension, cardiac symptoms, jaundice
- Mental status: affect, mood, behavioral changes, depression

Administer:
- Titrated dose; use lowest effective dose
- Oil solution deep in large muscle mass (IM), rotate sites
- With food or milk to decrease GI symptoms (PO)

Perform/provide:
- Storage in dark area

Evaluate:
- Therapeutic response: decreased abnormal uterine bleeding, absence of amenorrhea, decrease in size and growth of tumor

Teach patient/family:
- To avoid sunlight or use sunscreen; photosensitivity can occur
- About cushingoid symptoms
- To report breast lumps, vaginal bleeding, edema, jaundice, dark urine, clay-colored stools, dyspnea, headache, blurred vision, abdominal pain, numbness or stiffness in legs, chest pain; male to report impotence or gynecomastia
- To report suspected pregnancy

medrysone ophthalmic

See appendix c

megestrol (℞)

(me-jess'trole)

Megace, megestrol

Func. class.: Antineoplastic hormone

Chem. class.: Progestin

Action: Affects endometrium by antiluteinizing effect; this is thought to bring about cell death

Uses: Breast, endometrial cancer, renal cell cancer; cachexia anorexia weight loss in AIDs

Dosage and routes:

Endometrial/ovarian carcinoma

• *Adult:* **PO** 40-320 mg/day in divided doses

Breast carcinoma

• *Adult:* **PO** 40 mg qid or 160 mg qd

Anorexia (AIDS)

• *Adult:* **PO** 800 mg qd (oral susp)

Hot flashes (off label)

• *Adult:* **PO** 20 mg qd

Available forms: Tabs 20, 40 mg; oral susp 40 mg/ml

Side effects/adverse reactions:

GI: Nausea, vomiting, diarrhea, abdominal cramps, weight gain

GU: Gynecomastia, fluid retention, hypercalcemia, vaginal bleeding, discharge, impotence, decreased libido

CV: ***Thrombophlebitis, thromboembolism***

INTEG: Alopecia, rash, pruritus, purpura, itching

CNS: Mood swings

Contraindications: Hypersensitivity, pregnancy D (tabs); X (susp)

Do not confuse:

Megace/Reglan

Pharmacokinetics:

PO: Duration 1-3 days, half-life 60 min; metabolized in liver; excreted in feces, breast milk

Lab test interferences:

Increase: Alk phosphatase, urinary sodium, urinary pregnanediol, plasma amino acids

False positive: Urine glucose

Decrease: HDL, glucose tolerance test

NURSING CONSIDERATIONS

Assess:

• I&O ratio; weights

• Effects of alopecia on body image; discuss feelings about body changes

◆ Symptoms indicating severe allergic reaction: rash, pruritus, urticaria, purpuric skin lesions, itching, flushing

• Frequency of stools, characteristics: cramping, acidosis, signs of dehydration (rapid respirations, poor skin turgor, decreased urine output, dry skin, restlessness, weakness)

• Anorexia, nausea, vomiting, constipation, weakness, loss of muscle tone

◆ Thrombophlebitis: Homans' sign, edema, pain in calf, thigh, notify prescriber immediately

Administer:

• Oral susp for AIDS patients; shake well

• Tablets for carcinoma

Perform/provide:

• Nutritious diet with iron, vitamin supplements as ordered

• Storage in tight container at room temperature

Evaluate:

• Therapeutic response: decreased tumor size, spread of malignancy; weight gain in AIDS patients

Teach patient/family:

• To report vaginal bleeding

- That nonhormonal contraception should be used during and 4 mo after treatment
- That gynecomastia can occur; reversible after discontinuing treatment

◆ To recognize and report signs of fluid retention, thromboemboli and report immediately

meloxicam (℞)

(mel-ox'i-kam)

Mobic

Func. class.: Nonsteroidal antiinflammatory/nonopioid analgesic (NSAIDs)

Chem. class.: Oxicam

Action: Inhibits prostaglandin synthesis by decreasing an enzyme needed for biosynthesis; analgesic, antiinflammatory, antipyretic effects

Uses: Osteoarthritis

Dosage and routes:

- *Adult:* **PO** 7.5 mg qd, may increase to 15 mg qd

Available forms: Tabs 7.5 mg

Side effects/adverse reactions:

CV: Hypertension, angina, ***cardiac failure, MI,*** hypotension, palpitations, ***dysrhythmias,*** tachycardia

CNS: Dizziness, drowsiness, tremors, headache, nervousness, malaise, fatigue, insomnia, depression, ***seizures***

EENT: Tinnitus, hearing loss

GI: Pancreatitis, nausea, colitis, GERD, vomiting, diarrhea, constipation, flatulence, cramps, dry mouth, peptic ulcer, ***GI bleeding, perforation***

GU: ***Nephrotoxicity: dysuria, hematuria, oliguria, azotemia***

HEMA: ***Blood dyscrasias,*** anemia, prolonged bleeding

INTEG: Rash, urticaria, photosensitivity

SYST: ***Angioedema, anaphylaxis***

Contraindications: Hypersensitivity, asthma, severe renal disease, severe hepatic disease, peptic ulcer disease, L&D, lactation, CV bleeding; avoid in 2nd/3rd trimester

Precautions: Pregnancy (C), children, bleeding disorders, GI disorders, cardiac disorders, hypersensitivity to other antiinflammatory agents, elderly, CCr <25 ml/min

Pharmacokinetics:

PO: Peak 4-5 hr

IM: Peak 50 min, half-life 6 hr, enters breast milk, <50% metabolized by liver, excreted by kidneys

Interactions:

- ↑ meloxicam action: phenytoin, sulfonamides, salicylates
- ↓ meloxicam action: cholestyramine
- ↑ action of: aminoglycosides, hydantoins, diuretics, anticoagulants
- ↓ action of: β-blockers
- Nephrotoxicity: cycloSPORINE

🍃 ↑ gastric irritation: arginine, gossypol

🍃 ↑ NSAIDs effect: bearberry, bilberry

🍃 ↑ bleeding risk: bogbean, chondroitin

NURSING CONSIDERATIONS

Assess:

- Renal, hepatic, blood studies: BUN, creatinine, AST, ALT, Hgb before treatment, periodically thereafter
- Bleeding times; check for bruising, bleeding; test for occult blood in urine

◆ For anaphylaxis and angioedema; emergency equipment should be nearby

◆ Hepatic dysfunction: jaundice, yellow sclera and skin, clay-colored stools

• Audiometric, ophthalmic exam before, during, after treatment
• GI condition, hypertension, cardiac conditions

Administer:
• May take without regard to meals, to take with food for GI upset
• Take with full glass of water and sit upright for ½ hr

Perform/provide:
• Storage at room temperature

Evaluate:
• Therapeutic response: decreased pain, stiffness, swelling in joints, ability to move more easily

Teach patient/family:
• To report blurred vision or ringing, roaring in ears (may indicate toxicity)
• To avoid driving, other hazardous activities if dizziness or drowsiness occurs
• To report change in urine pattern, weight increase, edema, pain increase in joints, fever, blood in urine (indicates nephrotoxicity); to report rash, black stools, or continuing headache
• To avoid alcohol, aspirin, acetaminophen without consulting prescriber

---

HIGH ALERT

melphalan (℞)
(mel'fa-lan)
Alkeran, L-PAM, phenylalanine mustard
Func. class.: Antineoplastic, alkylating agent
Chem. class.: Nitrogen mustard

Action: Responsible for cross-linking DNA strands leading to cell death; activity is not cell cycle phase specific

Uses: Multiple myeloma, malignant melanoma, advanced ovarian cancer

Investigational uses: Breast, testicular, prostate carcinoma; osteogenic sarcoma, chronic myelogenous leukemia

Dosage and routes:
Multiple myeloma
• *Adult:* **PO** 150 mcg/kg/day × 1 wk, then 21 days after, then 50 mcg/kg/day or 100-150 mcg/kg/day or 250 mcg/kg/day × 4 days for 2-3 wk, then 2-4 wk after, then 2-4 mg/day or 7 mg/m^2 × 5 day q5-6wk
• *Adult:* **IV INF** 16 mg/m^2, reduce in renal insufficiency, give over 15-20 min, give at 2 wk intervals × 4 doses, then at 4 wk intervals
Ovarian carcinoma
• *Adult:* **PO** 200 mcg/kg/day for 5 days q4-5wk

Available forms: Tabs 2 mg, powder for inj 50 mg

Side effects/adverse reactions:
HEMA: ***Thrombocytopenia, neutropenia, leukopenia,*** anemia
GI: Nausea, vomiting, stomatitis, diarrhea
GU: Amenorrhea, hyperuricemia, gonadal suppression
INTEG: Rash, urticaria, alopecia, pruritus
RESP: ***Fibrosis, dysplasia***
SYST: ***Anaphylaxis,*** allergic reactions

Contraindications: Lactation, pregnancy (D), hypersensitivity to this drug or other nitrogen mustards

Precautions: Radiation therapy, bone marrow depression, infections, renal disease, children

Do not confuse:
melphalan/Myleran

Pharmacokinetics: Metabolized in liver, excreted in urine, half-life 1½ hr

Interactions:
• ↑ toxicity: antineoplastics, radiation

M

• ↓ antibody response: live virus vaccines
• ↑ pulmonary toxicity: carmustine
• ↑ renal failure risk: cycloSPORINE
• ↑ enterocolitis risk: nalidixic acid

NURSING CONSIDERATIONS

Assess:

• CBC, differential, platelet count qwk; withhold drug if WBC is <3000/mm^3 or platelet count is <100,000/mm^3; notify prescriber; recovery usually occurs in 6 wk
• Renal studies: BUN, serum uric acid, urine CCr before, during therapy
• I&O ratio; report fall in urine output to 30 ml/hr
• For infection: fever, cough, temp, sore throat, notify prescriber
• For bleeding: bruising, blood in urine, stools, emesis
• Hepatic studies before, during therapy (bilirubin, AST, ALT, LDH) as needed or monthly
• Bleeding: hematuria, guaiac, bruising or petechiae, mucosa or orifices q8h
• Jaundiced skin and sclera, dark urine, clay-colored stools, itchy skin, abdominal pain, fever, diarrhea
• Buccal cavity q8h for dryness, sores, ulceration, white patches, oral pain, bleeding, dysphagia
• Local irritation, pain, burning, discoloration at inj site
Symptoms indicating severe allergic reaction: rash, pruritus, urticaria, purpuric skin lesions, itching, flushing; assess allergy to chlorambucil, cross-sensitivity may occur

Administer:

• Antiemetic 30-60 min before giving drug to prevent vomiting

IV route

• Give by intermittent inf after reconstituting with 10 ml diluent provided (5 mg/ml), shake, dilute dose with 0.9% NaCl (≤0.45 mg/ml), give within 1 hr, run over ≥15 min

Y-site compatibilities: Acyclovir, amikacin, aminophylline, ampicillin, aztreonam, bleomycin, bumetanide, buprenorphine, butorphanol, calcium gluconate, carboplatin, carmustine, cefazolin, cefepime, cefoperazone, cefotaxime, cefotetan, ceftazidime, ceftizoxime, ceftriaxone, cefuroxime, cimetidine, cisplatin, clindamycin, cyclophosphamide, cytarabine, dacarbazine, dactinomycin, DAUNOrubicin, dexamethasone, diphenhydrAMINE, DOXOrubicin, doxycycline, droperidol, enalaprilat, etoposide, famotidine, floxuridine, fluconazole, fludarabine, fluorouracil, furosemide, gallium, ganciclovir, gentamicin, granisetron, haloperidol, heparin, hydrocortisone, hydrocortisone sodium phosphate, hydromorphone, hydrOXYzine, idarubicin, ifosfamide, imipenem-cilastatin, lorazepam, mannitol, mechlorethamine, meperidine, mesna, methotrexate, methylPREDNISolone, metoclopramide, metronidazole, miconazole, minocycline, mitomycin, mitoxantrone, morphine, nalbuphine, netilmicin, ondansetron, pentostatin, piperacillin, plicamycin, potassium chloride, prochlorperazine, promethazine, ranitidine, sodium bicarbonate, streptozocin, teniposide, thiotepa, ticarcillin, ticarcillin/clavulanate, tobramycin, trimethoprim-sulfamethoxazole, vancomycin, vinBLAStine, vinCRIStine, vinorelbine, zidovudine

Perform/provide:

• Storage in airtight, light-resistant container
• Strict medical asepsis, protective isolation if WBC levels are low
• Increase fluid intake to 2-3 L/day to prevent urate deposits, calculi formation
• Diet low in purines: organ meats (kidney, liver), dried beans, peas to maintain alkaline urine

• Rinsing of mouth tid-qid with water, club soda; brushing of teeth bid-tid with soft brush or cotton-tipped applicators for stomatitis; use unwaxed dental floss
• Warm compresses at inj site for inflammation

Evaluate:
• Therapeutic response: decreased tumor size, spread of malignancy

Teach patient/family:
• That sterility, amenorrhea can occur; reversible after discontinuing treatment
• To avoid foods with citric acid, hot or rough texture
• To report any bleeding, white spots, or ulcerations in mouth to prescriber; tell patient to examine mouth qd
• To report signs of infection: fever, sore throat, flulike symptoms
• To report suspected pregnancy; to use contraception during treatment
• To report signs of anemia: fatigue, headache, faintness, shortness of breath, irritability
• To avoid use of razors, commercial mouthwash
• To avoid use of aspirin products, NSAIDs, alcohol

menotropins (℞)

(men-oh-troe′pins)

Humegon, Pergonal, Repronex

Func. class.: Gonadotropin

Chem. class.: Exogenous gonadotropin

Action: In women, increases follicular growth, maturation; in men, when given with hCG, stimulates spermatogenesis

Uses: Infertility, anovulation in women, stimulates spermatogenesis in men

Dosage and routes:

Infertility
• *Men:* **IM** 1 ampule 3 × wk with hCG 2000 units 2 × wk × 4 mo
• *Women:* **IM** 75 international units FSH, LH qd × 9-12 days, then 10,000 units hCG 1 day after these drugs; repeat × 2 menstrual cycles, then increase to 150 international units FSH, LH qd × 9-12 days, then 10,000 units hCG 1 day after these drugs × 2 menstrual cycles

Anovulation
• *Women:* **IM** 75 international units FSH, LH qd × 9-12 days, then 10,000 units hCG 1 day after last dose of these drugs; repeat × 1-3 menstrual cycles

Available forms: Powder for inj lyophilized 75 international units FSH, LH activity 150 international units FSH, LH activity

Side effects/adverse reactions:
CNS: Fever
CV: ***Hypovolemia***
RESP: ***ARDS, pulmonary embolism, pulmonary infarction, pleural effusion***
SYST: ***Anaphylaxis***
GI: Nausea, vomiting, diarrhea, anorexia
GU: Ovarian enlargement, abdominal distention/pain, multiple births, ovarian hyperstimulation: sudden ovarian enlargement, ascites with or without pain; gynecomastia in men
HEMA: ***Hemoperitoneum, arterial thromboembolism***

Contraindications: Primary ovarian failure, abnormal bleeding, thyroid/adrenal dysfunction, organic intracranial lesion, ovarian cysts, primary testicular failure, pregnancy (X)

NURSING CONSIDERATIONS

Assess:
• Weight qd; notify prescriber if weight increases rapidly

• Estrogen excretion level; if >100 mcg/24 hr, drug is withheld; hyperstimulation syndrome may occur
• I&O ratio; be alert for decreasing urinary output
• Ovarian enlargement, abdominal distention/pain; report symptoms immediately

Administer:

IM route

• After reconstituting with 1-2 ml sterile saline inj; use immediately

Evaluate:

• Therapeutic response: ovulation, pregnancy

Teach patient/family:

• That multiple births are possible; if pregnancy occurs, usually 4-6 wk after start of treatment
• To keep appointment during treatment qd × 2 wk

HIGH ALERT

meperidine (℞)

(me-per′i-deen)

Demerol, meperidine, Pethidine

Func. class.: Opioid analgesic

Chem. class.: Phenylpiperidine derivative

Controlled Substance Schedule II

Action: Depresses pain impulse transmission at the spinal cord level by interacting with opioid receptors

Uses: Moderate to severe pain, preoperatively, postoperatively

Investigational uses: Rigors

Dosage and routes:

Pain

• *Adult:* **PO/SC/IM** 50-150 mg q3-4h prn; **IV** 15-35 mg/hr as a **CONT INF;** PCA 10 mg, then 1-5 mg incremental dose; lockout interval 6-10 min
• *Child:* **PO/SC/IM** 1 mg/kg q3-4h prn, not to exceed 100 mg q4h

Labor analgesia

• *Adult:* **SC/IM** 50-100 mg given when contractions are regularly spaced, repeat q1-3h prn

Preoperatively

• *Adult:* **IM/SC** 50-100 mg q30-90 min before surgery; dose should be reduced if given **IV**
• *Child:* **IM/SC** 1-2.2 mg/kg 30-90 min before surgery

Renal disease

• CCr 10-50 ml/min 75% of dose; CCr <10 ml/min 50% of dose

Available forms include: Inj 10, 25, 50, 75, 100 mg/ml; tabs 50, 100 mg; syr 50 mg/5 ml

Side effects/adverse reactions:

CNS: Drowsiness, dizziness, confusion, headache, sedation, euphoria, ***increased intracranial pressure, seizures***

CV: Palpitations, bradycardia, change in B/P, tachycardia (IV)

EENT: Tinnitus, blurred vision, miosis, diplopia, depressed corneal reflex

GI: Nausea, vomiting, anorexia, constipation, cramps

GU: Urinary retention, dysuria

INTEG: Rash, urticaria, bruising, flushing, diaphoresis, pruritus

RESP: ***Respiratory depression***

Contraindications: Hypersensitivity, addiction (opioid)

Precautions: Addictive personality, pregnancy (B), lactation, increased intracranial pressure, MI (acute), severe heart disease, respiratory depression, hepatic disease, renal disease, child <18 yr, elderly

Do not confuse:

Demerol/Dilaudid

meperidine/hydromorphone/meprobamate/morphine

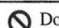

Pharmacokinetics: Absorption 50% (PO), well absorbed IM, SC

PO: Onset 15 min, peak ½-1 hr, duration 2-4 hr
SC/IM: Onset 10 min, peak ½-1 hr, duration 2-4 hr
IV: Onset 5 min, duration 2 hr
Metabolized by liver (to active/inactive metabolites), excreted by kidneys; crosses placenta, excreted in breast milk; half-life 3-4 hr; toxic by-product can result from regular use

Interactions:

- ↑ effects with: other CNS depressants, alcohol, opioids, sedative/hypnotics, antipsychotics, skeletal muscle relaxants
- ↑ adverse reactions: protease inhibitor antiretrovirals
- ↓ meperidine effect: phenytoin

May cause fatal reaction: MAOIs, procarbazine

↑ CNS depression: chamomile, hops, Jamaican dogwood, kava, lavender, mistletoe, nettle, pokeweed, poppy, senega, skullcap, valerian

Parsley may promote serotonin syndrome; avoid concurrent medicinal use

Lab test interferences:

Increase: Amylase, lipase

NURSING CONSIDERATIONS

Assess:

- Pain: location, type, character; give before pain becomes extreme; reassess after 60 min (IM, SC, PO) and 5-10 min (IV)
- Renal function prior to initiating therapy; poor renal function can lead to accumulation of toxic metabolite and seizures
- I&O ratio; check for decreasing output; may indicate urinary retention
- For constipation; increase fluids, bulk in diet; give laxatives if needed
- CNS changes: dizziness, drowsiness, hallucinations, euphoria, LOC, pupil reactions; at chronic or high-dose use
- Allergic reactions: rash, urticaria
- Respiratory dysfunction: depression, character, rate, rhythm; notify prescriber if respirations are <12/min
- CNS stimulation: occurs with chronic or high doses

Administer:

- Patient should remain recumbent for 1 hr after IM/SC route
- With antiemetic for nausea, vomiting
- When pain is beginning to return; determine dosage interval by patient response
- In gradually decreasing dose after long-term use; withdrawal symptoms may occur

IV route

- After diluting with 5 ml or more sterile H_2O or NS; give directly over 4-5 min; may be further diluted in sol to 1 mg/ml during anesthesia in D_5W or NS; if diluted in NS, may be given through patient-controlled inf device

Additive compatibilities: Cefazolin, DOBUTamine, ondansetron, scopolamine, succinylcholine, triflupromazine, verapamil

Syringe compatibilities: Atropine, benzquinamide, butorphanol, chlorproMAZINE, cimetidine, dimenhyDRINATE, diphenhydrAMINE, droperidol, fentanyl, glycopyrrolate, hydrOXYzine, ketamine, metoclopramide, midazolam, pentazocine, perphenazine, prochlorperazine, promazine, promethazine, ranitidine, scopolamine

Y-site compatibilities: Amifostine, amikacin, ampicillin, atenolol, aztreonam, bumetanide, cefamandole, cefazolin, cefmetazole, cefotaxime, cefotetan, cefoxitin, ceftazidime, ceftizoxime, ceftriaxone,

M

cefuroxime, cephalothin, cephapirin, chloramphenicol, cisatracurium, cladribine, clindamycin, dexamethasone, diltiazem, diphenhydrAMINE, DOBUTamine, DOPamine, DOXOrubicin liposome, doxycycline, droperidol, erythromycin, famotidine, filgrastim, fluconazole, fludarabine, gallium, gentamicin, granisetron, heparin, hydrocortisone, insulin (regular), kanamycin, labetalol, lidocaine, methyldopate, magnesium sulfate, melphalan, methylPREDNISolone, metoclopramide, metoprolol, metronidazole, moxalactam, ondansetron, oxacillin, oxytocin, paclitaxel, penicillin G potassium, piperacillin, potassium chloride, propofol, propranolol, ranitidine, remifentanil, sargramostim, teniposide, thiotepa, ticarcillin, ticarcillin/clavulanate, tobramycin, trimethoprim-sulfamethoxazole, vancomycin, verapamil, vinorelbine

Perform/provide:
- Storage in light-resistant container at room temperature
- Assistance with ambulation
- Safety measures: night-light, call bell within easy reach

Evaluate:
- Therapeutic response: decrease in pain

Teach patient/family:
- To report any symptoms of CNS changes, allergic reactions
- That physical dependency may result from extended use
- That drowsiness, dizziness may occur; to call for assistance
- That withdrawal symptoms may occur: nausea, vomiting, cramps, fever, faintness, anorexia
- To make position changes slowly; orthostatic hypotension can occur
- To avoid OTC medications, alcohol unless directed by prescriber

Treatment of overdose: Naloxone (Narcan) 0.2-0.8 mg IV, O_2, IV fluids, vasopressors

mercaptopurine (℞)

(mer-kap-toe-pyoor′een)
Purinethol, 6-MP

Func. class.: Antineoplastic-antimetabolite

Chem. class.: Purine analog

Action: Inhibits purine metabolism at multiple sites, which inhibits DNA and RNA synthesis, S phase of cell cycle specific

Uses: Chronic myelocytic or acute lymphoblastic leukemia in children, acute myelogenous leukemia

Investigational uses: Polycythemia vera, psoriatic arthritis, colitis, lymphoma

Dosage and routes:
- *Adult:* **PO** 80-100 mg/m^2 qd max 5 mg/kg/day; maintenance 1.5-2.5 mg/kg/day
- *Child:* 75 mg/m^2/day; maintenance 1.5-2.5 mg/kg/day

Available forms: Tabs 50 mg

Side effects/adverse reactions:

CNS: Fever, headache, weakness

HEMA: ***Thrombocytopenia, leukopenia, myelosuppression, anemia***

GI: Nausea, vomiting, anorexia, diarrhea, stomatitis, ***hepatotoxicity*** (high doses), jaundice, gastritis

GU: ***Renal failure,*** hyperuricemia, ***oliguria,*** crystalluria, ***hematuria***

INTEG: Rash, dry skin, urticaria

Contraindications: Patients with prior drug resistance, leukopenia (<2500/mm^3), thrombocytopenia (<100,000/mm^3), anemia, pregnancy (D), lactation

Precautions: Renal disease

Pharmacokinetics: Incompletely absorbed when taken orally; metabolized in liver, excreted in urine

Interactions:
• ↑ toxicity: radiation or other antineoplastics
• ↑ bone marrow depression: allopurinol, co-trimoxazole
• Reversal of neuromuscular blockade: nondepolarizing muscle relaxants
• ↑ or ↓ anticoagulant action: warfarin
• ↓ antibodies: live virus vaccines

NURSING CONSIDERATIONS
Assess:
• CBC, differential, platelet count qwk; withhold drug if WBC is <3500 or platelet count is <100,000; notify prescriber; drug should be discontinued
• Renal studies: BUN, serum uric acid, urine CCr, electrolytes before, during therapy
• I&O ratio; report fall in urine output to <30 ml/hr
• Monitor temp q4h; fever may indicate beginning infection; no rectal temps
• Hepatic studies before, during therapy: bilirubin, alk phosphatase, AST, ALT, qwk during beginning therapy
• Bleeding: hematuria, guaiac, bruising, petechiae; mucosa or orifices q8h
• Buccal cavity q8h for dryness, sores, ulceration, white patches, oral pain, bleeding, dysphagia
◆ Symptoms indicating severe allergic reaction: rash, urticaria, itching, flushing

Administer:
• Antacid before oral agent; give drug after evening meal before bedtime
• Allopurinol or sodium bicarbonate to maintain uric acid levels, alkalinization of urine

Perform/provide:
• Strict medical asepsis, protective isolation if WBC levels are low
• Increase fluid intake to 2-3 L/day to prevent urate deposits, calculi formation, unless contraindicated
• Diet low in purines: absence of organ meats (kidney, liver), dried beans, peas to maintain alkaline urine
• Rinsing of mouth tid-qid with water, club soda; brushing of teeth bid-tid with soft brush or cotton-tipped applicators for stomatitis; use unwaxed dental floss
• Nutritious diet with iron, vitamin supplements as ordered
• Storage in tightly closed container in cool environment

Evaluate:
• Therapeutic response: decreased size of tumor, spread of malignancy

Teach patient/family:
• To avoid foods with citric acid, hot or rough texture for stomatitis
• To report stomatitis: any bleeding, white spots, ulcerations in mouth; tell patient to examine mouth qd, report symptoms
• That contraceptive measures are recommended during therapy; to avoid breastfeeding
• To drink 10-12 (8 oz) glasses of fluid/day
• To notify prescriber of fever, chills, sore throat, nausea, vomiting, anorexia, diarrhea, bleeding, bruising, which may indicate blood dyscrasias
• To report signs of infection: fever, sore throat, flulike symptoms
• To report signs of anemia: fatigue, headache, faintness, shortness of breath, irritability
• To report bleeding: avoid use of razors, commercial mouthwash
• To avoid use of aspirin products, NSAIDs

meropenem (℞)

(mer-oh-pen′em)

Merrem IV

Func. class.: Antiinfective-misc.

Chem. class.: Carbapenem

Action: Interferes with cell wall replication of susceptible organisms; osmotically unstable cell wall swells, bursts from osmotic pressure

Uses: Serious infections caused by gram-positive bacteria: *Streptococcus pneumoniae,* group A β-hemolytic streptococci, enterococcus; gram-negative: *Klebsiella, Proteus, Escherichia coli, Pseudomonas aeruginosa;* appendicitis, peritonitis caused by *viridans* group streptococci; *Bacteroides fragilis, Bacterioides thetaiotamicron,* bacterial meningitis (≥3 mo)

Dosage and routes:

• *Adult:* **IV** 1 g q8h, given over 15-30 min or as an **IV BOL** 5-20 ml given over 3-5 min

• *Child ≥3 mo:* **IV** 20-40 mg/kg q8h (max 2g q8h meningitis)

• *Child >50 kg:* **IV** 1 g q8h (intraabdominal infection) or 2 g q8h (meningitis) given over 15-30 min or as an **IV BOL** 5-20 ml over 3-5 min

Renal disease

• *Adult:* **IV** CCr 26-50 ml/min 1 g q12h; CCr 10-25 ml/min 500 mg q12h; CCr <10 ml/min 500 mg q24h

Available forms: Inj 500 mg, 1 g

Side effects/adverse reactions:

CNS: Fever, somnolence, ***seizures,*** dizziness, weakness, myoclonia, *headache*

GI: Diarrhea, nausea, vomiting, ***pseudomembranous colitis, hepatitis,*** glossitis

CV: Hypotension, palpitations

HEMA: ***Eosinophilia, neutropenia,*** decreased Hgb, Hct

INTEG: *Rash,* urticaria, *pruritus,* pain at inj site, phlebitis, erythema at inj site

SYST: ***Anaphylaxis***

RESP: Chest discomfort, dyspnea, hyperventilation

Contraindications: Hypersensitivity to meropenem or imipenem

Precautions: Pregnancy (B), lactation, elderly, renal disease

Pharmacokinetics:

IV: Onset immediate, peak dose dependent, half-life 1 hr, hepatic metabolism

Interactions:

• ↑ meropenem plasma levels: probenecid

Lab test interferences:

Increase: AST, ALT, LDH, BUN, alk phosphatase, bilirubin, creatinine

False positive: Direct Coombs' test

NURSING CONSIDERATIONS

Assess:

• Sensitivity to carbapenem antibiotics, penicillins

• Renal disease: lower dose may be required

• Bowel pattern qd; if severe diarrhea occurs, drug should be discontinued; may indicate pseudomembranous colitis

• For infection: temp, sputum, characteristics of wound, before, during, and after treatment

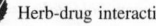

◆ Allergic reactions, anaphylaxis: rash, urticaria, pruritus; may occur few days after therapy begins

• Overgrowth of infection: perineal itching, fever, malaise, redness, pain, swelling, drainage, rash, diarrhea, change in cough, sputum

Administer:

• By IV inf or IV bol

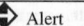

• After C&S is taken

• Reconstitute with 0.9% NaCl, D_5W, LR, dilute in 5-20 ml comp sol, give by direct IV over 3-5 min; give by intermittent inf, dilute in 5-20 ml of comp sol, give over 15-30 min

Additive compatibilities: Aminophylline, atropine, cimetidine, dexamethasone, DOBUTamine, DOPamine, enalaprilat, fluconazole, furosemide, gentamicin, heparin, insulin (regular), magnesium sulfate, metoclopramide, morphine, norepinephrine, phenobarbital, ranitidine, vancomycin

Y-site compatibilities: Aminophylline, atenolol, atropine, cimetidine, dexamethasone, digoxin, diphenhydrAMINE, enalaprilat, fluconazole, furosemide, gentamicin, heparin, insulin (regular), metoclopramide, morphine, norepinephrine, phenobarbital, vancomycin

Evaluate:

• Therapeutic response: negative C&S; absence of symptoms and signs of infection

Teach patient/family:

• To report severe diarrhea; may indicate pseudomembranous colitis

• To report sore throat, bruising, bleeding, joint pain; may indicate blood dyscrasias (rare)

• To report overgrowth of infection: black, furry tongue; vaginal itching; foul-smelling stools

• To avoid breastfeeding; drug is excreted in breast milk

Treatment of overdose: EpINEPHrine, antihistamines; resuscitate if needed (anaphylaxis)

mesalamine (℞)

(mez-al'a-meen)

Asacol, Canasa, Mesasal, Pentasa, Rowasa Salofalk✦

Func. class.: GI antiinflammatory

Chem. class.: 5-Aminosalicylic acid

Action: May diminish inflammation by blocking cyclooxygenase, inhibiting prostaglandin production in colon; local action only

Uses: Mild to moderate active distal ulcerative colitis, proctosigmoiditis, proctitis

Dosage and routes:

• *Adult:* **RECT** 60 ml (4 g) hs, retained for 8 hr × 3-6 wk; **PO** 800 mg tid × 6 wk; **SUPP** 500 mg bid × 3-6 wk

Available forms: Rect susp 4 g/60 ml; supp 500 mg; tab del rel 400 mg; con rel cap 250 mg (Pentasa)

Side effects/adverse reactions:

CV: Pericarditis, myocarditis

GI: Cramps, gas, nausea, diarrhea, rectal pain, constipation

CNS: Headache, fever, dizziness, insomnia, asthenia, weakness, fatigue

INTEG: Rash, itching, acne

SYST: Flulike symptoms, malaise, back pain, peripheral edema, leg and joint pain, arthralgia, dysmenorrhea, ***anaphylaxis,*** acute intolerance syndrome

EENT: Sore throat, cough, pharyngitis, rhinitis

Contraindications: Hypersensitivity to this drug or salicylates

Precautions: Renal disease, pregnancy (B), lactation, children, sulfite sensitivity

Do not confuse:

Asacol/Ansaid

Pharmacokinetics:

RECT: Primarily excreted in feces

M

but some in urine as metabolite; half-life 1 hr, metabolite half-life 5-10 hr
Interactions:
- ↑ mesalamine absorption: omeprazole

Lab test interferences:
Increase: AST, ALT, alk phosphatase, LDH, GGTP, amylase, lipase
NURSING CONSIDERATIONS
Assess:
- For allergy to salicylates, sulfonamides, if allergic reactions occur, discontinue drug
- Renal studies: BUN, creatinine before and during treatment
- GI symptoms: cramps, gas, nausea, diarrhea, rectal pain; if severe, drug should be discontinued
- I&O ratios, increase fluids to 1500 ml qd to prevent crystalluria

Administer:
- May give orally; tabs should be swallowed whole
- Rectally; drug should be given hs, retained until morning; empty bowel before insertion

Perform/provide:
- Storage at room temperature

Evaluate:
- Therapeutic response: absence of pain, bleeding from GI tract, decrease in number of diarrhea stools

Teach patient/family:
- That usual course of therapy is 3-6 wk
- To shake bottle well (rectal susp)
- Method of rectal administration
- To inform prescriber of GI symptoms

⃠ Not to break, crush, or chew tabs
- To report abdominal cramping, pain, diarrhea with blood, headache, fever, rash, chest pain; drug should be discontinued

metaproterenol (℞)
(met-a-proe-ter′e-nole)
Alupent
Func. class.: Bronchodilator-selective β_2-agonist

Action: Relaxes bronchial smooth muscle by direct action on β_2-adrenergic receptors with increased levels of cAMP with increased bronchodilation, diuresis, cardiac CNS stimulation
Uses: Bronchial asthma, bronchospasm
Dosage and routes:
- *Adult and child >12 yr:* **INH** 2-3 inhalations; may repeat q3-4h, not to exceed 12 inhalations/day
- *Adult:* **PO** 20 mg q6-8h
- *Geriatric:* **PO** 10 mg tid-qid, initially
- *Child >9 yr or >27 kg:* **PO** 20 mg q6-8h or 0.4-0.9 mg/kg tid
- *Child 6-9 yr or <27 kg:* **PO** 10 mg q6-8h or 0.4-0.9 mg/kg tid
- *Child 2-6 yr:* **PO** 1.3-2.6 mg/kg divided q6-8h

Available forms: Tabs 10, 20 mg; aerosol 0.65 mg/dose; syr 10 mg/5 ml; sol for inh 0.4%, 0.6%, 5%
Side effects/adverse reactions:
CNS: *Tremors,* anxiety, insomnia, headache, dizziness, stimulation
CV: Palpitations, tachycardia, hypertension, dysrhythmias, ***cardiac arrest*** (high dose)
GI: Nausea, vomiting, dry mouth
RESP: ***Paradoxical bronchospasm***
Contraindications: Hypersensitivity to sympathomimetics, narrow-angle glaucoma, cardiac dysrhythmias with tachycardia
Precautions: Pregnancy (C), cardiac disorders, hyperthyroidism, diabetes mellitus, prostatic hypertrophy, seizure disorder, elderly, child <6 yr (PO)

Do not confuse:
Alupent/Atrovent
Pharmacokinetics: Well absorbed (PO)
PO: Onset 15-30 min, peak 1 hr, duration 4 hr, excreted in urine as metabolites
INH: Onset 5 min, peak 1 hr, duration 1-6 hr
Interactions:
• ↑ effects of both drugs: other sympathomimetics, bronchodilators
• ↓ β-blockers action
Hypertensive crisis: MAOIs
↑ effect: black/green tea, coffee, cola nut, guarana, yerba maté
Lab test interferences:
Decrease: Potassium

NURSING CONSIDERATIONS
Assess:
• Respiratory function: vital capacity, forced expiratory volume, ABGs; also B/P; lung sounds, secretions before and after treatment
• Tolerance over long-term therapy; dose may have to be changed; check for rebound bronchospasm
Administer:
• 2 hr before hs to avoid sleeplessness
• PO with food for GI upset
Perform/provide:
• Storage at room temperature; do not use discolored sol
• Spacer device for elderly
Evaluate:
• Therapeutic response: absence of dyspnea, wheezing; improved ABGs
Teach patient/family:
• To increase fluid intake (2-3 L/day) to liquefy secretions
• Not to use OTC medications; excess stimulation may occur
• To notify prescriber of headaches, chest pain, weakness, dizziness, anxiety
• Use of inhaler; review package insert with patient
• To avoid getting aerosol in eyes
• To wash inhaler in warm water and dry qd
• All aspects of drug; avoid smoking, smoke-filled rooms, persons with respiratory infections

metformin (℞)
(met-for′min)
Glucophage, Glucophage XR, Novo-Metformin✤
Func. class.: Antidiabetic, oral
Chem. class.: Biguanide

Action: Inhibits hepatic glucose production and increases sensitivity of peripheral tissue to insulin
Uses: Stable adult-onset diabetes mellitus (type 2) (NIDDM)
Dosage and routes:
• *Adult:* **PO** 500 mg bid initially, then increase to desired response 1-3 g; dosage adjustment q2-3wk or 850 mg qd with morning meal with dosage increased every other wk, max 2500 mg/day, ext rel max 2000 mg/day
• *Geriatric:* **PO,** use lowest effective dose
Available forms: Tabs 500, 850, 1000 mg; ext rel tab 500 mg
Side effects/adverse reactions:
CNS: Headache, weakness, dizziness, drowsiness, tinnitus, fatigue, vertigo, *agitation*
GI: Nausea, vomiting, diarrhea, heartburn, anorexia, metallic taste
HEMA: ***Thrombocytopenia,*** decreased vit B_{12} concentration
INTEG: Rash
ENDO: ***Lactic acidosis,*** hypoglycemia
Contraindications: Hypersensitivity, hepatic, creatinine >1.5 mg/ml (males) ≥1.4 (females), CHF, alcoholism, cardiopulmonary disease, history of lactic acidosis

M

Precautions: Previous hypersensitivity, pregnancy (B), elderly, thyroid disease

Pharmacokinetics: Excreted by the kidneys unchanged 35%-50%, half-life 1½-5 hr, terminal 6-20 hr, peak 1-3 hr

Interactions:

- ↑ metformin level: cimetidine, digoxin, morphine, procainamide, quinidine, ranitidine, triamterene, vancomycin
- ↑ hypoglycemia: cimetidine, calcium channel blockers, corticosteroids, estrogens, oral contraceptives, phenothiazines, sympathomimetics, diuretics, phenytoin
- Do not give with radiologic contrast media; may cause renal failure

↑ metformin level: Quinine

Hyperglycemia: glucosamine

Hypoglycemia: chromium, coenzyme Q-10, fenugreek

↓ antidiabetic effect: bee pollen, blue cohosh, broom, chromium, elecampane, eucalyptus, gotu kola

↑ antidiabetic effect: alfalfa, aloe, basil, bay, bilberry, bitter melon, black catechu, buchu, burdock, coriander, dandelion, eyebright (po), fenugreek, garlic, ginseng, glucomannan, glucosamine, goat's rue, gymnema, horehound, horse chestnut, jambul, myrrh, myrtle

NURSING CONSIDERATIONS

Assess:

- For hypoglycemic reactions (sweating, weakness, dizziness, anxiety, tremors, hunger), hyperglycemic reactions soon after meals
- CBC (baseline, q3mo) during treatment; check LFTs periodically AST, LDH, renal studies: BUN, creatinine during treatment; glucose, glycosylated Hgb

For lactic acidosis: malaise, myalgia, abdominal distress; risk increases with age, poor renal function; monitor electrolytes, lactate, pyruvate, blood pH, ketones, glucose

Administer:

PO route

- Twice a day given with meals to decrease GI upset and provide best absorption, may also be taken as a single dose
- Tabs crushed and mixed with meal or fluids for patients with difficulty swallowing

Do not crush, chew, break ext rel tab

Perform/provide:

- Conversion from other oral hypoglycemic agents; change may be made without gradual dosage change; monitor serum or urine glucose and ketones tid during conversion
- Storage in tight container in cool environment

Evaluate:

- Therapeutic response: decrease in polyuria, polydipsia, polyphagia; clear sensorium; absence of dizziness; stable gait, blood glucose at normal level

Teach patient/family:

Lactic acidosis symptoms: hyperventilation, fatigue, malaise, chills, myalgia, somnolence; to notify prescriber immediately

- To use capillary blood glucose test or Chemstrip tid
- The symptoms of hypo/hyperglycemia, what to do about each
- That drug must be continued on daily basis; explain consequence of discontinuing drug abruptly
- To avoid OTC medications unless approved by prescriber
- That diabetes is a lifelong illness; that this drug is not a cure; only controls symptoms
- That all food included in diet plan must be eaten to prevent hypoglycemia

• To carry emergency ID and glucagon emergency kit for emergencies
• That Glucophage XR tab may appear in stool
Treatment of overdose: Glucose 25 g IV via dextrose 50% sol, 50 ml or 1 mg glucagon

---

HIGH ALERT

methadone (℞)

(meth'a-done)
Dolophine, methadone, Methadose
Func. class.: Opioid analgesic
Chem. class.: Synthetic diphenylheptane derivative

Controlled Substance Schedule II
Action: Depresses pain impulse transmission at the spinal cord level by interacting with opioid receptors, produce CNS depression
Uses: Severe pain, opioid withdrawal
Dosage and routes:
Severe pain
• *Adult:* **PO/SC/IM** 2.5-10 mg q3-4h prn
Opioid withdrawal
• *Adult:* **PO** 15-40 mg/day individualized initially, then 20-120 mg/day titrated to patient response
• *Child:* 0.05-0.1 mg/kg/dose q6-12h
Renal disease
• *Adult:* CCr 10-50 ml/min dose q8h; CCr <10 ml/min dose q8-12h
Available forms: Inj 10 mg/ml; tabs 5, 10 mg; oral sol 5, 10 mg/5 ml; dispersible tabs 40 mg; oral conc 10 mg/ml; oral sol 5 mg/5 ml, 10 mg/5 ml, 10 mg/10 ml
Side effects/adverse reactions:
CNS: Drowsiness, dizziness, confusion, headache, sedation, euphoria, ***seizures***
GI: Nausea, vomiting, anorexia, constipation, cramps, biliary tract spasm
GU: Increased urinary output, dysuria, urinary retention
INTEG: Rash, urticaria, bruising, flushing, diaphoresis, pruritus
EENT: Tinnitus, blurred vision, miosis, diplopia
CV: Palpitations, bradycardia, change in B/P, ***cardiac arrest, shock***
RESP: ***Respiratory depression, respiratory arrest***
Contraindications: Hypersensitivity to this drug or chlorobutanol (inj), addiction (opiate)
Precautions: Addictive personality, pregnancy (C), lactation, increased intracranial pressure, MI (acute), severe heart disease, respiratory depression, hepatic disease, renal disease, children <18 yr, elderly
Do not confuse:
methadone/methylphenidate
Pharmacokinetics:
PO: Onset 30-60 min, peak 1½-2 hr, duration 6-8 hr, cumulative 22-48 hr
SC/IM: Onset 10-20 min, peak 1½-2 hr, duration 4-6 hr, cumulative 22-48 hr
Metabolized by liver; excreted by kidneys; crosses placenta; excreted in breast milk; half-life 15-30 hr, extended interval with continued dosing; 90% bound to plasma proteins
Interactions:
• ↑ effects with other CNS depressants: alcohol, opiates, sedative/hypnotics, antipsychotics, skeletal muscle relaxants
• ↓ analgesia: rifampin, phenytoin, nalbuphine, pentazine
⬗Unpredictable reactions: MAOIs, do not use together
↑ CNS depression: chamomile,

M

hops, Jamaican dogwood, kava, lavender, mistletoe, nettle, pokeweed, poppy, senega, skullcap, valerian
↑ anticholinergic effect: corkwood

Lab test interferences:

Increase: Amylase, lipase

NURSING CONSIDERATIONS

Assess:

- For pain: type, location, intensity, grimacing before and 1½-2 hr after administration; use pain scoring
- I&O ratio; check for decreasing output; may indicate urinary retention
- CNS changes: dizziness, drowsiness, hallucinations, euphoria, LOC, pupil reaction
- Allergic reactions: rash, urticaria
- Respiratory dysfunction: respiratory depression, character, rate, rhythm; notify prescriber if respirations are <10/min
- For opioid detoxification: no analgesia occurs, only prevention of withdrawal symptoms
- B/P, pulse
- Bowel changes, bulk, fluids, laxatives should be used for constipation

Administer:

- With antiemetic if nausea/vomiting occurs
- When pain is beginning to return; determine dosage interval by patient response
- Rotating inj sites, give deep in large muscle mass (IM)

Perform/provide:

- Storage in light-resistant container at room temperature
- Assistance with ambulation
- Safety measures: night-light, call bell within easy reach

Evaluate:

- Therapeutic response: decrease in pain, successful opioid withdrawal

Teach patient/family:

- To report any symptoms of CNS changes, allergic reactions
- That physical dependency may result from extended use
- Withdrawal symptoms may occur: nausea, vomiting, cramps, fever, faintness, anorexia

Treatment of overdose: Naloxone (Narcan) 0.2-0.8 mg IV, O_2, IV fluids, vasopressors

methimazole (℞)

(meth-im'a-zole)

Tapazole

Func. class.: Thyroid hormone antagonist (antithyroid)

Chem. class.: Thioamide

Action: Inhibits synthesis of thyroid hormones by decreasing iodine use in manufacture of thyroglobin and iodothyronine; does not affect already formed hormones

Uses: Hyperthyroidism, preparation for thyroidectomy, thyrotoxic crisis, thyroid storm

Dosage and routes:

Hyperthyroidism

- *Adult:* **PO** 5-20 mg tid depending on severity of condition; continue until euthyroid; maintenance dose 5-15 mg qd-tid, maximal dose 150 mg qd
- *Child:* **PO** 0.4 mg/kg/day in divided doses q8h; continue until euthyroid; maintenance dose 0.2 mg/kg/day in divided doses q8h

Preparation and thyroidectomy

- *Adult and child:* **PO** same as above; iodine may be added × 10 days before surgery

Thyrotoxic crisis

- *Adult and child:* **PO** same as hyperthyroidism with iodine and propranolol

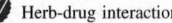

Available forms: Tabs 5, 10 mg

Side effects/adverse reactions:
ENDO: Enlarged thyroid
INTEG: Rash, urticaria, pruritus, alopecia, hyperpigmentation, lupus-like syndrome
GU: ***Nephritis***
CNS: Drowsiness, headache, vertigo, fever, paresthesias, neuritis
HEMA: ***Agranulocytosis, leukopenia, thrombocytopenia, hypothrombinemia, lymphadenopathy,*** bleeding, vasculitis
GI: Nausea, diarrhea, vomiting, ***jaundice, hepatitis,*** loss of taste
MS: Myalgia, arthralgia, nocturnal muscle cramps
Contraindications: Hypersensitivity, pregnancy (D), lactation
Precautions: Infection, bone marrow depression, hepatic disease
Pharmacokinetics:
PO: Onset 1 wk, duration is up to 10 wk, half-life 5-13 hr; excreted in urine, breast milk; crosses placenta
Interactions:
• ↑ bone marrow depression: radiation, antineoplastic agents
• ↓ effectiveness: amiodarone, potassium iodide
• Agranulocytosis: phenothiazines
• ↑ response to digitalis, warfarin
Lab test interferences:
Increase: PT, AST, ALT, alk phosphatase

NURSING CONSIDERATIONS
Assess:
• Pulse, B/P, temp
• I&O ratio; check for edema: puffy hands, feet, periorbits; indicate hypothyroidism
• Weight qd; same clothing, scale, time of day
• T_3, T_4, which are increased; serum TSH, which is decreased; free thyroxine index, which is increased if dosage is too low; discontinue drug 3-4 wk before RAIU
◆ Blood work: CBC for blood dyscrasias: leukopenia, thrombocytopenia, agranulocytosis, if these occur, drug should be discontinued and other treatment initiated; LFTs
• Hypersensitivity: rash, enlarged cervical lymph nodes; drug may have to be discontinued
• Hypoprothrombinemia: bleeding, petechiae, ecchymosis
• Clinical response: after 3 wk should include increased weight, pulse; decreased T_4
◆ Bone marrow depression: sore throat, fever, fatigue
Administer:
• With meals to decrease GI upset
• At same time each day to maintain drug level
• Lowest dose that relieves symptoms; discontinue before RAIU
Perform/provide:
• Storage in light-resistant container
• Fluids to 3-4 L/day, unless contraindicated
Evaluate:
• Therapeutic response: weight gain, decreased pulse, decreased T_4, B/P
Teach patient/family:
• Not to breastfeed
• To take pulse daily
• To report redness, swelling, sore throat, mouth lesions, fever, which indicate blood dyscrasias
• To keep graph of weight, pulse, mood
• To avoid OTC products that contain iodine
• That seafood, other iodine products may be restricted
• Not to discontinue this medication abruptly; thyroid crisis may occur; stress patient response
• That response may take several mo if thyroid is large
• The symptoms and signs of overdose: periorbital edema, cold intolerance, mental depression
• The symptoms of inadequate dose: tachycardia, diarrhea, fever, irritability

M

• To take medication as prescribed; do not skip or double dose

methocarbamol (℞)

(meth-oh-kar′ba-mole)

Carbacot, methocarbamol, Robaxin

Func. class.: Skeletal muscle relaxant, central acting

Chem. class.: Carbamate derivative

Action: Depresses multisynaptic pathways in the spinal cord, causing skeletal muscle relaxation

Uses: Adjunct for relief of spasm and pain in musculoskeletal conditions

Dosage and routes:

Pain

• *Adult:* **PO** 1.5 g × 2-3 days, then 1 g qid; **IM** 500 mg in each gluteal region, may repeat q8h; **IV BOL** 1-3 g/day at 3 ml/min; **IV INF** 1 g/250 ml D_5W or NS, not to exceed 3 g/day

• *Geriatric:* **PO** 500 mg qid, titrate to needed dose

Available forms: Tabs 500, 750 mg; inj 100 mg/ml

Side effects/adverse reactions:

CNS: Dizziness, weakness, drowsiness, headache, tremor, depression, insomnia; ***seizures*** (IV, IM use)

HEMA: Hemolysis, increased hemoglobin (IV only)

EENT: Diplopia, temporary loss of vision, blurred vision, nystagmus

CV: Postural hypotension, ***bradycardia***

GI: Nausea, vomiting, hiccups, anorexia, metallic taste

GU: Brown, black, green urine

INTEG: Rash, pruritus, fever, facial flushing, urticaria

SYST: ***Anaphylaxis*** (IM, IV)

Contraindications: Hypersensitivity, child <12 yr, intermittent porphyria

Precautions: Renal disease, hepatic disease, addictive personalities, pregnancy (C), myasthenia gravis, epilepsy

Pharmacokinetics:

IM/IV: Onset rapid

PO: Onset ½ hr, peak 1-2 hr, half-life 1-2 hr

Metabolized in liver, excreted in urine unchanged, crosses placenta

Interactions:

• ↑ CNS depression: alcohol, tricyclics, opioids, barbiturates, sedatives, hypnotics

• Considered incompatible with any drug in sol or syringe

↑ CNS depression: chamomile, hops, kava, skullcap, valerian

Lab test interferences:

False increase: VMA, urinary 5-HIAA

NURSING CONSIDERATIONS

Assess:

• Blood studies: CBC, WBC, differential; blood dyscrasias may occur

• During and after inj: CNS effects, rash, conjunctivitis, nasal congestion may occur

• Hepatic studies: AST, ALT, alk phosphatase; hepatitis may occur

• ECG in epileptic patients; poor seizure control has occurred

• Allergic reactions: rash, fever, respiratory distress

• Severe weakness, numbness in extremities

• Tolerance: increased need for medication, more frequent requests for medication, increased pain

• CNS depression: dizziness, drowsiness, psychiatric symptoms

Administer:

PO route

• With meals for GI symptoms

IM route
- IM deep in large muscle mass; rotate sites
- Do not give SC

IV route
- IV undiluted over 1 min or more, give 300 mg or less/1 min or longer; may be diluted in 250 ml or less D_5 or isotonic NaCl sol
- By slow IV to prevent phlebitis; keep recumbent for 15 min to prevent orthostatic hypotension; check for extravasation

Perform/provide:
- Storage in tight container at room temperature
- Assistance with ambulation if dizziness/drowsiness occurs
- Recumbent position after IV administration

Evaluate:
- Therapeutic response: decreased pain, spasticity

Teach patient/family:
- Not to discontinue medication quickly; insomnia, nausea, headache, spasticity, tachycardia will occur; drug should be tapered off over 1-2 wk
- That urine may turn green, black, or brown
- Not to take with alcohol, other CNS depressants
- To avoid altering activities while taking this drug
- To avoid hazardous activities if drowsiness, dizziness occurs
- To avoid using OTC medication: cough preparations, antihistamines, unless directed by prescriber

Treatment of overdose: Induce emesis of conscious patient, lavage, dialysis; have epINEPHrine, antihistamines, and corticosteroids available

HIGH ALERT

methotrexate (amethopterin, MTX) (℞)

(meth-oh-trex'ate)

Folex, Folex PFS, methotrexate, Rheumatrex

Func. class.: Antineoplastic-antimetabolite

Chem. class.: Folic acid antagonist

Action: Inhibits an enzyme that reduces folic acid, which is needed for nucleic acid synthesis in all cells; S phase of cell cycle specific; immunosuppressive

Uses: Acute lymphocytic leukemia, in combination for breast, lung, head, neck carcinoma; lymphosarcoma, gestational choriocarcinoma, hydatidiform mole, psoriasis, rheumatoid arthritis, mycosis fungoides

Investigational uses: Used investigationally to produce abortion

Dosage and routes:

Acute lymphocytic leukemia
- *Adult and child:* **PO/IM/IV** 3.3 mg/m^2/day × 4-6 wk until remission, then 20-30 mg/m^2 **PO/IM** qwk in 2 divided doses or 2.5 mg/kg **IV** × 2 wk

Choriocarcinoma
- *Adult and child:* **PO/IM** 15-30 mg/m^2 qd × 5 days, then off 1 wk; may repeat

Meningeal leukemia
- *Adult and child:* 12 mg/m^2 **INTRATHECALLY** q2-5 days until CSF is normal, then 1 additional dose, max 15 mg

Burkitt's lymphoma (stages I, II, III)
- *Adult:* **PO** 10-25 mg qd × 4-8 days with 7-day rest period

M

Lymphosarcoma (stage III)
• *Adult:* **PO/IM/IV** 0.625-2.5 mg/kg/day
Osteosarcoma
• *Adult and child:* **IV** 12 g/m^2 given over 4 hr, then leucovorin rescue
Mycosis fungoides
• *Adult:* **PO** 2.5-10 mg/day until cleared (may be many months); **IM** 50 mg qwk or 25 mg 2 × /wk
Psoriasis
• *Adult:* **PO/IM/IV** 10-25 mg qwk or 2.5 mg **PO** q12hr × 3 doses, may increase to 25 mg qwk
Breast cancer
• *Adult:* **IV** 40 mg/m^2 on days 1 and 8 with other antineoplastics
Rheumatoid arthritis
• *Adults:* **PO** 7.5 mg/wk or divided doses of 2.5 mg q12h × 3 given qwk; max 20 mg/wk
Polyarticular-course-juvenile RA
• *Child:* **PO** 10 mg/m^2 qwk
Available forms: Tabs 2.5, 5, 7.5, 10, 15 mg; inj 25 mg/ml; powder for inj 20, 25, 50, 100, 250 mg, 1 g
Side effects/adverse reactions:
HEMA: ***Leukopenia, thrombocytopenia, myelosuppression, anemia***
GI: Nausea, vomiting, anorexia, diarrhea, ulcerative stomatitis, ***hepatotoxicity,*** cramps, ulcer, gastritis, ***GI hemorrhage,*** abdominal pain, hematemesis, ***hepatic fibrosis, acute toxicity***
GU: Urinary retention, ***renal failure,*** menstrual irregularities, defective spermatogenesis, ***hematuria, azotemia, uric acid nephropathy***
INTEG: Rash, alopecia, dry skin, urticaria, photosensitivity, folliculitis, vasculitis, petechiae, ecchymosis, acne, alopecia, ***severe fatal skin reaction***
CNS: Dizziness, ***seizures, leukencephalopathy,*** headache, confusion, hemiparesis, malaise, fatigue, chills, fever; ***arachnoiditis*** (intrathecal)
RESP: ***Methotrexate-induced lung disease***
SYST: ***Sudden death, pneumocystis carinii***
Contraindications: Hypersensitivity, leukopenia (<3500/mm^3), thrombocytopenia (<100,000/mm^3), anemia, psoriatic patients with severe renal/hepatic disease, pregnancy (X), alcoholism, HIV
Precautions: Renal disease, lactation, children
Do not confuse:
methotrexate/metolazone
Pharmacokinetics:
PO: Readily absorbed
PO/IM/IV: Onset unknown; duration unknown
IT: Onset, peak, duration unknown
Not metabolized; excreted in urine (unchanged); crosses placenta, blood-brain barrier; 50% plasma protein bound
Interactions:
• ↑ toxicity: salicylates, sulfa drugs, other antineoplastics, radiation, alcohol, probenecid, NSAIDs, phenylbutazone, theophylline, penicillins
• ↓ effect of oral digoxin, vaccines, phenytoin, fosphenytoin
• ↑ hypoprothrombinemia: oral anticoagulants
• ↓ effect of methotrexate: folic acid supplements

NURSING CONSIDERATIONS
Assess:
PO
• Make sure that drug is taken weekly in RA, JRA
◆ CBC, differential, platelet count weekly; withhold drug if WBC is <3500/mm^3 or platelet count is <100,000/mm^3; notify prescriber; drug should be discontinued; WBC, platelet nadirs occur on day 7
• Renal studies: BUN, serum uric acid, urine CCr, electrolytes before, during therapy

• I&O ratio; report fall in urine output to <30 ml/hr
• Monitor temp q4h; fever may indicate beginning infection; no rectal temps
• Hepatic studies before and during therapy: bilirubin, alk phosphatase, AST, ALT; liver biopsy should be done before start of therapy (psoriasis patients)
• Bleeding time, coagulation time during treatment; bleeding: hematuria, guaiac, bruising or petechiae, mucosa or orifices q8h
• Effects of alopecia on body image; discuss feelings about body changes
⇔ Hepatotoxicity: jaundiced skin and sclera, dark urine, clay-colored stools, pruritus, abdominal pain, fever, diarrhea
• Monitor methotrexate levels, adjust leucovorin dose based on the level
• Buccal cavity q8h for dryness, sores, ulceration, white patches, oral pain, bleeding, dysphagia
⇔ Symptoms indicating severe allergic reaction: rash, urticaria, itching, flushing

Administer:

• Antacid before oral agent; give drug after evening meal before bedtime
• Antiemetic 30-60 min before giving drug
• Allopurinol or sodium bicarbonate to maintain uric acid levels, alkalinization of urine (pH >6.5), adequate fluids

IV route

• After diluting 5 mg/2 ml of sterile H_2O for inj; give through Y-tube or 3-way stopcock at 10 mg or less/min
⇔ Leucovorin calcium within 24 hr of this drug to prevent tissue damage; check agency policy, continue until methotrexate level $<10^{-8}$m
⇔ Give sodium bicarbonate tabs or IV fluids to prevent precipitation of drug at high doses; urine pH should be >7; may need to reduce dosage if BUN 20-30 mg/dl or creatinine is 1.2-2 mg/dl; stop drug if BUN >30 mg/dl or creatinine is >2 mg/dl

Additive compatibilities: Cephalothin, cyclophosphamide, cytarabine, fluorouracil, hydrOXYzine, mercaptopurine, ondansetron, sodium bicarbonate, vinCRIStine

Solution compatibilities: Amino acids, 4.25%/D_{25}, D_5W, sodium bicarbonate 0.05 mol/L, sodium chloride 0.9%

Syringe compatibilities: Bleomycin, cisplatin, cyclophosphamide, doxapram, DOXOrubicin, fluorouracil, furosemide, heparin, leucovorin, mitomycin, vinBLAStine, vinCRIStine

Y-site compatibilities: Allopurinol, amifostine, amphotericin B cholesteryl, asparaginase, aztreonam, bleomycin, cefepime, ceftriaxone, cimetidine, cisplatin, cyclophosphamide, cytarabine, DAUNOrubicin, dexchlorpheniramine, diphenhydrAMINE, DOXOrubicin, DOXOrubicin liposome, etoposide, famotidine, filgrastim, fludarabine, fluorouracil, furosemide, gallium, ganciclovir, granisetron, heparin, hydromorphone, imipenem/cilastatin, leucovorin, lorazepam, melphalan, mesna, methylPREDNISolone, metoclopramide, mitomycin, morphine, ondansetron, oxacillin, paclitaxel, piperacillin/tazobactam, prochlorperazine, ranitidine, sargramostim, teniposide, thiotepa, vinBLAStine, vinCRIStine, vinorelbine

Perform/provide:

• Strict medical asepsis and protective isolation if WBC levels are low
• Liquid diet: carbonated beverage,

M

Jell-O; dry toast, crackers may be added when patient is not nauseated or vomiting
- Increased fluid intake to 2-3 L/day to prevent urate deposits, calculi formation, unless contraindicated
- Diet low in purines: absence of organ meats (kidney, liver), dried beans, peas to maintain alkaline urine
- Rinsing of mouth tid-qid with water, club soda; brushing of teeth bid-tid with soft brush or cotton-tipped applicators for stomatitis; use unwaxed dental floss
- Nutritious diet with iron, vitamin supplements
- Storage in tightly closed container in cool environment; store injection, powder for inj in dark, dry area

Evaluate:
- Therapeutic response: decreased tumor size, spread of malignancy

Teach patient/family:
- To report any complaints, side effects to nurse or prescriber: black tarry stools, chills, fever, sore throat, bleeding, bruising, cough, shortness of breath, dark or bloody urine
- That hair may be lost during treatment; wig or hairpiece may make patient feel better; tell patient that new hair may be different in color, texture (alopecia is rare)
- To avoid foods with citric acid, hot or rough texture if stomatitis is present
- To report stomatitis: any bleeding, white spots, ulcerations in mouth to prescriber; tell patient to examine mouth qd, report symptoms to nurse, use good oral hygiene
- That contraceptive measures are recommended during therapy and for at least 8 wk following cessation of therapy, to discontinue breastfeeding; toxicity to infant may occur
- To drink 10-12 glasses of fluid/day
- To avoid alcohol, salicylates, live vaccines
- To avoid use of razors, commercial mouthwash
- To use sunblock to prevent burns

methylcellulose (OTC)

(meth-ill-sell'yoo-lose)

Citrucel

Func. class.: Laxative, bulk

Chem. class.: Hydrophilic semisynthetic cellulose derivative

Action: Attracts water, expands in intestine to increase peristalsis; also absorbs excess water in stool; decreases diarrhea

Uses: Chronic constipation

Dosage and routes:
- *Adult:* **PO** up to 6 g qd in divided doses
- *Child 6-12 yr:* **PO** 3 g qd in divided doses

Available forms: Powder 105 mg/g, 196 mg/g

Side effects/adverse reactions:

*GI: **Obstruction,*** abdominal distention

Contraindications: Hypersensitivity, GI obstruction, hepatitis

Do not confuse:

Citrucel/Citracal

Pharmacokinetics:

PO: Onset 12-24 hr, peak 1-3 days

Interactions:
- ↓ absorption: antibiotics, digitalis, nitrofurantoin, salicylates, tetracyclines, oral anticoagulants

↑ laxative action: flax senna

NURSING CONSIDERATIONS

Assess:
- Blood, urine electrolytes if used often
- I&O ratio to identify fluid loss
- Cause of constipation; lack of fluids, bulk, exercise

• Cramping, rectal bleeding, nausea, vomiting; drug should be discontinued

Administer:

PO route

• Alone for better absorption; do not take within 1 hr of other drugs

• In morning or evening (oral dose)

Evaluate:

• Therapeutic response: decrease in constipation

Teach patient/family:

⊘ To swallow tabs whole; do not break, crush, or chew

• To increase fluid intake

• That normal bowel movements do not always occur daily

• Not to use in presence of abdominal pain, nausea, vomiting

• To notify prescriber if constipation unrelieved or if symptoms of electrolyte imbalance occur: muscle cramps, pain, weakness, dizziness, excessive thirst

methyldopa/methyldopate (℞)

(meth-ill-doe′pa)

Aldomet, Apo-Methyldopa✦, Dopamet✦, methyldopa/methyldopate, Novamedopa✦, Nu-Medopa✦

Func. class.: Antihypertensive

Chem. class.: Centrally acting α-adrenergic inhibitor

Action: Stimulates central inhibitory α-adrenergic receptors or acts as false transmitter, resulting in reduction of arterial pressure

Uses: Hypertension, hypertensive crisis

Dosage and routes:

• *Adult:* **PO** 250-500 mg bid or tid, then adjusted q2d as needed, 0.5-2 g qd in 2-4 divided doses (maintenance), not to exceed 3 g/day; **IV** 250-500 mg in 100 ml D_5W q6h, run over 30-60 min, not to exceed 1 g q6h, switch to oral as soon as possible

• *Geriatric:* **PO** 125 mg bid-tid, increase q2d as needed, max 3 g/day

• *Child:* **PO** 10 mg/kg/day in 2-4 divided doses, not to exceed 65 mg/kg or 3 g/day, whichever is less; **IV** 20-40 mg/kg/day in 4 divided doses, not to exceed 65 mg/kg or 3g, whichever is less

Available forms: Methyldopa: tabs 125, 250, 500 mg; oral susp 50 mg/ml; methyldopate: inj 50 mg/ml

Side effects/adverse reactions:

ENDO: Breast enlargement, gynecomastia, lactation, amenorrhea

GI: Nausea, vomiting, diarrhea, constipation, ***hepatic dysfunction,*** sore or "black" tongue, ***pancreatitis,*** colitis, flatulence

CV: Bradycardia, ***myocarditis,*** orthostatic hypotension, angina, edema, weight gain, ***CHF,*** paradoxical pressor response (IV use)

CNS: Drowsiness, weakness, dizziness, sedation, headache, depression, psychosis paresthesias, parkinsonism, Bell's palsy, nightmares

EENT: Nasal congestion

HEMA: ***Leukopenia, thrombocytopenia, hemolytic anemia, granulocytopenia,*** positive Coombs' test

INTEG: Rash, ***toxic epidermal necrolysis,*** lupuslike syndrome

GU: Impotence, failure to ejaculate

Contraindications: Active hepatic disease, hypersensitivity

Precautions: Pregnancy (B) (PO); (C) (IV), hepatic disease, eclampsia, severe cardiac disease, renal disease

Do not confuse:

methyldopa/L-dopa (levodopa)

Pharmacokinetics:

PO: Peak 2-4 hr, duration 12-24 hr

IV: Peak 2 hr, duration 10-16 hr

M

Metabolized by liver, excreted in urine

Interactions:

• ↑ pressor effect: sympathomimetic amines, MAOIs

• ↑ hypotension, CNS toxicity: levodopa

• ↑ psychosis: haloperidol

• Lithium toxicity: lithium

• ↑ CNS depression: alcohol, antihistamines, antidepressants, analgesics, sedative/hypnotics

• ↑ B/P: phenothiazines, β-blockers, amphetamines, NSAIDs, tricyclics, barbiturates

• ↑ hypoglycemia: TOLBUTamide

↓ effect: capsicum, Indian snakeroot

↑ toxicity, death: aconite

↑ or ↓ antihypertensive effect: astragalus, cola tree

↑ antihypertensive effect: barberry, betony, black catechu, black cohosh, bloodroot, broom, burdock, cat's claw, dandelion, goldenseal, Irish moss, Jamaican dogwood, kelp, khella, mistletoe, parsley

↓ antihypertensive effect: coltsfoot, guarana, khat, licorice

Lab test interferences:

Interference: Urinary uric acid, serum creatinine, AST

False increase: Urinary catecholamines

NURSING CONSIDERATIONS

Assess:

• Blood studies: neutrophils, decreased platelets

• Direct Coombs' test before/after 6, 12 mo of therapy

• Baselines in renal, hepatic studies, before therapy begins

• B/P when beginning treatment, periodically thereafter, report significant changes

• Allergic reaction: rash, fever, pruritus, urticaria; drug should be discontinued if antihistamines fail to help

• CNS symptoms, especially in the elderly, depression, change in mental status

• Symptoms of CHF: edema, dyspnea, wet rales, B/P

• Renal symptoms: polyuria, oliguria, urinary frequency; I&O ratio, weight, report weight gain >5 lb

Administer:

PO route

• Shake susp before use

IV route

• After diluting with 100 ml D_5W; run over ½-1 hr

Additive compatibilities: Aminophylline, ascorbic acid, chloramphenicol, diphenhydrAMINE, heparin, magnesium sulfate, multivitamins, netilmicin, potassium chloride, promazine, sodium bicarbonate, succinylcholine, verapamil, vit B/C

Solution compatibilities: D_5W, D_5/0.9% NaCl, Ringer's, sodium bicarbonate 5%, 0.9% NaCl, amino acids 4.25%/D_{25}, Dextran$_6$/0.9% NaCl, Normosol R, Normosol M/D_5W

Y-site compatibilities: Esmolol, heparin, meperidine, morphine, theophylline

Perform/provide:

• Storage of tabs in tight container

Evaluate:

• Therapeutic response: decrease in B/P in hypertension

Teach patient/family:

• To avoid hazardous activities

• Not to discontinue drug abruptly, or withdrawal symptoms may occur: anxiety, increased B/P, headache, insomnia, increased pulse, tremors, nausea, sweating

• Not to use OTC (cough, cold, allergy) products unless directed by prescriber

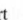

• To comply with dosage schedule even if feeling better

• To rise slowly to sitting or standing position to minimize orthostatic hypotension
• To notify prescriber of mouth sores, sore throat, fever, swelling of hands or feet, irregular heartbeat, chest pain, signs of angioedema
• That excessive perspiration, dehydration, vomiting, diarrhea may lead to fall in blood pressure; consult prescriber
• That dizziness, fainting, lightheadedness may occur during first few days of therapy
• That compliance is necessary; not to skip or stop drug unless directed by prescriber
• That drug may cause skin rash or impaired perspiration

Treatment of overdose: Gastric evacuation, sympathomimetics may be indicated; if severe, hemodialysis

methylergonovine (℞)

(meth-ill-er-goe-noe'veen)
Methergine,
methylergonovine
Func. class.: Oxytocic
Chem. class.: Ergot alkaloid

Action: Stimulates uterine, vascular, smooth muscle, causing contractions; decreases bleeding

Uses: Treatment of hemorrhage postpartum or postabortion, uterine contractions

Dosage and routes:
• *Adult:* **PO** 200-400 mcg q6-12hr × 2-7 days **IM/IV** 200 mcg q2-4hr for 1-5 doses

Available forms: Inj 200 mcg/ml; tabs 200 mcg

Side effects/adverse reactions:
RESP: Dyspnea
GU: Cramping
CNS: Headache, dizziness, ***seizures***
GI: Nausea, vomiting
CV: ***Hypotension,*** chest pain, palpitation, *hypertension,* ***dysrhythmias; CVA (IV)***
EENT: Tinnitus
INTEG: Sweating, rash, allergic reactions

Contraindications: Hypersensitivity to ergot preparations, indication of labor, before delivery of placenta, hypertension, pelvic inflammatory disease, respiratory disease, cardiac disease, peripheral vascular disease

Precautions: Pregnancy (C), severe hepatic disease, severe renal disease, jaundice, diabetes mellitus, convulsive disorders, sepsis

Pharmacokinetics:
PO: Onset 5-25 min, duration 3 hr
IM: Onset 2-5 min, duration 3 hr
IV: Onset immediate, duration 45 min
Metabolized in liver, excreted in urine

M

Interactions:
• ↑ vasoconstriction: vasopressors, nicotine

NURSING CONSIDERATIONS

Assess:
• B/P, pulse, character and amount of vaginal bleeding; watch for indications of hemorrhage
• Respiratory rate, rhythm, depth; notify prescriber of abnormalities
• For uterine relaxation; observe for severe cramping
◆ Ergot toxicity: tinnitus, hypertension, palpitations, chest pain, nausea, vomiting, weakness; cold, numb extremities

Administer:
• Only during fourth stage of labor; not to be used to augment labor
• IM in deep muscle mass; rotate injection sites of additional doses

IV route
• Undiluted through Y-tube or 3-way

stopcock; give 0.2 mg or less/min or diluted in 5 ml 0.9% NaCl given through Y-site

• With crash cart available on unit; IV route used only in emergencies

Y-site compatibilities: Heparin, hydrocortisone sodium succinate, potassium chloride, vit B/C

Evaluate:

• Therapeutic response: absence of hemorrhage

Teach patient/family:

• To report increased blood loss, severe abdominal cramps, fever or foul-smelling lochia

• To avoid smoking

methylphenidate (℞)

(meth-ill-fen′i-date)

Concerta, Metadate CD, Metadate ER, Methylin, Methylin SR, PMS-methylphenidate, Methidate, PMS-Methylphenidate♣, Riphenidate♣, Ritalin, Ritalin SR

Func. class.: Cerebral stimulant

Chem. class.: Piperidine derivative

Controlled Substance Schedule II

Action: Increases release of norepinephrine, DOPamine in cerebral cortex to reticular activating system; exact action not known

Uses: Attention deficit hyperactivity disorder, narcolepsy

Investigational uses: Depression in the elderly; cancer, post-stroke patients, HIV, brain injury, anesthesia-related hiccups

Dosage and routes:

Attention deficit hyperactivity disorder

• *Child >6 yr:* **PO** 5 mg before breakfast and lunch, increasing by 5-10 mg/wk, not to exceed 60 mg/day; sus rel 20 mg qd-tid

Narcolepsy

• *Adult:* **PO** 10 mg bid-tid, 30-45 min before meals, may increase up to 40-60 mg/day

Depression (elderly)

• *Geriatric:* **PO** 2.5 mg QAM, increase q 3rd day by 2.5 mg to desired dose, max 20 mg/day

Available forms: Tabs 5, 10, 20 mg; tabs ext rel 10, 20, mg; tabs, ext rel (Concerta): 18, 36, 54 mg; cap, ext rel 20 mg

Side effects/adverse reactions:

MISC: Fever, arthralgia, scalp hair loss

CNS: Hyperactivity, insomnia, restlessness, talkativeness, dizziness, drowsiness, toxic psychosis, headache, akathisia, dyskinesia, masking or worsening of Gilles de la Tourette's syndrome, ***seizures***

GI: Nausea, anorexia, dry mouth, weight loss, abdominal pain

CV: Palpitations, tachycardia, B/P changes, angina, ***dysrhythmias,*** palpitations

INTEG: ***Exfoliative dermatitis,*** urticaria, rash, erythema multiforme

ENDO: Growth retardation

HEMA: ***Leukopenia, anemia, thrombocytopenic purpura***

Contraindications: Hypersensitivity, anxiety, history of Gilles de la Tourette's syndrome; children <6 yr, glaucoma

Precautions: Hypertension, depression, pregnancy (C), seizures, lactation, drug abuse

Do not confuse:

methylphenidate/methadone

Pharmacokinetics:

PO: Onset ½-1 hr, duration 4-6 hr, metabolized by liver, excreted by kidneys

Interactions:
• Hypertensive crisis: MAOIs or within 14 days of MAOIs, vasopressors
• ↓ effect of: guanethidine
• ↑ effects of: tricyclics, anticonvulsants, SSRIs
• Drug/food: ↑ stimulation: caffeine
↑ CNS stimulation: cola nut, guarana, horsetail, yerba maté, yohimbe
Synergistic effect: melatonin

NURSING CONSIDERATIONS
Assess:
• VS, B/P; may reverse antihypertensives; check patients with cardiac disease more often for increased B/P
• CBC, urinalysis, in diabetes: blood glucose, urine glucose; insulin changes may have to be made, since eating will decrease
• Height, growth rate q3mo in children; growth rate may be decreased
• Mental status: mood, sensorium, affect, stimulation, insomnia, aggressiveness
Withdrawal symptoms: headache, nausea, vomiting, muscle pain, weakness
• Appetite, sleep, speech patterns
• For attention span, decreased hyperactivity in ADHD persons

Administer:
• At least 6 hr before hs to avoid sleeplessness (regular release); at least 10 hr (SR, ER)
• Gum, hard candy, frequent sips of water for dry mouth

Evaluate:
• Therapeutic response: decreased hyperactivity (ADHD) or ability to stay awake (narcolepsy)

Teach patient/family:
• To decrease caffeine consumption (coffee, tea, cola, chocolate); may increase irritability, stimulation; not to use guarana, yerba maté, cola nut
Not to break, crush, or chew time-released medication
• To avoid OTC preparations unless approved by prescriber
• To taper off drug over several wk, or depression, increased sleeping, lethargy will occur
• To avoid driving, hazardous activities if dizziness, blurred vision occur
• To avoid alcohol ingestion
• To avoid hazardous activities until stabilized on medication
• To get needed rest; patients will feel more tired at end of day
• That shell of Concerta tab may appear in stools

Treatment of overdose: Administer fluids; hemodialysis or peritoneal dialysis; antihypertensive for increased B/P; administer short-acting barbiturate before lavage

M

* methylPREDNISolone (℞)
(meth-il-pred-niss′oh-lone)
A-Methapred, depMedalone, Depoject, Depo-Medrol, Depopred, Depo-Predate, Medrol, Duralone, Medralone, Rep-Pred, Solu-Medrol
Func. class.: Corticosteroid
Chem. class.: Glucocorticoid, immediate acting

Action: Decreases inflammation by suppression of migration of polymorphonuclear leukocytes, fibroblasts; reversal of increased capillary permeability and lysosomal stabilization

Uses: Severe inflammation, shock, adrenal insufficiency, collagen disorders, management of acute spinal cord injury

Dosage and routes:

Adrenal insufficiency/inflammation

• *Adult:* **PO** 2-60 mg in 4 divided doses; **IM** 10-80 mg (acetate); **IM/IV** 10-250 mg (succinate); intraarticular 4-30 mg (acetate); **RECT** 40 mg 3-7 × wk for ≥2 wk

• *Child:* **IV** 117 mcg-1.66 mg/kg in 3-4 divided doses (succinate); **RECT** 0.5-1 mg/kg (15-30 mg/m^2) qd or qod × 1 wk or more

Shock

• *Adult:* **IV** 100-250 mg q2-6h or 30 mg/kg, then q4-6h prn, for 2-3 days (succinate)

Multiple sclerosis

• *Adult:* **PO** 160 mg/day × 1 wk, then 64 mg qod × 30 days

Available forms: Tabs 2, 4, 6, 8, 16, 24, 32 mg; inj 20, 40, 80 mg/ml acetate; inj 40, 125, 500, 1000, 2000 mg/vial succinate; susp for inj 20, 40, 80 mg/ml; dose pack 4 mg tabs; enema 40 mg

Side effects/adverse reactions:

CNS: Depression, flushing, sweating, headache, mood changes

CV: Hypertension, ***circulatory collapse, thrombophlebitis, embolism,*** tachycardia

EENT: Fungal infections, increased intraocular pressure, blurred vision, cataracts

GI: Diarrhea, nausea, abdominal distention, ***GI hemorrhage,*** increased appetite, pancreatitis

HEMA: ***Thrombocytopenia***

INTEG: Acne, poor wound healing, ecchymosis, petechiae

MS: Fractures, osteoporosis, weakness

Contraindications: Psychosis, hypersensitivity, idiopathic thrombocytopenia, acute glomerulonephritis, amebiasis, fungal infections, nonasthmatic bronchial disease, child <2 yr, AIDS, TB

Precautions: Pregnancy (C), lactation, diabetes mellitus, glaucoma, osteoporosis, seizure disorders, ulcerative colitis, CHF, myasthenia gravis, renal disease, esophagitis, peptic ulcer

Do not confuse:

methylPREDNISolone/predniSONE

methylPREDNISolone/medroxyPROGESTERone

methylPREDNISolone/methylTESTOSTERone

Pharmacokinetics: Well absorbed PO, IM

PO: Peak 1-2 hr, duration 1½ days

IM: Peak 4-8 days, duration 1-4 wk

Intraarticular: Peak 1 wk

Half-life >3½ hr; crosses placenta, enters breast milk in small amounts; metabolized in liver, excreted by kidneys (unchanged)

Interactions:

• ↓ methylPREDNISolone action: rifampin, phenytoin, theophylline

• ↓ effects of antidiabetics, vaccines, somatrem

• ↑ side effects: amphotericin B, diuretics

• ↑ methylPREDNISolone action: oral contraceptives

• Drug/food: do not use with grapefruit juice, level of methylPREDNISolone will be increased

↑ hypokalemia: aloe, buckthorn, cascara sagrada, Chinese rhubarb, senna

↑ corticosteroid effect: aloe, licorice, perilla

Lab test interferences:

Increase: Cholesterol, sodium, blood glucose, uric acid, calcium, urine glucose

Decrease: Ca, K, T_4, T_3, thyroid ^{131}I uptake test, urine 17-OHCS, 17-KS

False negative: Skin allergy tests

NURSING CONSIDERATIONS

Assess:

- Potassium depletion: parethesias, fatigue, nausea, vomiting, depression, polyuria, dysrhythmias, weakness
- Edema, hypertension, cardiac symptoms
- Mental status: affect, mood, behavioral changes, aggression
- Potassium, blood glucose, urine glucose while on long-term therapy; hypokalemia and hyperglycemia
- Joint mobility, pain, edema if given intraarticularly
- B/P q4h, pulse; notify prescriber of chest pain, rales
- I&O ratio; be alert for decreasing urinary output, increasing edema; weight daily; notify prescriber of weekly gain >5 lb
- Adrenal insufficiency: weight loss, nausea, vomiting, confusion, anxiety, hypotension, weakness
- Plasma cortisol levels during long-term therapy (normal level: 138-635 nmol/L SI units when drawn at 8 AM)
- Growth in children on long-term treatment

Administer:

- Titrated dose; use lowest effective dose
- IM inj deep in large muscle mass; rotate sites; avoid deltoid; use 21G needle; after shaking suspension (parenteral)
- In one dose in AM to prevent adrenal suppression; avoid SC administration; may damage tissue
- With food or milk to decrease GI symptoms (PO)

◆ Do not give Solu-Medrol intrathecally

IV route

- After diluting with diluent provided; agitate slowly; give 500 mg or less/1 min or longer; may be given as IV infusion in its own diluent over 10-20 min

Additive compatibilities: Chloramphenicol, cimetidine, clindamycin, DOPamine, granisetron, heparin, norepinephrine, penicillin G potassium, ranitidine, theophylline, verapamil

Syringe compatibilities: Granisetron, metoclopramide

Y-site compatibilities: Acyclovir, amifostine, amphotericin B cholesteryl, amrinone, aztreonam, cefepime, cisplatin, cladribine, cyclophosphamide, cytarabine, DOPamine, DOXOrubicin, enalaprilat, famotidine, fludarabine, granisetron, heparin, melphalan, meperidine, methotrexate, metronidazole, midazolam, morphine, piperacillin/tazobactam, remifentanil, sodium bicarbonate, tacrolimus, teniposide, theophylline, thiotepa

Perform/provide:

- Assistance with ambulation in patient with bone tissue disease to prevent fractures

Evaluate:

- Therapeutic response: ease of respirations, decreased inflammation; decreased symptoms of adrenal insufficiency
- Infection: increased temp, WBC, even after withdrawal of medication; drug masks infection

Teach patient/family:

- To increase intake of potassium, calcium, protein
- To carry emergency ID (steroid user)
- To notify prescriber if therapeutic response decreases; dosage adjustment may be needed
- Not to discontinue abruptly, or adrenal crisis can result
- To avoid OTC products: salicylates, alcohol in cough products, cold preparations unless directed by pre-

M

scriber; to avoid vaccinations, since immunosuppression occurs
- About cushingoid symptoms
- To recognize the symptoms of adrenal insufficiency: nausea, anorexia, fatigue, dizziness, dyspnea, weakness, joint pain

*methylPREDNISolone topical

See appendix c

methysergide (℞)

(meth-i-ser'jide)

Sansert

Func. class.: Adrenergic blocker, serotonin antagonist

Chem. class.: Ergot derivative

Action: Competitively blocks serotonin HT receptors in CNS and periphery; potent vasoconstrictor

Uses: Prophylaxis for migraine and other vascular headaches. If no improvement is noted in 3 wk, drug is unlikely to be beneficial

Dosage and routes:
- *Adult:* **PO** 2-4 mg bid with meals; 3-4 wk rest period after each 6 mo treatment

Available forms: Tabs 2 mg

Side effects/adverse reactions:

CNS: Tremors, anxiety, insomnia, headache, dizziness, euphoria, confusion, depersonalization, hallucination, paresthesias, drowsiness

CV: ***Retroperitoneal fibrosis,*** valvular thickening, palpitations, tachycardia, postural hypertension, angina, ***thrombophlebitis,*** ECG changes, ***cardiac fibrosis***

GI: Nausea, vomiting, weight gain

MS: Arthralgia, myalgia

INTEG: Flushing, rash, alopecia

HEMA: ***Blood dyscrasias***

Contraindications: Hypersensitivity to ergot, tartrazine, occlusion (peripheral, vascular), CAD, hepatic disease, renal disease, peptic ulcer, hypertension, connective tissue disease, fibrotic pulmonary disease, pregnancy (X)

Precautions: Lactation, children

Pharmacokinetics:

PO: Half-life 10 hr, metabolized by liver, excreted in urine (metabolites/unchanged drug)

Interactions:
- ↑ vasoconstriction: β-blockers, smoking
- ↓ effect of: opiates

NURSING CONSIDERATIONS

Assess:
- Weight daily; check for peripheral edema in feet, legs; B/P
- For stress, activity, recreation, coping mechanisms
- Neurologic status: LOC, blurring vision, nausea, vomiting, tingling in extremities that precedes headache
- Ingestion of tyramine foods (pickled products, beer, wine, aged cheese), food additives, preservatives, colorings, artificial sweeteners, chocolate, caffeine may precipitate these types of headaches

Administer:

PO route
- Give with or after meals to avoid GI symptoms
- Only to women who are not pregnant; harm to fetus may occur
- For less than 6 mo continuously, a 3-4 wk drug-free period must follow each 6 mo period

Perform/provide:
- Storage in dark area
- Quiet, calm environment with decreased stimulation such as noise, bright light, or excessive talking

Evaluate:
- Therapeutic response: decrease in frequency, severity of headache

Teach patient/family:

- Not to use OTC medications; serious interactions may occur
- To maintain dose at approved level, not to increase even if drug does not relieve headache
- To report side effects: increased vasoconstriction starting with cold extremities, then paresthesia, weakness
- That headaches may increase when drug discontinued after long-term use
- To keep drug out of reach of children; death may occur
- To report at once: dyspnea, paresthesias, urinary problems, pain in abdomen, chest, back, legs
- To use drug for less than 6 mo unless a 3-4 wk rest period has been taken
- That drug may cause drowsiness

metipranolol ophthalmic

See appendix c

metoclopramide (℞)

(met-oh-kloe-pra′mide)

Apo-Metoclop✤, Clopra, Emex✤, Maxeran✤, metoclopramide, Octamide-PFS, Reclomide, Reglan

Func. class.: Cholinergic, antiemetic

Chem. class.: Central dopamine receptor antagonist

Action: Enhances response to acetylcholine of tissue in upper GI tract, which causes contraction of gastric muscle; relaxes pyloric, duodenal segments; increases peristalsis without stimulating secretions, blocks dopamine in chemoreceptor trigger zone of CNS

Uses: Prevention of nausea, vomiting induced by chemotherapy, radiation, delayed gastric emptying, gastroesophageal reflux

Investigational uses: Hiccups, migraines

Dosage and routes:

Renal dose

- *Adult:* CCr <40 ml/min 50% of dose

Nausea/vomiting

- *Adult:* **IV** 1-2 mg/kg 30 min before administration of chemotherapy, then q2h × 2 doses, then q3h × 3 doses
- *Child:* **IV** 0.1-0.2 mg/kg/dose

Facilitate small bowel intubation, in radiologic exams

- *Adult and child >14 yr:* **IV** 10 mg over 1-2 min
- *Child <6 yr:* **IV** 0.1 mg/kg
- *Child 6-14 yr:* **IV** 2.5-5 mg

Diabetic gastroparesis

- *Adult:* **PO** 10 mg 30 min ac, hs × 2-8 wk
- *Geriatric:* **PO** 5 mg ½ hr ac hs, increase to 10 mg if needed

Hiccups

- *Adult:* **PO/IM** 10-20 mg qid **(PO);** may give 10 mg **IM**

Gastroesophageal reflux

- *Adult:* **PO** 10-15 mg qid 30 min ac
- *Child:* **PO** 0.4-0.8 mg/kg/day in 4 divided doses

Available forms: Tabs 5, 10 mg; syr 5 mg/5 ml; inj 5 mg/ml; conc sol 10 mg/ml

Side effects/adverse reactions:

CNS: Sedation, fatigue, restlessness, headache, sleeplessness, dystonia, dizziness, drowsiness, ***suicide ideation, seizures,*** EPS

GI: Dry mouth, constipation, nausea, anorexia, vomiting, diarrhea

GU: Decreased libido, prolactin secretion, amenorrhea, galactorrhea

CV: Hypotension, supraventricular tachycardia

INTEG: Urticaria, rash
HEMA: ***Neutropenia, leukopenia, agranulocytosis***
Contraindications: Hypersensitivity to this drug or procaine or procainamide, seizure disorder, pheochromocytoma, breast cancer (prolactin dependent), GI obstruction
Precautions: Pregnancy (B), lactation, GI hemorrhage, CHF, Parkinson's disease
Do not confuse:
metoclopramide/metolazone
Reglan/Megace
Pharmacokinetics:
IV: Onset 1-3 min, duration 1-2 hr
PO: Onset ½-1 hr, duration 1-2 hr
IM: Onset 10-15 min, duration 1-2 hr
Metabolized by liver, excreted in urine, half-life 4 hr
Interactions:
- ↓ action of metoclopramide: anticholinergics, opiates
- ↑ sedation: alcohol, other CNS depressants
- ↑ risk of EPS: haloperidol, phenothiazines
- Avoid use with MAOIs

Lab test interferences:
Increase: Prolactin, aldosterone, thyrotropin
NURSING CONSIDERATIONS
Assess:
- For EPS and tardive dyskinesia, more likely to occur in elderly patient
- Mental status: depression, anxiety, irritability
- GI complaints: nausea, vomiting, anorexia, constipation

Administer:
PO route
- ½-1 hr before meals for better absorption
- Gum, hard candy, frequent rinsing of mouth for dry oral cavity

IV route
- DiphenhydrAMINE IV for EPS
- Undiluted if dose is ≤10 mg; give over 2 min; more than 10 mg may be diluted in 50 ml or more D_5W, NaCl, Ringer's, LR and given over 15 min or more

Additive compatibilities: Clindamycin, meropenem, morphine, multivitamins, potassium acetate, potassium chloride, potassium phosphate, verapamil
Syringe compatibilities: Aminophylline, ascorbic acid, atropine, benztropine, bleomycin, butorphanol, chlorproMAZINE, cisplatin, cyclophosphamide, cytarabine, dexamethasone, dimenhyDRINATE, diphenhydrAMINE, DOXOrubicin, droperidol, fentanyl, fluorouracil, heparin, hydrocortisone, hydrOXYzine, insulin (regular), leucovorin, lidocaine, magnesium sulfate, meperidine, methotrimeprazine, methylPREDNISolone, midazolam, mitomycin, morphine, pentazocine, perphenazine, prochlorperazine, promazine, promethazine, ranitidine, scopolamine, sufentanil, vinBLAStine, vinCRIStine, vit B/C
Y-site compatibilities: Acyclovir, aldesleukin, amifostine, aztreonam, bleomycin, ciprofloxacin, cisatracurium, cisplatin, cladribine, cyclophosphamide, cytarabine, diltiazem, DOXOrubicin, droperidol, famotidine, filgrastim, fluconazole, fludarabine, fluorouracil, foscarnate, gallium, granisetron, heparin, idarubicin, leucovorin, melphalan, meperidine, meropenum, methotrexate, mitomycin, morphine, ondansetron, paclitaxel, piperacillin/tazobactam, propofol, remifentanil, sargramostim, sufentanil, tacrolimus, teniposide, thiotepa, vinBLAStine, vinCRIStine, vinorelbine, zidovudine

Perform/provide:
• Protect from light with aluminum foil during infusion
• Discard open ampules

Evaluate:
• Therapeutic response: absence of nausea, vomiting, anorexia, fullness

Teach patient/family:
• To avoid driving, other hazardous activities until patient is stabilized on this medication
• To avoid alcohol, other CNS depressants that will enhance sedating properties of this drug

metolazone (℞)
(me-tole'a-zone)
Mykrox, Zaroxolyn
Func. class.: Diuretic, antihypertensive
Chem. class.: Thiazide-like quinazoline derivative

Action: Acts on distal tubule and cortical thick ascending limb of the loop of Henle by increasing excretion of water, sodium, chloride, potassium, magnesium, bicarbonate

Uses: Edema, hypertension, CHF, nephrotic syndrome

Dosage and routes:
Edema
• *Adult:* **PO** 5-20 mg/day
Hypertension
• *Adult:* **PO** 2.5-5 mg/day (Zaroxolyn)
• *Child:* **PO** 0.2-0.4 mg/kg/day divided q12-24h
• *Adult:* **PO** 0.5 mg (Mykrox) qd in AM, may increase to 1 mg

Available forms: Tabs 0.5 (Mykrox), 2.5, 5, 10 mg

Side effects/adverse reactions:
GU: Urinary frequency, polyuria, ***uremia, glucosuria***
CNS: Drowsiness, paresthesia, anxiety, depression, headache, *dizziness, fatigue, weakness*
GI: Nausea, vomiting, anorexia, constipation, diarrhea, cramps, pancreatitis, GI irritation, ***hepatitis***
EENT: Blurred vision
INTEG: Rash, urticaria, purpura, photosensitivity, fever
META: Hyperglycemia, increased creatinine, BUN
HEMA: ***Aplastic anemia, hemolytic anemia, leukopenia, agranulocytosis, neutropenia***
CV: Irregular pulse, orthostatic hypotension, palpitations, volume depletion
ELECT: Hypokalemia, hypomagnesemia, hypercalcemia, hyponatremia, hypochloremia, hypophosphatemia

Contraindications: Hypersensitivity to thiazides or sulfonamides, anuria, lactation

Precautions: Hypokalemia, renal disease, hepatic disease, gout, COPD, lupus erythematosus, diabetes mellitus, pregnancy (B)

M

Do not confuse:
metolazone/methotrexate
metolazone/metoclopramide

Pharmacokinetics:
PO: Onset 1 hr, peak 2 hr, duration 12-24 hr; excreted unchanged by kidneys; crosses placenta; enters breast milk; half-life 8 hr

Interactions:
• ↓ action of metolazone: NSAIDs, salicylates
• ↑ hypokalemia: mezlocillin, piperacillin, amphotericin B, glucocorticoids, digoxin, stimulants, laxatives
• ↑ hypotension: alcohol (large amounts), nitrates, antihypertensives, barbiturates, opioids
• ↑ toxicity: lithium
↑ hypokalemia: aloe, buckthorn, cascara sagrada, rhubarb, senna
↑ toxicity, death: aconite

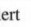

↑ or ↓ antihypertensive effect: astragalus, cola tree

↑ antihypertensive effect: barberry, betony, black catechu, black cohosh, bloodroot, broom, burdock, cat's claw, dandelion, goldenseal, Irish moss, Jamaican dogwood, kelp, khella, mistletoe, parsley

↓ antihypertensive effect: coltsfoot, guarana, khat, licorice

Lab test interferences:
Increase: BSP retention, calcium, amylase, parathyroid test
Decrease: PBI, PSP

NURSING CONSIDERATIONS
Assess:
- Weight, I&O daily to determine fluid loss; effect of drug may be decreased if used qd
- Rate, depth, rhythm of respiration, effect of exertion
- B/P lying, standing; postural hypotension may occur
- Electrolytes: K, Mg, Na, Cl; include BUN, blood glucose, CBC, serum creatinine, blood pH, ABGs, uric acid, calcium
- Improvement in edema of feet, legs, sacral area daily if medication is being used in CHF
- Improvement in CVP q8h
- Signs of metabolic alkalosis: drowsiness, restlessness
- Signs of hypokalemia: postural hypotension, malaise, fatigue, tachycardia, leg cramps, weakness
- Rashes, fever qd
- Confusion, especially in elderly; take safety precautions if needed

Administer:
- In AM to avoid interference with sleep if using drug as a diuretic
- Potassium replacement if potassium <3 mg/dl
- With food, if nausea occurs; absorption may be decreased slightly
- Extended product is Zaroxolyn; prompt product is Mykrox

Evaluate:
- Therapeutic response: decreased edema, B/P

Teach patient/family:
- To increase fluid intake to 2-3 L/day unless contraindicated, to rise slowly from lying or sitting position
- To notify prescriber of muscle weakness, cramps, nausea, dizziness
- That drug may be taken with food or milk
- To use sunscreen for photosensitivity
- That blood glucose may be increased in diabetics
- To take early in day to avoid nocturia

Treatment of overdose: Lavage if taken orally; monitor electrolytes; administer dextrose in saline; monitor hydration, CV, renal status

metoprolol (℞)
(meh-toe'proe-lole)
Betaloc♣, Betaloc Durules♣, Lopresor♣, Lopressor, Lopressor SR♣, Novometoprol♣, Toprol-XL

Func. class.: Antihypertensive, antianginal
Chem. class.: β_1-Blocker

Action: Lowers B/P by β-blocking effects; reduces elevated renin plasma levels; blocks β_2-adrenergic receptors in bronchial, vascular smooth muscle only at high doses

Uses: Mild to moderate hypertension, acute MI to reduce cardiovascular mortality, angina pectoris, NYHA class II, III heart failure

Investigational uses: Atrial ectopy, antipsychotic induced akathisia, rapid heart rate control, unstable angina, variceal bleeding in portal hypotension

Dosage and routes:

Hypertension

- *Adult:* **PO** 50 mg bid, or 100 mg qd; may give up to 200-450 mg in divided doses; **EXT REL** give qd
- *Geriatric:* **PO** 25 mg/day initially, increase weekly as needed

Myocardial infarction

- *Adult:* (early treatment) **IV BOL** 5 mg q2min × 3, then 50 mg **PO** 15 min after last dose and q6h × 48 hr; (late treatment) **PO** maintenance 100 mg bid for 3 mo

Angina

- *Adult:* **PO** 100 mg qd, increase qwk prn or 100 mg ext rel qd

Available forms: Tabs 50, 100 mg; inj 1 mg/ml; ext rel tab 25, 50, 100, 200 mg

Side effects/adverse reactions:

CV: Hypotension, ***bradycardia, CHF,*** *palpitations,* dysrhythmias, ***cardiac arrest, AV block, pulmonary edema, chest pain***

CNS: Insomnia, dizziness, mental changes, hallucinations, ***depression,*** anxiety, headaches, nightmares, confusion, fatigue

GI: Nausea, vomiting, colitis, cramps, *diarrhea,* constipation, flatulence, dry mouth, *hiccups*

INTEG: Rash, purpura, alopecia, dry skin, urticaria, pruritus

HEMA: ***Agranulocytosis, eosinophilia, thrombocytopenia, purpura***

EENT: Sore throat; dry, burning eyes

GU: Impotence

RESP: ***Bronchospasm,*** dyspnea, wheezing

Contraindications: Hypersensitivity to β-blockers, cardiogenic shock, heart block (2nd, 3rd degree), sinus bradycardia, bronchial asthma

Precautions: Major surgery, pregnancy (C), lactation, diabetes mellitus, renal disease, thyroid disease, COPD, CAD, nonallergic bronchospasm, hepatic disease, CHF

Do not confuse:

metoprolol/misoprostol

Pharmacokinetics:

PO: Peak 2-4 hr, duration 13-19 hr; half-life 3-4 hr; metabolized in liver (metabolites); excreted inurine; crosses placenta; enters breast milk

Interactions:

- ↑ hypotension, bradycardia: reserpine, hydrALAZINE, methyldopa, prazosin, amphetamines, epINEPHrine, H_2-antagonists, calcium channel blockers
- ↑ hypoglycemic effects: insulin oral antidiabetics
- Do not use with MAOIs
- ↓ antihypertensive effect: salicylates, NSAIDs
- ↑ effects of: benzodiazepines
- ↓ effects of DOPamine, DOBUTamine, xanthines
- Drug/food: ↑ absorption with food

↑ toxicity, death: aconite

↑ or ↓ antihypertensive effect: astragalus, cola tree

↑ antihypertensive effect: barberry, betony, black catechu, black cohosh, bloodroot, broom, burdock, cat's claw, dandelion, goldenseal, Irish moss, Jamaican dogwood, kelp, khella, mistletoe, parsley

↓ antihypertensive effect: coltsfoot, guarana, khat, licorice

Lab test interferences:

Increase: Renal, hepatic studies

NURSING CONSIDERATIONS

Assess:

- ECG directly when giving IV during initial treatment
- I&O, weight daily
- B/P during initial treatment, periodically thereafter; pulse q4h; note rate, rhythm, quality
- Apical/radial pulse before administration; notify prescriber of any significant changes or pulse <50 bpm

M

• Baselines in renal, hepatic studies before therapy begins
• Edema in feet, legs daily
• Skin turgor, dryness of mucous membranes for hydration status

Administer:

PO route

• PO ac, hs, tab may be crushed or swallowed whole, except for ext rel tab

IV route

• IV, undiluted, give over 1 min, × 3 doses at 2 min intervals; start **PO** 15 min after last IV dose

Y-site compatibilities: Alteplase, meperidine, morphine

Perform/provide:

• Storage in dry area at room temperature, do not freeze

Evaluate:

• Therapeutic response: decreased B/P after 1-2 wk

Teach patient/family:

• To take with or immediately after meals
• Not to discontinue drug abruptly; taper over 2 wk; may cause precipitate angina
• Not to use OTC products containing α-adrenergic stimulants (nasal decongestants, OTC cold preparations) unless directed by prescriber
• To report bradycardia, dizziness, confusion, depression, fever, sore throat, shortness of breath to prescriber
• To take pulse at home; advise when to notify prescriber
• To avoid alcohol, smoking, sodium intake
• To comply with weight control, dietary adjustments, modified exercise program
• To carry emergency ID to identify drug, allergies
• To avoid hazardous activities if dizziness is present
• To report symptoms of CHF: difficult breathing, especially on exertion or when lying down, night cough, swelling of extremities
• To take medication hs to prevent effect of orthostatic hypotension
• To wear support hose to minimize effects of orthostatic hypotension

Treatment of overdose: Lavage, IV atropine for bradycardia, IV theophylline for bronchospasm, digitalis, O_2, diuretic for cardiac failure, hemodialysis, hypotension administer vasopressor (norepinephrine)

metronidazole (℞)

(me-troe-ni′da-zole)

Apo-Metronidazole✦, Flagyl, Flagyl ER, Flagyl IV, Flagyl IV RTU, metronidazole, Novonidazole✦, Protostat, Trikacide✦

Func. class.: Antiinfective, misc

Chem. class.: Nitroimidazole derivative

Action: Direct-acting amebicide/trichomonacide binds, degrades DNA in organism

Uses: Intestinal amebiasis, amebic abscess, trichomoniasis, refractory trichomoniasis, bacterial anaerobic infections, giardiasis, septicemia, endocarditis, bone, joint infections, lower respiratory tract infections

Dosage and routes:

Trichomoniasis

• *Adult:* **PO** 250 mg tid × 7 days or 2 g in single dose; do not repeat treatment for 4-6 wk
• *Child:* **PO** 5 mg/kg tid × 7 days

Refractory trichomoniasis

• *Adult:* **PO** 250 mg bid × 10 days

Amebic hepatic abscess

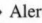

• *Adult:* **PO** 500-750 mg tid × 5-10 days

• *Child:* **PO** 35-50 mg/kg/day in 3 divided doses × 10 days

Intestinal amebiasis

• *Adult:* **PO** 750 mg tid × 5-10 days

• *Child:* **PO** 35-50 mg/kg/day in 3 divided doses × 10 days; then oral iodoquinol

Anaerobic bacterial infections

• *Adult:* **IV INF** 15 mg/kg over 1 hr, then 7.5 mg/kg **IV** or **PO** q6h, not to exceed 4 g/day; first maintenance dose should be administered 6 hr following loading dose

Giardiasis

• *Adult:* **PO** 250 mg tid × 5 days

• *Child:* **PO** 5 mg/kg tid × 5 days

Antibiotic-associated pseudomembranous colitis

• *Adult:* **PO** 250-500 mg 3-4 ×/day × 10-14 days

• *Child:* **PO** 20 mg/kg/day (max 2 g) divided q6h

Available forms: Tabs 250, 375, 500 mg; tab, ext rel 750 mg; inj 500 mg/100 ml; powder for inj 500 mg single dose

Side effects/adverse reactions:

CV: Flat T waves

CNS: Headache, dizziness, confusion, irritability, restlessness, ataxia, depression, fatigue, drowsiness, insomnia, paresthesia, peripheral neuropathy, ***seizures,*** incoordination, depression

EENT: Blurred vision, sore throat, retinal edema, dry mouth, metallic taste, furry tongue, glossitis, stomatitis

GI: Nausea, vomiting, diarrhea, epigastric distress, *anorexia,* constipation, *abdominal cramps,* metallic taste, ***pseudomembranous colitis***

GU: Darkened urine, vaginal dryness, polyuria, ***albuminuria,*** dysuria, cystitis, decreased libido, ***neurotoxicity,*** incontinence, dyspareunia

HEMA: ***Leukopenia, bone marrow, depression, aplasia***

INTEG: Rash, pruritus, urticaria, flushing

Contraindications: Hypersensitivity to this drug, renal disease, hepatic disease, contracted visual or color fields, blood dyscrasias, pregnancy (1st trimester), lactation, CNS disorders

Precautions: *Candida* infections, pregnancy (B) (2nd/3rd trimesters)

Pharmacokinetics:

IV: Onset immediate, peak end of inf

PO: Peak 1-2 hr, half-life 6-11 hr

Crosses placenta, enters breast milk, excreted in feces; absorbed PO (80%-85%)

Interactions:

• Disulfiram reaction: alcohol

• ↑ action of: anticoagulants

• ↓ metronidazole action: phenobarbital, phenytoin

• Toxicity: cimetidine, lithium

Lab test interferences:

Decrease: AST, ALT

NURSING CONSIDERATIONS

Assess:

• For infection: WBC, wound symptoms, fever, skin or vaginal secretions; start treatment after C&S

• Stools during entire treatment; should be clear at end of therapy; stools should be free of parasites for 1 yr before patient is considered cured (amebiasis)

• Vision by ophthalmic exam during, after therapy; vision problems often occur

• I&O; weight daily; stools for number, frequency, character

◆ Neurotoxicity: peripheral neuropathy, seizures, dizziness, uncoordination, pruritus, joint pains; drug may be discontinued

• Allergic reaction: fever, rash, itching, chills; drug should be discontinued if these symptoms occur

• Superinfection: fever, monilial growth, fatigue, malaise
• Renal and reproductive dysfunction: dysuria, polyuria, impotence, dyspareunia, decreased libido

Administer:

PO route

• PO with or after meals to avoid GI symptoms, metallic taste; crush tabs if needed

IV route

• Prediluted; metronidazole IV, dilute with 4.4 ml sterile H_2O or 0.9% NaCl; must be diluted further with 8 mg/ml or more 0.9% NaCl, D_5W, or LR; must neutralize with 5 mEq $NaCO_3$/500 mg; CO_2 gas will be generated and may require venting; run over 1 hr or more; primary IV must be discontinued; may be given as continuous infusion; do not use aluminum products; IV may require venting

Additive compatibilities: Amikacin, aminophylline, cefazolin, cefotaxime, ceftazidime, ceftizoxime, ceftriaxone, cefuroxime, chloramphenicol, ciprofloxacin, clindamycin, disopyramide, floxacillin, fluconazole, gentamicin, heparin, moxalactam, multielectrolyte concentrate, multivitamins, netilmicin, penicillin G potassium, tobramycin

Y-site compatibilities: Acyclovir, allopurinol, amifostine, amiodarone, cefepime, cisatracurium, cyclophosphamide, diltiazem, DOPamine, DOXOrubicin liposome, enalaprilat, esmolol, fluconazole, foscarnet, granisetron, heparin, hydromorphone, labetalol, lorazepam, magnesium sulfate, melphalan, meperidine, methylPREDNISolone, midazolam, morphine, perphenazine, piperacillin/tazobactam, remifentanil, sargramostim, tacrolimus, teniposide, theophylline, thiotepa, vinorelbine

Perform/provide:

• Storage in light-resistant container; do not refrigerate

Evaluate:

• Therapeutic response: decreased symptoms of infection

Teach patient/family:

• That urine may turn dark-reddish brown, drug may cause metallic taste
• Proper hygiene after BM; handwashing technique
• To notify physician for numbness or tingling of extremities
• To avoid hazardous activities, since dizziness can occur
• Need for compliance with dosage schedule, duration of treatment
• To use condoms if treatment for trichomoniasis, or cross-contamination may occur
• To use frequent sips of water, sugarless gum, candy for dry mouth
• That treatment of both partners is necessary in trichomoniasis
• Not to drink alcohol or use preparations containing alcohol during use or for 48 hr after use of drug; disulfiram-like reaction can occur

mexiletine (℞)

(mex-il′e-teen)

Mexitil

Func. class.: Antidysrhythmic (Class IB)

Chem. class.: Lidocaine analog

Action: Increases electrical stimulation threshold of ventricle, His-Purkinje system, which stabilizes cardiac membrane

Uses: Life-threatening ventricular tachycardia; because of proarrhythmic effects, use with lesser dysrhythmias not recommended

Investigational uses: Diabetic neuropathy, ventricular tachycardia, other ventricular dysrhythmias in acute phase of MI

Research note: Fluvoxamine given with mexiletine resulted in an increase of AUC and peak concentration of mexiletine[23]

Dosage and routes:

• *Adult:* **PO** 200-400 mg (loading dose), then 200 mg q8h, then 200-400 mg q8h

Diabetic neuropathy (off-label)

• *Adult:* **PO** 150 mg/day for 3 days, then 300 mg/day for 3 days, followed by 10 mg/kg/day

Available forms: Caps 100, 150, 200, 250 mg

Side effects/adverse reactions:

CNS: Headache, dizziness, confusion, ***seizures,*** tremors, psychosis, nervousness, paresthesias, weakness, fatigue, coordination difficulties, change in sleep habits

EENT: Blurred vision, tinnitus

GI: Nausea, vomiting, anorexia, diarrhea, abdominal pain, ***hepatitis,*** dry mouth, peptic ulcer, altered taste, ***GI bleeding,*** constipation

CV: Hypotension, bradycardia, angina, PVCs, ***heart block, cardiovascular collapse or arrest,*** sinus node slowing, ***left ventricular failure,*** syncope, ***cardiogenic shock, AV conduction disturbances, CHF, atrial dysrhythmias, palpitations, ventricular dysrhythmias***

RESP: Dyspnea

INTEG: Rash, alopecia, dry skin

HEMA: ***Thrombocytopenia, leukopenia, agranulocytosis***

GU: Urinary hesitancy, decreased libido

MISC: Edema, arthralgia, fever, systemic lupus erythematosus syndrome

Contraindications: Hypersensitivity, cardiogenic shock, severe heart block

Precautions: Pregnancy (C), lactation, children, hepatic disease, CHF, seizure disorder, hypotension

Pharmacokinetics:

PO: Peak 2-3 hr; half-life 12 hr, metabolized by liver, excreted unchanged by kidneys (10%), excreted in breast milk

Interactions:

• ↓ or ↑ mexiletine effects: cimetidine

• ↓ mexiletine levels: phenytoin, phenobarbital, rifampin, urinary acidifiers, aluminum/magnesium hydroxide, atropine, opiates

• ↑ mexiletine effects: metoclopramide, urinary alkalinizers

• ↑ levels of: caffeine, theophylline

• Drug/smoking: ↓ drug effect

↑ hypokalemia, ↑ antidysrhythmic action: aloe, buckthorn, cascara sagrada, rhubarb, senna

↑ toxicity, death: aconite

↑ effect: aloe, broom, chronic buckthorn use, cascara sagrada (chronic use), Chinese rhubarb, figwort, fumitory, goldenseal, kudzu, licorice

↓ effect: coltsfoot

↑ serotonin effect: horehound

Lab test interferences:

Increase: CPK

NURSING CONSIDERATIONS

Assess:

• ECG continuously for increased PR or QRS segments; discontinue or reduce rate; watch for increased ventricular ectopic beats; may have to rebolus

• Blood levels (therapeutic level 0.5-2 mcg/ml)

• B/P continuously for fluctuations in cardiac rate

• I&O ratio, electrolytes (K, Na, Cl), liver enzymes

Malignant hyperthermia: tachypnea, tachycardia, changes in B/P, fever

• Respiratory status: rate, rhythm, lung fields for rales, watch for respiratory depression

• CNS effects: dizziness, confu-

M

sion, psychosis, paresthesias, convulsions; drug should be discontinued
- Lung fields, bilateral rales may occur in CHF patient
- Increased respiration, increased pulse; drug should be discontinued

Administer:
- With food for GI upset

Evaluate:
- Therapeutic response: decreased dysrhythmias

Treatment of overdose: O_2, artificial ventilation, ECG; administer DOPamine for circulatory depression, diazepam or thiopental for convulsions, to acidify urine

mezlocillin (℞)

(mez-loe-sill'in)
Mezlin

Func. class.: Antiinfective, broad-spectrum
Chem. class.: Extended-spectrum penicillin

Action: Interferes with cell wall replication of susceptible organisms; osmotically unstable cell wall swells, bursts from osmotic pressure

Uses: Effective for gram-positive cocci *(Staphylococcus aureus, Streptococcus viridans, Streptococcus faecalis, Streptococcus pneumoniae),* gram-negative cocci *(Neisseria gonorrhoeae),* gram-positive bacilli *(Clostridium perfringens, Clostridium tetani),* gram-negative bacilli *(Bacteroides, Escherichia coli, Haemophilus influenzae, Klebsiella, Proteus mirabilis, Proteus vulgaris, Providencia rettgeri, Morganella morganii, Enterobacter, Serratia, Pseudomonas, Shigella, Citrobacter, Veillonella)*; and *Peptococcus, Peptostreptococcus*

Dosage and routes:
- *Adult:* **IM/IV** 200-300 mg/kg/day (serious infections) q4-6h or **IV** 500 mg q8h, may give up to 24 g/day for severe infections
- *Child:* **IM/IV** 50 mg/kg q4-6h
- *Infant >8 days (>2000 g):* 75 mg/kg q6h; *<2000 g:* 75 mg/kg q8h
- *Infant <8 days:* 75 mg/kg q12h

Renal dose
- Dose reduction indicated in renal impairment (CCr <30 ml/min)

Hepatic dose
- Hepatic dose give 50% of dose

Available forms: Powder for inj 1, 2, 3, 4, 20 g

Side effects/adverse reactions:
HEMA: Anemia, increased bleeding time, ***bone marrow depression, granulocytopenia***
GI: Nausea, vomiting, diarrhea; increased AST, ALT; abdominal pain, glossitis, colitis, abnormal taste
GU: Oliguria, proteinuria, hematuria, (vaginitis, moniliasis), ***glomerulonephritis,*** increased BUN, creatinine
CNS: Lethargy, hallucinations, anxiety, depression, twitching, ***coma, seizures***
META: Hyperkalemia, hypokalemia, alkalosis, hypernatremia

Contraindications: Hypersensitivity to penicillins

Precautions: Pregnancy (B), lactation, hypersensitivity to cephalosporins, neonates, renal disease

Do not confuse:
methicillin/mezlocillin

Pharmacokinetics:
IM: Peak 45 min
IV: Peak 5 min
Half-life 50-55 min; partially metabolized in liver; excreted in urine, bile, breast milk (small amount); crosses placenta

Interactions:
- ↓ effect of: oral contraceptives
- ↓ excretion of lithium

- ↑ hypokalemia: diuretics, digoxin
- ↑ mezlocillin concentrations: aspirin, probenecid

↓ absorption: khat, separate by ≥2 hr

Lab test interferences:
False positive: Urine glucose, urine protein

NURSING CONSIDERATIONS

Assess:

- I&O ratio; report hematuria, oliguria, since penicillin in high doses is nephrotoxic
- Any patient with compromised renal system, since drug is excreted slowly in poor renal system function; toxicity may occur rapidly
- Hepatic studies: AST, ALT
- Blood studies: WBC, RBC, Hct, Hgb, bleeding time
- Renal studies: urinalysis, protein, blood, BUN, creatinine
- C&S before drug therapy; drug may be given as soon as culture is taken
- Bowel pattern before and during treatment
- Skin eruptions after administration of penicillin to 1 wk after discontinuing drug
- Respiratory status: rate, character, wheezing, and tightness in chest
- Check IV site for thrombophlebitis
- For possible seizures; seizure precautions in those on high doses
- WBC, differential, hepatic, renal studies periodically for patients on long-term therapy
- Allergies before initiation of treatment, and reaction of each medication
- For signs, symptoms of vaginitis during therapy

Administer:

- Drug after C&S completed

IV route

- After diluting 1 g or less/10 ml of sterile H_2O, D_5, or 0.9% NaCl for inj; shake, dilute further with D_5W or 0.45 NaCl, and give over 3-5 min; may be given by intermittent inf over ½ hr, change site q48h

Solution compatibilities: $D_{10}W$, D_5W, 0.9% NaCl

Syringe compatibilities: Heparin

Y-site compatibilities: Amifostine, aztreonam, cyclophosphamide, DOXOrubicin liposome, famotidine, fludarabine, granisetron, hydromorphone, morphine, perphenazine, propofol, remifentanil, sargramostim, tacrolimus, teniposide, thiotepa

Perform/provide:

- Adrenaline, suction, tracheostomy set, endotracheal intubation equipment
- Adequate fluid intake (2 L) during diarrhea episodes
- Scratch test to assess allergy after securing order from prescriber; usually done when penicillin is only drug of choice
- Storage at room temperature; reconstituted sol is stable for 24 hr refrigerated

Evaluate:

- Therapeutic response: absence of fever, draining wounds

Teach patient/family:

- That culture may be taken after completed course of medication
- To report sore throat, fever, fatigue (may indicate superinfection)
- To wear or carry emergency ID if allergic to penicillins
- To report diarrhea, symptoms of *Candida* vaginitis

Treatment of anaphylaxis: Withdraw drug, maintain airway, administer epINEPHrine, aminophylline, O_2, IV corticosteroids

miconazole topical

See appendix c

miconazole vaginal antifungal

See appendix c

midazolam (℞)

(mid'ay-zoe-lam)

Versed

Func. class.: Sedative, hypnotic, antianxiety

Chem. class.: Benzodiazepine, short-acting

Controlled Substance Schedule IV

Action: Depresses subcortical levels in CNS; may act on limbic system, reticular formation; may potentiate γ-aminobutyric acid (GABA) by binding to specific benzodiazepine receptors

Uses: Preoperative sedation, general anesthesia induction, sedation for diagnostic endoscopic procedures, intubation

Investigational uses: Epileptic seizures, refractory status epilepticus

Dosage and routes:

Preoperative sedation

• *Adult:* **IM** 0.07-0.08 mg/kg ½-1 hr before general anesthesia

• *Child <6 mo:* **IM** 0.1-0.15 mg/kg, may give up to 0.5 mg/kg if needed

• *Child 6 mo-5 yr:* **PO** 0.25-1 mg/kg, max 20 mg as a single dose

• *Child 6 yr-16 yr:* 0.25-0.5 mg/kg, max 20 mg as a single dose

Induction of general anesthesia

• *Adult and child 12-16 yr:* **IV** (unpremedicated patients) 0.3-0.35 mg/kg over 30 sec, wait 2 min, follow with 25% of initial dose if needed; (premedicated patients) 0.15-0.35 mg/kg over 20-30 sec, allow 2 min for effect

• *Child 6-12 yr:* **IV** 0.025-0.05 mg/kg, total dose up to 0.4 mg/kg may be needed

• *Child 6 mo-5 yr:* **IV** 0.05-0.1 mg/kg, total dose up to 0.6 mg/kg may be needed

• *Child <6 mo:* Titrate with small increments

Continuous infusion for intubation (critical care)

• *Adult:* **IV** 0.01-0.05 mg/kg over several min; repeat at 10-15 min intervals, until adequate sedation; then 0.02-0.10 mg/kg/hr maintenance

• *Child:* **IV** 0.05-0.2 mg/kg over 2-3 min, then 0.06-0.12 mg/kg/hr by cont inf; adjust as needed

Available forms: Inj 1, 5 mg/ml, syr 2 mg/ml

Side effects/adverse reactions:

CNS: Retrograde amnesia, euphoria, confusion, headache, anxiety, insomnia, slurred speech, paresthesia, tremors, weakness, chills

RESP: Coughing, ***apnea, bronchospasm, laryngospasm,*** dyspnea, ***respiratory depression***

CV: Hypotension, PVCs, tachycardia, bigeminy, nodal rhythm, ***cardiac arrest***

EENT: Blurred vision, nystagmus, diplopia, blocked ears, loss of balance

GI: Nausea, vomiting, increased salivation, hiccups

INTEG: Urticaria, pain, swelling at inj site, rash, pruritus

Contraindications: Pregnancy (D), hypersensitivity to benzodiazepines, shock, coma, alcohol intoxication, acute narrow-angle glaucoma

Precautions: COPD, CHF, chronic renal failure, chills, elderly, debilitated, children, lactation

Do not confuse:

Versed/Vepesid

Versed/Vistaril

Pharmacokinetics:

IM: Onset 15 min, peak ½-1 hr

IV: Onset 3-5 min, onset of anes-

thesia 1½-2½ min; protein binding 97%; half-life 1.2-12.3 hr
Metabolized in liver; metabolites excreted in urine; crosses placenta, blood-brain barrier

Interactions:

- ↑ respiratory depression: other CNS depressants, alcohol, barbiturates, opiate analgesics, verapamil, ritonavir, indinavir, fluvoxamine
- ↓ midazolam metabolism: azole antifungals, cimetidine, erythromycin, ranitidine, theophylline
- Extended half-life: oral contraceptives
- Drug/food: ↑ midazolam effect: grapefruit juice

↑ hypotension: black cohosh
↑ CNS depression: catnip, chamomile, clary, cowslip, hops, kava, lavender, mistletoe, nettle, pokeweed, poppy, Queen Anne's lace, senega, skullcap, valerian

NURSING CONSIDERATIONS

Assess:

- Injection site for redness, pain, swelling
- Degree of amnesia in elderly; may be increased
- Anterograde amnesia
- Vital signs for recovery period in obese patient, since half-life may be extended
- Apnea, respiratory depression that may be increased in the elderly

Administer:

PO route

- Remove cap of press-in bottle adaptor and push adaptor into neck of bottle, close with cap, remove cap and insert tip of dispenser and insert into adaptor; turn upside-down and withdraw correct dose; place in mouth

IM route

- IM deep into large muscle mass

IV route

- May be given diluted or undiluted
- After diluting with D_5W or 0.9% NaCl to 0.25 mg/ml; give over 2 min (conscious sedation) or over 30 sec (anesthesia induction)

Additive compatibility: Hydromorphone

Syringe compatibilities: Atracurium, atropine, benzquinamide, buprenorphine, butorphanol, chlorproMAZINE, cimetidine, cisatracurium, diphenhydrAMINE, droperidol, fentanyl, glycopyrrolate, hydromorphone, hydrOXYzine, meperidine, metoclopramide, morphine, nalbuphine, promazine, promethazine, remifentanil, scopolamine, sufentanil, thiethylperazine, trimethobenzamide

Y-site compatibilities: Amikacin, amiodarone, atracurium, calcium gluconate, cefazolin, cefmetazole, cefotaxime, cimetidine, ciprofloxacin, clindamycin, digoxin, diltiazem, DOPamine, epINEPHrine, erythromycin, esmolol, etomidate, famotidine, fentanyl, fluconazole, gentamicin, haloperidol, heparin, hydromorphone, insulin (regular), labetalol, lorazepam, methylPREDNISolone, metronidazole, milrinone, morphine, niCARdipine, nitroglycerin, norepinephrine, pancuronium, piperacillin, potassium chloride, ranitidine, sodium nitroprusside, sufentanil, theophylline, tobramycin, vancomycin, vecuronium

Perform/provide:

- Assistance with ambulation until drowsy period relieved
- Storage at room temperature
- Immediate availability of resuscitation equipment, O_2 to support airway; do not give by rapid bolus

Evaluate:

- Therapeutic response: induction of sedation, general anesthesia

Teach patient/family:

- That amnesia occurs; events may not be remembered

M

Treatment of overdose: O_2, vasopressors, physostigmine, resuscitation

midodrine (℞)

(mye'doh-dreen)
ProAmatine
Func. class.: Vasopressor

Action: Activates α-adrenergic receptors of arteriolar, venous vasculature by increasing vascular tone
Uses: Orthostatic hypotension
Dosage and routes:
• *Adult:* **PO** 10 mg tid
Renal dose
• *Adult:* **PO** 2.5 mg tid
Available forms: Tabs 2.5, 5 mg
Side effects/adverse reactions:
CNS: Drowsiness, restlessness, headache, *paresthesia, pain,* chills, confusion
GI: Nausea, anorexia
EENT: Dry mouth, blurred vision
INTEG: Pruritus, piloerection, rash
GU: Dysuria
CV: ***Supine hypertension,*** vasodilation, flushing face
Contraindications: Hypersensitivity, severe organic heart disease, acute renal disease, urinary retention, pheochromocytoma, thyrotoxicosis, persistent/excessive supine hypertension
Precautions: Children, urinary retention, lactation, prostatic hypertrophy, pregnancy (C), hepatic function impairment, orthostatic diabetic patients
Do not confuse:
ProAmatine/Protamine
Pharmacokinetics:
PO: Peak 1-2 hr, half-life 3-4 hr
Interactions:
• ↑ bradycardia: β-blockers, psychotropics, cardiac glycosides
• ↑ pressor effects: α-agonist
• ↑ supine hypertension: fludrocortisone

NURSING CONSIDERATIONS
Assess:
• VS, B/P (standing, supine); notify prescriber if B/P supine is increased
• Observe for drowsiness, dizziness, LOC
Administer:
• Tablets may be swallowed whole, chewed, or allowed to dissolve
• Upon arising, midday, and late afternoon (no later than 6 PM)
• Avoid administering if patient is to be supine during day
Evaluate:
• Therapeutic response: decreased orthostatic hypotension
Teach patient/family:
• To avoid hazardous activities, activities requiring alertness; dizziness may occur; instruct patient to request assistance with ambulation
• To avoid alcohol, other depressants

mifepristone (℞)

(mif-ee-press'tone)
Mifeprex
Func. class.: Abortifacient
Chem. class.: Antiprogestational

Action: Stimulates uterine contractions, causing complete abortion
Uses: Abortion through 49 days' gestation
Investigational uses: Postcoital contraception/contragestation, intrauterine fetal death, endometriosis, Cushing's syndrome, unresectable meningioma
Dosage and routes:
• *Adult:* **PO** 600 mg day 1, 400 mcg misoprostol day 3
Available forms: Tabs 200 mg

Side effects/adverse reactions:

MISC: Fatigue, back pain, fever, viral infections, chills, sinusitis
CNS: Dizziness, insomnia, anxiety, syncope, fainting, headache
GI: Nausea, vomiting, diarrhea, dyspepsia
GU: Uterine cramping, uterine hemorrhage, vaginitis, pelvic pain

Contraindications: Hypersensitivity, severe hepatic disease, severe renal disease, IUD, ectopic pregnancy, chronic adrenal failure, bleeding disorder, inherited porphyrias, PID, respiratory disease, cardiac disease

Precautions: Asthma, anemia, jaundice, diabetes mellitus, convulsive disorders, women >35 yr/smoke ≥10 cigarettes/day, past uterine surgery, pregnancy (C)

Pharmacokinetics: Rapidly absorbed, peak 90 min, 98% bound to plasma proteins, albumin, glycoprotein, excretion via feces, urine

Interactions:

- ↓ metabolism of: erythromycin, ketoconazole, itraconazole
- Drug/food: ↓ metabolism of mifepristone: grapefruit juice
- ↓ by: St. John's wort

NURSING CONSIDERATIONS

Assess:

- B/P, pulse; watch for change that may indicate hemorrhage
- Respiratory rate, rhythm, depth; notify prescriber of abnormalities
- For length, duration of contraction; notify prescriber of contractions lasting over 1 min or absence of contractions
- For incomplete abortion, pregnancy must be terminated by another method; drug is teratogenic

Perform/provide:

- Emotional support before and after abortion

Evaluate:

- Therapeutic response: expulsion of fetus

Teach patient/family:

- To report increased blood loss, abdominal cramps, increased temp, foul-smelling lochia
- Some methods of comfort control and pain control
- Must continue with follow-up
- That cramping and vaginal bleeding will occur

miglitol (℞)

(mig'lih-tol)
Glyset
Func. class.: Oral hypoglycemic
Chem. class.: α-Glucosidase inhibitor

Action: Delays digestion of ingested carbohydrates, results in smaller rise in blood glucose after meals; does not increase insulin production

Uses: Non–insulin-dependent diabetes mellitus (NIDDM) type 2

Dosage and routes:

- *Adult:* **PO** 25 mg tid initially, with first bite of meal; maintenance dose may be increased to 50 mg tid; may be increased to 100 mg tid if needed (only in patients >60 kg) with dosage adjustment at 4-8 wk intervals

Available forms: Tabs 25, 50, 100 mg

Side effects/adverse reactions:

GI: Abdominal pain, diarrhea, flatulence, ***hepatotoxicity***
HEMA: Low iron
INTEG: Rash

Contraindications: Hypersensitivity, diabetic ketoacidosis, cirrhosis, inflammatory bowel disease, colonic ulceration, partial intestinal obstruction, chronic intestinal disease

Precautions: Pregnancy (B), renal

disease, lactation, children, hepatic disease

Pharmacokinetics: Peak 2-3 hr, not metabolized, excreted in urine as unchanged drug, half-life 2 hr

Interactions:

- ↓ levels of: digoxin, propranolol, ranitidine
- ↓ miglitol levels: digestive enzymes, intestinal adsorbents; do not use together
- Drug/food: ↑ diarrhea; carbohydrates

↓ hypoglycemic effect: broom, buchu, dandelion, juniper

↑ or ↓ hypoglycemic effect: chromium, fenugreek, ginseng

Improved glucose tolerance: karela

NURSING CONSIDERATIONS

Assess:

- Hypoglycemia, hyperglycemia; even though drug does not cause hypoglycemia, if patient is on sulfonylureas or insulin, hypoglycemia may be additive
- Blood glucose levels, glycosylated hemoglobin, LFTs

Administer:

- Tid with first bite of each meal

Perform/provide:

- Storage in tight container in cool environment

Evaluate:

- Therapeutic response: decreased signs/symptoms of diabetes mellitus (polyuria, polydipsia, polyphagia, clear sensorium, absence of dizziness, stable gait)

Teach patient/family:

- The symptoms of hypo/hyperglycemia, what to do about each, that during periods of stress, infection, surgery, insulin may be required
- That medication must be taken as prescribed; explain consequences of discontinuing medication abruptly
- To avoid OTC medications unless approved by health-care provider
- That diabetes is lifelong illness; that this drug is not a cure
- To carry emergency ID for emergency purposes
- That diet and exercise regimen must be followed

miglustat

See appendix a—selected new drugs

HIGH ALERT

milrinone (℞)

(mill'rih-nohn)

Primacor

Func. class.: Inotropic/vasodilator agent with phosphodiesterase activity

Chem. class.: Bipyridine derivative

Action: Positive inotropic agent, increases contractility of cardiac muscle with vasodilator properties; reduces preload and afterload by direct relaxation on vascular smooth muscle

Uses: Short-term management of advanced CHF that has not responded to other medication; can be used with digitalis

Dosage and routes:

- *Adult:* **IV BOL** 50 mcg/kg given over 10 min; start inf of 0.375-0.75 mcg/kg/min; reduce dose in renal impairment

Available forms: Inj 1 mg/ml; premixed inj 200 mcg/ml in D_5W

Side effects/adverse reactions:

HEMA: ***Thrombocytopenia***

MISC: Headache, hypokalemia, tremor

CV: ***Dysrhythmias,*** hypotension, chest pain

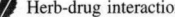

GI: Nausea, vomiting, anorexia, abdominal pain, ***hepatotoxicity, jaundice***

Contraindications: Hypersensitivity to this drug, severe aortic disease, severe pulmonic valvular disease, acute myocardial infarction

Precautions: Lactation, pregnancy (C), children, renal disease, hepatic disease, atrial flutter/fibrillation, elderly

Pharmacokinetics:

IV: Onset 2-5 min, peak 10 min, duration variable; half-life 2.4 hr; metabolized in liver; excreted in urine as drug (83%) and metabolites (12%)

NURSING CONSIDERATIONS

Assess:

◆ ECG continuously during IV, ventricular dysrhythmia can occur

- B/P and pulse q5min during infusion; if B/P drops 30 mm Hg, stop infusion and call prescriber
- Electrolytes: K, Na, Cl, Ca; renal studies: BUN, creatinine; blood studies: platelet count
- ALT, AST, bilirubin qd
- I&O ratio and weight qd; diuresis should increase with continuing therapy
- If platelets are <150,000/mm^3, drug is usually discontinued and another drug started
- Extravasation; change site q48h

Administer:

- Potassium supplements if ordered for potassium levels <3 mg/dl

IV route

- Give IV loading dose undiluted over 10 min
- Into running dextrose infusion through Y-connector or directly into tubing; dilute with 0.9% NaCl to 1-3 mg/ml; do not mix with glucose for long-term infusion
- By inf pump for doses other than bolus

Additive compatibilities: Quinidine

Syringe compatibilities: Atropine, calcium chloride, digoxin, epINEPHrine, lidocaine, morphine, propranolol, sodium bicarbonate, verapamil

Y-site compatibilities: Digoxin, diltiazem, DOBUTamine, DOPamine, epINEPHrine, fentanyl, heparin, hydromorphone, labetalol, lorazepam, midazolam, morphine, niCARdipine, nitroglycerin, norepinephrine, propranolol, quinidine, ranitidine, thiopental, vecuronium

Evaluate:

- Therapeutic response: increased cardiac output, decreased PCWP, adequate CVP, decreased dyspnea, fatigue, edema, ECG

Treatment of overdose: Discontinue drug, support circulation

minocycline (℞)

(min-oh-sye′kleen)

Dynacin, Minocin

Func. class.: Broad-spectrum antiinfective

Chem. class.: Tetracycline

Action: Inhibits protein synthesis, phosphorylation in microorganisms by binding to 30S ribosomal subunits, reversibly binding to 50S ribosomal subunits; bacteriostatic

Uses: Syphilis, *Chlamydia trachomatis,* gonorrhea, lymphogranuloma venereum, rickettsial infections, inflammatory acne, *Neisseria meningitidis, Neisseria gonorrheae, Treponema pallidum, Chlamydia trachomatis, Ureaplasma urealyticum, Mycoplasma pneumoniae, Nocardia,* periodontitis

Investigational uses: Rheumatoid arthritis

Dosage and routes:

- *Adult:* **PO/IV** 200 mg, then 100 mg q12h or 50 mg q6h, not to exceed 400 mg/24 hr **IV; SUBGINGIVAL** inserted into periodontal packet

• *Child >8 yr:* **PO/IV** 4 mg/kg then 4 mg/kg/day **PO** in divided doses q12h

Gonorrhea

• *Adult:* **PO** 200 mg, then 100 mg q12h × 4 days

Chlamydia trachomatis

• *Adult:* **PO** 100 mg bid × 7 days

Syphilis

• *Adult:* **PO** 200 mg, then 100 mg q12h × 10-15 days

Uncomplicated gonococcal urethritis in men

• *Adult:* **PO** 100 mg q12h × 5 days

Rheumatoid arthritis (off-label)

• *Adult:* **PO** 100 mg bid for ≤48 wk

Available forms: Caps 50, 75, 100 mg; oral susp 50 mg/5 ml; powder for inj 100 mg; caps, pellet filled 50, 100 mg

Side effects/adverse reactions:

CNS: Dizziness, fever, light-headedness, vertigo

HEMA: ***Eosinophilia, neutropenia, thrombocytopenia, hemolytic anemia***

EENT: Dysphagia, glossitis, decreased calcification of deciduous teeth, permanent discoloration of teeth, oral candidiasis

GI: Nausea, abdominal pain, *vomiting, diarrhea,* anorexia, enterocolitis, ***hepatotoxicity,*** flatulence, abdominal cramps, epigastric burning, stomatitis

CV: Pericarditis

GU: Increased BUN, polyuria, polydipsia, ***renal failure, nephrotoxicity***

INTEG: Rash, urticaria, photosensitivity, increased pigmentation, ***exfoliative dermatitis,*** pruritus, angioedema, blue-gray color of skin, mucous membranes

Contraindications: Hypersensitivity to tetracyclines, children <8 yr, pregnancy (D)

Precautions: Hepatic disease, lactation

Pharmacokinetics:

PO: Peak 2-3 hr, half-life 11-17 hr; excreted in urine, feces, breast milk; crosses placenta; 70%-75% protein bound

Interactions:

• ↓ effect of minocycline: antacids, sodium bicarbonate, alkali products, iron, kaolin/pectin, cimetidine

• ↑ effect: warfarin

• ↓ effect of barbiturates, carbamazepine, phenytoin, penicillins, oral contraceptives, calcium

Lab test interferences:

False negative: Urine glucose with Clinistix or Tes-Tape

NURSING CONSIDERATIONS

Assess:

• I&O ratio

• Blood tests: PT, CBC, AST, ALT, BUN, creatinine

• Signs of anemia: Hct, Hgb, fatigue

• Allergic reactions: rash, itching, pruritus, angioedema

• Nausea, vomiting, diarrhea; administer antiemetic, antacids as ordered

• Overgrowth of infection: fever, malaise, redness, pain, swelling, drainage, perineal itching, diarrhea, changes in cough or sputum, black, furry tongue

Administer:

• After C&S obtained

PO route

• 2 hr before or after laxative or ferrous products; 3 hr after antacid or kaolin-pectin product (PO)

IV route

• After diluting 100 mg/5 ml sterile H_2O for inj; further dilute in 500-1000 ml of NaCl, dextrose sol, LR, Ringer's sol; run 100 mg/6 hr

Y-site compatibilities: Aztreonam,

cisatracurium, cyclophosphamide, filgrastim, fludarabine, granisetron, heparin, hydrocortisone, magnesium sulfate, melphalan, perphenazine, potassium chloride, remifentanil, sargramostim, teniposide, vinorelbine, vit B/C

Perform/provide:

• Storage in airtight, light-resistant container at room temperature

Evaluate:

• Therapeutic response: decreased temp, absence of lesions, negative C&S

Teach patient/family:

• To avoid sunlight; sunscreen does not seem to decrease photosensitivity

• That all prescribed medication must be taken to prevent superinfection; not to use outdated product, Fanconi's syndrome may occur

• To take with a full glass of water; take with food for GI symptoms

minoxidil (℞)

(mi-nox'i-dill)

Loniten, minoxidil, Rogaine (top)

Func. class.: Antihypertensive

Chem. class.: Vasodilator, peripheral

Action: Directly relaxes arteriolar smooth muscle, causing vasodilation

Uses: Severe hypertension unresponsive to other therapy (use with diuretic); topically to treat alopecia

Dosage and routes:

Severe hypertension

• *Adult:* **PO** 2.5-5 mg/day not to exceed 100 mg daily, usual range 10-40 mg/day in single doses

• *Geriatric:* **PO** 2.5 mg qd, may be increased gradually

• *Child <12 yr:* **PO** (initial) 0.2 mg/kg/day; (effective range) 0.25-1 mg/kg/day; (max) 50 mg/day

Alopecia

• *Adult:* **TOP** 1 ml bid, rub into scalp daily, max 2 ml/day

Available forms: Tabs 2.5, 10 mg; top 2% sol

Side effects/adverse reactions:

Systemic

CV: Severe rebound hypertension on withdrawal in children, tachycardia, angina, increased T wave, ***CHF, pulmonary edema, pericardial effusion,*** edema, sodium, water retention

CNS: Headache, fatigue

GI: Nausea, vomiting

GU: Breast tenderness

INTEG: Pruritus, ***Stevens-Johnson syndrome,*** rash, hirsutism

HEMA: Hct, Hgb, erythrocyte count may decrease initially

Contraindications: Acute MI, dissecting aortic aneurysm, hypersensitivity, pheochromocytoma

Precautions: Pregnancy (C), lactation, children, renal disease, CAD, CHF, elderly

Do not confuse:

Loniten/Lotensin

minoxidil/Monopril

Pharmacokinetics:

PO: Onset 30 min, peak 2-3 hr, duration 75 hr; half-life 4.2 hr; metabolized in liver; metabolites excreted in urine, feces

Interactions:

• Orthostatic hypotension: antihypertensives

Lab test interferences:

Increase: Renal studies

Decrease: Hgb/Hct/RBC

NURSING CONSIDERATIONS

Assess:

• Monitor closely, usually given with β-blocker to prevent tachycardia and increased myocardial workload, usually given with diuretic to prevent serious fluid accumulation,

M

patient should be hospitalized during beginning treatment
• Nausea, edema in feet, legs daily
• Skin turgor, dryness of mucous membranes for hydration status
• Rales, dyspnea, orthopnea
• Electrolytes: K, Na, Cl, CO_2
• Renal studies: catecholamines, BUN, creatinine
• Hepatic studies: AST, ALT, alk phosphatase
• B/P, pulse
• Weight daily, I&O

Administer:

TOP route

• 1 ml no matter how much balding has occurred; increasing dosage does not speed growth

PO route

• With meals for better absorption, to decrease GI symptoms
• With β-blocker and/or diuretic for hypertension

Perform/provide:

• Storage protected from light and heat

Evaluate:

• Therapeutic response: decreased B/P or increased hair growth

Teach patient/family:

• That body hair will increase but is reversible after discontinuing treatment
• Not to discontinue drug abruptly
• To report pitting edema, dizziness, weight gain >5 lb, shortness of breath, bruising or bleeding, heart rate >20 beats/min over normal, severe indigestion, dizziness, lightheadedness, panting, new or aggravated symptoms of angina
• To take drug exactly as prescribed, or serious side effects may occur

Topical

• That for topical use, treatment must continue long-term or new hair will be lost
• Not to use except on scalp

Treatment of overdose: Administer normal saline IV, vasopressors

mirtazapine (℞)

(mer-ta'za-peen)

Remeron, Remeron Soltab

Func. class.: Antidepressant

Chem. class.: Tetracyclic

Action: Blocks reuptake of norepinephrine, serotonin into nerve endings, increasing action of norepinephrine, serotonin in nerve cells

Uses: Depression, dysthymic disorder, bipolar disorder—depressed, agitated depression

Dosage and routes:

• *Adult:* **PO** 15 mg/day at hs, maintenance to continue for 6 mo, titrate up to 45 mg/day; orally disintegrating tabs: open blister pack, place tab on tongue, allow to disintegrate, swallow
• *Geriatric:* **PO** 7.5 mg q hs, increase by 7.5 mg q1-2wk to desired dose, max 45 mg/day

Available forms: Tabs 15, 30 mg; orally disintegrating tab 15, 30, 45 mg

Side effects/adverse reactions:

HEMA: ***Agranulocytosis, thrombocytopenia, eosinophilia, leukopenia***

CNS: Dizziness, drowsiness, confusion, headache, anxiety, tremors, stimulation, weakness, insomnia, nightmares, EPS (elderly), increased psychiatric symptoms, ***seizures***

GI: Diarrhea, dry mouth, nausea, vomiting, ***paralytic ileus,*** increased appetite, cramps, epigastric distress, constipation, ***jaundice, hepatitis,*** stomatitis

GU: Urinary retention, ***acute renal failure***

INTEG: Rash, urticaria, sweating, pruritus, photosensitivity

CV: Orthostatic hypotension, ECG

*changes, tachycardia, **hypertension,*** palpitations
EENT: Blurred vision, tinnitus, mydriasis
SYST: Flulike symptoms
Contraindications: Hypersensitivity to tricyclics, recovery phase of MI, convulsive disorders, prostatic hypertrophy
Precautions: Suicidal patients, severe depression, increased intraocular pressure, narrow-angle glaucoma, urinary retention, cardiac disease, renal disease, hepatic disease, hypothyroidism, hyperthyroidism, electroshock therapy, elective surgery, elderly, pregnancy (C)
Pharmacokinetics:
PO: Peak 12 hr, metabolized by liver; excreted in urine, feces; crosses placenta; half-life 20-40 hr
Interactions:
- ↓ effects of clonidine, indirect-acting sympathomimetics (epHEDrine)
- ↑ CNS depression, alcohol, barbiturates, benzodiazepines, other CNS depressants

Hyperpyretic crisis, seizures, hypertensive episode: MAOIs
↑ anticholinergic effect: belladonna, henbane
↑ antidepressant action: scopolia
↑ CNS depression: chamomile, hops, kava, skullcap, valerian
Serotonin syndrome: SAM-e, St. John's wort
Lab test interferences:
Increase: Serum bilirubin, blood glucose, alk phosphatase
False increase: Urinary catecholamines
Decrease: VMA, 5-HIAA
NURSING CONSIDERATIONS
Assess:
- B/P (lying, standing), pulse q4h; if systolic B/P drops 20 mm Hg, hold drug, notify prescriber; take vital signs q4h in patients with cardiovascular disease
- Blood studies: CBC, leukocytes, differential, cardiac enzymes if patient is receiving long-term therapy
- Hepatic studies: AST, ALT, bilirubin, creatinine
- Weight qwk; appetite may increase with drug
- ECG for flattening of T wave, bundle branch block, AV block, dysrhythmias in cardiac patients
- EPS primarily in elderly: rigidity, dystonia, akathisia
- Mental status: mood, sensorium, affect, suicidal tendencies, increase in psychiatric symptoms: depression, panic
- Alcohol consumption; if alcohol is consumed, hold dose until morning

Administer:
- Increased fluids, bulk in diet for constipation, especially elderly
- With food, milk for GI symptoms
- Dosage hs if oversedation occurs during day; may take entire dose hs; elderly may not tolerate once/day dosing
- Gum, hard candy, or frequent sips of water for dry mouth
- Orally disintegrating tab: no water needed; allow to dissolve on tongue

Perform/provide:
- Storage in tight container at room temperature; do not freeze
- Assistance with ambulation during beginning therapy, since drowsiness/dizziness occurs
- Safety measures, including side rails, primarily in elderly
- Checking to see PO medication swallowed

Evaluate:
- Therapeutic response: decreased depression

M

Teach patient/family:

- That therapeutic effects may take 2-3 wk
- To use caution in driving, other activities requiring alertness, because of drowsiness, dizziness, blurred vision
- To report immediately urinary retention
- To avoid alcohol ingestion, other CNS depressants

Treatment of overdose: ECG monitoring, induce emesis; lavage, activated charcoal; administer anticonvulsant

misoprostol (℞)

(mye-soe-prost′ole)

Cytotec

Func. class.: Gastric mucosa protectant, antiulcer

Chem. class.: Prostaglandin E_1-analog

Action: Inhibits gastric acid secretion; may protect gastric mucosa; can increase bicarbonate, mucus production

Uses: Prevention of nonsteroidal antiinflammatory drug-induced gastric ulcers

Investigational uses: Used investigationally with methotrexate to produce abortion

Dosage and routes:

- *Adult:* **PO** 200 mcg qid with food for duration of nonsteroidal antiinflammatory therapy; if 200 mcg is not tolerated, 100 mcg may be given

Available forms: Tabs 100, 200 mcg

Side effects/adverse reactions:

GI: Diarrhea, nausea, vomiting, flatulence, constipation, dyspepsia, abdominal pain

GU: Spotting, cramps, hypermenorrhea, menstrual disorders

Contraindications: Hypersensitivity, pregnancy (X)

Precautions: Lactation, children, elderly, renal disease

Do not confuse:

cytotec/Cytoxan

misoprostol/metoprolol

Pharmacokinetics:

PO: Peak 12 min, plasma steady state achieved within 2 days, excreted in urine

Interactions:

- Drug/food: ↓ absorption when taken with food

NURSING CONSIDERATIONS

Assess:

- GI symptoms: hematemesis, occult or frank blood in stools, gastric aspirate, cramping, severe diarrhea
- Obtain a negative pregnancy test; miscarriages are common
- Gastric pH (>5 should be maintained)

Administer:

- PO with meals for prolonged drug effect; avoid use of magnesium antacids

Perform/provide:

- Storage at room temperature

Evaluate:

- Therapeutic response: absence of pain or GI complaints; prevention of ulcers

Teach patient/family:

- To take only as directed
- Not to take if pregnant (can cause miscarriage) and not to become pregnant while taking this medication; if pregnancy occurs during therapy, discontinue drug, notify prescriber; not to administer to nursing mothers
- Not to give drug to anyone else or take for more than 4 wk unless directed by prescriber
- To avoid OTC preparations: aspirin, cough, cold products; condition may worsen

HIGH ALERT

mitomycin (℞)

(mye-toe-mye'sin)

mitomycin, Mutamycin

Func. class.: Antineoplastic, antibiotic

Action: Inhibits DNA synthesis, primarily; derived from *Streptomyces caespitosus;* appears to cause cross-linking of DNA, a vesicant

Uses: Pancreas, stomach cancer, head and neck or breast cancer

Investigational uses: Palliative treatment of head, neck, colon, breast, biliary, cervical, lung malignancies

Dosage and routes:

• *Adult:* **IV** 10-20 mg/m^2 q6-8wk

Available forms: Inj 5, 20, 40 mg/vial

Side effects/adverse reactions:

HEMA: ***Thrombocytopenia, leukopenia, anemia***

GI: Nausea, vomiting, anorexia, stomatitis, ***hepatotoxicity,*** diarrhea

GU: Urinary retention, ***renal failure,*** edema

INTEG: Rash, alopecia, ***extravasation***

RESP: ***Fibrosis, pulmonary infiltrate,*** dyspnea

CNS: Fever, headache, confusion, drowsiness, syncope, fatigue

EENT: Blurred vision, drowsiness, syncope

MISC: ***Hemolytic uremic syndrome***

Contraindications: Hypersensitivity, pregnancy (D) (1st trimester), as a single agent, thrombocytopenia, coagulation disorders, lactation

Precautions: Renal disease, bone marrow depression

Pharmacokinetics: Half-life 1 hr, metabolized in liver, 10% excreted in urine (unchanged)

Interactions:

• ↑ toxicity: other antineoplastics, radiation

NURSING CONSIDERATIONS

Assess:

• CBC, differential, platelet count weekly; withhold drug if WBC is <2000/mm^3, granulocyte count <1000/mm^3, or platelet count is <100,000/mm^3; notify prescriber

• Pulmonary function tests, chest x-ray before, during therapy; chest x-ray should be obtained q2wk during treatment

⬌ Fatal hemolytic uremic syndrome: hypertension, thrombocytopenia, microangiopathic hemolytic anemia, occurs in those on long-term therapy

• Renal studies: BUN, serum uric acid, urine CCr, electrolytes before, during therapy

• I&O ratio; report fall in urine output to <30 ml/hr

• Monitor temp q4h; fever may indicate beginning infection

• Hepatic studies before, during therapy: bilirubin, AST, ALT, alk phosphatase as needed or monthly; check for jaundiced skin and sclera, dark urine, clay-colored stools, itchy skin, abdominal pain, fever, diarrhea

• Bleeding: hematuria, guaiac, bruising, petechiae, mucosa or orifices q8h

⬌ Pulmonary fibrosis: bronchospasm

• Dyspnea, rales, unproductive cough; chest pain, tachypnea, fatigue, increased pulse, pallor, lethargy

• Effects of alopecia on body image; discuss feelings about body changes

• Inflammation of mucosa, breaks in skin

• Buccal cavity q8h for dryness, sores, ulceration, white patches, oral pain, bleeding, dysphagia

M

• Local irritation, pain, burning at inj site
• GI symptoms: frequency of stools, cramping
• Acidosis, signs of dehydration: rapid respirations, poor skin turgor, decreased urine output, dry skin, restlessness, weakness

Administer:

IV route

• Apply ice compress for extravasation; stop infusion
• Antiemetic 30-60 min before giving drug to prevent vomiting
• IV after diluting 5 mg/10 ml or 10 mg/40 ml sterile H_2O for inj; shake, allow to stand, give through Y-tube or 3-way stopcock; give over 5-10 min, color of reconstituted sol is gray

Additive compatibilities: Dexamethasone, hydrocortisone

Solution compatibilities: LR, 0.3% NaCl, 0.5% NaCl

Syringe compatibilities: Bleomycin, cisplatin, cyclophosphamide, DOXOrubicin, droperidol, fluorouracil, furosemide, heparin, leucovorin, methotrexate, metoclopramide, vinBLAStine, vinCRIStine

Y-site compatibilities: Allopurinol, amifostine, bleomycin, cisplatin, cyclophosphamide, DOXOrubicin, droperidol, fluorouracil, furosemide, granisetron, heparin, leucovorin, melphalan, methotrexate, metoclopramide, ondansetron, teniposide, thiotepa, vinBLAStine, vinCRIStine

Perform/provide:

• Rinsing of mouth tid-qid with water; brushing of teeth with baking soda bid-tid with soft brush or cotton-tipped applicators for stomatitis; use unwaxed dental floss
• Storage at room temperature 1 wk after reconstituting or 2 wk refrigerated

Evaluate:

• Therapeutic response: decreased tumor size, spread of malignancy

Teach patient/family:

• To report any complaints, side effects to nurse or prescriber
• That hair may be lost during treatment and wig or hairpiece may make the patient feel better; tell patient that new hair may be different in color, texture
• To avoid foods with citric acid, hot or rough texture
• To report any bleeding, white spots, ulcerations in mouth; tell patient to examine mouth qd
• To avoid crowds, people with infections if granulocyte count is low

RARELY USED

mitotane (℞)

(mye'toe-tane)

Lysodren, p'-DDD

Func. class.: Antineoplastic

Uses: Adrenocortical carcinoma

Dosage and routes:

• *Adult:* **PO** 9-10 g/day in divided doses tid or qid; may have to decrease dose for severe reaction

Contraindications: Hypersensitivity

HIGH ALERT

mitoxantrone (℞)

(mye-toe-zan'trone)

Novantrone

Func. class.: Antineoplastic, antiinfective, immunomodulator

Chem. class.: Synthetic anthraquinone

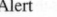

Action: DNA reactive agent, cytocidal effect on both proliferating and

nonproliferating cells, suggesting lack of cell cycle phase specificity (vesicant)
Uses: Acute nonlymphocytic leukemia (adult), relapsed leukemia, breast cancer; used with steroids to treat bone pain (advanced prostate cancer), multiple sclerosis (MS)
Investigational uses: Breast, liver malignancies, non-Hodgkin's lymphoma
Dosage and routes:
Induction
• *Adult:* **IV INF** 12 mg/m^2/day on days 1-3, and 100 mg/m^2 cytosine arabinoside × 7 days as a continuous 24 hr inf
Consolidation
• *Adult:* **IV** 12 mg/m^2 given as a short 5-15 min inf
Multiple sclerosis
• *Adult:* **IV INF** 12 mg/m^2 as a 5-15 min inf q 3 mos
Available forms: Inj 2 mg/ml
Side effects/adverse reactions:
CNS: Headache, ***seizures***
EENT: Conjunctivitis, blue/green sclera
GI: Nausea, vomiting, diarrhea, anorexia, mucositis, ***hepatotoxicity***
HEMA: ***Thrombocytopenia, leukopenia, myelosuppression, anemia***
INTEG: Rash, necrosis at inj site, dermatitis, thrombophlebitis at injection site, alopecia
CV: ***CHF, cardiopathy, dysrhythmias***
MISC: Fever
RESP: Cough, dyspnea
Contraindications: Hypersensitivity, pregnancy (D)
Precautions: Myelosuppression, lactation, cardiac disease, children; renal, hepatic disease; gout
Pharmacokinetics: Highly bound to plasma proteins, metabolized in liver, excreted via renal, hepatobiliary systems; half-life 24-72 hr

Interactions:
• Do not mix with heparin; precipitate will form
• Do not mix with any other drug
• ↑ bone marrow depression toxicity: radiation, other antineoplastics
• ↑ adverse reactions: live virus vaccines

NURSING CONSIDERATIONS
Assess:
• CBC, differential, platelet count qwk; withhold drug if WBC is <4000/mm^3 or platelet count is <75,000/mm^3; notify prescriber of these results
• Hepatic studies before, during therapy: bilirubin, AST, ALT, alk phosphatase prn or qmo
• Renal studies: BUN, serum uric acid, urine CCr, electrolytes before, during therapy
• Bleeding, hematuria, guaiac, bruising or petechiae, mucosa or orifices q8h
• Jaundiced skin and sclera, dark urine, clay-colored stools, itchy skin, abdominal pain, fever, diarrhea
◆ ECG, ECHO, chest x-ray RAI angiography to assess ejection fraction before and during treatment, cardiotoxic, may develop during treatment or months to years after treatment
• Acidosis, signs of dehydration: rapid respirations, poor skin turgor, decreased urine output, dry skin, restlessness, weakness
◆ For secondary acute myelogenous leukemia (AML) that can develop after taking this drug
◆ For MS: obtain MUGA, LVEF baselines; repeat LVEF if symptoms of CHF occur or if cumulative dose is >100 mg/m^2; do not administer to patients who have received a lifetime dose of ≥140 mg/m^2 or if LVEF <50% or significant LVEF
• Do not administer to patients with

M

MS if neutrophils <1500 cells/mm^3
• Obtain pregnancy test in all women of childbearing age, even if birth control is used

Administer:
• Medications by oral route if possible; avoid IM, SC, IV routes to prevent infections
• Antiemetic 30-60 min before giving drug to prevent vomiting

IV route
• IV after diluting with 50 ml or more NS or D_5W; give over 3-5 min, running IV of D_5W or NS; may be diluted further in D_5W, NS and run over 15-30 min; check for extravasation

Additive compatibilities: Cyclophosphamide, cytarabine, fluorouracil, hydrocortisone, potassium chloride

Solution compatibilities: D_5/0.9 NaCl, D_5W, 0.9% NaCl

Y-site compatibilities: Allopurinol, amifostine, cladribine, filgrastim, fludarabine, granisetron, melphalan, ondansetron, sargramostim, teniposide, thiotepa, vinorelbine

Perform/provide:
• Liquid diet: carbonated beverages, Jell-O; dry toast, crackers may be added if patient is not nauseated or vomiting
• Rinsing of mouth tid-qid with water, club soda; brushing of teeth bid-qid with soft brush or cotton-tipped applicators for stomatitis; use unwaxed dental floss

Evaluate:
• Therapeutic response: decreased tumor size, spread of malignancy

Teach patient/family:
• To report side effects to nurse or physician
• To avoid foods with citric acid, rough texture, or hot
• To report any bleeding, white spots, ulcerations in mouth; tell patient to examine mouth qd
• That sclera, urine may turn blue or green
• To notify prescriber if pregnancy is suspected or planned

HIGH ALERT

mivacurium (℞)

(miv-a-kure'ee-um)
Mivacron
Func. class.: Nondepolarizing neuromuscular blocker

Action: Inhibits transmission of nerve impulses by binding competitively with cholinergic receptor sites, antagonizing action of acetylcholine

Uses: Facilitation of endotracheal intubation, skeletal muscle relaxation during mechanical ventilation, surgery, or general anesthesia

Dosage and routes:
• *Adult:* **IV** 0.15 mg/kg; maintenance q15min
• *Child 2-12 yr:* **IV** 0.2 mg/kg for a 10 min block

Available forms: 5, 10 ml single-use vial (2 mg/ml); premixed infusion in D_5W 50-ml flex container

Side effects/adverse reactions:
CV: Decreased B/P, bradycardia, tachycardia
RESP: ***Prolonged apnea, bronchospasm, wheezing, respiratory depression***
EENT: Diplopia
MS: Weakness, prolonged skeletal muscle relaxation, ***paralysis***
INTEG: Rash, urticaria

Contraindications: Hypersensitivity

Precautions: Pregnancy (C), renal or hepatic disease, lactation, children <3 mo, fluid and electrolyte imbalances, neuromuscular disease, respiratory disease, obesity, elderly

Do not confuse:
Mivacron/Mazicon
Pharmacokinetics: Rapidly hydrolyzed by plasma cholinesterases, peak 2-3 min, reversal within 15-30 min
Interactions:
• ↑ neuromuscular blockade: aminoglycosides, quinidine, local anesthetics, polymyxin antibiotics, enflurane, isoflurane, tetracyclines, halothane, magnesium, colistin, procainamide, bacitracin, lincomycin, clindamycin, lithium
NURSING CONSIDERATIONS
Assess:
• For electrolyte imbalances (K, Mg); may lead to increased action of this drug
• VS (B/P, pulse, respirations, airway) until fully recovered; rate, depth, pattern of respirations, strength of hand grip
• I&O ratio; check for urinary retention, frequency, hesitancy
• Recovery: decreased paralysis of face, diaphragm, leg, arm, rest of body
• Allergic reactions: rash, fever, respiratory distress, pruritus; drug should be discontinued
Administer:
• Using nerve stimulator by anesthesiologist to determine neuromuscular blockade
• Anticholinesterase to reverse neuromuscular blockade
• By slow IV over 1-2 min (only by qualified persons, usually an anesthesiologist)
• Only fresh sol
Y-site compatibilities: Etomidate, thiopental
Perform/provide:
• Storage at room temperature; do not freeze
• Reassurance if communication is difficult during recovery from neuromuscular blockade
• Frequent (q2h) instillation of artificial tears and covering eyes to prevent drying of cornea
Evaluate:
• Therapeutic response: paralysis of jaw, eyelid, head, neck, rest of body
Treatment of overdose: Neostigmine, monitor VS; may require mechanical ventilation

---

RARELY USED

modafinil (℞)
(moh-daf'ih-nil)
Provigil
Func. class.: Cerebral stimulant

Controlled Substance Schedule IV
Uses: Narcolepsy
Dosage and routes:
• *Adult:* **PO** 200 mg qd in the AM, may increase to 400 mg qd if needed
Hepatic dose
• Reduce dose by 50%
Contraindications: Hypersensitivity, hyperthyroidism, hypertension, glaucoma, severe arteriosclerosis, drug abuse, cardiovascular disease, anxiety

moexipril (℞)
(moe-ex'ih-prill)
Univasc
Func. class.: Antihypertensive
Chem. class.: Angiotensin-converting enzyme inhibitor

Action: Selectively suppresses renin-angiotensin-aldosterone system; inhibits ACE; prevents conversion of angiotensin I to angiotensin II; results in dilation of arterial, venous vessels
Uses: Hypertension, alone or in combination with thiazide diuretics

M

Dosage and routes:
• *Adult:* **PO** 7.5 mg 1 hr ac initially, may be increased or divided depending on B/P response; maintenance dosage; 7.5-30 mg qd in 1-2 divided doses 1 hr ac
Renal dose
• *Adult:* **PO** CCr <40 ml/min 3.75 mg/day titrate to desired dose
Available forms: Tabs 7.5, 15 mg
Side effects/adverse reactions:
CV: Hypotension, postural hypotension
GU: Impotence, dysuria, nocturia, proteinuria, nephrotic syndrome, acute reversible renal failure, polyuria, oliguria, frequency
HEMA: ***Neutropenia***
INTEG: Rash
RESP: ***Bronchospasm,*** dyspnea, dry cough
META: Hypokalemia
GI: Loss of taste
CNS: Fever, chills
SYST: ***Angioedema, anaphylaxis***
Contraindications: Hypersensitivity, children, lactation, heart block, bilateral renal stenosis, potassium-sparing diuretics, pregnancy (D) 2nd/3rd trimester
Precautions: Dialysis patients, hypovolemia, leukemia, scleroderma, lupus erythematosus, blood dyscrasias, CHF, diabetes mellitus, renal disease, thyroid disease, COPD, asthma, pregnancy (C) (1st trimester)
Pharmacokinetics: Metabolized by liver (metabolites), excreted in urine; crosses placenta; excreted in breast milk
Interactions:
• ↑ hypotension: diuretics, other antihypertensives, ganglionic blockers, adrenergic blockers, phenothiazines
• Do not use with potassium-sparing diuretics, sympathomimetics, potassium supplements
• ↓ antihypertensive effect: NSAIDs
• ↑ toxicity: digoxin, lithium
• ↑ hyperkalemia: cycloSPORINE
Lab test interferences:
False positive: Urine acetone
NURSING CONSIDERATIONS
Assess:
• Blood tests: neutrophils, decreased platelets
• B/P
• Renal studies: protein, BUN, creatinine; watch for increased levels that may indicate nephrotic syndrome
• Baselines in renal, hepatic studies before therapy begins
• Potassium levels, although hyperkalemia rarely occurs
• Edema in feet, legs daily
• Allergic reaction: rash, fever, pruritus, urticaria; drug should be discontinued if antihistamines fail to help
• Symptoms of CHF; edema, dyspnea, wet rales, B/P
• Renal symptoms: polyuria, oliguria, frequency
Administer:
• PO 1 hr before meals
Perform/provide:
• Storage in tight container at 86° F (30° C) or less
Evaluate:
• Therapeutic response: decrease in B/P in hypertension
Teach patient/family:
• To take 1 hr ac
• Not to discontinue drug abruptly
• Not to use OTC (cough, cold, or allergy) products unless directed by prescriber
• To comply with dosage schedule, even if feeling better
• To rise slowly to sitting or standing position to minimize orthostatic hypotension
• To notify prescriber of mouth sores, sore throat, fever, swelling of hands or feet, irregular heart-

beat, chest pain, signs of angioedema
• That excessive perspiration, dehydration, vomiting, diarrhea may lead to fall in blood pressure; consult prescriber if these occur
• That dizziness, fainting, lightheadedness may occur during first few days of therapy
• That skin rash or impaired perspiration may occur
• How to take B/P
Treatment of overdose: 0.9% NaCl IV inf, hemodialysis

mometasone topical

See appendix c

montelukast (℞)

(mon-teh-loo'kast)
Singulair
Func. class.: Bronchodilator
Chem. class.: Leukotriene antagonist, cysteinyl

Action: Inhibits leukotriene (LTD_4) formation; leukotrienes exert their effects by increasing neutrophil, eosinophil migration; aggregation of neutrophils, monocytes; smooth muscle contraction, capillary permeability; these actions further lead to bronchoconstriction, inflammation, edema
Uses: Chronic asthma in adults and children
Investigational uses: Chronic urticaria
Dosage and routes:
Asthma
• *Adult and child ≥15 yr:* **PO** 10 mg qd PM
• *Child 6-14 yr:* **PO** 5 mg chew tab qd PM
• *Child 2-5 yr:* **PO** chew tab 4 mg qd
• *Child 12-23 mo:* **PO** 1 packet of granules taken PM
Available forms: Tabs 10 mg; tabs, chew 4, 5 mg; oral granules 4 mg/packet
Side effects/adverse reactions:
CNS: Dizziness, fatigue, headache
GI: Abdominal pain, dyspepsia
INTEG: Rash
MS: Asthenia
RESP: Influenza, cough, nasal congestion
Contraindications: Hypersensitivity
Precautions: Acute attacks of asthma, alcohol consumption, pregnancy (B), lactation, child <6 yr, aspirin sensitivity
Pharmacokinetics: Rapidly absorbed, peak 3-4 hr, half-life 2.7-5.5 hr; protein binding 99%; metabolized by liver, excreted via bile
Interactions:
• ↓ montelukast levels: phenobarbital, rifampin
↑ stimulation: black, green tea, guarana
Lab test interferences:
Increase: ALT, AST

NURSING CONSIDERATIONS
Assess:
Adult patients carefully for symptoms of Churg-Strauss syndrome (rare), including eosinophilia, vasculitic rash, worsening pulmonary symptoms, cardiac complications, and/or neuropathy
• CBC, blood chemistry, during treatment
• Respiratory rate, rhythm, depth; auscultate lung fields bilaterally; notify prescriber of abnormalities
• Allergic reactions: rash, urticaria; drug should be discontinued
Administer:
PO route
• In PM qd

M

Granules

• May give directly in the mouth or mixed with a spoonful of soft food (carrots, applesauce, ice cream, rice)

• Do not open packet until ready to use, mix whole dose, give within 15 min

Evaluate:

• Therapeutic response: ability to breathe more easily

Teach patient/family:

• To check OTC medications, current prescription medications for epHEDrine, which will increase stimulation; to avoid alcohol

• To avoid hazardous activities; dizziness may occur

• That drug is not to be used for acute asthma attacks

• If aspirin sensitivity is known, do not take NSAIDs while taking this product

• To continue to use inhaled beta-agonists if exercise-induced asthma occurs

moricizine (℞)

(more-i′siz-een)

Ethmozine

Func. class.: Antidysrhythmic, group 1A

Chem. class.: Phenothiazine

Action: Decreased rate of rise of action potential, prolonging refractory period and shortening the action potential duration; depression of inward influx if sodium mediates the effects; drug may slow atrial and AV nodal conduction

Uses: Life-threatening ventricular dysrhythmias

Dosage and routes:

Hospitalization is required when initiating therapy

• *Adult:* **PO** 10-15 mg/kg/day or 600-900 mg/day in 2-3 divided doses

Hepatic dose

• *Adult:* **PO** 600 mg or less qd

Available forms: Film-coated tabs 200, 250, 300 mg

Side effects/adverse reactions:

GI: Nausea, abdominal pain, vomiting, diarrhea

CNS: Dizziness, headache, fatigue, perioral numbness, euphoria, nervousness, sleep disorders, depression, tinnitus, fatigue, anxiety

RESP: Dyspnea, hyperventilation, ***apnea,*** asthma, pharyngitis, cough

GU: Sexual dysfunction, difficult urination, dysuria, incontinence, urinary retention

CV: Palpitations, chest pain, ***CHF,*** hypertension, syncope, dysrhythmias, bradycardia, ***MI, thrombophlebitis,*** ECG abnormalities, ***cardiac arrest***

MISC: Sweating, musculoskeletal pain, drug fever, blurred vision, dry mouth

Contraindications: 2nd/3rd degree AV block, right bundle branch block, cardiogenic shock, hypersensitivity

Precautions: CHF, hypokalemia, hyperkalemia, sick sinus syndrome, pregnancy (B), lactation, children, impaired hepatic and renal function, cardiac dysfunction

Pharmacokinetics: Half-life 1.5-3.5 hr; peak 0.5-2.2 hr; metabolized by the liver; metabolites excreted in feces and urine, protein binding >90%

Interactions:

• ↑ plasma levels of moricizine: cimetidine

• Digoxin or propranolol may enhance some cardiac effects of moricizine; moricizine may decrease effects of theophylline

• ↓ effects of: theophylline

↑ anticholinergic effect: henbane

↑ hypokalemia, ↑ antidysrhyth-

mic action: aloe, buckthorn, cascara sagrada, rhubarb, senna
↑ toxicity, death: aconite
↑ effect: aloe, broom, chronic buckthorn use, cascara sagrada (chronic use), Chinese rhubarb, figwort, fumitory, goldenseal, kudzu, licorice
↓ effect: coltsfoot
↑ serotonin effect: horehound
Lab test interferences:
Increase: CPK

NURSING CONSIDERATIONS
Assess:
- GI status: bowel pattern, number of stools
- Cardiac status: rate, rhythm, quality
- Chest x-ray, pulmonary function test during treatment
- I&O ratio; check for decreasing output
- B/P for fluctuations
- Lung fields: bilateral rales may occur in CHF patient
- Increased respirations, increased pulse; drug should be discontinued

Toxicity: fine tremors, dizziness, emesis, lethargy, coma, syncope, hypotension, conduction disturbances
- Cardiac status: respiration, rate, rhythm, character continuously

Administer:
- Initiate therapy in hospital
- Dosage adjustment should be ≥3 days

Evaluate:
- Therapeutic response: absence of dysrhythmias

Teach patient/family:
- To report side effects to prescriber

Treatment of overdose: O_2 artificial ventilation, ECG; administer DOPamine for circulatory depression, diazepam or thiopental for convulsions

HIGH ALERT

morphine (℞)

(mor'feen)
Astramorph, Astramorph PF, Duramorph, Epimorph✤, Infumorph, morphine sulfate, Morphitec✤, M.O.S.✤, M.O.S.-S.R.✤, MS Contin, MSIR, OMS Concentrate, Oramorph SR, RMS, Roxanol, Roxanol Rescudose, Roxanol-T, Statex
Func. class.: Opioid analgesic

Controlled Substance Schedule II
Action: Depresses pain impulse transmission at the spinal cord level by interacting with opioid receptors
Uses: Severe pain
Dosage and routes:
- *Adult:* **SC/IM** 5-20 mg q4h prn; **PO** 10-30 mg q4h prn; **EXT REL** 70-kg patient q8-12h; **RECT** 10-30 mg q4h prn; **IV** 4-10 mg diluted in 4-5 ml H_2O for injection, over 5 min
- *Child:* **SC/IV** 0.1-0.2 mg/kg, not to exceed 15 mg; **PO** 0.2-0.5 mg/kg q4-6h (reg rel), q12h (sus rel)

Available forms: Inj 0.5, 1, 2, 3, 4, 5, 8, 10, 15, 25, 50 mg/ml; sol tabs 10, 15, 30 mg; oral sol 10, 20 mg/5 ml, 20 mg/10 ml, 20 mg/ml; oral tabs 15, 30 mg; rect supp 5, 10, 20, 30 mg; ext rel tabs 15, 30, 60, 100, 200 mg; caps 15, 30 mg; syr 1, 5 mg/ml
Side effects/adverse reactions:
HEMA: ***Thrombocytopenia***
CNS: Drowsiness, dizziness, confusion, headache, sedation, euphoria
CV: Palpitations, ***bradycardia,*** change in B/P, ***shock, cardiac arrest***
EENT: Tinnitus, blurred vision, miosis, diplopia

M

GI: Nausea, vomiting, anorexia, constipation, cramps, biliary tract pressure
GU: Urinary retention
INTEG: Rash, urticaria, bruising, flushing, diaphoresis, pruritus
RESP: ***Respiratory depression, respiratory arrest, apnea***
Contraindications: Hypersensitivity, addiction (opioid), hemorrhage, bronchial asthma, increased intracranial pressure
Precautions: Addictive personality, pregnancy (C), lactation, acute MI, severe heart disease, elderly, respiratory depression, hepatic disease, renal disease, child <18 yr
Do not confuse:
morphine/hydromorphone
Roxanol/Roxicet
Pharmacokinetics:
PO: Onset variable, peak variable, duration variable
IM: Onset ½ hr, peak ½-1 hr, duration 3-7 hr
SC: Onset 15-20 min, peak 50-90 min, duration 3-5 hr
IV: Peak 20 min
RECT: Peak ½-1 hr, duration 4-5 hr
Intrathecal: Onset rapid, duration up to 24 hr
Metabolized by liver, crosses placenta; excreted in urine, breast milk; half-life 1½-2 hr
Interactions:
• Unpredictable reaction, avoid use: MAOIs
• ↑ effects with other CNS depressants: alcohol, opiates, sedative/hypnotics, antipsychotics, skeletal muscle relaxants
• ↓ morphine action: rifampin
↑ anticholinergic effect: corkwood
↑ CNS depression: chamomile, hops, Jamaican dogwood, kava, lavender, mistletoe, nettle, pokeweed, poppy, senega, skullcap, valerian
↓ morphine effect: cranberry juice (excessive amounts), oats
Lab test interferences:
Increase: Amylase
NURSING CONSIDERATIONS
Assess:
• Pain: location, type, character; give dose before pain becomes severe
• Bowel status; constipation common
• I&O ratio; check for decreasing output; may indicate urinary retention
• B/P, pulse, respirations (character, depth, rate)
• CNS changes: dizziness, drowsiness, hallucinations, euphoria, LOC, pupil reaction
• Allergic reactions: rash, urticaria
• Respiratory dysfunction: depression, character, rate, rhythm; notify prescriber if respirations are <12/min
Administer:
• With antiemetic for nausea, vomiting
• When pain is beginning to return; determine dosage interval by response; continuous dosing is more effective than prn
• May be given by patient: controlled analgesia
• Epidural cautiously in the elderly
IV route
• After diluting with 5 ml or more sterile H_2O or NS; give 15 mg or less over 4-5 min; give through Y-tube or 3-way stopcock; may be added to IV sol, each 0.1-1 mg diluted in 1 ml D_5W, $D_{10}W$, 0.9% NaCl, 0.45% NaCl, Ringer's, LR, given with inf pump titrated to patient response
Additive compatibilities: Alteplase, atracurium, baclofen, bupivacaine, DOBUTamine, fluconazole, furosemide, meropenem, metoclopramide, ondansetron, succinylcholine, verapamil

Syringe compatibilities: Atropine, benzquinamide, bupivacaine, butorphanol, cimetidine, dimenhyDRINATE, diphenhydrAMINE, droperidol, fentanyl, glycopyrrolate, hydrOXYzine, ketamine, metoclopramide, midazolam, milrinone, pentazocine, perphenazine, promazine, ranitidine, scopolamine

Y-site compatibilities: Allopurinol, amifostine, amikacin, aminophylline, amiodarone, ampicillin, ampicillin/sulbactam, amsacrine, atenolol, atracurium, aztreonam, bumetanide, calcium chloride, cefamandole, cefazolin, cefmetazole, cefoperazone, cefotaxime, cefotetan, cefoxitin, ceftazidime, ceftizoxime, ceftriaxone, cefuroxime, cephalothin, cephapirin, chloramphenicol, cisatracurium, cisplatin, cladribine, clindamycin, cyclophosphamide, cytarabine, dexamethasone, digoxin, diltiazem, DOBUTamine, DOPamine, doxycycline, enalaprilat, epINEPHrine, erythromycin, esmolol, etomidate, famotidine, fentanyl, filgrastim, fluconazole, fludarabine, foscarnet, gentamicin, granisetron, heparin, hydrocortisone, hydromorphone, IL-2, insulin (regular), kanamycin, labetalol, lidocaine, lorazepam, magnesium sulfate, melphalan, meropenem, methotrexate, methyldopate, methylPREDNISolone, metoclopramide, metoprolol, metronidazole, mezlocillin, midazolam, milrinone, moxalactam, nafcillin, niCARdipine, nitroglycerin, norepinephrine, ondansetron, oxacillin, oxytocin, paclitaxel, pancuronium, penicillin G potassium, piperacillin, piperacillin/tazobactam, potassium chloride, propofol, propranolol, ranitidine, remifentanil, sodium bicarbonate, sodium nitroprusside, teniposide, thiotepa, ticarcillin, ticarcillin/clavulanate, tobramycin, trimethoprim-sulfamethoxazole, vancomycin, vecuronium, vinorelbine, vit B/C, warfarin, zidovudine

Perform/provide:
- Storage in light-resistant container at room temperature
- Assistance with ambulation
- Safety measures: side rails, nightlight, call bell within easy reach
- Gradual withdrawal after long-term use

Evaluate:
- Therapeutic response; decrease in pain intensity

Teach patient/family:
- To change position slowly; orthostatic hypotension may occur
- To report any symptoms of CNS changes, allergic reactions
- That physical dependency may result from long-term use
- To avoid use of alcohol, CNS depressants
- That withdrawal symptoms may occur: nausea, vomiting, cramps, fever, faintness, anorexia

Treatment of overdose: Naloxone (Narcan) 0.2-0.8 mg IV, O_2, IV fluids, vasopressors

moxalactam

See cephalosporins—3rd generation

moxifloxacin

Avelox, Avelox IV

Func. class.: Antiinfective

Chem. class.: Fluoroquinolone

Action: Interferes with conversion of intermediate DNA fragments into high-molecular-weight DNA in bacteria; DNA gyrase inhibitor

Uses: Acute bacterial sinusitis: *Streptococcus pneumoniae, Hae-*

mophilus influenzae, Moraxella catarrhalis; acute bacterial exacerbation of chronic bronchitis: *S. pneumoniae, H. influenzae, Haemophilus parainfluenzae, Klebsiella pneumoniae, Staphylococcus aureus, M. catarrhalis;* community-acquired pneumonia: *S. pneumoniae, H. influenzae, Mycoplasma pneumoniae, Chlamydia pneumoniae, M. catarrhalis;* uncomplicated skin/skin structure infections: *S. aureus, Streptococcus pyogenes*

Dosage and routes:

Acute bacterial sinusitis

• *Adult:* **PO/IV** 400 mg q24h × 10 days

Acute bacterial exacerbation of chronic bronchitis

• *Adult:* **PO/IV** 400 mg q24h × 5 days

Community acquired pneumonia

• *Adult:* **PO/IV** 400 mg q24h × 7-14 days

Uncomplicated skin/skin structure infections

• *Adult:* **PO/IV** 400 mg q24h × 7 days

Available forms: Tabs 400 mg; inj premix 400 mg

Side effects/adverse reactions:

CV: Prolonged QT interval, ***dysrhythmias***

CNS: Headache, dizziness, fatigue, insomnia, depression, *restlessness,* ***seizures,*** confusion

GI: Nausea, diarrhea, increased ALT, AST, flatulence, heartburn, *vomiting,* oral candidiasis, dysphagia, ***pseudomembranous colitis***

INTEG: Rash, pruritus, urticaria, photosensitivity, flushing, fever, chills

MS: Tremor, arthralgia, tendon rupture

SYST: ***Anaphylaxis, Stevens-Johnson syndrome***

EENT: Blurred vision, tinnitus

Contraindications: Hypersensitivity to quinolones

Precautions: Pregnancy (C), lactation, children, renal disease, epilepsy, uncorrected hypokalemia, prolonged QT interval, patients receiving class IA, III antidysrhythmics

Pharmacokinetics: Excreted in urine as active drug, metabolites

Interactions:

• ↓ moxifloxacin absorption: magnesium antacids, aluminum hydroxide, zinc, iron, sucralfate, calcium, enteral feeding, didanosine

• ↑ moxifloxacin serum levels: probenecid

• ↑ toxicity: caffeine, theophylline, cycloSPORINE

• ↑ warfarin, cycloSPORINE effect

• Prolonged QT: antidysrythmics class IA, III

↑ antiinfective effect: cola tree

NURSING CONSIDERATIONS

Assess:

• CNS symptoms: headache, dizziness, fatigue, insomnia, depression, ***seizures***

• Renal, hepatic studies: BUN, creatinine, AST, ALT

• I&O ratio, urine pH <5.5 is ideal

Allergic reactions and anaphylaxis: fever, flushing, rash, urticaria, pruritus; keep epINEPHrine, emergency equipment nearby for anaphylaxis

Administer:

PO route

• 3 hr before or 3 hr after antacids, zinc, iron, calcium

IV route

• Discontinue primary IV while administering moxifloxacin

• Do not give SC, IM

Solution compatibilities: 0.9% NaCl, D_5, D_{10}, LR, sterile water for inj

Perform/provide:

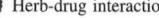

• Limited intake of alkaline foods, drugs: milk, dairy products, alkaline antacids, sodium bicarbonate

Evaluate:
- Therapeutic response: decreased pain, C&S; absence of infection

Teach patient/family:
- Not to take any products containing magnesium or calcium (such as antacids), iron, or aluminum with this drug or within 2 hr of drug
- That photosensitivity may occur; patient should avoid sunlight or use sunscreen to prevent burns
- To use frequent rinsing of mouth, sugarless candy or gum for dry mouth
- To take as prescribed, not to double or miss doses
- Not to use theophylline with this product, may cause toxicity; contact prescriber if taking theophylline
- That fluids must be increased to 3 L/day to avoid crystallization in kidneys
- If dizziness occurs, to ambulate, perform activities with assistance
- To complete full course of drug therapy
- To contact prescriber if adverse reaction occurs or if inflammation or pain in tendon occurs

multivitamins (OTC, ℞)

Adavite, Dayalets, LKV Drops, Multi-75, Multiday, One-A-Day, Optilets, Poly-Vi-sol, Quin tabs, Ru-Lets, Sesame Street Vitamins, Tab-A-Vite, Therabid, Theragram, Unicaps, Vita-Bob, Vita-Kid, many other brands

Func. class.: Vitamins, multiple

Action: Needed for adequate metabolism

Uses: Prevention and treatment of vitamin deficiencies

Dosage and routes:
- *Adult and child:* **PO/IV**—depends on brand

Available forms: Many

Side effects/adverse reactions: None known at recommended dosage

Precautions: Pregnancy (A)

Do not confuse:
Theragran/Phenergan

NURSING CONSIDERATIONS

Assess:
- Vitamin deficiency: usually more than one vitamin is deficient

Administer:
- Liquid multivitamins diluted or dropped into patient's mouth using dropper provided with some brands
- Chew tabs should be chewed, not swallowed whole
- Give by cont IV inf only after diluting 5-10 ml multivitamins/500-1000 ml of D_5W, $D_{10}W$, $D_{20}W$, LR, D_5/LR, D_5/0.9% NaCl, 0.9% NaCl, 3% NaCl
- Do not use sol with crystals, precipate, or color other than bright yellow

Additive compatibilities: Cefoxitin, isoproterenol, methyldopate, metoclopramide, metronidazole, netilmicin, norepinephrine, sodium bicarbonate, verapamil

Y-site compatibilities: Acyclovir, ampicillin, cefazolin, cephalothin, cephapirin, diltiazem, erythromycin, fludarabine, gentamicin, tacrolimus

Evaluate:
- Therapeutic response: check each individual vitamin for guidelines

Teach patient/family:
- That adequate nutrition must be maintained to prevent further deficiencies
- The drug interactions that should be avoided
- To comply with regimen
- To avoid presenting flavored mul-

M

tivitamins as candy; child may overdose
• To store out of children's reach

mupirocin topical

See appendix c

muromonab-CD3 (℞)

(mur-oo-mone'ab)
Orthoclone OKT3
Func. class.: Immunosuppressant
Chem. class.: Murine monoclonal antibody

Action: Reverses graft rejection by blocking T-cell function
Uses: Acute allograft rejection in renal, cardiac/hepatic transplant patients
Dosage and routes:
• *Adult:* **IV BOL** 5 mg/day × 10-14 days
• *Child:* **IV** 100 mcg/kg/day × 10-14 days
Cardiac/hepatic allograft rejection, steroid resistant
• *Adult:* **IV BOL** 5 mg/day × 10-14 days; begin when it is known that rejection has not been reversed by steroids
Available forms: Inj 5 mg/5 ml
Side effects/adverse reactions:
CNS: Pyrexia, chills, tremors, ***aseptic meningitis***
RESP: Dyspnea, wheezing, ***pulmonary edema***
CV: Chest pain
GI: Vomiting, nausea, diarrhea
MISC: ***Infection, cytokine release syndrome, anaphylaxis***
Contraindications: Hypersensitivity to murine origin, fluid overload
Precautions: Pregnancy (C), child <2 yr, fever
Pharmacokinetics: Trough level steady state 3-14 days
Interactions:
• ↑ immunosuppression: immunosuppressants
• ↑ infection risk: cycloSPORINE, corticosteroids, azathioprine
• ↑ CNS symptoms: indomethacin
• ↓ immune response: vaccines
Interference with immunosuppression: astragalus, echinacea, melatonin
↓ effect: ginseng, maitake, mistletoe, schisandra, St. John's wort, turmeric
NURSING CONSIDERATIONS
Assess:
For cytokine release syndrome (CRS): nausea, vomiting, chills, fever, joint pain, weakness, dizziness, diarrhea, tremors, abdominal pain
For hypersensitivity, ***anaphylaxis:*** dyspnea, bronchospasm, urticaria, tachycardia, angioedema; emergency equipment must be available
• Blood studies: Hgb, WBC, platelets during treatment qmo; if leukocytes are <3000/mm^3, drug should be discontinued; CD3, CD4, CD8, CD3 ≤25 cells/mm^3
• Hepatic studies: alk phosphatase, AST, ALT, bilirubin
Hepatotoxicity: dark urine, jaundice, itching, light-colored stools; drug should be discontinued
• For infection: sore throat, fever, chills, temp, notify prescriber immediately
For aseptic meningitis: fever, headache, photophobia
For fluid overload: increased weight, I&O, edema, rales
Administer:
• For several days before transplant surgery
• All medications PO if possible; avoid IM injection, since infection may occur

IV route

- IV undiluted; withdraw with a 0.2-0.22 low protein-binding µm filter, discard and use new needle for administration; give over 1 min
- Incompatible with any drug in syringe or sol

Evaluate:

- Therapeutic response: absence of graft rejection

Teach patient/family:

- To report fever, chills, sore throat, fatigue, since serious infection may occur; rash, dyspnea, fast heartbeat
- To use contraceptive measures during treatment
- To report cytokine release syndrome, give symptoms
- To avoid vaccinations during treatment
- To avoid persons with infections, crowds; infections may occur

mycophenolate (℞)

(mye-koe-phen'oh-late)

CellCept

Func. class.: Immunosuppressant

Action: Inhibits inflammatory responses that are mediated by the immune system; prolongs the survival of allogenic transplants

Uses: Organ transplants (to prevent rejection); prophylaxis of organ rejection in allogenic cardiac, hepatic, renal transplants

Investigational uses: Refractory uveitis, second-line therapy for Churg-Strauss syndrome, diffuse proliferative lupus nephritis (in combination)

Research note: When iron was administered with mycophenolate, a decreased absorption of mycophenolate resulted[24]

Dosage and routes:

Renal transplant

- *Adult:* **PO/IV** give initial dose 72 hr prior to transplantation; 1 g bid given to renal transplant patients in combination with corticosteroids, cycloSPORINE

Renal dose

- *Adult:* **PO/IV** GFR <25 ml/min, max 2 g/day

Cardiac transplant

- *Adult:* **PO/IV** 1.5 g bid, IV can be started ≤24 hr after transplant, switch to **PO** when able

Hepatic transplant

- *Adult:* **PO/IV** 1.5 g bid; give IV over ≥2 hr

Available forms: Caps 250 mg; tabs 250, 500 mg; inj (powder) 500 mg/20 ml vial; powder for oral susp 200 mg/ml

Side effects/adverse reactions:

GI: Diarrhea, constipation, nausea, vomiting, stomatitis, ***GI bleeding***

HEMA: ***Leukopenia, thrombocytopenia, anemia, pancytopenia***

INTEG: Rash

MS: Arthralgia, muscle wasting

RESP: Dyspnea, respiratory infection, increased cough, pharyngitis, bronchitis, pneumonia

CNS: Tremor, dizziness, insomnia, headache, fever

META: Peripheral edema, hypercholesterolemia, hypophosphatemia, edema, hyperkalemia, hypokalemia, hyperglycemia

GU: UTI, hematuria, ***renal tubular necrosis***

CV: Hypertension, chest pain

SYST: ***Lymphoma,*** *nonmelanoma skin carcinoma*

Contraindications: Hypersensitivity to this drug or mycophenolic acid

Precautions: Lymphomas, malignancies, neutropenia, renal disease, pregnancy (C), lactation

Pharmacokinetics: Rapidly and completely absorbed, metabolized to active metabolite (MPA), excreted in urine, feces

Interactions:

- ↑ concentration of both drugs: acyclovir, ganciclovir
- ↑ mycophenolate levels: probenecid, salicylate
- ↓ mycophenolate levels: antacids, cholestyramine
- ↓ protein binding of phenytoin, theophylline
- Avoid administration with azathioprine
- Drug/food: ↓ absorption if taken with food

Interference with immunosuppressant: astragalus, echinacea, melatonin

NURSING CONSIDERATIONS

Assess:

- Blood studies: CBC during treatment monthly
- Hepatic studies: alk phosphatase, AST, ALT, bilirubin

Administer:

- 72 hr prior to transplantation; may be given in combination with corticosteroids, cycloSPORINE
- Give alone for better absorption (PO)

IV route

- Do not give by rapid or bolus inj; reconstitute and dilute to 6 mg/ml with D_5W, give over ≥2 hr
- Do not admix with mycophenolate IV in infusion catheter or with other IV drugs or infusion admixtures

Evaluate:

- Therapeutic response: absence of graft rejection

Teach patient/family:

- To report fever, rash, severe diarrhea, chills, sore throat, fatigue, since serious infections may occur
- To reduce risk of infection by avoiding crowds

Not to break, crush, or chew tabs, do not open caps

- The need for repeated lab tests
- To limit exposure to sunlight/UV light
- To use contraception before, during, and 6 wk after therapy

nabumetone (℞)

(na-byoo'me-tone)

Relafen

Func. class.: Nonsteroidal antiinflammatory

Chem. class.: Acetic acid derivative

Action: Inhibits prostaglandin synthesis by decreasing enzyme needed for biosynthesis; analgesic, antiinflammatory

Uses: Osteoarthritis, rheumatoid arthritis, acute or chronic treatment

Dosage and routes:

- *Adult:* **PO** 1 g as a single dose; may increase to 2 g/day if needed; may give qd or bid as a divided dose

Available forms: Tabs 500, 750 mg

Side effects/adverse reactions:

CNS: Dizziness, headache, drowsiness, fatigue, tremors, confusion, insomnia, anxiety, depression, nervousness

GU: ***Nephrotoxicity, dysuria, hematuria, oliguria, azotemia,*** cystitis

GI: Nausea, anorexia, vomiting, diarrhea, jaundice, ***cholestatic hepatitis,*** constipation, flatulence, cramps, dry mouth, peptic ulcer, gastritis, ***ulceration, perforation***

CV: Tachycardia, peripheral edema, palpitations, dysrhythmias, ***CHF***

INTEG: Purpura, rash, pruritus, sweating, photosensitivity

HEMA: ***Blood dyscrasias***

EENT: Tinnitus, hearing loss, blurred vision

RESP: Dyspnea, pharyngitis, ***bronchospasm***

SYST: ***Anaphylaxis, angioneurotic edema***

Contraindications: Hypersensitivity to this drug or aspirin, iodides, NSAIDs, asthma, severe renal disease, severe hepatic disease, avoid in late pregnancy

Precautions: Pregnancy (C); lactation, children, bleeding disorders, GI disorders, cardiac disorders, renal disorders, hepatic dysfunction, elderly

Pharmacokinetics:

PO: Peak 2½-4 hr, plasma protein binding >90%, half-life 22-30 hr; metabolized in liver to active metabolite; excreted in urine (metabolites), breast milk

Interactions:

- ↓ effect of: diuretics, antihypertensives
- ↑ bleeding risk: anticoagulants, thrombolytics, valproic acid, cefamandole, cefotetan, cefoperazone, plicamycin, clopidogrel, eptifibatide, ticlopidine
- ↑ hematologic reactions risk: antineoplastics, radiation
- ↑ GI reactions: salicylates, NSAIDs, alcohol, potassium, corticosteroids

↑ gastric irritation: arginine, gossypol

↑ NSAIDs effect: bearberry, bilberry

↑ bleeding risk: bogbean, chondroitin

NURSING CONSIDERATIONS

Assess:

- Pain: frequency, intensity, characteristics; relief of pain after med
- Asthma, aspirin sensitivity or nasal polyps; increased hypersensitivity reactions
- Renal, hepatic studies: BUN, creatinine, AST, ALT, Hgb, LDH, blood glucose, WBC, platelets, CCr before treatment, periodically thereafter
- Audiometric, ophthalmic exam before, during, after treatment
- For eye, ear problems: blurred vision, tinnitus; may indicate toxicity

Administer:

- With food for GI symptoms

Perform/provide:

- Storage at room temperature

Evaluate:

- Therapeutic response: decreased pain and stiffness in joints

Teach patient/family:

- To avoid alcoholic beverages and aspirin
- To report blurred vision, ringing, roaring in ears; may indicate toxicity
- To avoid driving, other hazardous activities if dizziness, drowsiness occur
- To report change in urine pattern, increased weight, edema, increased pain in joints, fever, blood in urine; indicates nephrotoxicity
- That therapeutic effects may take up to 1 mo
- To take with a full glass of water to enhance absorption and sit upright
- To report dark stools; may indicate GI bleeding

nadolol (℞)

(nay-doe′lole)

Corgard, Syn-Nadolol✦

Func. class.: Antihypertensive, antianginal

Chem. class.: β-Adrenergic receptor blocker

Action: Long-acting, nonselective β-adrenergic receptor blocking agent; mechanism is similar to that of propranolol

Uses: Chronic stable angina pectoris, mild to moderate hypertension

Investigational uses: Tachydysrhythmias, aggression, anxiety, tremors, esophageal varices (rebleeding only), hyperthyroidism adjunctive therapy, prophylaxis of migraine headaches

Dosage and routes:

• *Adult:* **PO** 40 mg qd, increase by 40-80 mg q3-7d; maintenance 40-240 mg/day for angina, 40-320 mg/day for hypertension

• *Geriatric:* **PO** 20 mg/day, may increase by 20 mg until desired dose

Renal dose

• *Adult:* **PO** CCr 31-50 ml/min give q24-36h; CCr 10-30 ml/min give q24-48h; CCr < 10 ml/min give q40-60h

Available forms: Tabs 20, 40, 80, 120, 160 mg

Side effects/adverse reactions:

RESP: Dyspnea, respiratory dysfunction, ***bronchospasm,*** cough, wheezing, nasal stuffiness, pharyngitis, ***laryngospasm***

CV: ***Bradycardia,*** *hypotension,* ***CHF,*** palpitations, ***AV block,*** chest pain, peripheral ischemia, flushing, edema, vasodilation, conduction disturbances, ***pulmonary edema***

HEMA: ***Agranulocytosis, thrombocytopenia***

GI: Nausea, vomiting, diarrhea, colitis, constipation, cramps, dry mouth, flatulence, hepatomegaly, ***pancreatitis,*** taste distortion

INTEG: Rash, pruritus, fever, alopecia

CNS: Depression, hallucinations, dizziness, fatigue, lethargy, paresthesias, headache

EENT: Sore throat

GU: Impotence

Contraindications: Hypersensitivity to this drug, cardiac failure, cardiogenic shock, 2nd, 3rd degree heart block, bronchospastic disease, sinus bradycardia, CHF, COPD

Precautions: Diabetes mellitus, pregnancy (C), renal disease, lactation, hyperthyroidism, peripheral vascular disease, myasthenia gravis, major surgery, nonallergic bronchospasm

Do not confuse:

Corgard/Cognex

Pharmacokinetics:

PO: Onset variable, peak 3-4 hr, duration 17-24 hr; half-life 20-24 hr; not metabolized; excreted in urine (unchanged), bile, breast milk; protein binding 30%

Interactions:

• Peripheral ischemia: ergots

• ↓ antihypertensive effect: NSAIDs

• ↑ bradycardia: digoxin

• ↑ hypotension, bradycardia: clonidine, epINEPHrine

• Do not use with MAOIs, bradycardia may occur

• ↑ hypotensive effects: other hypotensive agents, oral contraceptives, phenothiazines

• ↓ β-blocking effect: thyroid hormones

↑ toxicity, death: aconite

↑ or ↓ antihypertensive effect: astragalus, cola tree

↑ antihypertensive effect: barberry, betony, black catechu, black cohosh, bloodroot, broom, burdock, cat's claw, dandelion, goldenseal, Irish moss, Jamaican dogwood, kelp, khella, mistletoe, parsley

↓ antihypertensive effect: coltsfoot, guarana, khat, licorice

Lab test interferences:

Increase: Serum potassium, serum uric acid, ALT, AST, alk phosphatase, LDH, blood glucose, cholesterol

NURSING CONSIDERATIONS

Assess:

• B/P, pulse, respirations during beginning therapy, orthostatic hypotension

• Weight qd; report gain of 5 lb

• I&O ratio, CCr if kidney damage is diagnosed

• qd, note need to be administered more often
• Pain: duration, time started, activity being performed, character
• Headache, light-headedness, decreased B/P; may indicate a need for decreased dosage

Administer:

PO route

• With 8 oz water

Evaluate:

• Therapeutic response: decreased B/P, symptoms of angina

Teach patient/family:

• That drug may mask signs of hypoglycemia or alter blood glucose in diabetics
◆ Not to discontinue abruptly, serious dysrhythmias may occur
• To avoid OTC drugs unless prescriber approves
• To avoid hazardous activities if dizziness occurs
• To comply with complete medical regimen
• To rise slowly to prevent orthostatic hypotension
• How and when to check B/P and pulse; to hold dose if pulse ≤50 bpm

nafarelin (℞)

(naf-ah-rell'in)

Synarel

Func. class.: Gonadotropin

Chem. class.: Analog of gonadotropin-releasing hormone

Action: Stimulates the release of LH and FSH, which increases ovarian steroid production; repeated dosing prevents stimulation of the pituitary gland

Uses: Endometriosis, gonadotropin-dependent precocious puberty

Dosage and routes:

• *Adult:* **NASAL** 400 mcg/day as one spray (200 mcg) into one nostril in morning and one spray into other nostril in evening; start treatment between days 2 and 4 of menstrual cycle; may increase to 800 mcg/day (one spray into each nostril twice a day); recommended duration of treatment is 6 mo
• *Child:* **NASAL** 2 sprays in each nostril AM and PM, may increase to 3 sprays alternating nostril tid

Available forms: Nasal spray 2 mg/ml (200 mcg/spray)

Side effects/adverse reactions:

GU: Decreased libido, vaginal dryness, breast tenderness, increased pubic hair

CNS: Headache, flushing, depression, insomnia, emotional lability, hot flashes

INTEG: Nasal irritation, acne

MISC: Body odor, seborrhea, rhinitis

SENSITIVITY: Shortness of breath, chest pain, urticaria, pruritus

Contraindications: Hypersensitivity, pregnancy (X), lactation, undiagnosed abnormal vaginal bleeding

Precautions: Children

Pharmacokinetics: Rapidly absorbed, peak 10-40 min, half-life 3 hr; 80% bound to plasma proteins

Interactions:

• ↓ nafarelin absorption: nasal decongestants (nasal sprays)

NURSING CONSIDERATIONS

Assess:

• Pain in endometriosis during treatment
• Endocrine studies, bone age, sex steroids, RHCG, GnRH, baseline q8wk
• For precocious puberty including secondary sex characteristics
• Test results: pituitary/hypothalamus dysfunction (decreased LH); postmenopausal (increased LH)

N

Administer:

NASAL route

• Repeated doses may be necessary to elevate pituitary gonadotropin reserve

Perform/provide:

• Storage at room temperature; protect from light

Evaluate:

• Therapeutic response: decreased symptoms of endometriosis; adequate resolution of central precocious puberty

Teach patient/family:

• To use nonhormonal contraception

• About correct nasal use, one spray in right nostril AM, one in left nostril PM

• That medication may cause hot flashes, decreased libido, vaginal dryness

nafcillin (℞)

(naf-sill'in)

nafcillin sodium, Nallpen, Unipen

Func. class.: Antiinfective, broad-spectrum

Chem. class.: Penicillinase-resistant penicillin

Action: Interferes with cell wall replication of susceptible organisms; osmotically unstable cell wall swells, bursts from osmotic pressure

Uses: Effective for gram-positive cocci *(Staphylococcus aureus, Streptococcus viridans, Streptococcus pneumoniae),* infections caused by penicillinase-producing *Staphylococcus*

Dosage and routes:

• *Adult:* **PO** 250-1000 mg q4-6h; **IM** 500 mg q4-6h; **IV** 500-1500 mg q4-6h

• *Child and infants, most infections:* **PO** 6.25-12.5 mg/kg q6h; pharyngitis **PO** 250 mg q8h; **IM** 25 mg/kg q12h; **IV** most infections 10-20 mg/kg q4h or 20-40 mg/kg q8h, max 200 mg/kg/day

• *Neonates:* **PO** 10 mg/kg q6-8h; **IM** 10 mg/kg q12h; **IV:** most infections 10-20 mg/kg q4h or 20-40 mg/kg q8h, max 200 mg/kg/day

Meningitis

• *Neonates ≥2 kg:* 50 mg/kg q8h × 1 wk of life, then 50 mg/kg q6h

• *Neonates <2 kg:* 25-50 mg/kg q12h × 1 wk of life, then 50 mg/kg q8h

Available forms: Caps 250 mg; tabs 500 mg; powder for inj 1, 2, 10 g

Side effects/adverse reactions:

HEMA: Anemia, increased bleeding time, ***bone marrow depression, granulocytopenia***

GI: Nausea, vomiting, diarrhea, increased AST, ALT, abdominal pain, glossitis, ***pseudomembranous colitis***

GU: Oliguria, ***proteinuria, hematuria,*** vaginitis, moniliasis, ***glomerulonephritis,*** interstitial nephritis

CNS: Lethargy, hallucinations, anxiety, depression, twitching, ***coma, seizures***

SYST: ***Anaphylaxis, serum sickness***

Contraindications: Hypersensitivity to penicillins

Precautions: Pregnancy (B), hypersensitivity to cephalosporins, neonates

Pharmacokinetics:

IM/PO: Peak 30-60 min, duration 4-6 hr, half-life 1 hr, metabolized by liver, excreted in bile, urine

Interactions:

• ↓ effect: oral contraceptives, anticoagulants

• ↑ nafcillin concentrations: aspirin, probenecid, disulfiram

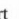

• Drug/food: ↓ absorption: food, carbonated drinks, citrus juice

↓ absorption: khat, separate by ≥2 hr

Do not use acidophilus with antiinfectives

Lab test interferences:

False-positive: Urine glucose, urine protein

NURSING CONSIDERATIONS

Assess:

• I&O ratio; report hematuria, oliguria, since penicillin in high doses is nephrotoxic

Any patient with compromised renal system, since drug is excreted slowly in poor renal system function; toxicity may occur rapidly

• Hepatic studies: AST, ALT

• Blood studies: WBC, RBC, H&H, bleeding time

• Renal studies: urinalysis, protein, blood, BUN, creatinine

• C&S before drug therapy; drug may be given as soon as culture is taken

• Bowel pattern before and during treatment

• Respiratory status: rate, character, wheezing, and tightness in chest

Allergies before initiation of treatment; monitor for anaphylaxis, dyspnea, rash, laryngeal edema; stop drug; keep emergency equipment nearby; skin eruptions after administration of penicillin to 1 wk after discontinuing drug

• Differential WBC in patients on long-term therapy

Administer:

PO route

• Drug after C&S has been completed

• Divided oral doses on empty stomach before meals; oral absorption is erratic

IM route

• IM deep in gluteal muscle

IV route

• After diluting 1 g/3.4 ml or 2 g/6.8 ml to 250 mg/ml sterile H_2O for inj; further dilute 15-30 ml sterile H_2O or NS sol; give through Y-tube or 3-way stopcock; 500 mg or less/5-10 min; may be further diluted and run over 24 hr

Additive compatibilities: Chloramphenicol, chlorothiazide, dexamethasone, diphenhydrAMINE, epHEDrine, heparin, hydrOXYzine, lidocaine, potassium chloride, prochlorperazine, sodium bicarbonate, sodium lactate

Syringe compatibilities: Cimetidine, heparin

Y-site compatibilities: Acyclovir, atropine, cyclophosphamide, diazepam, enalaprilat, esmolol, famotidine, fentanyl, fluconazole, foscarnet, hydromorphone, magnesium sulfate, morphine, perphenazine, propofol, theophylline, zidovudine

Perform/provide:

• Adrenalin, suction, tracheostomy set, endotracheal intubation equipment

• Adequate fluid intake (2 L) during diarrhea episodes

• Scratch test to assess allergy after securing order from prescriber; usually done when penicillin is only drug of choice

• Storage in tight container; refrigerate reconstituted sol

Evaluate:

• Therapeutic response: absence of fever, draining wounds

Teach patient/family:

• All aspects of drug therapy, including need to complete course of medication to ensure organism death (10-14 days); culture may be taken after completed course

• To report sore throat, fever, fatigue (may indicate superinfection)

• To wear or carry emergency ID if allergic to penicillins

• To notify nurse of diarrhea

Not to break, crush, or chew caps

N

Treatment of anaphylaxis: Withdraw drug; maintain airway; administer epINEPHrine, aminophylline, O_2, IV corticosteroids

naftifine topical

See appendix c

HIGH ALERT

nalbuphine (℞)

(nal'byoo-feen)

Nubain, nalbuphine HCl

Func. class.: Opioid analgesic

Chem. class.: Synthetic opioid agonist, antagonist

Action: Depresses pain impulse transmission at the spinal cord level by interacting with opioid receptors
Uses: Moderate to severe pain
Dosage and routes:
Analgesic
• *Adult:* **SC/IM/IV** 10-20 mg q3-6h prn, not to exceed 160 mg/day
Balanced anesthesia supplement
• *Adult:* **IV** 0.3-3 mg/kg given over 10-15 min, may give 0.25-0.5 mg/kg as needed for maintenance
Available forms: Inj 10, 20 mg/ml
Side effects/adverse reactions:
CNS: Drowsiness, dizziness, confusion, headache, sedation, euphoria, dysphoria (high doses), hallucinations, dreaming, tolerance, physical, psychological dependency
GI: Nausea, vomiting, anorexia, constipation, cramps
GU: Increased urinary output, dysuria, urinary retention, urgency
INTEG: Rash, urticaria, bruising, flushing, diaphoresis, pruritus
EENT: Tinnitus, blurred vision, miosis, diplopia
CV: Palpitations, bradycardia, change in B/P, orthostatic hypotension
RESP: ***Respiratory depression,*** pulmonary edema
Contraindications: Hypersensitivity, addiction (opiate)
Precautions: Addictive personality, pregnancy (C), lactation, increased intracranial pressure, MI (acute), severe heart disease, respiratory depression, hepatic disease, renal disease
Pharmacokinetics:
SC/IM/IV: Duration 3-6 hr; metabolized by liver, excreted by kidneys, half-life 5 hr
Interactions:
• ↑ effects with other CNS depressants: alcohol, opiates, sedative/hypnotics, antipsychotics, skeletal muscle relaxants
Avoid use with MAOIs, unpredictable reactions may occur
↑ CNS depression: chamomile, hops, Jamaican dogwood, kava, lavender, mistletoe, nettle, pokeweed, poppy, senega, skullcap, valerian
↑ anticholinergic effect: corkwood
Lab test interferences:
Increase: Amylase
NURSING CONSIDERATIONS
Assess:
• I&O ratio; check for decreasing output; may indicate urinary retention
For withdrawal reactions in opiate-dependent individuals: pulmonary embolus, vascular occlusion; abscesses, ulcerations, nausea, vomiting, seizures; however, there is a low potential for dependence
• CNS changes: dizziness, drowsiness, hallucinations, euphoria, LOC, pupil reaction
• Allergic reactions: rash, urticaria
• Respiratory dysfunction: respiratory depression, character, rate, rhythm; notify prescriber if respirations are <10/min

• Need for pain medication by pain sedation scoring, physical dependency

Administer:

• With antiemetic if nausea, vomiting occur

• When pain is beginning to return; determine dosage interval by response

IM route

• IM deep in large muscle mass, rotate inj sites

IV route

• Undiluted 10 mg or less over 3-5 min

Syringe compatibilities: Atropine, cimetidine, diphenhydrAMINE, droperidol, glycopyrrolate, hydrOXYzine, lidocaine, midazolam, prochlorperazine, ranitidine, scopolamine, trimethobenzamide

Y-site compatibilities: Amifostine, aztreonam, cefmetazole, cisatracurium, cladribine, filgrastim, fludarabine, granisetron, melphalan, paclitaxel, propofol, remifentanil, teniposide, thiotepa, vinorelbine

Perform/provide:

• Storage in light-resistant area at room temperature

• Assistance with ambulation

• Safety measures: night-light, call bell within easy reach

Evaluate:

• Therapeutic response: decrease in pain

Teach patient/family:

• To report any symptoms of CNS changes, allergic reactions

• That physical dependency may result from long-term use

• That withdrawal symptoms may occur: nausea, vomiting, cramps, fever, faintness, anorexia

Treatment of overdose: Naloxone (Narcan) 0.2-0.8 mg IV, O_2, IV fluids, vasopressors

nalidixic acid (℞)

(nal-i-dix′ik)

NegGram

Func. class.: Urinary tract anti-infective

Chem. class.: Quinolone

Action: Appears to inhibit DNA polymerization, primary target is single-stranded DNA precursors in late-stage chromosomal replication

Uses: UTIs (acute/chronic) caused by *Escherichia coli, Klebsiella, Enterobacter, Proteus mirabilis, Proteus vulgaris, Proteus morganii*

Dosage and routes:

• *Adult:* **PO** 1 g qid × 1-2 wk, 2 g/day for long-term treatment

• *Child >3 mo:* **PO** 55 mg/kg/day in 4 divided doses for 1-2 wk; 33 mg/kg/day in 4 divided doses for long-term treatment

Renal dose

• *Adult:* **PO** CCr <50 ml/min avoid use

Available forms: Tabs 250, 500 mg, 1 g; susp 250 mg/5 ml

Side effects/adverse reactions:

INTEG: Pruritus, rash, urticaria, photosensitivity

CNS: Dizziness, headache, drowsiness, insomnia, ***seizures***

GI: Nausea, vomiting, abdominal pain, diarrhea

EENT: Sensitivity to light, blurred vision, change in color perception

Contraindications: Hypersensitivity, CNS damage, hepatic failure, infants <3 mo, seizure disorder

Precautions: Elderly, renal disease, hepatic disease, pregnancy (C), lactation

Pharmacokinetics:

PO: Peak 1-2 hr, metabolized in liver, excreted in urine (unchanged/conjugates), crosses placenta, enters breast milk

Interactions:

- ↑ effects of oral coagulants, check for bleeding
- ↓ effect: nitrofurantoin
- ↑ stimulation: caffeine

Photosensitivity: dong quai, St. John's wort

Lab test interferences:

False positive: Urinary glucose

False increase: 17-OHCS, VMA

NURSING CONSIDERATIONS

Assess:

- Blood count for patients on chronic therapy
- I&O ratio; urine pH <5.5 is ideal
- Renal, hepatic function
- Photosensitivity: drug should be discontinued
- CNS symptoms: insomnia, vertigo, headache, drowsiness, convulsions
- Allergy: fever, flushing, rash, urticaria, pruritus

Administer:

PO route

- After clean-catch urine for C&S
- Two daily doses if urine output is high or if patient has diabetes
- 2 hr before or 2 hr after antacids

Perform/provide:

- Protection from freezing

Evaluate:

- Therapeutic response: decreased dysuria, negative culture

Teach patient/family:

- That photosensitivity occurs; that patient should avoid sunlight or use sunscreen to prevent burns
- To take medication with food or milk to decrease GI irritation; take 2 hr before or 2 hr after antacids
- To protect suspension from freezing, shake well before taking
- That drug may cause drowsiness; instruct client to seek aid in walking, other activities; advise client not to drive or operate machinery while on medication
- That diabetics should monitor blood glucose

naloxone (℞)

(nal-oks'one)

naloxone HCl, Narcan

Func. class.: Opioid antagonist, antidote

Chem. class.: Thebaine derivative

Action: Competes with opioids at opiate receptor sites

Uses: Respiratory depression induced by opioids, pentazocine, propoxyphene; refractory circulatory shock, asphyxia neonatorum

Dosage and routes:

Opioid-induced respiratory depression

- *Adult:* **IV/SC/IM** 0.4-2 mg; repeat q2-3min if needed
- *Child:* **IV/SC/IM** 0.5-2 mcg/kg as small frequent, q/min **BOL** or as **INF** titrated to response

Postoperative respiratory depression

- *Adult:* **IV** 0.1-0.2 mg q2-3min prn
- *Child:* **IV/IM/SC** 0.01 mg/kg q2-3min prn

Asphyxia neonatorum

- *Neonate:* **IV** 0.01 mg/kg given into umbilical vein after delivery; may repeat q2-3min × 3 doses

Available forms: Inj 0.02, 0.4 mg/ml

Side effects/adverse reactions:

CNS: Drowsiness, nervousness

CV: Rapid pulse, increased systolic B/P (high doses), ***ventricular tachycardia, fibrillation***

GI: Nausea, vomiting

RESP: Hyperpnea

Contraindications: Hypersensitivity, respiratory depression

Precautions: Pregnancy (B), chil-

dren, cardiovascular disease, opioid dependency, lactation
Do not confuse:
Narcan/Norcuron
Pharmacokinetics: Well absorbed IM, SC; metabolized by liver, crosses placenta; excreted in urine, breast milk; half-life 1 hr
IV: Onset 1 min, duration 45 min
IM/SC: Onset 2-5 min, duration 45-60 min
Interactions:
• ↓ effect of opioid analgesics
Lab test interferences:
Interference: Urine VMA, 5-HIAA, urine glucose
NURSING CONSIDERATIONS
Assess:
• Withdrawal: cramping, hypertension, anxiety, vomiting, signs of withdrawal in drug-dependent individuals may occur up to 2 hr after administration
• VS q3-5min
• ABGs including Po_2, Pco_2
• Cardiac status: tachycardia, hypertension; monitor ECG
• Respiratory dysfunction: respiratory depression, character, rate, rhythm; if respirations are <10/min, administer naloxone; probably due to opioid overdose; monitor LOC
• For pain: duration, intensity, location, before and after administration; may be used for respiratory depression
Administer:
• Only with resuscitative equipment, O_2 nearby
• Only sol prepared within 24 hr
IV route
• Undiluted with sterile H_2O for inj; may be further diluted with NS or D_5 and given as an inf; give 0.4 mg or less over 15 sec or titrate inf to response
Additive compatibilities: Verapamil
Syringe compatibilities: Benzquinamide, heparin
Y-site compatibilities: Propofol
Perform/provide:
• Dark storage at room temperature
Evaluate:
• Therapeutic response: reversal of respiratory depression; LOC-alert

naltrexone (℞)

(nal-trex'one)
ReVia, Trexan
Func. class.: Opioid antagonist
Chem. class.: Thebaine derivative

Action: Competes with opioids at opioid receptor sites
Uses: Blockage of opioid analgesics, used in treatment of opiate addiction
Investigational uses: Pruritus, alcohol dependence
Dosage and routes:
• *Adult:* **PO** 25 mg, may give 25 mg after 1 hr if no withdrawal symptoms; 50-150 mg may be given qd depending on need, maintenance 50 mg q24h; 100-150 mg may be given on alternate days or 3 days per wk
Pruritus (off-label)
• *Adult:* **PO** 50 mg qd
Available forms: Tabs 50 mg
Side effects/adverse reactions:
MISC: Increased thirst, chills, fever
MS: Joint and muscle pain
GU: Delayed ejaculation, decreased potency
CNS: Stimulation, drowsiness, dizziness, confusion, ***seizures,*** headache, flushing, hallucinations, nervousness, irritability, ***suicidal ideation***
GI: Nausea, vomiting, diarrhea, heartburn, anorexia, ***hepatitis,*** constipation
INTEG: Rash, urticaria, bruising, oily skin, acne, pruritus

N

EENT: Tinnitus, hearing loss, blurred vision
CV: Rapid pulse, ***pulmonary edema,*** hypertension
RESP: Wheezing, hyperpnea, nasal congestion, rhinorrhea, sneezing, sore throat
Contraindications: Hypersensitivity, opioid dependence, hepatic failure, hepatitis
Precautions: Pregnancy (C), hepatic disease, lactation, children
Pharmacokinetics:
PO: Onset 15-30 min, peak 1-2 hr, duration is dose dependent
Metabolized by liver, excreted by kidneys; crosses placenta, excreted in breast milk; half-life 4 hr; extensive first-pass metabolism

NURSING CONSIDERATIONS
Assess:
- VS q3-5min
- ABGs including Po_2, Pco_2
- Signs of withdrawal in drug-dependent individuals
- Cardiac status: tachycardia, hypertension
- Respiratory dysfunction: respiratory depression, character, rate, rhythm; if respirations are <10/min, respiratory stimulant should be administered

Administer:
- Only if resuscitative equipment is nearby

Perform/provide:
- Storage in tight container

Evaluate:
- Therapeutic response: blocking opiate ingestion

Teach patient/family:
- That they must be drug-free to start treatment
- That using opioid while taking this drug could prove fatal because high dose is needed to overcome this antagonist
- To carry emergency ID stating med used
- If surgery is needed, all involved should be aware of this drug

nandrolone (℞)

(nan′droe-lone)
Deca-Durabolin, Hybolin Decanoate, Kabolin
Func. class.: Androgenic anabolic steroid, antianemic
Chem. class.: Halogenated testosterone derivative

Action: Increases weight by building body tissue, increases potassium, phosphorus, chloride, nitrogen levels, increases bone development
Uses: Tissue building, severe disease, refractory anemias, metastatic breast cancer
Dosage and routes:
Tissue building (possibly effective)
- *Adult:* **IM** 50-100 mg q3-4wk (decanoate)
- *Child 2-13 yr:* **IM** 25-50 mg q3-4wk (decanoate)

Severe disease/refractory anemias
- *Adult:* **IM** 100-200 mg qwk (decanoate)

Breast cancer
- *Adult:* **IM** 50-100 mg qwk (phenpropionate)

Available forms: Inj 100, 200 mg/ml
Side effects/adverse reactions:
INTEG: Rash, acneiform lesions, oily hair, skin, flushing, sweating, acne vulgaris, alopecia, hirsutism
CNS: Dizziness, headache, fatigue, tremors, paresthesias, flushing, sweating, anxiety, lability, insomnia, carpal tunnel syndrome, chills
MS: Cramps, spasms
CV: Increased B/P
GU: ***Hematuria,*** amenorrhea, vaginitis, decreased libido, decreased breast size, clitoral hypertrophy, testicular atrophy, priapism

GI: Nausea, vomiting, constipation, weight gain, ***cholestatic jaundice***
EENT: Conjunctival edema, nasal congestion
ENDO: Abnormal GTT

Contraindications: Severe renal, severe cardiac, severe hepatic disease, hypersensitivity, pregnancy (X), lactation, abnormal genital bleeding, males with cancer of breast, prostate

Precautions: Diabetes mellitus, CV disease, MI

Pharmacokinetics:

IM: Metabolized in liver, crosses placenta, excreted in breast milk, urine

Interactions:

- ↑ effects of oral antidiabetics
- ↑ bleeding risk: anticoagulants, NSAIDs, salicylates
- Edema: ACTH, adrenal steroids
- ↓ effects of insulin

Lab test interferences:

Increase: Serum cholesterol, blood glucose, urine glucose
Decrease: Serum calcium, serum potassium, T_4, T_3, thyroid ^{131}I uptake test, urine 17-OHCS, 17-KS, PBI, BSP

NURSING CONSIDERATIONS

Assess:

- Anemia symptoms: dyspnea, fatigue, weakness, pallor
- Weight daily; notify prescriber if weekly weight gain is >5 lb
- B/P q4h
- I&O ratio; be alert for decreasing urinary output, increasing edema
- Growth rate in children, since growth rate may be uneven (linear/bone growth) with extended use
- Electrolytes: K, Na, Cl, Ca; cholesterol
- Hepatic studies: ALT, AST, bilirubin
- Edema, hypertension, cardiac symptoms, jaundice
- Mental status: affect, mood, behavioral changes, aggression
- Signs of masculinization in female: increased libido, deepening of voice, decreased breast tissue, enlarged clitoris, menstrual irregularities; male: gynecomastia, impotence, testicular atrophy
- Hypercalcemia: lethargy, polyuria, polydipsia, nausea, vomiting, constipation, drug may have to be decreased
- Hypoglycemia in diabetics, since oral antidiabetic action is increased

Administer:

IM route

- Titrated dose; use lowest effective dose
- Inject deeply, use large muscle mass

Perform/provide:

- Diet with increased calories, protein; decrease sodium if edema occurs

Evaluate:

- Therapeutic response: increased appetite, increased stamina

Teach patient/family:

- That drug must be combined with complete health plan: diet, rest, exercise
- To notify prescriber if therapeutic response decreases
- Not to discontinue abruptly
- About changes in sex characteristics
- That females should report menstrual irregularities
- That 1-3 mo course is necessary for response in breast cancer

naphazoline nasal agent

See appendix c

naphazoline ophthalmic

See appendix c

naproxen (OTC, ℞)

(na-prox'en)

Apo-Naproxen🍁, EC-Naprosyn, Naprelan, Napron X, Naprosyn, Naprosyn-E🍁, Naprosyn-SR🍁, Naxen🍁, Novo-Naprox🍁, Nu-Naprox🍁

naproxen sodium

Aleve, Anaprox, Anaprox DS, Apo-Napro-Na🍁, Apo-Napro-Na DS, Naprelan, Novo-Naprox Sodium🍁, Novo-Naprox Sodium DS🍁, Synflex🍁, Synflex DS🍁

Func. class.: Nonsteroidal antiinflammatory, nonopioid analgesic

Chem. class.: Propionic acid derivative

Action: Inhibits prostaglandin synthesis by decreasing an enzyme needed for biosynthesis; analgesic, antiinflammatory, antipyretic

Uses: Mild to moderate pain, osteoarthritis, rheumatoid, gouty arthritis, juvenile arthritis, primary dysmenorrhea

Dosage and routes:

- *Adult:* **PO** 250-500 mg bid, not to exceed 1 g/day (base); 550 mg, then 275 mg q6-8h prn, not to exceed 1375 mg (sodium)
- *Child:* **PO** 10 mg/kg in 2 divided doses

Available forms: Tabs, naproxen: 250, 375, 500 mg; tabs, del rel 375, 500 mg; tabs, oral susp 125 mg/5 ml; naproxen sodium tabs, cont rel 421.5, 550 mg; tabs 275, 550 mg

Side effects/adverse reactions:

GI: Nausea, anorexia, vomiting, diarrhea, jaundice, ***cholestatic hepatitis,*** constipation, flatulence, cramps, dry mouth, peptic ulcer, ***GI ulceration, bleeding, perforation***

CNS: Dizziness, drowsiness, fatigue, tremors, confusion, insomnia, anxiety, depression

CV: Tachycardia, peripheral edema, palpitations, dysrhythmias

INTEG: Purpura, rash, pruritus, sweating

GU: ***Nephrotoxicity: dysuria, hematuria, oliguria, azotemia***

HEMA: ***Blood dyscrasias***

EENT: Tinnitus, hearing loss, blurred vision

SYST: ***Anaphylaxis***

Contraindications: Hypersensitivity, asthma, severe renal disease, severe hepatic disease, ulcer disease, avoid in 2nd/3rd trimester pregnancy

Precautions: Pregnancy (B) 1st trimester, lactation, children <2 yr, bleeding disorders, GI disorders, cardiac disorders, hypersensitivity to other antiinflammatory agents, elderly, CCr <25 ml/min

Pharmacokinetics:

PO: Peak 2-4 hr, half-life 3-3½ hr; metabolized in liver; excreted in urine (metabolites), breast milk; 99% protein binding

Interactions:

- ↑ bleeding risk: oral anticoagulants, thrombolytic agents, eptifibatide, tirofiban, cefamandole, cefotetan, cefoperazone, clopidogrel, ticlopidine, plicamycin, valproic acid
- ↓ effect of: antihypertensives, diuretics
- ↑ GI side effects risk: aspirin, corticosteroids, alcohol, NSAIDs
- Possible renal impairment: ACE inhibitors
- Toxicity risk: methotrexate, lithium, antineoplastics, radiation treatment

Bleeding risk: anise, arnica,

chamomile, clove, dong quai, fenugreek, feverfew, garlic, ginger, ginkgo, ginseng *(Panax),* licorice

↑ gastric irritation: arginine, gossypol

↑ NSAIDs effect: bearberry, bilberry

↑ bleeding risk: bogbean, chondroitin

Lab test interferences:
Increase: BUN, alk phosphatase
False increase: 5-HIAA, 17KGS

NURSING CONSIDERATIONS

Assess:

• Pain: frequency, characteristics, intensity; relief prior to and 1-2 hr after med

Asthma, aspirin hypersensitivity or nasal polyps, increased risk of hypersensitivity

• Renal, hepatic, blood studies: BUN, creatinine, AST, ALT, Hgb, LDH, blood glucose, Hct, WBC, platelets CCr before treatment, periodically thereafter

• Audiometric, ophthalmic exam before, during, after treatment

• For eye, ear problems: blurred vision, tinnitus (may indicate toxicity)

Administer:

• With food to decrease GI symptoms; take on empty stomach to facilitate absorption

Perform/provide:

• Storage at room temperature

Evaluate:

• Therapeutic response: decreased pain, stiffness, swelling in joints, ability to move more easily

Teach patient/family:

• To use sunscreen to prevent photosensitivity

• To report blurred vision, ringing, roaring in ears (may indicate toxicity)

• To avoid driving, other hazardous activities if dizziness or drowsiness occurs

• To report change in urine pattern, weight increase, edema (face, lower extremities), pain increase in joints, fever, blood in urine (indicates nephrotoxicity); black stools, flulike symptoms

• That therapeutic effects may take up to 1 mo

• To avoid ASA, alcohol, steroids

naratriptan (℞)

(nair′ah-trip-tan)

Amerge

Func. class.: Antimigraine agent

Chem. class.: 5-HT_1 receptor agonist

Action: Binds selectively to the vascular 5-HT_1 receptor subtype, exerts antimigraine effect; causes vasoconstriction in cranial arteries

Uses: Acute treatment of migraine with or without aura

Dosage and routes:

• *Adult:* **PO** 1 or 2.5 mg with fluids, if headache returns, repeat once after 4 hr, max 5 mg/24 hr

Hepatic/renal dose

Max 2.5 mg/24 hr

Available forms: Tab 1, 2.5 mg

Side effects/adverse reactions:

GI: Nausea, vomiting

MS: Weakness, neck stiffness, myalgia

CNS: Dizziness, sedation, fatigue

CV: Increased B/P, palpitations, ***tachydysrhythmias, PR, QTc prolongation, ST/T wave changes, PVCs, atrial flutter/fibrillation, coronary vasospasm***

EENT: EENT infections, photophobia

MISC: Temperature change sensations; tightness, pressure sensations

Contraindications: Angina pectoris, history of MI, documented silent ischemia, ischemic heart disease, concurrent ergotamine-containing

N

preparations, uncontrolled hypertension, CV syndromes, hemiplegic or basilar migraines, hypersensitivity, severe renal disease (CCr <15 ml/min); severe hepatic disease (Child-Pugh grade C)

Precautions: Postmenopausal women, men >40 yr, risk factors for CAD, hypercholesterolemia, obesity, diabetes, impaired hepatic or renal function, pregnancy (C), lactation, children, elderly, peripheral vascular disease

Pharmacokinetics: Peak 2-3 hr, 28%-31% plasma protein binding, half-life 6 hr, metabolized in the liver (metabolite), excreted in urine, feces; may be excreted in breast milk

Interactions:
- ↑ vasospastic effects: ergot, ergot derivatives, other 5-HT_1 agonists
- ↑ adverse reactions risk: MAOIs, do not use together
- Weakness, hyperreflexia, incoordination: SSRIs (fluoxetine, fluvoxamine, paroxetine, sertraline)

Serotonin syndrome: SAM-e, St. John's wort

↑ effect: butterbur

NURSING CONSIDERATIONS

Assess:
- For stress level, activity, recreation, coping mechanisms
- Neurologic status: LOC blurred vision, nausea, vomiting, tingling in extremities preceding headache

Administer:
- With fluids as soon as symptoms appear, may take another dose after 4 hr; do not take >5 mg in any 24-hr period

Perform/provide:
- Quiet, calm environment with decreased stimulation for noise, bright light, excessive talking

Evaluate:
- Therapeutic response: decrease in frequency, severity of headache

Teach patient/family:
- To report pain, tightness in chest, neck, throat, or jaw; notify prescriber immediately if sudden, severe abdominal pain occurs
- Not to use if another 5-HT_1 agonist or an ergot preparation has been used in the past 24 hr
- Advise patient to notify prescriber if pregnancy is planned or suspected

natamycin ophthalmic

See appendix c

nedocromil (℞)

(ned-o-kroe′mill)

Tilade

Func. class.: Antiasthmatic

Chem. class.: Mast cell stabilizer

Action: Stabilizes the membrane of the sensitized mast cell, preventing release of chemical mediators after an antigen-IgE interaction

Uses: Severe perennial bronchial asthma, exercise-induced bronchospasm (prevention), prevention of acute bronchospasm induced by environmental pollutants; *not* for treatment of acute asthma attacks

Dosage and routes:
- *Adult and child >12 yr:* **INH** 2 inhalations 2-4 ×/day at regular intervals to provide 14 g/day

Available forms: 1.75 mg nedocromil sodium per activation in 16.2 g canisters providing at least 112 metered inhalations

Side effects/adverse reactions:

EENT: Throat irritation, cough, nasal congestion, burning eyes, rhinitis

CNS: Headache, dizziness, neuritis, dysphonia

GI: Nausea, vomiting, anorexia, dry mouth, bitter taste
MISC: ***Anaphylaxis***
Contraindications: Hypersensitivity to this drug or lactose, status asthmaticus
Precautions: Pregnancy (B), lactation, children
Pharmacokinetics:
INH: Peak 15 min, duration 4-6 hr; excreted unchanged in urine; half-life 80 min

NURSING CONSIDERATIONS
Assess:
• Pulmonary function testing baseline (asthma)
• Respiratory status: rate, rhythm, characteristics, cough, wheezing, dyspnea
Administer:
• By inhalation only, with spacer device if needed
• Gargle, sip of water to decrease irritation in throat
Evaluate:
• Therapeutic response: decrease in asthmatic symptoms, congested, runny nose
Teach patient/family:
• To clear mucus before using
• The proper technique: exhale; using inhaler, inhale deeply with head tipped back to open airway; remove, hold breath, exhale; use Halermatic or Spinhaler with Intal caps
• That therapeutic effect may take up to 4 wk
• That drug is preventive only, not restorative

nefazodone (℞)
(ne-faz′o-done)
Serzone
Func. class.: Antidepressant—misc
Chem. class.: Phenylpiperazine

Action: Selectively inhibits serotonin uptake by brain, potentiates behavorial changes, occupies central $S\text{-}H_2$ receptors
Uses: Major depression
Research note: Clozapine given with nefazodone resulted in an increase of clozapine[25]
Dosage and routes:
• *Adult:* **PO** 200 mg/day (100 mg bid); dose may be increased to 300 mg/day (150 mg bid), max 600 mg/day
• *Elderly:* 100 mg/day (50 mg bid); increase to 100 mg bid after 2 wk to desired dose
Available forms: Tabs 50, 100, 150, 200, 250 mg
Side effects/adverse reactions:
CNS: Somnolence, dizziness, *headache, insomnia*
GI: Nausea, constipation, dry mouth
GU: Urinary frequency, retention, UTI
CV: Postural hypotension
RESP: Pharyngitis, cough
EENT: Blurred vision, abnormal vision
Contraindications: Hypersensitivity to this drug or phenylpiperazines
Precautions: Pregnancy (C), lactation, children, elderly, cardiovascular disease, seizure disorder, history of taking digoxin, recent MI, mania, renal disease
Do not confuse:
Serozone/Seroquel
Pharmacokinetics: Metabolized in liver extensively to metabolites; excreted in urine, breast milk; peak 1-3 hr; half-life triphasic 2-4 hr
Interactions:
• ↑ effect: CNS depressants, alcohol
• ↑ plasma concentrations: benzodiazepines
⬌ Hypertensive crisis: MAOIs
• ↑ toxicity: triazolam, alprazolam, midazolam, phenytoin, MAOIs, carbamazepine, digoxin

N

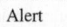

Serotonin syndrome: SAM-e, St. John's wort

↑ CNS depression: chamomile, hops, kava, lavender, skullcap, valerian

↑ anticholinergic effect: corkwood, jimsonweed

NURSING CONSIDERATIONS

Assess:

- B/P (lying, standing), pulse q4h; if systolic B/P drops 20 mm Hg, hold drug, notify prescriber; take vital signs q4h in patients with cardiovascular disease
- Blood studies: CBC, leukocytes, differential, cardiac enzymes (long-term therapy)
- Hepatic studies: AST, ALT, bilirubin; if levels at >3 × upper limit of normal, discontinue drug
- Mental status: mood, sensorium, affect, suicidal tendencies; increase in psychiatric symptoms: depression, panic
- Urinary retention, constipation; constipation is more likely in children, elderly
- Alcohol consumption; hold dose until morning

Administer:

- With food, milk for GI symptoms
- Crushed if patient cannot swallow whole

Perform/provide:

- Storage at room temperature; do not freeze

Evaluate:

- Therapeutic response: decrease in depression; absence of suicidal thoughts

Teach patient/family:

- That therapeutic effects may take 3-4 wk
- To use caution in driving, other activities requiring alertness because of drowsiness, dizziness; to avoid rising quickly from sitting to standing, especially elderly
- To avoid alcohol ingestion, other CNS depressants, benzodiazepines
- To increase bulk in diet for constipation, especially elderly
- To take gum, hard sugarless candy, frequents sips of water for dry mouth
- To report immediately urinary retention

Treatment of overdose: ECG monitoring; induce emesis; lavage, activated charcoal; administer anticonvulsant

nelfinavir (℞)

(nell-fin'a-ver)

Viracept

Func. class.: Antiretroviral

Chem. chass.: HIV protease inhibitor

Action: Inhibits human immunodeficiency virus (HIV) protease, which prevents maturation of the infectious virus

Uses: HIV in combination with other antiretrovirals

Dosage and routes:

- *Adult and child >13 yr:* **PO** 750 mg tid or 1250 mg bid
- *Child 2-13 yr:* **PO** 20-30 mg/kg tid, max 750 mg tid

Available forms: Tabs 250, 625 mg; powder, oral 50 mg/g

Side effects/adverse reactions:

HEMA: ***Anemia, leukopenia, thrombocytopenia, Hgb abnormalities***

GI: Diarrhea, anorexia, dyspepsia, *nausea, flatulence*

CNS: Headache, asthenia, poor concentration, ***seizures***

INTEG: Rash, dermatitis

MS: Pain, arthralgia, myalgia, myopathy

CV: Bleeding

ENDO: Hypoglycemia, hyperlipidemia

Contraindications: Hypersensitivity to protease inhibitors
Precautions: Hepatic disease, pregnancy (B), lactation, renal disease, hemophilia, PKU
Pharmacokinetics: Half-life 3½-5 hr
Interactions:
Serious dysrhythmias: ergots, midazolam, triazolam, amiodarone, quinidine
- ↓ effect of: oral contraceptives
- ↑ effect: rifabutin
- ↑ nelfinavir levels: ketoconazole, indinavir, ritonavir
- ↓ nelfinavir levels: rifamycins, nevirapine, phenobarbital, phenytoin, carbamazepine
- Drug/food: ↑ absorption with food

↓ antiretroviral effect: St. John's wort

NURSING CONSIDERATIONS
Assess:
- Signs of infection, anemia
- Hepatic studies: ALT, AST
- C&S before drug therapy; drug may be taken as soon as culture is taken; repeat C&S after treatment; determine the presence of other sexually transmitted diseases
- Bowel pattern before, during treatment; if severe abdominal pain with bleeding occurs, drug should be discontinued; monitor hydration
- Skin eruptions, rash, urticaria, itching
- Allergies before treatment, reaction of each medication; place allergies on chart
- Viral load, CD4 cell counts baseline and throughout treatment

Administer:
- With food
- Oral powder mixed with fluids if desired, do not mix with juice or acidic fluids, stable mixed for 6 hr

Teach patient/family:
- To avoid taking with other medications unless directed by prescriber
- That drug does not cure, but does manage symptoms, and does not prevent transmission of HIV to others
- To use a nonhormonal form of birth control while taking this drug
- If dose is missed, to take as soon as remembered up to 1 hr before next dose; do not double dose
- To take with food

neomycin (℞)

(nee-oh-mye'sin)
Mycifradin, Myciguent
Func. class.: Antiinfective
Chem. class.: Aminoglycoside

Action: Interferes with protein synthesis in bacterial cell by binding to 30S ribosomal subunit, causing inaccurate peptide sequence to form in protein chain, causing bacterial death
Uses: Severe systemic infections of CNS, respiratory, GI, urinary tract, eye, bone, skin, soft tissues caused by *Pseudomonas aeruginosa, Escherichia coli, Enterobacter, Klebsiella pneumoniae, Proteus vulgaris;* also used for hepatic coma, preoperatively to sterilize bowel, infectious diarrhea caused by enteropathogenic *E. coli*
Dosage and routes:
Hepatic encephalopathy
- *Adult:* **PO** 4-12 g/day in divided doses × 5-6 days
- *Child:* **PO** 50-100 mg/kg/day in divided doses

Preoperative intestinal antisepsis
- *Adult:* **PO** on 3rd day of a 3-day regimen, give 1 g early PM, repeat in 1 hr, repeat at hs (given with erythromycin); give saline cathartic before giving this drug
- *Child:* **PO** 14.7 mg/kg or 4.7 mg/m² q4h × 3 days

N

Available forms: Tabs 500 mg; oral sol 125 mg/5 ml

Side effects/adverse reactions:

GU: ***Oliguria, hematuria, renal damage, azotemia, renal failure, nephrotoxicity***

CNS: Confusion, depression, numbness, tremors, ***seizures,*** muscle twitching, ***neurotoxicity,*** dizziness, vertigo

EENT: ***Ototoxicity,*** deafness, visual disturbances, tinnitus

HEMA: ***Agranulocytosis, thrombocytopenia,*** leukopenia, eosinophilia, anemia

GI: Nausea, vomiting, anorexia; increased ALT, AST, bilirubin; hepatomegaly, ***hepatic necrosis,*** splenomegaly

CV: Hypotension, hypertension, palpitation

INTEG: Rash, burning, urticaria, photosensitivity, dermatitis, alopecia

Contraindications: Bowel obstruction (oral use), severe renal disease, hypersensitivity, infants, children

Precautions: Mild renal disease, pregnancy (C), hearing deficits, lactation, myasthenia gravis, Parkinson's disease

Pharmacokinetics:

PO: Onset rapid, peak 1-2 hr

Plasma half-life 2-3 hr; not metabolized, excreted unchanged in feces, crosses placenta

Interactions:

- ↑ ototoxicity, neurotoxicity, nephrotoxicity: other aminoglycosides, amphotericin B, polymyxin, vancomycin, ethacrynic acid, furosemide, mannitol, methoxyflurane, cisplatin, cephalosporins, bacitracin
- ↑ effects: nondepolarizing muscle relaxants, succinylcholine, oral anticoagulants when given with oral neomycin
- ↓ effects of digoxin, penicillin V when given with oral neomycin

Toxicity: lysine (large amounts)

Do not use acidophilus with antiinfectives

NURSING CONSIDERATIONS

Assess:

- Weight before treatment; calculation of dosage is usually based on ideal body weight, but may be calculated on actual body weight
- I&O ratio, urinalysis qd for proteinuria, cells, casts; report sudden change in urine output
- Urine pH if drug is used for UTI; urine should be kept alkaline
- Renal impairment by securing urine for CCr testing, BUN, serum creatinine; lower dosage should be given in renal impairment
- Deafness by audiometric testing, ringing, roaring in ears, vertigo; assess hearing before, during, after treatment
- Dehydration: high specific gravity, decrease in skin turgor, dry mucous membranes, dark urine
- Overgrowth of infection: fever, malaise, redness, pain, swelling, perineal itching, diarrhea, stomatitis, change in cough, sputum
- C&S before starting treatment to identify infecting organism
- Vestibular dysfunction: nausea, vomiting, dizziness, headache; drug should be discontinued if severe
- Injection sites for redness, swelling, abscesses; use warm compresses at site

Administer:

- Drug in evenly spaced doses to maintain blood level
- Bicarbonate to alkalinize urine if ordered in treating UTI, as drug is most active in alkaline environment

Perform/provide:

- Adequate fluids of 2 L/day unless contraindicated to prevent irritation of tubules
- Supervised ambulation, other safety measures, with vestibular dysfunction

Evaluate:
- Therapeutic response: absence of fever, draining wounds, negative C&S after treatment

Teach patient/family:
- To report headache, dizziness, symptoms of overgrowth of infection, renal impairment
- To report loss of hearing, ringing, roaring in ears or a feeling of fullness in head
- To take all of medication, to take a missed dose as soon as remembered, do not double doses

Treatment of overdose: Hemodialysis; monitor serum levels of drug

neomycin otic
See appendix c

neomycin topical
See appendix c

neostigmine (℞)
(nee-oh-stig′meen)
neostigmine, Prostigmin
Func. class.: Cholinergic stimulant; anticholinesterase
Chem. class.: Quaternary compound

Action: Inhibits destruction of acetylcholine, which increases concentration at sites where acetylcholine is released; this facilitates transmission of impulses across myoneural junction

Uses: Myasthenia gravis, nondepolarizing neuromuscular blocker antagonist, bladder distention, postoperative ileus

Dosage and routes:

Renal dose
- CCr 10-50 ml/min 50% of dose; CCr <10 ml/min 25% of dose

Myasthenia gravis
- *Adult:* **PO** 15 mg q3-4h, may increase to 375 mg/day; **IM/IV** 0.5-2 mg q1-3h
- *Child:* **PO** 2 mg/kg/day q3-4h

Nondepolarizing neuromuscular blocker antagonist
- *Adult:* **IV** 0.5-2 mg slowly, may repeat if needed (give 0.6-1.2 mg atropine before this drug)
- *Infant/child:* **IV** 0.025-0.1 mg/kg/dose

Abdominal distention/postoperative ileus
- *Adult:* **IM/SC** 0.25-1 mg (1:4000) q4-6h depending on condition × 2-3 days

Available forms: Tabs 15 mg; inj 1:1000, 1:2000, 1:4000

Side effects/adverse reactions:
INTEG: Rash, urticaria, flushing
CNS: Dizziness, headache, sweating, weakness, ***convulsions,*** incoordination, ***paralysis,*** drowsiness, loss of consciousness
GI: Nausea, diarrhea, vomiting, cramps, increased peristalsis, salivary and gastric secretions
CV: Tachycardia, dysrhythmias, bradycardia, hypotension, AV block, ECG changes, ***cardiac arrest,*** syncope
GU: Urinary frequency, incontinence, urgency
RESP: ***Respiratory depression, bronchospasm, constriction, laryngospasm, respiratory arrest,*** dyspnea
EENT: Miosis, blurred vision, lacrimation, visual changes

Contraindications: Obstruction of intestine, renal system, bromide sensitivity, peritonitis

Precautions: Bradycardia, pregnancy (C), hypotension, seizure disorders, bronchial asthma, coronary occlusion, hyperthyroidism, dysrhythmias, peptic ulcer, megacolon, poor GI motility, lactation, children

Pharmacokinetics:
PO: Onset 45-75 min, duration 2½-4 hr
IM/SC: Onset 10-30 min, duration 2½-4 hr
IV: Onset 4-8 min; duration 2-4 hr; metabolized in liver, excreted in urine

Interactions:
- ↑ action of decamethonium, succinylcholine
- ↓ neostigmine action: antihistamines, antidepressants, atropine, haloperidol, phenothiazines, quinidine, disopyramide

↑ effect: pill-bearing spurge

NURSING CONSIDERATIONS

Assess:
- VS, respiration q8h
- I&O ratio; check for urinary retention or incontinence

For bradycardia, hypotension, bronchospasm, headache, dizziness, convulsions, respiratory depression; drug should be discontinued if toxicity occurs

Administer:
- Only with atropine sulfate available for cholinergic crisis
- Only after all other cholinergics have been discontinued
- Increased doses, as ordered if tolerance occurs
- Larger doses after exercise or fatigue, as ordered

PO route
- On empty stomach for better absorption

IV route
- Undiluted, give through Y-tube or 3-way stopcock; give 0.5 mg or less over 1 min

Additive compatibilities: Netilmicin

Syringe compatibilities: Glycopyrrolate, heparin, pentobarbital, thiopental

Y-site compatibilities: Heparin, hydrocortisone, potassium chloride, vit B/C

Perform/provide:
- Storage at room temperature

Evaluate:
- Therapeutic response: increased muscle strength, hand grasp, improved gait, absence of labored breathing (if severe)

Teach patient/family:
- That drug is not a cure; it only relieves symptoms
- To wear emergency ID specifying myasthenia gravis, drugs taken

Treatment of overdose: Respiratory support, atropine 1-4 mg (IV)

nesiritide (℞)

(neh-seer'ih-tide)
Natrecor
Func. class.: Vasodilator
Chem. class.: Human B-type natriuretic peptide

Action: Uses DNA technology; human B-type natriuretic peptide binds to the receptor in vascular smooth muscle and endothelial cells, leading to smooth muscle relaxation

Uses: Acutely decompensated CHF

Dosage and routes:
- *Adult:* **IV BOL** 2 mcg/kg, then **IV INF** 0.01 mcg/kg/min

Available forms: Powder for inj, 1.5 mg single-use vial

Side effects/adverse reactions:
CNS: Headache, insomnia, dizziness, anxiety, confusion, paresthesia, tremor
CV: Hypotension, ***tachycardia,*** dysrhythmias, bradycardia, ventricular tachycardia, ventricular extrasystoles, atrial fibrillation
GI: Vomiting, nausea
INTEG: Rash, sweating, pruritus, inj site reaction
MISC: Abdominal pain, back pain

RESP: Increased cough, hemoptysis, ***apnea***
Contraindications: Hypersensitivity, cardiogenic shock or B/P <90 mm Hg as primary therapy
Precautions: Pregnancy (C); mitral stenosis; significant valvular stenosis, restriction, or obstructive cardiomyopathy, or any condition that is dependent upon venous return; renal disease, lactation, children
Pharmacokinetics: Half-life 18 min
Interactions:

- ↑ symptomatic hypotension with ACE inhibitors

NURSING CONSIDERATIONS
Assess:

- PCWP, RAP, cardiac index, MPAP
- B/P, pulse during treatment until stable

Administer:

IV route

- Do not administer nesiritide through a central heparin-coated catheter; heparin should be administered through a separate catheter
- Prime IV fluid with infusion of 25 ml before connecting to patient's vascular access port and before bolus dose or IV infusion
- Reconstitute one 1.5 mg vial/5 ml of diluent from prefilled 250-ml plastic IV bag with diluent of choice (D_5, 0.9% NaCl, D_5/½ NaCl, D_5/0.2% NaCl); do not shake vial, roll gently; use only clear sol
- Withdraw all contents of reconstituted vial and add to the 250-ml plastic IV bag (6 mcg/ml), invert bag several times
- Use within 24 hr of reconstituting

Evaluate:

- Therapeutic response: improvement in CHF with improved PCWP, RAP, MPAP

Teach patient/family:

- To explain purpose of medication and expected results

nevirapine

(ne-veer′a-peen)
Viramune
Func. class.: Antiretroviral
Chem. class.: Non-nucleoside reverse transcriptase inhibitor (NNRTI)

Action: Binds directly to reverse transcriptase and blocks RNA, DNA, causing a disruption of the enzyme's site
Uses: HIV-1 in combination with other highly active antiretroviral treatments (HAART)
Research note: Nevirapine given with warfarin resulted in decreased warfarin action[26]
Dosage and routes:

- *Adult:* **PO** 200 mg qd × 2 wk, then 200 mg bid in combination
- *Child ≥8 yr:* **PO** 4 mg/kg/qd × 2 wk, then 4 mg/kg/bid
- *Child 2 mo-8 yr:* **PO** 4 mg/kg qd × 2 wk, then 7 mg/kg bid

Available forms: Tabs 200 mg; oral susp 50 mg/5 ml
Side effects/adverse reactions:

GI: Diarrhea, abdominal pain, *nausea, stomatitis,* ***hepatotoxicity***
CNS: Paresthesia, headache, fever, peripheral neuropathy
INTEG: Rash, toxic epidermal necrolysis
MS: Pain, myalgia
HEMA: ***Neutropenia, anemia, thrombocytopenia***
MISC: ***Stevens-Johnson syndrome***
Contraindications: Hypersensitivity
Precautions: Hepatic disease, pregnancy (C), lactation, children, renal disease
Do not confuse
nevirapine/nelfinavir
viramune/viracept
Pharmacokinetics: Rapidly ab-

sorbed, 60% bound to plasma proteins, metabolized by liver; metabolized by hepatic P450 enzyme system

Interactions:

- ↓ nevirapine levels: rifamycins
- ↑ nevirapine levels: cimetidine, macrolide antiinfectives
- ↓ effects of protease inhibitors, oral contraceptives, ketoconazole, methadone

↓ action of antiretroviral: St. John's wort, do not use concurrently

NURSING CONSIDERATIONS

Assess:

- Signs of infection, anemia
- Hepatic, blood studies during treatment: ALT, AST, viral load, CD4; renal studies; if LFTs are elevated significantly, drug should be withheld
- C&S before drug therapy; drug may be taken as soon as culture is taken; repeat C&S after treatment; determine the presence of other sexually transmitted disease
- Bowel pattern before, during treatment; if severe abdominal pain with bleeding occurs, drug should be discontinued; monitor hydration

Allergies before treatment, reaction to each medication; skin eruptions; rash, urticaria, itching; if rash is severe or systemic symptoms occur, discontinue immediately

Administer:

- Without regard to meals

Teach patient/family:

To report any right quadrant pain, jaundice, rash immediately

- That drug may be taken with food, antacids, didanosine
- To take as prescribed; if dose is missed, take as soon as remembered up to 1 hr before next dose; do not double dose
- That drug is not a cure, controls symptoms of HIV
- To avoid OTC agents unless approved by prescriber
- To use a nonhormonal form of contraception during treatment
- That drug must be taken in equal intervals around the clock to maintain blood levels for duration of therapy

niacin (OTC, ℞)

(nye'a-sin)

Edur-Acin, Nia-Bid, Niac, Niacels, Niacor, Niaspan, Nicobid, Nico-400, Nicolar, Nicotinex

nicotinic acid (OTC, ℞)

Novo-Niacin✤, Slo-Niacin, vitamin B

niacinamide (OTC, ℞)

nicotinamide (OTC, ℞)

Func. class.: Vit B_3, antihyperlipidemic

Chem. class.: Water-soluble vitamin

Action: Needed for conversion of fats, protein, carbohydrates, by oxidation reduction; acts directly on vascular smooth muscle, causing vasodilation, reduces LDL, HDL, triglycerides and lipoprotein A

Uses: Pellagra, hyperlipidemias (types 4, 5), peripheral vascular disease who present a risk for pancreatitis

Dosage and routes:

Niacin deficiency

- *Adult:* **PO** 100-500 mg/day in divided doses; **IM/SC** 5-100 mg 5 or more ×/day; **IV** 25-100 mg bid or tid

Adjunct in hyperlipidemia

- *Adult:* **PO** 250 mg after evening meal; may increase dose at 1-4 wk intervals to 1-2 g tid, max 6 g/day;

ext rel 500 mg HS, × 4 wk, then 1000 mg HS for wk 5-8, do not increase by more than 500 mg q4wk, max 2000 mg/day

Pellagra

• *Adult:* **PO** 300-500 mg qd in divided doses

• *Child:* **PO** 100-300 mg qd in divided doses

Peripheral vascular disease

• *Adult:* **PO** 250-800 mg qd in divided doses

Available forms: Niacin tabs 25, 50, 100, 250, 500, 1000 mg; caps, time rel 250, 500 mg; tabs, timed rel 250, 500, mg; cap, ext rel 250, 400, mg; sus rel tabs 500 mg; cont rel tabs 250, 500, 750 mg; sus rel cap 125, 500 mg; elix 50 mg/5 ml; nicotinamide—tabs 100, 250, 500 mg

Side effects/adverse reactions:

CNS: Paresthesias, headache, dizziness, anxiety

GI: Nausea, vomiting, anorexia, ***jaundice, hepatotoxicity,*** diarrhea, peptic ulcer, dyspepsia

GU: Hyperuricemia, ***glycosuria, hypoalbuminemia***

CV: Postural hypotension, vasovagal attacks, dysrhythmias, vasodilation

EENT: Blurred vision, ptosis

INTEG: Flushing, dry skin, rash, pruritus, itching, tingling

Contraindications: Hypersensitivity, peptic ulcer, hepatic disease, lactation, hemorrhage, severe hypotension

Precautions: Glaucoma, cardiovascular disease, CAD, diabetes mellitus, gout, schizophrenia, pregnancy (C), lactation

Do not confuse:

Nicobid/Nitro-Bid

Pharmacokinetics:

PO: Peak 30-70 min, half-life 45 min; metabolized in liver; 30% excreted unchanged in urine

Interactions:

• Myopathy, rhabdomyolysis: HMG-CoA reductase inhibitors

• Postural hypotension: ganglionic blockers

• ↑ flushing, pruritus: alcohol, avoid use

Lab test interferences:

Increase: Bilirubin, alk phosphatase, hepatic enzymes, LDH, uric acid

Decrease: Cholesterol

False increase: Urinary catecholamines

False-positive: Urine glucose

NURSING CONSIDERATIONS

Assess:

• Hepatic studies: AST, ALT, bilirubin, uric acid, alk phosphatase; blood glucose before and during treatment

• Cardiac status: rate, rhythm, quality; postural hypotension, dysrhythmias

• Nutritional status: liver, yeast, legumes, organ meat, lean poultry; fat in diet

• Hepatic dysfunction: clay-colored stools, itching, dark urine, jaundice

• CNS symptoms: headache, paresthesias, blurred vision

• For symptoms of niacin deficiency: nausea, vomiting, anemia, poor memory, confusion, dermatitis

• For lipid, triglyceride, cholesterol level, if using for hyperlipidemia

Administer:

• With meals for GI symptoms, and 325 mg aspirin or NSAIDs ½ hr before dose to decrease flushing

Evaluate:

• Therapeutic response: decreased lipids, warm extremities, absence of numbness in extremities

Teach patient/family:

• That flushing and increase in feelings of warmth will occur several hr after taking drug (PO); after 2 wk of therapy, these side effects diminish

• To remain recumbent if postural hypotension occurs; to rise slowly to prevent orthostatic hypotension
• To abstain from alcohol if drug is prescribed for hyperlipidemia
• To avoid sunlight if skin lesions are present
Not to break, crush, or chew ext rel tabs, caps
To report clay-colored stools, anorexia, jaundiced sclera, skin; dark urine, hepatotoxicity may occur

*niCARdipine (℞)

(nye-card'i-peen)
Cardene, Cardene IV, Cardene SR
Func. class.: Calcium channel blocker, antianginal, antihypertensive
Chem. class.: Dihydropyridine

Action: Inhibits calcium ion influx across cell membrane during cardiac depolarization; produces relaxation of coronary vascular smooth muscle, peripheral vascular smooth muscle; dilates coronary vascular arteries; increases myocardial oxygen delivery in patients with vasospastic angina
Uses: Chronic stable angina pectoris, hypertension
Research note: Grapefruit juice given with niCARdipine resulted in increased niCARdipine levels[28]
Dosage and routes:
Hypertension
• *Adult:* **PO** 20 mg tid initially, may increase after 3 days (range 20-40 mg tid) or 30 mg bid sus rel, may increase to 60 mg bid; **IV** 0.5-2.2 mg/hr
Angina
• *Adult:* **PO** 20 mg tid, may be adjusted q3d, may use 20-40 mg tid
Renal dose
• *Adult:* **PO** 20 mg tid; or 30 mg bid (sus rel)
Hepatic dose
• *Adult:* **PO** 20 mg bid
Available forms: Caps 20, 30 mg; caps sus rel 30, 45, 60 mg; inj 2.5 mg/ml
Side effects/adverse reactions:
CV: Edema, bradycardia, hypotension, palpitations, ***pulmonary edema,*** chest pain, tachycardia, increased angina
GI: Nausea, vomiting, gastric upset, constipation, ***hepatitis,*** abdominal cramps
GU: Nocturia, polyuria, ***acute renal failure***
INTEG: Rash
CNS: Headache, dizziness, anxiety, depression, confusion, paresthesia, somnolence
OTHER: Blurred vision, flushing, sweating, shortness of breath,
Contraindications: Sick sinus syndrome, 2nd-/3rd-degree heart block, hypersensitivity
Precautions: CHF, hypotension, hepatic injury, pregnancy (C), lactation, children, renal disease, elderly
Do not confuse:
niCARdipine/NIFEdipine
Cardene/Cardizem
Cardene SR/Cardizem SR
Pharmacokinetics:
PO: Onset 30 min, peak 1-2 hr, duration 8 hr
PO-SR: Onset unknown, peak 2-6 hr, duration 10-12 hr, half-life 2-5 hr
Metabolized by liver, excreted in urine 60%, 35% feces
Interactions:
• ↑ effects of digitalis, neuromuscular blocking agents, theophylline, other antihypertensives, nitrates, alcohol, quinidine
• ↑ niCARdipine effects: cimetidine

• ↓ antihypertensive effect: NSAIDs, rifampin
• ↑ toxicity risk: cycloSPORINE, prazosin, carbamazepine, quinidine, propranolol
• Food/drug: ↑ hypotensive effect: grapefruit juice
↑ effect: barberry, betel palm, burdock, goldenseal, khat, khella, lily of the valley, plantain
↓ effect: yohimbe

NURSING CONSIDERATIONS

Assess:

Cardiac status: B/P, pulse, respiration, ECG during long-term treatment
• Anginal pain: intensity, location, duration, alleviating factors
• Potassium, renal, hepatic studies, periodically
CHF: weight gain, rales, jugular venous distention, dyspnea, I&O

Administer:

PO route

Do not open, break, crush, chew sus rel cap
• Without regard to meals

IV route

• Dilute each 25 mg/240 ml of compatible sol (0.1 mg/ml), give slowly
• Stable at room temperature 24 hr

Y-site compatibilities: Diltiazem, DOBUTamine, DOPamine, epINEPHrine, fentanyl, hydromorphone, labetalol, lorazepam, midazolam, milrinone, morphine, nitroglycerin, norepinephrine, ranitidine, vecuronium

Evaluate:

• Therapeutic response: decreased anginal pain, decreased B/P

Teach patient/family:

• To avoid hazardous activities until stabilized on drug, dizziness is no longer a problem
• To limit caffeine consumption, take no alcohol products
• To avoid OTC drugs unless directed by prescriber
• To comply in all areas of medical regimen: diet, exercise, stress reduction, drug therapy
To notify prescriber of irregular heartbeat, shortness of breath, swelling of feet and hands, pronounced dizziness, constipation, nausea, hypotension

Treatment of overdose: Defibrillation, β-agonists, IV calcium, diuretics, atropine for AV block, vasopressor for hypotension

nicotine (OTC, ℞)

(nik'o-teen)

nicotine chewing gum (OTC, ℞)

Nicorette

nicotine inhaler (OTC, ℞)

Nicotrol Inhaler

nicotine nasal spray (℞)

Nicotrol NS

nicotine transdermal (℞)

Clear Nicoderm CQ, Habitrol, Nicoderm CQ, Nicotrol

Func. class.: Smoking deterrent
Chem. class.: Ganglionic cholinergic agonist

Action: Agonist at nicotinic receptors in peripheral, central nervous systems; acts at sympathetic ganglia, on chemoreceptors of aorta, carotid bodies; also affects adrenalin-releasing catecholamines

Uses: Deter cigarette smoking

Investigational uses: Gilles de la Tourette's syndrome

Dosage and routes:

Nicotine chewing gum

• *Adult:* Gum 1 piece chewed × ½ hr as needed to abstain from smoking, not to exceed 30/day

Nicotine inhaler

• *Adult:* **INH** 6 cartridges/day for first 3-6 wk, max 16/day × 12 wk

Nicotine nasal spray

• *Adults:* 1 spray in each nostril 1-2 ×/hr, max 5 ×/hr or 40 ×/day, max 3 mo

Nicotine transdermal/inhaler system

• *Habitrol, Nicoderm:* 21 mg/day × 4-8 wk; 14 mg/day × 2-4 wk; 7 mg/day × 2-4 wk

• *Nicotrol:* 15 mg/day × 12 wk; 10 mg/day × 2 wk; 5 mg/day × 2 wk

• *Nicotrol Inhaler:* delivers 30% of what a smoker receives from an actual cigarette

Gilles de la Tourette's syndrome (off-label)

• *Adult/child:* Chewing gum: 2 mg chewed × ½ hr bid for 1-6 mo; TD: 7 or 10 mg patch qd × 2 days

Available forms: Transdermal patch delivering 7, 14, 21 mg/day (Habitrol, Nicoderm, nicotine transdermal system); 5, 10, 15 mg/day (Nicoderm); nicotine inhaler: 4 mg delivered; nasal spray: 0.5 mg nicotine/actuation; gum: 2 mg/piece

Side effects/adverse reactions:

RESP: Breathing difficulty, cough, hoarseness, sneezing, wheezing

EENT: Jaw ache, irritation in buccal cavity

CNS: Dizziness, vertigo, insomnia, headache, confusion, convulsions, depression, euphoria, numbness, tinnitus, strange dreams

GI: Nausea, vomiting, anorexia, indigestion, diarrhea, abdominal pain, constipation, eructation

CV: Dysrhythmias, tachycardia, palpitations, edema, flushing, hypertension

Contraindications: Hypersensitivity, immediate post MI recovery period, severe angina pectoris, pregnancy (X), gum; (D), transdermal

Precautions: Vasospastic disease, dysrhythmias, diabetes mellitus, hyperthyroidism, pheochromocytoma, coronary disease, esophagitis, peptic ulcer, lactation, hepatic/renal disease

Pharmacokinetics: Onset 15-30 min, metabolized in liver, excreted in urine, half-life 2-3 hr, 30-120 hr (terminal)

Interactions:

• ↓ absorption: glutethimide

• ↑ absorption: SC insulin

• ↓ metabolism of propoxyphene

• Smoking cessation ↑ diuretic effects of furosemide

• ↑ blood levels with cessation of smoking: caffeine, theophylline, pentazocine, imipramine, oxazepam, propranolol, acetaminophen

↑ effect: blue cohosh, lobelia

↓ effect: oats

NURSING CONSIDERATIONS

Assess:

• Adverse reaction: irritation of buccal cavity, dislike of taste, jaw ache

Evaluate:

• Therapeutic response: decrease in urge to smoke, decreased need for gum after 3-6 mo

Teach patient/family:

Gum

• To chew gum slowly for 30 min to promote buccal absorption of the drug; do not chew over 45 min

• To begin drug withdrawal after 3 mo use; not to exceed 6 mo

• All aspects of drug use; give package insert to patient and explain

• That gum will not stick to dentures, dental appliances

• That gum is as toxic as cigarette; to be used only to deter smoking

• Not to use during pregnancy; birth defects may occur

• ***Transdermal patch***

• That patch is as toxic as cigarettes; to be used only to deter smoking

• Not to use during pregnancy; birth defects may occur
• To keep used and unused system out of reach of children and pets
• To apply once a day to a nonhairy, clean, dry area of skin on upper body or upper outer arm; to rotate sites to prevent skin irritation
• To stop smoking immediately when beginning patch treatment
• To apply promptly after removing from protective patch; system may lose strength

Inhaler

• That puffing on mouthpiece delivers nicotine through the mouth lining

*NIFEdipine (℞)

(nye-fed'i-peen)

Adalat, Adalat CC, Apo-Nifed✤, NIFEdipine, Novo-Nifedin✤, Nu-Nifedin✤, Procardia, Procardia XL

Func. class.: Calcium-channel blocker, antianginal, antihypertensive

Chem. class.: Dihydropyridine

Action: Inhibits calcium ion influx across cell membrane during cardiac depolarization; relaxes coronary vascular smooth muscle; dilates coronary arteries; increases myocardial oxygen delivery in patients with vasospastic angina; dilates peripheral arteries

Uses: Chronic stable angina pectoris, vasospastic angina, hypertension

Investigational uses: Migraines, CHF, Raynaud's disease, anal fissures

Dosage and routes:

• *Adult:* **PO** immediate release 10 mg tid, increase in 10 mg increments q7-14d, not to exceed 180 mg/24 hr or single dose of 30 mg; sus rel 30-60 mg/qd, may increase q7-14d, doses >120 mg not recommended
• *Child:* **PO** 0.25-0.5 mg/kg/dose q4-6h, max 1-2 mg/kg/day

Anal fissures (off-label)

• *Adult:* **TOP** 0.2% gel q12h × 21 days

Available forms: Caps 5, 10, 20 mg; tabs, ext rel 10, 20, 30, 60, 90 mg; tabs 10 mg, gel 0.2%

Side effects/adverse reactions:

CNS: Headache, fatigue, drowsiness, dizziness, anxiety, depression, weakness, insomnia, light-headedness, paresthesia, tinnitus, blurred vision, nervousness, tremor

CV: ***Dysrhythmias,*** edema, hypotension, palpitations, tachycardia

GI: Nausea, vomiting, diarrhea, gastric upset, constipation, increased LFTs, dry mouth, flatulence

GU: Nocturia, polyuria

INTEG: Rash, pruritus, flushing, hair loss

MISC: Sexual difficulties, cough, fever, chills

SYST: ***Stevens-Johnson syndrome***

Contraindications: Hypersensitivity

Precautions: CHF, hypotension, sick sinus syndrome, 2nd-, 3rd-degree heart block, hypotension less than 90 mm Hg systolic, hepatic injury, pregnancy (C), lactation, children, renal disease

Do not confuse:

NIFEdipine/niCARdipine

Pharmacokinetics:

Well-absorbed PO

PO-ER: Duration 24 hr

PO: Onset 20 min, peak 0.5-6 hr, duration 6-8 hr, half-life 2-5 hr

Metabolized by liver, excreted in urine 60-80%; feces 15%

Interactions:

• ↓ antihypertensive effect: NSAIDs

- ↑ toxicity risk: cimetidine, propranolol, cycloSPORINE, prazosin, carbamazepine, digoxin
- ↑ effects of theophylline, β-blockers, antihypertensives
- ↓ effects of quinidine
- Food/drug: ↑ NIFEdipine level: grapefruit juice

↑ effect: barberry, betel palm, burdock, goldenseal, khat, khella, lily of the valley, plantain

↓ effect: yohimbe

Lab test interferences:
Positive: ANA, direct Coombs' test

NURSING CONSIDERATIONS

Assess:
- Anginal pain: location, intensity, duration, character, alleviating, aggravating factors
- Cardiac status: B/P, pulse, respiration, ECG
- Potassium, renal/hepatic studies periodically during treatment

Administer:
- Without regard to meals
- SL: may puncture cap and squeeze drug into buccal pouch

Evaluate:
- Therapeutic response: decreased anginal pain, B/P, activity tolerance

Teach patient/family:
- To avoid hazardous activities until stabilized on drug, dizziness is no longer a problem
- To limit caffeine consumption; take no alcohol products
- To avoid OTC drugs unless directed by a prescriber
- That ext rel nonabsorbable shell may appear in stools
- To comply with all areas of medical regimen: diet, exercise, stress reduction, drug therapy
- To change position slowly; orthostatic hypotension is common

Not to break, crush, or chew ext rel tabs

To notify prescriber of dyspnea, edema of extremities, nausea, vomiting, severe ataxia, severe rash

Treatment of overdose: Defibrillation, atropine for AV block, vasopressor for hypotension

nilutamide
(nye-loo'ta-mide)
Anandron✦, Nilandron
Func. class.: Antineoplastic-hormone
Chem. class.: Antiandrogen

Action: Interferes with testosterone uptake in the nucleus or testosterone activity in target tissues; arrests tumor growth in androgen-sensitive tissue (e.g., prostate gland); prostatic carcinoma is androgen-sensitive, so tumor growth is arrested

Uses: Metastatic prostatic carcinoma, stage D2 in combination with surgical castration

Dosage and routes:
- *Adult:* **PO** 300 mg qd × 30 days, then 150 mg qd

Available forms: Tabs 100✦, 150 mg

Side effects/adverse reactions:
CNS: Hot flashes, drowsiness, insomnia, dizziness, hyperthesia, depression
GU: Decreased libido, impotence, testicular atrophy, UTI, hematuria, nocturia, gynecomastia
GI: Diarrhea, nausea, vomiting, increased liver function studies, constipation, dyspepsia, ***hepatotoxicity***
INTEG: Rash, sweating, alopecia, dry skin
RESP: Dyspnea, URI, pneumonia, ***interstitial pneumonitis***
HEMA: Anemia
EENT: Delay in adaptation to dark
MISC: Edema

Contraindications: Hypersensitiv-

ity, severe hepatic impairment, severe respiratory disease, women
Precautions: Pregnancy (C)
Pharmacokinetics: Rapidly and completely absorbed; excreted in urine and feces as metabolites
Interactions:
- ↑ toxicity of vit K, phenytoin, theophylline

NURSING CONSIDERATIONS
Assess:
- ⬥ Hepatic studies: AST, ALT, alk phosphatase, which may be elevated; if elevated 3× normal, discontinue drug
- For CNS symptoms: drowsiness, insomnia, dizziness
- Chest x-rays, routinely, baseline pulmonary function studies, dyspnea, cough, which may indicate interstitial pneumonitis; discontinue treatment if this condition is suspected
- For hyperglycemia, increased BUN, creatinine, alk phosphatase leukopenia

Administer:
- Without regard to meals

Perform/provide:
- Storage at room temperature

Evaluate:
- Therapeutic response: decrease in prostatic tumor size, decrease in spread of cancer

Teach patient/family:
- ⬥ To report side effects: decreased libido, impotence, breast enlargement, hot flashes, diarrhea, dyspnea, cough, shortness of breath; if SOB occurs notify prescriber immediately
- ⬥ To report signs of hepatotoxicity: dark urine, abdominal pain, clay-colored stools, jaundice eyes, skin
- To wear tinted lens to alleviate delay in adapting to the dark
- That drug is started on day of or day after surgical castration
- To avoid alcohol consumption

Treatment of overdose: Induce vomiting, provide supportive care

nisoldipine

(nye-sole'dih-peen)
Sular
Func. class.: Calcium channel blocker, antihypertensive
Chem. class.: Dihydropyridine

Action: Inhibits calcium ion influx across cell membrane, resulting in dilation of peripheral arteries
Uses: Essential hypertension, alone or with other antihypertensives
Dosage and routes:
- *Adult:* **PO** 20 mg qd initially, may increase by 10 mg/wk, usual dose 20-40 mg qd, max 60 mg/day
- *Geriatric/hepatic dose:* **PO** 10 mg/day, increase by 10 mg/wk

Available forms: Tabs, ext rel 10, 20, 30, 40 mg
Side effects/adverse reactions:
CV: Dysrhythmia, edema, CHF, hypotension, palpitations, ***MI, pulmonary edema,*** tachycardia, syncope, AV block, angina, chest pain, ECG abnormalities
GI: Nausea, vomiting, diarrhea, gastric upset, constipation, increased LFTs, dry mouth, dyspepsia, dysphagia, flatulence
GU: Nocturia, hematuria, dysuria
INTEG: Rash, pruritus
MISC: Sexual difficulties, cough, nasal congestion, SOB, wheezing, epistaxis, dyspnea, gingival hyperplasia, chills, fever, gout, sweating
CNS: Headache, fatigue, drowsiness, dizziness, anxiety, depression, nervousness, insomnia, lightheadedness, paresthesia, tinnitus, psychosis, somnolence, ataxia, confusion, malaise, migraine
HEMA: Anemia, leukopenia, petechia
Contraindications: Hypersensitiv-

N

ity, sick sinus syndrome, 2nd-, 3rd-degree heart block
Precautions: CHF, hypotension <90 mm Hg systolic, hepatic injury, pregnancy (C), lactation, children, renal disease, elderly
Pharmacokinetics: Metabolized by liver, excreted in urine, peak 6-12 hr, highly protein bound
Interactions:

- ↑ effects of β-blockers, antihypertensives, digitalis
- ↑ nisoldipine level: cimetidine, ranitidine, azole antifungals
- ↓ nisoldipine effect: hydantoins
- Drug/food: ↑ nisoldipine level: high-fat foods; increased hypotensive effect: grapefruit juice

↑ effect: barberry, betel palm, burdock, goldenseal, khat, khella, lily of the valley, plantain
↓ effect: yohimbe

NURSING CONSIDERATIONS
Assess:

- Cardiac status: B/P, pulse, respiration, ECG
- I&O ratios, weight qd
- For CHF: weight gain, jugular vein distention, edema, rales

Administer:

- Once daily as whole tablet; avoid high-fat foods, grapefruit juice

Evaluate:

- Therapeutic response: decreased B/P

Teach patient/family:

To swallow whole; not to break, crush, or chew
- To avoid hazardous activities until stabilized on drug, dizziness is no longer a problem
- To report nausea, dizziness, edema, shortness of breath, palpitations
- To limit caffeine consumption
- To avoid OTC drugs unless directed by a prescriber
- The importance of complying with all areas of medical regimen: diet, exercise, stress reduction, drug therapy
- To rise slowly to prevent orthostatic hypotension

Treatment of overdose: Defibrillation, atropine for AV block, vasopressor for hypotension

nitazoxanide (℞)

(nye-taz-ox'a-nide)
Alinia
Func. class.: Antiprotozoal

Action: Interferes with DNA/RNA synthesis in protozoa
Uses: Diarrhea caused by *Cryptosporidium parvum* or *Giardia lamblia*
Dosage and routes:

- *Child 4-11 yr:* **PO** 10 ml q12h × 3 days
- *Child 12-47 mos:* **PO** 5 ml q12h × 3 days

Available forms: Powder for oral susp 100 mg/5 ml
Side effects/adverse reactions:
CV: Hypotension
HEMA: Anemia, ***leukopenia,*** neutropenia
INTEG: Pruritus, sweating
GI: Nausea, anorexia, flatulence, increased appetite, enlarged salivary glands, abdominal pain, diarrhea, vomiting
CNS: Dizziness, fever, headache
MISC: Increased creatinine, pale yellow eye discoloration, rhinitis, discolored urine, infection, malaise
Contraindications: Hypersensitivity
Precautions: Renal, hepatic disease, pregnancy (B), lactation, child <1 yr or >11 yr
Pharmacokinetics: Excreted in urine, bile, feces; hydrolyzed to active metabolite, which undergoes conjugation; metabolite protein binding >99%

NURSING CONSIDERATIONS
Assess:
- Signs of infection
- Bowel pattern before, during treatment

Administer:

PO route
- With food

Evaluate:
- Therapeutic response: C&S negative for organism

Teach patient/family:
- To take with food; shake susp well before e ach dose

nitrofurantoin (℞)

(nye-troe-fyoor'an-toyn)
Apo-Nitrofurantoin✤, Furadantin, Macrobid, Macrodantin, nitrofurantoin
Func. class.: Urinary tract anti-infective
Chem. class.: Synthetic nitrofuran derivative

Action: Appears to inhibit bacterial enzymes
Uses: Urinary tract infections caused by *Escherichia coli, Klebsiella, Pseudomonas, Proteus vulgaris, Proteus morganii, Serratia, Citrobacter, Staphylococcus aureus, Staphylococcus epidermidis, Enterococcus, Salmonella, Shigella*
Dosage and routes:
Active infections
- *Adult and child >12 yr:* **PO** 50-100 mg qid pc or 50-100 mg hs for long-term treatment
- *Child 1 mo-3 yr:* **PO** 5-7 mg/kg/day in 4 divided doses; 1-3 mg/kg/day for long-term treatment

Chronic suppression
- *Adult:* **PO** 50-100 mg QPM
- *Child:* **PO** 1 mg/kg/day QPM

Available forms: Caps 25, 50, 100 mg; tabs 50, 100 mg; susp 25 mg/5 ml; ext rel caps 100 mg; macrocrystal caps (Macrodantin) 25, 50, 100 mg
Side effects/adverse reactions:
INTEG: Pruritus, rash, urticaria, angioedema, alopecia, tooth staining
CNS: Dizziness, headache, drowsiness, peripheral neuropathy, chills
GI: Nausea, vomiting, abdominal pain, diarrhea, ***cholestatic jaundice,*** loss of appetite, ***pseudomembranous colitis***
Contraindications: Hypersensitivity, anuria, severe renal disease, infants <1 mo
Precautions: Pregnancy (B), lactation, G-6-PD deficiency, elderly, CCr <40
Pharmacokinetics:
PO: Half-life 20-60 min; crosses blood-brain barrier, placenta; enters breast milk; excreted as inactive metabolites in liver, unchanged in urine
Interactions:
- ↑ levels of nitrofurantoin: probenecid
- Antagonistic effect: norfloxacin
- ↓ absorption of magnesium trisilicate antacid

NURSING CONSIDERATIONS
Assess:
- Blood count during chronic therapy
- I&O ratio; urine pH <5.5 is ideal; C&S before treatment, after completion; symptoms of UTI
- CNS symptoms: insomnia, vertigo, headache, drowsiness, convulsions
- Allergy: fever, flushing, rash, urticaria, pruritus

Administer:

PO route
- After clean-catch urine for C&S
- Two daily doses if urine output is high or if patient has diabetes

Evaluate:
- Therapeutic response: decreased dysuria, fever; neg C&S

Teach patient/family:

- To take with food or milk; avoid alcohol
- To protect susp from freezing and shake well before taking
- That drug may cause drowsiness; instruct client to seek aid in walking and other activities; advise client not to drive or operate machinery while on medication
- That diabetics should monitor blood glucose level

⊘ Not to crush tabs, open caps

- That drug may turn urine rust-yellow to brown

⬥ To notify prescriber of symptoms of pseudomembranous colitis: fever, diarrhea with mucous, pus, or blood

nitrofurazone topical

See appendix c

nitroglycerin (℞)

(nye-troe-gli'ser-in)

transmucosal tablets (℞)

Nitrogard, Nitrogard SR

sustained release (℞)

Nitrocot, Nitroglyn E-R, Nitropar, Nitro-Time, Nitrong

IV (℞)

Nitro-Bid I.V., Tridil

ointment (℞)

Nitro-Bid, Nitrol

SL (℞)

Nitrostat, NitroQuick

spray (℞)

Nitrolingual Translingual Spray

transdermal (℞)

Deponit, Minitran, Nitrek, Nitrocine, Nitrodisc, Nitro-Dur, Transderm-Nitro

translingual nitrolingual

Func. class.: Coronary vasodilator, antianginal

Chem. class.: Nitrate

Action: Decreases preload, afterload, which is responsible for decreasing left ventricular end-diastolic pressure, systemic vascular resistance; dilates coronary arteries, improves blood flow through coronary vasculature, dilates arterial, venous beds systemically

Uses: Chronic stable angina pectoris, prophylaxis of angina pain, CHF associated with acute MI, controlled hypotension in surgical procedures

Dosage and routes:

- *Adult:* **SL** dissolve tab under tongue when pain begins; may repeat q5min until relief occurs; take no more than 3 tabs/15 min; use 1 tab prophylactically 5-10 min before activities; **SUS CAP** q6-12h on empty stomach; **TOP** 1-2 in q8h, increase to 4 in q4h as needed; **IV** 5 mcg/min, then increase by 5 mcg/min q3-5min; if no response after 20 mcg/min, increase by 10-20 mcg/min until desired response; **TRANS** apply a pad qd to a site free of hair; remove patch hs to provide 10-12h nitrate-free interval to avoid tolerance

• *Child:* **IV** initial: 0.25-0.5 mcg/kg/min, titrate to patient response, usual dose 1-3 mcg/kg/min transmucosal

Available forms: Buccal tabs 1, 2, 3 mg; translingual aero 0.4 mg/metered spray; sus rel caps 2.5, 6.5, 9, 13 mg; tabs, sus rel 2.6, 6.5, 9 mg; SL tabs 0.3, 0.4, 0.6 mg; oint 2%; trans syst 0.1, 0.2, 0.3, 0.4, 0.6, 0.8 mg/hr; inj sol 25 mg/250 ml, 50 mg/250 ml, 100 mg/250 ml, 200 mg/500 ml, 100 mg/500 ml, 200 mg/500 ml

Side effects/adverse reactions:

CV: Postural hypotension, tachycardia, ***collapse,*** syncope, palpitations

GI: Nausea, vomiting

INTEG: Pallor, sweating, rash

CNS: Headache, flushing, dizziness

Contraindications: Hypersensitivity to this drug or nitrites, severe anemia, increased intracranial pressure, cerebral hemorrhage, closed angle glaucoma

Precautions: Postural hypotension, pregnancy (C), lactation, children, severe hepatic/renal disease

Do not confuse:

Nitro-Bid/Nicobid

Pharmacokinetics:

SUS REL: Onset 20-45 min, duration 3-8 hr

SL: Onset 1-3 min, duration 30 min

TRANSDERMAL: Onset ½-1 hr, duration 12-24 hr

IV: Onset 1-2 min, duration 3-5 min

TRANSMUC: Onset 1-2 min, duration 3-5 hr

AEROSOL: Onset 2 min, duration 30-60 min

TOP OINT: Onset 30-60 min, duration 2-12 hr

Metabolized by liver, excreted in urine, half-life 1-4 min

Interactions:

• ↑ effects of β-blockers, diuretics, antihypertensives, calcium channel blockers

• ↓ heparin: IV nitroglycerin

• ↑ hypotension: sildenafil

• Severe hypotension, CV collapse: alcohol

• ↑ nitrate level: aspirin

NURSING CONSIDERATIONS

Assess:

• Orthostatic B/P, pulse

• Pain: duration, time started, activity being performed, character

• Tolerance if taken over long period

• Headache, light-headedness, decreased B/P; may indicate a need for decreased dosage

Administer:

PO route

• With 8 oz H_2O on empty stomach (oral tablet) 1 hr before or 2 hr after meals

Transdermal route

• Transmucosal tab should be placed between cheek and gum line

• Topical ointment should be measured on papers supplied

• Apply a new TD patch qd and remove after 12-14 hr to prevent tolerance

IV route

• Diluted in amount specified D_5, D_5W, 0.9% NaCl for infusion; use glass infusion bottles, non–polyvinyl chloride infusion tubing; titrate to patient response; do not use filters

Additive compatibilities: Alteplase, aminophylline, DOBUTamine, DOPamine, enalaprilat, furosemide, lidocaine, verapamil

Y-site compatibilities: Amiodarone,

amphotericin B cholesteryl, amrinone, atracurium, cefmetazole, cisatracurium, diltiazem, DOBUTamine, DOPamine, epINEPHrine, esmolol, famotidine, fentanyl, fluconazole, furosemide, haloperidol, heparin, hydromorphone, insulin (regular), labetalol, lidocaine, lorazepam, midazolam, milrinone, morphine, niCARdipine, norepinephrine, pancuronium, propofol, ranitidine, remifentanil, sodium nitroprusside, streptokinase, tacrolimus, theophylline, thiopental, vecuronium, warfarin

Evaluate:

• Therapeutic response: decrease, prevention of anginal pain

Teach patient/family:

• To place buccal tab between lip and gum above incisors or between cheek and gum

⃠ That sus rel must be swallowed whole, not chewed, broken, crushed

• That SL should be dissolved under tongue, not swallowed

• That aerosol should be sprayed under tongue, not inhaled

• To keep tabs in original container

• If 3 SL tabs in 15 min do not relieve pain, to seek immediate medical attention

• To avoid alcohol

• That drug may cause headache; tolerance usually develops; use nonopioid analgesic

• That drug may be taken before stressful activity: exercise, sexual activity

• That SL may sting when drug comes in contact with mucous membranes

• To avoid hazardous activities if dizziness occurs

• To comply with complete medical regimen

• To make position changes slowly to prevent fainting

HIGH ALERT

nitroprusside (℞)

(nye-troe-pruss'ide)

Nitropress, sodium nitroprusside

Func. class.: Antihypertensive, vasodilator

Action: Directly relaxes arteriolar, venous smooth muscle, resulting in reduction in cardiac preload, afterload

Uses: Hypertensive crisis, to decrease bleeding by creating hypotension during surgery, acute CHF

Dosage and routes:

• *Adult:* **IV INF** dissolve 50 mg in 2-3 ml of D_5W, then dilute in 250-1000 ml of D_5W; run at 0.5-8 mcg/kg/min

• *Child:* **IV** 0.3-0.5 mcg/kg/min, titrate to response

Available forms: Inj 50 mg

Side effects/adverse reactions:

GI: Nausea, vomiting, abdominal pain

CNS: Dizziness, headache, agitation, twitching, decreased reflexes, restlessness

INTEG: Pain, irritation at inj site, sweating

CV: Bradycardia, ECG changes, tachycardia

MISC: ***Cyanide, thiocyanate toxicity,*** flushing, hypothyroidism

Contraindications: Hypersensitivity, hypertension (compensatory) due to aortic coarctation or AV shunting, acute CHF associated with reduced peripheral vascular resistance

Precautions: Pregnancy (C), lactation, children, fluid, electrolyte imbalances, hepatic disease, renal disease, hypothyroidism, elderly

Pharmacokinetics:

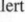

IV: Onset 1-2 min, duration 1-10 min, half-life 3 days in patients with

abnormal renal function, circulating half-life 2 min; metabolized in liver, excreted in urine

Interactions:

• Severe hypotension: ganglionic blockers, volatile liquid anesthetics, halothane, enflurane, circulatory depressants

↑ toxicity, death: aconite

↑ or ↓ antihypertensive effect: astragalus, cola tree

↑ antihypertensive effect: barberry, betony, black catechu, black cohosh, bloodroot, broom, burdock, cat's claw, dandelion, goldenseal, Irish moss, Jamaican dogwood, kelp, khella, mistletoe, parsley

↓ antihypertensive effect: coltsfoot, guarana, khat, licorice

NURSING CONSIDERATIONS

Assess:

• Electrolytes: K, Na, Cl, CO_2, CBC, serum glucose, serum methemoglobin if pulmonary O_2 levels are decreased

• Renal studies: catecholamines, BUN, creatinine

• Hepatic studies: AST, ALT, alk phosphatase

• B/P by direct means if possible; check ECG continuously; pulse, jugular vein distention; PCWP; rebound hypertension may occur after nitroprusside is discontinued

• Weight qd, I&O

Thiocyanate, lactate, cyanide levels if on long-term treatment, thiocyanate level should be ≤1 mmol/L

• Nausea, vomiting, diarrhea

• Edema in feet, legs daily; skin turgor, dryness of mucous membranes for hydration status

• Rales, dyspnea, orthopnea q30min

• For decrease in bicarbonate, Pco_2 blood pH, acidosis

Administer:

IV route

• Depending on B/P reading q15min

• IV after diluting 50 mg/2-3 ml of D_5W, further dilute in 250 ml of D_5W; use an infusion pump only; wrap bottle with aluminum foil to protect from light; observe for color change in the infusion; discard if highly discolored (blue, green, dark red); titrate to patient response

Syringe compatibilities: Heparin

Y-site compatibilities: Amrinone, atracurium, diltiazem, DOBUTamine, DOPamine, enalaprilat, famotidine, lidocaine, nitroglycerin, pancuronium, tacrolimus, theophylline, vecuronium

Evaluate:

• Therapeutic response: decreased B/P, absence of bleeding

Teach patient/family:

• To report headache, dizziness, loss of hearing, blurred vision, dyspnea, faintness, dizziness

Treatment of overdose: Administer amyl nitrate inhalation until 3% sodium nitrate solution can be prepared for IV administration, then inject sodium thiosulfate IV, correct drop in B/P with vasopressor

N

nizatidine (OTC, ℞)

(ni-za'ti-deen)

Axid, Axid AR

Func. class.: H_2-Receptor antagonist

Chem. class.: Substituted thiazole

Action: Blocks H_2-receptors, thereby reducing gastric acid output

Uses: Benign gastric and duodenal ulceration, prevention of duodenal ulcer recurrence, symptomatic relief of gastroesophageal reflux, heartburn prevention

Dosage and routes:

Renal dose

• *Adult:* **PO** CCr 20-50 ml/min give 150 mg/day; CCr <20 ml/min give 150 mg qod

Gastric and duodenal ulcer

• *Adult:* **PO** 300 mg at night or 150 mg bid for 4-8 wk; maintenance 150 mg at night

Prophylaxis of duodenal ulcer

• *Adult:* **PO** 150 mg qd hs

Gastroesophageal reflux

• *Adult:* **PO** 150 mg bid

Heartburn prevention

• *Adult:* **PO** 75 mg before eating

Available forms: Caps 150, 300 mg; tabs 75 mg

Side effects/adverse reactions:

CNS: Headache, somnolence, confusion, abnormal dreams, dizziness

ENDO: Gynecomastia

HEMA: ***Thrombocytopenia, agranulocytosis, aplastic anemia***

INTEG: Pruritus, sweating, urticaria, ***exfoliative dermatitis***

MS: Myalgia

RESP: ***Bronchospasm, laryngeal edema***

METAB: Hyperuricemia

GI: Elevated hepatic enzymes, ***hepatitis,*** jaundice, nausea

CV: ***Cardiac dysrhythmias, cardiac arrest***

Contraindications: Hypersensitivity

Precautions: Renal or hepatic impairment (reduce dose in renal impairment), pregnancy (B), lactation

Pharmacokinetics: Partially metabolized by liver, excreted by kidneys, plasma half-life 1½ hr, 70% absorbed orally, small amount (0.1% of plasma concentration) enters breast milk, 35% bound to plasma proteins

NURSING CONSIDERATIONS

Assess:

◆CBC with differential if on long-term therapy, agranulocytosis may occur

• Gastric pH (>5 should be maintained)

• Fluid balance, I&O

Administer:

PO route

• With meals for prolonged drug effect; antacids 1 hr before or 1 hr after drug

Evaluate:

• Mental status, confusion, dizziness, depression, anxiety, weakness, tremors, psychosis, diarrhea, jaundice, report immediately

• For GI symptoms: nausea, vomiting, diarrhea, cramps

Teach patient/family:

• That gynecomastia, impotence may occur, are reversible

• To avoid driving or other hazardous activities until patient is stabilized on this medication; dizziness may occur

• To avoid black pepper, caffeine, alcohol, harsh spices, extremes in temp of food

• To avoid OTC preparations: aspirin, cough, cold preparations

Treatment of overdose: Symptomatic and supportive therapy is recommended; activated charcoal, emesis or lavage may reduce absorption

---

HIGH ALERT

norepinephrine (℞)

(nor-ep-i-nef′rin)

Levophed

Func. class.: Adrenergic

Chem. class.: Catecholamine

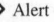

Action: Causes increased contractility and heart rate by acting on β-receptors in heart; also acts on α-receptors, causing vasoconstriction in blood vessels; B/P is elevated, coronary blood flow improves, cardiac output increases

Uses: Acute hypotension, shock

Dosage and routes:

• *Adult:* **IV INF** 8-12 mcg/min titrated to B/P

• *Child:* **IV INF** 0.05-0.1 mcg/kg/min titrated to B/P

Available forms: Inj 1 mg/ml

Side effects/adverse reactions:

CNS: Headache, anxiety, dizziness, insomnia, restlessness, tremor

CV: Palpitations, tachycardia, hypertension, ectopic beats, angina

GI: Nausea, vomiting

INTEG: Necrosis, tissue sloughing with extravasation, ***gangrene***

RESP: Dyspnea

GU: Decreased urine output

Contraindications: Hypersensitivity, ventricular fibrillation, tachydysrhythmias, pheochromocytoma

Precautions: Lactation, arterial embolism, peripheral vascular disease, hypertension, hyperthyroidism, elderly, heart disease, pregnancy (C)

Pharmacokinetics:

IV: Onset 1-2 min; metabolized in liver; excreted in urine (inactive metabolites); crosses placenta

Interactions:

• Severe hypertension: guanethidine

⬍ Do not use within 2 wk of MAOIs, antihistamines, ergots, methyldopa, oxytocics, tricyclic antidepressants, guanethidine, or hypertensive crisis may result

• Dysrhythmias: general anesthetics, bretylium

• ↓ norepinephrine action: α-blockers

• ↑ B/P: oxytocics

• ↑ pressor effect: tricyclics, MAOIs

• Incompatible with alkaline solutions: sodium, HCO_3^-

NURSING CONSIDERATIONS

Assess:

• I&O ratio; notify prescriber if output <30 ml/hr

• ECG during administration continuously; if B/P increases, drug is decreased

• B/P and pulse q2-3min after parenteral route

• CVP or PWP during infusion if possible

• For paresthesias and coldness of extremities; peripheral blood flow may decrease

• Injection site: tissue sloughing; administer phentolamine mixed with 0.9% NaCl

• Sulfite sensitivity, which may be life-threatening

Administer:

• Plasma expanders for hypovolemia

• IV after diluting with 500-1000 ml D_5W or D_5/0.9% NaCl; average dilution is 4 mg/1000 ml diluent (4 μg base/ml); give as infusion 2-3 ml/min; titrate to response

• Using 2-bottle setup so drug may be discontinued while IV is still running; use infusion pump

Additive compatibilities: Amikacin, calcium chloride, calcium gluconate, cimetidine, corticotropin, dimenhyDRINATE, DOBUTamine, heparin, hydrocortisone, magnesium sulfate, meropenem, methylPREDNISolone, multivitamins, netilmicin, potassium chloride, succinylcholine, verapamil, vit B/C

Syringe compatibilities: Heparin

Y-site compatibilities: Amiodarone, amrinone, cisatracurium, diltiazem, DOBUTamine, DOPamine, epINEPHrine, esmolol, famotidine, fentanyl, furosemide, haloperidol, heparin, hydrocortisone, hydromorphone, labetalol, lorazepam, meropenem, midazolam, milrinone, morphine, niCARdipine, nitroglycerin, potassium chloride, propofol, ranitidine, remifentanil, vecuronium, vit B/C

N

Perform/provide:
- Storage of reconstituted sol if refrigerated no longer than 24 hr
- Do not use discolored sol

Evaluate:
- Therapeutic response: increased B/P with stabilization

Teach patient/family:
- The reason for drug administration and to report dyspnea, dizziness, chest pain

Treatment of overdose: Administer fluids, electrolyte replacement

norethindrone (℞)

(nor-eth-in′drone)

Micronor, Nor-QD

Func. class.: Progestogen

Chem. class.: Progesterone derivative

Action: Inhibits secretion of pituitary gonadotropins, which prevents follicular maturation, ovulation; stimulates growth of mammary tissue; antineoplastic action against endometrial cancer

Uses: Uterine bleeding (abnormal), amenorrhea, endometriosis, contraception

Dosage and routes:
- *Adult:* **PO** 5-20 mg qd days 5-25 of menstrual cycle

Endometriosis
- *Adult:* **PO** 10 mg qd × 2 wk, then increased by 5 mg qd × 2 wk, up to 30 mg qd

Available forms: Tabs 5 mg

Side effects/adverse reactions:

CNS: Dizziness, headache, migraines, depression, fatigue

CV: Hypotension, ***thrombophlebitis,*** edema, ***thromboembolism, stroke, pulmonary embolism, MI***

GI: Nausea, vomiting, anorexia, cramps, increased weight, ***cholestatic jaundice***

EENT: Diplopia

GU: Amenorrhea, cervical erosion, breakthrough bleeding, dysmenorrhea, vaginal candidiasis, breast changes, (gynecomastia, testicular atrophy, impotence), endometriosis, ***spontaneous abortion***

INTEG: Rash, urticaria, acne, hirsutism, alopecia, oily skin, seborrhea, purpura, melasma

META: Hyperglycemia

Contraindications: Breast cancer, hypersensitivity, thromboembolic disorders, reproductive cancer, genital bleeding (abnormal, undiagnosed), pregnancy (X)

Precautions: Lactation, hypertension, asthma, blood dyscrasias, gallbladder disease, CHF, diabetes mellitus, bone disease, depression, migraine headache, convulsive disorders, hepatic disease, renal disease, family history of breast or reproductive tract cancer

Pharmacokinetics:

PO: Duration 24 hr, excreted in urine, feces, metabolized in liver

Interactions:

↓ contraception: St. John's wort

↑ stimulation: black/green tea, coffee, cola nut, guarana, yerba maté

Lab test interferences:

Increase: Alk phosphatase, nitrogen (urine), pregnanediol, amino acids, factors VII, VIII, IX, X

Decrease: GTT, HDL

NURSING CONSIDERATIONS

Assess:
- Weight qd: notify prescriber of weekly weight gain >5 lb
- B/P at beginning of treatment and periodically
- I&O ratio; be alert for decreasing urinary output, increasing edema
- Hepatic studies: ALT, AST, bilirubin, periodically during long-term therapy

• Edema, hypertension, cardiac symptoms, jaundice, thromboembolism
• Mental status: affect, mood, behavioral changes, depression
• Hypercalcemia

Administer:
• Titrated dose; use lowest effective dose
• In one dose in AM
• With food or milk to decrease GI symptoms

Perform/provide:
• Storage in dark area

Evaluate:
• Therapeutic response: decreased abnormal uterine bleeding, absence of amenorrhea

Teach patient/family:
• About cushingoid symptoms
• To report breast lumps, vaginal bleeding, amenorrhea, edema, jaundice, dark urine, clay-colored stools, dyspnea, headache, blurred vision, abdominal pain, numbness or stiffness in legs, chest pain; male to report impotence or gynecomastia
• To report suspected pregnancy immediately

norfloxacin (℞)

(nor-flox′-a-sin)

Noroxin

Func. class.: Urinary antiinfective

Chem. class.: Fluoroquinolone

Action: Interferes with conversion of intermediate DNA fragments into high-molecular-weight DNA in bacteria, inhibits DNA gyrase

Uses: Adult urinary tract infections (including complicated) caused by *Escherichia coli, Enterobacter cloacae, Proteus mirabilis, Klebsiella pneumoniae,* group D strep, indole-positive *Proteus, Citrobacter freundii, Staphylococcus aureus;* uncomplicated gonorrhea

Dosage and routes:

Renal dose
• *Adult:* **PO** CCr ≤30 ml/min 400 mg **PO** qd

Uncomplicated infections
• *Adult:* **PO** 400 mg bid × 3-10 days 1 hr before or 2 hr after meals

Complicated infections
• *Adult:* **PO** 400 mg bid × 10-21 days; 400 mg qd × 7-10 days in impaired renal function

Uncomplicated gonorrhea
• *Adult:* **PO** 800 mg as a single dose

Ocular infection
• *Adult and child:* **OPHTH** 1 gtt qid, may increase to 1 gtt q2h for severe infections

Prostatitis
• *Adult:* **PO** 400 mg bid × 4 wk

Available forms: Tabs 400 mg

Side effects/adverse reactions:
CNS: Headache, dizziness, fatigue, somnolence, depression, insomnia
GI: Nausea, constipation, increased ALT, AST, flatulence, heartburn, vomiting, diarrhea, dry mouth
INTEG: Rash
EENT: Visual disturbances

Contraindications: Hypersensitivity to quinolones

Precautions: Pregnancy (C), lactation, children, renal disease, seizure disorders

Pharmacokinetics: Peak 1 hr, half-life 3-4 hr; steady state 2 days; excreted in urine as active drug, metabolites

Interactions:
• ↓ norfloxacin effect: antacids, iron products, sucralfate; give 2 hr apart
• ↑ serum concentrations of: cycloSPORINE, probenecid
• Antagonizes effects of norfloxacin: nitrofurantoin, monitor closely
• ↑ anticoagulation: oral anticoagulants

N

- Possible ↑ levels, toxicity: theophylline, do not use together

Lab test interferences:
Increase: AST, ALT, BUN, creatinine, alk phosphatase

NURSING CONSIDERATIONS
Assess:
- Renal, hepatic studies: BUN, creatinine, AST, ALT
- I&O ratio; urine pH <5.5 is ideal
- CNS symptoms: insomnia, vertigo, headache, agitation, confusion
- Allergic reactions: fever, flushing, rash, urticaria, pruritus

Administer:
PO route
- After clean-catch urine for C&S
- Two daily doses if urine output is high or if patient has diabetes

Evaluate:
- Therapeutic response: decreased pain, frequency, urgency, C&S, absence of infection

Teach patient/family:
- That fluid intake must be 3 L/day to avoid crystallization in kidneys
- That if dizziness occurs, to walk, perform activities with assistance
- To complete full course of drug therapy, to take at same time of day
- To contact prescriber if adverse reaction occurs
- To take 1 hr before or 2 hr after meals; not to take antacids with or within 2 hr of this drug; to sip water or use hard candy for dry mouth

norfloxacin ophthalmic
See appendix c

norgestrel (℞)
(nor-jess'trel)
Ovrette
Func. class.: Progestogen
Chem. class.: Progesterone derivative

Action: Inhibits secretion of pituitary gonadotropins, which prevents follicular maturation, ovulation, stimulates growth of mammary tissue, antineoplastic action against endometrial cancer

Uses: Female contraception

Dosage and routes:
- *Adult:* **PO** 1 tab qd

Available forms: Tabs 0.075 mg

Side effects/adverse reactions:
CNS: Dizziness, headache, migraines, depression, fatigue
CV: Hypotension, ***thrombophlebitis,*** edema, ***thromboembolism, stroke, pulmonary embolism, myocardial infarction***
GI: *Nausea,* vomiting, anorexia, cramps, increased weight, ***cholestatic jaundice***
EENT: Diplopia
GU: Amenorrhea, cervical erosion, breakthrough bleeding, dysmenorrhea, vaginal candidiasis, breast changes, *gynecomastia, testicular atrophy, impotence,* endometriosis, ***spontaneous abortion***
INTEG: Rash, urticaria, acne, hirsutism, alopecia, oily skin, seborrhea, purpura, melasma
META: Hyperglycemia

Contraindications: Breast cancer, hypersensitivity, thromboembolic disorders, reproductive cancer, genital bleeding (abnormal, undiagnosed), cerebral hemorrhage, pregnancy (X)

Precautions: Lactation, hypertension, asthma, blood dyscrasias, gallbladder disease, CHF, diabetes mellitus, bone disease, depression, migraine headache, convulsive disorders, hepatic disease, renal disease, family history of breast or reproductive tract cancer

Pharmacokinetics:

PO: Duration 24 hr; excreted in urine, feces; metabolized in liver

Lab test interferences:

Increase: Alk phosphatase, nitrogen (urine), pregnanediol, amino acids, factors VII, VIII, IX, X

Decrease: GTT, HDL

NURSING CONSIDERATIONS

Assess:

• Weight qd; notify prescriber of weekly weight gain >5 lb

• B/P at beginning of treatment and periodically

• I&O ratio; be alert for decreasing urinary output, increasing edema

• Hepatic studies: ALT, AST, bilirubin, periodically during long-term therapy

• Edema, hypertension, cardiac symptoms, jaundice

• Mental status: affect, mood, behavioral changes, depression

• Hypercalcemia

Administer:

• Titrated dose; use lowest effective dose

• In one dose in AM

• With food or milk to decrease GI symptoms

• After warming to dissolve crystals

Perform/provide:

• Storage in dark area

Evaluate:

• Therapeutic response: absence of pregnancy

Teach patient/family:

• About cushingoid symptoms

• To report breast lumps, vaginal bleeding, edema, jaundice, dark urine, clay-colored stools, dyspnea, headache, blurred vision, abdominal pain, numbness or stiffness in legs, chest pain

• To report suspected pregnancy

• To monitor blood glucose if diabetic

nortriptyline (℞)

(nor-trip′ti-leen)

Aventyl, Pamelor

Func. class.: Antidepressant, tricyclic

Chem. class.: Dibenzocycloheptene—secondary amine

Action: Blocks reuptake of norepinephrine, serotonin into nerve endings, increasing action of norepinephrine, serotonin in nerve cells

Uses: Major depression

Investigational uses: Chronic pain management

Dosage and routes:

• *Adult:* **PO** 25 mg tid or qid; may increase to 150 mg/day; may give daily dose hs

• *Geriatric:* **PO** 10-25 mg q hs, increase by 10-25 mg at weekly intervals to desired dose; usual maintenance 75 mg

Available forms: Caps 10, 25, 50, 75 mg; sol 10 mg/5 ml

Side effects/adverse reactions:

HEMA: ***Agranulocytosis, thrombocytopenia, eosinophilia, leukopenia***

CNS: Dizziness, drowsiness, confusion, headache, anxiety, tremors, stimulation, weakness, insomnia, nightmares, EPS (elderly), increased psychiatric symptoms

GI: Constipation, dry mouth, nausea, vomiting, ***paralytic ileus,*** increased appetite, cramps, epigastric distress, jaundice, ***hepatitis,*** stomatitis

GU: Urinary retention, ***acute renal failure***

N

INTEG: Rash, urticaria, sweating, pruritus, photosensitivity
CV: Orthostatic hypotension, ECG changes, tachycardia, ***hypertension,*** palpitations
EENT: Blurred vision, tinnitus, mydriasis
Contraindications: Hypersensitivity to tricyclics, recovery phase of MI, convulsive disorders, prostatic hypertrophy
Precautions: Suicidal patients, severe depression, increased intraocular pressure, narrow-angle glaucoma, urinary retention, cardiac disease, hepatic disease, hyperthyroidism, electroshock therapy, elective surgery, pregnancy (C), lactation, children
Do not confuse:
nortriptyline/amitriptyline
Pharmacokinetics:
PO: Steady state 4-19 days; metabolized by liver; excreted by kidneys; crosses placenta; excreted in breast milk; half-life 18-28 hr
Interactions:
• ↓ effects of guanethidine, clonidine, indirect-acting sympathomimetics (epHEDrine)
• ↑ effects of direct-acting sympathomimetics (epINEPHrine), alcohol, barbiturates, benzodiazepines, CNS depressants
Hyperpyretic crisis, convulsions, hypertensive episode: MAOI
• Heavy smoking: ↓ drug effect
↑ anticholinergic effect: belladonna, corkwood, henbane, jimsonweed
↑ antidepressant action: scopolia
↑ CNS effect: hops, lavender
Serotonin syndrome: SAM-e, St. John's wort
Lab test interferences:
Increase: Serum bilirubin, blood glucose, alk phosphatase
False increase: Urinary catecholamines
Decrease: VMA, 5-HIAA

NURSING CONSIDERATIONS

Assess:
• B/P (lying, standing), pulse q4h; if systolic B/P drops 20 mm Hg, hold drug, notify prescriber; take vital signs q4h in patients with cardiovascular disease
• Blood studies: CBC, leukocytes, differential, cardiac enzymes if patient is receiving long-term therapy
• Hepatic studies: AST, ALT, bilirubin
• Weight qwk; appetite may increase with drug
• ECG for flattening of T wave, bundle branch block, AV block, dysrhythmias in cardiac patients
• EPS primarily in elderly: rigidity, dystonia, akathisia
• Mental status changes: mood, sensorium, affect, suicidal tendencies, increase in psychiatric symptoms, depression, panic
• Urinary retention, constipation; constipation is more likely to occur in children
Withdrawal symptoms: headache, nausea, vomiting, muscle pain, weakness; do not usually occur unless drug was discontinued abruptly
• Alcohol intake; if alcohol is consumed, hold dose until AM
Administer:
• Increased fluids, bulk in diet if constipation occurs
• With food, milk for GI symptoms
• Dosage hs for oversedation during day; may take entire dose hs; elderly may not tolerate once/day dosing
• Gum, hard candy, frequent sips of water for dry mouth
• Concentrate with fruit juice, water, or milk to disguise taste

Perform/provide:

- Storage in tight, light-resistant container at room temperature
- Assistance with ambulation during beginning therapy, since drowsiness/dizziness occurs
- Safety measures including side rails, primarily for elderly
- Checking to see if PO medication swallowed

Evaluate:

- Therapeutic response: decreased depression

Teach patient/family:

- That therapeutic effects may take 2-3 wk
- To use caution in driving, other activities requiring alertness because of drowsiness, dizziness, blurred vision
- To avoid alcohol ingestion, other CNS depressants
- Not to discontinue medication quickly after long-term use; may cause nausea, headache, malaise
- To wear sunscreen or large hat, since photosensitivity occurs
- To report immediately urinary retention

Treatment of overdose: ECG monitoring; induce emesis; lavage, activated charcoal; administer anticonvulsant

nystatin (℞)

(nye-stat'in)

Mycostatin, Nadostine✤, Nilstat, Nystex, PMS-Nystatin✤, Pastilles, nystatin

Func. class.: Antifungal

Chem. class.: Amphoteric polyene

Action: Interferes with fungal DNA replication; binds sterols in fungal cell membrane, which increases permeability, leaking of cell nutrients

Uses: *Candida* species causing oral, vaginal, intestinal infections

Dosage and routes:

Oral infection

- *Adult:* **SUSP** 400,000-600,000 units qid, use ½ dose in each side of mouth, swish and swallow

Infants: 200,000 units qid (100,000 units in each side of mouth)

- *Newborn and premature infant:* **SUSP** 100,000 units qid
- *Adult and child:* Troches 200,000-400,000 units qid × up to 2 wk

GI infection

- *Adult:* **PO** 500,000-1,000,000 units tid

Available forms: Tabs 500,000 units; powder 50 million, 150 million, 500 million, 1 billion, 2 billion, 5 billion units; susp 100,000 units per ml; troches 200,000 units

Side effects/adverse reactions:

INTEG: Rash, urticaria (rare)

GI: Nausea, vomiting, anorexia, diarrhea, cramps

Contraindications: Hypersensitivity

Precautions: Pregnancy (B)

Pharmacokinetics:

PO: Little absorption, excreted in feces

NURSING CONSIDERATIONS

Assess:

- For allergic reaction: rash, urticaria; drug may have to be discontinued
- For predisposing factors: antibiotic therapy, pregnancy, diabetes mellitus, sexual partner infection (vaginal infections)

Administer:

- Oral susp dose by placing ½ in each cheek, then swallow
- Topical dose after cleansing area; mouth may be swabbed

Perform/provide:

- Storage in refrigerator for oral susp; tabs in tight, light-resistant containers at room temperature

N

Evaluate:

- Therapeutic response: culture negative for *Candida*

Teach patient/family:

- That long-term therapy may be needed to clear infection; to complete entire course of medication
- Proper hygiene: changing socks if feet are infected; using no commercial mouthwashes for mouth infection
- Shake susp before measuring each dose
- To avoid getting preparation on hands
- To wear light-day pad for vaginal preparations
- To avoid tight shoes, bandages when using on feet
- To avoid sexual contact during treatment to minimize reinfection
- To notify prescriber of irritation; drug may have to be discontinued
- That relief from itching may occur after 24-72 hr

nystatin topical

See appendix c

nystatin vaginal antifungal

See appendix c

octreotide (℞)

(ok-tree'oh-tide)

Sandostatin, Sandostatin LAR Depot

Func. class.: Hormone, antidiarrheal

Chem. class.: Octapeptide

Action: A potent growth hormone similar to somatostatin

Uses: Sandostatin: acromegaly, carcinoid tumors, vasoactive intestinal peptide tumors (VIPomas); LAR Depot: long-term maintenance of acromegaly, carcinoid tumors, VIPomas

Investigational uses: GI fistula, variceal bleeding, diarrheal conditions, pancreatic fistula, irritable bowel syndrome, dumping syndrome

Dosage and routes:

Acromegaly

- *Adult:* **SC/IV** 50-100 mcg tid, adjust q2wk based on growth hormone levels (Sandostatin), or **IM** 20 mg q4wk × 3 mo, adjust by growth hormone levels (Sandostatin LAR)

VIPomas

- *Adult:* **SC/IV** 0.2-0.3 mg qd in 2-4 doses for 2 wk, not to exceed 0.45 mg qd (Sandostatin), or **IM** 20 mg q2wk × 2 mo, adjust dose (Sandostatin LAR)

Carcinoid tumors

- *Adult:* **SC/IV** 0.1-0.6 mg qd in 2-4 doses for 2 wk, titrated to patient response (Sandostatin), or **IM** 20 mg q4wk × 2 mo, adjust dose (Sandostatin LAR)

GI fistula

- *Adult:* **SC** 50-200 mcg q8h

Antidiarrheal in AIDS patients

- *Adult:* **SC/IV** 100-1800 mcg/day

Irritable bowel syndrome

- *Adult:* **SC** 100 mcg single dose to 125 mcg bid

Dumping syndrome
• *Adult:* **SC** 50-150 mcg/day
Variceal bleeding
• *Adult:* **IV** 25-50 mcg/hr CONT **IV** INF for 18 hr-5 days
Available forms: Sandostatin: inj 0.05, 0.1, 0.2, 0.5, 1 mg/ml; LAR depot: inj 10, 20, 30 mg/5 ml
Side effects/adverse reactions:
CNS: Headache, dizziness, fatigue, weakness, depression, anxiety, tremors, ***seizure,*** paranoia
CV: Sinus bradycardia, conduction abnormalities, ***dysrhythmias,*** chest pain, SOB, thrombophlebitis, ischemia, ***CHF,*** hypertension, palpitations
ENDO: Hyperglycemia, ketosis, hypothyroidism, hypoglycemia, galactorrhea, diabetes insipidus
GI: Diarrhea, nausea, abdominal pain, vomiting, flatulence, distention, constipation, ***hepatitis,*** increased LFTs, ***GI bleeding, pancreatitis***
GU: UTI, pollakiuria
HEMA: Hematoma of inj site, bruise
INTEG: Rash, urticaria, pain; inflammation at inj site
MS: Joint and muscle pain
Contraindications: Hypersensitivity
Precautions: Diabetes mellitus, hypothyroidism, pregnancy (B), elderly, lactation, children, renal disease
Pharmacokinetics: Absorbed rapidly, completely, peak ½ hr, half-life 1.7 hr, duration 12 hr, excreted unchanged in urine
Interactions:
• CycloSPORINE: Possible ↑ rejection
• Drug/food: ↓ absorption of dietary fat, decreased vit B_{12} levels
NURSING CONSIDERATIONS
Assess:
• Growth hormone antibodies, IGF-1, 1-4 hr intervals for 8-12 hr post dose in acromegaly; 5-HIAA, plasma serotonin, plasma substance P in carcinoid; VIP in VIPomas
• Thyroid function tests: T_3, T_4, T_7, TSH to identify hypothyroidism
• Fecal fat, serum carotene
• Allergic reaction: rash, itching, fever, nausea, wheezing
• For cardiac status: bradycardia, conduction abnormalities, dysrhythmias; monitor ECG for QT prolongation, low voltage, axis shifts, early repolarization, R/S transition, early wave progression
Administer:
SC route
• Rotate inj site, use hip, thigh, abdomen
• Avoid using medication that is cold; allow to reach room temperature
IM route
• Reconstitute with diluent provided; give into gluteal
IV route
• May use IV bolus if required; give over 3 min
• To use by intermittent infusion, dilute in 50-200 ml D_5W, 0.9% NaCl; give 15-30 min
Perform/provide:
• Storage in refrigerator for unopened amps, vials; or room temperature for 2 wk, protect from light; do not use discolored or cloudy sol
Evaluate:
• Therapeutic response: relief of diarrhea in AIDS, suppression of tumor growth in carcinoid or VIP tumors, decreasing symptoms of acromegaly
Teach patient/family:
• Regular assessments are required
• Regarding SC inj if patient or other persons will be giving inj
• To change position slowly to prevent orthostatic hypotension

ofloxacin (℞)

(o-flox'a-sin)

Floxin

Func. class.: Antiinfective

Chem. class.: Fluoroquinolone

Action: Interferes with conversion of intermediate DNA fragments into high-molecular-weight DNA in bacteria, inhibits DNA gyrase

Uses: Treatment of lower respiratory tract infections (pneumonia, bronchitis), genitourinary infections (prostatitis, UTIs) caused by *Escherichia coli, Klebsiella pneumoniae, Chlamydia trachomatis, Neisseria gonorrhoeae;* skin and skin structure infections; conjunctivitis (ophthalmic) (refer to Appendix C)

Dosage and routes:

Renal dose

- *Adult:* **PO** CCr 10-50 ml/min give q24h; CCr <10 ml/min give ½ of dose q24h

Lower respiratory tract infections/ skin and skin structure infections

- *Adult:* **PO, IV** 400 mg q12h × 10 days

Cervicitis, urethritis

- *Adult:* **PO, IV** 300 mg q12h × 7 days

Prostatitis

- *Adult:* **PO, IV** 300 mg q12h × 6 wk

Acute, uncomplicated gonorrhea

- *Adult:* **PO, IV** 400 mg as a single dose

Urinary tract infection

- *Adult:* **PO, IV** 200-400 mg q12h × 3-10 days

Available forms: Tabs 200, 300, 400 mg; inj 20, 40 mg/ml

Side effects/adverse reactions:

CNS: Dizziness, headache, fatigue, somnolence, depression, insomnia, lethargy, malaise, ***seizures***

GI: Diarrhea, nausea, vomiting, anorexia, flatulence, heartburn, dry mouth, increased AST, ALT, abdominal pain, constipation, ***pseudomembranous colitis***

INTEG: Rash, pruritus

EENT: Visual disturbances

SYST: ***Anaphylaxis, Stevens-Johnson syndrome***

Contraindications: Hypersensitivity to quinolones

Precautions: Pregnancy (C), lactation, children, elderly, renal disease, seizure disorders, excessive sunlight

Pharmacokinetics:

PO: Peak 1-2 hr, half-life 9 hr, steady state 2 days; excreted in urine as active drug, metabolites; 90%-95% bioavailability

Interactions:

- ↓ absorption: antacids with aluminum, magnesium, iron products, sucralfate, zinc products; separate by 2 hr
- May alter blood glucose levels: antidiabetics
- ↑ CNS stimulation, seizures: NSAIDs
- ↑ anticoagulation: oral anticoagulants
- Possible theophylline toxicity: theophylline, do not use together
- Drug/food: ↓ absorption

↑ effect: cola nut

NURSING CONSIDERATIONS

Assess:

- Renal, hepatic studies: BUN, creatinine, AST, ALT
- I&O ratio; urine pH <5.5 is ideal
- CNS symptoms: insomnia, vertigo, headache, agitation, confusion
- Allergic reactions: rash, flushing, urticaria, pruritus

Administer:

PO route

- 2 hr before or 2 hr after antacids, calcium, iron, zinc products
- After clean-catch urine for C&S

IV route

• Dilute to 4 mg/ml with 0.9% NaCl, D_5W, D_5/LR, $D_5/0.9\%$ NaCl, 5% $NaCO_3$, D_5 plasmalyte 56, sodium lactate; give over 1 hr or more

Additive compatibilities: Ceftazidime, clindamycin, gentamicin, piperacillin, tobramycin, vancomycin

Syringe compatibilities: Cefotaxime

Y-site compatibilities: Ampicillin, cisatracurium, docetaxel, etoposide, gemcitabine, granisetron, linezolid, propofol, remifentanil, thiotepa

Perform/provide:

• Storage for 2 wk refrigerated or 6 mo frozen after reconstitution

Evaluate:

• Therapeutic response: urine culture, absence of symptoms of infection

Teach patient/family:

• That fluid intake must be 3 L/day to avoid crystallization in kidneys
• That if dizziness or lightheadedness occurs, ambulate, perform activities with assistance
• To complete full course of therapy
• To notify prescriber of adverse reactions or tendon pain
• To avoid iron- or mineral-containing supplements within 2 hr before or after dose
• To prevent sun exposure, photosensitivity can occur

olanzapine

(oh-lanz'a-peen)

Zyprexa, Zyprexa, Zydis

Func. class.: Antipsychotic, neuroleptic

Chem. class.: Thienbenzodiazepine

Action: Unknown; may mediate antipsychotic activity by both dopamine and serotonin type 2 (5-HT2) antagonist; also, may antagonize muscarinic receptors, histaminic (H_1)- and α-adrenergic receptors

Uses: Schizophrenia, acute manic episodes in bipolar disorder

Investigational uses: Dementia related to Alzheimer's disease

Research note: One case of writer's cramp has been attributed to olanzapine use[29]

Dosage and routes:

Schizophrenia

• *Adult:* **PO** 5-10 mg initially qd, may increase dosage by 5 mg at 1 wk or more intervals; orally disintegrating tabs: open blister pack, place tab on tongue, let disintegrate, swallow
• *Elderly:* **PO** 5 mg, may increase cautiously at 1 wk intervals

Bipolar mania

• *Adult:* **PO** 10-15 mg qd, may increase dose >24 hr, by 5 mg

Available forms: Tab 2.5, 5, 7.5, 10, 15 mg; orally disintegrating tabs 5, 10, 15, 20 mg

Side effects/adverse reactions:

GI: Dry mouth, nausea, vomiting, anorexia, constipation, abdominal pain, weight gain

GU: Urinary retention, urinary frequency, enuresis, impotence, amenorrhea, gynecomastia, breast engorgement, premenstrual syndrome

INTEG: Rash

CNS: EPS: pseudoparkinsonism, akathisia, dystonia, tardive dyskinesia, seizures, headache, ***neuroleptic malignant syndrome (rare),*** somnolence, agitation, nervousness, hostility, dizziness, hypertonia, tremor, euphoria

MS: Joint pain, twitching

Contraindications: Hypersensitivity

O

Precautions: Pregnancy (C), lactation, hypertension, hepatic disease, cardiac disease, elderly

Pharmacokinetics: Well absorbed, peak 6 hr, metabolized by liver, excreted in urine, 93% bound to plasma proteins

Interactions:

• Oversedation: other CNS depressants, alcohol, barbiturate anesthetics, antihistamines, sedatives/hypnotics, antidepressants

• ↓ olanzapine levels: carbamazepine, omeprazole, rifampin

• ↑ hypotension: antihypertensives, alcohol, diazepam

• ↓ antiparkinson activity: levodopa, bromocriptine, other DOPamine agonists

• ↑ anticholinergic effects: anticholinergics

↑ EPS: betel palm, kava

↑ effect: cola tree, hops, nettle, nutmeg

Lab test interferences:

Increase: LFTs, prolactin, CPK

NURSING CONSIDERATIONS

Assess:

• Mental status: orientation, mood, behavior, presence of hallucinations and type before initial administration and monthly

• Swallowing of PO medication: check for hoarding or giving of medication to other patients

• I&O ratio; palpate bladder if low urinary output occurs, urinary retention may be the cause especially in elderly

• Bilirubin, CBC

• Urinalysis recommended before, during prolonged therapy

• Affect, orientation, LOC, reflexes, gait, coordination, sleep pattern disturbances

• B/P sitting, standing, lying: take pulse and respirations q4h during initial treatment; establish baseline before starting treatment; report drops of 30 mm Hg; obtain baseline ECG

• Dizziness, faintness, palpitations, tachycardia on rising

For neuroleptic malignant syndrome: hyperpyrexia, muscle rigidity, increased CPK, altered mental status, for acute dystonia (check chewing, swallowing, eyes, pill rolling)

• EPS, including akathisia (inability to sit still, no pattern to movements), tardive dyskinesia (bizarre movements of the jaw, mouth, tongue, extremities), pseudoparkinsonism (rigidity, tremors, pill rolling, shuffling gait)

• Skin turgor daily

• Constipation, urinary retention daily; increase bulk, H_2O in diet

Administer:

• Antiparkinsonian agent for EPS

• Decreased dose in elderly

• PO with full glass of water, milk; or with food to decrease GI upset

• Orally disintegrating tabs: open blister pack, place tab on tongue until dissolved, swallow; no water needed

Perform/provide:

• Decreased stimuli by dimming light, avoiding loud noises

• Supervised ambulation until stabilized on medication; do not involve in strenuous exercise program because fainting is possible; patient should not stand still for long periods

• Increased fluids, bulk in diet to prevent constipation

• Sips of water, candy, gum for dry mouth

• Storage in tight, light-resistant container

Evaluate:

• Therapeutic response: decrease in emotional excitement, hallucinations, delusion, paranoia, reorganization of patterns of thought, speech

Teach patient/family:

- To use good oral hygiene; frequent rinsing of mouth, sugarless gum, candy, ice chips for dry mouth
- To avoid hazardous activities until drug response is determined
- That orthostatic hypotension occurs often and to rise from sitting or lying position gradually
- To avoid hot tubs, hot showers, tub baths, since hypotension may occur
- To avoid abrupt withdrawal of this drug, or EPS may result; drug should be withdrawn slowly
- To avoid OTC preparations (cough, hay fever, cold) unless approved by prescriber, since serious drug interactions may occur; avoid use with alcohol, CNS depressants; increased drowsiness may occur
- That in hot weather, heat stroke may occur; take extra precautions to stay cool

Treatment of overdose: Lavage if orally ingested; provide airway; do not induce vomiting or use epINEPHrine

olmesartan medoxomil (℞)

(ol-meh-sar'tan)

Benicar

Func. class.: Antihypertensive

Chem. class.: Angiotensin II receptor (type AT_1) antagonist

Action: Blocks the vasoconstrictor and aldosterone-secreting effects of angiotensin II; selectively blocks the binding of angiotensin II to the AT_1 receptor found in tissues

Uses: Hypertension, alone or in combination with other antihypertensives

Dosage and routes:

- *Adult:* **PO,** single agent 20 mg qd initially in patients who are not volume depleted, may be increased to 40 mg qd if needed after 2 wk

Available forms: Tabs 5, 20, 40 mg

Side effects/adverse reactions:

CNS: Dizziness, fatigue, headache, insomnia

GI: Diarrhea, abdominal pain

MS: Arthralgia, pain

RESP: Upper respiratory infection, bronchitis

SYST: ***Angioedema***

CV: Chest pain, peripheral edema, tachycardia

EENT: Sinusitis, rhinitis, pharyngitis

Contraindications: Hypersensitivity, pregnancy (D) 2nd/3rd trimesters

Precautions: Hypersensitivity to ACE inhibitors; pregnancy (C) 1st trimester, lactation; children; elderly; hepatic disease

Pharmacokinetics: Excreted in urine and feces

Interactions:

↑ toxicity, death: aconite

↑ or ↓ antihypertensive effect: astragalus, cola tree

↑ antihypertensive effect: barberry, betony, black catechu, black cohosh, bloodroot, broom, burdock, cat's claw, dandelion, goldenseal, Irish moss, Jamaican dogwood, kelp, khella, mistletoe, parsley

↓ antihypertensive effect: coltsfoot, guarana, khat, licorice

NURSING CONSIDERATIONS

Assess:

- For pregnancy, this drug can cause fetal death when given in pregnancy
- Response and adverse reactions especially in renal disease
- B/P, pulse q4h; note rate, rhythm, quality; electrolytes: K, Na, Cl; baselines in renal, hepatic studies before therapy begins

• Skin turgor, dryness of mucous membranes for hydration status; for angioedema: facial swelling, dyspnea

Administer:

• Without regard to meals

Evaluate:

• Therapeutic response: decreased B/P

Teach patient/family:

• To comply with dosage schedule, even if feeling better

• To notify prescriber of mouth sores, fever, swelling of hands or feet, irregular heartbeat, chest pain

• That excessive perspiration, dehydration, vomiting, diarrhea may lead to fall in blood pressure; to consult prescriber if these occur

• That drug may cause dizziness, fainting; light-headedness may occur

• To rise slowly to sitting or standing position to minimize orthostatic hypotension

• To notify prescriber immediately if pregnant; not to use during lactation

• To avoid all OTC medications, unless approved by prescriber

• To inform all health-care providers of medication use

• To use proper technique for obtaining B/P and acceptable parameters

olopatadine ophthalmic

See appendix c

olsalazine (℞)

(ohl-sal′ah-zeen)

Dipentum ♣

Func. class.: Antiinflammatory

Chem. class.: Salicylate derivative

Action: Bioconverted to 5-aminosalicylic acid, which decreases inflammation

Uses: Maintenance of remission of ulcerative colitis in patients intolerant to sulfasalazine

Dosage and routes:

• *Adult:* **PO** 500 mg bid

Available forms: Caps 250 mg

Side effects/adverse reactions:

GI: Nausea, vomiting, abdominal pain, ***hepatitis,*** diarrhea, bloating

CNS: Headache, hallucinations, depression, vertigo, fatigue, dizziness

HEMA: ***Leukopenia, neutropenia, thrombocytopenia, agranulocytosis, anemia***

INTEG: Rash, dermatitis, urticaria

Contraindications: Hypersensitivity to salicylates

Precautions: Pregnancy (C), child <14 yr, lactation; impaired hepatic, renal function; severe allergy; bronchial asthma

Pharmacokinetics:

PO: Partially absorbed, peak 1½ hr, half-life 5-10 hr, excreted in urine as 5-aminosalicylic acid and metabolites, crosses placenta

Lab test interferences:

False positive: Urinary glucose test

NURSING CONSIDERATIONS

Assess:

◆ Blood dyscrasias: skin rash, fever, sore throat, bruising, bleeding, fatigue, joint pain (rare)

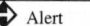

• Allergic reaction: rash, dermatitis, urticaria, pruritus, dyspnea, bronchospasm

Administer:
- Medication after C&S; repeat C&S after full course of medication
- Total daily dose evenly spaced to minimize GI intolerance, with food

Perform/provide:
- Storage in tight, light-resistant container at room temperature

Evaluate:
- Therapeutic response: absence of fever, mucus in stools

omeprazole (℞)

(oh-mep′ray-zole)

Losec♣, Prilosec

Func. class.: Antiulcer, proton pump inhibitor

Chem. class.: Benzimidazole

Action: Suppresses gastric secretion by inhibiting hydrogen/potassium ATPase enzyme system in gastric parietal cell; characterized as gastric acid pump inhibitor, since it blocks final step of acid production

Uses: Gastroesophageal reflux disease (GERD), severe erosive esophagitis, poorly responsive systemic GERD, pathologic hypersecretory conditions (Zollinger-Ellison syndrome, systemic mastocytosis, multiple endocrine adenomas); treatment of active duodenal ulcers with or without antiinfectives for *Helicobacter pylori*

Investigational uses: Posterior laryngitis, enhancing pancreatin

Dosage and routes:

Active duodenal ulcers
- *Adult:* **PO** 20 mg qd × 4-8 wk; associated with *H. pylori* 40 mg q AM and clarithromycin 500 mg tid on day 1-14, then 20 mg qd on day 15-28

Severe erosive esophagitis/poorly responsive GERD
- *Adult:* **PO** 20 mg qd × 4-8 wk

Pathologic hypersecretory conditions
- *Adult:* **PO** 60 mg/day; may increase to 120 mg tid; daily doses >80 mg should be divided

Gastric ulcer
- *Adult:* **PO** 40 mg qd 4-8 wk
- *Elderly:* ≤20 mg/day

Laryngitis (unlabeled)
- *Adult:* **PO** 20-40 mg qhs × 6-24 wk or 20 mg bid × 4-12 wk

Available forms: Caps, delayed rel 10, 20, 40 mg

Side effects/adverse reactions:

CNS: Headache, dizziness, asthenia

GI: Diarrhea, abdominal pain, vomiting, nausea, constipation, flatulence, acid regurgitation, abdominal swelling, anorexia, irritable colon, esophageal candidiasis, dry mouth

RESP: Upper respiratory infections, cough, epistaxis

INTEG: Rash, dry skin, urticaria, pruritus, alopecia

META: Hypoglycemia, increased hepatic enzymes, weight gain

EENT: Tinnitus, taste perversion

CV: Chest pain, angina, tachycardia, bradycardia, palpitations, peripheral edema

GU: UTI, urinary frequency, increased creatinine, ***proteinuria, hematuria,*** testicular pain, glycosuria

HEMA: ***Pancytopenia, thrombocytopenia, neutropenia, leukocytosis,*** anemia

MISC: Back pain, fever, fatigue, malaise

Contraindications: Hypersensitivity

Precautions: Pregnancy (C), lactation, children

Do not confuse:

Prilosec/Prinivil

Prilosec/Prozac

Prilosec/predniSONE

Pharmacokinetics: Peak ½-3½ hr, half-life ½-1 hr, protein binding

95%, eliminated in urine as metabolites and in feces; in elderly elimination rate decreased, bioavailability increased; metabolized by CYP450 enzyme system
Interactions:
• ↑ serum levels of: diazepam, phenytoin, flurazepam, triazolam, cycloSPORINE, disulfiram
• Possible ↑ bleeding: warfarin
• Delayed absorption of: ampicillin, iron salts, digoxin, ketoconazole, cyanocobalamin

NURSING CONSIDERATIONS
Assess:
• GI system: bowel sounds q8h, abdomen for pain, swelling, anorexia
• Hepatic enzymes: AST, ALT, alk phosphatase during treatment
Administer:
⊘ Before eating; swallow capsule whole; do not break, crush, or chew
Evaluate:
• Therapeutic response: absence of epigastric pain, swelling, fullness
Teach patient/family:
• To report severe diarrhea; drug may have to be discontinued
• That diabetic patient should know hypoglycemia may occur
• To avoid hazardous activities; dizziness may occur
• To avoid alcohol, salicylates, ibuprofen; may cause GI irritation

ondansetron (℞)
(on-dan-seh'tron)
Zofran
Func. class.: Antiemetic
Chem. class.: 5-HT_3 receptor antagonist

Action: Prevents nausea, vomiting by blocking serotonin peripherally, centrally, and in the small intestine
Uses: Prevention of nausea, vomiting associated with cancer chemotherapy, radiotherapy, and prevention of postoperative nausea, vomiting
Investigational uses: Bulimia; pruritus (rectal use)
Dosage and routes:
Hepatic dose
• *Adult:* **PO/IM/IV** Max dose 8 mg qd
Prevention of nausea/vomiting of cancer chemotherapy
• *Adult and child 4-18 yr:* **IV** 0.15 mg/kg infused over 15 min, 30 min before start of cancer chemotherapy; 0.15 mg/kg given 4 hr and 8 hr after first dose or 32 mg as a single dose; dilute in 50 ml of D_5 or 0.9% NaCl before giving; rectal use (off-label) 16 mg qd 2 hr prior to chemotherapy
• *Adult:* **IV** 0.15 mg/kg 15-30 min prior to chemotherapy, repeat 4, 8 hr later or 32 mg single dose ½ hr prior to chemotherapy; **PO** 8 mg ½ hr prior to chemotherapy, repeat 8 hr later
• *Child 4-18 yr:* **IV** 0.15 mg/kg ½ hr prior to chemotherapy, repeat 4, 8 hr later
Prevention of nausea/vomiting of radiotherapy
• *Adult:* **PO** 8 mg tid, may repeat q8hr
Prevention of postoperative nausea/vomiting
• *Adult:* **IV/IM** 4 mg undiluted over >30 sec prior to induction of anesthesia
• *Child 2-12 yr:* **IV** 0.1 mg/kg (≤40 kg); **IV** 4 mg (≥40 kg) give ≥30 sec
Bulimia (unlabeled)
• *Adult:* **PO** 4 mg tid (base dose); prn during bingeing/purging
Pruritus (unlabeled)
• *Adult:* **PO** 4 mg bid
Available forms: Inj 2 mg/ml, 32 mg/50 ml (premixed); tabs 4, 8 mg; oral sol 4 mg/5 ml; oral disintegrating tabs 4, 8 mg

Side effects/adverse reactions:
GI: Diarrhea, constipation, abdominal pain
CNS: Headache, dizziness, drowsiness, fatigue, EPS
MISC: Rash, ***bronchospasm*** (rare), *musculoskeletal pain, wound problems, shivering, fever, hypoxia, urinary retention*
Contraindications: Hypersensitivity
Precautions: Pregnancy (B), lactation, children, elderly
Do not confuse:
Zofran/Zantac
Pharmacokinetics:
IV: Mean elimination half-life 3.5-4.7 hr, plasma protein binding 70%-76%; extensively metabolized in the liver

NURSING CONSIDERATIONS

Assess:
- For absence of nausea, vomiting during chemotherapy
- Hypersensitivity reaction: rash, bronchospasm
- For EPS: shuffling gait, tremors, grimacing, rigidity

Administer:
IV route
- After diluting a single dose in 50 ml NS or D_5W, 0.45% NaCl or NS; give over 15 min

Additive compatibilities: Cisplatin, cyclophosphamide, cytarabine, dacarbazine, dexamethasone, DOXOrubicin, etoposide, fluconazole, hydromorphone, meperidine, methotrexate, morphine
Solution compatibilities: May also be diluted with D_5W, lactated Ringer's, D_5/0.9% NaCl, D_5/0.45% NaCl
Y-site compatibilities: Aldesleukin, amifostine, amikacin, aztreonam, bleomycin, carboplatin, carmustine, cefazolin, cefmetazole, cefotaxime, cefoxitin, ceftazidime, ceftizoxime, cefuroxime, chlorproMAZINE, cimetidine, cisatracurium, cisplatin, cladribine, clindamycin, cyclophosphamide, cytarabine, dacarbazine, dactinomycin, DAUNOrubicin, dexamethasone, diphenhydrAMINE, DOPamine, DOXOrubicin, DOXOrubicin liposome, doxycycline, droperidol, etoposide, famotidine, filgrastim, floxuridine, fluconazole, fludarabine, gallium, gentamicin, haloperidol, heparin, hydrocortisone, hydromorphone, hydrOXYzine, ifosfamide, imipenem/cilastatin, magnesium sulfate, mannitol, mechlorethamine, melphalan, meperidine, mesna, methotrexate, metoclopramide, miconazole, mitomycin, mitoxantrone, morphine, paclitaxel, pentostatin, piperacillin/tazobactam, potassium chloride, prochlorperazine, promethazine, ranitidine, remifentanil, streptozocin, teniposide, thiotepa, ticarcillin, ticarcillin/clavulanate, vancomycin, vinBLAStine, vinCRIStine, vinorelbine, zidovudine
Perform/provide:
- Storage at room temperature 48 hr after dilution

Evaluate:
- Therapeutic response: absence of nausea, vomiting during cancer chemotherapy

Teach patient/family:
- To report diarrhea, constipation, rash, or changes in respirations or discomfort at insertion site

oral contraceptives (℞)

Func. class.: Hormone
Chem. class.: Estrogen, progestin combinations

Action: Prevents ovulation by suppressing FSH, LH; *monophasic:* estrogen/progestin (fixed dose) used during a 21-day cycle; ovulation is inhibited by suppression of FSH and LH; thickness of cervical mucus and endometrial lining prevents pregnancy; *biphasic:* ovulation is inhibited by suppression of FSH and LH; alteration of cervical mucus, endometrial lining prevents pregnancy; *triphasic:* ovulation is inhibited by suppression of FSH and LH; change of cervical mucus, endometrial lining prevents pregnancy; variable doses of estrogen/progestin combinations may be similar to natural hormonal fluctuations; *progestin-only pill and implant:* change of cervical mucus and endometrial lining prevents pregnancy; ovulation may be suppressed

Uses: To prevent pregnancy, endometriosis, hypermenorrhea

Dosage and routes:

- *Adult:* **PO** 1 qd starting on day 5 of menstrual cycle; day 1 is 1st day of period

21 tablet packs

- *Adult:* **PO** 1 qd starting on day 7 of menstrual cycle; day 1 is 1st day of period, then on 20 or 21 days, off 7 days

28 tablet packs

- *Adult:* **PO** 1 qd continuously

Biphasic

- *Adult:* 1 qd × 10 days, then next color 1 qd × 11 days

Triphasic

- *Adult:* 1 qd; check package insert

Implant

- *Adult:* Subdermal 6 cap implanted during 1st wk of menses

Endometriosis

- *Adult:* **PO** 1 qd × 20 days from day 5 to 24 of cycle

Available forms: Check specific brand

Side effects/adverse reactions:

GI: Nausea, vomiting, cramps, diarrhea, bloating, constipation, change in appetite, ***cholestatic jaundice***

INTEG: Chloasma, melasma, acne, rash, urticaria, erythema, pruritus, hirsutism, alopecia, photosensitivity

CV: Increased B/P, ***cerebral hemorrhage, thrombosis, pulmonary embolism,*** fluid retention, edema

ENDO: Decreased glucose tolerance, increased TBG, PBI, T_4, T_3

GU: Breakthrough bleeding, amenorrhea, spotting, dysmenorrhea, galactorrhea, endocervical hyperplasia, vaginitis, cystitis-like syndrome, breast change

CNS: Depression, fatigue, dizziness, nervousness, anxiety, headache

EENT: Optic neuritis, retinal thrombosis, cataracts

HEMA: Increased fibrinogen, clotting factor

Contraindications: Pregnancy (X), lactation, reproductive cancer, thrombophlebitis, MI, hepatic tumors, hepatic disease, CAD, women 40 and over, CVA

Precautions: Depression, hypertension, renal disease, seizure disorders, lupus erythematosus, rheumatic disease, migraine headache, amenorrhea, irregular menses, breast cancer (fibrocystic), gallbladder disease, diabetes mellitus, heavy smoking, acute mononucleosis, sickle cell disease

Pharmacokinetics: Excreted in breast milk

Interactions:

- ↓ oral contraceptives effectiveness: anticonvulsants, rifampin, analgesics, antibiotics, antihistamines, griseofulvin
- ↓ oral anticoagulants action
- Drug/food: ↑ peak level: grapefruit juice

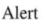

↓ oral contraceptives effect: saw palmetto, St. John's wort

Altered action: alfalfa, black cohosh, chaste tree

Lab test interferences:
Increase: PT; clotting factors VII, VIII, IX, X; TBG, PBI, T_4, platelet aggregability, BSP, triglycerides, bilirubin, AST, ALT
Decrease: T_3, antithrombin III, folate, metyrapone test, GTT, 17-OHCS

NURSING CONSIDERATIONS
Assess:
• Glucose, thyroid function, LFTs
• Reproductive changes: change in breasts, tumors, positive Pap smear; drug should be discontinued
Administer:
• PO with food for GI symptoms; give at same time each day
• Subdermal implant of 6 caps effective for 5 yr; then should be removed
• IM inj deep in large muscle mass after shaking suspension; ensure patient not pregnant if inj are 2 wk or more apart
Evaluate:
• Therapeutic response: absence of pregnancy, endometriosis, hypermenorrhea
Teach patient/family:
• About detection of clots using Homan's sign
• To use sunscreen or avoid sunlight; photosensitivity can occur
• To take at same time each day to ensure equal drug level
• To report GI symptoms that occur after 4 mo
• To use another birth control method during 1st week of oral contraceptive use
• To take another tablet as soon as possible if one is missed
• That after drug is discontinued, pregnancy may not occur for several months
• To report abdominal pain, change in vision, shortness of breath, change in menstrual flow, spotting, breakthrough bleeding, breast lumps, swelling, headache, severe leg pain
• That continuing medical care is needed: Pap smear and gynecologic examinations q6mo
• To notify health care providers and dentists of oral contraceptive

orlistat (℞)

(or'lih-stat)
Xenical
Func. class.: Weight control agent
Chem. class.: Lipase inhibitor

Action: Inhibits the absorption of dietary fats
Uses: Obesity management
Dosage and routes:
• *Adult:* **PO** 120 mg tid with each main meal containing fat
Available forms: Caps 120 mg
Side effects/adverse reactions:
MS: Back pain, arthritis, myalgia, tendinitis
CNS: Insomnia, depression, anxiety, dizziness, headache, fatigue
GI: Oily spotting, flatus with discharge, fecal urgency, fatty/oily stool, oily evacuation, fecal incontinence, nausea, vomiting, abdominal pain, infectious diarrhea, rectal pain, tooth disorder
GU: UTI, vaginitis, menstrual irregularity
RESP: Influenza, URI, LRI, EENT symptoms
INTEG: Dry skin, rash
Contraindications: Hypersensitivity, malabsorption syndrome, cholestasis, lactation
Precautions: Hypothyroidism, other organic causes of obesity, children, pregnancy (B)
Pharmacokinetics: Minimal absorption, peak 8 hr, 99% protein binding, excretion in feces, half-life 1-2 hr

Interactions:
• ↓ absorption: fat-soluble vitamins, cycloSPORINE
• ↑ lipid-lowering effect: pravastatin

NURSING CONSIDERATIONS
Assess:
• Weight weekly, diabetic patients may need reduction in oral hypoglycemics
• For misuse in certain population (anorexia nervosa, bulimia)

Administer:
• For obesity only if patient is on weight-reduction program that includes dietary changes, exercise; patient should be on a diet with 30% of calories from fat, omit dose of orlistat if a meal contains no fat

Evaluate:
• Therapeutic response: decrease in weight

Teach patient/family:
• Safety and effectiveness beyond 2 yr have not been determined
• By instructing patient to read patient's information sheet, discuss unpleasant GI side effects
• To take a multivitamin containing fat-soluble vitamins 2 hr before or after orlistat; phyllium taken with each dose or at bedtime may decrease GI symptoms
• To avoid hazardous activities until stabilized on medication, discuss unpleasant side effects
• To notify prescriber if pregnancy is planned or suspected

oseltamivir (℞)

(oss-el-tam'ih-veer)
Tamiflu
Func. class.: Antiviral
Chem. class.: Neuramidase inhibitor

Action: Inhibits influenza virus neuraminidase with possible alteration of virus particle aggregation and release

Uses: Prevention/treatment of influenza type A

Dosage and routes:
Treatment
• *Adult/child >40 kg:* **PO** 75 mg bid × 5 days, begin treatment within 2 days of onset of symptoms
• *Child 23-40 kg and ≥1 yr:* **PO** 60 mg bid
• *Child 15-23 kg and ≥1 yr:* **PO** 45 mg bid
• *Child ≤15 kg/≥1 yr:* **PO** 30 mg bid
• *Adult renal dose:* **PO** CCr <30 ml/min 75 mg qd × 5 days

Prevention
• *Adult/child ≥13 yr:* **PO** 75 mg qd × ≥7 days
• *Adult/child ≥13 yr renal dose:* **PO** CCr 10-30 ml/min 75 mg qod

Available forms: Caps 75 mg; powder for oral susp 12 mg/ml after reconstitution

Side effects/adverse reactions:
CNS: Headache, dizziness, fatigue, *insomnia*
GI: Nausea, vomiting, diarrhea, abdominal pain
RESP: Cough

Contraindications: Hypersensitivity

Precautions: Hepatic disease, renal disease, elderly, pregnancy (C)

Pharmacokinetics: Rapidly absorbed, protein binding low, converted to oseltamivir carboxylate, half-life 1-3 hr

NURSING CONSIDERATIONS
Assess:
• Bowel pattern before, during treatment
• Signs of infection; fever, fatigue, sore throat, headache, muscle soreness, aches

Administer:
• Within 2 days of symptoms of influenza; continue for 5 days

• At least 4 hr before hs to prevent insomnia

Perform/provide:
• Storage in tight, dry container

Evaluate:
• Therapeutic response: absence of fever, malaise, cough, dyspnea in infection

Teach patient/family:
• About aspects of drug therapy
• To avoid hazardous activities if dizziness occurs
• To take missed dose as soon as remembered within 2 hr of next dose

oxacillin (℞)

(ox-a-sill'in)

Bactocill, oxacillin sodium

Func. class.: Broad-spectrum antiinfective

Chem. class.: Penicillinase-resistant penicillin

Action: Interferes with cell wall replication of susceptible organisms; osmotically unstable cell wall swells, bursts from osmotic pressure

Uses: Effective for gram-positive cocci *(Staphylococcus aureus, Streptococcus pneumoniae),* infections caused by penicillinase-producing *Staphylococcus*

Dosage and routes:
• *Adult:* **PO** 2-6 g/day in divided doses q4-6h; **IM/IV** 2-12 g/day in divided doses q4-6h
• *Child:* **PO** 50-100 mg/kg/day in divided doses q6h; **IM/IV** 50-100 mg/kg/day in divided doses q4-6h

Available forms: Caps 250, 500 mg; powder for oral susp 250 mg/5 ml; powder for inj 250, 500 mg, 1, 2, 4, 10 g

Side effects/adverse reactions:
SYST: ***Anaphylaxis, serum sickness***
HEMA: Anemia, increased bleeding time, ***bone marrow depression, granulocytopenia***
GI: Nausea, vomiting, diarrhea, increased AST, ALT, abdominal pain, glossitis, colitis, ***pseudomembranous colitis***
GU: ***Oliguria, proteinuria, hematuria,*** *vaginitis, moniliasis,* ***glomerulonephritis***
CNS: Lethargy, hallucinations, anxiety, depression, twitching, ***coma, seizures***

Contraindications: Hypersensitivity to penicillins

Precautions: Pregnancy (B), hypersensitivity to cephalosporins, neonates

Do not confuse:
Bactocil/Pathocil

Pharmacokinetics:
PO/IM: Peak 30-60 min, duration 4-6 hr
IV: Peak 5 min, duration 4-6 hr, half-life 30-60 min
Metabolized in the liver; excreted in urine, bile, breast milk; crosses placenta

Interactions:
• ↓ oxacillin antimicrobial effectiveness: tetracyclines, rifampin, erythromycins, chloramphenicol, cholestyramine, colestipol
• ↓ oral contraceptives effect
• ↑ oxacillin concentrations: aspirin, probenecid, disulfiram
↓ absorption: khat, separate by ≥2 hr
Do not use acidophilus with antiinfectives

Lab test interferences:
False positive: Urine glucose, urine protein

NURSING CONSIDERATIONS

Assess:
• I&O ratio; report hematuria, oliguria, since penicillin in high doses is nephrotoxic
Any patient with compromised renal system, since drug is excreted slowly in poor renal system function; toxicity may occur rapidly

• Hepatic studies: AST, ALT
• Blood studies: WBC, RBC, Hct/Hgb, bleeding time
• Renal studies: urinalysis, protein
• C&S before therapy; drug may be given as soon as culture is taken
• Bowel pattern before and during treatment
• Skin eruptions after administration of penicillin to 1 wk after discontinuing drug
• Respiratory status: rate, character, wheezing, tightness in chest
• Allergies before initiation of treatment, and reaction of each medication

Administer:
• Drug after C&S completed
• PO with full glass of water 1 hr before or 2 hr after meals
• IM inj deep in gluteal muscle

IV route
• After diluting 500 mg or less/5 ml sterile H_2O or NaCl for inj; may dilute further in D_5W, NS, LR and give 1 g over 10 min; may be given as infusion over 6 hr

Additive compatibilities: Cephapirin, chloramphenicol, DOPamine, potassium chloride, sodium bicarbonate

Y-site compatibilities: Acyclovir, cyclophosphamide, diltiazem, famotidine, fluconazole, foscarnet, heparin, hydrocortisone, hydromorphone, labetalol, magnesium sulfate, meperidine, methotrexate, morphine, perphenazine, potassium chloride, tacrolimus, vit B/C, zidovudine

Perform/provide:
• Adrenalin, suction, tracheostomy set, endotracheal intubation equipment
• Scratch test to assess allergy, after securing order from prescriber; usually done when penicillin is only drug of choice
• Storage in airtight container; refrigerate reconstituted sol up to 2 wk

Evaluate:
• Therapeutic response: absence of fever, draining wounds

Teach patient/family:
• All aspects of drug therapy, including need to complete course of medication to ensure organism death (10-14 days); culture may be taken after completed course
• To report sore throat, fever, fatigue (may indicate superinfection); persistent diarrhea
• To wear or carry emergency ID if allergic to penicillins
• To take on empty stomach with a full glass of water

Treatment of anaphylaxis: Withdraw drug, maintain airway, administer epINEPHrine, aminophylline, O_2, IV corticosteroids

oxaliplatin (℞)
(ox-al-i′plat-in)
Eloxitan

Func. class.: Antineoplastic
Chem. class.: Platinum coordination complex

Action: Forms crosslinks, inhibiting DNA replication and transcription, cell-cycle nonspecific

Uses: Metastatic carcinoma of the colon or rectum in combination with 5-FU/leucovorin

Dosage and routes:
Dosage protocols may vary
• *Adult:* **IV INF** *Day 1:* oxaliplatin 85 mg/m^2 in 250-500 ml D_5W and leucovorin 200 mg/m^2 in D_5W, give both over 2 hr at the same time in separate bags using a Y-line, followed by 5-FU 400 mg/m^2 **IV BOL** over 2-4 min, then 5-FU 600 mg/m^2 **IV INF** in 500 ml D_5W as a 22-hr

CONT INF; *Day 2:* leucovorin 200 mg/m^2 **IV INF** over 2 hr, then 5-FU 400 mg/m^2 **IV BOL** over 2-4 min, then 5-FU 600 mg/m^2 **IV INF** in 500 D_5W as a 22-hr **CONT INF;** repeat cycle q2wk

Available forms: Powder for inj 50, 100 mg single-use vials

Side effects/adverse reactions:
EENT: Decreased visual acuity, tinnitus, hearing loss
HEMA: ***Thrombocytopenia, leukopenia, pancytopenia, neutropenia, anemia, hemolytic uremic syndrome***
CV: Cardiac abnormalities
GI: Severe nausea, vomiting, diarrhea, weight loss, stomatitis, anorexia, gastroesophageal reflux, constipation, dyspepsia, mucositis, flatulence
GU: Hematuria, dysuria, creatinine
INTEG: Alopecia, rash, flushing, extravasation, redness, swelling, pain at inj site
CNS: Peripheral neuropathy, fatigue, headache, dizziness, insomnia
RESP: ***Fibrosis,*** dyspnea, cough, rhinitis, URI, pharyngitis
META: Hypokalemia
SYST: ***Anaphylaxis, angioedema***

Contraindications: Hypersensitivity to this drug or other platinum products, radiation therapy or chemotherapy within 1 mo, thrombocytopenia, smallpox vaccination, pregnancy (D)

Precautions: Pneumococcus vaccination, lactation, children, elderly

Pharmacokinetics: Metabolized in liver, excreted in urine; after administration, 15% of platinum is in systemic circulation, 85% is either in tissues or being eliminated in urine

Interactions:
- Risk of bleeding: aspirin, NSAIDs, alcohol
- ↓ antibody response: live virus vaccines
- ↑ myelosuppression: myelosuppressive agents, radiation
- ↑ nephrotoxicity: aminoglycosides, loop diuretics

NURSING CONSIDERATIONS

Assess:

For bone marrow depression
- CBC, differential, platelet count weekly; withhold drug if WBC is <4000 or platelet count is <100,000; notify prescriber of results
- Renal studies: BUN, creatinine, serum uric acid, urine CCr before, electrolytes during therapy; dose should not be given if BUN <25 mg/dl; creatinine <1.5 mg/dl; I&O ratio; report fall in urine output of <30 ml/hr
- For anaphylaxis: wheezing, tachycardia, facial swelling, fainting; discontinue drug and report to prescriber; resuscitation equipment should be nearby
- Monitor temp q4h (may indicate beginning infection)
- Hepatic studies before, during therapy (bilirubin, AST, ALT, LDH) as needed or monthly
- Bleeding: hematuria, guaiac, bruising or petechiae, mucosa or orifices q8h; obtain prescription for viscous lidocaine (Xylocaine)
- Effects of alopecia on body image; discuss feelings about body changes
- Jaundice of skin, sclera; dark urine; clay-colored stools; itchy skin; abdominal pain; fever; diarrhea
- Edema in feet, joint pain, stomach pain, shaking

Administer:

IV route
- Do not reconstitute or dilute with sodium chloride or any chloride-containing solutions
- Do not use aluminum equipment during any preparation or adminis-

tration, will degrade platinum; do not refrigerate unopened powder or solution
• Prepare in biologic cabinet using gown, gloves, mask, do not allow drug to come in contact with skin, use soap and water if contact occurs
• Hydrate patient with 0.9% NaCl over 8-12 hr before treatment
• EpINEPHrine, antihistamines, corticosteroids for hypersensitivity reaction
• Antiemetic 30-60 min before giving drug and prn
• Allopurinol to maintain uric acid levels, alkalinization of urine
• Diuretic (furosemide 40 mg IV) or mannitol after infusion

Perform/provide:
• Comprehensive oral hygiene
• All medications PO, if possible, avoid IM inj when platelets <100,000/mm^3
• Increase fluid intake to 2-3 L/day to prevent urate deposits, calculi formation; elimination of drug

Evaluate:
• Therapeutic response: decreased tumor size, spread of malignancy

Teach patient/family:
• To report signs of infection: increased temp, sore throat, flulike symptoms
• To report signs of anemia: fatigue, headache, faintness, shortness of breath, irritability
• To report bleeding: avoid use of razors, commercial mouthwash
• To avoid aspirin, ibuprofen, NSAIDs, alcohol; may cause GI bleeding
• To report any complaints or side effects to nurse or prescriber
• To report any changes in breathing, coughing
• That hair may be lost during treatment; a wig or hairpiece may make patient feel better; new hair may be different in color, texture
• To report numbness, tingling in face or extremities, poor hearing or joint pain, swelling
• Not to receive vaccines during treatment
• To use contraception during treatment and 4 mo after; this drug may cause infertility

oxaprozin (℞)

(ox-a-proe′zin)
Daypro
Func. class.: Nonsteroidal antiinflammatory, antirheumatics
Chem. class.: Propionic acid derivative

Action: May inhibit prostaglandin synthesis by decreasing enzyme needed for biosynthesis; analgesic, antiinflammatory

Uses: Acute and long-term management of osteoarthritis, rheumatoid arthritis

Dosage and routes:
• *Adult:* **PO** 600-1200 mg qd; maximum dose 1800 mg/day or 26 mg/kg, whichever is lower

Available forms: Tabs 600 mg

Side effects/adverse reactions:
MISC: ***Anaphylaxis, angioneurotic edema***
GI: Nausea, anorexia, vomiting, diarrhea, jaundice, ***cholestatic hepatitis,*** constipation, flatulence, cramps, dry mouth, peptic ulcer, ***GI bleeding***
CNS: Dizziness, headache, drowsiness, fatigue, tremors, confusion, insomnia, anxiety, depression
CV: Tachycardia, peripheral edema, palpitations, dysrhythmias
INTEG: Purpura, rash, pruritus, sweating
GU: ***Nephrotoxicity: dysuria, hematuria, oliguria, azotemia***
HEMA: ***Increased bleeding time***

EENT: Tinnitus, hearing loss, blurred vision

Contraindications: Hypersensitivity, asthma, patients in whom aspirin and iodides have induced symptoms of allergic reactions or asthma

Precautions: Pregnancy (C), avoid in late pregnancy, lactation, children, bleeding disorders, GI disorders, cardiac disorders, hypersensitivity to other antiinflammatory agents, severe renal and hepatic disease, elderly, CHF

Do not confuse:

Daypro/Diupres

Pharmacokinetics:

PO: Onset 1 wk, peak unknown, duration unknown, half-life 40-50 hr; metabolized in liver; excreted in urine (metabolites), breast milk; 99% plasma protein binding

Interactions:

• ↑ toxicity: aspirin, cycloSPORINE, methotrexate

• ↑ bleeding risk: oral anticoagulants, thrombolytics, cefamandole, cefotetan, cefoperazone, clopidogrel, eptifibatide, plicamycin, ticlopidine, tirofiban

• ↑ levels of phenytoin, lithium, avoid concomitant use

• ↓ effect: antihypertensives, diuretics

• ↑ GI side effects: aspirin, corticosteroids, NSAIDs, alcohol, potassium supplements

↑ bleeding risk: anise, arnica, chamomile, clove, dong quai, fenugreek, feverfew, garlic, ginger, ginkgo, ginseng *(Panax)*, licorice

↑ gastric irritation: arginine, gossypol

NSAIDs effect: bearberry, bilberry

↑ bleeding risk: bogbean, chondroitin

NURSING CONSIDERATIONS

Assess:

• Pain: frequency, intensity, characteristics; relief of pain after med

Asthma, aspirin hypersensitivity, oronasal polyps; increased hypersensitivity reactions

• Renal, hepatic, blood studies: BUN, creatinine, AST, ALT, Hgb, before treatment, periodically thereafter

• Audiometric, ophthalmic exam before, during, after treatment

• For eye, ear problems: blurred vision, tinnitus; may indicate toxicity

Administer:

• With food, antacids to decrease GI symptoms

Perform/provide:

• Storage at room temperature

Evaluate:

• Therapeutic response: decreased pain, stiffness in joints, decreased swelling in joints, ability to move more easily

Teach patient/family:

To report blurred vision, ringing, roaring in ears; may indicate toxicity

• To avoid driving, other hazardous activities if dizziness/drowsiness occurs

To report change in urine pattern, increased weight, edema, increased pain in joints, fever, blood in urine; indicates nephrotoxicity

• That therapeutic effects may take up to 1 mo

• To take with a full glass of water to enhance absorption, sit upright for ½ hr after dose

oxazepam (℞)

(ox-ay′ze-pam)

Apo-Oxazepam♣, Novoxapam♣, oxazepam, Serax

Func. class.: Sedative/hypnotic; antianxiety

Chem. class.: Benzodiazepine

Controlled Substance Schedule IV

Action: Potentiates the actions of GABA, especially in limbic system and reticular formation

Uses: Anxiety, alcohol withdrawal

Dosage and routes:

Anxiety

• *Adult:* **PO** 10-30 mg tid-qid

Alcohol withdrawal

• *Adult:* **PO** 15-30 mg tid-qid

Available forms: Caps 10, 15, 30 mg; tabs 10, 15, 30 mg

Side effects/adverse reactions:

CNS: Dizziness, drowsiness, confusion, headache, anxiety, tremors, fatigue, depression, insomnia, hallucinations, paradoxical excitement, transient amnesia

GI: Nausea, vomiting, anorexia

INTEG: Rash, dermatitis, itching

CV: Orthostatic hypotension, ***ECG changes, tachycardia,*** hypotension

EENT: Blurred vision, tinnitus, mydriasis

HEMA: Leukopenia

Contraindications: Hypersensitivity to benzodiazepines, narrow-angle glaucoma, psychosis, pregnancy (D), lactation, child <12 yr

Precautions: Elderly, debilitated, hepatic disease, renal disease

Pharmacokinetics:

PO: Peak 2-4 hr, metabolized by liver, excreted by kidneys, half-life 5-15 hr

Interactions:

• ↓ oxazepam effects: oral contraceptives, valproic acid

• ↑ oxazepam effects: CNS depressants, alcohol, disulfiram, oral contraceptives

↑ CNS depression: catnip, chamomile, clary, cowslip, hops, kava, lavender, mistletoe, nettle, pokeweed, poppy, Queen Anne's lace, senega, skullcap, valerian

↑ hypotension: black cohosh

Lab test interferences:

Increase: AST, ALT, serum bilirubin

Decrease: RAIU

False increase: 17-OHCS

NURSING CONSIDERATIONS

Assess:

• B/P (lying, standing), pulse; if systolic B/P drops 20 mm Hg, hold drug, notify prescriber

• Blood studies: CBC during long-term therapy; blood dyscrasias have occurred rarely

• Hepatic studies: AST, ALT, bilirubin, creatinine, LDH, alk phosphatase if taking long term

• Mental status: mood, sensorium, affect, sleeping pattern, drowsiness, dizziness

Physical dependency, withdrawal symptoms: headache, nausea, vomiting, muscle pain, weakness, tremors, convulsions (long-term use)

• Suicidal tendencies

Administer:

PO route

• With food, milk for GI symptoms

• Sugarless gum, hard candy, frequent sips of water for dry mouth

Perform/provide:

• Assistance with ambulation during beginning therapy; drowsiness/dizziness occurs

• Safety measures, including side rails

• Check to see if PO medication has been swallowed

Evaluate:

• Therapeutic response: decreased anxiety, restlessness, insomnia

Teach patient/family:

- That drug may be taken with food
- That medication is not to be used for everyday stress or used longer than 4 mo unless directed by prescriber; not to take more than prescribed dose; may be habit forming
- To avoid OTC preparations (cough, cold, hay fever) unless approved by prescriber
- To avoid driving, activities that require alertness, since drowsiness may occur
- To avoid alcohol ingestion, other psychotropic medications unless directed by prescriber
- Not to discontinue medication abruptly after long-term use
- To rise slowly, or fainting may occur, especially elderly
- That drowsiness may worsen at beginning of treatment

Treatment of overdose: Lavage, VS, supportive care, flumazenil

oxcarbazepine (℞)

(ox′kar-baz′uh-peen)

Trileptal

Func. class.: Anticonvulsant

Action: May inhibit nerve impulses by limiting influx of sodium ions across cell membrane in motor cortex

Uses: Partial seizures

Investigational uses: Trigeminal neuralgia, atypical panic disorder

Dosage and routes:

Seizures, adjunctive therapy

- *Adult:* **PO** 300 mg bid, may be increased to 600 mg/day in divided doses bid; maintenance 1200 mg/day
- *Child 4-16 yr:* **PO** 8-10 mg/kg/day divided bid, max 600 mg/day; dose is determined by weight

Conversion to monotherapy in partial seizures

- *Adult:* **PO** 300 mg bid with reduction in other anticonvulsants, increase oxcarbazepine to max 600 mg/day q1wk over 2-4 wk; withdraw other anticonvulsants over 3-6 wk

Initiation of monotherapy in partial seizures

- *Adult:* **PO** 300 mg bid, increase by 300 mg/day q3days to 1200 mg divided bid

Renal dose

- *Adult:* **PO** CCr <30 ml/min 150 mg bid and increase slowly

Available forms: Tabs, film-coated, 150, 300, 600 mg

Side effects/adverse reactions:

CNS: Headache, dizziness, confusion, fatigue, feeling abnormal, ataxia, abnormal gait, tremors, anxiety, agitation, ***worsening of seizures***

CV: Hypotension, chest pain, edema

EENT: Blurred vision, diplopia, nystagmus, rhinitis, sinusitis

GI: Nausea, constipation, diarrhea, anorexia, vomiting, abdominal pain, gastritis, dry mouth, thirst, ***rectal hemorrhage***

GU: Frequency, UTI, vaginitis

INTEG: Purpura, rash, acne

Contraindications: Hypersensitivity

Precautions: Hypersensitivity to carbamazepine, pregnancy (C), lactation, child <4 yr, renal disease, fluid restriction

Pharmacokinetics:

PO: Onset unknown, peak unknown, metabolized by liver to active metabolite; terminal half-life 9 hr metabolite

Interactions:

- ↓ oxcarbazepine levels: phenobarbital, phenytoin, valproic acid, verapamil
- ↑ CNS depression: alcohol

• ↓ effects: felodipine, oral contraceptive, carbamazepine

↓ anticonvulsant effect: ginseng, santonica

↑ anticonvulsant effect: ginkgo

NURSING CONSIDERATIONS

Assess:

• Description of seizures: frequency, duration, aura

• Mental status: mood, sensorium, affect, behavioral changes; if mental status changes, notify prescriber

• Eye problems: need for ophthalmic exams before, during, after treatment (slit lamp, funduscopy, tonometry)

Administer:

PO route

• With food, milk to decrease GI symptoms

Perform/provide:

• Storage at room temperature

• Hard candy, gum, frequent rinsing for dry mouth

• Assistance with ambulation during early part of treatment; dizziness occurs

Evaluate:

• Therapeutic response: decreased seizure activity

Teach patient/family:

• To carry emergency ID stating patient's name, drugs taken, condition, prescriber's name and phone number

• To avoid driving, other activities that require alertness

• Not to discontinue medication quickly after long-term use

• To inform prescriber if hypersensitive to carbamazepine

• To avoid use of alcohol while taking this medication

• To use alternative contraception if using hormonal method

oxiconazole topical

See appendix c

oxtriphylline (℞)

(ox-trye'fi-lin)

Choledyl SA

Func. class.: Bronchodilator, spasmolytic

Chem. class.: Choline salt of theophylline

Action: Relaxes smooth muscle of respiratory system by blocking phosphodiesterase, which increases cAMP; 64% theophylline

Uses: Acute bronchial asthma, reversible bronchospasm in chronic bronchitis and COPD

Dosage and routes:

• *Adult and child >16 yr:* **PO** 4.7 mg/kg q8h or ext action q12h

• *Child 9-16 yr and smokers (adult):* 4.7 mg/kg q6h

• *Child 1-9 yr:* 6.2 mg/kg q6h

Available forms: Elix 100 mg/5 ml🍁; syr 50 mg/5 ml; tabs 100, 200 mg; ext rel tabs 400, 600 mg

Side effects/adverse reactions:

CNS: Anxiety, restlessness, insomnia, dizziness, ***convulsions,*** headache, light-headedness

CV: Palpitations, ***sinus tachycardia,*** hypotension

GI: Nausea, vomiting, anorexia, diarrhea, bitter taste, dyspepsia

RESP: Increased rate, ***respiratory arrest***

INTEG: Flushing, urticaria, alopecia

Contraindications: Hypersensitivity to xanthines, tachydysrhythmias, active peptic ulcer

Precautions: Elderly, CHF, cor pulmonale, hepatic disease, diabetes mellitus, hyperthyroidism, hypertension, children, pregnancy (C)

Pharmacokinetics:
ELIXIR: Peak 1 hr
PO-ER: Peak 4-7 hr, duration 8-12 hr
Metabolized in liver; excreted in urine, breast milk; crosses placenta

Interactions:
• ↑ toxicity: fluoroquinolones, β-blockers, cimetidine, oral contraceptives, corticosteroids, fluvoxamine, disulfiram, allopurinol, calcium channel blockers, oral contraceptives
• ↑ effects of: anticoagulants, coffee (caffeine items)
• ↓ lithium effect
• ↓ oxtriphylline level: rifampin, phenytoin, barbiturates, ketoconazole, smoking
• Drug/food: caffeine: ↑ effect
• ↓ effect: charbroiled foods, smoking
↑ action of both: cola tree
↑ oxtriphylline toxicity: cayenne
↓ oxtriphylline level: St. John's wort

NURSING CONSIDERATIONS

Assess:
• Therapeutic blood levels; toxicity may occur with small increase above therapeutic level; therapeutic theophylline levels: 11-20 mcg/ml; watch for toxicity: nausea, vomiting, diarrhea, restlessness, tachycardia
• Smoking: reduces effects of theophyllines, requiring larger doses
• Respiratory rate, rhythm, depth; auscultate lung fields bilaterally; notify prescriber of abnormalities
• Allergic reactions: rash, urticaria; drug should be discontinued
• I&O ratios, increase in weight
• Pulmonary function studies baseline and during treatment

Administer:
• PO after meals to decrease GI symptoms; absorption may be affected

Perform/provide:
• Storage in closed container away from heat; protect elixir from light

Evaluate:
• Therapeutic response: absence of dyspnea, wheezing

Teach patient/family:
Not to break, crush, or chew tab
• To check OTC medications, prescription medications for ephedrine, which will increase stimulation
• To avoid hazardous activities; dizziness may occur
• If GI upset occurs, to take drug with 8 oz water; avoid food; absorption may be decreased
To notify prescriber of toxicity: nausea, vomiting, anxiety, convulsions, insomnia, rapid pulse
• To notify prescriber of change in smoking habit; may need to change dose; encourage not to smoke

oxybutynin (℞)
(ox-i-byoo′ti-nin)
Ditropan, Ditropan XL, oxybutynin
Func. class.: Anticholinergic
Chem. class.: Synthetic tertiary amine

Action: Relaxes smooth muscles in urinary tract by inhibiting acetylcholine at postganglionic sites

Uses: Antispasmodic for neurogenic bladder

Dosage and routes:
• *Adult:* **PO** 5 mg bid-tid, not to exceed 5 mg qid; ER 5 mg qd, may increase by 5 mg, max 30 mg/day
• *Geriatric:* **PO** 2.5-5 mg tid, increase by 2.5 mg q several days
• *Child >5 yr:* **PO** 5 mg bid, not to exceed 5 mg tid
• *Child 1-5 yr:* **PO** 0.2 mg/kg/dose 2-4 ×/day

Available forms: Syr 5 mg/5 ml; tabs 5 mg; tabs, ext rel 5, 10, 15 mg

Side effects/adverse reactions:

CNS: Anxiety, restlessness, dizziness, ***convulsions,*** headache, drowsiness, confusion

CV: Palpitations, sinus tachycardia, hypotension

GI: Nausea, vomiting, anorexia, abdominal pain, constipation

GU: Dysuria, urinary retention, hesitancy

EENT: Blurred vision, increased intraocular tension, dry mouth, throat

Contraindications: Hypersensitivity, GI obstruction, GI hemorrhage, GU obstruction, glaucoma, severe colitis, myasthenia gravis, unstable CV status in acute hemorrhage

Precautions: Pregnancy (B), lactation, suspected glaucoma, children <12 yr, elderly

Do not confuse:

Ditropan/diazepam

Pharmacokinetics: Onset ½-1 hr, peak 3-4 hr, duration 6-10 hr; metabolized by liver, excreted in urine

Interactions:

- ↑ levels of atenolol, digoxin, nitrofurantoin
- ↓ levels of acetaminophen, haloperidol, levodopa
- ↑ or ↓ levels of phenothiazines

↑ constipation: black catechu

↓ anticholinergic effect: jaborandi tree, pill-bearing spurge

↑ anticholinergic action: butterbur, jimsonweed, scopolia

NURSING CONSIDERATIONS

Assess:

- Urinary patterns: distention, nocturia, frequency, urgency, incontinence
- Allergic reactions: rash, urticaria; if these occur, drug should be discontinued
- CNS effects: confusion, anxiety; anticholinergic effects in the elderly

Administer:

- Without regard to meals

Evaluate:

- Urinary status: dysuria, frequency, nocturia, incontinence

Teach patient/family:

- To avoid hazardous activities; dizziness, blurred vision may occur
- To avoid OTC medications with alcohol, other CNS depressants
- To prevent photophobia by wearing sunglasses
- Avoid hot weather, strenuous activity, drug decreases perspiration

HIGH ALERT

oxycodone (℞)

(ox-i-koe'done)

Endocodone, M-oxy, Oxy Contin, OxyFAST, OxyIR, Roxicodone, Roxicodone Supeudol✦

oxycodone/aspirin

Endodan✦, Oxycodan✦, Percodan, Percodan-Demi, Roxiprin

oxycodone/acetaminophen

Endocet✦, Oxycocet✦, Percocet, Roxicet, Roxilox, Tylox

Func. class.: Opiate analgesic

Chem. class.: Semisynthetic derivative

Controlled Substance Schedule II

Action: Inhibits ascending pain pathways in CNS, increases pain threshold, alters pain perception

Uses: Moderate to severe pain

Investigational uses: Postherpetic neuralgic (cont rel)

Dosage and routes:

- *Adult:* **PO** 10-30 mg q4hr (5 mg q6h for OxyIR, OxyFast) **OxyFast**

Conc Sol is extremely concentrated; do not use interchangeably
• *Child:* **PO** 0.05-0.15 mg/kg/dose up to 5 mg/dose q4-6h; not recommended in children
Available forms: Oxycodone tabs, cont rel 10, 20, 40, 80, 160 mg; tabs, immediate rel 15, 30 mg; tabs 5 mg; caps, immediate rel 5 mg; oral sol 5 mg/5 ml, 20 mg/ml; oxycodone with acetaminophen tabs 5 mg/325 mg; cap 5 mg/500 mg; oral sol 5 mg/325 mg/5 ml; oxycodone with aspirin 2.44 mg/325 mg, 4.88/325 mg
Side effects/adverse reactions:
CNS: Drowsiness, dizziness, confusion, headache, sedation, euphoria
GI: Nausea, vomiting, anorexia, constipation, cramps
GU: Increased urinary output, dysuria, urinary retention
INTEG: Rash, urticaria, bruising, flushing, diaphoresis, pruritus
EENT: Tinnitus, blurred vision, miosis, diplopia
CV: Palpitations, bradycardia, change in B/P
RESP: ***Respiratory depression***
Contraindications: Hypersensitivity, addiction (opiate)
Precautions: Addictive personality, pregnancy (B), lactation, increased intracranial pressure, MI (acute), severe heart disease, respiratory depression, hepatic disease, renal disease, child <18 yr
Do not confuse:
Percodan/Decadron
Roxicet/Roxanol
Tylox/Xanax
Tylox/Trimox
Tylox/Wymox
Pharmacokinetics:
PO: Onset 15-30 min, peak 1 hr, duration 4-6 hr; detoxified by liver, excreted in urine, crosses placenta, excreted in breast milk

Interactions:
• ↑ effects with other CNS depressants: alcohol, opioids, sedative/hypnotics, antipsychotics, skeletal muscle relaxants
↑ anticholinergic effect: corkwood
↑ sedative effect: Jamaican dogwood, lavender, mistletoe, nettle, pokeweed, poppy, senega, valerian
Lab test interferences:
Increase: Amylase

NURSING CONSIDERATIONS

Assess:
• I&O ratio; check for decreasing output; may indicate urinary retention
• CNS changes: dizziness, drowsiness, hallucinations, euphoria, LOC, pupil reaction
• Allergic reactions: rash, urticaria
• Respiratory dysfunction: respiratory depression, character, rate, rhythm; notify prescriber if respirations are <10/min
• Need for pain medication by pain, sedation scoring; physical dependence
Administer:
• 80, 160 mg cont rel tabs only in opioid-tolerant patients
• With antiemetic if nausea, vomiting occur
• When pain is beginning to return; determine dosage interval by response
Do not break, crush, or chew controlled release tabs
Perform/provide:
• Storage in light-resistant area at room temperature
• Assistance with ambulation
• Safety measures: night-light, call bell within easy reach
Evaluate:
• Therapeutic response: decrease in pain

Teach patient/family:
- To report any symptoms of CNS changes, allergic reactions
- That physical dependency may result from extended use
- That withdrawal symptoms may occur: nausea, vomiting, cramps, fever, faintness, anorexia

Treatment of overdose: Naloxone (Narcan) 0.2-0.8 mg IV, O_2, IV fluids, vasopressors

oxymetazoline nasal agent

See appendix c

oxymetazoline ophthalmic

See appendix c

HIGH ALERT

oxymorphone (℞)

(ox-i-mor′fone)

Numorphan

Func. class.: Opiate analgesic

Chem. class.: Semisynthetic phenanthrene derivative

Controlled Substance Schedule II

Action: Inhibits ascending pain pathways in CNS, increases pain threshold, alters pain perception

Uses: Moderate to severe pain

Dosage and routes:
- *Adult:* **IM/SC** 1-1.5 mg q4-6h prn; **IV** 0.5 mg q4-6h prn; **RECT** 5 mg q4-6h prn

Labor analgesia
- *Adult:* **IM:** 0.5-1 mg

Available forms: Inj 1, 1.5 mg/ml; supp 5 mg

Side effects/adverse reactions:

CNS: Drowsiness, dizziness, confusion, headache, sedation, ***seizures,*** *euphoria (elderly)*

GI: Nausea, vomiting, anorexia, constipation, cramps

GU: Increased urinary output, dysuria, urinary retention

INTEG: Rash, urticaria, bruising, flushing, diaphoresis, pruritus

EENT: Tinnitus, blurred vision, miosis, diplopia

CV: Palpitations, ***bradycardia,*** change in B/P

RESP: ***Respiratory depression***

Contraindications: Hypersensitivity, addiction (opiate)

Precautions: Addictive personality, pregnancy (B) (short-term), lactation, increased intracranial pressure, MI (acute), severe heart disease, respiratory depression, hepatic disease, renal disease, child <18 yr

Pharmacokinetics:

SC/IM: Onset 10-15 min, peak 1½ hr, duration, 3-6 hr

IV: Onset 5-10 min, peak 15-30 min, duration 3-6 hr

RECT: Onset 15-30 min, duration 3-6 hr

Metabolized by liver, excreted in urine, crosses placenta

Interactions:
- ↑ effects with other CNS depressants: alcohol, opiates, sedative/hypnotics, antipsychotics, skeletal muscle relaxants
- ↑ anticholinergic effect: corkwood
- ↑ sedative effect: Jamaican dogwood, lavender, mistletoe, nettle, pokeweed, poppy, senega, valerian

Lab test interferences:

Increase: Amylase

NURSING CONSIDERATIONS

Assess:
- I&O ratio for decreasing output; may indicate urinary retention

• CNS changes: dizziness, drowsiness, hallucinations, euphoria, LOC, pupil reaction
• Allergic reactions: rash, urticaria
• Respiratory dysfunction: respiratory depression, character, rate, rhythm; notify prescriber if respirations are <10/min
• Need for pain medication, physical dependence

Administer:
• With antiemetic for nausea, vomiting
• When pain is beginning to return; determine interval by response

IV route
• After diluting with 5 ml sterile H_2O or NS for inj; give over 2-5 min through Y-tube or 3-way stopcock

Syringe compatibilities: Glycopyrrolate, hydrOXYzine, ranitidine

Perform/provide:
• Storage in light-resistant area at room temperature
• Assistance with ambulation
• Safety measures: night-light, call bell within easy reach

Evaluate:
• Therapeutic response: decrease in pain

Teach patient/family:
• To report any symptoms of CNS changes, allergic reactions
• That physical dependency may result from extended use
• That withdrawal symptoms may occur: nausea, vomiting, cramps, fever, faintness, anorexia

Treatment of overdose: Naloxone (Narcan) 0.2-0.8 mg IV, O_2, IV fluids, vasopressors

HIGH ALERT

oxytocin (℞)

(ox-i-toe'sin)

Pitocin, Syntocinon

Func. class.: Oxytocic

Chem. class.: Hormone

Action: Acts directly on myofibrils, producing uterine contraction; stimulates milk ejection by the breast

Uses: Stimulation, induction of labor; missed or incomplete abortion; postpartum bleeding

Dosage and routes:

Postpartum hemorrhage
• *Adult:* **IV** 10 units infused at 20-40 mU/min
• *Adult:* **IM** 10 units after delivery of placenta

Fetal stress test
• *Adult:* **IV** 0.5 mU/min, increase q20min until 3 contractions within 10 min

Stimulation of labor
• *Adult:* **IV** 1-2 mU/min, increase by 1-2 mU q15-60 min until contractions occur; then decrease dose

Incomplete abortion
• *Adult:* **IV INF** 10 units/500 ml D_5W or 0.9% NaCl at 20-40 mU/min

Available forms: Inj 10 units/ml

Side effects/adverse reactions:

CNS: ***Convulsions, tetanic contractions***

CV: Hypotension, hypertension, dysrhythmias, increased pulse, bradycardia, tachycardia, PVC

FETUS: Dysrhythmias, jaundice, hypoxia, ***intracranial hemorrhage***

GI: Anorexia, nausea, vomiting, constipation

GU: ***Abruptio placentae, decreased uterine blood flow***

HEMA: Increased hyperbilirubinemia

INTEG: Rash
RESP: ***Asphyxia***
Contraindications: Hypersensitivity, serum toxemia, cephalopelvic disproportion, fetal distress, hypertonic uterus
Precautions: Cervical/uterine surgery, uterine sepsis, primipara >35 yr, 1st, 2nd stage of labor
Pharmacokinetics:
IM: Onset 3-7 min, duration 1 hr, half-life 12-17 min
IV: Onset 1 min, duration 30 min, half-life 12-17 min
Interactions:
- Hypertension: vasopressors

Hypertension: ephedra
NURSING CONSIDERATIONS
Assess:
- I&O ratio
- Respiration
- B/P, pulse; watch for changes that may indicate hemorrhage
- Respiratory rate, rhythm, depth; notify prescriber of abnormalities
- Length, intensity, duration of contraction; notify prescriber of contractions lasting over 1 min or absence of contractions; turn patient on her side
- FHTs, fetal distress; watch for acceleration, deceleration; notify prescriber if problems occur; fetal presentation, pelvic dimensions; turn patient on left side if FHT change in rate

For signs and symptoms of water intoxication; confusion, anuria, drowsiness, headache
Administer:
Labor induction
- After diluting 10 units/L of 0.9% NS or D_5 NS run at 1-2 mU/min at 15-30 min intervals to begin normal labor; dilute 10-40 mU/min, titrate to control postpartum bleeding; dilute 10 units/500 ml sol; run 10 units-20 mU/ml; administer by only 1 route at a time; use inf pump; rotate inf to provide mixing; do not shake

Control of postpartum bleeding
- Dilute 10-40 units/1 L of sol, run at 10-20 mU/min; adjust rate as needed
- With crash cart available on unit (Mg^+SO_4 at bedside)

Additive compatibilities: Chloramphenicol, metaraminol, netilmicin, sodium bicarbonate, thiopental, verapamil
Y-site compatibilities: Heparin, hydrocortisone, insulin (regular), meperidine, morphine, potassium chloride, vit B/C, warfarin
Evaluate:
- Therapeutic response: stimulation of labor, control of postpartum bleeding

Teach patient/family:
- To report increased blood loss, abdominal cramps, fever, foul-smelling lochia
- That contractions will be similar to menstrual cramps, gradually increasing in intensity

paclitaxel (℞)
(pa-kli-tax'el)
Onxol, Taxol
Func. class.: Misc. antineoplastic
Chem. class.: Antimicrotubule, natural diterpene

Action: Inhibits reorganization of microtubule network needed for interphase and mitotic cellular functions; also causes abnormal bundles of microtubules during cell cycle and multiple esters of microtubules during mitosis
Uses: Taxol: metastatic carcinoma of the ovary, breast; AIDS-related Kaposi's sarcoma (2nd-line), non–

small cell lung cancer (1st-line), adjuvant treatment for node-positive breast cancer; Onxol: failure of other treatment in breast cancer, advanced carcinoma in ovarian cancer

Investigational uses: Advanced head, neck, small cell lung cancer; non-Hodgkin's lymphoma, adenocarcinoma of the upper GI tract, hormone-refractory prostate cancer

Dosage and routes:

Ovarian carcinoma

• *Adult:* **IV INF** 135 mg/m^2 given over 24 hr q3wk then cisplatin 75 mg/m^2; or 175 mg/m^2 over 3 hr q3wk; or 175 mg/m^2 over 3 hr

Advanced ovarian carcinoma

• *Adult:* **IV/INF** 175 mg/m^2 with cisplatin 75 mg/m^2 using a 3-hr regimen q3wk

Breast carcinoma

• *Adult:* **IV INF** 175 mg/m^2 over 3 hr q3wk × 4 courses

AIDS-related Kaposi's sarcoma

• *Adult:* **IV INF** 135 mg/m^2 over 3 hr q3wk or 100 mg/m^2 over 3 hr q2wk

1st-line non–small cell lung cancer

• *Adult:* **IV INF** 135 mg/m^2/24 hr inf with cisplatin 75 mg/m^2 × 3 wk

Available forms: Inj 30 mg/5 ml vial (6 mg/ml)

Side effects/adverse reactions:

HEMA: ***Neutropenia, leukopenia, thrombocytopenia, anemia,*** bleeding, infections

SYST: Hypersensitivity reactions, ***anaphylaxis***

CV: Bradycardia, *hypotension,* abnormal ECG

NEURO: Peripheral neuropathy

MS: Arthralgia, myalgia

GI: Nausea, vomiting, diarrhea, mucositis, increased bilirubin, alk phosphatase, AST

INTEG: Alopecia

Contraindications: Hypersensitivity to paclitaxel or other drugs with polyoxyethylated castor oil, neutropenia of <1500/mm^3, pregnancy (D)

Precautions: Children, lactation; hepatic, cardiovascular disease; CNS disorder

Do not confuse:

paclitaxel/paroxetine
paclitaxel/Paxil
Taxol/Paxil
Taxol/Taxotera

Pharmacokinetics: 89%-98% of drug is serum protein bound, metabolized in liver, excreted in bile and urine; terminal half-life 5.3-17.4 hr

Interactions:

• ↑ myelosuppression: other antineoplastics, radiation

• ↓ paclitaxel metabolism: ketoconazole, verapamil, diazepam, cycloSPORINE, teniposide, etoposide, quinidine, dexamethasone, vinCRIStine, testosterone

• ↑ DOXOrubicin levels: DOXOrubicin

• ↓ immune response: live virus vaccines

NURSING CONSIDERATIONS

Assess:

• CBC, differential, platelet count prior to and qwk; withhold drug if WBC is <1500/mm^3 or platelet count is <100,000/mm^3, notify prescriber

• Monitor temp q4h (may indicate beginning infection)

• Hepatic studies before, during therapy (bilirubin, AST, ALT, LDH, bilirubin) prn or qmo, check for jaundiced skin and sclera, dark urine, clay-colored stool, itchy skin, abdominal pain, fever, diarrhea

• VS during 1st hr of infusion, check IV site for signs of infiltration

◆ Hypersensitive reactions, anaphylaxis including hypotension, dyspnea, angioedema, generalized urticaria; discontinue infusion immediately

P

• Bleeding: hematuria, guaiac, bruising or petechiae, mucosa or orifices q8h; obtain prescription for viscous lidocaine (Xylocaine)
• Effects of alopecia on body image; discuss feelings about body changes

Administer:
• Antiemetic 30-60 min before giving drug and prn

IV route
• After diluting in 0.9% NaCl, D_5, D_5 and 0.9% NaCl, D_5LR to a concentration of 0.3-1.2 mg/ml
• Using an in-line filter ≤0.22 μm
• After premedicating with dexamethasone 20 mg PO 12 hr and 6 hr before paclitaxel, diphenhydrAMINE 50 mg IV ½-1 hr before paclitaxel and cimetidine 300 mg or ranitidine 50 mg IV ½-1 hr before paclitaxel
• Using only glass bottles, polypropylene, polyolefin bags and administration sets; do not use PVC infusion bags or sets
• Using gloves and cytotoxic handling precautions

Y-site compatibilities: Acyclovir, amikacin, aminophylline, ampicillin/sulbactam, bleomycin, butorphanol, calcium chloride, carboplatin, cefepime, cefotetan, ceftazidime, ceftriaxone, cimetidine, cisplatin, cladribine, cyclophosphamide, cytarabine, dacarbazine, dexamethasone, diphenhydrAMINE, DOXOrubicin, droperidol, etoposide, famotidine, floxuridine, fluconazole, fluorouracil, furosemide, ganciclovir, gentamicin, granisetron, haloperidol, heparin, hydrocortisone, hydromorphone, ifosfamide, lorazepam, magnesium sulfate, mannitol, meperidine, mesna, methotrexate, metoclopramide, morphine, nalbuphine, ondansetron, pentostatin, potassium chloride, prochlorperazine, propofol, ranitidine, sodium bicarbonate, thiotepa, vancomycin, vinBLAStine, vinCRIStine, zidovudine

Perform/provide:
• Confirmation that dexamethasone was given 12 hr and 6 hr before infusion begins
• Storage of prepared sol up to 27 hr in refrigeration

Evaluate:
• Therapeutic response: decreased tumor size, spread of malignancy

Teach patient/family:
• To report signs of infection: fever, sore throat, flulike symptoms
• To report signs of anemia: fatigue, headache, faintness, shortness of breath, irritability
• To report bleeding; avoid use of razors, commercial mouthwash
• To avoid use of aspirin, ibuprofen
• To report any complaints or side effects to nurse or prescriber
• That hair may be lost during treatment; a wig or hairpiece may make patient feel better; new hair may be different in color, texture
• That pain in muscles and joints 2-5 days after infusion is common
• To use nonhormonal type of contraception
• To avoid receiving vaccinations while on this drug

palivizumab (℞)

(pal-ih-viz'uh-mab)

Synagis

Func. class.: Monoclonal antibody

Action: A humanized monoclonal antibody that exhibits neutralizing and fusion-inhibitory activity against respiratory syncytial virus (RSV)

Uses: Prevention of serious lower respiratory tract disease caused by RSV in pediatric patients

Dosage and routes:

• *Child:* **IM** 15 mg/kg, those patients who develop RSV should receive monthly doses during RSV season

Available forms: Lyophilized inj 100 mg

Side effects/adverse reactions:

GI: Nausea, vomiting, diarrhea, increased AST

RESP: URI, ***apnea***

EENT: Otitis media, rhinitis, pharyngitis

INTEG: Rash, inj site reaction

SYST: ***Anaphylaxis***

Contraindications: Hypersensitivity, adults, cyanotic congenital heart disease

Precautions: Thrombocytopenia, coagulation disorders, established RSV, congenital heart disease, chronic lung disease, systemic allergic reactions, pregnancy (C)

Pharmacokinetics: Mean half-life 20 days

NURSING CONSIDERATIONS

Assess:

• For presence of RSV infection, drug is given to prevent infection For side effects; report if allergic reaction is evident

• For anaphylaxis: difficulty breathing; drug should be discontinued and have emergency equipment nearby

Administer:

• IM only

• After adding 1 ml of sterile water for inj per 100 mg vial, gently swirl, let stand at room temperature for 20 min until sol clarifies; given within 6 hr of reconstitution

Teach patient/family:

• To report upper respiratory infections, earaches, rash, sore throat

pamidronate (℞)

(pam-i-drone'ate)

Aredia

Func. class.: Bone-resorption inhibitor, electrolyte modifier

Chem. class.: Bisphosphonate

Action: Inhibits bone resorption, apparently without inhibiting bone formation and mineralization; absorbs calcium phosphate crystals in bone and may directly block dissolution of hydroxyapatite crystals of bone

Uses: Moderate to severe Paget's disease associated with malignancy with or without bone metastases, osteolytic bone metastases in breast cancer, multiple myeloma patients

Dosage and routes:

Hypercalcemia of malignancy

• *Adult:* **IV INF** 60-90 mg in moderate hypercalcemia, 90 mg in severe hypercalcemia over 24 hr

Osteolytic lesions from multiple myeloma

• *Adult:* **IV** 90 mg over 4 hr, qmo

Paget's disease

• *Adult:* **IV** 90-180 mg/treatment, may use 30 mg qd × 3 days

Available forms: Inj 30, 60, 90 mg/vial

Side effects/adverse reactions:

INTEG: Redness, swelling, induration, pain on palpation at site of catheter insertion

RESP: Coughing, dyspnea, URI

META: Anemia, hypokalemia, hypomagnesemia, hypophosphatemia, hypocalcemia

GI: Abdominal pain, anorexia, constipation, nausea, vomiting, diarrhea, dyspepsia

MS: Bone pain, myalgia

CV: Hypertension

GU: UTI, fluid overload

Contraindications: Hypersensitiv-

P

ity to bisphosphonates, pregnancy (D)
Precautions: Children, nursing mothers, renal dysfunction
Do not confuse:
Aredia/Adriamycin
Pharmacokinetics: Rapidly cleared from circulation and taken up mainly by bones, primarily in areas of high bone turnover, eliminated primarily by kidneys
Interactions:
• Hypomagnesemia, hypokalemia: digoxin
• ↓ pamidronate effect: calcium, vit D
• Do not mix with calcium-containing infusion sol such as Ringer's sol
NURSING CONSIDERATIONS
Assess:
• Renal studies, Ca, P, Mg, K
• For hypercalcemia: paresthesia, twitching, laryngospasm, Chvostek's, Trousseau's signs
Administer:
IV route
• After reconstituting by adding 10 ml of sterile water for inj to each vial (30 mg/10 ml, or 60 mg/10 ml, or 90 mg/10 ml depending on vial used), then add to 1000 ml of sterile 0.45%, 0.9% NaCl, D_5W, run over 24 hr for hypercalcemia or 60 mg ≥4 hr, 90 mg over 24 hr; dilute reconstituted sol in 500 ml of 0.9% NaCl, 0.45% NaCl, or D_5W, give over 4 hr (multiple myeloma, Paget's disease)
Perform/provide:
• Storage of infusion sol up to 24 hr at room temperature
• Reconstituted sol with sterile water may be stored under refrigeration for up to 24 hr
Evaluate:
• Therapeutic response: decreased calcium levels
Teach patient/family
• To report hypercalcemic relapse: nausea, vomiting, bone pain, thirst
• To continue with dietary recommendations including calcium and vit D

pancreatin (℞)
(pan'kree-a-tin)
Creon, Donnazyne, Hi-Vegi-Lip, 4x Pancreatin 600 mg, 8x Pancreatin 900 mg, Pancrezyme 4x
Func. class.: Digestant
Chem. class.: Pancreatic enzyme concentrate—bovine/porcine

Action: Pancreatic enzyme needed for breakdown of substances released from the pancreas
Uses: Exocrine pancreatic secretion insufficiency, cystic fibrosis (digestive aid)
Dosage and routes:
• *Adult:* **PO** 8000-24,000 USP units with meals
Available forms: Tabs 650, 2000, 12,000 units, others in combination
Side effects/adverse reactions:
GI: Anorexia, nausea, vomiting, diarrhea, glossitis, anal soreness
GU: Hyperuricuria, hyperuricemia
INTEG: Rash, hypersensitivity
EENT: Buccal soreness
Contraindications: Hypersensitivity to pork, chronic pancreatic disease
Precautions: Pregnancy (C), lactation
Interactions:
• ↓ absorption: cimetidine, antacids, oral iron
NURSING CONSIDERATIONS
Assess:
• I&O ratio; watch for increasing urinary output
• Fecal fat, nitrogen, PT, calcium during treatment

- For polyuria, polydipsia, polyphagia (may indicate diabetes mellitus)
- For allergy to pork

Administer:

PO route

- After antacid or H_2-blockers; decreased pH inactivates drug
- ⃠ Whole; do not break, crush, or chew (enteric coated)
- Low-fat diet for GI symptoms

Perform/provide:

- Storage in tight container at room temperature

Evaluate:

- Therapeutic response: relief of GI symptoms

pancrelipase (℞)

(pan-kre-li'pase)

Cotazym, Cotazym-65B✤, Cotazym E.C.S. 8, Cotazym E.C.S. 20, Cotazym Capsules, Cotazym-S, Creon, Ilozyme, Ku-Zyme HP, Lipram-PN16, Lipram-CR20, Lipram-UL12, Lipram-PN10, Pancrease Capsules, Pancrease MT 4, Pancrease MT 10, Pancrease MT 16, Protilase, Ultrase MT 12, Ultrase MT 20, Viokase, Zymase

Func. class.: Digestant

Chem. class.: Pancreatic enzyme—bovine/porcine

Action: Pancreatic enzyme needed for breakdown of substances released from the pancreas

Uses: Exocrine pancreatic secretion insufficiency, cystic fibrosis (digestive aid), steatorrhea, pancreatic enzyme deficiency

Dosage and routes:

- *Adult and child:* **PO** 1-3 caps/tabs ac or with meals, or 1 cap/tab with snack or 1-2 powder pkt ac

Available forms: Powder: 16,800 units lipase/70,000 units protease and amylase; caps: 8000 units lipase/30,000 units protease and amylase; cap, delayed rel 4000 units lipase/12,000 units protease and amylase, 4000 units lipase/25,000 units protease/20,000 units amylase, 5000 units lipase/20,000 units protease and amylase, 10,000 units lipase/30,000 units protease and amylase, 12,000 units lipase/24,000 units protease and amylase, 12,000 units lipase/39,000 units protease and amylase, 16,000 units lipase/48,000 units protease and amylase, 20,000 units lipase/65,000 units protease and amylase, 24,000 units lipase/78,000 units protease and amylase

Side effects/adverse reactions:

GI: Anorexia, nausea, vomiting, diarrhea

GU: Hyperuricuria, hyperuricemia

Contraindications: Allergy to pork

Precautions: Pregnancy (C)

Interactions:

- ↓ absorption: cimetidine, antacids, oral iron

NURSING CONSIDERATIONS

Assess:

- For appropriate height, weight development; may be delayed
- I&O ratio; watch for increasing urinary output
- Fecal fat, nitrogen, PT during treatment
- For polyuria, polydipsia, polyphagia (may indicate diabetes mellitus)
- For pork sensitivity, cross-sensitivity may occur

Administer:

- After antacid or cimetidine; decreased pH inactivates drug
- Powder mixed in prepared fruit juice for infants, children
- Low-fat diet for GI symptoms

P

Perform/provide:
- Storage in tight container at room temperature

Evaluate:
- Therapeutic response: improved digestion of carbohydrates, protein, fat; absence of steatorrhea

Teach patient/family:
- Not to inhale powder; may be very irritating to mucous membranes; some powder may irritate skin
- To take with 8 oz water or more, not to allow to sit in mouth, have patient sit up during administration
- To notify prescriber of allergic reactions, abdominal pain, cramping, or blood in the urine

---

HIGH ALERT

pancuronium (℞)

(pan-kyoo-roe′nee-um)

pancuronium bromide,
Pavulon

Func. class.: Neuromuscular blocker (nondepolarizing)

Chem. class.: Synthetic curariform

Action: Inhibits transmission of nerve impulses by binding with cholinergic receptor sites, antagonizing action of acetylcholine

Uses: Facilitation of endotracheal intubation, skeletal muscle relaxation during mechanical ventilation, surgery, or general anesthesia

Dosage and routes:
- *Adult:* **IV** 0.04-0.1 mg/kg, then 0.01 mg/kg q½-1h
- *Child >10 yr:* **IV** 0.04-0.1 mg/kg, then ⅕ initial dose q½-1h

Available forms: Inj 1, 2 mg/ml

Side effects/adverse reactions:

CV: Bradycardia; tachycardia; increased, decreased B/P; ventricular extrasystoles

RESP: ***Prolonged apnea, bronchospasm, cyanosis, respiratory depression***

EENT: Increased secretions

MS: Weakness to prolonged skeletal muscle relaxation

INTEG: Rash, flushing, pruritus, urticaria, sweating, salivation

SYST: ***Anaphylaxis***

Contraindications: Hypersensitivity to bromide ion

Precautions: Pregnancy (C), renal disease, cardiac disease, lactation, children <2 yr, electrolyte imbalances, dehydration, neuromuscular disease, respiratory disease

Pharmacokinetics:

IV: Onset 3-5 min, dose dependent, peak 3-5 min; metabolized (small amounts), excreted in urine (unchanged), crosses placenta

Interactions:
- ↑ neuromuscular blockade: aminoglycosides, clindamycin, enflurane, isoflurane, lincomycin, lithium, local anesthetics, opioid analgesics, polymyxin anti-infectives, quinidine, thiazides
- Dysrhythmias: theophylline

Lab test interferences:

Decrease: Cholinesterase

NURSING CONSIDERATIONS

Assess:
- For electrolyte imbalances (K, Mg); may lead to increased action of this drug
- VS (B/P, pulse, respirations, airway) until fully recovered; rate, depth, pattern of respirations, strength of hand grip
- I&O ratio; check for urinary retention, frequency, hesitancy
- Recovery: decreased paralysis of face, diaphragm, leg, arm, rest of body; allow to recover fully before neuro assessment

 Allergic reactions, anaphylaxis: rash, fever, respiratory distress, pruritus; drug should be discontinued

Administer:

IV direct route

• With diazepam or morphine when used for therapeutic paralysis; this drug provides no sedation

• Using nerve stimulator by anesthesiologist to determine neuromuscular blockade

• Atropine to counteract muscarinic effects

• After succinylcholine effects subside

• Anticholinesterase to reverse neuromuscular blockade

• IV undiluted, give over 1-2 min (only by qualified persons)

Additive compatibilities: Verapamil

Syringe compatibilities: Heparin

Y-site compatibilities: Aminophylline, cefazolin, cefuroxime, cimetidine, DOBUTamine, DOPamine, epINEPHrine, esmolol, fentanyl, fluconazole, gentamicin, heparin, hydrocortisone, isoproterenol, lorazepam, midazolam, morphine, nitroglycerin, nitroprusside, ranitidine, trimethoprim-sulfamethoxazole, vancomycin

Perform/provide:

• Storage in refrigerator; do not store in plastic; use only fresh sol

• Reassurance if communication is difficult during recovery from neuromuscular blockade

• Frequent (q2h) instillation of artificial tears and covering eyes to prevent drying of cornea

Evaluate:

• Therapeutic response: paralysis of jaw, eyelid, head, neck, rest of body

Treatment of overdose: Edrophonium or neostigmine, atropine, monitor VS; may require mechanical ventilation

pantoprazole (℞)

(pan-toe-pray′zole)

Protonix, Prontonix IV

Func. class.: Proton pump inhibitor

Chem. class.: Benzimidazole

Action: Suppresses gastric secretion by inhibiting hydrogen/potassium ATPase enzyme system in gastric parietal cell; characterized as gastric acid pump inhibitor, since it blocks final step of acid production

Uses: Gastroesophageal reflux disease (GERD), severe erosive esophagitis, maintenance, long-term pathologic hypersecretory conditions including Zollinger-Ellison syndrome

Dosage and routes:

GERD

• *Adult:* **PO** 40 mg qd × 8 wk, may repeat course

Erosive esophagitis

• *Adult:* **IV** 40 mg qd × 7-10 day **PO** 40 mg qd × 8 wk; may repeat **PO** course

Pathological hypersecretory conditions

• *Adult:* **IV** 80 mg q12h; max 240 mg/day

Available forms: Tabs, delayed rel 20, 40 mg; powder for inj, freeze-dried 40 mg/vial

Side effects/adverse reactions:

CNS: Headache, insomnia

GI: Diarrhea, abdominal pain, flatulence

INTEG: Rash

META: Hyperglycemia

Contraindications: Hypersensitivity

Precautions: Pregnancy (C), lactation, children

Pharmacokinetics: Peak 2.4 hr, duration >24 hr, half-life 1.5 hr, pro-

P

tein binding 97%, eliminated in urine as metabolites and in feces; in elderly elimination rate decreased

Interactions:

• ↑ pantoprazole serum levels: diazepam, phenytoin, flurazepam, triazolam, clarithromycin

• ↑ bleeding: warfarin

• May ↓ absorption: sucralfate

NURSING CONSIDERATIONS

Assess:

• GI system: bowel sounds q8h, abdomen for pain, swelling, anorexia

• Hepatic studies: AST, ALT, alk phosphatase during treatment

Administer:

PO route

⊘ Do not crush del rel tabs, swallow whole

• May take with or without food

IV route

• Reconstitute with 10 ml 0.9% NaCl, further dilute with 80 ml LR, D_5, 0.9% NaCl (0.8 mg/ml), give over 15 min (≤6 mg/min) using in-line filter provided

Evaluate:

• Therapeutic response: absence of epigastric pain, swelling, fullness

Teach patient/family:

• To report severe diarrhea; drug may have to be discontinued

• That diabetic patient should know hypoglycemia may occur

• To avoid hazardous activities; dizziness may occur

• To avoid alcohol, salicylates, ibuprofen; may cause GI irritation

---

RARELY USED

papaverine (℞)

(pa-pav′er-een)

Func. class.: Peripheral vasodilator

Uses: Arterial spasm resulting in cerebral and peripheral ischemia; myocardial ischemia associated with vascular spasm or dysrhythmias; angina pectoris; peripheral pulmonary embolism; visceral spasm as in ureteral, biliary, GI colic, peripheral vascular disease

Dosage and routes:

• *Adult:* **SUS REL** 150-300 mg q8-12h; **IM/IV** 30-120 mg

Contraindications: Hypersensitivity, complete AV heart block

RARELY USED

paraldehyde (℞)

(par-al′de-hyde)

Func. class.: Anticonvulsant

Uses: Refractory seizures, status epilepticus, sedation, insomnia, alcohol withdrawal, tetanus, eclampsia

Dosage and routes:

Seizures

• *Adult:* **IM** 5-10 ml; divide 10 ml into 2 inj; **IV** 0.2-0.4 ml/kg in **NS** inj

• *Child:* **IM** 0.15 ml/kg; **RECT** 0.3 ml/kg q4-6h or 1 ml/yr of age, not to exceed 5 ml; may repeat in 1 hr prn; **IV** 5 ml/90 ml **NS** inj; begin infusion at 5 ml/hr; titrate to patient response

Alcohol withdrawal

• *Adult:* **PO/RECT** 5-10 ml, not to exceed 60 ml; **IM** 5 ml q4-6h × 24 hr, then q6h on following days, not to exceed 30 ml

Sedation

• *Adult:* **PO/REC** 4-10 ml; **IM** 5 ml; **IV** 3-5 ml in emergency only; Child: **PO/REC/IM** 0.15 ml/kg

Tetanus

• *Adult:* **IV** 4-5 ml or 12 ml by gastric tube q4h diluted with water; **IM** 5-10 ml prn

Contraindications: Hypersensitivity, gastroenteritis with ulceration

RARELY USED

paramethadione (℞)

(par-a-meth-a-dye′one)

Func. class.: Anticonvulsant

Uses: Refractory absence (petit mal) seizures

Dosage and routes:

- *Adult:* **PO** 300 mg tid; may increase by 300 mg/wk, not to exceed 600 mg qid
- *Child >6 yr:* **PO** 0.9 g/day in divided doses tid or qid
- *Child 2-6 yr:* **PO** 0.6 g/day in divided doses tid or qid
- *Child <2 yr:* **PO** 0.3 g/day in divided doses tid or qid

Contraindications: Hypersensitivity, blood dyscrasias, pregnancy (D), lactation

paricalcitol (℞)

(par-ih-cal′sih-tol)

Zemplar

Func. class.: Vit D analong

Chem. class.: Fat-soluble vitamin

Action: Reduces parathyroid hormone (PTH) levels; suppresses PTH levels in patients with chronic renal failure with absence of hypercalcemia/hyperphosphatemia. Serum PO_4, calcium, CaXP may increase

Uses: Hyperparathyroidism in chronic renal failure

Dosage and routes:

- *Adult:* **IV BOL** 0.04-0.1 mcg/kg (2.8-7 mcg) no more than qod during dialysis; may increase by 2-4 mcg q2-4wk until target serum intact Pth (1.5 – 3 × non-uremic upper limit of normal) is achieved

Available forms: Inj 5 mcg/ml

Side effects/adverse reactions:

GI: Nausea, vomiting, anorexia, dry mouth

CNS: Lightheadedness

CV: Palpitations

OTHER: Pneumonia, edema, chills, fever, flu, *sepsis*

Contraindications: Hypersensitivity, hypercalcemia

Precautions: Cardiovascular disease, renal calculi, pregnancy (C), elderly, lactation, children

Interactions:

- Digitalis toxicity: digitalis

NURSING CONSIDERATIONS

Assess:

- Ca, PO_4, q2×/wk during initial therapy; after dose is established take calcium and phosphorus qmo

Administer:

IV route

- By IV bolus only

Evaluate:

- Decreased hypoparathyroidism in chronic renal disease

Teach patient/family:

- To report weakness, lethargy, headache, anorexia, loss of weight
- To report nausea, vomiting, palpitations

RARELY USED

paromomycin (℞)

(par-oh-moe-mye′sin)

Func. class.: Amebicide

Uses: Intestinal amebiasis, adjunct in hepatic coma

Dosage and routes:

Intestinal amebiasis

- *Adult and child:* **PO** 25-35 mg/kg/day in 3 divided doses × 5-10 day pc

P

Hepatic coma
• *Adult:* 4 g qd in divided doses × 5-6 day
Contraindications: Hypersensitivity, renal disease, GI obstruction

paroxetine (℞)
(par-ox'e-teen)
Paxil, Paxil CR
Func. class.: Antidepressant, SSRI
Chem. class.: Phenylpiperidine derivative

Action: Inhibits CNS neuron uptake of serotonin but not of norepinephrine or DOPamine
Uses: Major depressive disorder, obsessive-compulsive disorder, panic disorder, generalized anxiety disorder
Investigational uses: Diabetic neuropathy, headaches, premature ejaculation, premenstrual disorders, bipolar depression with lithium, fibromyalgia, posttraumatic stress
Research note: Risperidone given with paroxetine resulted in an increase of risperidone levels[30]
Research note: One study has shown a decrease in thyroxine during treatment with paroxetine[31]
Dosage and routes:
Depression
• *Adult:* **PO** 20 mg qd in AM; after 4 wk if no clinical improvement is noted, dose may be increased by 10 mg/day qwk to desired response, not to exceed 60 mg/day or **CONTROLLED REL** 25 mg/day, may increase by 12.5 mg/day weekly up to 62.5 mg/day
• *Geriatric:* **PO** 10 mg qd, increase by 10 mg to desired dose, max 40 mg/day
Renal dose
• *Adult:* **PO** 10 mg qd in AM, may increase by 10 mg/day qwk, max 50 mg qd or **CONTROLLED REL** 12.5 mg/day, max 50 mg/day
Obsessive-compulsive disorder
• *Adult:* **PO** 40 mg/day in AM, start with 20 mg/day, increase 10 mg/day increments, max 60 mg/day
Panic disorder
• *Adult:* **PO** 40 mg/day, start with 10 mg/day and increase in 10 mg/day increments, max 60 mg/day or **CONTROLLED REL** 12.5 mg/day, max 75 mg/day
Premenstrual disorders (off-label)
• *Adult:* **PO** 10-30 mg qd
Available forms: Tabs 10, 20, 30, 40 mg; oral susp 10 mg/5 ml; controlled rel 12.5, 25, 37.5 mg
Side effects/adverse reactions:
CNS: Headache, nervousness, insomnia, drowsiness, anxiety, tremor, dizziness, fatigue, sedation, abnormal dreams, agitation, apathy, euphoria, hallucinations, delusions, psychosis
GI: Nausea, diarrhea, dry mouth, anorexia, dyspepsia, constipation, cramps, vomiting, taste changes, flatulence, decreased appetite
INTEG: Sweating, rash
RESP: Infection, pharyngitis, nasal congestion, sinus headache, sinusitis, cough, dyspnea
CV: Vasodilation, postural hypotension, palpitations
MS: Pain, arthritis, myalgia, myopathy, myosthenia
GU: Dysmenorrhea, decreased libido, urinary frequency, UTI, amenorrhea, cystitis, impotence, abnormal ejaculation (male)
EENT: Visual changes
SYST: Asthenia, fever
Contraindications: Hypersensitivity, patients taking MAOIs, alcohol use
Precautions: Pregnancy (B), lactation, children, elderly, seizure his-

tory, patients with history of mania, renal and hepatic disease

Do not confuse:

paroxetine/paclitaxel

Paxil/paclitaxel

Paxil/Taxol

Pharmacokinetics:

PO: Peak 5.2 hr; metabolized in liver by CPY50 enzyme system, unchanged drugs and metabolites excreted in feces and urine; half-life 21 hr; protein binding 95%

Interactions:

• ↑ bleeding: warfarin

Do not use with MAOIs, thioridazine potentially fatal reactions can occur

• ↑ paroxetine plasma levels: cimetidine

• ↑ agitation: L-tryptophan

• ↓ paroxetine levels: phenobarbital and phenytoin

• ↑ side effects: highly protein-bound drugs

• Paroxetine may ↓ digoxin levels

• ↑ theophylline levels: theophylline

Possible serotonin syndrome: SAM-e, St. John's wort

↑ anticholinergic effect: corkwood, jimsonweed

Hypertensive crisis: ephedra

↑ sedative: hops, lavender

↑ CNS stimulation: yohimbe

Lab test interferences:

Increase: Serum bilirubin, blood glucose, alk phosphatase

Decrease: VMA, 5-HIAA

False increase: Urinary catecholamines

NURSING CONSIDERATIONS

Assess:

• Mental status: mood, sensorium, affect, suicidal tendencies, increase in psychiatric symptoms, depression, panic

• B/P (lying/standing), pulse q4h; if systolic B/P drops 20 mm Hg, hold drug, notify prescriber; take vital signs q4h in patients with cardiovascular disease

• Blood studies: CBC, leukocytes, differential, cardiac enzymes if patient is receiving long-term therapy

• Hepatic studies: AST, ALT, bilirubin, creatinine

• Weight qwk; appetite may decrease with drug

• ECG for flattening of T wave, bundle branch, AV block, dysrhythmias in cardiac patients

• EPS primarily in elderly: rigidity, dystonia, akathisia

• Urinary retention, constipation

• Withdrawal symptoms: headache, nausea, vomiting, muscle pain, weakness; not usual unless drug discontinued abruptly

• Alcohol intake; if alcohol is consumed, hold dose until morning

Administer:

• Increased fluids, bulk in diet for constipation, urinary retention

• With food, milk for GI symptoms

• Crushed if patient is unable to swallow medication whole

• Dosage hs for oversedation during day; may take entire dose hs; elderly may not tolerate once/day dosing

• Gum, hard candy, frequent sips of water for dry mouth

Perform/provide:

• Storage at room temperature; do not freeze

• Assistance with ambulation during therapy, since drowsiness, dizziness occur

• Safety measures primarily in elderly

• Checking to see if PO medication swallowed

Evaluate:

• Therapeutic response: decreased depression

Teach patient/family:

• That therapeutic effect may take 1-4 wk

• To use caution in driving, other activities requiring alertness because of drowsiness, dizziness, blurred vision

• Not to discontinue medication quickly after long-term use; may cause nausea, headache, malaise

• To avoid alcohol ingestion, other CNS depressants

Treatment of overdose: Airway, for seizures give diazepam, symptomatic treatment

---

HIGH ALERT

pegaspargase (℞)

(peg-as′per-gase)

Oncaspar, PEG-L-asparaginase

Func. class.: Antineoplastic

Chem. class.: Escherichia coli enzyme

Action: Indirectly inhibits protein synthesis in tumor cells; without amino acid, DNA, RNA synthesis is halted; asparagine, protein synthesis is halted; G_1 phase; cell-cycle specific; a nonvesicant; a modified version of L-asparaginase

Uses: Acute lymphocytic leukemia in combination with other antineoplastics

Dosage and routes:

In combination

• *Adult and child with BSA ≥0.6 m²:* **IV/IM** 2500 international units/m² q14d, run **IV** over 1-2 hr in 100 ml of NaCl or D_5 through a running **IV**; **IM** should be no more than 2 ml in one inj site

• *Child with BSA <0.6 m²:* **IV/IM** 82.5 international units/kg q14d

Sole induction

• *Adult:* **IV** 2500 international units/m² q14 days

Available forms: Inj 750 international units/ml in a phosphate buffered saline sol

Side effects/adverse reactions:

SYST: ***Anaphylaxis, hypersensitivity***

HEMA: ***Thrombocytopenia, leukopenia, myelosuppression, anemia, decreased clotting factors, pancytopenia***

GI: Nausea, vomiting, anorexia, cramps, stomatitis, ***hepatotoxicity, pancreatitis,*** *diarrhea*

GU: Urinary retention, ***renal failure,*** glycosuria, polyuria, azotemia, uric acid neuropathy

INTEG: Rash, urticaria, chills, fever

ENDO: Hyperglycemia

RESP: ***Fibrosis, pulmonary infiltrate, severe bronchospasm***

CV: Chest pain, ***hypertension***

CNS: Neuritis, dizziness, headache, ***coma,*** depression, fatigue, confusion, hallucinations, ***seizures***

Contraindications: Hypersensitivity, infant, lactation, pancreatitis

Precautions: Renal disease, hepatic disease, pregnancy (C), CNS disease

Pharmacokinetics: Half-life 5½ days, onset rapid, duration 2 wk, metabolized in reticuloendothelial system

Interactions:

• ↓ action of methotrexate

• Do not use with radiation

• Coagulation factor imbalances: heparin, warfarin, aspirin, NSAIDs

NURSING CONSIDERATIONS

Assess:

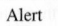

◆ For signs and symptoms of pancreatitis (nausea, vomiting, severe abdominal pain), anaphylaxis (bronchospasm, dyspnea), cyanosis

• CBC, differential, platelet count qwk; withhold drug if WBC count is <4000 or platelet count is <75,000; notify prescriber of results
• Pulmonary function tests, chest x-ray studies before and during therapy; chest x-ray film should be obtained q2wk during treatment, watch for severe bronchospasm, fibrosis, pulmonary infiltrate
• Renal studies: BUN, serum uric acid, ammonia, urine CCr, electrolytes before and during therapy
• I&O ratio; report fall in urine output of 30 ml/hr, may indicate renal failure
• Temp q4h (may indicate beginning infection)
• Hepatic studies before and during therapy (bilirubin, AST, ALT, LDH) as needed or monthly, hepatotoxicity can occur; check for jaundiced skin, sclera; dark urine, clay-colored stools, itchy skin, abdominal pain, fever, diarrhea
• RBC, Hct, Hgb; may be decreased
• Serum, urine glucose levels, glycosuria can occur
• Bleeding: hematuria, stool guaiac, bruising or petechiae, mucosa or orifices q8h
• Dyspnea, rales, nonproductive cough, chest pain, tachypnea, fatigue, increased pulse, pallor, lethargy, swelling around eyes or lips; anaphylaxis may occur
• B/P, since hypertension can occur
• Local irritation, pain, burning, discoloration at inj site
• Symptoms of severe allergic reaction: rash, pruritus, urticaria, purpuric skin lesions, itching, flushing, dyspnea
• Frequency of stools, characteristics; cramping, acidosis; signs of dehydration: rapid respirations, poor skin turgor, decreased urine output, dry skin, restlessness, weakness

Administer:
• Antispasmodic if GI symptoms occur
• Allopurinol or sodium bicarbonate to reduce uric acid levels, alkalinization of urine

IV INF route
• Using 21, 23, 25G needle; administer by slow IV infusion via Y-tube or 3-way stopcock of flowing D_5W or NS infusion over 2 hr after diluting
• Considered incompatible with other drugs in syringe or sol

Perform/provide:
• Deep-breathing exercises with patient tid-qid; place in semi-Fowler's position
• Increase fluid intake to 2-3 L/day to prevent urate deposits, calculi formation
• Diet low in purines: no organ meats (kidney, liver), dried beans, peas to maintain alkaline urine
• Rinsing of mouth tid-qid with water, club soda; brushing of teeth bid-tid with soft brush or cotton-tipped applicator for stomatitis; use unwaxed dental floss
• Warm compresses at inj site for inflammation
• Nutritious diet with iron, vitamin supplements
• HOB raised to facilitate breathing

Evaluate:
• Therapeutic response: decreased exacerbations in acute lymphocytic leukemia

Teach patient/family:
• To report nausea, vomiting, bruising, bleeding, stomatitis, severe diarrhea, jaundice, chest pain, abdominal pain, trouble breathing, rash
• To avoid vaccinations without advice of prescriber
• Not to use hard-bristled toothbrush, razors
• To avoid OTC medications, alcohol

P

Treatment of anaphylaxis: Administer epINEPHrine, diphenhydrAMINE, IV corticosteroids

pegfilgrastim (℞)

(peg-fill-grass′stim)

Neulasta

Func. class.: Hematopoietic agent

Chem. class.: Granulocyte colony-stimulating factor

Action: Stimulates proliferation and differentiation of neutrophils

Uses: To decrease infection in patients receiving antineoplastics that are myelosuppressive; to increase WBC in patients with drug-induced neutropenia

Dosage and routes:

• *Adult:* **SC** 6 mg give once per chemotherapy cycle

Available forms: Sol for inj 10 mg/ml

Side effects/adverse reactions:

RESP: Respiratory distress syndrome

CNS: Fever, fatigue, headache, dizziness, insomnia, peripheral edema

HEMA: ***Leukocytosis, granulocytopenia***

INTEG: Alopecia

MS: Skeletal pain

GI: Nausea, vomiting, diarrhea, mucositis, anorexia, constipation, dyspepsia, abdominal pain, stomatitis

Contraindications: Hypersensitivity to proteins of *E. coli,* filgrastim; ARDS

Precautions: Pregnancy (C), lactation, children, myeloid malignancies, sickle cell disease

Pharmacokinetics: Half life: 15-80 hr

Interactions:

• Do not use this drug concomitantly or 2 wk before or 24 hr after administration of cytotoxic chemotherapy

• ↑ release of neutrophils: lithium

Lab test interferences:

Increase: Uric acid, LDH, alk phosphatase

NURSING CONSIDERATIONS

Assess:

◆ Allergic reactions, anaphylaxis: rash, urticaria; discontinue this drug, have emergency equipment nearby

• Blood studies: CBC, platelet count before treatment and twice weekly; neutrophil counts may be increased for 2 days after therapy

• B/P, respirations, pulse before and during therapy

• Bone pain, give mild analgesics

Administer:

• Using single-use vials; after dose is withdrawn, do not reenter vial

• Do not use 6 mg fixed dose in infants, children, or others <45 kg

• Inspect sol for discoloration, particulates; if present, do not use

• Do not administer in the period 14 days before and 24 hr after cytotoxic chemotherapy

Perform/provide:

• Storage in refrigerator; do not freeze; may store at room temperature up to 6 hr, avoid shaking, protect from light

Evaluate:

• Therapeutic response: absence of infection

Teach patient/family:

• The technique for self-administration: dose, side effects, disposal of containers and needles; provide instruction sheet

peginterferon alfa-2a (℞)

(peg-in-ter-feer'on)
Pegasys
Func. class.: Immunomodulator

Action: Stimulates genes to modulate many biologic effects, including inhibition of viral replication; inhibits ion cell proliferation, immunomodulation, stimulates effector proteins, decreases leukocyte, platelet counts
Uses: Chronic hepatitis C infections in adults with compensated liver disease
Dosage and routes:
• *Adult:* **SC** 180 mcg qwk × 48 wk; if poorly tolerated, reduce dose to 135 mcg qwk; in some cases reduction to 90 mcg may be needed
Available forms: Inj 180 mcg/ml
Side effects/adverse reactions:
CNS: Headache, insomnia, dizziness, anxiety, hostility, lability, nervousness, depression, fatigue, poor concentration, pyrexia
GI: Abdominal pain, nausea, diarrhea, anorexia, vomiting, dry mouth
MS: Back pain, myalgia, arthralgia
INTEG: Alopecia, pruritus, rash, dermatitis
HEMA: ***Thrombocytopenia,*** neutropenia
Contraindications: Hypersensitivity to interferons, neonates, infants, autoimmune hepatitis, decompensated hepatic disease prior to use of this drug
Precautions: Thyroid disorders, myelosuppression, hepatic, cardiac disease, lactation, children <18 yr, depression/suicide, preexisting ophthalmologic disorders, pancreatitis, renal disease, pregnancy (C), elderly
Pharmacokinetics: Half-life 15-80 hr, large variability in other pharmacokinetics
Interactions:
• Use caution when giving with theophylline, myelosuppressive agents
NURSING CONSIDERATIONS
Assess:
• ALT, HCV viral load; patients who show no reduction in ALT, HCV are unlikely to show benefit of treatment after 6 mo
• Platelet counts, heme concentration, ANC, serum creatinine concentration, albumin, bilirubin, TSH, T_4, AFP
• For myelosuppression, hold dose if neutrophil count is $<500 \times 10^6$/L or if platelets are $<50 \times 10^9$/L
• For hypersensitivity: discontinue immediately if hypersensitivity occurs
Evaluate:
• Therapeutic response: decreased chronic hepatitis C signs/symptoms, undetectable viral load
Teach patient/family:
• Provide patient or family member with written, detailed information about drug
• Instructions for home use if appropriate
• Take in evening to reduce discomfort, sleep through some side effects

pegvisomant

See appendix a—selected new drugs

pemoline (℞)

(pem'oh-leen)
Cylert, Pem ADD, pemoline
Func. class.: Cerebral stimulant
Chem. class.: Oxazolidinone derivative

P

Controlled Substance Schedule IV
Action: Exact mechanism unknown; may act through dopaminergic mechanisms; produces CNS stimulation and a paradoxic effect in ADHD
Uses: Attention deficit hyperactivity disorder when other treatment has failed
Investigational uses: Narcolepsy, fatigue, excessive daytime sleepiness
Dosage and routes:
- *Child >6 yr:* **PO** 37.5 mg in AM, increasing by 18.75 mg/wk, not to exceed 112.5 mg/day

Available forms: Tabs 18.75, 37.5, 75 mg; chewable tabs 37.5 mg
Side effects/adverse reactions:
MISC: Rashes, growth suppression in children
CNS: Hyperactivity, insomnia, restlessness, dizziness, depression, headache, stimulation, irritability, aggressiveness, hallucinations, ***seizures, masking or worsening of Gilles de la Tourette's syndrome,*** drowsiness, dyskinetic movements
GI: Nausea, anorexia, diarrhea, abdominal pain, increased liver enzymes, ***hepatitis,*** jaundice, weight loss, ***life-threatening hepatic failure***
CV: Tachycardia
Contraindications: Hypersensitivity, hepatic insufficiency
Precautions: Renal disease, pregnancy (B), lactation, drug abuse, child <6 yr, psychosis, tics, seizure disorder
Pharmacokinetics:
PO: Peak 2-4 hr, duration 8 hr, metabolized (50%) by liver, excreted (40%) by kidneys, half-life 10-30 hr
Interactions:
- ↑ CNS stimulation: other CNS stimulants
- ↓ seizure threshold: anticonvulsants

↑ CNS stimulation: horsetail, yohimbe
Synergistic effect: melatonin

NURSING CONSIDERATIONS
Assess:
- For attention span, decreased hyperactivity in ADHD persons
- Hepatic studies: ALT, AST, bilirubin; renal, creatinine, prior to treatment and periodically thereafter; if life-threatening, hepatic failure has occurred; discontinue drug if hepatic symptoms occur
- Height, growth rate q3mo in child; growth rate may be decreased
- Mental status: mood, sensorium, affect, stimulation, insomnia, aggressiveness

PO route
- In AM

Evaluate:
- Therapeutic response: decreased hyperactivity

Teach patient/family:
- To decrease caffeine consumption (coffee, tea, cola, chocolate); may increase irritability, stimulation
- To avoid OTC preparations unless approved by prescriber
- To withdraw over several wk
- To avoid alcohol ingestion
- To avoid hazardous activities until patient is stabilized
- That therapeutic effect may take 2-4 wk
- To notify prescriber if tremors, insomnia, palpitations, restlessness, jaundice, bleeding, dark urine occur
- Regarding the possibility of hepatotoxicity and need for blood work

penciclovir topical
See appendix c

PENICILLINS

penicillin G benzathine (℞)

(pen-i-sill'in)

Bicillin L-A, Megacillin✤, Permapen

penicillin G (℞)

Penicillin G Potassium, Pfizerpen

penicillin G procaine (℞)

Ayercillin✤, Wycillin

penicillin V potassium (℞)

Apo-Pen-VK✤, Beepen-VK, Nadopen-V✤, Novopen-VK✤, Pen-Vee K✤, PVF K✤, Veetids

Func. class.: Broad-spectrum antiinfective

Chem. class.: Natural penicillin

Action: Interferes with cell wall replication of susceptible organisms; osmotically unstable cell wall swells, bursts from osmotic pressure, results in cell death

Uses: Respiratory infections, scarlet fever, erysipelas, otitis media, pneumonia, skin and soft tissue infections, gonorrhea; effective for gram-positive cocci *(Staphylococcus, Streptococcus pyogenes, S. viridans, S. faecalis, S. bovis, S. pneumoniae)*, gram-negative cocci *(Neisseria gonorrhoeae)*, gram-positive bacilli *(Actinomyces, Bacillus anthracis, Clostridium perfringens, C. tetani, Corynebacterium diphtheriae, Listeria monocytogenes)*, gram-negative bacilli *(Escherichia coli, Proteus mirabilis, Salmonella, Shigella, Enterobacter, Streptobacillus moniliformis)*, spirochetes *(Treponema pallidum)*

Dosage and routes:

Penicillin G benzathine

Early syphilis

- *Adult:* **IM** 2.4 million units in single dose

Congenital syphilis

- *Child <2 yr:* **IM** 50,000 units/kg in single dose

Prophylaxis of rheumatic fever, glomerulonephritis

- *Adult and child:* **IM** 1.2 million units in single dose qmo or 600,000 units q2wk

Upper respiratory infections (group A streptococcal)

- *Adult:* **IM** 1.2 million units in single dose
- *Child >27 kg:* **IM** 900,000 units in single dose
- *Child <27 kg:* **IM** 300,000-600,000 g in single dose

Available forms: Inj 300,000 units/ml; 600,000; 1,200,000; 2,400,000 units/dose

Penicillin G

- Dosage reduction indicated in renal impairment (CCr <50 ml/min)

Pneumococcal/streptococcal infections (serious)

- *Adult:* **IM/IV** 5-24 million units in divided doses q4-6h
- *Child <12 yr:* **IV** 150,000 units/kg/day in 4-6 divided doses

Available forms: Powder for inj 1, 5, 20 million units/vial; inj 1, 2, 3 million units/50 ml

Penicillin G procaine

Renal dose

- CCr 10-30 ml/min give q8-12h; CCr <10 ml/min give q12-18h

Moderate to severe infections

- *Adult and child:* **IM** 600,000-1.2 million units in 1 or 2 doses/day for 10 days to 2 wk
- *Newborn:* 50,000 units/kg **IM** once daily (avoid use in newborns)

Gonorrhea
• *Adult and child >12 yr:* **IM** 4.8 million units in two inj given 30 min after probenecid 1 g
Pneumococcal pneumonia
• *Adult and child >12 yr:* **IM** 600,000-1.2 million units/day × 7-10 days
Available forms: Inj 300,000, 500,000, 600,000, 1,200,000, 2,400,000 units/unit dose
Penicillin V potassium
• Dosage reduction indicated in renal impairment (CCr <50 ml/min)
Pneumococcal/staphylococcal infections
• *Adult:* **PO** 250-500 mg q6h
• *Child <12 yr:* **PO** 25-50 mg/kg/day in divided doses q6-8h
Streptococcal infections
• *Adult:* **PO** 125-250 mg q6-8h × 10 days
Prevention of recurrence of rheumatic fever/chorea
• *Adult:* **PO** 125 mg bid continuously
• *Child <5 yr:* **PO** 125 mg bid
• *Child >5 yr:* **PO** 250 mg bid
Vincent's gingivitis/pharyngitis
• *Adult:* **PO** 250 mg q6-8h
Available forms: Tabs 125, 250, 500 mg; powder for oral sol 125, 250 mg/5 ml

Side effects/adverse reactions:
HEMA: Anemia; increased bleeding time; ***bone marrow depression, granulocytopenia***
GI: Nausea, vomiting, diarrhea, increased AST, ALT, abdominal pain, glossitis, colitis
GU: ***Oliguria, proteinuria, hematuria,*** *vaginitis, moniliasis,* ***glomerulonephritis***
CNS: Lethargy, hallucinations, anxiety, depression, twitching, ***coma, seizures***
META: Hyperkalemia, hypokalemia, alkalosis, hypernatremia
MISC: ***Anaphylaxis, serum sickness,*** *local pain,* tenderness and fever with IM inj

Contraindications: Hypersensitivity to penicillins; neonates

Precautions: Hypersensitivity to cephalosporins, pregnancy (B), lactation, severe renal disease

Pharmacokinetics:
Penicillin G benzathine
IM: Very slow absorption, duration 21-28 days, half-life 30-60 min; excreted in urine, feces, breast milk; crosses placenta
Penicillin G
IV: Peak immediate
IM: Peak ¼-½ hr
PO: Peak 1 hr, duration 6 hr
Excreted in urine unchanged, excreted in breast milk, crosses placenta, half-life 30-60 min
Penicillin G procaine
IM: Peak 1-4 hr, duration 15 hr, excreted in urine
Penicillin V potassium
PO: Peak 30-60 min, duration 6-8 hr, half-life 30 min, excreted in urine, breast milk

Interactions:
• ↓ antimicrobial effect of penicillin: tetracyclines
• ↑ penicillin concentrations: aspirin, probenecid
• ↓ effect of oral contraceptives
• ↑ effect of heparin
↓ absorption of penicillin: khat
Do not use acidophilus with antiinfectives

Lab test interferences:
False positive: Urine glucose, urine protein

NURSING CONSIDERATIONS
Assess:
• For infection: temp, characteristics of sputum, wounds, urine, stools before, during, and after treatment
• I&O ratio; report hematuria, oliguria, since penicillin in high doses is nephrotoxic

⬥ Any patient with compromised renal system, since drug is excreted slowly in poor renal system function; toxicity may occur rapidly
• Hepatic studies: AST, ALT
• Blood studies: WBC, RBC, Hct, Hgb, bleeding time
• Renal tests: urinalysis, protein, blood
• C&S before therapy; drug may be given as soon as culture is taken
• Bowel pattern before and during treatment
• Skin eruptions after administration of penicillin to 1 wk after discontinuing drug
• Respiratory status: rate, character, wheezing, tightness in chest
⬥ Allergies before initiation of treatment, reaction of each medication; because of prolonged action, allergic reaction may be prolonged and severe; watch for anaphylaxis: rash, dyspnea, pruritus, laryngeal edema

Administer:

Penicillin G benzathine
• Drug after C&S completed
• After shaking well, deep IM inj in large muscle mass; avoid intravascular inj, aspirate

Penicillin G
• Drug after C&S

Solution compatibility: Sterile H_2O for inj

Additive compatibilities: Ascorbic acid, calcium chloride, calcium gluconate, cephapirin, chloramphenicol, cimetidine, clindamycin, colistimethate, corticotropin, dimenhyDRINATE, diphenhydrAMINE, epHEDrine, erythromycin, furosemide, hydrocortisone, kanamycin, lidocaine, magnesium sulfate, methicillin, methylprednisolone, metronidazole, polymyxin B, predniso-LONE, potassium chloride, procaine, prochlorperazine, ranitidine, verapamil

Syringe compatibilities: Heparin

Y-site compatibilities: Acyclovir, amiodarone, cyclophosphamide, diltiazem, enalaprilat, esmolol, fluconazole, foscarnet, heparin, hydromorphone, labetalol, magnesium sulfate, meperidine, morphine, perphenazine, potassium chloride, tacrolimus, theophylline, verapamil, vit B/C

Penicillin G procaine
• Drug after C&S
• Deep IM inj avoid intravascular inj, aspirate

Penicillin V potassium
• Orally on empty stomach for best absorption
• Drug after C&S

Perform/provide:
• Adrenaline, suction, tracheostomy set, endotracheal intubation equipment
• Adequate fluid intake (2 L) during diarrhea episodes
• Scratch test to assess allergy after securing order from prescriber; usually done when penicillin is only drug of choice
• Storage in dry, tight container; oral susp refrigerated 2 wk, 1 wk at room temperature

Evaluate:
• Therapeutic response: absence of fever, draining wounds
• Allergies before initiation of treatment, reaction of each medication; highlight allergies on chart; hypersensitivity reaction may be delayed

Teach patient/family:
• To report sore throat, fever, fatigue; may indicate superinfection
• To wear or carry emergency ID if allergic to penicillins
• To report diarrhea, prevent dehydration
• To shake susp well before each dose; store in refrigerator for up to 2 wk

• To use all medication prescribed
• To use additional contraception if using any of these drugs

Treatment of anaphylaxis: Withdraw drug; maintain airway; administer epINEPHrine, aminophylline, O_2, IV corticosteroids

pentamidine (℞)

(pen-tam′i-deen)

Nebupent, Pentam 300, Pentacarinat*, Pneumopent*

Func. class.: Antiprotozoal

Chem. class.: Aromatic diamide derivative

Action: Interferes with DNA/RNA synthesis in protozoa

Uses: Treatment/prevention of *Pneumocystis carinii* infections

Dosage and routes:

• *Adult and child:* **IV/IM** 4 mg/kg/day × 2-3 wk; **NEB** 300 mg via specific nebulizer given q4wk for prevention

Available forms: Inj, aerosol 300 mg/vial; sol for aerosol 60 mg/vial*

Side effects/adverse reactions:

CV: Hypotension, ventricular tachycardia, ECG abnormalities, ***dysrhythmias***

HEMA: Anemia, ***leukopenia, thrombocytopenia***

INTEG: Sterile abscess, pain at injection site, pruritus, urticaria, *rash*

GU: ***Acute renal failure, increased serum creatinine, renal toxicity***

GI: Nausea, vomiting, anorexia; increased AST, ALT; ***acute pancreatitis,*** metallic taste

CNS: Disorientation, hallucinations, *dizziness,* confusion

RESP: Cough, shortness of breath, ***bronchospasm*** (with aerosol)

MISC: Fatigue, chills, night sweats, ***anaphylaxis, Stevens-Johnson syndrome***

META: Hyperkalemia, hypocalcemia, hypoglycemia

Precautions: Blood dyscrasias, hepatic disease, renal disease, diabetes mellitus, cardiac disease, hypocalcemia, pregnancy (C), hypertension, hypotension, lactation, children

Pharmacokinetics: Excreted unchanged in urine (66%)

Interactions:

• Nephrotoxicity: aminoglycosides, amphotericin B, colistin, cisplatin, foscarnet, methoxyflurane, polymyxin B, vancomycin

Fatal dysrhythmias: erythromycin IV

• ↑ myelosuppression: antineoplastics, radiation

NURSING CONSIDERATIONS

Assess:

• Blood tests, blood glucose, CBC, platelets, calcium, magnesium
• I&O ratio; report hematuria, oliguria
• ECG for cardiac dysrhythmias
• Patient should be lying down when receiving drug; severe hypotension may develop; monitor B/P during administration and until B/P stable

Any patient with compromised renal system; drug is excreted slowly in poor renal system function; toxicity may occur rapidly

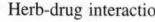

• Hepatic studies: AST, ALT
• Renal studies: urinalysis, BUN, creatinine; nephrotoxicity may occur
• Signs of infection, anemia
• Bowel pattern before, during treatment
• Sterile abscess, pain at inj site
• Respiratory status: rate, character, wheezing, dyspnea
• Dizziness, confusion, hallucination
• Allergies before treatment, reaction of each medication; place allergies on chart in bright red letters; notify all people giving drugs

Administer:

INH route

• Through nebulizer; mix contents in 6 ml of sterile H_2O; do not use low pressure (<20 psi); flow rate should be 5-7 L/min (40-50 psi) air or O_2 source over 30-45 min until chamber is empty

IM route

• 300 mg diluted in 3 ml sterile H_2O; give deep IM by Z-track; painful by this route

IV route

• Reconstitute 300 mg/3-5 ml of sterile water for inj, D_5W, withdraw dose and further dilute in 50-250 ml D_5W, give over 1-2 hr

Y-site compatibilities: Diltiazem, zidovudine

Perform/provide:

• Storage in refrigerator protected from light

Evaluate:

• Therapeutic response: decreased temp, increased ability to breathe

Teach patient/family:

• To report sore throat, fever, fatigue (may indicate superinfection)
• To maintain adequate fluid intake

HIGH ALERT

pentazocine (℞)

(pen-taz'oh-seen)

Talwin, Talwin NX

Func. class.: Opiate analgesic, antagonist

Chem. class.: Synthetic benzomorphan

Controlled Substance Schedule IV

Action: Inhibits ascending pain pathways in CNS, increases pain threshold, alters pain perception

Uses: Moderate to severe pain

Dosage and routes:

• *Adult:* **PO** 50-100 mg q3-4h prn, not to exceed 600 mg/day; **IV/IM/SC** 30 mg q3-4h prn, not to exceed 360 mg/day

Labor

• *Adult:* **IM** 60 mg; **IV** 30 mg q2-3h when contractions are regular

Renal dose

• CCr 10-50 ml/min give q24-36h; CCr <10 ml/min give q48h

Available forms: Inj 30 mg/ml; tabs 50 mg

Side effects/adverse reactions:

CNS: Drowsiness, dizziness, confusion, headache, sedation, euphoria, hallucinations, dreaming

GI: Nausea, vomiting, anorexia, constipation, *cramps,* dry mouth

GU: Increased urinary output, dysuria, urinary retention

INTEG: Rash, urticaria, bruising, flushing, diaphoresis, pruritus, severe irritation at inj sites

EENT: Tinnitus, blurred vision, miosis, diplopia

CV: Palpitations, bradycardia, change in B/P, tachycardia, increased B/P (high doses)

RESP: ***Respiratory depression***

Contraindications: Hypersensitivity, addiction (opiate)

Precautions: Addictive personality, pregnancy (C), lactation, increased intracranial pressure, MI (acute), severe heart disease, respiratory depression, hepatic disease, renal disease, seizure disorder, child <18 yr, head trauma

Pharmacokinetics:

SC/IM: Onset 15-30 min, peak 1-2 hr, duration 2-4 hr

IV: Onset 2-3 min, duration 4-6 hr

Metabolized by liver, excreted by kidneys, crosses placenta, half-life 2-3 hr, extensive first-pass metabolism with less than 20% entering circulation

Interactions:

⬥ Unpredictable reactions: MAOIs
• ↑ effects: CNS depressants; alco-

P

hol, sedative/hypnotics, antipsychotics, skeletal muscle relaxants
• ↓ effects: opiates

Lab test interferences:
Increase: Amylase

NURSING CONSIDERATIONS
Assess:
• For pain: intensity, duration, location prior to and 1 hr after dose
• I&O ratio; check for decreasing output; may indicate urinary retention
• For withdrawal symptoms in opiate-dependent patients
• Pulmonary embolism, abscesses, ulcerations, vascular occlusion, WBC
• CNS changes: dizziness, drowsiness, hallucinations, euphoria, LOC, pupil reaction
• Allergic reactions: rash, urticaria
• Respiratory dysfunction: respiratory depression, character, rate, rhythm; notify prescriber if respirations are <10/min
• Need for pain medication, physical dependence

Administer:
• With antiemetic if nausea, vomiting occur
• When pain is beginning to return; determine dosage interval by patient response

SC/IM route
• Give IM deeply into large muscle mass, rotate sites; SC may cause necrosis with repeated inj

IV route
• Undiluted or diluted 5 mg/ml of sterile H_2O for inj; give 5 mg or less over 1 min

Syringe compatibilities: Atropine, benzquinamide, butorphanol, chlorproMAZINE, cimetidine, dimenhyDRINATE, diphenhydrAMINE, droperidol, fentanyl, hydromorphone, hydrOXYzine, meperidine, metoclopramide, morphine, perphenazine, prochlorperazine, promazine, promethazine, ranitidine, scopolamine

Y-site compatibilities: Heparin, hydrocortisone, potassium chloride, vit B/C

Perform/provide:
• Storage in light-resistant area at room temperature
• Assistance with ambulation
• Safety measures: night-light, call bell within easy reach

Evaluate:
• Therapeutic response: decrease in pain

Teach patient/family:
• To report any symptoms of CNS changes, allergic reactions
• That physical dependency may result from extended use
• That withdrawal symptoms may occur: nausea, vomiting, cramps, fever, faintness, anorexia

Treatment of overdose: Naloxone (Narcan) 0.2-0.8 mg IV, O_2, IV fluids, vasopressors

HIGH ALERT

pentobarbital (℞)

(pen-toe-bar′bi-tal)
Nembutal, Novopentobarb🍁, Nova-Rectal🍁, pentobarbital sodium

Func. class.: Sedative/hypnotic barbiturate; anticonvulsant
Chem. class.: Barbitone, short acting

Controlled Substance Schedule II (USA), Schedule G (Canada)

Action: Depresses activity in brain cells, primarily in reticular activating system in brain stem; selectively depresses neurons in posterior hypothalamus, limbic structures

Uses: Insomnia, sedation, preoperative medication, increased intracranial pressure, dental anesthetic

Dosage and routes:

Insomnia

- *Adult:* **PO** 100-200 mg hs; **IM** 150-200 mg hs; **IV** 100 mg initially, then up to 500 mg; **RECT** 120-200 mg hs
- *Child:* **IM** 2-6 mg/kg, not to exceed 100 mg; **PO** 2-6 mg/kg/day in divided doses; **PO** preoperatively 2-6 mg/kg, max 100 mg/dose; **IV** 100 mg (hypnotic/anticonvulsant)

Available forms: Caps 50, 100 mg; elix 20 mg/5 ml; rect supp 25, 30, 50, 60, 120, 200 mg; inj 50 mg/ml

Side effects/adverse reactions:

CNS: Lethargy, drowsiness, hangover, dizziness, paradoxical stimulation in elderly and children, lightheadedness, dependence, ***CNS depression,*** mental depression, slurred speech

GI: Nausea, vomiting, diarrhea, constipation

INTEG: Rash, urticaria, pain, abscesses at inj site, angioedema, thrombophlebitis, ***Stevens-Johnson syndrome***

CV: Hypotension, bradycardia

RESP: ***Respiratory depression, apnea, laryngospasm, bronchospasm***

HEMA: ***Agranulocytosis, thrombocytopenia, megaloblastic anemia*** (long-term treatment)

Contraindications: Hypersensitivity to barbiturates, pregnancy (D), respiratory depression, addiction to barbiturates; severe liver, renal impairment; porphyria, uncontrolled pain

Precautions: Anemia, lactation, hepatic disease, renal disease, hypertension, elderly, acute/chronic pain

Do not confuse:

pentobarbital/phenobarbital

Pharmacokinetics:

PO: Onset 15-30 min, duration 4-6 hr

RECT: Onset slow, duration 4-6 hr

Metabolized by liver, excreted by kidneys (metabolites); half-life 15-48 hr

Interactions:

- ↑ CNS depression: alcohol, MAOIs, sedatives, other CNS depressants, antihistamines, opiates
- ↓ effect of oral anticoagulants, corticosteroids, griseofulvin, quinidine
- ↑ half-life of doxycycline

↑ pentobarbital levels: eucalyptus, Jamaican dogwood, kava, lemon balm nettle, pill-bearing spurge, poppy, quinine, senega, valerian

Lab test interferences:

False increase: Sulfobromophthalein

NURSING CONSIDERATIONS

Assess:

- VS q30min after parenteral route for 2 hr
- Blood studies: Hct, Hgb, RBCs, serum folate, vit D (long-term therapy); PT in patients receiving anticoagulants
- Hepatic studies: AST, ALT, bilirubin; if increased, drug is usually discontinued
- Mental status: mood, sensorium, affect, memory (long, short)
- Physical dependency: more frequent requests for medication, shakes, anxiety

Barbiturate toxicity: hypotension; pupillary constriction; cold, clammy skin; cyanosis of lips; insomnia; nausea; vomiting; hallucinations; delirium; weakness; coma; mild symptoms may occur in 8-12 hr without drug

- Respiratory changes: respiratory depression, character, rate, rhythm; hold drug if respirations are <10/min or if pupils are dilated
- Blood dyscrasias: fever, sore throat, bruising, rash, jaundice, epistaxis

P

Administer:
• For <14 days, since not effective after that; tolerance develops
• After removal of cigarettes to prevent fires
• After trying conservative measures for insomnia

PO route
• Use elixir alone or diluted in fluids
• ½-1 hr before hs for sleeplessness
• On empty stomach for best absorption
• Crushed or whole
• Alone; do not mix with other drugs or inject if there is precipitate

IM route
• Inj deep in large muscle mass to prevent tissue sloughing and abscesses; do not inject more than 5 ml in one site

IV route
• IV undiluted or dilute in sterile H_2O, LR, NaCl, give 50 mg or less/min; titrate to patient response; use only clear sol; avoid extravasation
• IV only with resuscitative equipment available; administer at <100 mg/min (only by qualified personnel)

Additive compatibilities: Amikacin, aminophylline, calcium chloride, cephapirin, chloramphenicol, dimenhyDRINATE, erythromycin lactobionate, lidocaine, thiopental, verapamil

Syringe compatibilities: Aminophylline, epHEDrine, hydromorphone, neostigmine, scopolamine, sodium bicarbonate, thiopental

Y-site compatibilities: Acyclovir, insulin (regular), propofol

Perform/provide:
• Assistance with ambulation after receiving dose
• Safety measures: night-light, call bell within easy reach
• Checking to see if PO medication has been swallowed
• Storage of suppositories in refrigerator; do not use aqueous solutions that contain precipitate

Evaluate:
• Therapeutic response: ability to sleep at night, less early morning awakening if taking drug for insomnia, or decrease in number, severity of seizures if taking drug for seizure disorder

Teach patient/family:
• That hangover is common
• That drug is indicated only for short-term treatment of insomnia; probably ineffective after 2 wk
• That physical dependency may result from extended use (45-90 days depending on dose)
• To avoid driving, other activities requiring alertness
• To avoid alcohol ingestion, CNS depressants; serious CNS depression may result
• Not to discontinue medication quickly after long-term use; drug should be tapered over 1-2 wk
• To tell all prescribers that a barbiturate is being taken
• That withdrawal insomnia may occur after short-term use; not to start using drug again; insomnia will improve in 1-3 nights
• That effects may take 2 nights for benefits to be noticed
• Alternative measures to improve sleep (reading, exercise several hr before hs, warm bath, warm milk, TV, self-hypnosis, deep breathing)

Treatment of overdose: Lavage, activated charcoal, warming blanket, vital signs, hemodialysis, I&O ratio

HIGH ALERT

pentostatin (℞)

(pen-toh-stat′in)

Nipent

Func. class.: Antineoplastic, enzyme inhibitor

Chem. class.: Streptomyces antibioticus derivative

Action: Inhibits the enzyme adenosine deaminase (ADA), which is able to block DNA synthesis and some RNA synthesis

Uses: α-Interferon-refractory hairy cell leukemia, chronic lymphocytic leukemia

Dosage and routes:

- *Adult:* **IV** 4 mg/m^2 every other wk; may be given **IV BOL,** or diluted in a larger volume and given over 20-30 min

Available forms: Inj 10 mg/vial

Side effects/adverse reactions:

CNS: Headache, anxiety, confusion, depression, dizziness, insomnia, nervousness, paresthesia

RESP: Cough, upper respiratory infection, bronchitis, dyspnea, epistaxis, pneumonia, pharyngitis, rhinitis, sinusitis

SYST: Fever, infection, fatigue, pain, allergic reaction, chills, ***death, sepsis,*** chest pain, flulike symptoms

HEMA: ***Leukopenia, anemia, thrombocytopenia,*** *ecchymosis,* ***lymphadenopathy,*** petechiae

GI: Nausea, vomiting, anorexia, diarrhea, constipation, flatulence, stomatitis, elevated LFTs

INTEG: Rash, eczema, dry skin, pruritus, sweating, herpes simplex/zoster

GU: ***Hematuria,*** dysuria, increased BUN/creatinine

Contraindications: Hypersensitivity to this drug or mannitol, pregnancy (D)

Precautions: Renal disease, lactation, children, bone marrow depression

Pharmacokinetics:

IV: Elimination half-life 5.7 hr, low protein binding, 90% excreted in urine unchanged or as metabolites

Interactions:

⬥ Fatal pulmonary toxicity: fludarabine

- ↑ adverse reactions: vidarabine

Lab test interferences:

Increase: Uric acid

NURSING CONSIDERATIONS

Assess:

- CBC, differential, platelet count qwk; withhold drug if WBC is <2000/mm^3 or platelet count is <75,000/mm^3; notify prescriber
- Renal studies; BUN, serum uric acid, urine CCr, electrolytes before, during therapy
- I&O ratio; report fall in urine output to <30 ml/hr
- Monitor temp q4h; fever may indicate beginning infection
- Hepatic studies before, during therapy: bilirubin, AST, ALT, alk phosphatase, prn or qmo; check for jaundiced skin and sclera, dark urine, clay-colored stools, itchy skin, abdominal pain, fever, diarrhea
- Bleeding: hematuria, guaiac stools, bruising, petechiae, mucosa or orifices q8h
- Effects of alopecia on body image; discuss feelings about body changes
- Inflammation of mucosa, breaks in skin
- Buccal cavity q8h for dryness, sores, ulceration, white patches, oral pain, bleeding, dysphagia
- Local irritation, pain, burning at inj site

P

• Symptoms of severe allergic reaction: rash, pruritus, urticaria, purpuric skin lesions, itching, flushing
• GI symptoms: frequency of stools, cramping
• Acidosis, signs of dehydration; rapid respiration, poor skin turgor, decreased urine output, dry skin, restlessness, weakness

Administer:
• Antiemetic 30-60 min before giving drug to prevent vomiting
• Antibiotics as ordered for prophylaxis of infection

IV route
• After diluting, use with 5 ml sterile H_2O for injection and mix thoroughly (2 mg/ml); may be given by bolus or diluted in 25-50 ml 5% dextrose, or 0.9% NaCl (0.33 or 0.18 mg/ml)

Solution compatibilities: D_5W, 0.9% NaCl, LR

Y-site compatibilities: Fludarabine, melphalan, ondansetron, paclitaxel, sargramostim

Perform/provide:
• Hydrocortisone, sodium thiosulfate to infiltration area, and ice compress after stopping infusion
• Strict hand-washing technique, gloves, protective covering
• Liquid diet: carbonated beverages; gelatin may be added if patient is not nauseated or vomiting
• Rinsing of mouth tid-qid with water, club soda; brushing of teeth bid-qid with soft brush or cotton-tipped applicators for stomatitis; use unwaxed dental floss
• Storage in refrigerator; reconstituted or diluted sol may be stored at room temperature up to 8 hr

Evaluate:
• Therapeutic response: decrease in tumor size, spread of malignancy

Teach patient/family:
• To report any complaints, side effects to nurse or prescriber
• That hair may be lost during treatment and wig or hairpiece may make patient feel better; tell patient that new hair may be different in color, texture
• To avoid foods with citric acid, hot or rough texture
• To report any bleeding, white spots, ulcerations in mouth to prescriber; tell patient to examine mouth qd
• To avoid crowds and sources of infection when granulocyte count is low

pentoxifylline (℞)

(pen-tox′ih-fill-in)

Trental

Func. class.: Hemorrheologic agent

Chem. class.: Dimethylxanthine derivative

Action: Decreases blood viscosity, stimulates prostacyclin formation, increases blood flow by increasing flexibility of RBCs; decreases RBC hyperaggregation; reduces platelet aggregation, decreases fibrinogen concentration

Uses: Intermittent claudication related to chronic occlusive vascular disease

Investigational uses: Cerebrovascular insufficiency, diabetic neuropathies, TIAs, leg ulcers, strokes, aphthous stomatitis

Dosage and routes:
• *Adult:* **PO** 400 mg tid with meals

Stomatitis (off-label)
• *Adult:* **PO** 400 mg tid × 1-6 mo

Available forms: Tabs, cont release 400 mg; tab ext rel 400 mg

Side effects/adverse reactions:

MISC: Epistaxis, flulike symptoms, laryngitis, nasal congestion, ***leukopenia,*** malaise, weight changes

EENT: Blurred vision, earache, increased salivation, sore throat, conjunctivitis
CNS: Headache, anxiety, *tremors,* confusion, *dizziness*
GI: Dyspepsia, nausea, vomiting, anorexia, bloating, belching, constipation, cholecystitis, dry mouth, thirst, bad taste
INTEG: Rash, pruritus, urticaria, brittle fingernails
CV: Angina, dysrhythmias, palpitation, hypotension, chest pain, dyspnea, edema
Contraindications: Hypersensitivity to this drug or xanthines, retinal/cerebral hemorrhage
Precautions: Pregnancy (C), angina pectoris, cardiac disease, lactation, children, impaired renal function, recent surgery, peptic ulceration
Pharmacokinetics:
PO: Peak 1 hr, half-life ½-1 hr, degradation in liver, excreted in urine
Interactions:
• ↑ risk of bleeding: warfarin, salicylates, NSAIDs, thrombolytics, plicamycin, valproic acid
• ↑ theophylline level: theophylline
• ↑ hypotension: antihypertensives, nitrates
↑ bleeding potential: anise, arnica, chamomile, clove, dong quai, fenugreek, feverfew, garlic, ginger, ginkgo, ginseng *(Panax),* licorice
NURSING CONSIDERATIONS
Assess:
• B/P, respirations of patient also taking antihypertensives; intermittent claudication baseline and throughout
Administer:
• With meals to prevent GI upset
Do not break, crush, or chew ext rel tabs
Evaluate:
• Therapeutic response: decreased pain, cramping, increased ambulation
Teach patient/family:
• That therapeutic response may take 2-4 wk
• To observe feet for arterial insufficiency
• To use cotton socks, well-fitted shoes; not to go barefoot
• To watch for bleeding, bruises, petechiae, epistaxis
• To avoid smoking, to prevent blood vessel constriction

RARELY USED

perflutren lipid microsphere (℞)

(per-flu'tren)
Definity
Func. class.: Diagnostic drug

Uses: Contrast enhancement during echocardiographic procedures
Dosage and routes:
Use only after activation in the Vialmix apparatus
• *Adult:* **IV BOL** 10 μl/kg of the activated product within 30-60 sec, followed by 10-ml saline flush, may repeat
• *Adult:* **IV INF** 1.3 ml/50 ml preservative-free saline, give at 4 ml/min, not to exceed 10 ml/min
Contraindications: Hypersensitivity to octafluoropropane, known cardiac shunts, administration by direct intraarterial inj

perindopril (℞)

(per-in'doe-pril)

Aceon

Func. class.: Antihypertensive

Chem. class.: Angiotensin-converting enzyme inhibitor

Action: Selectively suppresses renin-angiotensin-aldosterone system; inhibits ACE; prevents conversion of angiotensin I to angiotensin II, dilation of arterial, venous vessels

Uses: Hypertension

Dosage and routes:

Hypertension

• *Adult:* **PO** 4 mg/day, may increase or decrease to desired response range 4-8 mg/day; may give in 2 divided doses or as a single dose

Patients on diuretics

• Discontinue diuretic 2-3 days prior to perindopril then resume diuretic if needed

Renal impairment

• *Adult:* **PO** CCr <30 ml/min 2 mg/day, max 8 mg/day

Available forms: Tabs scored 2, 4, 8 mg

Side effects/adverse reactions:

CV: Hypotension, chest pain, tachycardia, dysrhythmias, syncope

CNS: Insomnia, dizziness, paresthesias, headache, fatigue, anxiety

GI: Nausea, vomiting, colitis, cramps, diarrhea, constipation, flatulence, dry mouth, loss of taste

INTEG: Rash, purpura, alopecia, hyperhidrosis

HEMA: ***Agranulocytosis, neutropenia***

SYST: ***Angioedema***

EENT: Tinnitus, visual changes, sore throat, double vision, dry burning eyes

GU: ***Proteinuria, renal failure,*** increased frequency of polyuria or oliguria

RESP: Dyspnea, dry cough, rales

META: Hyperkalemia

Contraindications: Hypersensitivity, history of angioedema, pregnancy (D) 2nd/3rd trimester

Precautions: Renal disease, hyperkalemia, pregnancy (C) 1st trimester, lactation, hepatic failure, dehydration, bilateral renal artery stenosis

Pharmacokinetics: Metabolized by liver, excreted in urine

Interactions:

• Hypersensitivity: allopurinol

• Severe hypotension: diuretics, other antihypertensives

• Hyperkalemia: salt substitutes, potassium-sparing diuretics, potassium supplements

• May ↑ effects of neuromuscular blocking agents, antihypertensives, lithium

• Effects may be ↑ by diuretics

↑ toxicity, death: aconite

↑ or ↓ antihypertensive effect: astragalus, cola tree

↑ antihypertensive effect: barberry, betony, black catechu, black cohosh, bloodroot, broom, burdock, cat's claw, dandelion, goldenseal, Irish moss, Jamaican dogwood, kelp, khella, mistletoe, parsley

↓ antihypertensive effect: coltsfoot, guarana, khat, licorice

Lab test interferences:

Interference: Glucose/insulin tolerance tests

NURSING CONSIDERATIONS

Assess:

• B/P, pulse q4h; note rate, rhythm, quality

• Electrolytes: K, Na, Cl during 1st 2 wk of therapy

• Baselines in renal, hepatic studies before therapy begins and 1 wk into therapy

• Edema in feet, legs daily

• Skin turgor, dryness of mucous membranes for hydration status
• Symptoms of CHF: edema, dyspnea, wet rales
Administer:
• **PO** as a single dose or in 2 divided doses
Evaluate:
• Therapeutic response: decreased B/P
Teach patient/family:
• Not to use OTC (cough, cold, or allergy) products unless directed by prescriber; to avoid salt substitutes
• To avoid sunlight or wear sunscreen for photosensitivity
• To comply with dosage schedule, even if feeling better
• To notify prescriber of mouth sores, sore throat, fever, swelling of hands or feet, irregular heartbeat, chest pains, signs of angioedema
• That excessive perspiration, dehydration, vomiting, diarrhea may lead to fall in blood pressure; consult prescriber if these occur
• That drug may cause dizziness, fainting; light-headedness may occur during 1st few days of therapy
• That drug may cause skin rash or impaired perspiration; angioedema may occur and to D/C if it occurs
• Not to discontinue drug abruptly
• That CV adverse reactions may reoccur
• To rise slowly to sitting or standing position to minimize orthostatic hypotension
Treatment of overdose: Lavage, IV atropine for bradycardia, IV theophylline for bronchospasm, digitalis, O_2, diuretic for cardiac failure

RARELY USED

permethrin (OTC, ℞)
(per-meth′rin)
Acticin, Elimite, Nix
Func. class.: Pediculicide

Uses: Lice, nits, ticks, flea nits
Dosage and routes:
Lice (head)
• *Adult and child:* Wash hair, towel dry; apply liberally to hair, leave on 10 min, rinse with water
Scabies
• *Adult and child:* **TOP** 5% cream applied and massaged into all skin surfaces; leave cream on 8-14 hr, then wash
Contraindications: Hypersensitivity

perphenazine (℞)
(per-fen′a-zeen)
Apo-Perphenazine♣, perphenazine, PMS Perphenazine♣, Trilafon, Trilafon Concentrate
Func. class.: Antipsychotic, neuroleptic
Chem. class.: Phenothiazine piperidine

Action: Depresses cerebral cortex, hypothalamus, limbic system, which control activity, aggression; blocks neurotransmission produced by dopamine at synapse; exhibits strong α-adrenergic, anticholinergic blocking action; as antiemetic inhibits medullary chemoreceptor trigger zone; mechanism for antipsychotic effects is unclear
Uses: Psychotic disorders, schizophrenia, nausea, vomiting
Dosage and routes:
• *Geriatric:* **PO** 2-4 mg qd-bid, increase by 2-4 mg/wk to desired dose

P

Nausea/vomiting

• *Adult and child >12 yr:* **IM** 5-10 mg prn, max 15 mg in ambulatory patients, 30 mg in hospitalized patients; **PO** 8-16 mg/day in divided doses, up to 24 mg; **IV** not to exceed 5 mg, give diluted or slow **IV** drip

Psychiatric use in hospitalized patients

• *Adult:* **PO** 8-16 mg bid-qid, gradually increased to desired dose, not to exceed 64 mg/day; **IM** 5 mg q6h, not to exceed 30 mg/day

• *Child >12 yr:* **PO** 6-12 mg in divided doses

Nonhospitalized patients

• *Adult:* **PO** 4-8 mg tid

Available forms: Tabs 2, 4, 8, 16 mg; oral sol 16 mg/5 ml; inj 5 mg/ml; syr 2 mg/5 ml

Side effects/adverse reactions:

RESP: ***Laryngospasm,*** dyspnea, ***respiratory depression***

CNS: EPS: pseudoparkinsonism, akathisia, dystonia, tardive dyskinesia, ***seizures,*** *headache,* ***neuroleptic malignant syndrome,*** dizziness

HEMA: Anemia, ***leukopenia, leukocytosis, agranulocytosis***

INTEG: Rash, photosensitivity, dermatitis

EENT: Blurred vision, glaucoma

GI: Dry mouth, nausea, vomiting, anorexia, constipation, diarrhea, jaundice, weight gain

GU: Urinary retention, urinary frequency, enuresis, impotence, amenorrhea, gynecomastia

CV: Orthostatic hypotension (elderly), ***cardiac arrest,*** ECG changes, ***tachycardia***

Contraindications: Hypersensitivity, blood dyscrasias, coma, child <12 yr, brain damage, bone marrow depression

Precautions: Pregnancy (C), lactation, seizure disorders, hypertension, hepatic disease, cardiac disease, elderly, narrow-angle glaucoma

Pharmacokinetics:

Metabolized by liver; excreted in urine, breast milk; crosses placenta

PO: Onset erratic, peak 2-4 hr

IM: Onset 10 min, peak 1-2 hr; duration 6 hr, occasionally 12-24 hr

Interactions:

• Oversedation: other CNS depressants, alcohol, barbiturate anesthetics

• Toxicity: epINEPHrine

• ↓ absorption: aluminum hydroxide or magnesium hydroxide antacids

• ↑ risk of EPS: lithium

• ↑ effects of both drugs: β-adrenergic blockers, alcohol

• ↑ anticholinergic effects: anticholinergics

• ↓ antiparkinson effect: levodopa

↑ anticholinergic effect: henbane leaf

↑ EPS: betel palm, kava

↑ action: cola tree, hops, nettle, nutmeg

Lab test interferences:

Increase: LFTs, cardiac enzymes, cholesterol, blood glucose, prolactin, bilirubin, PBI, cholinesterase, ^{131}I

Decrease: Hormones (blood, urine)

False positive: Pregnancy tests, PKU

False negative: Urinary steroids, 17-OHCS

NURSING CONSIDERATIONS

Assess:

• Mental status before initial administration

• Swallowing of PO medication; check for hoarding or giving of medication to other patients

• I&O ratio; palpate bladder if urinary output is low, urinary retention may be the cause

• Bilirubin, CBC, LFTs qmo

• Urinalysis is recommended before and during prolonged therapy

• Affect, orientation, LOC, reflexes, gait, coordination, sleep pattern disturbances
• B/P standing and lying; also include pulse, respirations q4h during initial treatment; establish baseline before starting treatment; report drops of 30 mm Hg
• Dizziness, faintness, palpitations, tachycardia on rising
• EPS including akathisia (inability to sit still, no pattern to movements), tardive dyskinesia (bizarre movements of jaw, mouth, tongue, extremities), pseudoparkinsonism (rigidity, tremors, pill rolling, shuffling gait)
• Skin turgor daily
◆ For neuroleptic malignant syndrome: hyperthermia, altered mental status, increased CPK, muscle rigidity
• Constipation, urinary retention daily; increase bulk, water in diet

Administer:

• Antiparkinsonian agent on order from prescriber for EPS

PO route

• Concentrate mixed in water, orange, pineapple, apricot, prune, tomato, grapefruit juice; do not mix with caffeine beverages (coffee, cola), tannics (tea), or pectinates (apple juice), since incompatibility may result; use 60 ml diluent for each 5 ml of concentrate

IM route

• IM inj into large muscle mass

IV route

• After diluting each 5 mg/9 ml of NaCl, shake, give 0.5 mg or less (1 ml = 0.5 mg) over 1 min; may be further diluted and infused

Additive compatibilities: Ascorbic acid, ethacrynate, netilmicin

Syringe compatibilities: Atropine, benztropine, butorphanol, chlorproMAZINE, cimetidine, dimenhyDRINATE, diphenhydrAMINE, droperidol, fentanyl, hydrOXYzine, meperidine, methotrimeprazine, metoclopramide, morphine, pentazocine, prochlorperazine, promethazine, ranitidine, scopolamine

Y-site compatibilities: Acyclovir, amikacin, ampicillin, azlocillin, cefamandole, cefazolin, cefotaxime, cefoxitin, cefuroxime, cephalothin, cephapirin, chloramphenicol, clindamycin, doxycycline, erythromycin, famotidine, gentamicin, kanamycin, metronidazole, mezlocillin, minocycline, moxalactam, nafcillin, oxacillin, penicillin G potassium, piperacillin, tacrolimus, ticarcillin, ticarcillin/clavulanate, tobramycin, trimethoprim-sulfamethoxazole, vancomycin

Perform/provide:

• Decreased sensory input by dimming lights, avoiding loud noises
• Supervised ambulation until stabilized on medication; do not involve in strenuous exercise program because fainting is possible; patient should not stand still for long periods
• Increased fluids, bulk in diet to prevent constipation
• Sips of water, sugarless candy, gum, ice chips for dry mouth
• Storage in tight, light-resistant container

Evaluate:

• Therapeutic response: decrease in emotional excitement, hallucinations, delusions, paranoia, reorganization of patterns of thought, speech

Teach patient/family:

• That orthostatic hypotension occurs frequently and to rise from sitting or lying position gradually; to avoid hazardous activities until stabilized on medication
• To remain lying down after IM inj for at least 30 min

• To avoid hot tubs, hot showers, tub baths, since hypotension may occur
• To avoid abrupt withdrawal of this drug, or EPS may result; drug should be withdrawn slowly
• To avoid OTC preparations (cough, hay fever, cold) unless approved by prescriber, since serious drug interactions may occur; avoid use with alcohol or CNS depressants; increased drowsiness may occur
• To use a sunscreen
• About compliance with drug regimen
• About necessity for meticulous oral hygiene, since oral candidiasis may occur
• To report sore throat, malaise, fever, bleeding, mouth sores; if these occur, CBC should be drawn and drug discontinued
• In hot weather, that heat stroke may occur; to take extra precautions to stay cool

Treatment of overdose: Lavage if orally ingested; provide an airway; *do not induce vomiting*

RARELY USED

phenacemide (℞)

(fe-nass′e-mide)

Func. class.: Anticonvulsant

Uses: Refractory, generalized tonic-clonic (grand mal), complex-partial (psychomotor), absence (petit mal), atypical seizures

Dosage and routes:

• *Adult:* **PO** 500 mg tid, may increase by 500 mg/wk, not to exceed 5 g/day
• *Child 5-10 yr:* **PO** 250 mg tid, may increase by 250 mg/wk, not to exceed 1.5 g/day prn

Contraindications: Hypersensitivity, psychiatric condition, pregnancy (D), lactation

phenazopyridine (℞, OTC)

(fen-az-oh-peer′i-deen)

Azo-Standard, Baridium, Eridium, Geridium, Phenazo✚, phenazopyridine, Phenazodine, Prodium, Pyridiate, Pyridium, Urodine, Urogesic, Viridium

Func. class.: Nonopioid analgesic (urinary system)

Chem. class.: Azodye

Action: Exerts analgesic, anesthetic action on the urinary tract mucosa

Uses: Urinary tract irritation, infection used with a urinary antiinfective

Dosage and routes:

• *Adult:* **PO** 200 mg tid × 2 days or less when used with antibacterial for UTI
• *Child 6-12 yr:* **PO** 4 mg/kg tid × 2 days

Renal dose

• Do not use in CCr <50 ml/min

Available forms: Tabs 100, 200 mg

Side effects/adverse reactions:

HEMA: ***Thrombocytopenia, agranulocytosis, leukopenia, neutropenia, hemolytic anemia, methemoglobinemia***

CNS: Headache

GI: Nausea, vomiting, diarrhea, heartburn, anorexia, ***hepatic toxicity***

INTEG: Rash, skin pigmentation, pruritus

GU: ***Renal toxicity,*** *orange-red urine*

Contraindications: Hypersensitivity, renal insufficiency

Precautions: Pregnancy (B), lactation, children <12 yr

Pharmacokinetics:
Metabolized by liver, excreted by kidneys, crosses placenta, duration 6-8 hr
Lab test interferences:
Interference: Urinalysis
NURSING CONSIDERATIONS
Assess:
• Urinary status: burning, pain, itching, urgency, frequency, hematuria, before/after treatment completed
• Hepatic studies: AST, ALT, bilirubin if patient is on long-term therapy
◆ Hepatotoxicity: dark urine, clay-colored stools, jaundiced skin and sclera, itching, abdominal pain, fever, diarrhea if patient is on long-term therapy
• Allergic reactions: rash, urticaria; drug may have to be discontinued
Administer:
PO route
• To patient crushed or whole; chewable tablets may be chewed
• With food or milk to decrease gastric symptoms
Evaluate:
• Therapeutic response: decrease in urinary pain
Teach patient/family:
• Not to exceed recommended dosage and to take with meals
• To discontinue after pain is relieved but continue to take concurrent prescribed antiinfective until finished
• That urine may turn red-orange; may stain clothing or contact lenses
Treatment of overdose: Methylene blue 1-2 mg/kg IV or 100-200 mg vit C PO

RARELY USED

phendimetrazine (℞)
(fen-dye-me′tra-zeen)
Func. class.: Anorexiant

Uses: Exogenous obesity
Dosage and routes:
• *Adult:* **PO** 35 mg bid-tid 1 hr ac, not to exceed 70 mg tid; **SUS REL** 105 mg qd ac AM
Contraindications: Hypersensitivity, hyperthyroidism, hypertension, glaucoma, severe arteriosclerosis, severe cardiovascular disease, children <12 yr, agitated states, drug abuse, MAOI use within 14 days

phenelzine (℞)
(fen′el-zeen)
Nardil
Func. class.: Antidepressant, MAOI
Chem. class.: Hydrazine

Action: Increases concentrations of endogenous epINEPHrine, norepinephrine, serotonin, DOPamine in storage sites in CNS by inhibition of MAO; increased concentration reduces depression
Uses: Depression, when uncontrolled by other means
Dosage and routes:
• *Adult:* **PO** 45 mg/day in divided doses; may increase to 60 mg/day; dose should be reduced to 15 mg/day, not to exceed 90 mg/day
• *Geriatric:* **PO** 7.5 mg qd, increase by 7.5-15 mg q3-4 days; usual dose 15-60 mg/day in divided doses
Available forms: Tabs 15 mg
Side effects/adverse reactions:
HEMA: ***Anemia***
CNS: Dizziness, drowsiness, confusion, headache, anxiety, tremors,

P

stimulation, weakness, hyperreflexia, mania, insomnia, fatigue, weight gain
GI: Constipation, dry mouth, nausea, vomiting, *anorexia,* diarrhea, weight gain
GU: Change in libido, urinary frequency
INTEG: Rash, flushing, increased perspiration
CV: Orthostatic hypotension, hypertension, dysrhythmias, ***hypertensive crisis,*** tachycardia, peripheral edema
EENT: Blurred vision
ENDO: ***SIADH-like syndrome***

Contraindications: Hypersensitivity to MAOIs, hypertension, CHF, severe hepatic disease, pheochromocytoma, severe renal disease, severe cardiac disease, active alcoholism

Precautions: Suicidal patients, convulsive disorders, severe depression, schizophrenia, hyperactivity, diabetes mellitus, pregnancy (C), child <16 yr

Pharmacokinetics: Metabolized by liver, excreted by kidneys

Interactions:
• ↑ hypotension: thiazide diuretics
• Confusion, shivering, hyperreflexia: L-tryptophan
• Toxicity: sumatriptan, sulfonamides
• ↓ serotonin, norepinephrine: rauwolfia alkaloids
• ↑ pressor effects: guanethidine, clonidine, indirect-acting or mixed sympathomimetics (epHEDrine)
• ↑ effects of direct-acting sympathomimetics (epINEPHrine): alcohol, barbiturates, benzodiazepines, CNS depressants, levodopa
⬥Hyperpyretic crisis, convulsions, hypertensive episode: tricyclics, SSRIs, meperidine, methylphenidate, amphetamines, nasal decongestants, sinus medications, appetite suppressants, asthma inhalants
• ↑ hypoglycemic effect: antidiabetics
• Drug/food: avoid tyramine foods, caffeine
🍃 ↑ sympathomimetic action: betel palm, butcher's broom, capsicum peppers, galanthamine, green tea (large amounts), guarana (large amounts), night-blooming cereus
🍃 Hypertension: brewer's yeast
🍃 Tension headaches, irritability, visual hallucinations, mania: ginseng
🍃 ↑ effect: ginkgo, nutmeg, yohimbe
🍃 ↑ anticholinergic effect: jimsonweed
🍃 Serotonin syndrome: parsley, St. John's wort
🍃 ↓ effect: valerian

NURSING CONSIDERATIONS

Assess:
• B/P (lying, standing), pulse; if systolic B/P drops 20 mm Hg, hold drug, notify prescriber
• Blood studies: CBC, leukocytes, cardiac enzymes (long-term therapy)
• Hepatic studies: ALT, AST, bilirubin; hepatotoxicity may occur
⬥Toxicity: increased headache, palpitation; discontinue drug immediately; prodromal signs of hypertensive crisis
• Mental status changes: mood, sensorium, affect, memory (long, short); increase in psychiatric symptoms
• Urinary retention, constipation, edema; take weight qwk
• Withdrawal symptoms: headache, nausea, vomiting, muscle pain, weakness

Administer:

PO route
• Increased fluids, bulk in diet for constipation

• With food, milk for GI symptoms
• Crushed if patient cannot swallow medication whole
• Dosage hs for oversedation during day
• Gum, hard candy, or frequent sips of water for dry mouth
• Phentolamine for severe hypertension

Perform/provide:
• Storage in tight container in cool environment
• Ambulation assistance at start of therapy, since drowsiness/dizziness occurs, especially elderly
• Safety measures including side rails
• Checking to see if PO medication swallowed

Evalute:
• Therapeutic response: decreased depression

Teach patient/family:
• That therapeutic effects may take 1-4 wk
• To avoid driving, other activities requiring alertness
• To avoid alcohol ingestion, CNS depressants, OTC medications: cold, weight loss, hay fever, cough syrup
• To rise slowly to prevent orthostatic hypotension
• Not to discontinue medication quickly after long-term use
• To avoid high-tyramine foods: cheese (aged), sour cream, beer, wine, pickled products, liver, raisins, bananas, figs, avocados, meat tenderizers, chocolate, yogurt; provide complete list of tyramine-containing foods; increased caffeine
• To report headache, palpitation, neck stiffness, dizziness, constriction in chest, throat, rash, insomnia, change in strength, changes in urinary patterns, color of urine

Treatment of overdose: Lavage, activated charcoal, monitor electrolytes, vital signs, diazepam IV, $NaHCO_3$

HIGH ALERT

phenobarbital (℞)

(fee-noe-bar'bi-tal)

Ancalixir✤, Barbita, Luminal, phenobarbital sodium, Solfoton

Func. class.: Anticonvulsant
Chem. class.: Barbiturate

Controlled Substance Schedule IV

Action: Decreases impulse transmission; increases seizure threshold at cerebral cortex level

Uses: All forms of epilepsy, status epilepticus, febrile seizures in children, sedation, insomnia

Investigational uses: Hyperbilirubinemia, chronic cholestasis

Dosage and routes:

Seizures
• *Adult:* **PO** 60-200 mg/day in divided doses tid or total dose hs
• *Child:* **PO** 4-6 mg/kg/day in divided doses q12h; may be given as single dose

Status epilepticus
• *Adult:* **IV INF** 10 mg/kg; run no faster than 50 mg/min; may give up to 20 mg/kg
• *Child:* **IV INF** 5-10 mg/kg; may repeat q10-15min up to 20 mg/kg; run no faster than 50 mg/min

Insomnia
• *Adult:* **PO/IM** 100-320 mg
• *Child:* **PO/IM** 3-5 mg/kg

Sedation
• *Adult:* **PO** 30-120 mg/day in 2-3 divided doses
• *Child:* **PO** 3-5 mg/kg/day in 3 divided doses

P

Preoperative sedation
• *Adult:* **IM** 100-200 mg 1-1½ hr before surgery
• *Child:* **IM** 16-100 mg or **PO/IM/IV** 1-3 mg/kg 1-1½ hr before surgery

Available forms: Caps 15 mg; elix 20 mg/5 ml; tabs 8, 15, 30, 60, 100 mg; inj 30, 60, 65, 130 mg/ml

Side effects/adverse reactions:
CNS: Paradoxic excitement (elderly), drowsiness, lethargy, hangover headache, flushing, hallucinations, ***coma***
GI: Nausea, vomiting, diarrhea, constipation
INTEG: Rash, urticaria, ***Stevens-Johnson syndrome, angioedema,*** local pain, swelling, necrosis, ***thrombophlebitis***

Contraindications: Hypersensitivity to barbiturates, porphyria, hepatic disease, respiratory disease, nephritis, hyperthyroidism, diabetes mellitus, elderly, lactation, pregnancy (D)

Precautions: Anemia

Do not confuse:
phenobarbital/pentobarbital

Pharmacokinetics:
IV: Onset 5 min, peak 30 min, duration 4-6 hr
IM/SC: Onset 10-30 min, duration 4-6 hr
PO: Onset 20-60 min, peak 8-12 hr, duration 6-10 hr
Metabolized by liver; crosses placenta; excreted in urine, breast milk; half-life 53-118 hr

Interactions:
• ↑ effects: CNS depressants, alcohol, chloramphenicol, valproic acid, disulfiram, nondepolarizing skeletal muscle relaxants, sulfonamides
• ↓ effects: theophylline, oral anticoagulants, corticosteroids, metronidazole, doxycycline, quinidine
• ↑ orthostatic hypotension: furosemide
↑ phenobarbital levels: quinine
↑ CNS depression: chamomile, eucalyptus, hops, Jamaican dogwood, kava, lemon balm, nettle, pill-bearing spurge, poppy, senega, skullcap, valerian
↓ barbiturate effect: St. John's wort

NURSING CONSIDERATIONS

Assess:
• Mental status: mood, sensorium, affect, memory (long, short)
• For respiratory depression
• Blood dyscrasias: fever, sore throat, bruising, rash, jaundice
• Convulsion activity: type, duration, precipitating factors
• Blood studies, LFTs during long-term treatment
• Therapeutic blood level periodically: 15-40 mcg/ml
• Respiratory status: rate, rhythm, depth

Administer:

IM route
• IM inj deep in large muscle mass to prevent tissue sloughing; use <5 ml in each site

IV route
• Slow IV after dilution with at least 10 ml sterile H_2O for inj regardless of dose; give 65 mg or less/min; titrate to patient response

Additive compatibilities: Amikacin, aminophylline, calcium chloride, calcium gluconate, cephapirin, colistimethate, dimenhyDRINATE, meropenem, polymyxin B, sodium bicarbonate, thiopental, verapamil

Solution compatibilities: D_5W, $D_{10}W$, 0.45% NaCl, 0.9% NaCl, Ringer's, dextrose/saline combinations, dextrose/Ringer's, dextrose/LR combinations, sodium lactate

Syringe compatibilities: Heparin

Y-site compatibilities: Enalaprilat, meropenem, propofol, sufentanil

Perform/provide:
• Supervision of ambulation for dizziness, drowsiness
Evaluate:
• Therapeutic response: decreased seizures, increased sedation
Teach patient/family:
• To use exactly as ordered
• To avoid other CNS depressants, including alcohol
• To avoid hazardous activities until stabilized on drug; drowsiness may occur
• Never to withdraw drug abruptly; withdrawal symptoms may occur
• That therapeutic effects (PO) may not be seen for 2-3 wk
Treatment of overdose: Lavage, activated charcoal, warming blanket, vital signs, hemodialysis, I&O ratio

RARELY USED

phenoxybenzamine (℞)

(fen-ox-ee-ben′za-meen)
Func. class.: Antihypertensive

Uses: Pheochromocytoma
Dosage and routes:
• *Adult:* **PO** 10 mg qd, increase by 10 mg qod, usual range: 20-40 mg bid-tid
• *Child:* **PO** 0.2 mg/kg or 6 mg/m^2/day, max 10 mg; may increase q4d; maintenance dose 0.4-1.2 mg/kg/day or 12-36 mg/m^2/day divided doses tid or qid
Contraindications: Hypersensitivity, CHF, angina, cerebral vascular insufficiency, coronary arteriosclerosis

phentolamine (℞)

(fen-tole′a-meen)
Regitine, Rogitine✤
Func. class.: Antihypertensive
Chem. class.: α-Adrenergic blocker

Action: α-Adrenergic blocker, binds to α-adrenergic receptors, dilating peripheral blood vessels, lowering peripheral resistances, lowering blood pressure
Uses: Hypertension, pheochromocytoma, prevention, treatment of dermal necrosis following extravasation of norepinephrine or DOPamine
Investigational uses: Impotence, hypertensive crisis due to MAOIs
Dosage and routes:
Treatment of hypertensive episodes in pheochromocytoma
• *Adult:* **IV/IM,** 5 mg, repeat if necessary
• *Child:* **IV/IM,** 1 mg, repeat if necessary
Diagnosis of pheochromocytoma
• *Adult:* **IV** 25 mg; if negative, repeat with 5 mg IV
• *Child:* **IV** 0.5 mg; if negative, repeat with 1 mg IV
Treatment of necrosis
• *Adult:* 5-10 mg/10 ml **NS** injected into area of norepinephrine extravasation within 12 hr
• *Child:* 0.1-0.2 mg/kg, max 10 mg
Prevention of necrosis
• *Adult:* 10 mg/L of norepinephrine-containing sol
• *Child:* **IV** 0.1-0.2 mg/kg, max 10 mg
Available forms: Inj 5 mg/ml
Side effects/adverse reactions:
GI: Dry mouth, nausea, vomiting, diarrhea, abdominal pain
CV: Hypotension, tachycardia, angina, dysrhythmias, ***MI***

P

CNS: Dizziness, flushing, weakness, ***cerebrovascular spasm***
EENT: Nasal congestion
Contraindications: Hypersensitivity, MI, coronary insufficiency, angina
Precautions: Pregnancy (C), lactation
Pharmacokinetics:
IV: Peak 2 min, duration 10-15 min
IM: Peak 15-20 min, duration 3-4 hr
Metabolized in liver, excreted in urine
Interactions:
• ↑ effects of epINEPHrine, antihypertensives
↑ toxicity, death: aconite
↑ or ↓ antihypertensive effect: astragalus, cola tree
↑ antihypertensive effect: barberry, betony, black catechu, black cohosh, bloodroot, broom, burdock, cat's claw, dandelion, goldenseal, Irish moss, Jamaican dogwood, kelp, khella, mistletoe, parsley
↓ antihypertensive effect: coltsfoot, guarana, khat, licorice

NURSING CONSIDERATIONS
Assess:
• Electrolytes: K, Na, Cl, CO_2; weight qd, I&O
• B/P lying, standing before starting treatment, q4h after
• Nausea, vomiting, diarrhea, edema in feet, legs daily; skin turgor, dryness of mucous membranes for hydration status, postural hypotension, cardiac system: pulse, ECG
Administer:
• Gum, frequent rinsing of mouth, or hard candy for dry mouth
• With vasopressor available
• After discontinuing all medication for 24 hr
IV route
• After diluting 5 mg/1 ml sterile H_2O for inj; give 5 mg or less/min; patient to remain recumbent during administration
CONT INF route
• Dilute 5-10 mg/500 ml D_5W, titrate to patient response
• 10 mg/L may be added to norepinephrine in IV sol for prevention of dermal necrosis
Additive compatibilities: DOBUTamine, verapamil
Syringe compatibilities: Papaverine
Y-site compatibilities: Amiodarone
Evaluate:
• Therapeutic response: decreased B/P
Teach patient/family:
• That bed rest is required during treatment, 1 hr after
Treatment of overdose: Administer norepinephrine; discontinue drug

phenylephrine (℞)
(fen-ill-ef'rin)
Neo-Synephrine
Func. class.: Adrenergic, direct-acting
Chem. class.: Substituted phenylethylamine

Action: Powerful and selective (α_1) receptor agonist causing contraction of blood vessels
Uses: Hypotension, paroxysmal supraventricular tachycardia, shock, maintain B/P for spinal anesthesia
Dosage and routes:
Hypotension
• *Adult:* **SC/IM** 2-5 mg, may repeat q10-15 min if needed, do not exceed initial dose; **IV** 50-100 mcg, may repeat q10-15 min if needed, do not exceed initial dose
• *Child:* **IM/SC** 0.1 mg/kg/dose q1-2h prn
Supraventricular tachycardia
• *Adult:* **IV BOL** 0.5-1 mg given rapidly, not to exceed prior dose by >0.1 mg, total dose ≤1 mg

Shock

• *Adult:* **IV INF** 10 mg/500 ml D_5W given 100-180 mcg/min (if 20 gtt/ml inf device), then maintenance of 40-60 mcg/min (if 20 gtt/ml inf device)

• *Child:* **IV BOL** 5-20 mcg/kg/dose q10-15 min; **IV INF** 0.1-0.5 mcg/kg/min

Available forms: Inj 1% (10 mg/ml)

Side effects/adverse reactions:

CNS: Headache, anxiety, tremor, insomnia, dizziness

CV: Palpitations, tachycardia, hypertension, ectopic beats, angina, reflex bradycardia, ***dysrhythmias***

GI: Nausea, vomiting

INTEG: Necrosis, tissue sloughing with extravasation, ***gangrene***

SYST: ***Anaphylaxis***

Contraindications: Hypersensitivity, ventricular fibrillation, tachydysrhythmias, pheochromocytoma, narrow-angle glaucoma, severe hypertension

Precautions: Pregnancy (C), lactation, arterial embolism, peripheral vascular disease, elderly, hyperthyroidism, bradycardia, myocardial disease, severe arteriosclerosis, partial heart block

Pharmacokinetics:

IV: Duration 20-30 min

IM/SC: Duration 45-60 min

Interactions:

⬧Do not use within 2 wk of MAOIs, or hypertensive crisis may result

• Dysrhythmias: general anesthetics, digoxin, bretylium

• ↓ phenylephrine action: α-blockers

• ↑ in B/P: oxytocics

• ↑ pressor effect: tricyclics, β-blockers, H_1 antihistamines

NURSING CONSIDERATIONS

Assess:

• I&O ratio; notify prescriber if output <30 ml/hr

• ECG during administration continuously; if B/P increases, drug is decreased

• B/P and pulse q5min after parenteral route

• CVP or PWP during inf if possible

• For paresthesias and coldness of extremities; peripheral blood flow may decrease

Administer:

IV route

• Plasma expanders for hypovolemia

• IV after diluting 1 mg/9 ml sterile H_2O for inj; give dose over ½-1 min; may be diluted 10 mg/500 ml of D_5W or NS; titrate to response (normal B/P); check for extravasation, check site for infiltration, use infusion pump

Additive compatibilities: Chloramphenicol, DOBUTamine, lidocaine, potassium chloride, sodium bicarbonate

Y-site compatibilities: Amiodarone, amrinone, cisatracurium, famotidine, haloperidol, remifentanil, zidovudine

Perform/provide:

• Storage of reconstituted sol if refrigerated for no longer than 24 hr

• Discard discolored sol

Evaluate:

• Therapeutic response: increased B/P with stabilization

Teach patient/family:

• The reason for administration

• To report pain at infusion site or other adverse reactions immediately

Treatment of overdose: Administer an α-blocker

phenylephrine nasal agent

See appendix c

phenylephrine ophthalmic

See appendix c

phenytoin (℞)

(fen'i-toh-in)

Dilantin, Dilantin Infatab, Dilantin Kapseals, Dilantin-125, diphenylhydantoin, DPH, Phenytex

Func. class.: Anticonvulsant; antidysrhythmic (IB)

Chem. class.: Hydantoin

Action: Inhibits spread of seizure activity in motor cortex by altering ion transport; increases AV conduction

Uses: Generalized tonic-clonic seizures; status epilepticus; nonepileptic seizures associated with Reye's syndrome or after head trauma; migraines, trigeminal neuralgia, Bell's palsy, ventricular dysrhythmias uncontrolled by antidysrhythmics

Dosage and routes:

Renal dose

• Do not use loading dose CCr <10 ml/min or hepatic failure

Seizures

• *Adult:* **PO** 1 g or 20 mg/kg (ext rel) in 3-4 divided doses given q2h, or 400 mg, then 300 mg q2h × 2 doses, maintenance 300-400 mg/day, max 600 mg/day; **IV** 15-20 mg/kg, max 25-50 mg/min, then 100 mg q6-8h

• *Child:* **PO** 5 mg/kg/day in 2-3 divided doses, maintenance 4-8 mg/kg/day in 2-3 divided doses, max 300 mg/day; **IV** 15-20 mg/kg at 1-3 mg/kg/min

Status epilepticus

• *Adult:* **IV** 10-15 mg/kg, max 25-50 mg/min, may give 100 mg q6-8h thereafter

• *Child:* **IV** 15-20 mg/kg, max in divided doses 1-3 mg/kg/min

Neuritic pain

• *Adult:* **PO** 200-600 mg/day in divided doses

Ventricular dysrhythmias

• *Adult:* **PO** loading dose 1 g divided over 24 hr, then 500 mg/day × 2 days; **IV** 250 mg over 5 min until dysrhythmias subside or until 1 g is given, or 100 mg q15min until dysrhythmias subside or until 1 g given

• *Child:* **PO** 3-8 mg/kg or 250 mg/m^2/day as single dose or 2 divided doses; **IV** 3-8 mg/kg over several min, or 250 mg/m^2/day as single dose or 2 divided doses

Available forms: Susp 30, 125 mg/5 ml; tabs, chewable 50 mg; inj 50 mg/ml; caps ext rel 30, 100 mg; caps prompt rel 30, 100 mg

Side effects/adverse reactions:

CNS: Drowsiness, dizziness, insomnia, paresthesias, depression, suicidal tendencies, aggression, headache, confusion, slurred speech

CV: Hypotension, ***ventricular fibrillation***

EENT: Nystagmus, diplopia, blurred vision

GI: Nausea, vomiting, constipation, anorexia, weight loss, ***hepatitis,*** jaundice, gingival hyperplasia

GU: ***Nephritis,*** urine discoloration

HEMA: ***Agranulocytosis, leukopenia, aplastic anemia, thrombocytopenia, megaloblastic anemia***

ENDO: Diabetes insipidus

INTEG: Rash, ***lupus erythematosus, Stevens-Johnson syndrome,*** hirsutism

SYST: Hypocalcemia

Contraindications: Hypersensitivity, psychiatric condition, bradycardia, SA and AV block, Stokes-Adams syndrome, hepatic failure, acute intermittent porphyria

Precautions: Allergies, hepatic disease, renal disease, elderly, petit mal seizures, pregnancy (C), hypotension, myocardial insufficiency

Pharmacokinetics:

PO-ER: Onset 2-24 hr, peak 4-12 hr, duration 12-36 hr

IV: Onset 1-2 hr, duration 12-24 hr

PO: Onset 2-24 hr, peak 1½-2½ hr, duration 6-12 hr

Metabolized by liver, excreted by kidneys; highly protein-bound, half-life 22 hr, dose dependent

Interactions:

- ↓ phenytoin effects: alcohol (chronic use), antacids, barbiturates, carbamazepine, diazoxide, rifampin, folic acid
- ↑ phenytoin effect: benzodiazepines, cimetidine, tricyclics, salicylates, valproate, cycloSERINE, diazepam, chloramphenicol

↑ potassium loss, ↑ antidysrhythmic action: aloe, buckthorn, cascara sagrada, senna

↓ anticonvulsant effect: ginseng, santonica, valerian

↑ action: ginkgo

Lab test interferences:

Decrease: Dexamethasone, metyrapone test serum, PBI, urinary steroids

Increase: Glucose, alk phosphatase, BSP

NURSING CONSIDERATIONS

Assess:

For phenytoin hypersensitivity syndrome 3-12 wk after start of treatment: rash, temp, lymphadenopathy; may cause hepatotoxicity, renal failure, rhabdomyolysis

For beginning rash that may lead to Stevens-Johnson syndrome or toxic epidermal necrolysis; phenytoin should not be used again

- Drug level: toxic level 30-50 mcg/ml, ther level: 7.5-20 mcg/ml, wait ≥1 wk to draw levels
- For seizures: duration, type, intensity precipitating factors
- Blood studies: CBC, platelets q2wk until stabilized, then qmo × 12, then q3mo; discontinue drug if neutrophils <1600/mm^3; renal function: albumin conc
- Mental status: mood, sensorium, affect, memory (long, short)
- Respiratory depression; rate, depth, character
- Blood dyscrasias: fever, sore throat, bruising, rash, jaundice

Administer:

- Do not interchange chewable product with caps, not equivalent; only ext rel caps are to be used for once a day dosing
- Shake susp well before each dose

G tube/NG tube: dilute susp prior to administration, flush tube with 20 ml H_2O after dose

IV route

- After diluting with diluent provided (2.2 ml/100 mg, 5.2 ml/250 mg, 1 ml/50 mg); shake; place vial in warm water to dissolve powder; give through Y-tube or 3-way stopcock; inject slowly <50 mg/min; clear IV tubing first with NS sol; use in-line filter; discard 4 hr after preparation; inject into large veins to prevent purple glove syndrome

Additive compatibilities: Bleomycin, sodium bicarbonate, verapamil

Y-site compatibilities: Esmolol, famotidine, fluconazole, foscarnet, tacrolimus

Evaluate:

- Therapeutic response; decrease in severity of seizures, ventricular dysrhythmias

Teach patient/family:

- To take PO doses divided with or after meals to decrease adverse effects
- That if diabetic, urine glucose should be monitored
- That urine may turn pink
- Not to discontinue drug abruptly; seizures may occur

P

• Proper brushing of teeth using a soft toothbrush, flossing to prevent gingival hyperplasia; need to see dentist frequently
• To avoid hazardous activities until stabilized on drug
• To carry emergency ID stating drug use
• That heavy use of alcohol may diminish effect of drug; to avoid OTC medications; not to use antacids or antidiarrheals within 2 hr of this product
• Not to change brands or forms once stabilized on therapy; brands may vary

RARELY USED

physostigmine (℞)

(fi-zoe-stig′meen)
Antilirium
Func. class.: Antidote, reversible anticholinesterase

Uses: To reverse CNS effects of diazepam; anticholinergic, tricyclics, Alzheimer's disease, hereditary ataxia
Dosage and routes:
Overdose of anticholinergics
• *Adult:* **IM/IV** 2 mg; give no more than 1 mg/min; may repeat
• *Child:* **IM/IV** inj 0.02 mg/kg, not more than 0.5 mg/min; may repeat at 5-10 min intervals until max dose of 2 mg
Postanesthesia
• *Adult:* **IM/IV** 0.5-1 mg; give no more than 1 mg/min **(IV);** can repeat at 10 to 30 min intervals
Contraindications: Hypotension, obstruction of intestine or renal system , asthma, gangrene, CV disease, choline esters, depolarizing neuromuscular blocking agents, diabetes

physostigmine ophthalmic

See appendix c

phytonadione (vit K_1) (℞)

(fye-toe-na-dye′one)
AquaMEPHYTON, Mephyton
Func. class.: Vit K_1, fat-soluble vitamin

Action: Needed for adequate blood clotting (factors II, VII, IX, X)
Uses: Vit K malabsorption, hypoprothrombinemia, prevention of hypoprothrombinemia caused by oral anticoagulants, prevention of hemorrhagic disease of the newborn
Dosage and routes:
Hypoprothrombinemia caused by vit K malabsorption
• *Adult:* **PO/IM** 2.5-25 mg, may repeat or increase to 50 mg
• *Child:* **PO/IM** 5-10 mg
• *Infant:* **PO/IM** 2 mg
Prevention of hemorrhagic disease of the newborn
• *Neonate:* **IM** 0.5-1 mg within 1 hr after birth, repeat in 2-3 wk if required
Hypoprothrombinemia caused by oral anticoagulants
• *Adult and child:* **PO/SC/IM** 2.5-10 mg, may repeat 12-48 hr after **PO** dose or 6-8 hr after **SC/IM** dose, based on PT
Available forms: Tabs 5 mg; inj 2 mg, 10 ml aqueous colloidal; inj aqueous dispersion 10 mg/ml (IM)
Side effects/adverse reactions:
CNS: Headache, ***brain damage*** (large doses)
GI: Nausea, decreased LFTs
HEMA: ***Hemolytic anemia, hemoglobinuria, hyperbilirubinemia***
INTEG: Rash, urticaria

Contraindications: Hypersensitivity, severe hepatic disease, last few wk of pregnancy
Precautions: Pregnancy (C), neonates
Pharmacokinetics:
PO/INJ: Metabolized, crosses placenta
Interactions:
- ↓ action of phytonadione: cholestyramine, mineral oil
- ↓ action of oral anticoagulants
- Drug/food: Olestra, ↓ vit K levels

NURSING CONSIDERATIONS
Assess:
- For bleeding: emesis, stools, urine
- PT during treatment (2-sec deviation from control time, bleeding time, and clotting time); monitor for bleeding, pulse, and B/P
- Nutritional status: liver (beef), spinach, tomatoes, coffee, asparagus, broccoli, cabbage, lettuce, greens

Administer:
IV route
- After diluting with D_5NS 10 ml or more; give 1 mg/min or more
- ⬥ IV only when other routes not possible (deaths have occurred)

Additive compatibilities: Amikacin, calcium gluceptate, cephapirin, chloramphenicol, cimetidine, netilmicin, sodium bicarbonate
Syringe compatibilities: Doxapram
Y-site compatibilities: Ampicillin, epINEPHrine, famotidine, heparin, hydrocortisone, potassium chloride, tolazoline, vit B/C
Perform/provide:
- Storage in tight, light-resistant container

Evaluate:
- Therapeutic response: decreased bleeding tendencies, decreased PT, decreased clotting time

Teach patient/family:
- Not to take other supplements unless directed by prescriber
- The necessary foods for diet
- To avoid IM inj, use soft toothbrush, do not floss, use electric razor until coagulation defect corrected
- To report symptoms of bleeding
- Not to use OTC medications unless approved by prescriber
- The importance of frequent lab tests to monitor coagulation factors

pilocarpine ophthalmic
See appendix c

pimecrolimus topical
See appendix c

pindolol (℞)
(pin'doe-lole)
Novo-Pindol✦, Syn-Pindolol✦, Visken
Func. class.: Antihypertensive
Chem. class.: Nonselective β-blocker

Action: Competitively blocks stimulation of β-adrenergic receptor within vascular smooth muscle; decreases rate of SA node discharge, increases recovery time, slows conduction of AV node, decreases heart rate, which decreases O_2 consumption in myocardium; also decreases renin-aldosterone-angiotensin system, at high doses inhibits $β_2$ receptors in bronchial system
Uses: Mild to moderate hypertension
Dosage and routes:
- *Adult:* **PO** 5 mg bid, usual dose 15 mg/day (5 mg tid), may increase by 10 mg/day q3-4wk to a max of 60 mg/day

• *Geriatric:* **PO** 5 mg qd, increase by 5 mg q3-4wk

Available forms: Tabs 5, 10 mg

Side effects/adverse reactions:

CV: Hypotension, bradycardia, ***CHF,*** edema, chest pain, palpitation, claudication, tachycardia, ***AV block, pulmonary edema, bradycardia, dysrhythmias***

CNS: Insomnia, dizziness, hallucinations, anxiety, fatigue, headache, depression

GI: Nausea, vomiting, ***ischemic colitis,*** diarrhea, *abdominal pain,* ***mesenteric arterial thrombosis,*** flatulence, constipation

INTEG: Rash, alopecia, pruritus, fever

HEMA: ***Agranulocytosis, thrombocytopenia, purpura***

EENT: Visual changes, sore throat, *double vision;* dry, burning eyes, nasal stuffiness

GU: Impotence, urinary frequency

RESP: ***Bronchospasm,*** *dyspnea,* cough, rales

MISC: Joint pain, muscle pain

Contraindications: Hypersensitivity to β-blockers, cardiogenic shock; 2nd-, 3rd-degree heart block; sinus bradycardia, CHF, cardiac failure, bronchial asthma, severe COPD

Precautions: Major surgery, pregnancy (B), lactation, diabetes mellitus, renal disease, thyroid disease, COPD, well-compensated heart failure, CAD, nonallergic bronchospasm, peripheral vascular disease, hepatic disease

Do not confuse:

pindolol/Parlodel

pindolol/Plendil

Pharmacokinetics:

PO: Peak 2-4 hr; half-life 3-4 hr, excreted 30%-45% unchanged; 60%-65% metabolized by liver; excreted in breast milk; protein binding 40%

Interactions:

• ↑ hypotension, bradycardia: reserpine, hydrALAZINE, methyldopa, prazosin, anticholinergics

• ↓ antihypertensive effects: NSAIDs, sympathomimetics, thyroid

• ↑ effects of: β-blockers, calcium channel blockers

• ↓ hypoglycemic effect: sulfonylureas

• ↓ bronchodilation: theophyllines, β_2-agonists

↑ toxicity, death: aconite

↑ or ↓ antihypertensive effect: astragalus, cola tree

↑ antihypertensive effect: barberry, betony, black catechu, black cohosh, bloodroot, broom, burdock, cat's claw, dandelion, goldenseal, Irish moss, Jamaican dogwood, kelp, khella, mistletoe, parsley

↓ antihypertensive effect: coltsfoot, guarana, khat, licorice

Lab test interferences:

Increase: Renal, hepatic studies

Interference: Glucose, insulin tolerance test

NURSING CONSIDERATIONS

Assess:

• I&O, weight qd

• B/P during initial treatment, periodically thereafter; pulse q4h, note rate, rhythm, quality; apical, radial pulse before administration; notify prescriber of any significant changes

• Baselines in renal, hepatic studies before therapy begins

• Skin turgor, dryness of mucous membranes for hydration status; edema in feet, legs qd

Administer:

• PO ac, hs; tablet may be crushed or swallowed whole

Perform/provide:

• Storage in dry area at room temperature; do not freeze

Evaluate:
• Therapeutic response: decreased B/P after 1-2 wk

Teach patient/family:
• To take with or immediately after meals if GI symptoms occur
• Not to discontinue drug abruptly; taper over 2 wk; may cause precipitate angina
• Not to use OTC products containing α-adrenergic stimulants (nasal decongestants, OTC cold preparations) unless directed by prescriber
• To report bradycardia, dizziness, confusion, depression, fever, sore throat, shortness of breath to prescriber
• To take pulse at home; to notify prescriber if pulse <60 bpm
• To avoid alcohol, smoking, sodium
• To comply with weight control, dietary adjustments, modified exercise program
• To carry emergency ID to identify drug, allergies
• To avoid hazardous activities if dizziness is present
• To report symptoms of CHF: difficult breathing, especially on exertion or when lying down, night cough, swelling of extremities
• To take medication at bedtime to prevent orthostatic hypotension
• To wear support hose to minimize effects of orthostatic hypotension

Treatment of overdose: Lavage, IV atropine for bradycardia, IV theophylline for bronchospasm, digitalis, O_2, diuretic for cardiac failure, hemodialysis, hypotension; give vasopressor (norepinephrine)

pioglitazone (℞)
(pie-oh-glye'ta-zone)
Actos
Func. class.: Antidiabetic, oral
Chem. class.: Thiazolidinedione

Action: Improves insulin resistance by hepatic glucose metabolism, insulin receptor kinase activity, insulin receptor phosphorylation

Uses: Stable adult-onset diabetes mellitus (type 2) NIDDM

Dosage and routes:

Monotherapy
• *Adult:* **PO** 15-30 qd, may increase to 45 mg/day

Combination therapy
• *Adult:* **PO** 15-30 mg qd with a sulfonylurea, metformin, or insulin. Decrease sulfonylurea dose if hypoglycemia occurs. Decrease insulin dose by 10%-25% if hypoglycemia occurs or if plasma glucose is <100 mg/dl, max 45 mg/day

Hepatic dose
• Do not use in active hepatic disease or if ALT >2.5 times ULN

Available forms: Tabs 15, 30, 45 mg

Side effects/adverse reactions:
MISC: Myalgia, sinusitis, URI, pharyngitis
CNS: Headache
ENDO: Aggravated diabetes mellitus

Contraindications: Hypersensitivity to thiazolidinedione, lactation, children, diabetic ketoacidosis

Precautions: Pregnancy (C), elderly, thyroid disease, hepatic, renal disease, edema, CHF

Pharmacokinetics: Maximal reduction in FBS after 12 wk; half-life 3-7 hr, terminal 16-24 hr

P

Interactions:

• ↓ effect of: oral contraceptives, use an alternative contraceptive method

• ↓ pioglitazone effort: ketoconazole

↑ hypoglycemia: chromium, coenzyme Q-10, fenugreek

Poor blood glucose control: glucosamine

↓ antidiabetic effect: bee pollen, blue cohosh, broom, chromium, elecampane, eucalyptus, gotu kola

↑ antidiabetic effect: alfalfa, aloe, basil, bay, bilberry, bitter melon, black catechu, buchu, burdock, coriander, dandelion, eyebright (po), fenugreek, garlic, ginseng, glucomannan, glucosamine, goat's rue, gymnema, horehound, horse chestnut, jambul, myrrh, myrtle

NURSING CONSIDERATIONS

Assess:

• For hypoglycemic reactions (sweating, weakness, dizziness, anxiety, tremors, hunger), hyperglycemic reactions soon after meals

• CBC (baseline, q3mo) during treatment; check LFTs periodically AST, LDH, renal studies: BUN, creatinine, urinary glucose

• FBS, glycosylated Hgb, fasting plasma insulin, plasma lipids/lipoproteins, B/P, body weight during treatment

Administer:

• Once a day; give with meals to decrease GI upset and provide best absorption

• Tabs crushed and mixed with food or fluids for patients with difficulty swallowing

Perform/provide:

• Conversion from other oral hypoglycemic agents; change may be made without gradual dosage change; monitor serum or urine glucose and ketones tid during conversion

• Storage in tight container in cool environment

Teach patient/family:

• To use capillary blood glucose test or Chemstrip tid; that periodic LFTs are mandatory

• The symptoms of hypo/hyperglycemia, what to do about each

• That the drug must be continued on daily basis; explain consequence of discontinuing drug abruptly

• To avoid OTC medications or herbal preparations unless approved by prescriber

• That diabetes is lifelong illness; that this drug is not a cure; only controls symptoms

• That all food included in diet plan must be eaten to prevent hypoglycemia

• To carry emergency ID and glucagon emergency kit for emergencies

• To notify prescriber if oral contraceptives are used

• Not to use if breast-feeding

Evaluate:

• Therapeutic response: Decrease in polyuria, polydipsia, polyphagia; clear sensorium; absence of dizziness; stable gait, blood glucose at normal level

---

HIGH ALERT/RARELY USED

pipecuronium (℞)

(pip-e-kyoor-oh′nee-um)

Arduran

Func. class.: Neuromuscular blocker (nondepolarizing)

Uses: Facilitation of endotracheal intubation; skeletal muscle relaxation during mechanical ventilation, surgery, or general anesthesia

Dosage and routes:
• *Adult:* **IV** dosage is individualized; in patients with normal renal function who are not obese, initial dose is 70-85 mcg/kg; maintenance dose ranges from 10-15 mcg/kg
• *Child 1-14 yr:* **IV** 57 mcg/kg
• *Child 3 mo-1 yr:* **IV** 40 mcg/kg
Contraindications: Hypersensitivity to bromide ion

piperacillin (℞)

(pip'er-ah-sill'in)
Pipracil
Func. class.: Broad-spectrum antiinfective
Chem. class.: Extended-spectrum penicillin

Action: Interferes with cell wall replication of susceptible organisms; osmotically unstable cell wall swells and bursts from osmotic pressure
Uses: Respiratory, skin, urinary tract, bone infections; gonorrhea; pneumonia; effective for gram-positive cocci *(Staphylococcus aureus, Streptococcus pyogenes, Streptococcus viridans, Streptococcus faecalis, Streptococcus bovis, Streptococcus pneumoniae),* gram-negative cocci *(Neisseria gonorrhoeae, Neisseria meningitidis),* gram-positive bacilli *(Acinetobacter, Clostridium perfringens, Clostridium tetani),* gram-negative bacilli *(Bacteroides, Citrobacter, Enterobacter, Escherichia coli, Eubacterium, Fusobacterium nucleatum, Klebsiella, Morganella morganii, Peptococcus, Peptostreptococcus, Proteus mirabilis, Proteus vulgaris, Providencia rettgeri, Pseudomonas aeruginosa, Serratia)*

Dosage and routes:
Renal dose
• *Adult:* **IV** CCr 20-40 ml/min give q8h; CCr <20 ml/min give q12h; CCr 10-50 ml/min give q6-8h; CCr <10 ml/min give q8h
Urinary tract infections
• *Adult:* **IV** 8-16 g/day (125-200 mg/kg/day) in divided doses q6-8h
Serious systemic infections
• *Adult and child >12 yr:* **IM/IV** 2-4 g q4-6h (2 g/site **IM**)
• *Child <12 yr:* **IM/IV** 200-300 mg/kg/day in divided doses q4-6h
• *Neonates <36 wk:* **IV** 75 mg/kg q12h in the 1st wk of life, then q8h in 2nd wk
• *Full-term infants:* **IV** 75 mg/kg q8h in 1st wk of life; q6h thereafter
Prophylaxis of surgical infections
• *Adult:* **IV** 2 g ½-1 hr before procedure; may be repeated during surgery or after surgery
Available forms: Powder for inj 2, 3, 4, 40 g
Side effects/adverse reactions:
HEMA: Anemia, increased bleeding time, ***bone marrow depression,*** thrombocytopenia
GI: Nausea, vomiting, diarrhea; increased AST, ALT; abdominal pain, glossitis, ***pseudomembranous colitis***
GU: ***Oliguria, proteinuria, hematuria,*** *vaginitis, moniliasis,* ***glomerulonephritis***
CNS: Lethargy, hallucinations, anxiety, depression, twitching, ***coma, seizures***
META: Hypokalemia, hypernatremia
SYST: ***Serum sickness, anaphylaxis***
Contraindications: Hypersensitivity to penicillins, neonates
Precautions: Pregnancy (B), lactation, hypersensitivity to cephalosporins; CHF, renal disease, seizures
Pharmacokinetics:
IM: Peak 30-50 min

P

IV: Peak 20-30 min

Half-life 0.7-1.33 hr; excreted in urine, bile, breast milk; crosses placenta

Interactions:

• ↓ antimicrobial effect of piperacillin: tetracyclines (with high concentrations of piperacillin), aminoglycosides

• ↓ effect of: oral contraceptives

• ↑ piperacillin concentrations: aspirin, probenecid

↓ absorption: khat

Do not use acidophilus with antiinfectives

Lab test interferences:

False positive: Urine glucose, urine protein, Coombs' test

NURSING CONSIDERATIONS

Assess:

• For infection: temp, WBC, sputum, stools, urine, wounds

• I&O ratio; report hematuria, oliguria, since penicillin in high doses is nephrotoxic

Any patient with compromised renal system, since drug is excreted slowly in poor renal system function; toxicity may occur rapidly

• Hepatic studies: AST, ALT

• Blood studies: WBC, RBC, Hgb, Hct, bleeding time prior to and periodically during treatment

• Renal studies: urinalysis, protein, blood, BUN, creatinine prior to and periodically during treatment

• C&S before drug therapy; drug may be taken as soon as culture is taken

• Bowel pattern before and during treatment

• Skin eruptions after administration of penicillin to 1 wk after discontinuing drug

• Respiratory status: rate, character, wheezing, tightness in chest

• Allergies before initiation of treatment, reaction of each medication

Administer:

• Drug after C&S completed

IM route

• 2 g/4 ml, 3 g/6 ml, 4 g/8 ml of sterile water, 0.9% NaCl max 2 g/site

IV route

• After diluting 1 g or less/5 ml or more sterile H_2O or 0.9% NaCl; shake; give dose over 3-5 min; may further dilute to 50-100 ml with D_5W, 0.9% NS, and give over ½ hr; discontinue primary IV

Additive compatibilities: Ciprofloxacin, clindamycin, fluconazole, hydrocortisone, ofloxacin, potassium chloride, verapamil

Syringe compatibilities: Heparin

Y-site compatibilities: Acyclovir, allopurinol, amifostine, aztreonam, ciprofloxacin, cyclophosphamide, diltiazem, DOXOrubicin liposome, enalaprilat, esmolol, famotidine, fludarabine, foscarnet, gallium, granisetron, heparin, hydromorphone, IL-2, labetalol, lorazepam, magnesium sulfate, melphalan, meperidine, midazolam, morphine, perphenazine, propofol, ranitidine, remifentanil, tacrolimus, teniposide, theophylline, thiotepa, verapamil, zidovudine

Perform/provide:

• Adrenaline, suction, tracheostomy set, endotracheal intubation equipment on unit

• Adequate intake of fluids (2 L) during diarrhea episodes

• Scratch test to assess allergy after securing order from prescriber; usually done when penicillin is only drug of choice

• Storage of reconstituted sol 24 hr at room temperature or 7 days refrigerated

Evaluate:

• Therapeutic response: absence of fever, purulent drainage, redness, inflammation

Teach patient/family:
- That culture may be taken after completed course of medication
- To report sore throat, fever, fatigue; may indicate superinfection
- To wear or carry emergency ID if allergic to penicillins
- To notify nurse of diarrhea

Treatment of anaphylaxis: Withdraw drug, maintain airway, administer epINEPHrine, aminophylline, O_2, IV corticosteroids

piperacillin/tazobactam (℞)

(pip′er-ah-sill′in & ta-zoe-bak′tam)

Zosyn

Func. class.: Antiinfective, broad-spectrum

Chem. class.: Extended-spectrum penicillin, β-lactamase inhibitor

Action: Interferes with cell wall replication of susceptible organisms; osmotically unstable cell wall swells and bursts from osmotic pressure

Uses: Moderate to severe infections: piperacillin-resistant, β-lactamase-producing strains causing infections in respiratory, skin, urinary tract, bone, gonorrhea, pneumonia; effective for resistant *Staphylococcus aureus,* resistant *Escherichia coli, Bacteroides fragilis, Bacteroides ovatus, Bacteroides thetaiotaomicron, Bacteroides vulgatus, Haemophilus influenzae*

Dosage and routes:

Renal dose
- *Adult:* **IV** CCr 20-40 ml/min give 2.25 g q6h; CCr <20 ml/min give 2.25 g q8h

Nosocomial pneumonia
- *Adult:* **IV** 3.375g q6-8h with an aminoglycoside × 1-2 wk; continue aminoglycoside only if *Pseudomonas aeruginosa* is isolated

Other infections
- *Adult:* **IV INF** 6-12 g/day given 2.25 g q8h to 3.375 g q6h over 30 min × 7-10 days

Available forms: Powder for inj 2 g piperacillin/0.25 g tazobactam, 3 g piperacillin/0.375 g tazobactam, 4 g piperacillin/0.5 g tazobactam, 36 g piperacillin/4.5 g tazobactam

Side effects/adverse reactions:

CNS: Lethargy, hallucinations, anxiety, depression, twitching, insomnia, headache, fever, dizziness

GI: Nausea, vomiting, diarrhea; increased AST, ALT; abdominal pain, glossitis, ***pseudomembranous colitis,*** constipation

GU: ***Oliguria, proteinuria, hematuria,*** *vaginitis, moniliasis,* ***glomerulonephritis***

HEMA: Anemia, increased bleeding time, ***bone marrow depression***

META: Hypokalemia, hypernatremia

INTEG: Rash, pruritus

SYST: ***Serum sickness, anaphylaxis***

Contraindications: Hypersensitivity to penicillins, neonates

Precautions: Pregnancy (B), lactation, hypersensitivity to cephalosporins, CHF, renal insufficiency in children, seizures

Pharmacokinetics:

IV: Peak completion of IV, duration 6 hr

Half-life 0.7-1.2 hr; excreted in urine, bile, breast milk; crosses placenta; 33% bound to plasma proteins

Interactions:
- ↑ effect of neuromuscular blockers, oral anticoagulants

P

• ↓ antimicrobial effect of piperacillin: tetracyclines, aminoglycosides IV
• ↓ effect of: oral contraceptives
• ↑ piperacillin concentrations: aspirin, probenecid
↓ absorption: khat
Do not use acidophilus with antiinfectives

Lab test interferences:
False positive: Urine glucose, urine protein, Coombs' test
Decrease: Hct, Hgb, electrolytes
Increase: Platelet count, eosinophilia, neutropenia, leukopenia, serum creatinine, PTT, AST, ALT, alk phosphatase, bilirubin, BUN, electrolytes

NURSING CONSIDERATIONS
Assess:
• For infection: temp, stools, urine, sputum, wounds
• I&O ratio; report hematuria, oliguria, since penicillin in high doses is nephrotoxic
Any patient with compromised renal system, since drug is excreted slowly in poor renal system function; toxicity may occur rapidly
• Hepatic studies: AST, ALT prior to and periodically thereafter
• Blood studies: WBC, RBC, Hct, Hgb, bleeding time prior to and periodically thereafter
• Renal studies: urinalysis, protein, blood, BUN, creatinine prior to and periodically thereafter
• C&S before drug therapy; drug may be given as soon as culture is taken
• Bowel pattern before and during treatment
• Skin eruptions after administration of penicillin to 1 wk after discontinuing drug
• Respiratory status: rate, character, wheezing, tightness in chest
• Allergies before initiation of treatment, reaction of each medication

Administer:
• Drug after C&S is complete

IV route
• After diluting 5 ml 0.9% NaCl for injection or sterile H_2O for injection, dextran 6% in NS, dextrose 5%, KCl 40 mEq, bacteriostatic saline/parabens, bacteriostatic saline/benzyl alcohol, bacteriostatic H_2O/benzyl alcohol per 1 g piperacillin; shake well; further dilute in at least 50 ml compatible IV sol and run as int inf over at least 30 min

Y-site compatibilities: Aminophylline, aztreonam, bleomycin, bumetanide, buprenorphine, butorphanol, calcium gluconate, carboplatin, carmustine, cefepime, cimetidine, clindamycin, cyclophosphamide, cytarabine, dexamethasone, diphenhydrAMINE, DOPamine, enalaprilat, etoposide, floxuridine, fluconazole, fludarabine, fluorouracil, furosemide, gallium, granisetron, heparin, hydrocortisone, hydromorphone, ifosfamide, leucovorin, lorazepam, magnesium sulfate, mannitol, meperidine, mesna, methotrexate, methylPREDNISolone, metoclopramide, metronidazole, morphine, ondansetron, plicamycin, potassium chloride, ranitidine, remifentanil, sargramostim, sodium bicarbonate, thiotepa, trimethoprim-sulfamethoxazole, vinBLAStine, vinCRIStine, zidovudine

Perform/provide:
• Adrenaline, suction, tracheostomy set, endotracheal intubation equipment on unit
• Adequate intake of fluids (2 L) during diarrhea episodes
• Scratch test to assess allergy on order from prescriber; usually when penicillin is only drug of choice
• Discard after 24 hr if stored at room temperature or after 48 hr if refrigerated; use single-dose vials

immediately after reconstitution; stable in ambulatory IV pump for 12 hr

Evaluate:

- Therapeutic response: absence of fever, purulent drainage, redness, inflammation; culture shows decreased organisms

Teach patient/family:

- That culture may be taken after completed course of medication
- To report sore throat, fever, fatigue (may indicate superinfection)
- To wear or carry emergency ID if allergic to penicillins
- To notify nurse of diarrhea

Treatment of overdose: Withdraw drug, maintain airway, administer epINEPHrine, aminophylline, O_2, IV corticosteroids for anaphylaxis

pirbuterol (℞)

(peer-byoo′ter-ole)

Maxair

Func. class.: Bronchodilator

Chem. class.: β-Adrenergic agonist

Action: Causes bronchodilation with little effect on heart rate by action on β-receptors, causing increased cAMP and relaxation of smooth muscle

Uses: Reversible bronchospasm (prevention, treatment) including asthma; may be given with theophylline or steroids

Dosage and routes:

- *Adult and child >12 yr:* **INH** 1-2 puffs (0.4 mg) q4-6h; max 12 **INH**/day

Available forms: Aerosol delivery 0.2 mg pirbuterol/actuation

Side effects/adverse reactions:

CNS: Tremors, anxiety, insomnia, headache, dizziness, stimulation, restlessness, hallucinations, drowsiness, irritability

EENT: Dry nose and mouth, irritation of nose, throat

CV: Palpitations, tachycardia, hypertension, angina, hypotension, dysrhythmias

GI: Gastritis, nausea, vomiting, anorexia

MS: Muscle cramps

RESP: ***Paradoxical bronchospasm,*** dyspnea, coughing

Contraindications: Hypersensitivity to sympathomimetics, tachycardia

Precautions: Lactation, pregnancy (C), cardiac disorders, hyperthyroidism, diabetes mellitus, prostatic hypertrophy

Pharmacokinetics:

INH: Onset 3 min, peak ½-1 hr, duration 5 hr

Interactions:

- ↑ action of other aerosol bronchodilators
- ↑ pirbuterol action: tricyclics, antihistamines, levothyroxine
- ↓ pirbuterol action: β-blockers

Hypertensive crisis: MAOIs

↑ action of both: cola nut, guarana, yerba maté

↑ effect: green tea (large amounts), guarana

NURSING CONSIDERATIONS

Assess:

- Respiratory function: vital capacity, forced expiratory volume, ABGs, B/P, lung sounds, pulse, characteristics of sputum

Paradoxical bronchospasm, that can occur rapidly, hold drug, notify prescriber

Administer:

- After shaking; exhale, place mouthpiece in mouth, inhale slowly, hold breath, remove, exhale slowly
- Gum, sips of water for dry mouth

Perform/provide:

- Storage in light-resistant container; do not expose to temperatures over 86° F (30° C)

P

Evaluate:

- Therapeutic response: absence of dyspnea, wheezing over 1 hr

Teach patient/family:

- Not to use OTC medications; extra stimulation may occur
- Use of inhaler; review package insert with patient
- To avoid getting aerosol in eyes
- To wash inhaler in warm water and dry qd, rinse mouth after use; if used with inhalers containing glucocorticosteroids, wait 5 min before using steroid inhaler
- About all aspects of drug; avoid smoking, smoke-filled rooms, persons with respiratory infections
- To keep fluid intake >2 L/day to liquefy thick secretions

Treatment of overdose: Administer a β-adrenergic blocker

piroxicam (℞)

(peer-ox'i-kam)

Apo-Piroxicam✱, Feldene, Novopirocam✱, Nu-Pirox, PMS-Piroxicam✱

Func. class.: Nonsteroidal antiinflammatory

Chem. class.: Oxicam derivative

Action: Inhibits prostaglandin synthesis by decreasing an enzyme needed for biosynthesis; has analgesic, antiinflammatory, antipyretic properties

Uses: Mild to moderate pain, osteoarthritis, rheumatoid arthritis

Dosage and routes:

- *Adult:* **PO** 20 mg qd or 10 mg bid

Available forms: Caps 10, 20 mg

Side effects/adverse reactions:

GI: Nausea, anorexia, vomiting, diarrhea, jaundice, ***cholestatic hepatitis,*** constipation, flatulence, cramps, dry mouth, peptic ulcer, ***bleeding, ulceration, perforation***

CNS: Dizziness, *drowsiness,* fatigue, tremors, confusion, insomnia, anxiety, depression, *headache*

CV: Tachycardia, peripheral edema, palpitations, dysrhythmias

INTEG: Purpura, rash, pruritus, sweating, photosensitivity

GU: ***Nephrotoxicity: dysuria, hematuria, oliguria, azotemia***

HEMA: ***Blood dyscrasias***

EENT: Tinnitus, hearing loss, blurred vision

SYST: ***Anaphylaxis***

Contraindications: Hypersensitivity, asthma, severe renal disease, severe hepatic disease, ulcer disease, cardiac disease

Precautions: Pregnancy (B), avoid in late pregnancy, lactation, children, bleeding disorders, GI disorders, cardiac disorders, hypersensitivity to other antiinflammatory agents, CHF

Pharmacokinetics:

PO: Peak 2 hr; duration 48-72 hr, half-life 30-80 hr; metabolized in liver; excreted in urine (metabolites), breast milk; 99% protein binding

Interactions:

- ↑ toxicity: cycloSPORINE, methotrexate, lithium, alcohol, oral anticoagulants, aspirin, corticosteroids
- ↓ effects of: antihypertensives, diuretics
- Hypoglycemia: oral antidiabetics

(Herb) ↑ gastric irritation: arginine, gossypol

(Herb) ↑ NSAIDs effect: bearberry, bilberry

(Herb) ↑ bleeding risk: bogbean, chondroitin

NURSING CONSIDERATIONS

Assess:

- For pain: location, duration, type, ROM before and 1-2 hr after administration

• Renal, hepatic, blood studies: BUN, creatinine, AST, ALT, Hgb, before treatment, periodically thereafter
• Audiometric, ophthalmic exam before, during, after treatment
• For eye, ear problems: blurred vision, tinnitus (may indicate toxicity)
⬥ Those with aspirin sensitivity, asthma, nasal polyps may develop allergic reactions

Administer:
• With food to decrease GI symptoms; take on empty stomach to facilitate absorption; take drug same time qd

Perform/provide:
• Storage at room temperature

Evaluate:
• Therapeutic response: decreased pain, stiffness, swelling in joints; ability to move more easily

Teach patient/family:
⊘ Not to break, crush, or chew caps
• To report blurred vision or ringing, roaring in ears (may indicate toxicity)
• To avoid driving, other hazardous activities if dizzy or drowsy
• That patient should drink at least 6-8 glasses of water/day
• To report change in urine pattern, weight increase, edema, pain increase in joints, fever, blood in urine (indicates nephrotoxicity)
• That therapeutic effects may take up to 1 mo
• To avoid ASA, other OTC meds, alcohol; advise patient to use sunscreen

plasma protein fraction (℞)

Plasmanate, Plasma Plex, Plasmatein, Protenate

Func. class.: Blood derivative

Chem. class.: Human plasma in NaCl

Action: Exerts similar oncotic pressure as human plasma, expands blood volume

Uses: Hypovolemic shock, hypoproteinemia, ARDS, preoperative cardiopulmonary bypass, acute hepatic failure, nephrotic syndrome

Dosage and routes:

Hypovolemia
• *Adult:* **IV INF** 250-500 ml (12.5-25 g protein), not to exceed 10 ml/min
• *Child:* **IV INF** 22-33 ml/kg at 5-10 ml/min

Hypoproteinemia
• *Adult:* **IV INF** 1000-1500 ml qd, not to exceed 8 ml/min

Available forms: Inj 5%

Side effects/adverse reactions:
GI: Nausea, vomiting, increased salivation
INTEG: Rash, urticaria, cyanosis
CNS: Fever, chills, headache, paresthesias, flushing
RESP: Altered respirations, dyspnea, ***pulmonary edema***
CV: ***Fluid overload,*** hypotension, erratic pulse

Contraindications: Hypersensitivity, CHF, severe anemia, renal insufficiency

Precautions: Decreased salt intake, decreased cardiac reserve, lack of albumin deficiency, hepatic disease, renal disease, pregnancy (C)

Pharmacokinetics: Metabolized as a protein/energy source

Lab test interferences:
False increase: Alk phosphatase

P

NURSING CONSIDERATIONS

Assess:

• Blood studies: Hct, Hgb, electrolytes, serum protein; if serum protein declines, dyspnea, hypoxemia can result

• B/P (decreased), pulse (erratic), respiration during infusion

• I&O ratio; urinary output may decrease

• CVP, pulmonary wedge pressure (increases if overload occurs), jugular vein distention

• Allergy: fever, rash, itching, chills, flushing, urticaria, nausea, vomiting, or hypotension requires discontinuation of infusion; use new lot if therapy reinstituted, premedicate with diphenhydrAMINE

Increased CVP reading: distended neck veins indicate circulatory overload; SOB, anxiety, insomnia, expiratory rales, frothy blood-tinged cough, cyanosis indicate pulmonary overload

Administer:

IV route

• No dilution required; use infusion pump, use large-gauge needle (≥20G), discard unused portion, infuse slowly

• Within 4 hr of opening

Additive compatibilities: Carbohydrate and electrolyte sol, whole blood, packed red blood cells, chloramphenicol, tetracycline

Perform/provide:

• Adequate hydration before administration

• Storage—check type of albumin, date; may have to refrigerate

Evaluate:

• Therapeutic response: increased B/P, decreased edema, increased serum albumin

HIGH ALERT

plicamycin (℞)

(ply-ka-my′sin)

Mithramycin, Mithracin

Func. class.: Antineoplastic, antibiotic; hypocalcemic

Chem. class.: Crystalline aglycone

Action: Inhibits DNA, RNA, protein synthesis; derived from *Streptomyces plicatus;* replication is decreased by binding to DNA; demonstrates calcium-lowering effect not related to its tumoricidal activity; also acts on osteoclasts and blocks action of parathyroid hormone; a vesicant

Uses: Testicular cancer, hypercalcemia, hypercalciuria, symptomatic treatment of advanced neoplasms

Dosage and routes:

Testicular tumors

• *Adult:* **IV** 25-30 mcg/kg/day × 8-10 days, not to exceed 30 mcg/kg/day

Hypercalcemia/hypercalciuria

• *Adult:* **IV** 25 mcg/kg/day × 3-4 days, repeat at intervals of 1 wk

Available forms: Inj 2500 mcg/vial powder

Side effects/adverse reactions:

META: Decreased serum Ca, P, K

HEMA: ***Hemorrhage, thrombocytopenia,*** decreased PT, WBC count

GI: Nausea, vomiting, anorexia, diarrhea, stomatitis, increased liver enzymes

GU: Increased BUN, creatinine; ***proteinuria***

INTEG: Rash, cellulitis, ***extravasation,*** facial flushing

CNS: Drowsiness, weakness, lethargy, headache, flushing, fever, depression

Contraindications: Hypersensitiv-

ity, thrombocytopenia, bone marrow depression, bleeding disorders, pregnancy (X), lactation, child <15 yr

Precautions: Renal disease, hepatic disease, electrolyte imbalances, lactation

Pharmacokinetics: Crosses blood-brain barrier, excreted in urine; little known about pharmacokinetics

Interactions:

- ↑ toxicity: other antineoplastics or radiation
- ↑ bleeding risk: anise, arnica, chamomile, clove, dong quai, fenugreek, garlic, ginger, ginkgo, ginseng *(Panax),* licorice

NURSING CONSIDERATIONS

Assess:

- CBC, differential, platelet count qwk; withhold drug if WBC is $<4000/mm^3$ or platelet count is $<50{,}000/mm^3$; notify prescriber
- Renal studies: BUN, serum uric acid, urine CCr, electrolytes before, during therapy
- I&O ratio; report urine output <30 ml/hr
- Monitor temp q4h; fever may indicate beginning infection
- Hepatic studies before, during therapy: bilirubin, AST, ALT, alk phosphatase prn or qmo; jaundiced skin, sclera; dark urine, clay-colored stools, itchy skin, abdominal pain, fever, diarrhea
- Alkalosis if severe vomiting is present
- Toxicity: facial flushing, epistaxis, increased PT, thrombocytopenia; drug should be discontinued
- Bleeding: hematuria, guaiac stools, bruising or petechiae, mucosa or orifices q8h; may progress to severe bleeding
- Inflammation of mucosa, breaks in skin
- Buccal cavity q8h for dryness, sores, ulceration, white patches, oral pain, bleeding, dysphagia
- Local irritation, pain, burning at inj site
- Frequency of stools, characteristics, cramping
- Acidosis, signs of dehydration: rapid respirations, poor skin turgor, decreased urine output, dry skin, restlessness, weakness

Administer:

- Antiemetic 30-60 min before giving drug and 4-10 hr after treatment to prevent vomiting
- Transfusion for anemia
- Antispasmodic for diarrhea, phenothiazine for nausea and vomiting

IV route

- Dilute 2.5 mg/4.9 ml of sterile H_2O; (500 mcg/ml) dilute single dose in 1000 ml of D_5W run over 4-6 hr
- EDTA for extravasation, apply ice compress
- Slow IV infusion using 20G, 21G needle

Y-site compatibilities: Allopurinol, amifostine, aztreonam, filgrastim, granisetron, melphalan, piperacillin/tazobactam, teniposide, thiotepa, vinorelbine

Perform/provide:

- Liquid diet: carbonated beverages; gelatin may be added if patient is not nauseated or vomiting
- Rinsing of mouth tid-qid with water; brushing of teeth with baking soda bid-tid with soft brush or cotton-tipped applicator for stomatitis; unwaxed dental floss
- Usage immediately after mixing

Evaluate:

- Therapeutic response: decreased tumor size, spread of malignancy

Teach patient/family:

- To report any complaints or side effects to nurse or prescriber
- To avoid foods with citric acid, hot or rough texture

P

• To report to prescriber any bleeding, white spots, ulcerations in the mouth; tell patient to examine mouth qd
• To avoid driving, activities requiring alertness; drowsiness may occur
• To report leg cramps, tingling of fingertips, weakness; may indicate hypocalcemia
• To avoid crowds, persons with infections when granulocyte count is low

polymyxin B ophthalmic

See appendix c

RARELY USED

poractant alfa (℞)

Curosurf

Func. class.: Lung surfactant extract

Uses: Treatment (rescue) of respiratory distress syndrome in premature infants

Dosage and routes:

• **INTRATRACHEAL INSTILL: Premature**

• *Infant:* 2.5 ml/kg birth weight up to 2 subsequent doses of 1.25 ml/kg birth weight can be administered at 12-hr intervals, max 5 ml/kg

porfimer (℞)

(pour′fih-mur)

Photofrin

Func. class.: Antineoplastic-miscellaneous

Action: Used in photodynamic treatment of tumors (PDT); antitumor and cytotoxic actions are light and O_2 dependent; used with 630 nm laser light

Uses: Esophageal cancer (completely obstructing), endobronchial non–small cell lung cancer

Dosage and routes:

• Refer to Optiguide for complete instructions

• *Adult:* **IV** 2 mg/kg, then illumination with laser light 40-50 hr after inj; a second laser light application may be given 96-120 hr after inj; may repeat q30 days × 3

Endobronchial cancer

• *Adult:* 200 joules/cm of tumor length

Available forms: Cake/powder for inj 75 mg

Side effects/adverse reactions:

CV: Hypotension, hypertension, atrial fibrillation, ***cardiac failure,*** *tachycardia*

GI: Abdominal pain, constipation, diarrhea, dyspepsia, dysphagia, eructation, esophageal edema/bleeding, hematemesis, melena, nausea, vomiting, anorexia

CNS: Anxiety, confusion, insomnia

RESP: ***Pleural effusion,*** pneumonia, dyspnea, respiratory insufficiency, ***tracheoesophageal fistula***

MISC: Dehydration, weight decrease, anemia, photosensitivity reaction, UTI, moniliasis

Contraindications: Porphyria, porphyrin allergy (porfimer); tracheoesophageal, bronchoesophageal fistula; major blood vessels with eroding tumors (PDT)

Precautions: Elderly, pregnancy (C), lactation, children

Pharmacokinetics: Half-life 250 hr, 90% protein bound

Interactions:

• ↑ photosensitivity: tetracyclines, sulfonamides, phenothiazines, sulfonylureas, thiazides

NURSING CONSIDERATIONS

Assess:

• Ocular sensitivity: sensitivity to sun, bright lights, car headlights, patients should wear dark sunglasses with an average light transmittance of <4%

• Chest pain: may be so severe as to necessitate opiate analgesics

• For extravasation at inj site: take care to protect from light

Administer:

• As a single slow IV inj over 3-5 min at 2 mg/kg; reconstitute each vial with 31.8 ml D_5 or 0.9% NaCl (2.5 mg/ml), shake well; do not mix with other drugs or sol; protect from light and use immediately

• Laser light is initiated 630 nm wave length laser light

Perform/provide:

• Wiping of spills with damp cloth, avoid skin/eye contact, use rubber gloves, eye protection, dispose of material in polyethylene bag according to policy

Teach patient/family:

• To report chest pain, eye sensitivity

• To wear sunglasses; avoid exposure to sunlight or bright light for 30 days

potassium acetate

potassium bicarbonate (OTC, ℞)

K+ Care ET, K-Electrolyte, K-Ide, Klor-Con EF, K-Lyte, K-Vescent

potassium bicarbonate and potassium chloride (OTC, ℞)

Klorvess, Klorvess Effervescent Granules, K-Lyte/Cl, Neo-K✦

potassium bicarbonate and potassium citrate (OTC, ℞)

Effer-K, K-Lyte DS

potassium chloride (OTC, ℞)

Apo-K✦, Cena-K, Gen-K, K+ Care, K+ 10, Kalium Durules✦, Kaochlor, Kaochlor S-F, Kaon-Cl, Kay Ciel, KCl, K-Dur, K-Lease, K-Long✦, K-Lor, Klor-Con, Klorvess, Klotrix, K-Lyte/C1 powder, K-med, K-Norm, K-Sol, K-tab, Micro-K, Micro-LS, Potasalan, Roychlor, Rum-K, Slow-K, Ten-K

potassium chloride/ potassium bicarbonate/ potassium citrate (OTC, ℞)

Kaochlor Eff

potassium gluconate (OTC, ℞)

Kaon, Kaylixir, K-G Elixir, Potassium-Rougier✦

potassium gluconate/ potassium chloride (OTC, ℞)

Kolyum

potassium gluconate/ potassium citrate (OTC, ℞)

Twin-K

Func. class.: Electrolyte, mineral replacement

Chem. class.: Potassium

Action: Needed for adequate transmission of nerve impulses and cardiac contraction, renal function, intracellular ion maintenance

Uses: Prevention and treatment of hypokalemia

Dosage and routes:

Potassium acetate—hypokalemia

• *Adult and child:* **PO** 40-100 mEq/day in divided doses 2-4 days

Potassium bicarbonate

• *Adult:* **PO** dissolve 25-50 mEq in water qd-qid

Hypokalemia (prevention)

• *Adult and child:* **PO** 20 mEq/day in 2-4 divided doses

Potassium chloride

• *Adult:* **PO** 40-100 mEq in divided doses tid-qid; **IV** 20 mEq/hr when diluted as 40 mEq/1000 ml, not to exceed 150 mEq/day

• *Child:* **PO** 2-4 mEq/kg/day

Potassium gluconate

• *Adult:* **PO** 40-100 mEq in divided doses tid-qid

Potassium phosphate

• *Adult:* **IV** 1 mEq/hr in sol of 60 mEq/L, not to exceed 150 mEq/day; **PO** 40-100 mEq/day in divided doses

• *Child:* **IV** max rate of inf 1 mEq/kg/hr

Available forms: Tabs for sol 6.5, 25 mEq; caps, ext rel 8, 10 mEq; powder for sol 3.3, 5, 6.7, 10, 13.3 mEq/5 ml; tabs 2, 4, 5, 13.4 mEq; tabs, ext rel 6.7, 8, 10 mEq; elix 6.7 mEq/5 ml; oral sol 2.375 mEq/5 ml; inj for prep of IV 1.5, 2, 2.4, 3, 3.2, 4.4, 4.7 mEq/ml

Side effects/adverse reactions:

CNS: Confusion

CV: Bradycardia, ***cardiac depression, dysrhythmias, arrest, peaking T waves, lowered R and depressed RST, prolonged P-R interval, widened QRS complex***

GI: Nausea, vomiting, cramps, pain, *diarrhea,* ulceration of small bowel

GU: Oliguria

INTEG: Cold extremities, rash

Contraindications: Renal disease (severe), severe hemolytic disease, Addison's disease, hyperkalemia, acute dehydration, extensive tissue breakdown

Precautions: Cardiac disease, potassium-sparing diuretic therapy, systemic acidosis, pregnancy (C)

Pharmacokinetics:

PO: Excreted by kidneys and in feces; onset of action ≈30 min

IV: Immediate onset of action

Interactions:

• Hyperkalemia: potassium phosphate IV and products containing calcium or magnesium; potassium-sparing diuretic, or other potassium products, ACE inhibitors

NURSING CONSIDERATIONS

Assess:

• ECG for peaking T waves, lowered R, depressed RST, prolonged P-R interval, widening QRS complex, hyperkalemia; drug should be reduced or discontinued

• Potassium level during treatment (3.5-5 mg/dl is normal level)

• I&O ratio; watch for decreased urinary output; notify prescriber immediately

• Cardiac status: rate, rhythm, CVP, PWP, PAWP, if being monitored directly

Administer:

PO route

• With meal or pc; dissolve effervescent tabs, powder in 8 oz cold water or juice; do not give IM, SC

⊘ Do not crush, break or chew ext rel tabs/caps or enteric products

IV route

• Through large-bore needle to decrease vein inflammation; check for extravasation

• In large vein, avoiding scalp vein in child (IV)

• IV after diluting in large volume of IV sol and give as an inf, slowly by IV inf to prevent toxicity; never give IV bolus or IM

Potassium acetate
Additive compatibilities: Metoclopramide
Y-site compatibilities: Ciprofloxacin
Potassium chloride
Additive compatibilities: Aminophylline, amiodarone, atracurium, bretylium, calcium gluconate, cefepime, cephalothin, cephapirin, chloramphenicol, cimetidine, ciprofloxacin, cisatracurium, clindamycin, cloxacillin, corticotropin, cytarabine, dimenhyDRINATE, DOPamine, DOXOrubicin liposome, enalaprilat, erythromycin, floxacillin, fluconazole, fosphenytoin, furosemide, heparin, hydrocortisone, isoproterenol, lidocaine, metaraminol, methicillin, methyldopate, metoclopramide, mitoxantrone, nafcillin, netilmicin, norepinephrine, oxacillin, penicillin G potassium, phenylephrine, piperacillin, ranitidine, sodium bicarbonate, thiopental, vancomycin, verapamil, vit B/C
Y-site compatibilities: Acyclovir, aldesleukin, allopurinol, amifostine, aminophylline, amiodarone, ampicillin, amrinone, atropine, aztreonam, betamethasone, calcium gluconate, cefmetazole, cephalothin, cephapirin, chlordiazepoxide, chlorproMAZINE, ciprofloxacin, cladribine, cyanocobalamin, dexamethasone, digoxin, diltiazem, diphenhydrAMINE, DOBUTamine, DOPamine, droperidol, edrophonium, enalaprilat, epINEPHrine, esmolol, estrogens, ethacrynate, famotidine, fentanyl, filgrastim, fludarabine, fluorouracil, furosemide, gallium, granisetron, heparin, hydrALAZINE, idarubicin, indomethacin, insulin (regular), isoproterenol, kanamycin, labetalol, lidocaine, lorazepam, magnesium sulfate, melphalan, meperidine, methicillin, methoxamine, methylergonovine, midazolam, minocycline, morphine, neostigmine, norepinephrine, ondansetron, oxacillin, oxytocin, paclitaxel, penicillin G potassium, pentazocine, phytonadione, piperacillin/tazobactam, prednisoLONE, procainamide, prochlorperazine, propofol, propranolol, pyridostigmine, remifentanil, sargramostim, scopolamine, sodium bicarbonate, succinylcholine, tacrolimus, teniposide, theophylline, thiotepa, trimethaphan, trimethobenzamide, vinorelbine, warfarin, zidovudine

Perform/provide:
- Storage at room temperature

Evaluate:
- Therapeutic response: absence of fatigue, muscle weakness; decreased thirst and urinary output; cardiac changes

Teach patient/family:
- To add potassium-rich foods to diet: bananas, orange juice, avocados; whole grains, broccoli, carrots, prunes, cocoa after this medication is discontinued
- To avoid OTC products: antacids, salt substitutes, analgesics, vitamin preparations, unless specifically directed by prescriber
- To report hyperkalemia symptoms (lethargy, confusion, diarrhea, nausea, vomiting, fainting, decreased output) or continued hypokalemia symptoms (fatigue, weakness, polyuria, polydipsia, cardiac changes)
- To take capsules with full glass of liquid
- To dissolve powder or tablet completely in at least 120 ml water or juice
- Importance of regular follow-up visits

potassium iodide (℞)

Pima, potassium iodide solution, SSKI, Thyro-Block

Func. class.: Thyroid hormone antagonist

Chem. class.: Iodine product

Action: Inhibits secretion of thyroid hormone, fosters colloid accumulation in thyroid follicles, decreases vascularity of gland

Uses: Preparation for thyroidectomy, thyrotoxic crisis, neonatal thyrotoxicosis, radiation protectant, thyroid storm

Dosage and routes:

Thyrotoxic crisis

• *Adult and child:* **PO** 1 ml in water tid after meals (strong iodine sol)

Preparation for thyroidectomy

• *Adult and child:* **PO** 0.1-0.3 ml tid (strong iodine sol) or 5 gtt in water tid pc × 2-3 wk before surgery (potassium iodide sol)

Available forms: Sol 5%, 10%, 21 mg/gtt; tabs 130, 300 mg; inj 10%, 20%; oral syr 325 mg/5 ml; tabs 130 mg✤

Side effects/adverse reactions:

ENDO: Hypothyroidism, hyperthyroid adenoma

INTEG: Rash, urticaria, ***angineurotic edema,*** acne, mucosal hemorrhage, fever

CNS: Headache, confusion, paresthesias

GI: Nausea, diarrhea, vomiting, small-bowel lesions, upper gastric pain

MS: Myalgia, arthralgia, weakness

EENT: Metallic taste, stomatitis, salivation, periorbital edema, sore teeth and gums, cold symptoms

Contraindications: Hypersensitivity to iodine, pulmonary edema, pulmonary TB, pregnancy (D)

Precautions: Lactation, children

Pharmacokinetics:

PO: Onset 24-48 hr, peak 10-15 days after continuous therapy, uptake by thyroid gland or excreted in urine; crosses placenta

Interactions:

• Hypothyroidism: lithium, other antithyroid agents

Lab test interferences:

Interference: Urinary 17-OHCS

NURSING CONSIDERATIONS

Assess:

• Pulse, B/P, temp

• I&O ratio; check for edema: puffy hands, feet, periorbit; indicate hypothyroidism

• Weight qd; same clothing, scale, time of day

• T_3, T_4, which is increased; serum TSH, which is decreased; free thyroxine index, which is increased if dosage is too low; discontinue drug 3-4 wk before RAIU

◆ Overdose: peripheral edema, heat intolerance, diaphoresis, palpitations, dysrhythmias, severe tachycardia, fever, delirium, CNS irritability

• Hypersensitivity: rash; enlarged cervical lymph nodes may indicate drug should be discontinued

• Hypoprothrombinemia: bleeding, petechiae, ecchymosis

• Clinical response: after 3 wk should include increased weight, pulse; decreased T_4

Administer:

• Strong iodine solution after diluting with water or juice to improve taste

• Through straw to prevent tooth discoloration

• With meals to decrease GI upset

• At same time each day to maintain drug level

• Lowest dose that relieves symptoms, discontinue before RAIU

Perform/provide:
• Fluids to 3-4 L/day, unless contraindicated
Evaluate:
• Therapeutic response: weight gain, decreased pulse, T_4, size of thyroid gland
Teach patient/family:
• To abstain from breastfeeding after delivery
• To keep graph of weight, pulse, mood
• To avoid OTC products that contain iodine
• That seafood, other iodine products may be restricted
• Not to discontinue this medication abruptly; thyroid crisis may occur; stress response
• That response may take several mo if thyroid is large
• To discontinue drug, notify prescriber of fever, rash, metallic taste, swelling of throat; burning of mouth, throat; sore gums, teeth; severe GI distress, enlargement of thyroid, cold symptoms

---

RARELY USED

pralidoxime (℞)
(pra-li-dox′eem)
Protopam Chloride
Func. class.: Cholinesterase reactivator

Uses: Cholinergic crisis in myasthenia gravis, organophosphate poisoning antidote (early), relief of paralysis of respiratory muscles; used as an adjunct to systemic atropine administration
Dosage and routes:
Anticholinesterase overdose
• *Adult:* **IV** 1-2 g, then 250 mg q5min until desired response
Organophosphate poisoning
• *Adult:* **IV INF** 1-2 g/100 ml 0.9% NaCl over 15-30 min; may repeat in 1 hr; **PO** 1-3 g q5h
• *Child:* **IV INF** 20-40 mg/kg/dose diluted in 100 ml 0.9% NaCl over 15-30 min
Contraindications: Hypersensitivity, carbamate insecticide poisoning

pramipexole (℞)
(pra-mi-pex′ol)
Mirapex
Func. class.: Antiparkinson agent
Chem. class.: Dopamine-receptor agonist, non-ergot

Action: Selective agonist for D_2 receptors (presynaptic/postsynaptic sites); binding at D_3 receptor contributes to antiparkinson effects
Uses: Parkinsonism
Investigational uses: Restless leg syndrome
Dosage and routes:
Initial treatment
• *Adult:* **PO** from a starting dose of 0.375 mg/day given in 3 divided doses; increase gradually by 0.125 mg/dose at 5-7 day intervals until total daily dose of 4.5 mg is reached
Maintenance treatment
• *Adult:* **PO** 1.5-4.5 mg qd in 3 divided doses
Renal dose
• *Adult:* **PO** CCr 35-59 ml/min-0.125 mg bid, may increase q5-7 days to 1.5 mg bid; CCr 15-34 ml/min 0.125 mg qd, increase q5-7 days to 1.5 mg qd
Restless leg syndrome (off-label)
• *Adult:* **PO** 0.125-0.375 mg 1-2 hr prior to hs, increase gradually

P

Available forms: Tabs 0.125, 0.25, 1, 1.5 mg

Side effects/adverse reactions:

HEMA: ***Hemolytic anemia, leukopenia, agranulocytosis***

CNS: Agitation, insomnia, psychosis, hallucination, depression, dizziness, headache, confusion, ***sleep attacks***

GI: Nausea, anorexia, constipation, dysphagia, dry mouth

CV: Orthostatic hypotension, edema, syncope, tachycardia

GU: Impotence, urinary frequency

EENT: Blurred vision

Contraindications: Hypersensitivity

Precautions: Renal disease, cardiac disease, MI with dysrhythmias, affective disorders, psychosis, pregnancy (C), preexisting dyskinesias

Pharmacokinetics: Minimally metabolized, peak 2 hr, half-life 8 hr, 12-14 hr in elderly

Interactions:

- ↑ pramipexole levels: levodopa, cimetidine, ranitidine, diltiazem, triamterene, verapamil, quinidine
- ↓ pramipexole levels: DOPamine antagonists, phenothiazines, metoclopramide, butyrophenones

↓ effect of pramipexole: chaste tree fruit, kava

NURSING CONSIDERATIONS

Assess:

- Renal studies
- Involuntary movements in parkinsonism: akinesia, tremors, staggering gait, muscle rigidity, drooling
- B/P, ECG, respiration during initial treatment; hypo/hypertension should be reported
- Mental status: affect, mood, behavioral changes, depression; complete suicide assessment

For sleep attacks: may fall asleep during activities without warning; may need to discontinue medication

Administer:

- Adjust dosage to patient response
- With meals to minimize GI symptoms

Perform/provide:

- Assistance with ambulation during beginning therapy
- Testing for diabetes mellitus, acromegaly if on long-term therapy

Evaluate:

- Therapeutic response: decrease in akathisia, increased mood

Teach patient/family:

- That therapeutic effects may take several wk to a few mo
- To change positions slowly to prevent orthostatic hypotension
- To use drug exactly as prescribed: if drug is discontinued abruptly, parkinsonian crisis may occur, avoid alcohol, OTC sleeping products
- To notify prescriber if pregnancy is planned or suspected

pramoxine topical

See appendix c

pravastatin (℞)

(pra′va-sta-tin)

Pravachol

Func. class.: Antilipidemic

Chem. class.: HMG-CoA reductase enzyme

Action: Inhibits HMG-CoA reductase enzyme, which reduces cholesterol synthesis

Uses: As an adjunct in primary hypercholesterolemia (types IIa, IIb, III, IV), to reduce the risk of recurrent MI, atherosclerosis, primary/secondary CV events

Dosage and routes:

- *Adult:* **PO** 40-80 mg qd at hs (range 20-80 mg qd)

• *Elderly/renal/hepatic disease:* **PO** 10 mg/day initially
Available forms: Tabs 10, 20, 40, 80 mg
Side effects/adverse reactions:
INTEG: Rash, pruritus, photosensitivity
GI: Nausea, constipation, diarrhea, flatus, abdominal pain, heartburn, ***hepatic dysfunction,*** pancreatitis, ***hepatitis***
EENT: Lens opacities
RESP: Common cold, rhinitis, cough
MS: Muscle cramps, myalgia, ***myositis, rhabdomyolysis***
CNS: Headache, dizziness, fatigue
MISC: Chest pain, rash, pruritus, photosensitivity
Contraindications: Hypersensitivity, pregnancy (X), lactation, active liver disease
Precautions: Past hepatic disease, alcoholism, severe acute infections, trauma, severe metabolic disorders, electrolyte imbalances
Do not confuse:
Pravachol/Prevacid
Pharmacokinetics: Peak 1-1½ hr; metabolized by the liver, protein binding 80%; excreted in urine 20%, feces 70%, breast milk; crosses placenta
Interactions:
• ↑ myopathy risk: erythromycin, niacin, cycloSPORINE, gemfibrozil, clofibrate, clarithromycin, itraconazole, protease inhibitors
• ↑ effects of warfarin, digoxin
• ↓ bioavailability of pravastatin: bile acid sequestrants
↑ effect: glucomannan
↓ effect: gotu kola
Lab test interferences:
Increase: CPK, LFTs
Altered: thyroid function tests
NURSING CONSIDERATIONS
Assess:
• Fasting lipid profile: LDL, HDL, TG, cholesterol q8wk, then q3-6mo when stable; obtain diet history
• Hepatic studies: baseline, q6wk during the first 3 mo, q8wk for remainder of yr, then q6mo; AST, ALT, LFTs may increase
• Ophthalmic status qyr
• Renal studies in patients with compromised renal system: BUN, I&O ratio, creatinine
For muscle tenderness, pain, obtain CPK, rhabdomyolysis may occur, therapy should be discontinued
Administer:
• Without regard to meals, hs
• Give 1 hr ac or 2 hr pc bile acid sequestrants
Perform/provide:
• Storage in cool environment in tight container protected from light
Evaluate:
• Therapeutic response: decrease in cholesterol to desired level after 8 wk
Teach patient/family:
• That blood work will be necessary during treatment
To report blurred vision, severe GI symptoms, dizziness, headache, muscle pain, weakness, fever
• That regimen will continue: low-cholesterol diet, exercise program
• To report suspected, planned pregnancy, not to use during pregnancy
• To use sunscreen protective clothing to prevent burns

prazosin (℞)
(pray'zoe-sin)
Minipress, prazosin
Func. class.: Antihypertensive
Chem. class.: α_1-Adrenergic blocker

Action: Blocks α-mediated vasoconstriction of adrenergic receptors, inducing peripheral vasodilation

P

Uses: Hypertension, refractory CHF, Raynaud's vasospasm
Investigational uses: Benign prostatic hypertrophy to decrease urine outflow obstruction
Dosage and routes:
Hypertension
• *Adult:* **PO** 1 mg bid or tid, increasing to 20 mg qd in divided doses if required; usual range 6-15 mg/day, not to exceed 1 mg initially; max 20-40 mg/day
• *Child:* **PO** 0.5-7 mg tid
Benign prostatic hyperplasia
• *Adult:* **PO** 1-5 mg bid
Available forms: Caps 1, 2, 5 mg
Side effects/adverse reactions:
CV: Palpitations, orthostatic hypotension, tachycardia, edema, rebound hypertension
CNS: Dizziness, headache, drowsiness, anxiety, depression, vertigo, weakness, fatigue
GI: Nausea, vomiting, diarrhea, constipation, abdominal pain
GU: Urinary frequency, incontinence, impotence, priapism, H_2O, sodium retention
EENT: Blurred vision, epistaxis, tinnitus, dry mouth, red sclera
Contraindications: Hypersensitivity
Precautions: Pregnancy (C), children, lactation
Pharmacokinetics:
PO: Onset 2 hr, peak 1-3 hr, duration 6-12 hr; half-life 2-3 hr, metabolized in liver, excreted via bile, feces (>90%), in urine (<10%), protein binding 97%
Interactions:
• ↑ hypotensive effects: β-blockers, nitroglycerin, alcohol, verapamil
• ↓ antihypertensive effect: NSAIDs, clonidine
↑ toxicity, death: aconite
↑ or ↓ antihypertensive effect: astragalus, cola tree
↑ antihypertensive effect: barberry, betony, black catechu, black cohosh, bloodroot, broom, burdock, cat's claw, dandelion, goldenseal, Irish moss, Jamaican dogwood, kelp, khella, mistletoe, parsley
↓ antihypertensive effect: coltsfoot, guarana, khat, licorice
Lab test interferences:
Increase: Urinary norepinephrine, VMA

NURSING CONSIDERATIONS
Assess:
• B/P (sitting, standing) during initial treatment, periodically thereafter; pulse, jugular venous distention q4h
• BUN, uric acid if on long-term therapy
• Weight qd, I&O; edema in feet, legs qd
• Skin turgor, dryness of mucous membranes for hydration status
• Rales, dyspnea, orthopnea q30min
Perform/provide:
• Storage in tight container in cool environment
Evaluate:
• Therapeutic response: decreased B/P
Teach patient/family:
• That fainting occasionally occurs after 1st dose; do not drive or operate machinery for 4 hr after 1st dose, or take 1st dose at bedtime
• To change positions slowly, to prevent orthostatic hypotension
• To avoid OTC medications unless approved by prescriber
Treatment of overdose: Administer volume expanders or vasopressors, discontinue drug, place in supine position

prednicarbate topical
See appendix c

*prednisoLONE (℞)

(pred-niss'oh-lone)

Articulose-50, Delta-Cortef, Hydeltrasol, Hydeltra-T.B.A., Key-Pred 25, Key-Pred 50, Key-Pred-SP, Orapred, Pediapred, Predaject-50, Predalone 50, Predalone-T.B.A., Predcor-25, Predcor-50, prednisoLONE, PrednisoLONE Acetate, Prednisol TBA, Prelone

Func. class.: Corticosteroid

Chem. class.: Glucocorticoid, immediate acting

Action: Decreases inflammation by suppression of migration of polymorphonuclear leukocytes, fibroblasts; reversal to increase capillary permeability and lysosomal stabilization

Uses: Severe inflammation, immunosuppression, neoplasms

Dosage and routes:

• *Adult:* **PO** 2.5-15 mg bid-qid; **IM** 2-30 mg (acetate, phosphate) q12h; **IV** 2-30 mg (phosphate) q12h; 2-30 mg in joint or soft tissue (phosphate), 4-40 mg in joint of lesion (tebutate)

Asthma/antiinflammatory

• *Child:* **PO** 1-2 mg/kg/day; **IV** 2-4 mg/kg/day

Available forms: Tabs 5 mg; syr 5 mg/5 ml, 15 mg/15 ml; acetate: inj 25, 50 mg/ml; tebutate: inj 20 mg/ml; phosphate: inj 20 mg/ml, oral liquid 5 mg/ml, tabs 1, 2.5, 5, 10, 20, 50 mg, oral sol 5 mg/ml, 5 mg/5 ml, syr 5 mg/5 ml

Side effects/adverse reactions:

INTEG: Acne, poor wound healing, ecchymosis, petechiae

CNS: Depression, flushing, sweating, headache, mood changes

CV: Hypertension, ***circulatory collapse, thrombophlebitis, embolism,*** tachycardia

HEMA: ***Thrombocytopenia***

MS: Fractures, osteoporosis, weakness

GI: Diarrhea, nausea, abdominal distention, ***GI hemorrhage,*** increased appetite, ***pancreatitis***

EENT: Fungal infections, increased intraocular pressure, blurred vision

Contraindications: Psychosis, hypersensitivity, idiopathic thrombocytopenia, acute glomerulonephritis, amebiasis, fungal infections, nonasthmatic bronchial disease, child <2 yr

Precautions: Pregnancy (C), diabetes mellitus, glaucoma, osteoporosis, seizure disorders, ulcerative colitis, CHF, myasthenia gravis

Do not confuse:

prednisoLONE/predniSONE

Pharmacokinetics:

PO: Peak 1-2 hr, duration 2 days

IM: Peak 3-45 hr

Interactions:

• ↓ prednisoLONE action: cholestyramine, colestipol, barbiturates, rifampin, epHEDrine, phenytoin, theophylline

• ↓ effects of anticoagulants, anticonvulsants, antidiabetics, ambenonium, neostigmine, isoniazid, toxoids, vaccines, anticholinesterases, salicylates, somatrem

• ↑ side effects: alcohol, salicylates, indomethacin, amphotericin B, digitalis, cycloSPORINE, diuretics

• ↑ prednisoLONE action: salicylates, estrogens, indomethacin, oral contraceptives, ketoconazole, macrolide antibiotics

Hypokalemia: aloe, buckthorn, cascara sagrada, Chinese rhubarb, senna

↑ effect: aloe, licorice, perilla

P

Lab test interferences:
Increase: Cholesterol, sodium, blood glucose, uric acid, calcium, urine glucose
Decrease: Calcium, potassium, T_4, T_3, thyroid ^{131}I uptake test, urine 17-OHCS, 17-KS, PBI
False negative: Skin allergy tests

NURSING CONSIDERATIONS

Assess:
- Potassium, blood glucose, urine glucose while on long-term therapy; hypokalemia and hyperglycemia
- Weight qd; notify prescriber if weekly gain >5 lb
- B/P q4h, pulse; notify prescriber if chest pain occurs
- I&O ratio; be alert for decreasing urinary output, increasing edema
- Plasma cortisol levels (long-term therapy) (normal level: 138-635 nmol/L SI units when drawn at 8 AM)
- Infection: increased temp, WBC, even after withdrawal of medication; drug masks infection
- Potassium depletion: paresthesias, fatigue, nausea, vomiting, depression, polyuria, dysrhythmias, weakness
- Edema, hypertension, cardiac symptoms
- Mental status: affect, mood, behavioral changes, aggression

Administer:

IM route
- After shaking suspension (parenteral)
- Titrated dose; use lowest effective dose
- IM inj deep in large muscle mass; rotate sites; avoid deltoid; use 21G needle
- In 1 dose in AM to prevent adrenal suppression; avoid SC administration; may damage tissue
- With food or milk to decrease GI symptoms

IV route
- Undiluted or added to NaCl or D_5 and given by IV inf; give 10 mg or less/1 min; decrease rate if burning occurs

Additive compatibilities: Ascorbic acid, cephalothin, cytarabine, erythromycin, fluorouracil, heparin, methicillin, penicillin G potassium, penicillin G sodium, vit B/C

Y-site compatibilities: Ciprofloxacin, heparin/hydrocortisone, potassium chloride, vit B/C

Perform/provide:
- Assistance with ambulation to patient with bone tissue disease to prevent fractures

Evaluate:
- Therapeutic response: ease of respirations, decreased inflammation

Teach patient/family:
- That emergency ID as steroid user should be carried
- To notify prescriber if therapeutic response decreases; dosage adjustment may be needed
- Not to discontinue abruptly; adrenal crisis can result; take exactly as prescribed
- To avoid OTC products: salicylates, cough products with alcohol, cold preparations unless directed by prescriber
- About cushingoid symptoms
- The symptoms of adrenal insufficiency: nausea, anorexia, fatigue, dizziness, dyspnea, weakness, joint pain

prednisoLONE ophthalmic

See appendix c

*predniSONE (℞)

(pred'ni-sone)

Apo-Prednisone♣, Deltasone♣, Liquid Pred, Meticorten, Orasone, Panasol-S, Prednicen-M, PredniSONE, Sterapred, Winpred

Func. class.: Corticosteroid

Chem. class.: Intermediate-acting glucocorticoid

Action: Decreases inflammation by suppression of migration of polymorphonuclear leukocytes, fibroblasts, reversal to increase capillary permeability, and lysosomal stabilization

Uses: Severe inflammation, immunosuppression, neoplasms, multiple sclerosis, collagen disorders, dermatologic disorders

Dosage and routes:

• *Adult:* **PO** 5-60 mg qd or divided bid-qid

• *Child:* **PO** 0.05-2 mg/kg/day divided 1-4 ×/day

Nephrosis

• *Child 18 mo-4 yr:* 7.5-10 mg qid initially

• *Child 4-10 yr:* 15 mg qid initially

• *Child >10 yr:* 20 mg qid initially

Multiple sclerosis

• *Adult:* **PO** 200 mg/day × 1 wk, then 80 mg qod × 1 mo

Available forms: Tabs 1, 2.5, 5, 10, 20, 50 mg; oral sol 5 mg/5 ml; syr 5 mg/5 ml

Side effects/adverse reactions:

CNS: Depression, flushing, sweating, headache, mood changes

CV: Hypertension, ***circulatory collapse, thrombophlebitis, embolism,*** tachycardia

EENT: Fungal infections, increased intraocular pressure, blurred vision

GI: Diarrhea, nausea, abdominal distention, ***GI hemorrhage,*** increased appetite, pancreatitis

HEMA: ***Thrombocytopenia***

INTEG: Acne, poor wound healing, ecchymosis, petechiae

MS: Fractures, osteoporosis, weakness

Contraindications: Psychosis, hypersensitivity, idiopathic thrombocytopenia, acute glomerulonephritis, amebiasis, fungal infections, nonasthmatic bronchial disease, child <2 yr, AIDS, TB

Precautions: Pregnancy (C), diabetes mellitus, glaucoma, osteoporosis, seizure disorders, ulcerative colitis, CHF, myasthenia gravis, renal disease, esophagitis, peptic ulcer

Do not confuse:

predniSONE/methylPREDNISolone

predniSONE/prednisoLONE

predniSONE/Prilosec

Pharmacokinetics:

PO: Well absorbed PO, peak 1-2 hr, duration 1-1½ days, half-life 3½-4 hr

Crosses placenta, enters breast milk, metabolized by liver after conversion

Interactions:

• ↓ predniSONE action: cholestyramine, colestipol, barbiturates, rifampin, epHEDrine, phenytoin, theophylline

• ↓ effects of anticoagulants, anticonvulsants, antidiabetics, ambenonium, neostigmine, isoniazid, toxoids, vaccines, anticholinesterases, salicylates, somatrem

• ↑ side effects: alcohol, salicylates, indomethacin, amphotericin B, digitalis, cycloSPORINE, diuretics

• ↑ predniSONE action: salicylates, estrogens, indomethacin, oral contraceptives, ketoconazole, macrolide antiinfectives

P

Hypokalemia: aloe, buckthorn, Chinese rhubarb, senna

↑ effect: aloe, licorice, perilla

Lab test interferences:

Increase: Cholesterol, sodium, blood glucose, uric acid, calcium, urine glucose

Decrease: Calcium, potassium, T_4, T_3, thyroid ^{131}I uptake test, urine 17-OHCS, 17-KS, PBI

False negative: Skin allergy tests

NURSING CONSIDERATIONS

Assess:

- Adrenal insufficiency: nausea, vomiting, anorexia, confusion, hypotension
- Potassium, blood glucose, urine glucose while on long-term therapy; hypokalemia and hyperglycemia
- Weight qd; notify prescriber of weekly gain >5 lb
- B/P q4h, pulse; notify prescriber of chest pain; monitor for rales, crackles, dyspnea if edema is present
- I&O ratio; be alert for decreasing urinary output, increasing edema
- Plasma cortisol (long-term therapy) (normal: 138-635 nmol/L SI units drawn at 8 AM)
- Infection: increased temp, WBC, even after withdrawal of medication; drug masks infection
- Potassium depletion: paresthesias, fatigue, nausea, vomiting, depression, polyuria, dysrhythmias, weakness
- Edema, hypertension, cardiac symptoms
- Mental status: affect, mood, behavioral changes, aggression

Administer:

- For long-term use, alternate-day therapy is recommended, to decrease adverse reactions
- Titrated dose; use lowest effective dose
- With food or milk to decrease GI symptoms

Perform/provide:

- Assistance with ambulation to patient with bone tissue disease to prevent fractures

Evaluate:

- Therapeutic response: ease of respirations, decreased inflammation

Teach patient/family:

- That emergency ID as steroid user should be carried; information on drug being taken and condition
- To notify prescriber if therapeutic response decreases; dosage adjustment may be needed
- To avoid vaccinations
- Not to discontinue abruptly, or adrenal crisis can result
- To avoid OTC products: salicylates, cough products with alcohol, cold preparations unless directed by prescriber
- About cushingoid symptoms: moon face, weight gain
- That drug causes immunosuppression; to report any symptoms of infection (fever, sore throat, cough)
- The symptoms of adrenal insufficiency: nausea, anorexia, fatigue, dizziness, dyspnea, weakness, joint pain

primaquine (℞)

(prim′a-kween)

Func. class.: Antimalarial

Chem. class.: Synthetic 8-aminoquinolone

Action: Unknown; thought to destroy exoerythrocytic forms by gametocidal action

Uses: Malaria caused by *Plasmodium vivax,* in combination with clindamycin for *Pneumocystis carinii* pneumonia

Dosage and routes:

- *Adult:* **PO** 15 mg (base) qd × 2 wk; 26.3-mg tab is 15-mg base

• *Child:* **PO** 0.5 mg/kg (0.3 mg/base/day) qd × 2 wk
Available forms: Tabs 26.3 mg, powder
Side effects/adverse reactions:
INTEG: Pruritus, skin eruptions, pallor, weakness
CNS: Headache, dizziness
EENT: Blurred vision, difficulty focusing
GI: Nausea, vomiting, anorexia, cramps
CV: Hypertension
HEMA: ***Agranulocytosis, granulocytopenia, leukopenia, hemolytic anemia, leukocytosis,*** mild anemia, ***methemoglobinemia***
Contraindications: Hypersensitivity, anemia, lupus erythematosus, methemoglobinemia, porphyria, rheumatoid arthritis, methemoglobin reductase deficiency, G6PD deficiency, iodine hypersensitivity
Precautions: Pregnancy (C), bone marrow suppression
Pharmacokinetics:
PO: Metabolized by liver (metabolites), half-life 3.7-9.6 hr
Interactions:
• Toxicity: quinacrine
NURSING CONSIDERATIONS
Assess:
• Ophthalmic test if long-term treatment or drug dosage >150 mg/day
• Hepatic studies qwk: AST, ALT, bilirubin, if on long-term therapy
• Blood studies: CBC; blood dyscrasias occur
• Allergic reactions: pruritus, rash, urticaria
• Blood dyscrasias: malaise, fever, bruising, bleeding (rare)
• For renal status: dark urine, hematuria, decreased output
◆ For hemolytic reaction: chills, fever, chest pain, cyanosis; drug should be discontinued immediately
Administer:
PO route
• Before or after meals at same time each day to maintain drug level
Evaluate:
• Therapeutic response: decreased symptoms of malaria
Teach patient/family:
• To report visual problems, fever, fatigue, dark urine, bruising, bleeding; may indicate blood dyscrasias
• To complete full course of therapy

primidone (℞)

(pri′mi-done)
Apo-Primidone✤, Mysoline, PMS-Primidone✤, primidone, Sertan✤
Func. class.: Anticonvulsant
Chem. class.: Barbiturate derivative

Action: Raises seizure threshold by conversion of drug to phenobarbital, decreases neuron firing
Uses: Generalized tonic-clonic (grand mal), complex-partial psychomotor seizures
Dosage and routes:
• *Adult and child >8 yr:* **PO** 100-125 mg hs on days 1, 2, 3; then 100-125 mg bid on days 4, 5, 6; then 100-125 mg tid on days 7, 8, 9, then maintenance 250 mg tid-qid, max 2 g/day in divided doses
• *Child <8 yr:* **PO** 50 mg hs on days 1, 2, 3; then 50 mg bid on days 4, 5, 6; then 100 mg bid on days 7, 8, 9, maintenance 125-250 mg tid or 10-25 mg/kg/day in divided doses
Available forms: Tabs 50, 250 mg; susp 250 mg/5 ml; chew tabs 125 mg✤
Side effects/adverse reactions:
HEMA: ***Thrombocytopenia, leukopenia, neutropenia, eosinophilia, megaloblastic anemia,*** decreased serum folate level, lymphadenopathy

CNS: Stimulation, drowsiness, irritability, psychosis, ataxia, vertigo, fatigue, emotional disturbances, mood changes, paranoia
GI: Nausea, vomiting, anorexia, ***hepatitis***
INTEG: Rash, edema, alopecia, lupuslike syndrome
EENT: Diplopia, nystagmus, edema of eyelids
GU: Impotence
Contraindications: Hypersensitivity, porphyria, pregnancy (D)
Precautions: COPD, hepatic disease, renal disease, hyperactive children
Pharmacokinetics:
PO: Peak 4 hr; excreted by kidneys, in breast milk; half-life 3-24 hr
Interactions:
• Primidone levels are ↓ by acetaZOLAMIDE, succinimides, carbamazepine
• Primidone levels are ↑ by: isoniazid, nicotinamide, hydantoins
• ↑ primidone levels: alcohol, heparin, CNS depressants, isoniazid, phenytoin, phenobarbital
• May ↓ effect of: oral contraceptives, acebutolol, metoprolol, propranolol, tricyclics, phenothiazines
↑ effect: ginkgo
↓ effect: ginseng, santonica
NURSING CONSIDERATIONS
Assess:
• For seizures: location, duration, type; folic acid deficiency; fatigue, weakness, neuropathy, depression
• Drug level: therapeutic level 5-12 mcg/ml; CBC should be done q6mo
• Mental status: mood, sensorium, affect, memory (long, short)
• Respiratory depression, wheezing
• Blood dyscrasias: fever, sore throat, bruising, rash, jaundice
Administer:
PO route
• After shaking liquid susp well
• With food for GI upset
• Tablets crushed and mixed with food or fluid for swallowing difficulties
Evaluate:
• Therapeutic response: decreased seizures
Teach patient/family:
• Not to withdraw drug quickly; withdrawal symptoms may occur
• To avoid hazardous activities until stabilized on drug; drowsiness, dizziness may occur
• To carry emergency ID with condition and medication
• To recognize the signs of blood dyscrasias; when to notify prescriber
• To avoid alcohol, CNS depressants

probenecid (℞)
(proe-ben′e-sid)
Benemid, Benuryl✦, probenecid, Probalan
Func. class.: Uricosuric
Chem. class.: Sulfonamide derivative

Action: Inhibits tubular reabsorption of urates, with increased excretion of uric acids
Uses: Hyperuricemia in gout, gouty arthritis, adjunct to cephalosporin or penicillin treatment
Dosage and routes:
Renal dose
• Avoid use if CCr <30 ml/min
Gonorrhea
• *Adult:* **PO** 1 g with 3.5 g ampicillin or 1 g ½ hr before 4.8 million units of aqueous penicillin G procaine injected into 2 sites **IM**
Gout/gouty arthritis
• *Adult:* **PO** 250 mg bid for 1 wk, then 500 mg bid, not to exceed 2

g/day; maintenance: 500 mg/day × 6 mo

Adjunct in penicillin/cephalosporin treatment

• *Adult and child >50 kg:* **PO** 500 mg qid

• *Child <50 kg:* **PO** 25 mg/kg, then 40 mg/kg in divided doses qid

Available forms: Tabs 0.5 g

Side effects/adverse reactions:

CNS: Drowsiness, headache

CV: Bradycardia

GU: Glycosuria, thirst, frequency, ***nephrotic syndrome***

GI: Gastric irritation, nausea, vomiting, anorexia, ***hepatic necrosis***

INTEG: Rash, dermatitis, pruritus, fever

META: Acidosis, hypokalemia, hyperchloremia, hyperglycemia

RESP: ***Apnea,*** irregular respirations

Contraindications: Hypersensitivity, severe hepatic disease, severe renal disease, CCr <50 mg/min, history of uric acid calculus

Precautions: Pregnancy (B), child <2 yr

Pharmacokinetics:

PO: Peak 2-4 hr, duration 8 hr, half-life 5-8 hr; metabolized by liver; excreted in urine

Interactions:

• ↑ effect of acyclovir, barbiturates, allopurinol, benzodiazepines, dyphylline, zidovudine

• ↑ toxicity: sulfa drugs, dapsone, clofibrate, indomethacin, rifampin, naproxen, methotrexate

• ↓ action of probenecid: salicylates

Lab test interferences:

False positive: Urine glucose with copper sulfate test (Clinitest)

Increase: BSP/urinary PSP, theophylline levels

NURSING CONSIDERATIONS

Assess:

• Uric acid levels (3-7 mg/dl); mobility, joint pain, swelling

• Respiratory rate, rhythm, depth; notify prescriber of abnormalities

• Electrolytes, CO_2 before, during treatment

• Urine pH, output, glucose during beginning treatment

⬥ For CNS symptoms: confusion, twitching, hyperreflexia, stimulation, headache; may indicate overdose

Administer:

• After meals or with milk if GI symptoms occur

• Increase fluid intake to 2-3 L/day to prevent urinary calculi

Evaluate:

• Therapeutic response: absence of pain, stiffness in joints

Teach patient/family:

• To avoid OTC preparations (aspirin) unless directed by prescriber; increase water intake, avoid alcohol, caffeine

procainamide (℞)

(proe-kane-ah'mide)

procainamide, Procanbid, Promine, Pronestyl, Pronestyl-SR

Func. class.: Antidysrhythmic (Class IA)

Chem. class.: Procaine HCl amide analog

Action: Depresses excitability of cardiac muscle to electrical stimulation and slows conduction in atrium, bundle of His, and ventricle increases refractory period

Uses: Life threatening ventricular dysrhythmias

Dosage and routes:

Atrial fibrillation/PAT

• *Adult:* **PO** 1-1.25 g; may give another 750 mg if needed; if no response, 500 mg-1 g q2h until de-

P

sired response; maintenance 50 mg/kg in divided doses q6h

Ventricular tachycardia

• *Adult:* **PO** 1 g; maintenance 50 mg/kg/day given in 3-hr intervals; sus rel tab 500 mg-1.25 g q6h

Other dysrhythmias

• *Adult:* **IV BOL** 100 mg q5min, given 25-50 mg/min, not to exceed 500 mg; or 17 mg/kg total then **IV INF** 2-6 mg/min

Renal dose

• *Adult:* **IV** CCr 10-50 ml/min give q6-12h; CCr <10 ml/min give q8-24h

Available forms: Caps 250, 375, 500 mg; tabs 250, 375, 500 mg; tabs sus rel 500, 750, 1000 mg; inj 100, 500 mg/ml

Side effects/adverse reactions:

CNS: Headache, dizziness, confusion, psychosis, restlessness, irritability, weakness

GI: Nausea, vomiting, anorexia, diarrhea, hepatomegaly, pain, bitter taste

CV: Hypotension, ***heart block, cardiovascular collapse, arrest***

HEMA: SLE syndrome, ***agranulocytosis, thrombocytopenia, neutropenia, hemolytic anemia***

INTEG: Rash, urticaria, edema, swelling (rare), pruritus, flushing

Contraindications: Hypersensitivity, severe heart block, lupus erythematosus, torsades de pointes

Precautions: Pregnancy (C), lactation, children, renal disease, hepatic disease, CHF, respiratory depression, cytopenia, bone marrow failure, dysrhythmia associated with digitalis toxicity, myasthenia gravis

Pharmacokinetics:

PO: Peak 1-2 hr, duration 3 hr (8 hr extended)

IM: Peak 10-60 min, duration 3 hr half-life 3 hr

Metabolized in liver to active metabolites, excreted unchanged by kidneys (60%)

Interactions:

• $\uparrow$ effects of neuromuscular blockers

• $\uparrow$ procainamide effects: cimetidine, quinidine, trimethoprim, β-blockers, ranitidine

• $\uparrow$ toxicity: other antidysrhythmics, thioridazine, quinolones

$\uparrow$ anticholinergic effect: henbane

$\uparrow$ toxicity, death: aconite

$\uparrow$ effect: aloe, broom, chronic buckthorn use, cascara sagrada (chronic use), Chinese rhubarb, figwort, fumitory, goldenseal, kudzu, licorice

$\downarrow$ effect: coltsfoot

$\uparrow$ serotonin effect: horehound

Lab test interferences:

$\uparrow$ ALT, AST, alk phosphatase, LDH, bilirubin

NURSING CONSIDERATIONS

Assess:

ECG continuously if using IV to determine increased PR or QRS segments; discontinue immediately; watch for increased ventricular ectopic beats, maximum need to rebolus

• Blood levels, 3-10 mcg/ml or NAPA levels 10-20 mcg/ml

CBC q2wk × 3 mo; leukocyte, neutrophil, platelet counts may be decreased, treatment may need to be discontinued

• I&O ratio; electrolytes (K, Na, Cl)

Toxicity: confusion, drowsiness, nausea, vomiting, tachydysrhythmias, oliguria

• ANA titer, during long-term treatment, watch for lupuslike symptoms

• Cardiac rate, rhythm, character, B/P continuously for fluctuations

• Respiratory status: rate, rhythm, character, lung fields; bilateral rales may occur in CHF patient; watch for respiratory depression

◆ CNS effects: dizziness, confusion, psychosis, paresthesias, seizures; drug should be discontinued

Administer:

PO route

⊘ Do not break, crush, chew sus rel tabs

IM route

- IM inj in deltoid; aspirate to avoid intravascular administration

IV route

- After diluting 100 mg/ml of D_5W or sterile H_2O for inj; give 20 mg or less/1 min; may dilute 1 g/250-500 ml D_5W, run at 2-6 mg/min
- Check IV site q8h for infiltration or extravasation

Additive compatibilities: Amiodarone, atracurium, DOBUTamine, flumazenil, lidocaine, netilmicin, verapamil

Solution compatibilities: D_5W, D_5/0.9% NaCl, 0.45% NaCl, 0.9% NaCl, water for inj

Y-site compatibilities: Amiodarone, cisatracurium, famotidine, heparin, hydrocortisone, potassium chloride, ranitidine, remifentanil, vit B/C

Evaluate:

- Therapeutic response: decreased dysrhythmias

Teach patient/family:

- That wax matrix may appear in stools
- Not to discontinue without health-care provider's advice

◆ To notify prescriber immediately if lupuslike symptoms appear (joint pain, butterfly rash, fever, chills, dyspnea)

◆ To notify prescriber of leukopenia (sore mouth, gums, throat) or thrombocytopenia (bleeding, bruising)

- How to take pulse and when to report to prescriber

Treatment of overdose: O_2 artificial ventilation, ECG, administer DOPamine for circulatory depression, diazepam or thiopental for convulsions, isoproterenol

procaine (℞)

(proe'kane)

Novocain, Unicaine

Func. class.: Local anesthetic

Chem. class.: Ester

Action: Competes with calcium for sites in nerve membrane that control sodium transport across cell membrane; decreases rise of depolarization phase of action potential

Uses: Spinal anesthesia, epidural, peripheral nerve block, perineum, lower extremities, infiltration

Dosage and routes:

Vary by route of anesthesia

Available forms: Inj 1%, 2%, 10%

Side effects/adverse reactions:

CNS: Anxiety, restlessness, ***convulsions, loss of consciousness,*** drowsiness, disorientation, tremors, shivering

CV: ***Myocardial depression, cardiac arrest, dysrhythmias,*** bradycardia, hypotension, hypertension, fetal bradycardia

GI: Nausea, vomiting

EENT: Blurred vision, tinnitus, pupil constriction

INTEG: Rash, urticaria, allergic reactions, edema, burning, skin discoloration at inj site, tissue necrosis

RESP: ***Status asthmaticus, respiratory arrest, anaphylaxis***

Contraindications: Hypersensitivity, child <12 yr, severe hepatic disease

Precautions: Elderly, severe drug allergies, pregnancy (C)

Pharmacokinetics: Onset 2-5 min, duration 1 hr; metabolized by liver, excreted in urine (metabolites)

Interactions:

• Dysrhythmias: epINEPHrine, halothane, enflurane

• Hypertension: MAOIs, tricyclics, phenothiazines

• ↓ action of procaine: chloroprocaine

NURSING CONSIDERATIONS

Assess:

• B/P, pulse, respiration during treatment

• Fetal heart tones if drug is used during labor

• Allergic reactions: rash, urticaria, itching

• Cardiac status: ECG for dysrhythmias, pulse, B/P during anesthesia

Administer:

• Only drugs that are not cloudy, do not contain precipitate

• Only with crash cart, resuscitative equipment nearby

• Only drugs without preservatives for epidural or caudal anesthesia

Additive compatibilities: Ascorbic acid, cephalothin, hydrocortisone, methicillin, penicillin G potassium, penicillin G sodium, vit B/C

Syringe compatibilities: Ampicillin, cloxacillin, glycopyrrolate, hydroxyzine, methicillin

Perform/provide:

• Use of new sol; discard unused portions

Evaluate:

• Therapeutic response: anesthesia necessary for procedure

Treatment of overdose: Airway, O_2, vasopressor, IV fluids, anticonvulsants for seizures

procarbazine (℞)

(proe-kar′ba-zeen)

Matulane, Natulan✱

Func. class.: Antineoplastic, alkylating agent

Chem. class.: Hydrazine derivative

Action: Inhibits DNA, RNA, protein synthesis; has multiple sites of action; a nonvesicant

Uses: Lymphoma, Hodgkin's disease, cancers resistant to other therapy

Investigational uses: Brain, lung malignancies, other lymphomas, multiple myeloma, malignant melanoma, polycythemia vera

• *Adult:* **PO** 2-4 mg/kg/day for first wk; maintain dosage of 4-6 mg/kg/day until platelets and WBC fall; after recovery, 1-2 mg/kg/day

• *Child:* **PO** 50 mg/m²/day for 7 days, then 100 mg/m² until desired response, leukopenia, or thrombocytopenia occurs; 50 mg/day is maintenance after bone marrow recovery

Available forms: Caps 50 mg

Side effects/adverse reactions:

HEMA: ***Thrombocytopenia, anemia, leukopenia, myelosuppression, bleeding tendencies,*** purpura, petechiae, epistaxis

GI: Nausea, vomiting, anorexia, diarrhea, constipation, dry mouth, stomatitis

EENT: Retinal hemorrhage, nystagmus, photophobia, diplopia

INTEG: Rash, pruritus, dermatitis, alopecia, herpes, hyperpigmentation

CNS: Headache, dizziness, insomnia, hallucinations, confusion, ***coma,*** pain, chills, fever, sweating, paresthesias, ***seizures***

RESP: Cough, pneumonitis

MS: Arthralgias, myalgias
GU: Azoospermia, cessation of menses
Contraindications: Hypersensitivity, pregnancy (D), thrombocytopenia, bone marrow depression
Precautions: Renal disease, hepatic disease, radiation therapy
Pharmacokinetics: Half-life 1 hr; concentrates in liver, kidney, skin; metabolized in liver, excreted in urine
Interactions:
• ↑ CNS depression: barbiturates, antihistamines, opioids, hypotensive agents, phenothiazines
• Hypotension: meperidine, do not use together
• Disulfiram-like reaction: alcohol, MAOIs, tricyclics, tyramine foods, sympathomimetic drugs
• Hypertension: guanethidine, levodopa, methyldopa, reserpine, caffeine
• ↑ hypoglycemia: insulin, oral hypoglycemics
• Life-threatening hypertension: sympathomimetics
• Drug/food: Hypertensive crisis: tyramine foods

NURSING CONSIDERATIONS
Assess:
• CBC, differential, platelet count qwk; withhold drug if WBC is <4000/mm^3 or platelet count is <100,000/mm^3; notify prescriber
• Renal studies: BUN, serum uric acid, urine CCr, electrolytes before, during therapy
• I&O ratio, report fall in urine output to <30 ml/hr
• Monitor temp q4h; fever may indicate beginning infection
• Hepatic studies before, during therapy: bilirubin, AST, ALT, alk phosphatase prn or qmo
• CNS changes: confusion, paresthesias, neuropathies, drug should be discontinued
◆ For tyramine foods in diet, hypertensive crisis can occur
◆ Toxicity: facial flushing, epistaxis, increased PT, thrombocytopenia; drug should be discontinued
• Bleeding: hematuria, guaiac stools, bruising or petechiae, mucosa or orifices q8h
• Effects of alopecia on body image; discuss feelings about body changes
• Jaundiced skin, sclera; dark urine, clay-colored stools, itchy skin, abdominal pain, fever, diarrhea
• Buccal cavity q8h for dryness, sores or ulceration, white patches, oral pain, bleeding, dysphagia
• Alkalosis if vomiting is severe
• GI symptoms: frequency of stools, cramping
• Acidosis, signs of dehydration: rapid respirations, poor skin turgor, decreased urine output, dry skin, restlessness, weakness

Administer:
• In divided doses and at hs to minimize nausea and vomiting
• Nonphenothiazine antiemetic 30-60 min before giving drug and 4-10 hr after treatment to prevent vomiting
• Transfusion for anemia
• Antispasmodic for GI symptoms

Perform/provide:
• Liquid diet: carbonated beverages; gelatin may be added if patient is not nauseated or vomiting
• Storage in tight, light-resistant container in cool environment

Evaluate:
• Therapeutic response: decreased tumor size, spread of malignancy

Teach patient/family:
• To report any complaints, side effects to nurse or prescriber; cough, shortness of breath, fever, chills, sore throat, bleeding, bruising, vomiting blood; black, tarry stools

P

• That hair may be lost during treatment and wig or hairpiece may make patient feel better; tell patient that new hair may be different in color, texture
• To avoid sunlight, or UV exposure, wear sunscreen or protective clothing
• To avoid foods with citric acid, hot or rough texture
• To report any bleeding, white spots, ulcerations in mouth to prescriber; tell patient to examine mouth qd
• To avoid driving, activities requiring alertness; dizziness may occur
• That contraceptive measures are recommended during therapy
• To avoid ingestion of alcohol, caffeine, tyramine-containing foods; cold, hay fever, weight-reducing products may cause serious drug interactions
• To avoid crowds, persons with infections if granulocytes are low

prochlorperazine (℞)

(proe-klor-pair′a-zeen)
Chlorpazine, Compa-Z, Compazine, Contranzine, Provacin ✱, Stemetil ✱, Ultrazine
Func. class.: Antiemetic, antipsychotic
Chem. class.: Phenothiazine, piperazine derivative

Action: Acts centrally by blocking chemoreceptor trigger zone, which in turn acts on vomiting center
Uses: Nausea, vomiting, psychotic disorders
Dosage and routes:
Postoperative nausea/vomiting
• *Adult:* **IM** 5-10 mg 1-2 hr before anesthesia; may repeat in 30 min; **IV** 5-10 mg 15-30 min before anesthesia; **IV INF** 20 mg/L D_5W or **NS** 15-30 min before anesthesia, not to exceed 40 mg/day
Severe nausea/vomiting
• *Adult:* **PO** 5-10 mg tid-qid; **SUS REL** 15 mg qd in AM or 10 mg q12h; **RECT** 25 mg/bid; **IM** 5-10 mg; may repeat q4h, not to exceed 40 mg/day
• *Child 18-39 kg:* **PO** 2.5 mg tid or 5 mg bid, not to exceed 15 mg/day; **IM** 0.132 mg/kg
• *Child 14-17 kg:* **PO/RECT** 2.5 mg bid-tid, not to exceed 10 mg/day; **IM** 0.132 mg/kg
• *Child 9-13 kg:* **PO/RECT** 2.5 mg qd-bid, not to exceed 7.5 mg/day; **IM** 0.132 mg/kg
Antipsychotic
• *Adult and child ≥12 yr:* **PO** 5-10 mg tid-qid; may increase q2-3day, max 150 mg/day; **IM** 10-20 mg q2-4hr up to 4 doses, then 10-20 mg q4-6h, max 200 mg/day; **RECT** 10 mg tid-qid, may increase by 5-10 mg q2-3 days as needed
• *Child 2-12 yr:* **PO** 2.5 mg bid-tid; **IM** 0.132 mg/kg
Antianxiety
• *Adult and child ≥12 yr:* 5 mg tid-qid, max 20 mg/day or >12 wk; **IM** 5-10 mg q3-4hr, max 40 mg/day; **IV** 2.5-10 mg; max 40 mg/day
• *Child 2-12 yr:* **IM** 132 mcg/kg
Available forms: Syr 5 mg/ml; inj 5 mg/ml; tabs 5, 10, 25 mg; caps, sus rel 10, 15 mg; supp 2.5, 5, 25 mg
Side effects/adverse reactions:
CNS: ***Neuroleptic malignant syndrome,*** *extrapyramidal reactions, tardive dyskinesia, euphoria,* ***depression,*** drowsiness, restlessness, tremor, dizziness
GI: Nausea, vomiting, anorexia, dry mouth, diarrhea, constipation, weight loss, metallic taste, cramps
HEMA: ***Agranulocytosis***
CV: ***Circulatory failure, tachycardia***

RESP: ***Respiratory depression***
EENT: Blurred vision
Contraindications: Hypersensitivity to phenothiazines, coma, seizure, encephalopathy, bone marrow depression, narrow-angle glaucoma
Precautions: Children <2 yr, pregnancy (C), elderly, lactation
Do not confuse:
Compazine/Coumadin
prochlorperazine/
chlorproMAZINE
Pharmacokinetics:
PO: Onset 30-40 min, duration 3-4 hr
SUS REL: Onset 30-40 min, duration 10-12 hr
RECT: Onset 60 min, duration 3-4 hr
IM: Onset 10-20 min, duration 12 hr
Metabolized by liver; excreted in urine, breast milk; crosses placenta
Interactions:
• ↓ prochlorperazine effect: barbiturates, antacids
• ↑ anticholinergic action: anticholinergics, antiparkinson drugs, antidepressants
↑ CNS depression: chamomile, cola nut, hops, kava, nettle, nutmeg, skullcap, valerian
↑ anticholinergic effect: henbane, jimsonweed, scopolia
↑ EPS: betel palm, kava
Lab test interferences:
Increase: LFTs, cardiac enzymes, cholesterol, blood glucose, prolactin, bilirubin, PBI, ^{131}I, alk phosphatase, leukocytes, granulocytes, platelets
Decrease: Hormones (blood and urine)
False-positive: Pregnancy tests, urine bilirubin
False-negative: Urinary steroids, 17-OHCS, pregnancy tests

NURSING CONSIDERATIONS
Assess:
• EPS: abnormal movement, tardive dyskinesia, akathisia
• VS, B/P; check patients with cardiac disease more often
For neuroleptic malignant syndrome: seizures, hyper/hypotension, fever, tachycardia, dyspnea, fatigue, muscle stiffness, loss of bladder control; notify prescriber immediately
CBC, LFTs during course of treatment, blood dyscrasias, hepatotoxicity may occur
• Respiratory status before, during, after administration of emetic; check rate, rhythm, character; respiratory depression can occur rapidly with elderly or debilitated patients
Administer:
IM route
• IM inj in large muscle mass; aspirate to avoid IV administration
• Keep patient recumbent for ½ hr
IV route
• IV after diluting 5 mg/9 ml of NaCl for inj (0.5 mg/ml); give 5 mg or less/min; may dilute 10-20 mg/L NaCl and give as infusion; can cause contact dermatitis
Additive compatibilities: Amikacin, ascorbic acid, dexamethasone, dimenhyDRINATE, erythromycin, ethacrynate, lidocaine, nafcillin, sodium bicarbonate, vit B/C
Syringe compatibilities: Atropine, butorphanol, chlorproMAZINE, cimetidine, diamorphine, diphenhydrAMINE, droperidol, fentanyl, glycopyrrolate, hydrOXYzine, meperidine, metoclopramide, nalbuphine, pentazocine, perphenazine, promazine, promethazine, ranitidine, scopolamine, sufentanil
Y-site compatibilities: Amsacrine, calcium gluconate, cisatracurium, cisplatin, cladribine, cyclophosphamide, cytarabine, DOXOrubicin, DOXOrubicin liposome, fluconazole, granisetron, heparin, hydrocortisone, melphalan, methotrexate, ondansetron, paclitaxel, potassium chloride, propofol, remifentanil,

P

sargramostim, sufentanil, teniposide, thiotepa, vinorelbine, vit B/C

Evaluate:

- Therapeutic response: absence of nausea, vomiting; reduced anxiety, agitation, excitability

Teach patient/family:

- To avoid hazardous activities, activities requiring alertness; dizziness may occur
- To avoid alcohol, other CNS depressants
- Not to double or skip doses
- That urine may be pink to reddish brown
- To report dark urine, clay-colored stools, bleeding, bruising, rash, blurred vision
- To avoid sun or wear sunscreen, protective clothing

progesterone (℞)

(proe-jess'ter-one)

Crinone, progesterone, Prometrium

Func. class.: Progestogen

Chem. class.: Progesterone derivative

Action: Inhibits secretion of pituitary gonadotropins, which prevents follicular maturation, ovulation; stimulates growth of mammary tissue; antineoplastic action against endometrial cancer

Uses: Contraception, amenorrhea, premenstrual syndrome, abnormal uterine bleeding, endometrial hyperplasia prevention

Investigational uses: Corpus luteum dysfunction

Dosage and routes:

Infertility

- *Adult:* **VAG** 90 mg qd

Amenorrhea/uterine bleeding

- *Adult:* **IM** 5-10 mg qd × 6-8 doses

Endometrial hyperplasia prevention

- *Adult:* **PO** 200 mg/day

Available forms: Inj 50 mg/ml; powder micronized, vag gel 8%; caps 100, 200 mg

Side effects/adverse reactions:

CNS: Dizziness, headache, migraines, depression, fatigue

CV: Hypotension, ***thrombophlebitis,*** edema, ***thromboembolism, stroke, pulmonary embolism, MI***

GI: Nausea, vomiting, anorexia, cramps, increased weight, ***cholestatic jaundice***

EENT: Diplopia, retinal thrombosis

GU: Amenorrhea, cervical erosion, breakthrough bleeding, dysmenorrhea, vaginal candidiasis, breast changes, *gynecomastia, testicular atrophy, impotence,* endometriosis, ***spontaneous abortion***

INTEG: Rash, urticaria, acne, hirsutism, alopecia, oily skin, seborrhea, purpura, melasma

META: Hyperglycemia

SYST: ***Angioedema, anaphylaxis***

Contraindications: Breast cancer, hypersensitivity, thromboembolic disorders, reproductive cancer, genital bleeding (abnormal, undiagnosed), cerebral hemorrhage, pregnancy (D)

Precautions: Lactation, hypertension, asthma, blood dyscrasias, gallbladder disease, CHF, diabetes mellitus, bone disease, depression, migraine headache, convulsive disorders, hepatic disease, renal disease, family history of breast or reproductive tract cancer

Pharmacokinetics:

IM, Rect, Vag: Duration 24 hr

Excreted in urine, feces; metabolized in liver

Interactions:

- ↓ progesterone effect: barbiturates, phenytoin
- ↑ hormonal effect: alfalfa

Lab test interferences:
Increase: Alk phosphatase, nitrogen (urine), pregnanediol, amino acids, factors VII, VIII, IX, X
Decrease: GTT, HDL

NURSING CONSIDERATIONS
Assess:
• Weight qd; notify prescriber of weekly weight gain >5 lb
• B/P at beginning of treatment and periodically
• I&O ratio; be alert for decreasing urinary output, increasing edema
• Hepatic studies: ALT, AST, bilirubin periodically during long-term therapy
• Edema, hypertension, cardiac symptoms, jaundice, thromboembolism
• Mental status: affect, mood, behavioral changes, depression
• Hypercalcemia

Administer:
• Titrated dose; use lowest effective dose
• After warming to dissolve crystals
• In one dose in AM
• With food or milk to decrease GI symptoms

Perform/provide:
• Storage in dark area

Evaluate:
• Therapeutic response: decreased abnormal uterine bleeding, absence of amenorrhea

Teach patient/family:
◆ To report breast lumps, vaginal bleeding, edema, jaundice, dark urine, clay-colored stools, dyspnea, headache, blurred vision, abdominal pain, numbness or stiffness in legs, chest pain
• To report suspected pregnancy
• To monitor blood glucose if diabetic

promethazine (℞)
(proe-meth'a-zeen)
Anergan, Antinaus, Histanil ✦, Pentazine, Phenazine, Phenecen-50, Phenergan, Phenergan Fortis, Phenergan Plain, Phenerzine, Phenoject, Pro-50, Promacot, Pro-med, Promet, promethazine HCl, Prorex, Shogan, V-Gan

Func. class.: Antihistamine, H_1-receptor antagonist
Chem. class.: Phenothiazine derivative

Action: Acts on blood vessels, GI, respiratory system by competing with histamine for H_1-receptor site; decreases allergic response by blocking histamine

Uses: Motion sickness, rhinitis, allergy symptoms, sedation, nausea, preoperative and postoperative sedation

Dosage and routes:
Nausea
• *Adult:* **PO/IM/IV/REC** 10-25 mg; may repeat 12.5-25 mg q4-6h
• *Child >2 yr:* **PO/IM/IV/REC** 0.25-0.5 mg/kg q4-6h

Motion sickness
• *Adult:* **PO** 25 mg bid, give ½-1 hr before departure
• *Child >2 yr:* **PO/IM/RECT** 12.5-25 mg bid, give ½-1 hr before departure

Allergy/rhinitis
• *Adult:* **PO** 12.5 mg qid, or 25 mg hs
• *Child >2 yr:* **PO** 6.25-12.5 mg tid or 25 mg hs

Sedation
• *Adult:* **PO/IM** 25-50 mg hs
• *Child >2 yr:* **PO/IM/RECT** 12.5-25 mg hs

P

Sedation (preoperative/postoperative)
- *Adult:* **PO/IM/IV** 25-50 mg
- *Child >2 yr:* **PO/IM/IV** 12.5-25 mg

Available forms: Tabs 10, 12.5, 25, 50 mg; supp 2.5, 5, 25 mg; inj 25, 50 mg/ml, syr 6.25 mg/5 ml, 10 mg/5 ml, 25 mg/5 ml

Side effects/adverse reactions:
CNS: Dizziness, drowsiness, poor coordination, fatigue, anxiety, euphoria, confusion, paresthesia, neuritis, EPS, ***neuroleptic malignant syndrome***
CV: Hypotension, palpitations, tachycardia
RESP: Increased thick secretions, wheezing, chest tightness, ***apnea in neonates, infants, young children***
HEMA: ***Thrombocytopenia, agranulocytosis, hemolytic anemia***
GI: Constipation, dry mouth, nausea, vomiting, anorexia, diarrhea
INTEG: Rash, urticaria, photosensitivity
GU: Urinary retention, dysuria, frequency
EENT: Blurred vision, dilated pupils, tinnitus, nasal stuffiness; dry nose, throat, mouth; photosensitivity

Contraindications: Hypersensitivity to H_1-receptor antagonist, acute asthma attack, lower respiratory tract disease

Precautions: Increased intraocular pressure, renal disease, cardiac disease, hypertension, bronchial asthma, seizure disorder, stenosed peptic ulcers, hyperthyroidism, prostatic hypertrophy, bladder neck obstruction, pregnancy (C)

Do not confuse:
Phenergan/Theragran

Pharmacokinetics:
PO: Onset 20 min, duration 4-6 hr; metabolized in liver; excreted by kidneys, GI tract (inactive metabolites)

Interactions:
- ↑ CNS depression: barbiturates, opioids, hypnotics, tricyclics, alcohol
- ↓ oral anticoagulants effect: heparin
- ↑ promethazine effect: MAOIs

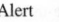

↑ anticholinergic effect: henbane, jimsonweed, scopolia

Lab test interferences:
False negative: Skin allergy test
False positive: Urine pregnancy test

NURSING CONSIDERATIONS

Assess:
- I&O ratio; be alert for urinary retention, frequency, dysuria; drug should be discontinued

CBC during long-term therapy; blood dyscrasias may occur
- Respiratory status: rate, rhythm, increase in bronchial secretions, wheezing, chest tightness
- Cardiac status: palpitations, increased pulse, hypotension

Administer:

PO route
- With meals for GI symptoms; absorption may slightly decrease
- When used for motion sickness, 30 min before travel

IM route
- IM inj deep in large muscle; rotate site

IV route
- After diluting each 25-50 mg/9 ml of NaCl for inj; give 25 mg or less/2 min

Additive compatibilities: Amikacin, ascorbic acid, chloroquine, hydromorphone, netilmicin, vit B/C

Syringe compatibilities: Atropine, butorphanol, chlorproMAZINE, cimetidine, dimenhyDRAMINE, droperidol, fentanyl, glycopyrrolate, hydromorphone, hydrOXYzine, meperidine, metoclopramide, midazolam, pentazocine, perphenazine, prochlorperazine, promazine, ranitidine, scopolamine

Y-site compatibilities: Amifostine, amsacrine, aztreonam, ciprofloxacin, cisatracurium, cisplatin, cladribine, cyclophosphamide, cytarabine, DOXOrubicin, filgrastim, fluconazole, fludarabine, granisetron, melphalan, ondansetron, remifentanil, sargramostim, teniposide, thiotepa, vinorelbine

Perform/provide:
- Hard candy, gum, frequent rinsing of mouth for dryness
- Storage in tight, light-resistant container

Evaluate:
- Therapeutic response: absence of running, congested nose, rashes, absence of motion sickness, nausea; sedation

Teach patient/family:
- That drug may cause photosensitivity; to avoid prolonged sunlight
- To notify prescriber of confusion, sedation, hypotension
- To avoid driving, other hazardous activity if drowsy
- To avoid concurrent use of alcohol, other CNS depressants

Treatment of overdose: Administer ipecac syrup or lavage, diazepam, vasopressors, barbiturates (short-acting)

propafenone (℞)

(pro-paff'e-nown)

Rythmol

Func. class.: Antidysrhythmic (Class IC)

Action: Slows conduction velocity; reduces membrane responsiveness; inhibits automaticity; increases ratio of effective refractory period to action potential duration; β-blocking activity

Uses: Life-threatening dysrhythmias, sustained ventricular tachycardia

Dosage and routes:
- *Adult:* **PO** 150 mg q8h; allow a 3-4 day interval before increasing dose, max 900 mg/day

Available forms: Tabs 150, 225, 300 mg

Side effects/adverse reactions:

INTEG: Rash

CV: ***Supraventricular dysrhythmia, ventricular dysrhythmia, bradycardia,*** pro-dysrhythmia, palpitations, AV block, intraventricular conduction delay, AV dissociation, hypotension, chest pain

HEMA: ***Leukopenia, agranulocytosis, granulocytopenia, thrombocytopenia,*** anemia, bruising

CNS: Headache, dizziness, abnormal dreams, syncope, confusion, ***seizures***

GI: Nausea, vomiting, constipation, dyspepsia, cholestasis, ***hepatitis,*** abnormal hepatic studies, dry mouth

RESP: Dyspnea

EENT: Blurred vision, altered taste, tinnitus

Contraindications: 2nd-, 3rd-degree AV block, right bundle branch block, cardiogenic shock, hypersensitivity, bradycardia, uncontrolled CHF, sick-sinus syndrome, marked hypotension, bronchospastic disorders

Precautions: CHF, hypokalemia, hyperkalemia, recent MI, nonallergic bronchospasm, pregnancy (C), lactation, children, hepatic or renal disease, elderly

Pharmacokinetics: Peak 3-5 hr, half-life 2-10 hr; metabolized in liver; excreted in urine (metabolite)

Interactions:
- ↑ anticoagulation: warfarin
- ↑ CNS effects: local anesthetics
- ↑ digoxin level: digoxin

P

• ↑ β-blocker effect: propranolol, metoprolol
• ↑ cycloSPORINE levels: cycloSPORINE
• ↓ propafenone effect: rifampin, cimetidine, quinidine
Hypokalemia, ↑ antidysrhythmic action: aloe, buckthorn, cascara sagrada, senna pod/leaf
↑ toxicity, death: aconite
↑ effect: aloe, broom, chronic buckthorn use, cascara sagrada (chronic use), Chinese rhubarb, figwort, fumitory, goldenseal, kudzu, licorice
↓ effect: coltsfoot
↑ serotonin effect: horehound

Lab test interferences:
Increase: CPK

NURSING CONSIDERATIONS

Assess:
• GI status: bowel pattern, number of stools
Cardiac status: rate, rhythm, quality; ECG or Holter monitor prior to and during therapy; watch for PR, QT prolongation
• Chest x-ray film, pulmonary function test during treatment
• I&O ratio; check for decreasing output; daily weight
• B/P for fluctuations
• Lung fields; bilateral rales, dyspnea, peripheral edema, weight gain, jugular venous distention may occur in CHF patient
Toxicity: fine tremors, dizziness, hypotension, drowsiness, abnormal heart rate
• Cardiac function: respiratory rate, rhythm, character continuously

Evaluate:
• Therapeutic response: absence of dysrhythmias

Teach patient/family:
• To avoid hazardous activities until response is known
• To report fever, chills, sore throat, bleeding, shortness of breath
• To carry emergency ID identifying medication and prescriber

Treatment of overdose: O_2, artificial ventilation, defibrillation ECG; administer dopamine for circulatory depression, diazepam or thiopental for convulsions, isoproterenol

propantheline (℞)

(proe-pan'the-leen)
Pro-Banthine, Propanthel♣,
Func. class.: GI anticholinergic, antiulcer agent
Chem. class.: Synthetic quaternary ammonium compound

Action: Inhibits muscarinic actions of acetylcholine at postganglionic parasympathetic neuroeffector sites

Uses: Treatment of peptic ulcer disease, irritable bowel syndrome, duodenography, urinary incontinence

Investigational uses: Antispasmodic uses

Dosage and routes:
• *Adult:* **PO** 15 mg tid ac, 30 mg hs
• *Elderly, small patients:* **PO** 7.5 mg tid ac
• *Child:* 0.375 mg/kg (10 mg/m^2) qid

Available forms: Tabs 7.5, 15 mg

Side effects/adverse reactions:
CNS: Confusion, stimulation in elderly, headache, insomnia, dizziness, drowsiness, anxiety, weakness, hallucinations
GI: Dry mouth, constipation, ***paralytic ileus,*** heartburn, nausea, vomiting, dysphagia, absence of taste
GU: Urinary hesitancy, retention, impotence
CV: Palpitations, tachycardia, orthostatic hypotension (elderly)
EENT: Blurred vision, photophobia, mydriasis, cycloplegia, increased ocular tension

INTEG: Urticaria, rash, pruritus, anhidrosis, fever, allergic reactions
Contraindications: Hypersensitivity to anticholinergics, narrow-angle glaucoma, GI obstruction, myasthenia gravis, paralytic ileus, GI atony, toxic megacolon
Precautions: Hyperthyroidism, coronary artery disease, dysrhythmias, CHF, ulcerative colitis, hypertension, hiatal hernia, hepatic disease, renal disease, pregnancy (C), urinary retention, prostatic hypertrophy, elderly
Pharmacokinetics:
PO: Onset 30-45 min, duration 6 hr; metabolized by liver, GI system; excreted in urine, bile
Interactions:
- ↑ anticholinergic effect: amantadine, tricyclics, MAOIs, H_1-antihistamines
- ↓ effect of phenothiazines, levodopa, ketoconazole

↑ anticholinergic effect: henbane, jimsonweed, scopolia

NURSING CONSIDERATIONS
Assess:
- VS, cardiac status: checking for dysrhythmias, increased rate, palpitations
- I&O ratio; check for urinary retention or hesitancy
- GI complaints: pain, bleeding (frank or occult), nausea, vomiting, anorexia

Administer:
- ½-1 hr ac for better absorption
- Decreased dose to elderly patients; metabolism may be slowed
- Gum, hard candy, frequent rinsing for dry mouth

Perform/provide:
- Storage in tight container protected from light
- Increased fluids, bulk, exercise to decrease constipation

Evaluate:
- Therapeutic response: absence of epigastric pain, bleeding, nausea, vomiting

Teach patient/family:
- To avoid driving, other hazardous activities until stabilized on medication; may cause blurred vision; to use caution when standing due to orthostatic hypotension
- To avoid alcohol, other CNS depressants; will enhance sedating properties of this drug
- To drink plenty of fluids
- To report dysphagia

proparacaine ophthalmic
See appendix c

HIGH ALERT

propofol (℞)
(pro′poh-fole)
Diprivan, Disoprofol
Func. class.: General anesthetic

Action: Produces dose-dependent CNS depression; action is unknown
Uses: Induction or maintenance of anesthesia as part of balanced anesthetic technique; sedation in mechanically ventilated patients
Dosage and routes:
Induction
- *Adult:* **IV** 2-2.5 mg/kg, approximately 40 mg q10sec until induction onset
- *Child ≥3 yr:* **IV** 2.5-3.5 mg/kg over 20-30 sec
- *Elderly:* **IV** 1-1.5 mg/kg, approximately 20 mg q10sec until induction onset

Maintenance
- *Adult:* **IV** 0.1-0.2 mg/kg/min (6-12 mg/kg/hr)

• *Child ≥3 yr:* **IV** 0.125-0.3 mg/kg/min (7.5-18 mg/kg/hr)
• *Elderly:* **IV** 0.05-0.1 mg/kg/min (3-6 mg/kg/hr)

ICU sedation

• *Adult:* **IV** 5 mcg/kg/min over 5 min; may give 5-10 mcg/kg/min over 5-10 min until desired response

Available forms: Inj 10 mg/ml in 20 ml ampule, 50 ml and 100 ml vials

Side effects/adverse reactions:

CNS: Movement, headache, jerking, fever, dizziness, shivering, tremor, confusion, somnolence, paresthesia, agitation, abnormal dreams, euphoria, fatigue

GI: Nausea, vomiting, abdominal cramping, dry mouth, swallowing, hypersalivation

MS: Myalgia

GU: Urine retention, green urine

EENT: Blurred vision, tinnitus, eye pain, strange taste

CV: Bradycardia, hypotension, hypertension, PVC, PAC, tachycardia, abnormal ECG, ST segment depression, ***asystole***

RESP: ***Apnea,*** *cough, hiccups,* dyspnea, hypoventilation, sneezing, wheezing, tachypnea, hypoxia

INTEG: Flushing, phlebitis, hives, burning/stinging at injection site

Contraindications: Hypersensitivity to drug or soybean oil, egg; hyperlipidemia

Precautions: Elderly, respiratory depression, severe respiratory disorders, cardiac dysrhythmias, pregnancy (B), labor and delivery, lactation, children

Pharmacokinetics: Onset 40 sec, rapid distribution, half-life 1-8 min, terminal elimination half-life 5-10 hr; 70% excreted in urine; metabolized in liver by conjugation to inactive metabolites

Interactions:

• ↑ CNS depression: alcohol, opioids, sedative/hypnotics, antipsychotics, skeletal muscle relaxants, inhalational anesthetics
• Do not administer with other drugs

NURSING CONSIDERATIONS

Assess:

• Injection site: phlebitis, burning, stinging
• ECG for changes: PVC, PAC, ST segment changes; monitor VS
• CNS changes: movement, jerking, tremors, dizziness, LOC, pupil reaction
• Allergic reactions: hives
• Respiratory dysfunction: respiratory depression, character, rate, rhythm; notify prescriber if respirations are <10/min

Administer:

IV route

• Shake well before use; if diluted, use only D_5W to not less than 2 mg/ml; give over 3-5 min, titrate to needed level of sedation; use only glass containers when mixing, not stable in plastic
• May be given by cont inf; give by inf pump
• Alone; do not mix with other agents before using
• Only with resuscitative equipment available
• Only by qualified persons trained in anesthesia

Y-site compatibilities: Acyclovir, alfentanil, amikacin, aminophylline, ampicillin, amrinone, aztreonam, bumetanide, buprenorphine, butorphanol, calcium gluconate, carboplatin, cefazolin, cefonicid, cefoperazone, cefotaxime, cefotetan, cefoxitin, ceftazidime, ceftizoxime, ceftriaxone, cefuroxime, chlorproMAZINE, cimetidine, ciprofloxacin, cisplatin, clindamycin, cyclophosphamide, cycloSPORINE, cytarabine, dexamethasone, digoxin, diphenhydrAMINE, DOBUTamine, DOPamine, DOXOrubicin, doxycycline, droperidol, enalaprilat, epHEDrine, epINEPHrine, esmolol, famotidine, fentanyl, fluconazole, fluorouracil, furosemide, ganciclovir, glycopyrrolate, granisetron, haloperidol, heparin, hydrocortisone, hydromorphone, hydrOXYzine, ifosfamide, imipenem/cilastatin, insulin, isoproterenol, ketamine, labetalol, levorphanol, lidocaine, lorazepam, magnesium sulfate, mannitol, meperidine, metoclopramide, mezlocillin, miconazole, morphine, nafcillin, nalbuphine, naloxone, nitroglycerin, norepinephrine, ofloxacin, paclitaxel, pentobarbital, phenobarbital, piperacillin, potassium chloride, prochlorperazine, propranolol, ranitidine, scopolamine, sodium bicarbonate, sodium nitroprusside, succinylcholine, sufentanil, ticarcillin, ticarcillin/clavulanate, vancomycin, vecuronium, verapamil

Solution compatibilities: D_5W, D_5LR, LR, D_5/0.45% NaCl, D_5/0.2% NaCl

Perform/provide:

• Storage in light-resistant area at room temperature, use within 6 hr of opening

Evaluate:

• Therapeutic response: induction of anesthesia

Teach patient/family:

• That this medication will cause dizziness, drowsiness, sedation

Treatment of overdose: Discontinue drug; administer vasopressor agents or anticholinergics, artificial ventilation

HIGH ALERT

propoxyphene (℞)

(proe-pox′i-feen)

Darvon, Darvon-N, Dolene, Novapropoxyn✦

Func. class.: Opiate analgesic

Chem. class.: Synthetic opiate

Controlled Substance Schedule IV

Action: Depresses pain impulse transmission at the spinal cord level by interacting with opioid receptors

Uses: Mild to moderate pain

Dosage and routes:

• *Adult:* **PO** 65 mg q4h prn (HCl)

• *Adult:* **PO** 100 mg q4h prn (napsylate)

Available forms: Propoxyphene HCl Caps 32, 65 mg; propoxyphene napsylate tabs 100 mg; oral susp 50 mg/5 ml

Side effects/adverse reactions:

CNS: Drowsiness, dizziness, confusion, headache, sedation, euphoria, ***seizures, hyperthermia*** (elderly)

GI: Nausea, vomiting, anorexia, constipation, cramps

GU: Urinary retention, dysuria

INTEG: Rash, urticaria, bruising, flushing, diaphoresis, pruritus

EENT: Tinnitus, blurred vision, miosis, diplopia

CV: Palpitations, bradycardia, change in B/P, ***dysrhythmias***

RESP: ***Respiratory depression***

Contraindications: Hypersensitivity to ASA products (some preparations), addiction (opioid)

Precautions: Addictive personality, pregnancy (C), lactation, increased intracranial pressure, MI (acute), severe heart disease, respiratory depression, hepatic disease, renal disease, child <18 yr, elderly

P

Pharmacokinetics:
PO: Onset ½-1 hr, peak 2-2½ hr, duration 4-6 hr
Metabolized by liver, excreted by kidneys (as metabolites), crosses placenta, excreted in breast milk, half-life 6-12 hr (metabolites)

Interactions:
Possible fatal reactions: MAOIs, alcohol
• ↑ effects with other CNS depressants: opioids, sedative/hypnotics, antipsychotics, skeletal muscle relaxants
↑ CNS depression: chamomile, hops, Jamaican dogwood, kava, lavender, mistletoe, nettle, pokeweed, poppy, senega, skullcap, valerian
↑ anticholinergic effect: corkwood

Lab test interferences:
Increase: Amylase

NURSING CONSIDERATIONS
Assess:
• For pain: duration, location, type
• I&O ratio; check for decreasing output; may indicate retention
• CNS changes: dizziness, drowsiness, hallucinations, euphoria, loss of consciousness, pupil reaction
• Allergic reactions: rash, urticaria
• Respiratory dysfunction: respiratory depression, character, rate, rhythm; notify prescriber if respirations are <10/min
• Need for pain medication; physical dependence

Administer:
• With antiemetic for nausea, vomiting
• When pain is beginning to return; determine dosage interval by response

Perform/provide:
• Storage in light-resistant area at room temperature
• Assistance with ambulation

Evaluate:
• Therapeutic response: decrease in pain

Teach patient/family:
• To report any symptoms of CNS changes, allergic reactions
• That physical dependency may result when used for extended periods; not to exceed dose
• That withdrawal symptoms may occur: nausea, vomiting, cramps, fever, faintness, anorexia

Treatment of overdose: Naloxone (Narcan) 0.2-0.8 mg IV, O_2, IV fluids, vasopressors

propranolol (℞)
(proe-pran′oh-lole)
Apo-Propranolol♣, Betaclinron E-R♣, Detensol♣, Inderal, Inderal LA, NovoPranol♣, propranolol HCl, PMS-Propranolol

Func. class.: Antihypertensive, antianginal, antidysrhythmic (class II)

Chem. class.: β-Adrenergic blocker

Action: Nonselective β-blocker with negative inotropic, chronotropic, dromotropic properties

Uses: Chronic stable angina pectoris, hypertension, supraventricular dysrhythmias, migraine, prophylaxis, MI, pheochromocytoma, essential tremor, cyanotic spells related to hypertrophic subaortic stenosis

Investigational uses: Anxiety; Parkinson's tremor, prevention of variceal bleeding caused by portal hypertension, akathisia induced by antipsychotics

Dosage and routes:
Dysrhythmias
• *Adult:* **PO** 10-30 mg tid-qid; **IV**

BOL 0.5-3 mg give 1 mg/min; may repeat in 2 min, may repeat q4h thereafter

• *Child:* **PO** 1 mg/kg/day divided in 2 doses; **IV** 0.01-0.1 mg/kg over 5 min

Hypertension

• *Adult:* **PO** 40 mg bid or 80 mg qd (sus rel) initially; usual dose 120-240 mg/day bid-tid or 120-160 mg qd (sus rel)

• *Child:* **PO** 0.5-1 mg/kg/day divided q6-12h

Angina

• *Adult:* **PO** 80-320 mg in divided doses bid-qid or 80 mg qd (sus rel); usual dose 160 mg qd (sus rel)

MI prophylaxis

• *Adult:* **PO** 180-240 mg/day tid-qid starting 5 day to 2 wk after MI

Pheochromocytoma

• *Adult:* **PO** 60 mg/day × 3 days preoperatively in divided doses or 30 mg/day in divided doses (inoperable tumor)

Migraine

• *Adult:* **PO** 80 mg/day (sus rel) or in divided doses; may increase to 160-240 mg/day in divided doses

• *Child:* **PO** 0.6-1.5 mg/kg/day divided q8h **PO**

Essential tremor

• *Adult:* **PO** 40 mg bid; usual dose 120 mg/day

Available forms: Caps, sus rel 60, 80, 120, 160 mg; tabs 10, 20, 40, 60, 80, 90 mg; inj 1 mg/ml; oral sol 4 mg/ml, 8 mg/ml; conc oral sol 80 mg/ml

Side effects/adverse reactions:

RESP: Dyspnea, respiratory dysfunction, *bronchospasm,* cough

CV: ***Bradycardia,*** hypotension, ***CHF,*** palpitations, AV block, peripheral vascular insufficiency, vasodilation, cold extremities, ***pulmonary edema, dysrhythmias***

HEMA: ***Agranulocytosis, thrombocytopenia***

GI: Nausea, vomiting, diarrhea, colitis, constipation, cramps, dry mouth, hepatomegaly, gastric pain, acute pancreatitis

GU: Impotence, decreased libido, UTIs

MS: Joint pain, arthralgia, muscle cramps, pain

MISC: Facial swelling, weight change, Raynaud's phenomenon

INTEG: Rash, pruritus, fever

CNS: Depression, hallucinations, dizziness, fatigue, lethargy, paresthesias, bizarre dreams, disorientation

EENT: Sore throat, ***laryngospasm,*** blurred vision, dry eyes

META: Hyperglycemia, hypoglycemia

Contraindications: Hypersensitivity to this drug; cardiac failure; cardiogenic shock, 2nd-, 3rd-degree heart block; bronchospastic disease; sinus bradycardia; CHF

Precautions: Diabetes mellitus, pregnancy (C), renal disease, lactation, hyperthyroidism, COPD, hepatic disease, children, myasthenia gravis, peripheral vascular disease, hypotension, CHF

Do not confuse:

Inderal/Toradol

Inderal/LA/IMDUR

Pharmacokinetics:

PO: Onset 30 min, peak 1-1½ hr, duration 6-12 hr

PO-ER: Peak 6 hr, duration 24 hr, half-life 8-11 hr

IV: Onset 2 min, peak 15 min, duration 3-6 hr; metabolized by liver; crosses placenta, blood-brain barrier; excreted in breast milk, protein binding 90%

Interactions:

• ↑ effect of: calcium channel blockers, neuromuscular blocker

• ↑ negative inotropic effects: disopyramide

P

- ↓ β-blocking effects: barbiturates
- ↑ β-blocking effect: cimetidine
- ↑ hypotension: quinidine, haloperidol, prazosin

↑ toxicity, death: aconite

↑ or ↓ antihypertensive effect: astragalus, cola tree

↑ antihypertensive effect: barberry, betony, black catechu, black cohosh, bloodroot, broom, burdock, cat's claw, dandelion, goldenseal, Irish moss, Jamaican dogwood, kelp, khella, mistletoe, parsley

↓ antihypertensive effect: coltsfoot, guarana, khat, licorice

Lab test interferences:
Increase: Serum potassium, serum uric acid, ALT, AST, alk phosphatase, LDH
Decrease: Blood glucose
Interference: Glaucoma testing

NURSING CONSIDERATIONS
Assess:
- B/P, pulse, respirations during beginning therapy; notify prescriber if pulse <50 bpm
- Weight qd; report gain of 5 lb

I&O ratio, CCr if kidney damage is diagnosed; watch for fluid overload: fatigue, weight gain, jugular distention, dyspnea, peripheral edema, rales, crackles

ECG continuously if using as antidysrhythmic, IV, PCWP, CVP

- Hepatic enzymes: AST, ALT, bilirubin
- Angina pain: duration, time started, activity being performed, character
- Tolerance (long-term use)
- Headache, light-headedness, decreased B/P; may indicate a need for decreased dosage

Administer:
PO route

Not to open, chew, crush ext rel cap

- May mix oral sol with liquid or semisolid food, rinse container to get entire dose
- With 8 oz water on empty stomach, food enhances bioavailability
- Do not give with aluminum-containing antacid; may decrease GI absorption

IV route
- IV undiluted or diluted 10 ml D_5W for inj; give 1 mg or less/min; may be diluted in 50 ml NaCl and run 1 mg over 10-15 min

Additive compatibilities: DOBUTamine, verapamil

Solution compatibilities: 0.9% NaCl, 0.45 NaCl, Ringer's, D_5W, D_5/0.9% NaCl, D_5/0.45% NaCl

Syringe compatibilities: Inamrinone, milrinone

Y-site compatibilities: Alteplase, amrinone, heparin, hydrocortisone, meperidine, milrinone, morphine, potassium chloride, propofol, tacrolimus, vit B/C

Perform/provide:
- Protection from light (injection)

Evaluate:
- Therapeutic response: decreased B/P, dysrhythmias

Teach patient/family:

Not to discontinue abruptly, may precipitate life-threatening dysrhythmias; to take drug at same time each day; to decrease dosage over 2 wk to prevent cardiac damage

- To avoid OTC drugs unless approved by prescriber
- To avoid hazardous activities if dizzy
- The importance of compliance with complete medical regimen
- To make position changes slowly to prevent fainting
- That sensitivity to cold may occur

propylthiouracil (℞)

(proe-pill-thye-oh-yoor'a-sill)
propylthiouracil, Propyl-Thyracil♣, PTU

Func. class.: Thyroid hormone antagonist (antithyroid)
Chem. class.: Thioamide

Action: Blocks synthesis peripherally of T_3, T_4 (triiodothyronine, thyroxine), inhibits organification of iodine

Uses: Preparation for thyroidectomy, thyrotoxic crisis, hyperthyroidism, thyroid storm

Dosage and routes:

Thyrotoxic crisis

• *Adult and child:* **PO** same as hyperthyroidism with iodine and propranolol

Preparation for thyroidectomy

• *Adult:* 600-1200 mg/day

• *Child:* 10 mg/kg/day in divided doses

Hyperthyroidism

• *Adult:* **PO** 100 mg tid increasing to 300 mg q8h if condition is severe; continue to euthyroid state, then 100 mg qd-tid

• *Child >10 yr:* **PO** 100 mg tid; continue to euthyroid state, then 25 mg tid to 100 mg bid

• *Child 6-10 yr:* **PO** 50-150 mg in divided doses q8h

• *Neonate:* **PO** 10 mg/kg/day in divided doses

Available forms: Tabs 50, 100 mg

Side effects/adverse reactions:

INTEG: Rash, urticaria, pruritus, alopecia, hyperpigmentation, lupus-like syndrome

GU: ***Nephritis***

CNS: Drowsiness, headache, vertigo, fever, paresthesias, neuritis

HEMA: ***Agranulocytosis, leukopenia, thrombocytopenia, hypothrombinemia, lymphadenopathy,*** bleeding, vasculitis, periarteritis

GI: Nausea, diarrhea, vomiting, ***jaundice, hepatitis,*** loss of taste

MS: Myalgia, arthralgia, nocturnal muscle cramps, osteoporosis

Contraindications: Hypersensitivity, pregnancy (D), lactation

Precautions: Infection, bone marrow depression, hepatic disease

Pharmacokinetics:

PO: Onset up to 3 wk, peak 6-10 wk, duration 1 wk to 1 mo, half-life 1-2 hr; excreted in urine, bile, breast milk; crosses placenta; concentration in thyroid gland

Interactions:

• ↑ anticoagulant effect: heparin, oral anticoagulants

• Bone marrow depression: radiation, antineoplastics

• ↑ effects: potassium/sodium iodide, lithium

• Agranulocytosis: phenothiazines

Lab test interferences:

Increase: PT, AST, ALT, alk phosphatase

NURSING CONSIDERATIONS

Assess:

• Pulse, B/P, temp

• I&O ratio; check for edema: puffy hands, feet, periorbits; indicates hypothyroidism

• Weight qd; same clothing, scale, time of day

• T_3, T_4, which are increased; serum TSH, which is decreased; free thyroxine index, which is increased if dosage is too low; discontinue drug 3-4 wk before RAIU

• Blood studies: CBC for blood dyscrasias: leukopenia, thrombocytopenia, agranulocytosis; LFTs

• Overdose: peripheral edema, heat intolerance, diaphoresis, palpitations, dysrhythmias, severe tachycardia, increased temp, delirium, CNS irritability

Hypersensitivity: rash, enlarged cervical lymph nodes; drug may have to be discontinued
- Hypoprothrombinemia: bleeding, petechiae, ecchymosis
- Clinical response: after 3 wk should include increased weight, pulse; decreased T_4
- Bone marrow depression: sore throat, fever, fatigue

Administer:
- With meals to decrease GI upset
- At same time each day to maintain drug level
- Lowest dose that relieves symptoms

Perform/provide:
- Storage in light-resistant container
- Fluids to 3-4 L/day, unless contraindicated

Evaluate:
- Therapeutic response: weight gain, decreased pulse, decreased T_4, decreased B/P

Teach patient/family:
- To abstain from breastfeeding after delivery
- To take pulse qd
- To report redness, swelling, sore throat, mouth lesions, which indicate blood dyscrasias
- To keep graph of weight, pulse, mood
- To avoid OTC products that contain iodine
- That seafood, other iodine products may be restricted
- Not to discontinue this medication abruptly; thyroid crisis may occur; stress response
- That response may take several months if thyroid is large
- The symptoms/signs of overdose: periorbital edema, cold intolerance, mental depression
- The symptoms of inadequate dose: tachycardia, diarrhea, fever, irritability
- To take medication as prescribed; not to skip or double dose; missed doses should be taken when remembered up to 1 hr before next dose
- To carry emergency ID listing condition, medication

protamine (℞)

(proe'ta-meen)

Func. class.: Heparin antagonist

Chem. class.: Low-molecular-weight protein

Action: Binds heparin, making it ineffective

Uses: Heparin overdose

Dosage and routes:
- *Adult and child:* **IV** 1 mg of protamine/90-115 units heparin given; administer slowly 1-3 min; not to exceed 50 mg/10 min

Available forms: Inj 10 mg/ml

Side effects/adverse reactions:

CV: Hypotension, bradycardia, ***circulatory collapse***

GI: Nausea, vomiting, anorexia

INTEG: *Rash,* dermatitis, urticaria

CNS: Lassitude

HEMA: Bleeding

RESP: Dyspnea, ***pulmonary edema, severe respiratory distress***

SYST: ***Anaphylaxis, angioedema***

Contraindications: Hypersensitivity

Precautions: Pregnancy (C), lactation, children, allergy to salmon

Pharmacokinetics:

IV: Onset 5 min, duration 2 hr

NURSING CONSIDERATIONS

Assess:

Hypersensitivity: urticuria, cough, wheezing, have emergency equipment nearby
- Blood studies (Hct, platelets, occult blood in stools) q3mo

• Coagulation tests (APTT, ACT) 15 min after dose, then in several hours
• VS, B/P, pulse after 30 min; plus 3 hr after dose
• Skin rash, urticaria, dermatitis
◆ Allergy to fish; use with caution; men that have had a vasectomy may be more prone to hypersensitivity

Administer:

IV route

• After diluting 50 mg/5 ml sterile bacteriostatic H_2O for inj; shake, give 20 mg or less over 1-3 min; may further dilute with equal volume of NaCl or D_5W and run over 2-3 hr; titrate to APTT, ACT; use infusion pump

Additive compatibilities: Cimetidine, ranitidine, verapamil

Perform/provide:

• Storage at 36°-46° F (2°-8° C)

Evaluate:

• Therapeutic response: reversal of heparin overdose

pseudoephedrine (OTC, ℞)

(soo-doh-eh-fed'rin)

Afrin, Allermed, Canafed, Cenafed, Children's Congestion Relief, Children's Silfedrine, Congestion Relief, Decofed Syrup, DeFed-60, Dorcol Children's Decongestant, Drixoral Non-Drowsy Formula, Dynafed, Efidac/24, Eltor♣, Genaphed, Halofed, Mini Thin Pseudo, PediaCare Infant's Decongestant, Pseudo, pseudoephedrine HCl, Pseudogest, Seudotabs, Sinustop Pro, Sudafed, Sudafed 12 Hour, Sudex, Triaminic AM Decongestant Formula

Func. class.: Adrenergic

Chem. class.: Substituted phenylethylamine

Action: Primary activity through α-effects on respiratory mucosal membranes reducing congestion hyperemia, edema; minimal bronchodilation secondary to β-effects

Uses: Nasal decongestant, adjunct in otitis media; with antihistamines

Dosage and routes:

• *Adult:* **PO** 60 mg q6h; ext rel 120 mg q12h or 240 mg q24h
• *Geriatric:* **PO** 30-60 mg q6h prn
• *Child 6-12 yr:* **PO** 30 mg q6h, not to exceed 120 mg/day
• *Child 2-6 yr:* **PO** 15 mg q6h, not to exceed 60 mg/day

Available forms: Caps, ext rel 120, 240 mg; oral sol 15 mg, 30 mg/5 ml; drops 7.5 mg/0.8 ml; tabs 30, 60 mg; caps 60 mg; tabs, ext rel 120, 240 mg

Side effects/adverse reactions:

CNS: Tremors, anxiety, insomnia, headache, dizziness, hallucinations, ***seizures*** (elderly)

EENT: Dry nose, irritation of nose and throat
CV: Palpitations, tachycardia, hypertension, chest pain, ***dysrhythmias, CV collapse***
GI: Anorexia, nausea, vomiting, dry mouth
GU: Dysuria
Contraindications: Hypersensitivity to sympathomimetics, narrow-angle glaucoma
Precautions: Pregnancy (C), cardiac disorders, hyperthyroidism, diabetes mellitus, prostatic hypertrophy, lactation, hypertension
Pharmacokinetics:
PO: Onset 15-30 min, duration 4-6 hr, 8-12 hr (ext rel); metabolized in liver, excreted in feces and breast milk
Interactions:
Do not use with MAOIs or tricyclics; hypertensive crisis may occur
- ↓ effect of this drug: methyldopa, urinary acidifiers, rauwolfia alkaloids
- ↑ effect of this drug: urinary alkalizers

NURSING CONSIDERATIONS
Assess:
- For nasal congestion; auscultate lung sounds; check for tenacious bronchial secretions
- B/P, pulse throughout treatment
- For CNS side effects in the elderly: excitation, seizures, hallucinations

Perform/provide:
- Storage at room temperature

Evaluate:
- Therapeutic response: decreased nasal congestion

Teach patient/family:
- The reason for drug administration
- Not to use continuously, or more than recommended dose; rebound congestion may occur
- To notify prescriber immediately of anxiety; slow, fast heart rate; dyspnea; seizures
- To check with prescriber before using other drugs, as drug interactions may occur
- To avoid taking near hs; stimulation can occur
- Not to use if stimulation, restlessness, or tremors occur
- That use in children may cause excessive agitation

psyllium (OTC, ℞)
(sill'ee-um)
Alramucil, Fiberall, Fiberall Natural Flavor and Orange Flavor, Genifiber, Hydrocil Instant, Karacil ♣, Konsyl, Konsyl Orange, Maalox Daily Fiber Therapy, Metamucil, Metamucil Lemon Lime, Metamucil Orange Flavor, Metamucil Sugar Free, Metamucil Sugar Free Orange Flavor, Modane Bulk, Mylanta Natural Fiber Supplement, Natural Fiber Laxative, Natural Fiber Laxative Sugar Free, Natural Vegetable Reguloid, Perdiem, Prodiem Plain ♣, Reguloid Natural, Reguloid Orange, Reguloid Sugar Free Orange, Reguloid Sugar Free Regular, Restore, Restore Sugar Free, Serutan, Syllact, V-Lax
Func. class.: Bulk laxative
Chem. class.: Psyllium colloid

Action: Bulk-forming laxative
Uses: Chronic constipation, ulcerative colitis, irritable bowel syndrome
Dosage and routes:
- *Adult:* **PO** 1-2 tsp in 8 oz H_2O bid or tid, then 8 oz H_2O or 1 premea-

sured packet in 8 oz H_2O bid or tid, then 8 oz H_2O
• *Child >6 yr:* **PO** 1 tsp in 4 oz H_2O hs
Available forms: Chew pieces 1.7, 3.4 g/piece; effervescent powder 3.4, 3.7 g/packet; powder 3.3, 3.4, 3.5, 4.94 g/tsp; granules 2.5, 4.03 g/tsp; wafers 3.4 g/wafer
Side effects/adverse reactions:
GI: Nausea, vomiting, anorexia, diarrhea, cramps, intestinal esophageal blockage
Contraindications: Hypersensitivity, intestinal obstruction, abdominal pain, nausea/vomiting, fecal impaction
Precautions: Pregnancy (C)
Pharmacokinetics: Excreted in feces, not absorbed in GI tract
Interactions:
• ↓ absorption of: cardiac glycosides, oral anticoagulants, salicylates
↑ laxative effect: flax, senna

NURSING CONSIDERATIONS
Assess:
• Blood, urine electrolytes if used often
• I&O ratio to identify fluid loss
• Cause of constipation; fluids, bulk, exercise missing
• Cramping, rectal bleeding, nausea, vomiting; drug should be discontinued

Administer:
PO route
• Alone for better absorption
• In morning or evening (oral dose)
• Immediately after mixing with H_2O
• With 8 oz H_2O or juice followed by another 8 oz of fluid

Evaluate:
• Therapeutic response: decrease in constipation or decreased diarrhea in colitis

Teach patient/family:
• To maintain adequate fluid consumption
• That normal bowel movements do not always occur daily
• Not to use in presence of abdominal pain, nausea, vomiting
• To notify prescriber if constipation unrelieved or if symptoms of electrolyte imbalance occur: muscle cramps, pain, weakness, dizziness, excessive thirst

pyrantel (OTC)

(pie-ran′tel)
Antiminth, Combantrin ♣, Pin-Rid, Pin-X, Reese's Pinworm
Func. class.: Anthelmintic
Chem. class.: Pyrimidine derivative

Action: Causes paralysis in worm by neuroblockade via stimulation of ganglionic receptors; worms expelled by normal peristalsis
Uses: Pinworms, roundworms, hookworms
Dosage and routes:
• *Adult and child >2 yr:* **PO** 11 mg/kg as single dose, not to exceed 1 g; repeat in 2 wk for pinworms
Available forms: Oral susp 50 mg/ml; liquid 50 mg/ml; caps, soft gel 180 mg
Side effects/adverse reactions:
INTEG: Rash
CNS: Dizziness, headache, drowsiness, insomnia, fever, weakness
GI: Nausea, vomiting, anorexia, diarrhea, distention, abdominal cramps
Contraindications: Hypersensitivity
Precautions: Seizure disorders, hepatic disease, dehydration, anemia, child <2 yr, pregnancy (C), malnutrition

P

Pharmacokinetics:

PO: Peak 1-3 hr; metabolized in liver; excreted in feces, urine (unchanged/ metabolites)

Interactions:

• Antagonizes effect of pyrantel: piperazine

NURSING CONSIDERATIONS

Assess:

• Stools during entire treatment; specimens must be sent to lab while still warm

• For diarrhea during expulsion of worms

• For allergic reaction: rash

Administer:

PO route

• After meals to avoid GI symptoms

• After shaking suspension

Perform/provide:

• Storage in tight, light-resistant container in cool environment

Evaluate:

• Therapeutic response: expulsion of worms, 3 negative stool cultures after completion of treatment

Teach patient/family:

• Proper hygiene after BM, including hand-washing technique; tell patient not to put fingers in mouth

• That infected person should sleep alone; not to shake bed linen; to change bed linen qd, wash in hot water; that all family members should be treated for pinworms; treat dogs/cats; keep children away from animal's feces

• To clean toilet qd with disinfectant (green soap solution)

• The need for compliance with dosage schedule, duration of treatment

• To drink fruit juice to help expel worms

• To wear shoes, wash all fruits, vegetables well before eating

pyrazinamide (℞)

(peer-a-zin'a-mide)

PMS Pyrazinamide♣, pyrazinamide, Tebrazid♣

Func. class.: Antitubercular agent

Chem. class.: Pyrazinoic acid amine, nicoturimide analog

Action: Bactericidal interference with lipid, nucleic acid biosynthesis

Uses: Tuberculosis, as an adjunct when other drugs are not feasible

Dosage and routes:

• *Adult and child:* **PO** 15-30 mg/kg/day not to exceed 2 g/day

Available forms: Tabs 500 mg

Side effects/adverse reactions:

INTEG: Photosensitivity, urticaria

CNS: Headache

GI: ***Hepatotoxicity,*** abnormal hepatic studies, peptic ulcer, nausea, vomiting, anorexia, cramps, diarrhea

GU: Urinary difficulty, increased uric acid

HEMA: ***Hemolytic anemia***

Contraindications: Hypersensitivity, severe hepatic damage, acute gout

Precautions: Pregnancy (C), child <13 yr, renal failure, diabetes, porphyria, chronic gout

Pharmacokinetics:

PO: Peak 2 hr, half-life 9-10 hr; metabolized in liver, excreted in urine (metabolites/unchanged drug)

Lab test interferences:

Increase: PBI

Decrease: 17-KS

NURSING CONSIDERATIONS

Assess:

• Signs of anemia: Hct, Hgb, fatigue

• Temp; if >101° F (38° C), drug should be reduced

❖Hepatic studies qwk: ALT, AST, bilirubin
• Renal status before, qmo: BUN, creatinine, output, sp gr, urinalysis, uric acid
• Hepatic status: decreased appetite, jaundice, dark urine, fatigue

Administer:

PO route
• With meals for GI symptoms
• After C&S is completed; qmo to detect resistance

Evaluate:
• Therapeutic response: decreased symptoms of TB, culture negative

Teach patient/family:
• That compliance with dosage schedule, length is necessary
• To avoid alcohol
• To report fever, loss of appetite, malaise, nausea, vomiting, darkened urine, pale stools

pyridostigmine (℞)

(peer-id-oh-stig′meen)
Mestinon, Mestinon SR, Mestinon Timespan, Regonol
Func. class.: Cholinergic; anticholinesterase
Chem. class.: Tertiary amine carbamate

Action: Inhibits destruction of acetylcholine, which increases concentration at sites where acetylcholine is released; this facilitates transmission of impulses across myoneural junction

Uses: Nondepolarizing muscle relaxant antagonist, myasthenia gravis

Dosage and routes:

Myasthenia gravis
• *Adult:* **PO** 60-180 mg bid-qid, not to exceed 1.5 g/day; **IM/IV** 2 mg or 1/30 of **PO** dose; **SUS REL** 180-540 mg qd or bid at intervals of at least 6 hr
• *Child:* 7 mg/kg/day in 5-6 divided doses

Nondepolarizing neuromuscular blocker antagonist
• *Adult:* 0.6-1.2 mg **IV** atropine, then 10-30 mg
• *Child:* **IV** 0.1-0.25 mg/kg/dose

Available forms: Tabs 60 mg; tabs, ext rel 180 mg; syr 60 mg/5 ml; inj 5 mg/ml

Side effects/adverse reactions:
INTEG: Rash, urticaria, flushing
CNS: Dizziness, headache, sweating, weakness, ***seizures,*** incoordination, ***paralysis,*** drowsiness, LOC
GI: Nausea, diarrhea, vomiting, cramps, increased salivary and gastric secretions, peristalsis
CV: Tachycardia, dysrhythmias, bradycardia, AV block, hypotension, ECG changes, ***cardiac arrest,*** syncope
GU: Urinary frequency, incontinence, urgency
RESP: ***Respiratory depression, bronchospasm, constriction, laryngospasm, respiratory arrest***
EENT: Miosis, blurred vision, lacrimation, visual changes

Contraindications: Bradycardia; hypotension; obstruction of intestine, renal system; bromide sensitivity

Precautions: Seizure disorders, bronchial asthma, coronary occlusion, hyperthyroidism, dysrhythmias, peptic ulcer, megacolon, poor GI motility, pregnancy (C)

Pharmacokinetics:
PO: Onset 20-30 min, duration 3-6 hr
IM/IV/SC: Onset 2-15 min, duration 2½-4 hr; metabolized in liver, excreted in urine

P

Interactions:

• ↓ action: gallamine, metocurine, pancuronium, tubocurarine, atropine

• ↑ action: decamethonium, succinylcholine

• ↓ pyridostigmine action: aminoglycosides, anesthetics, procainamide, quinidine, mecamylamine, polymyxin, magnesium, corticosteroids, antidysrhythmics

↑ effect: jaborandi tree, pill-bearing spurge

NURSING CONSIDERATIONS

Assess:

• VS, respiration q8h

• I&O ratio; check for urinary retention or incontinence

• Bradycardia, hypotension, bronchospasm, headache, dizziness, convulsions, respiratory depression; drug should be discontinued if toxicity occurs

Administer:

• Only with atropine sulfate available for cholinergic crisis

• Only after all other cholinergics have been discontinued

• Increased doses for tolerance, as ordered

• Larger doses after exercise or fatigue, as ordered

• On empty stomach for better absorption

IV route

• Undiluted, give through Y-tube or 3-way stopcock, give 0.5 mg or less/min

Syringe compatibilities: Glycopyrrolate

Y-site compatibilities: Heparin, hydrocortisone, potassium chloride, vit B/C

Perform/provide:

• Storage at room temperature

Evaluate:

• Therapeutic response: increased muscle strength, hand grasp, improved gait, absence of labored breathing (if severe)

Teach patient/family:

Not to break, crush, or chew sus rel tabs

• That drug is not a cure, only relieves symptoms

• To wear emergency ID specifying myasthenia gravis, drugs taken

Treatment of overdose: Discontinue drug, atropine 1-4 mg IV

pyridoxine (vit B_6)

(℞, OTC)

(peer-i-dox′een)

Beesix, Doxine, Nestrex, pyridoxine HCl, Pyri, Rodex, Vitabee 6, vitamin B_6

Func. class.: Vit B_6, water soluble

Action: Needed for fat, protein, carbohydrate metabolism; enhances glycogen release from liver and muscle tissue; needed as coenzyme for metabolic transformations of a variety of amino acids

Uses: Vit B_6 deficiency of inborn errors of metabolism, seizures, isoniazid therapy, oral contraceptives, alcoholic polyneuritis

Investigational uses: Palmar-Plantar erythrodysesthesia syndrome

Dosage and routes:

RDA

• *Adult:* **PO** male 1.7-2 mg; female 1.4-1.6 mg

Vit B_6 deficiency

• *Adult:* **PO/IM/IV** 5-25 mg qd × 3wk

• *Child:* **PO/IM/IV** 100 mg until desired response

Deficiency caused by isoniazid, cycloserine, hydralazine, penicillamine

• *Adult:* **PO** 6-100 mg qd

• *Child:* **PO** 5-25 mg/day

Prevention of deficiency caused by isoniazid, cycloserine, hydralazine, penicillamine
- *Adult:* **PO** 6-50 mg qd
- *Child:* **PO** 0.5-1.5 mg qd
- *Infant:* **PO** 0.1-0.5 mg qd

Palmar-Plantar erythrodysesthesia syndrome (off-label)
- *Adult:* **PO** 50-150 mg qd

Available forms: Tabs 10, 25, 50, 100 mg; tabs, ext rel 100 mg; inj 100 mg/ml; ext rel cap 150 mg

Side effects/adverse reactions:

CNS: Paresthesia, flushing, warmth, lethargy (rare with normal renal function)

INTEG: Pain at inj site

Contraindications: Hypersensitivity

Precautions: Pregnancy (A), lactation, children, Parkinson's disease, patients taking levodopa should avoid supplemental vitamins with >5 mg pyridoxine

Pharmacokinetics:

PO/Inj: Half-life 2-3 wk, metabolized in liver, excreted in urine

Interactions:
- ↓ effects of levodopa
- ↓ effects of pyridoxine: oral contraceptives, isoniazid, cycloSERINE, hydrALAZINE, penicillamine, chloramphenicol, immunosuppressants

NURSING CONSIDERATIONS

Assess:
- Pyridoxine levels throughout treatment
- Nutritional status: yeast, liver, legumes, bananas, green vegetables, whole grains

Administer:

PO route

⊘ Do not crush, break, chew ext rel tabs, caps

IM route
- Rotate sites; burning or stinging at site may occur
- Z-track to minimize pain

IV route
- Undiluted or added to most IV sol; give 50 mg or less/1 min if undiluted

Syringe compatibilities: Doxapram

Perform/provide:
- Storage in tight, light-resistant container

Evaluate:
- Therapeutic response: absence of nausea, vomiting, anorexia, skin lesions, glossitis, stomatitis, edema, seizures, restlessness, paresthesia

Teach patient/family:
- To avoid vitamin supplements unless directed by prescriber
- To keep out of children's reach
- To increase meat, bananas, potatoes, lima beans, whole grain cereals in diet
- To discuss birth control status with prescriber

pyrimethamine (℞)

(peer-i-meth'a-meen)

Daraprim, Fansidar (with sulfadoxine)

Func. class.: Antimalarial

Chem. class.: Folic acid antagonist

Action: Inhibits folic acid metabolism in parasite, prevents transmission by stopping growth of fertilized gametes

Uses: Malaria prophylaxis, *Plasmodium vivax*

Investigational uses: *Pneumocystis carinii* pneumonia as an adjunct

Dosage and routes:

Prophylaxis of malaria
- *Adult and child >10 yr:* **PO** 25 mg qwk
- *Child 4-10 yr:* **PO** 12.5 mg qwk
- *Child <4 yr:* **PO** 6.25 mg qwk

P

Toxoplasmosis
• *Adult:* **PO** 100 mg, then 25 mg qd × 4-5 wk, with 1 g sulfadoxine q6h
• *Child:* **PO** 1 mg/kg/day in 2 divided doses or 2 mg/kg/day × 3 days, then 1 mg/kg/day or divided twice qd × 4 wk, max 25 mg/day
Toxoplasmosis in AIDS patients
• *Adult:* **PO** 100-200 mg/day × 1-2 days, then 50-100 mg/day × 3-6 wk, then 25-50 mg/day for life (given with clindamycin or sulfADIAZINE)
Available forms: Tabs 25 mg; combo tabs 500 mg sulfadoxine/25 mg pyrimethamine
Side effects/adverse reactions:
RESP: ***Respiratory failure***
INTEG: Skin eruptions, photosensitivity
CNS: Stimulation, irritability, ***seizures,*** tremors, ataxia, fatigue
GI: Nausea, vomiting, cramps, anorexia, diarrhea, atrophic glossitis, gastritis
CV: ***Dysrhythmias***
HEMA: ***Thrombocytopenia, leukopenia, pancytopenia, megaloblastic anemia,*** decreased folic acid, ***agranulocytosis***
Contraindications: Hypersensitivity, chloroquine-resistant malaria, megaloblastic anemia caused by folate deficiency
Precautions: Blood dyscrasias, seizure disorder, pregnancy (C), lactation, G6PD disease, renal, hepatic disease
Pharmacokinetics:
PO: Peak 2 hr, half-life 111 hr; metabolized in liver, highly protein bound, excreted in urine (metabolites)
Interactions:
• Synergistic action: folic acid
• ↑ bone marrow suppression: bone marrow depressants, radiation therapy

NURSING CONSIDERATIONS
Assess:
• Folic acid level; megaloblastic anemia occurs
⬘ Blood studies, CBC, platelets, since blood dyscrasias occur; twice weekly if dosage is increased
⬘ For toxicity: vomiting, anorexia, seizure, blood dyscrasia, glossitis; drug should be discontinued immediately
Administer:
• Leucovorin IM 3-9 mg/day × 3 days if folic acid deficiency occurs
• Before or after meals at same time each day to maintain drug level, to decrease GI symptoms
Perform/provide:
• Storage in tight, light-resistant container
Evaluate:
• Therapeutic response: decreased symptoms of malaria
Teach patient/family:
• To report visual problems, fever, fatigue, bruising, bleeding; may indicate blood dyscrasias
Treatment of overdose: Gastric lavage, short-acting barbiturate, leucovorin, respiratory support if needed

quetiapine (℞)
(kwe-tie'a-peen)
Seroquel
Func. class.: Antipsychotic

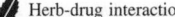

Action: Functions as an antagonist at multiple neurotransmitter receptors in the brain including $5HT_{1A}$, $5HT_2$, DOPamine D_1, D_2, H_1, and adrenergic α_1, α_2 receptors
Uses: Psychotic disorders
Research note: Increased dose of quetiapine may be necessary when used with phenytoin[33]
Dosage and routes:
• *Adult:* **PO** 25 mg bid, with incre-

mental increases of 25 mg bid-tid on days 2 and 3 to a dose of 300-400 mg qd given bid-tid, max 800 mg/day

Available forms: Tabs 25, 100, 200, 300 mg

Side effects/adverse reactions:

CNS: EPS, pseudoparkinsonism, akathisia, dystonia, tardive dyskinesia; drowsiness, insomnia, agitation, anxiety, *headache,* ***seizures, neuroleptic malignant syndrome,*** *dizziness*

CV: Orthostatic hypotension, ***tachycardia***

GI: Nausea, anorexia, constipation, abdominal pain, dry mouth

RESP: Rhinitis

INTEG: Rash

MISC: Asthenia, back pain, fever, ear pain

Contraindications: Hypersensitivity

Precautions: Children, pregnancy (C), hepatic disease, elderly, breast cancer, lactation, long-term use, seizures, dementia

Pharmacokinetics:

PO: Extensively metabolized by liver half-life ≥6 hr; peak 1½ hr; inhibits P450 CYP3A4 enzyme system

Interactions:

- ↑ CNS depression: alcohol, opioid analgesics, sedative/hypnotics, antihistamines
- ↓ quetiapine clearance of cimetidine
- ↑ quetiapine clearance of phenytoin, thioridazine, barbiturates, glucocorticoids, carbamazepine, rifampin
- ↓ effects of: DOPamine agonists, levodopa, lorazepam
- ↑ by erythromycin, fluconazole, itraconazole, ketoconazole

↑ action: cola tree, hops, nettle, nutmeg

↑ EPS: betel palm, kava

NURSING CONSIDERATIONS

Assess:

- Mental status before initial administration
- Swallowing of PO medication: check for hoarding or giving of medication to other patients
- I&O ratio; palpate bladder if urinary output is low
- Bilirubin, CBC, hepatic studies qmo
- Urinalysis before, during prolonged therapy
- Affect, orientation, LOC, reflexes, gait, coordination, sleep pattern disturbances
- B/P standing and lying; also pulse, respirations; take these q4h during initial treatment; establish baseline before starting treatment; report drops of 30 mm Hg; watch for ECG changes
- Dizziness, faintness, palpitations, tachycardia on rising
- EPS, including akathisia (inability to sit still, no pattern to movements), tardive dyskinesia (bizarre movements of the jaw, mouth, tongue, extremities), pseudoparkinsonism (rigidity, tremors, pill rolling, shuffling gait)

For neuroleptic malignant syndrome: hyperthermia, increased CPK, altered mental status, muscle rigidity, seizures, tachycardia, diaphoresis, hyper/hypotension, fatigue; notify prescriber immediately if symptoms occur

- Skin turgor qd
- Constipation, urinary retention qd; if these occur, increase bulk and water in the diet

Administer:

- Reduced dose in elderly
- Antiparkinsonian agent on order from prescriber, to be used for EPS

Perform/provide:

- Decreased stimulus by dimming lights, avoiding loud noises

• Supervised ambulation until patient is stabilized on medication; do not involve in strenuous exercise program because fainting is possible; patient should not stand still for a long time
• Sips of water, sugarless candy, gum for dry mouth
• Storage in tight, light-resistant container

Evaluate:
• Therapeutic response: decrease in emotional excitement, hallucinations, delusions, paranoia; reorganization of patterns of thought, speech

Teach patient/family:
• To rise slowly, to prevent orthostatic hypotension
• To take medication only as prescribed
• If drowsiness occurs, avoid hazardous activities such as driving
• To avoid use of CNS depressants and OTC meds unless directed by prescriber
• To notify prescriber if pregnancy is planned, suspected
• To notify prescriber immediately of fever, difficulty breathing, fatigue

quinapril (℞)

(kwin′a-pril)
Accupril
Func. class.: Antihypertensive
Chem. class.: Angiotensin-converting enzyme (ACE) inhibitor

Action: Selectively suppresses renin-angiotensin-aldosterone system; inhibits ACE, prevents conversion of angiotensin I to angiotensin II; results in dilation of arterial, venous vessels

Uses: Hypertension, alone or in combination with thiazide diuretics; systolic CHF

Dosage and routes:

Renal dose
• *Adult:* **PO** CCr 30-60 ml/min 5 mg/day initially; CCr <30 ml/min 2.5 mg/day initially

Hypertension (monotherapy)
• *Adult:* **PO** 10-20 mg qd initially, then 20-80 mg/day divided bid or qd
• *Geriatric:* **PO** 10 mg qd, titrate to desired response

Congestive heart failure
• *Adult:* **PO** 5 mg bid, may increase qwk until 20-40 mg/day in 2 divided doses

Available forms: Tabs 5, 10, 20, 40 mg

Side effects/adverse reactions:
CV: Hypotension, postural hypotension, syncope, palpitations, angina pectoris, ***MI, tachycardia,*** vasodilation
GU: Increased BUN, creatinine, decreased libido, impotence
HEMA: ***Thrombocytopenia, agranulocytosis***
INTEG: ***Angioedema,*** rash, sweating, photosensitivity, pruritus
RESP: Cough, pharyngitis, dyspnea
META: Hyperkalemia
GI: Nausea, diarrhea, constipation, vomiting, gastritis, ***GI hemorrhage,*** dry mouth
CNS: Headache, dizziness, fatigue, somnolence, depression, malaise, nervousness, vertigo
MISC: Back pain, amblyopia
MS: Myalgia

Contraindications: Hypersensitivity to ACE inhibitors, pregnancy (D) 2nd, 3rd trimester, children

Precautions: Impaired renal, hepatic function, dialysis patients, hypovolemia, blood dyscrasias, COPD, asthma, elderly, lactation, pregnancy (C) 1st trimester

Pharmacokinetics:

PO: Peak ½-1 hr, serum protein binding 97%, half-life 2 hr, metabolized by liver (active metabolites), metabolites excreted in urine (60%)/ feces (37%)

Interactions:

- ↑ hypotension: diuretics, other antihypertensives, ganglionic blockers, adrenergic blockers, phenothiazines, nitrates, acute alcohol ingestion
- Use caution with vasodilators, hydrALAZINE, prazosin, potassium-sparing diuretics, sympathomimetics, potassium supplements
- ↓ absorption of tetracycline
- ↓ hypotensive effect of quinapril: indomethacin
- ↑ toxicity of: lithium, digoxin

↑ toxicity, death: aconite

↑ or ↓ antihypertensive effect: astragalus, cola tree

↑ antihypertensive effect: barberry, betony, black catechu, black cohosh, bloodroot, broom, burdock, cat's claw, dandelion, goldenseal, Irish moss, Jamaican dogwood, kelp, khella, mistletoe, parsley

↓ antihypertensive effect: coltsfoot, guarana, khat, licorice

Lab test interferences:

False positive: Urine acetone, ANA titer

NURSING CONSIDERATIONS

Assess:

Blood studies: neutrophils, decreased platelets; WBC with differential baseline and periodically q3mo; if neutrophils $<1000/mm^3$, discontinue treatment

- B/P, orthostatic hypotension, syncope
- Renal studies: protein, BUN, creatinine; watch for increased levels; may indicate nephrotic syndrome
- Baselines in renal, hepatic studies before therapy begins and periodically; increased LFTs; uric acid and glucose may be increased
- Potassium levels; hyperkalemia is rare
- Edema in feet, legs qd, weight daily in CHF

Allergic reactions: rash, fever, pruritus, urticaria; drug should be discontinued if antihistamines fail to help

- Renal symptoms: oliguria, urinary frequency, dysuria

Administer:

PO route

- Tabs may be crushed if necessary

Evaluate:

- Therapeutic response: decrease in B/P

Teach patient/family:

- Not to discontinue drug abruptly
- Not to use OTC products (cough, cold, allergy); not to use salt substitutes containing potassium unless directed by prescriber
- To comply with dosage schedule, even if feeling better
- To rise slowly to sitting or standing position to minimize orthostatic hypotension
- To notify prescriber of mouth sores, sore throat, fever, swelling of hands or feet, irregular heartbeat, chest pain, persistent dry cough
- To report excessive perspiration, dehydration, vomiting, diarrhea; may lead to fall in B/P
- That drug may cause dizziness, fainting, light-headedness; may occur during first few days of therapy
- That drug may cause skin rash or impaired taste perception
- How to take B/P, and normal readings for age-group

Treatment of overdose: 0.9% NaCl IV inf

Q

quinidine (℞)

(kwin'i-deen)

quinidine gluconate

Quinaglute Dura-Tabs, Quinalan, Quinate♣

quinidine polygalacturonate

cardioquin

quinidine sulfate

Apo-Quinidine♣, Cin-Quin, Novoquinidine♣, Quinidex Extentabs, Quinora

Func. class.: Antidysrhythmic (Class IA)

Chem. class.: Quinine dextroisomer

Action: Prolongs duration of action potential and effective refractory period, thus decreasing myocardial excitability; anticholinergic properties

Uses: PVCs, atrial fibrillation, PAT, ventricular tachycardia, atrial flutter, malaria/IV quinidine gluconate

Dosage and routes:

Quinidine sulfate

Atrial fibrillation/flutter

• *Adult:* **PO** 200 mg q2-3h × 5-8 doses; may increase qd until sinus rhythm is restored; max 4 g/day given only after digitalization, maintenance 200-300 mg tid-qid or 300-600 mg q8-12h (sus rel)

Paroxysmal supraventricular tachycardia

• *Adult:* **PO** 400-600 mg q2-3h, then 200-300 mg q6-8h or 300-600 mg q8-12h (sus rel)

Premature atrial/ventricular contraction

• *Adult:* **PO** 200-300 mg q6-8h or 300-600 mg (sus rel) q8-12h; max 4 g/day

• *Child:* **PO** 30 mg/kg/day or 900 mg/m²/day in 5 divided doses

Quinidine gluconate

• *Adult:* **PO** 324-660 mg q6-12h (sus rel); **IM** 600 mg, then 400 mg q2h; **IV** give 16 mg/min

Available forms: *Gluconate* tabs sus rel 324, 330 mg; inj gluconate 80 mg/ml; *sulfate* tabs 200, 300 mg; tabs sus rel 300 mg; *polygalacturonate* tabs 275 mg

Side effects/adverse reactions:

CNS: Headache, dizziness, involuntary movement, confusion, psychosis, restlessness, irritability, syncope, excitement, depression, ataxia

EENT: Cinchonism: tinnitus, blurred vision, hearing loss, mydriasis, disturbed color vision

GI: Nausea, vomiting, anorexia, abdominal pain, *diarrhea,* ***hepatotoxicity***

CV: ***Hypotension,*** *bradycardia,* PVCs, ***heart block, cardiovascular collapse, arrest,*** torsades de pointes, widening QRS complex, ***ventricular tachycardia***

HEMA: ***Thrombocytopenia,*** hemolytic anemia, agranulocytosis, hypoprothrombinemia

RESP: Dyspnea, ***respiratory depression***

INTEG: Rash, urticaria, ***angioedema,*** swelling, photosensitivity, flushing with severe pruritus

Contraindications: Hypersensitivity, or idiosyncratic response, digitalis toxicity, history of long QT syndrome, drug-induced torsades de pointe, blood dyscrasias, severe heart block, myasthenia gravis

Precautions: Pregnancy (C), lactation, children, renal disease, potassium imbalance, liver disease, CHF, respiratory depression, elderly

Pharmacokinetics:

PO: Peak 0.5-6 hr, duration 6-8 hr; half-life 6-7 hr, metabolized in liver, excreted unchanged (10%-50%) by kidneys, protein bound (80%-90%)

Interactions:

- ↑ effects of neuromuscular blockers, digoxin, warfarin, tricyclics, propranolol
- ↑ quinidine effects: cimetidine, sodium bicarbonate, carbonic anhydrase inhibitors, antacids, hydroxide suspensions, amiodarone, verapamil
- ↓ quinidine effects: barbiturates, phenytoin, rifampin, nifedipine, sucralfate, cholinergics
- Additive vagolytic effect: anticholinergic blockers
- Additive cardiac depression: other antidysrhythmics, phenothiazines, reserpine
- Food/drug: delayed absorption, ↓ metabolism: grapefruit juice

Hypokalemia, ↑ antidysrhythmic action: aloe, buckthorn, cascara sagrada, senna

↑ toxicity, death: aconite

↑ effect: aloe, broom, chronic buckthorn use, cascara sagrada (chronic use), Chinese rhubarb, figwort, fumitory, goldenseal, kudzu, licorice

↓ effect: coltsfoot

↑ serotonin effect: horehound

Lab test interferences:

Increase: CPK

Interference: Triamterene therapy interferes with quinidine test levels

NURSING CONSIDERATIONS

Assess:

- ECG continuously to determine increased PR or QRS segments, QT interval; discontinue or reduce dose
- Blood levels (therapeutic level 2-7 mcg/ml)
- B/P continuously for fluctuations
- For cinchonism: tinnitus, headache, nausea, dizziness, fever, vertigo, tremor; may lead to hearing loss
- Cardiac status: rate, rhythm, character, continuously
- Respiratory status: rate, rhythm, lung fields for rales; increased respiration, increased pulse; drug should be discontinued
- CNS effects: dizziness, confusion, psychosis, paresthesias, convulsions; drug should be discontinued

Administer:

- AV node blocker (digoxin) before starting quinidine to avoid increased ventricular rate

PO route

- With a full glass of water, on empty stomach

Do not break, crush, chew ext rel products

- Sus rel forms not interchangeable

IM route

- IM inj in deltoid; aspirate to avoid intravascular administration

IV route

- After diluting 800 mg/50 ml or more D_5; give 16 mg or less over 1 min as inf; use infusion pump

Additive compatibilities: Bretylium, cimetidine, milrinone, ranitidine, verapamil

Y-site compatibilities: Diazepam, milrinone

Evaluate:

- Therapeutic response: decreased dysrhythmias

Teach patient/family:

- That if dizziness, drowsiness occur, avoid driving or hazardous activities
- To use sunglasses; may cause sensitivity to light
- To carry emergency ID stating disease and medication use
- How to take pulse and when to notify prescriber

quinine (OTC, ℞)

(kwye'nine)

Novoquine✦, quinine sulfate

Func. class.: Antimalarial

Chem. class.: Cinchona tree alkaloid

Action: Inhibits parasite replications, transcription of DNA to RNA by forming complexes with DNA of parasite

Uses: *Plasmodium falciparum,* malaria, nocturnal leg cramps

Dosage and routes:

- *Adult:* **PO** 650 mg q8h × 10 days, given with pyrimethamine 25 mg q12h × 3 days, with sulfADIAZINE 500 mg qid × 5 days
- *Child:* **PO** 25 mg/kg/day divided q8h for 3-7 days in conjunction with another agent

Leg cramps

- *Adult:* **PO** 250-300 mg hs

Available forms: Caps 200, 300, 325 mg; tabs 260, 325 mg

Side effects/adverse reactions:

RESP: Dyspnea

INTEG: Pruritus, pigmentary changes, skin eruptions, lichen planuslike eruptions, flushing, facial edema, sweating

HEMA: ***Thrombocytopenia, purpura, hypothrombinemia, hemolysis***

CNS: Headache, stimulation, fatigue, irritability, ***seizures,*** bad dreams, dizziness, fever, confusion, anxiety

EENT: Blurred vision, corneal changes, retinal changes, difficulty focusing, tinnitus, vertigo, deafness, photophobia, diplopia, night blindness

GU: Renal tubular damage, ***anuria***

GI: Nausea, vomiting, anorexia, diarrhea, epigastric pain

CV: Angina, dysrhythmias, tachycardia, hypotension, ***acute circulatory failure***

ENDO: Hypoglycemia

MISC: ***Hemolytic uremic syndrome***

Contraindications: Hypersensitivity, G6PD deficiency, retinal field changes, pregnancy (X)

Precautions: Blood dyscrasias, severe GI disease, neurologic disease, severe hepatic disease, psoriasis, cardiac dysrhythmias, tinnitus

Pharmacokinetics:

PO: Peak 1-3 hr, metabolized in liver, excreted in urine, half-life 8-14 hr

Interactions:

- Toxicity: $NaHCO_3$, acetaZOLAMIDE
- ↓ absorption: magnesium or aluminum salts
- ↑ levels of digoxin, digitoxin, neuromuscular blockers, other anticoagulants

Lab test interferences:

Increase: 17-KS

Interference: 17-OHCS

NURSING CONSIDERATIONS

Assess:

- B/P, pulse, watch for hypotension, tachycardia
- Hepatic studies qwk: ALT, AST, bilirubin
- Blood studies, CBC, since blood dyscrasias occur
- For cinchonism: nausea, blurred vision, tinnitus, headache, difficulty focusing

Administer:

- Before or after meals at same time each day to maintain level

Perform/provide:

- Storage in tight, light-resistant container

Evaluate:

- Therapeutic response: decreased symptoms of malaria

Teach patient/family:

- To avoid OTC preparations: cold preparations, tonic water

rabeprazole (℞)

(rah-bep′rah-zole)

Aciphex

Func. class.: Antiulcer, proton pump inhibitor

Chem. class.: Benzimidazole

Action: Suppresses gastric secretion by inhibiting hydrogen/potassium ATPase enzyme system in gastric parietal cell; characterized as gastric acid pump inhibitor, since it blocks final step of acid production

Uses: Gastroesophageal reflux disease (GERD), severe erosive esophagitis, poorly responsive systemic GERD, pathologic hypersecretory conditions (Zollinger-Ellison syndrome, systemic mastocytosis, multiple endocrine adenomas); treatment of active duodenal ulcers with or without antiinfectives for *Helicobacter pylori;* daytime, nighttime heartburn

Dosage and routes:

Healing of duodenal ulcers

• *Adult:* **PO** 20 mg qd × ≤4 wk to be taken after breakfast

Healing of erosive esophagitis or ulcerative GERD

• *Adult:* **PO** 20 mg qd × 4-8 wk

Pathologic hypersecretory conditions

• *Adult:* **PO** 60 mg/day; may increase to 120 mg in 2 divided doses

Available forms: Tabs, del rel 20 mg

Side effects/adverse reactions:

CNS: Headache, dizziness, asthenia

GI: Diarrhea, abdominal pain, vomiting, nausea, constipation, flatulence, acid regurgitation, abdominal swelling, anorexia, irritable colon, esophageal candidiasis, dry mouth

RESP: Upper respiratory infections, cough, epistaxis

INTEG: Rash, dry skin, urticaria, pruritus, alopecia

META: Hypoglycemia, increased hepatic enzymes, weight gain

EENT: Tinnitus, taste perversion

CV: Chest pain, angina, tachycardia, bradycardia, palpitations, peripheral edema

GU: UTI, urinary frequency, increased creatinine, ***proteinuria, hematuria,*** testicular pain, glycosuria

HEMA: ***Pancytopenia, thrombocytopenia, neutropenia, leukocytosis,*** anemia

MISC: Back pain, fever, fatigue, malaise

Contraindications: Hypersensitivity

Precautions: Pregnancy (C), lactation, children

Pharmacokinetics: Eliminated in urine as metabolites and in feces

Interactions:

• ↑ serum levels of rabeprazole: benzodiazepines, phenytoin, clarithromycin

• ↓ levels of rabeprazole: sucralfate

NURSING CONSIDERATIONS

Assess:

• GI system: bowel sounds q8h, abdomen for pain, swelling, anorexia

• Hepatic studies: AST, ALT, alk phosphatase during treatment

Administer:

⊘ After breakfast qd; do not crush, break, chew delayed rel tab

Evaluate:

• Therapeutic response: absence of epigastric pain, swelling, fullness

Teach patient/family:

• To report severe diarrhea, drug may have to be discontinued

• That diabetic patient should know hypoglycemia may occur

• To avoid hazardous activities; dizziness may occur

R

• To avoid alcohol, salicylates, NSAIDs; may cause GI irritation
• To wear sunscreen, protective clothing to prevent burns

radioactive iodine (sodium iodide) ^{131}I (℞)

Func. class.: Antithyroid
Chem. class.: Radiopharmaceutical

Action: Converted to protein-bound iodine by thyroid gland for use when needed
Uses: *High dose:* Thyroid cancer, hyperthyroidism
Low dose: Visualization to determine thyroid cancer, diagnostic aid in thyroid function studies
Dosage and routes:
Thyroid cancer
• *Adult:* **PO** 50-150 mCi, may repeat depending on clinical status
Hyperthyroidism
• *Adult:* **PO** 4-10 mCi, depending on serum thyroxine level
Available forms: Caps 1-50, 0.8-100 mCi; oral sol 7.05 mCi/ml, 3.5-150 mCi/vial
Side effects/adverse reactions:
ENDO: Hypothyroidism, ***hyperthyroid adenoma,*** transient thyroiditis
INTEG: Alopecia
HEMA: ***Eosinophilia, lymphedema, leukemia, bone marrow depression, leukopenia,*** anemia
GI: Nausea, diarrhea, vomiting
EENT: Sore throat, cough
Contraindications: Recent MI, lactation, large nodular goiter, pregnancy (X), age <30 yr, vomiting/diarrhea, acute hyperthyroidism, use of thyroid drugs, lactation
Pharmacokinetics:
PO: Onset 3-6 days; excreted in urine, sweat, feces, breast milk; crosses placenta; excreted in 56 days
Interactions:
• Hypothyroidism: lithium
• ↓ uptake if recent intake of stable iodine, thyroid, antithyroid drugs

NURSING CONSIDERATIONS
Assess:
• Weight qd with same clothing, scale, time of day
• Blood work, including CBC for blood dyscrasias (leukopenia, thrombocytopenia, agranulocytosis)
• Overdose: peripheral edema, heat intolerance, diaphoresis, palpitations, dysrhythmias, severe tachycardia, increased temp, delirium, CNS irritability
• Hypersensitivity: rash, enlarged cervical lymph nodes; drug may have to be discontinued
• Hypoprothrombinemia: bleeding, petechiae, ecchymosis
• Clinical response: after 3 wk should include increased weight, pulse; decreased T_4
• Bone marrow depression: sore throat, fever, fatigue
Administer:
• Only after discontinuing all other antithyroid agents × 5-7 days
• After NPO overnight, food delays action
• During or within 10 days after menstruation
Perform/provide:
• Limited contact with patient ½ hr/day for each person
• Adequate rest after treatment
• Fluids to 3-4 L/day for 48 hr to remove agent from body
Evaluate:
• Therapeutic response: weight gain, decreased pulse, decreased T_4, B/P
Teach patient/family:
• To empty bladder often during treatment; avoid irradiation of gonads
• To report redness, swelling, sore

throat, mouth lesions; indicate blood dyscrasias
• To avoid extended contact with children, spouse for 1 wk
• That bathroom may be used by entire family
• Not to take antithyroid agents but propranolol, which decreases hyperthyroid symptoms, until total effect of taking ^{131}I has occurred (about 6 wk)
• To avoid coughing, expectorating for 24 hr (saliva and vomitus are highly radioactive for 6-8 hr)

raloxifene (℞)

(ral-ox'ih-feen)

Evista

Func. class.: Bone resorption inhibitor, selective estrogen receptor modulator (SERM)

Chem. class.: Benzothiophene

Action: Reduces resorption of bone and decreases bone turnover; mediated through estrogen receptor binding

Uses: Prevention, treatment of osteoporosis in postmenopausal women

Dosage and routes:
• *Adult:* **PO** 60 mg qd

Available forms: Tabs 60 mg

Side effects/adverse reactions:

CNS: Insomnia, migraines, depression

CV: Hot flashes

GI: Nausea, vomiting, diarrhea, anorexia, cramps

GU: Vaginitis, UTI, leukorrhea, cystitis, *hot flashes*

INTEG: Rash, sweating

META: Weight gain, peripheral edema

MS: Arthralgia, myalgia, *leg cramps,* arthritis

RESP: Sinusitis, pharyngitis, increased cough, pneumonia, laryngitis, rhinitis, bronchitis

Contraindications: Hypersensitivity, pregnancy (X), lactation, women with active or history of venous thromboembolic events

Precautions: Venous thromboembolic events, hepatic disease

Pharmacokinetics: Elimination half-life 28-32 hr; excreted in feces; excreted in breast milk; highly bound to plasma proteins

Interactions:
• ↓ action of: anticoagulants
• ↓ action of raloxifene: ampicillin, cholestyramine
• Administer cautiously with other highly protein-bound drugs

Lab test interferences:

Increase: Apolipoprotein A_1, corticosteroid-binding globulin, thyroxine-binding globulin (TBG)

Decrease: Calcium, total protein, albumin, platelets, B, lipoprotein, fibrinogen, LDL cholesterol, total cholesterol

NURSING CONSIDERATIONS

Assess:
• Weight daily, notify prescriber of weekly weight gain >5 lb
• B/P q4h, watch for increase caused by H_2O and sodium retention
• I&O ratio; decreasing urinary output, increasing edema
• Hepatic studies, including AST, ALT, bilirubin, alk phosphatase
• Bone density test baseline and throughout treatment, bone-specific alk phosphatase, osteocalcin, collagen breakdown

Administer:

PO route
• Without regard to meals, Vit D
• Add calcium supplement if inadequate

Evaluate:
• Therapeutic response: prevention, treatment of osteoporosis

R

Teach patient/family:

- To weigh weekly, report gain >5 lb
- To discontinue 72 hr before prolonged bedrest; advise to avoid one position for long periods
- To take calcium supplements, vit D if intake is inadequate
- To increase exercise using weights
- To stop smoking and to decrease alcohol consumption
- That this drug does not help control hot flashes
- To report fever, acute migraine, insomnia, emotional distress; urinary tract infection, or vaginal burning/itching; swelling, warmth, or pain in calves

ramipril (℞)

(ra-mi'pril)

Altace

Func. class.: Antihypertensive

Chem. class.: Angiotensin-converting enzyme inhibitor (ACE)

Action: Selectively suppresses renin-angiotensin-aldosterone system; inhibits ACE, prevents conversion of angiotensin I to angiotensin II; results in dilation of arterial, venous vessels

Uses: Hypertension, alone or in combination with thiazide diuretics; CHF (post MI), reduction in risk of MI, stroke, death from CV disorders

Dosage and routes:

Hypertension

- *Adult:* **PO** 2.5 mg qd initially, then 2.5-20 mg/day divided bid or qd; ***renal impairment:*** 1.25 mg qd with CCr <40 ml/min/1.73 m^2, increase as needed to max of 5 mg/day

CHF post-MI

- *Adult:* **PO** 1.25-2.5 mg bid; may increase to 5 mg bid

Reduction in risk of MI, stroke, death

- *Adult:* **PO** 2.5 mg qd × 7 days, then 5 mg qd × 21 days; then may increase to 10 mg/day

Renal dose

- *Adult:* **PO** CCr <40 ml/min 1.73 m^2

Available forms: Caps 1.25, 2.5, 5, 10 mg

Side effects/adverse reactions:

CV: Hypotension, chest pain, palpitations, angina, syncope, dysrhythmia

GU: ***Proteinuria,*** increased BUN, creatinine, impotence

HEMA: Decreased Hct, Hgb, ***eosinophilia, leukopenia***

INTEG: Rash, sweating, photosensitivity, pruritus

RESP: Cough, dyspnea

META: Hyperkalemia

GI: Nausea, constipation, vomiting, dyspepsia, dysphagia, anorexia, diarrhea, abdominal pain

CNS: Headache, dizziness, anxiety, insomnia, paresthesia, fatigue, depression, malaise, vertigo, ***seizures***

EENT: Hearing loss

MISC: ***Angioedema***

MS: Arthralgia, arthritis, myalgia

Contraindications: Hypersensitivity to ACE inhibitors, pregnancy (D) 2nd/3rd trimester, lactation, children

Precautions: Impaired renal, hepatic function; dialysis patients, hypovolemia, blood dyscrasias, CHF, COPD, asthma, elderly, renal artery stenosis, pregnancy (C) 1st trimester

Do not confuse:

Altace/alteplase

Altace/Artane

ramipril/enalapril

Pharmacokinetics:

PO: Peak ½-1 hr, serum protein binding 73%, half-life 1-2 hr, 13-17 hr for active metabolite, metabolized by liver (metabolites excreted in urine, feces)

Interactions:

• ↑ hypotension: diuretics, other antihypertensives, ganglionic blockers, adrenergic blockers, nitrates, acute alcohol ingestion

• ↑ toxicity: vasodilators, hydrALAZINE, prazosin, potassium-sparing diuretics, sympathomimetics, potassium supplements

• ↓ absorption: antacids

• ↓ antihypertensive effect: indomethacin

• ↑ serum levels of digoxin, lithium

↑ toxicity, death: aconite

↑ or ↓ antihypertensive effect: astragalus, cola tree

↑ antihypertensive effect: barberry, betony, black catechu, black cohosh, bloodroot, broom, burdock, cat's claw, dandelion, goldenseal, Irish moss, Jamaican dogwood, kelp, khella, mistletoe, parsley

↓ antihypertensive effect: coltsfoot, guarana, khat, licorice

Lab test interferences:

False positive: Urine acetone, ANA titer

NURSING CONSIDERATIONS

Assess:

Blood studies: neutrophils, decreased platelets; WBC with diff baseline and periodically q3mo, if neutrophils <1000/mm^3, discontinue treatment

• B/P, orthostatic hypotension, syncope

• Renal studies: protein, BUN, creatinine; increased levels may indicate nephrotic syndrome

• Baselines in renal, hepatic function tests before therapy begins and periodically; increased LFTs; uric acid and glucose may be increased

• Potassium levels, although hyperkalemia rarely occurs

• Dipstick of urine for protein qd in first morning specimen; if protein is increased, a 24-hr urinary protein should be collected

• Edema in feet, legs qd, weight daily in CHF

Allergic reactions: rash, fever, pruritus, urticaria; drug should be discontinued if antihistamines fail to help

• Renal symptoms: polyuria, oliguria, urinary frequency, dysuria

Administer:

• Caps can be opened and added to food

Perform/provide:

• Storage in tight container at 86° F (30° C) or less

• Supine position for severe hypotension

Evaluate:

• Therapeutic response: decrease in B/P

Teach patient/family:

• Not to discontinue drug abruptly

• Not to use OTC products (cough, cold, allergy) unless directed by prescriber; not to use salt substitutes containing potassium without consulting prescriber

• To comply with dosage schedule, even if feeling better

• To rise slowly to sitting or standing position to minimize orthostatic hypotension

• To notify prescriber of mouth sores, sore throat, fever, swelling of hands or feet, irregular heartbeat, chest pain

• To report excessive perspiration, dehydration, vomiting, diarrhea; may lead to fall in B/P

• That drug may cause dizziness, fainting, light-headedness; may occur during first few days of therapy

• That drug may cause skin rash or impaired perspiration

• How to take B/P, and normal readings for age group

Treatment of overdose: 0.9% NaCl IV inf, hemodialysis

ranitidine (℞, OTC)

(ra-nit′i-deen)

Apo-Ranitidine♣, Zantac, Zantac C♣, Zantac EFFERdose, Zantac GELdose

ranitidine bismuth citrate

Tritec

Func. class.: H_2-histamine receptor antagonist

Action: Inhibits histamine at H_2-receptor site in parietal cells, which inhibits gastric acid secretion

Uses: Duodenal ulcer, Zollinger-Ellison syndrome, gastric ulcers, hypersecretory conditions, gastroesophageal reflux disease, stress ulcers, erosive esophagitis (maintenance), active duodenal ulcers with *Helicobacter pylori* in combination with clarithromycin

Investigational uses: Prevention of aspiration pneumonitis, stress ulcers, upper GI bleeding

Dosage and routes:

Ranitidine

Renal dose

• *Adult:* CCr <50 ml/min give **PO** q24h give **IM/IV** q8-24h

Duodenal ulcer

• *Adult:* **PO** 150 mg bid, maintenance 150 mg hs

Zollinger-Ellison syndrome

• *Adult:* **PO** 150 mg bid, may increase if needed

Gastric ulcer

• *Adult:* **PO** 150 mg bid × 6 wk, then 150 mg hs

GERD

• *Adult:* **PO** 150 mg bid

Erosive esophagitis

• *Adult:* **PO** 150 mg bid, 300 mg hs; **IM** 50 mg q6-8h; **IV BOL** 50 mg diluted to 20 ml over 5 min q6-8h; **IV INT INF** 50 mg/100 ml D_5 over 15-20 min q6-8h

• *Child:* **PO** 4-5 mg/kg/day divided q8-12h, max 6 mg/kg/day or 300 mg; **IV** 2-4 mg/kg/day divided q6-8h

ranitidine bismuth citrate

• *Adult:* **PO** 400 mg bid × 4 wk with clarithromycin 500 mg tid × 1st 2 wk

Available forms: Tabs 75, 150, 300 mg; sol for inj 25 mg/ml; tabs, effervescent 75, 150 mg; inj 25 mg/ml; caps 150, 300 mg; syr 15 mg/ml; granules, effervescent 150 mg/packet; ranitidine bismuth citrate: tabs 400 mg

Side effects/adverse reactions:

CNS: Headache, sleeplessness, dizziness, confusion, agitation, depression, hallucination (elderly)

GI: Constipation, abdominal pain, diarrhea, nausea, vomiting, ***hepatotoxicity***

GU: Impotence, gynecomastia

CV: Tachycardia, bradycardia, PVCs

EENT: Blurred vision, increased ocular pressure

INTEG: Urticaria, rash, fever

Contraindications: Hypersensitivity

Precautions: Pregnancy (B), lactation, child <12 yr, hepatic disease, renal disease

Do not confuse:

Zantac/Xanax

Zantac/Zofran

ranitidine/amantadine

Pharmacokinetics:

PO: Peak 2-3 hr, duration 8-12 hr; metabolized by liver; excreted in urine, breast milk; half-life 2-3 hr

Interactions:

• ↑ absorption, toxicity: anticoagulants, sulfonylureas, procainamide

• ↓ absorption of ranitidine: antacids, diazepam, anticholinergics, metoclopramide

Lab test interferences:
Increase: AST, ALT, alk phosphatase, creatinine, LDH, bilirubin
False positive: Urine protein

NURSING CONSIDERATIONS
Assess:
• Gastric pH (>5 should be maintained)
• I&O ratio, BUN, creatinine
• Mental status: confusion, dizziness, depression, anxiety, weakness, tremors, psychosis, diarrhea, abdominal discomfort, jaundice; report immediately
• GI complaints: nausea, vomiting, diarrhea, cramps

Administer:
PO route
• With meals for prolonged effect
• Antacids 1 hr before or 1 hr after ranitidine

IV route
• IV after diluting 50 mg/20 ml 0.9% NaCl, D_5W, $D_{10}W$, LR, $NaCO_3$ 5% and give 50 mg or less/5 min or more; may dilute 50 mg/50-100 ml of 0.9% NaCl, D_5W, $D_{10}W$, LR, $NaCO_3$ 5% and give over 15-20 min

Additive compatibilities: AcetaZOLAMIDE, amikacin, aminophylline, chloramphenicol, chlorothiazide, ciprofloxacin, colistimethate, dexamethasone, digoxin, DOBUTamine, DOPamine, doxycycline, epINEPHrine, erythromycin, floxacillin, fluconazole/ondansetron, flumazenil, furosemide, gentamicin, heparin, insulin (regular), isoproterenol, lidocaine, lincomycin, meropenem, methylPREDNISolone, moxalactam, penicillin G potassium, penicillin G sodium, polymyxin B, potassium chloride, protamine, quinidine, sodium nitroprusside, ticarcillin, tobramycin, vancomycin

Syringe compatibilities: Atropine, cyclizine, dexamethasone, dimenhyDRINATE, diphenhydrAMINE, DOBUTamine, DOPamine, fentanyl, glycopyrrolate, hydromorphone, isoproterenol, meperidine, metoclopramide, morphine, nalbuphine, oxymorphone, pentazocine, perphenazine, prochlorperazine, promethazine, scopolamine

Y-site compatibilities: Acyclovir, aldesleukin, allopurinol, amifostine, aminophylline, amsacrine, atracurium, aztreonam, bretylium, cefepime, cefmetazole, ceftazidime, ciprofloxacin, cisatracurium, cisplatin, cladribine, cyclophosphamide, cytarabine, diltiazem, DOBUTamine, DOPamine, DOXOrubicin, DOXOrubicin liposome, enalaprilat, epINEPHrine, esmolol, fentanyl, filgrastim, fluconazole, fludarabine, foscarnet, furosemide, gallium, granisetron, heparin, hydromorphone, idarubicin, labetalol, lorazepam, melphalan, meperidine, methotrexate, midazolam, milrinone, morphine, niCARdipine, nitroglycerin, norepinephrine, ondansetron, paclitaxel, pancuronium, piperacillin, piperacillin/tazobactam, procainamide, propofol, remifentanil, sargramostim, tacrolimus, teniposide, theophylline, thiopental, thiotepa, vecuronium, vinorelbine, warfarin, zidovudine

Perform/provide:
• Storage at room temperature

Evaluate:
• Therapeutic response: decreased abdominal pain

Teach patient/family:
• That gynecomastia, impotence may occur but are reversible
• To avoid driving, other hazardous activities until stabilized on this medication
• To avoid black pepper, caffeine, alcohol, harsh spices, extremes in temperature of food
• That drug must be continued for prescribed time to be effective

R

rasburicase (℞)

(rass-burr′i-case)

Elitek

Func. class.: Antineoplastic, antimetabolite

Chem. class.: Recombinant urate-oxidase enzyme

Action: Catalyzes enzymatic oxidation of uric acid into an inactive and a soluble metabolite

Uses: To reduce uric acid levels in children with leukemia, lymphoma, solid tumor malignancies who are receiving chemotherapy

Dosage and routes:

• *Adult:* **IV INF** 0.15 or 0.2 mg/kg as a single daily dose given as **IV INF** over ½ hr

Available forms: Powder for inj 1.5 mg/vial

Side effects/adverse reactions:

HEMA: ***Neutropenia with fever***

GI: Nausea, vomiting, anorexia, diarrhea, abdominal pain, constipation, dyspepsia, mucositis

SYST: Anaphylaxis, hemolysis, ***methemoglobinemia, sepsis***

CNS: Headache

Contraindications: Hypersensitivity, G6PD deficiency, hemolytic reactions, or methemoglobinemia reactions to this drug

Precautions: Lactation, children <2 yr, pregnancy (C)

Pharmacokinetics: Elimination half-life 18 hr

NURSING CONSIDERATIONS

Assess:

• Renal studies: BUN, serum uric acid, urine creatinine clearance, electrolytes before and during therapy

• Monitor temp q4h; fever may indicate beginning infection; no rectal temps

• Anaphylaxis, have emergency equipment nearby

• For G6PD deficiency, hemolytic reactions, methemoglobinemia; these patients should not be given this agent

• For toxicity: severe diarrhea, nausea, vomiting

• GI symptoms: frequency of stools, cramping, if severe diarrhea occurs, fluid and electrolytes may need to be given

Administer:

• Antiemetic 30-60 min before giving drug and prn

Evaluate:

• Therapeutic response: decreased uric acid levels

Teach patient/family:

• Reason for therapy, expected results

HIGH ALERT

remifentanil (℞)

(rem-ih-fin′ta-nill)

Ultiva

Func. class.: Opiate agonist analgesic

Chem. class.: μ-Opioid agonist

Controlled Substance Schedule II

Action: Inhibits ascending pain pathways in limbic system, thalamus, midbrain, hypothalamus

Uses: In combination with other drugs in general anesthesia to provide analgesia

Dosage and routes:

• *Adult:* Induction **IV** 0.5-1 mcg/kg/min with a hypnotic or volative agent; maintenance with isoflurane (0.4-1.5 MAC) or propofol (100-200 mcg/kg/min); CONT INF 0.25-0.4 mcg/kg/min

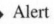

Available forms: Powder for inj-lyophilized 1 mg/ml after reconstitution

Side effects/adverse reactions:
CNS: Drowsiness, *dizziness,* confusion, *headache,* sedation, euphoria, delirium, agitation, anxiety
GI: Nausea, vomiting, anorexia, constipation, cramps, dry mouth
GU: Urinary retention, dysuria
INTEG: Rash, urticaria, bruising, flushing, diaphoresis, pruritus
EENT: Tinnitus, blurred vision, miosis, diplopia
CV: Palpitations, *bradycardia,* change in B/P, facial flushing, syncope, ***asystole***
RESP: ***Respiratory depression, apnea***
MS: Rigidity

Contraindications: Child <12 yr, hypersensitivity

Precautions: Pregnancy (C), lactation, increased intracranial pressure, acute MI, severe heart disease, renal disease, hepatic disease, asthma, respiratory conditions, convulsive disorders, elderly

Pharmacokinetics: Unknown

Interactions:
- Respiratory depression, hypotension, profound sedation: alcohol, sedatives, hypnotics, or other CNS depressants; antihistamines, phenothiazines

↑ CNS depression: kava

NURSING CONSIDERATIONS

Assess:
- I&O ratio, check for decreasing output; may indicate urinary retention, especially in elderly
- CNS changes; dizziness, drowsiness, hallucinations, euphoria, LOC, pupil reaction
- Allergic reactions: rash, urticaria
- Respiratory dysfunction: respiratory depression, character, rate, rhythm; notify prescriber if respirations are <12/min; CV status; bradycardia, syncope
- Use pain scoring to determine pain perception

Administer:
- Direct IV over 1½-3 min; use tuberculin syringe
- Interruption of infusion results in rapid reversal (no residual opioid effect within 5-10 min)

Y-site compatibilities: Acyclovir, alfentanil, amikacin, aminophylline, ampicillin, ampicillin/sulbactam, amrinone, aztreonam, bretylium, bumetanide, buprenorphine, butorphanol, calcium gluconate, cefazolin, cefotaxime, cefotetan, cefoxitin, ceftazidime, ceftizoxime, ceftriaxone, cefuroxime, cimetidine, ciprofloxacin, cisatracurium, clindamycin, dexamethasone, digoxin, diphenhydrAMINE, DOBUTamine, DOPamine, doxycycline, droperidol, enalaprilat, epINEPHrine, esmolol, famotidine, fentanyl, fluconazole, furosemide, ganciclovir, gentamicin, haloperidol, heparin, hydrocortisone sodium succinate, hydromorphone, hydrOXYzine, imipenem/cilastatin, isoproterenol, ketorolac, lidocaine, lorazepam, magnesium sulfate, mannitol, meperidine, methylPREDNISolone, sodium succinate, metoclopramide, metronidazole, mezlocillin, midazolam, minocycline, morphine, nalbuphine, netilmicin, nitroglycerin, norepinephrine, ofloxacin, ondansetron

Perform/provide:
- Storage in light-resistant area at room temperature

Evaluate:
- Therapeutic response: maintenance of anesthesia

Teach patient/family:
- To call for assistance when ambulating or smoking; drowsiness, dizziness may occur
- To make position changes slowly to prevent orthostatic hypotension

repaglinide (℞)

(re-pag'lih'nide)
Prandin
Func. class.: Antidiabetic
Chem. class.: Meglitinide

Action: Causes functioning β-cells in pancreas to release insulin, leading to drop in blood glucose levels; closes ATP-dependent potassium channels in the β-cell membrane; this leads to opening of calcium channels; increased calcium influx induces insulin secretion

Uses: Stable adult-onset diabetes mellitus (type 2) NIDDM

Research note: Repaglinide given with rifampin resulted in the decrease of repaglinide levels[34]

Dosage and routes:
• *Adult:* **PO** 1-2 mg with each meal, max 16 mg/day, adjust at weekly intervals

Available forms: Tabs 0.5, 1, 2 mg

Side effects/adverse reactions:
CNS: Headache, weakness, paresthesia
ENDO: ***Hypoglycemia***
GI: Nausea, vomiting, diarrhea, constipation, dyspepsia
INTEG: Rash, allergic reactions
MS: Back pains, arthralgia
RESP: URI, sinusitis, rhinitis, bronchitis

Contraindications: Hypersensitivity to meglitinides, diabetic ketoacidosis, type 1 diabetes

Precautions: Pregnancy (C), elderly, cardiac disease, severe renal disease, severe hepatic disease, thyroid disease, severe hypoglycemic reactions, lactation, children

Pharmacokinetics:
PO: Competely absorbed by GI route; onset 30 min, peak 1-1½ hr, duration <4 hr; half-life 1 hr; metabolized in liver; excreted in urine, feces (metabolites); crosses placenta; 98% plasma protein bound

Interactions:
• ↑ repaglinide metabolism: rifampin, barbiturates, carbamazepine
• ↓ repaglinide metabolism: antifungals (ketoconazole, miconazole), erythromycin
• ↑ repaglinide effect: NSAIDs, salicylates, sulfonamides, chloramphenicol, MAOIs, coumarins, β-blockers, probenecid
• ↓ repaglinide action: calcium channel blockers, corticosteroids, oral contraceptives, thizide diuretics, thyroid preparations, estrogens, phenothiazines, phenytoin, rifampin, isoniazid, phenobarbital, sympathomimetics
↓ hypoglycemic effect: broom, buchu, dandelion, juniper
↑ or ↓ hypoglycemic effect: chromium, fenugreek, ginseng
↓ glucose tolerance: karela
↓ antidiabetic effect: bee pollen, blue cohosh, broom, chromium, elecampane, eucalyptus, gotu kola
↑ antidiabetic effect: alfalfa, aloe, basil, bay, bilberry, bitter melon, black catechu, buchu, burdock, coriander, dandelion, eyebright (po), fenugreek, garlic, ginseng, glucomannan, glucosamine, goat's rue, gymnema, horehound, horse chestnut, jambul, myrrh, myrtle

NURSING CONSIDERATIONS

Assess:
Hypo/hyperglycemic reaction that can occur soon after meals: dizziness, weakness, headache, tremor, anxiety, tachycardia, hunger, sweating, abdominal pain
• Glycosylated Hgb, fasting glucose during treatment

Administer:
• Up to 15 min before meals; 2, 3, or 4×/day preprandially

• Skip dose if meal is skipped; add dose if meal is added

Perform/provide:

• Storage in tight container in cool environment

Evaluate:

• Therapeutic response: decrease in polyuria, polydipsia, polyphagia, clear sensorium, absence of dizziness, stable gait

Teach family/patient:

• To use a capillary blood glucose test while on this drug

• The symptoms of hypo/hyperglycemia; what to do about each

• That drug must be continued on daily basis; explain consequences of discontinuing drug abruptly

• To avoid OTC medications unless ordered by prescriber

• That diabetes is a lifelong illness; drug will not cure disease

• That all food included in diet plan must be eaten to prevent hypoglycemia; to have glucagon emergency kit available

• To carry emergency ID

• To avoid alcohol, explain disulfiram-like reaction

Treatment of overdose: Glucose 25 g IV via dextrose 50% solution, 50 ml or 1 mg glucagon

RARELY USED

reserpine (℞)

(re-ser'peen)

Novoreserpine✦, Reserfia✦, reserpine

Func. class.: Antihypertensive, antiadrenergic agent, peripheral action

Uses: Hypertension

Dosage and routes:

• *Adult:* **PO** 0.25-0.5 mg qd × 1-2 wk, then 0.1-0.25 mg qd maintenance

• *Geriatric:* **PO** 0.05 mg qd, increase by 0.05 weekly to desired dose

Contraindications: Hypersensitivity, depression, suicidal patients, active peptic ulcer disease, ulcerative colitis, pregnancy (D), Parkinson's disease

Rh_o(D) immune globulin standard dose IM_o (℞)

Gamulin Rh, HydroRho-D, Rho-GAM

Rh_o(D) globulin microdose IM (℞)

HypRho-D Mini-Dose, MiCRhoGAM, Mini-Gamulin

Rh_o(D) globulin IV (℞)

WinRho SD, WinRho SDF

Func. class.: Immune globulins

Action: Suppresses immune response of nonsensitized Rh_o (D or D^u)-negative patients who are exposed to Rh_o (D or D^u)-positive blood

Uses: Prevention of isoimmunization in Rh-negative women given Rh-positive blood after abortions, miscarriages, amniocentesis

Dosage and routes:

Prior delivery

• *Adult:* **IM** 1 vial (standard dose) at 26-28 wk, 1 vial (standard dose) 72 hr after delivery

Pregnancy termination <13 wk

• *Adult:* **IM** 1 vial (microdose) within 72 hr

Pregnancy termination >13 wks

• *Adult:* **IM** 1 vial (standard dose) within 72 hr

R

Fetal-maternal hemorrhage

• *Adult:* **IM** packed RBCs volume of hemorrhage/15 = needed vials (standard dose)

Following delivery

• *Adult:* **IM** 1 vial (standard dose) if fetal-packed RBCs <15 ml, or 2 vials if fetal-packed RBCs >15 ml; given within 72 hr of delivery or miscarriage

Transfusion error

• *Adult:* **IM** (standard dose) give within 72 hr

After 34 wk gestation

• *Adult:* **IM/IV** 120 mcg given within 72 hr (IV dose)

Available forms: Inj single-dose vial (50 mcg/vial-microdose; 300 mcg/vial-standard); inj 120, 300 mcg Rh_o (D) immune globulin IV, human

Side effects/adverse reactions:

INTEG: Irritation at inj site, fever

CNS: Lethargy

MS: Myalgia

Contraindications: Previous immunization with this drug, Rh_o (O)-positive/D^u-positive patient

Precautions: Pregnancy (C)

Do not confuse:

Gamulin Rh/MICRh_oGAM

Interactions:

• ↓ antibody response: live virus vaccines

NURSING CONSIDERATIONS

Assess:

• Allergies, reactions to immunizations; previous immunization with this drug

• For intravascular hemolysis: back pain, chills, hemoglobinuria, renal insufficiency

• Type, crossmatch mother and newborn's cord blood; if mother is Rh_o (D) negative, D^u-negative and newborn Rh_o (D) positive, this medication should be given

Administer:

IM route

• Reconstitute Rh_o(D) immune globulin IV using 1.25 ml of 0.9% NaCl, swirl

• IM inj in deltoid; aspirate within 3 hr if possible

• Only equal lot numbers of drug, cross-match

• Only MICRhoGAM for abortions or miscarriages <12 wk unless fetus or father is Rh negative; unless patient is Rh_o (D)-positive, D^u-positive, Rh antibodies are present

• Do not use Rh_o(D) immune globulin or Rh_o(D) immune globulin micro dose by IV

IV direct route

• Reconstitute Rh_o(D) immune globulin IV using 2.5 ml of 0.9% NaCl, swirl, give over 3-5 min

Perform/provide:

• Storage in refrigerator

Evaluate:

• Rh_o (D) sensitivity in transfusion error, prevention of erythroblastosis fetalis for normal vision

Teach patient/family:

• How drug works; that drug must be given after subsequent deliveries if subsequent babies are Rh positive

riboflavin (vit B_2)

(OTC)

(rye'boh-flay-vin)

Func. class.: Vit B_2, water soluble

Action: Needed for respiratory reactions by catalyzing proteins and

Uses: Vit B_2 deficiency or polyneuritis; cheilosis adjunct with thiamine

Dosage and routes:

Deficiency

• *Adult and child >12 yr:* **PO** 5-25 mg qd

• *Child <12 yr:* **PO** 2-10 mg qd, then 0.6 mg/1000 calories ingested

RDA

• *Adult:* males 1.4-1.8 mg, females 1.2-1.3 mg

Available forms: Tabs 5, 10, 25, 50, 100, 250 mg

Side effects/adverse reactions:

GU: Yellow discoloration of urine (large doses)

Precautions: Pregnancy (A)

Pharmacokinetics:

PO: Half-life 65-85 min, 60% protein bound, unused amounts excreted in urine (unchanged)

Interactions:

• ↓ action of: tetracyclines

• ↑ riboflavin need: alcohol, probenecid, tricyclics, phenothiazines

Lab test interferences:

• May cause false elevations of urinary catecholamines

NURSING CONSIDERATIONS

Assess:

• Nutritional status: liver, eggs, dairy products, yeast, whole grain, green vegetables

Administer:

• With food for better absorption

Perform/provide:

• Storage in airtight, light-resistant container

Evaluate:

• Therapeutic response: absence of headache, GI problems, cheilosis, skin lesions, depression, burning, itchy eyes, anemia

Teach patient/family:

• That urine may turn bright yellow

• About addition of needed foods that are rich in riboflavin

• To avoid alcohol

rifabutin (℞)

(riff'a-byoo-ten)

Mycobutin

Func. class.: Antimycobacterial agent

Chem. class.: Rifamycin S derivative

Action: Inhibits DNA-dependent RNA polymerase in susceptible strains of *Escherichia coli* and *Bacillus subtilis;* mechanism of action against *Mycobacterium avium* unknown

Uses: Prevention of *Mycobacterium avium* complex (MAC) in patients with advanced HIV infection

Investigational uses: *Helicobacter pylori* that has not responded to other treatment

Dosage and routes:

• *Adult:* 300 mg qd (may take as 150 mg bid)

Available forms: Caps 150 mg

Side effects/adverse reactions:

INTEG: Rash

MS: Asthenia, arthralgia, myalgia

MISC: Flulike symptoms, shortness of breath, chest pressure

GI: Nausea, vomiting, anorexia, diarrhea, heartburn, ***hepatitis,*** discolored saliva

GU: Hematuria, *discolored urine*

CNS: Headache, fatigue, anxiety, confusion, insomnia

HEMA: ***Hemolytic anemia, eosinophilia, thrombocytopenia, leukopenia***

Contraindications: Hypersensitivity, active TB, WBC <1000/mm^3 or platelet count <50,000/mm^3

Precautions: Pregnancy (B), lactation, hepatic disease, blood dyscrasias, children

Do not confuse:

rifabutin/rifampin

R

Pharmacokinetics:
PO: Peak 2-3 hr, duration >24 hr, half-life 3 hr; metabolized in liver (active/inactive metabolites), excreted in urine primarily as metabolites

Interactions:
• ↓ action of: amprenavir, anticoagulants, β-blockers, barbiturates, clofibrate, corticosteroids, cycloSPORINE, dapsone, delavirdine, digoxin, disopyramide, efavirenz, estrogens, fluconazole, indinavir, ketoconazole, nelfinavir, nevirapine, opioid analgesic, oral contraceptives, phenytoin, quinidine, saquinavir, sulfonylureas, theophylline, tocainide, verapamil, zidovudine
• ↑ levels of rifabutin: ritonavir
• Drug/food: high-fat diet ↓ absorption

Lab test interferences:
Interference: Folate level, vit B_{12}, BSP, gallbladder studies

NURSING CONSIDERATIONS

Assess:
• CBC for neutropenia, thrombocytopenia, eosinophilia
• For acute TB: chest x-ray, sputum culture, blood culture, biopsy of lymph nodes, PPD; drug should not be given for active TB
• Signs of anemia: Hct, Hgb, fatigue
• Hepatic studies qwk: ALT, AST, bilirubin
• Renal status before, qmo: BUN, creatinine, output, specific gravity, urinalysis
• Hepatic status: decreased appetite, jaundice, dark urine, fatigue

Administer:
• With food if GI upset occurs; better to take on empty stomach 1 hr ac or 2 hr pc, high-fat foods slow absorption
• Antiemetic if vomiting occurs
• After C&S is completed; qmo to detect resistance

Evaluate:
• Therapeutic response: not used for active TB because of risk of development of resistance to rifampin; culture negative

Teach patient/family:
• That patients using oral contraceptives should consider using nonhormonal methods of birth control, since rifabutin may decrease their efficacy
• That compliance with dosage schedule, duration is necessary
• That scheduled appointments must be kept; relapse may occur
• That urine, feces, saliva, sputum, sweat, tears may be colored red-orange; soft contact lenses may be permanently stained
• To report flulike symptoms: excessive fatigue, anorexia, vomiting, sore throat; unusual bleeding, yellowish discoloration of skin, eyes
• To report myositis: muscle or bone pain

rifampin (℞)
(rif'am-pin)
Rifadin, Rimactane, Rofact✱
Func. class.: Antitubercular
Chem. class.: Rifamycin B derivative

Action: Inhibits DNA-dependent polymerase, decreases tubercle bacilli replication

Uses: Pulmonary tuberculosis, meningococcal carriers (prevention)

Research note: Repaglinide given with rifampin resulted in the decrease of repaglinide levels[35]

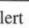

Dosage and routes:
Tuberculosis
• *Adult:* **PO/IV** max 600 mg/day as single dose 1 hr ac or 2 hr pc or 10 mg/kg/day 2-3 ×/wk
• *Child >5 yr:* **PO/IV** 10-20 mg/kg/day as single dose 1 hr ac or 2 hr

pc, not to exceed 600 mg/day, with other antituberculars

• 6-mo regimen: 2 mo treatment of isoniazid, rifampin, pyrazinamide and possibly streptomycin or ethambutol; then rifampin and isoniazid × 4 mo

• 9-mo regimen: rifampin and isoniazid supplemented with pyrazinamide, or streptomycin or ethambutol

Meningococcal carriers

• *Adult:* **PO/IV** 600 mg bid × 2 days

• *Child >5 yr:* **PO/IV** 10-20 mg/kg not to exceed 600 mg/dose

• *Infant 3 mo-1 yr:* 5 mg/kg **PO** bid for 2 days

Prevention of H. influenzae type B infection

• *Adult:* **PO** 600 mg/day × 4 days

• *Child:* **PO** 20 mg/kg/day × 4 days

Available forms: Caps 150, 300 mg; powder for inj 600 mg/vial

Side effects/adverse reactions:

INTEG: Rash, pruritus, urticaria

EENT: Visual disturbances

MS: Ataxia, weakness

MISC: Flulike symptoms, menstrual disturbances, edema, shortness of breath

GI: Nausea, vomiting, anorexia, diarrhea, ***pseudomembranous colitis,*** *heartburn,* sore mouth and tongue, ***pancreatitis,*** increased LFTs

GU: ***Hematuria, acute renal failure, hemoglobinuria***

CNS: Headache, fatigue, anxiety, drowsiness, confusion

HEMA: ***Hemolytic anemia, eosinophilia, thrombocytopenia, leukopenia***

Contraindications: Hypersensitivity

Precautions: Pregnancy (C), lactation, hepatic disease, blood dyscrasias

Do not confuse:
rifampin/rifabutin

Pharmacokinetics:

PO: Peak 2-3 hr, duration >24 hr, half-life 3 hr; metabolized in liver (active/inactive metabolites), excreted in urine as free drug (30% crosses placenta) and breast milk

Interactions:

• ↓ action of: acetaminophen, alcohol, anticoagulants, antidiabetics, β-blockers, barbiturates, benzodiazepines, chloramphenicol, clofibrate, corticosteroids, cycloSPORINE, dapsone, digoxin, diltiazem, doxycycline, fluoroquinolones, haloperidol, hormones, imidazole antifungals, NIFEdipine, oral contraceptives, phenytoin, protease inhibitors, sulfonamides, theophylline, verapamil, zidovudine

• Lithium toxicity: lithium

• Hepatotoxicity: isoniazid

• Incompatible with sodium lactate

Lab test interferences:

Interference: Folate level, vit B_{12}, gallbladder studies, dexamethasone suppression test

False positive: Direct Coombs' test

NURSING CONSIDERATIONS

Assess:

• For infection: sputum culture, lung sounds

• Signs of anemia: Hct, Hgb, fatigue

• Hepatic studies qmo: ALT, AST, bilirubin

• Renal status before, qmo: BUN, creatinine, output, specific gravity, urinalysis

• Hepatic status: decreased appetite, jaundice, dark urine, fatigue

Administer:

• After C&S is completed; qmo to detect resistance

PO route

• On empty stomach, 1 hr ac or 2 hr pc with a full glass of water

• Antiemetic if vomiting occurs

IV route

• After diluting each 600 mg/10 ml of sterile water for inj (60 mg/ml), agitate, withdraw dose and dilute in 100 ml or 500 ml of D_5W or 0.9% NaCl given as an inf over 3 hr, or if diluted in 100 ml, give over ½ hr; do not admix with other sol or medications

Evaluate:

• Therapeutic response: decreased symptoms of TB, culture negative

Teach patient/family:

• That compliance with dosage schedule, duration is necessary
• That scheduled appointments must be kept; relapse may occur
• To avoid alcohol, hepatotoxicity may occur
• That urine, feces, saliva, sputum, sweat, tears may be colored red-orange; soft contact lenses may be permanently stained
• To report flulike symptoms: excessive fatigue, anorexia, vomiting, sore throat; unusual bleeding, yellowish discoloration of skin, eyes
• To use nonhormonal form of birth control

rifapentine (℞)

(riff'ah-pen-teen)
Priftin
Func. class.: Antitubercular
Chem. class.: Rifamycin derivative

Action: Inhibits DNA-dependent polymerase, decreases tubercle bacilli replication

Uses: Pulmonary tuberculosis, must be used with at least one other antitubercular

Dosage and routes:

Intensive phase

• *Adult:* **PO** 600 mg (four 150 mg tabs 2×/wk), with an interval of 72 hr between doses × 2 mo; must be given with at least one other antitubercular

Continuation phase

• *Adult:* **PO** 600 mg qwk × 4 mo in combination with isoniazid or other appropriate antitubercular

Available forms: Tabs 150 mg

Side effects/adverse reactions:

INTEG: Rash, pruritus, urticaria, acne
EENT: Visual disturbances
MS: Gout, arthrosis
MISC: Edema, aggressive reaction, increased B/P
GI: Nausea, vomiting, anorexia, diarrhea, bilirubinemia, hepatitis, increased ALT, AST, *heartburn,* ***pancreatitis***
GU: ***Hematuria,*** pyuria, ***proteinuria,*** urinary casts, urine discoloration
CNS: Headache, fatigue, anxiety, dizziness
HEMA: ***Thrombocytopenia, leukopenia, neutropenia, lymphopenia,*** anemia, ***leukocytosis,*** purpura, hematoma

Contraindications: Hypersensitivity to rifamycins, porphyria

Precautions: Pregnancy (C), lactation, hepatic disease, blood dyscrasias, children <12 yr, HIV, elderly

Pharmacokinetics:

PO: Peak 5-6 hr, half-life 13 hr; metabolized in liver (active/inactive metabolites), excreted in urine and feces, excreted in breast milk, protein binding 97%, steady state 10 days

Interactions:

• Use with extreme caution with protease inhibitors
• ↓ action of: amitriptyline, anticoagulants, antidiabetics, barbiturates, β-blockers, chloramphenicol, clarithromycin, clofibrate, corticosteroids, cycloSPORINE, dapsone, delavirdine, diazepam, digoxin, diltiazem, disopyramide, doxycycline, fentanyl, fluconazole, fluoroquino-

lones, haloperidol, indinavir, itraconazole, ketoconazole, methadone, mexiletine, nelfinavir, NIFEdipine, nortriptyline, oral contraceptives, phenothiazines, phenytoin, progestins, quinidine, quinine, ritonavir, saquinavir, sildenafil, tacrolimus, theophylline, thyroid preparations, tocainide, verapamil, warfarin, zidovudine

• Drug/food: ↑ absorption with food

Lab test interferences:
Interference: Folate level, vit B_{12}

NURSING CONSIDERATIONS

Assess:
• Baselines in CBC, AST, ALT, bilirubin, platelets
• For infection: sputum culture, lung sounds
• Signs of anemia: Hct, Hgb, fatigue
• Hepatic studies qmo: ALT, AST, bilirubin
• Renal status qmo: BUN, creatinine, output, specific gravity, urinalysis
• Hepatic status: decreased appetite, jaundice, dark urine, fatigue

Administer:
PO route
• May give with food for GI upset
• Antiemetic if vomiting occurs
• After C&S is completed; qmo to detect resistance

Evaluate:
• Therapeutic response: decreased symptoms of TB, culture negative

Teach patient/family:
• That compliance with dosage schedule, duration is necessary
• That scheduled appointments must be kept; relapse may occur
• That urine, feces, saliva, sputum, sweat, tears may be colored red-orange; soft contact lenses, dentures may be permanently stained
• To use alternative method of contraception, oral contraceptive action may be decreased
• To report flulike symptoms: excessive fatigue, anorexia, vomiting, sore throat; unusual bleeding, yellowish discoloration of skin, eyes

riluzole (℞)

(rill'you-zole)
Rilutek
Func. class.: ALS agent
Chem. class.: Benzathiazole

Action: Unknown; may act by inhibiting glutamate, interfering with binding of amino acid receptors, and inactivating of voltage-dependent sodium channels

Uses: Amyotropic lateral sclerosis (ALS)

Dosage and routes:
• *Adult:* **PO** 50 mg q12h, take 1 hr ac or 2 hr pc

Available forms: Tabs 50 mg

Side effects/adverse reactions:
GI: Nausea, vomiting, dyspepsia, anorexia, diarrhea, flatulence, stomatitis, dry mouth
HEMA: ***Neutropenia***
CNS: Hypertonia, depression, dizziness, insomnia, somnolence, vertigo
INTEG: Pruritus, eczema, alopecia, ***exfoliative dermatitis***
RESP: Decreased lung function, rhinitis, increased cough
CV: Hypertension, tachycardia, phlebitis, palpitation, postural hypertension
GU: UTI, dysuria

Contraindications: Hypersensitivity

Precautions: Neutropenia, renal disease, hepatic disease, elderly, pregnancy (C), lactation, children

Pharmacokinetics: Well absorbed, extensively metabolized by the liver, excretion in urine/feces

Interactions:

- ↓ elimination of riluzole: caffeine, theophylline, amitriptyline, quinolones
- ↑ elimination of riluzole: cigarette smoking, rifampin, omeprazole, charcoal-broiled food
- Drug/food: high fat meal: ↓ absorption

NURSING CONSIDERATIONS

Assess:

- Hepatic studies: AST, ALT, bilirubin, GGT, baseline and qmo × 3 mo, then q3mo; monitor liver chemistries
- For neutropenia <500/mm

Administer:

- 1 hr ac or 2 hr pc; a high-fat meal decreases absorption

Teach patient/family:

- To report febrile illness, which may indicate neutropenia
- The reason for drug and expected results

rimantadine (℞)

(ri-man′tah-deen)

Flumadine

Func. class.: Synthetic antiviral

Chem. class.: Tricyclic amine

Action: Prevents uncoating of nucleic acid in viral cell, preventing penetration of virus to host; causes release of dopamine from neurons

Uses: Prophylaxis or treatment of influenza type A

Dosage and routes:

Renal/hepatic dose

- Reduce dose as needed

Influenza type A

Prophylaxis

- *Adult and child >10 yr:* **PO** 100 mg bid; in renal, hepatic disease, lower dose to 100 mg/day
- *Child <10 yr:* **PO** 5 mg/kg/day, not to exceed 150 mg

Treatment

- *Adult:* **PO** 100 mg bid; in renal or hepatic disease, lower dose to 100 mg/day; start treatment at onset of symptoms, continue for at least 1 wk
- *Geriatric:* **PO** 100 mg/day

Available forms: Tabs 100 mg; syr 50 mg/5 ml

Side effects/adverse reactions:

CNS: Headache, dizziness, fatigue, depression, hallucinations, tremors, ***seizures,*** insomnia, *poor concentration,* asthenia, gait abnormalities, *anxiety, confusion*

CV: Pallor, palpitations, *hypotension, edema*

EENT: Tinnitus, taste abnormality, eye pain

GI: Nausea, vomiting, constipation, dry mouth, anorexia, abdominal pain, diarrhea, dyspepsia

INTEG: Rash

Contraindications: Hypersensitivity to drugs of adamantance class (this drug, amantadine)

Precautions: Epilepsy, hepatic disease, renal disease, pregnancy (C), lactation, children <1 yr

Do not confuse:

rimantadine/amantadine

Pharmacokinetics:

PO: Peak 6 hr, elimination half-life 25½ hr, plasma protein binding (40%)

Interactions:

- ↓ peak concentration of rimantadine: acetaminophen, aspirin
- ↑ rimantadine concentration: cimetidine

NURSING CONSIDERATIONS

Assess:

- Assess for seizures; if seizures occur, drug should be discontinued
- I&O ratio; report urinary frequency, hesitancy in renal disease
- Bowel pattern before, during treatment
- CNS effect in elderly or patients with severe hepatic/renal disease

• Skin eruptions, photosensitivity after administration of drug
• Respiratory status: rate, character, wheezing, tightness in chest
• Allergies before initiation of treatment, reaction of each medication; list allergies on chart in bright red letters
• Signs of infection

Administer:
• Within 48 hr of exposure to influenza; continue for 10 days after contact
• At least 4 hr before hs to prevent insomnia
• After meals for better absorption, to decrease GI symptoms
• In divided doses to prevent CNS disturbances: headache, dizziness, fatigue, drowsiness

Perform/provide:
• Storage in tight, dry container

Evaluate:
• Therapeutic response: absence of fever, malaise, cough, dyspnea in infection

Teach patient/family:
• About aspects of drug therapy: need to report dyspnea, dizziness, poor concentration, behavioral changes
• To avoid hazardous activities if dizziness occurs

Treatment of overdose: Withdraw drug, maintain airway, administer epINEPHrine, aminophylline, O_2, IV corticosteroids, physostigmine

rimexolone ophthalmic

See appendix c

risedronate (℞)

(rih-sed'roh-nate)
Actonel
Func. class.: Bone resorption inhibitor
Chem. class.: Bisphosphonate

Action: Inhibits bone resorption, absorbs calcium phosphate crystal in bone and may directly block dissolution of hydroxyapatite crystals of bone

Uses: Paget's disease, prevention, treatment of osteoporosis in postmenopausal women, glucocorticoid-induced osteoporosis

Dosage and routes:

Paget's disease
• *Adult:* **PO** 30 mg qd × 2 mo; patients with Paget's disease should receive calcium and vit D if dietary intake is lacking; if relapse occurs, retreatment is advised

Postmenopausal osteoporosis
• *Adult:* **PO** 5 mg qd or 35 mg qwk

Glucocorticoid osteoporosis
• *Adult:* **PO** 5 mg qd

Available forms: Tabs 5, 30, 35 mg

Side effects/adverse reactions:
CNS: Dizziness, headache, depression
GI: Abdominal pain, anorexia, diarrhea, nausea, constipation
MS: Bone pain, arthralgia
CV: Chest pain, hypertension
MISC: Rash, UTI, pharyngitis

Contraindications: Hypersensitivity to bisphosphonates, inability to stand or sit upright for ≥30 min

Precautions: Children, lactation, pregnancy (C), renal disease, active upper GI disorders

Pharmacokinetics: Rapidly cleared from circulation, taken up mainly by bones, eliminated primarily through kidneys

R

Interactions:
• ↓ absorption of risedronate: calcium supplements, antacids
• ↑ GI irritation: NSAIDs, salicylates
• Drug/food: ↓ bioavailability: take ½ hr before food or drinks other than water

NURSING CONSIDERATIONS
Assess:
• Symptoms of Paget's disease: headache, bone pain, increased head circumference
• Electrolytes: renal function studies; Ca, P, Mg, K
• For hypercalcemia: paresthesia, twitching, laryngospasm, Chvostek's, Trousseau's signs

Administer:
• PO for 2 months to be effective in Paget's disease
• With a full glass of water, patient should be in upright position for ½ hr
• Supplemental calcium and vit D in Paget's disease
• Give qd ≥30 min ac

Perform/provide:
• Storage in cool environment, out of direct sunlight

Evaluate:
• Therapeutic response: increased bone mass, absence of fractures

Teach patient/family:
• To sit upright for ½ hr after dose to prevent irritation
• To comply with diet
• To notify prescriber if pregnancy is suspected

risperidone (℞)

(ris-pehr'ih-dohn)
Risperdal
Func. class.: Antipsychotic
Chem. class.: Benzisoxazole derivative

Action: Unknown; may be mediated through both DOPamine type 2 (D_2) and serotonin type 2 ($5\text{-}HT_2$) antagonism

Uses: Psychotic disorders

Research note: Risperidone given with paroxetine resulted in an increase of risperidone levels[36]

Dosage and routes:
• *Adult:* **PO** 1 mg bid, with incremental increases of 1 mg bid on days 2 and 3 to a dose of 3 mg bid by day 3; then do not increase dose for at least 1 wk
• *Geriatric:* **PO** 0.5 mg qd-bid, increase by 1 mg qwk

Hepatic/renal dose
• *Adult:* **PO** 0.5 mg bid, increase by 0.5 mg bid, increase to 1.5 mg bid

Available forms: Tabs 1, 2, 3, 4 mg; oral sol 1 mg/ml

Side effects/adverse reactions:
CNS: EPS, pseudoparkinsonism, akathisia, dystonia, tardive dyskinesia; drowsiness, insomnia, agitation, anxiety, headache, ***seizures, neuroleptic malignant syndrome,*** dizziness
CV: Orthostatic hypotension, ***tachycardia***
EENT: Blurred vision
GI: Nausea, vomiting, *anorexia, constipation,* jaundice, weight gain
RESP: Rhinitis

Contraindications: Hypersensitivity, lactation, seizure disorders

Precautions: Children, renal disease, pregnancy (C), hepatic disease, elderly, breast cancer

Do not confuse:
Risperdal/reserpine

Pharmacokinetics:
PO: Extensively metabolized by liver to a major active metabolite, plasma protein binding 90%

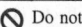

Interactions:
• ↑ sedation: other CNS depressants, alcohol
• ↑ EPS: other antipsychotics

• ↑ risperidone excretion: carbamazepine
• ↓ levodopa effect: levodopa
↑ CNS depression: kava
↑ action: cola tree, hops, nettle, nutmeg
↑ EPS: betel palm, kava

Lab test interferences:
Increase: Prolactin levels

NURSING CONSIDERATIONS

Assess:
• Mental status before initial administration
• Swallowing of PO medication; check for hoarding or giving of medication to other patients
• I&O ratio; palpate bladder if urinary output is low
• Bilirubin, CBC, hepatic studies qmo
• Urinalysis before, during prolonged therapy
• Affect, orientation, LOC, reflexes, gait, coordination, sleep pattern disturbances
• B/P standing and lying; also pulse, respirations; take these q4h during initial treatment; establish baseline before starting treatment; report drops of 30 mm Hg; watch for ECG changes
• Dizziness, faintness, palpitations, tachycardia on rising
• EPS, including akathisia (inability to sit still, no pattern to movements), tardive dyskinesia (bizarre movements of the jaw, mouth, tongue, extremities), pseudoparkinsonism (rigidity, tremors, pill rolling, shuffling gait)
For neuroleptic malignant syndrome: hyperthermia, increased CPK, altered mental status, muscle rigidity
• Skin turgor qd
• Constipation, urinary retention qd; if these occur, increase bulk and water in diet

Administer:
• Reduced dose in elderly
• Antiparkinsonian agent on order from prescriber, to be used for EPS

Perform/provide:
• Decreased stimulus by dimming lights, avoiding loud noises
• Supervised ambulation until patient is stabilized on medication; do not involve in strenuous exercise program because fainting is possible; patient should not stand still for a long time
• Increased fluids to prevent constipation
• Sips of water, candy, gum for dry mouth
• Storage in tight, light-resistant container

Evaluate:
• Therapeutic response: decrease in emotional excitement, hallucinations, delusions, paranoia; reorganization of patterns of thought, speech

Teach patient/family:
• That orthostatic hypotension may occur and to rise from sitting or lying position gradually
• To avoid hot tubs, hot showers, tub baths; hypotension may occur
• To avoid abrupt withdrawal of this drug; EPS may result; drug should be withdrawn slowly
• To avoid OTC preparations (cough, hay fever, cold) unless approved by prescriber, since serious drug interactions may occur; avoid use with alcohol, CNS depressants; increased drowsiness may occur
• To avoid hazardous activities if drowsy or dizzy
• Compliance with drug regimen
• To report impaired vision, tremors, muscle twitching
• In hot weather, that heat stroke may occur; take extra precautions to stay cool

R

• To use contraception, inform prescriber if pregnancy is planned or suspected

Treatment of overdose: Lavage if orally ingested; provide airway; *do not induce vomiting*

ritodrine (℞)

(rih'toh-dreen)

ritodrine, Yutopar

Func. class.: Tocolytic, uterine relaxant

Chem. class.: β_2-Adrenergic agonist

Action: Reduces frequency, intensity of uterine contractions by stimulation of the β_2-receptors in uterine smooth muscle

Uses: Management of preterm labor

Dosage and routes:

• *Adult:* **IV INF** 150 mg/500 ml (0.3 mg/ml) given 0.1 mg/min, increased gradually by 0.05 mg/min q10min until desired response, max 0.35 mg/min

Available forms: Inj 10 mg/ml, 15 mg/ml

Side effects/adverse reactions:

MISC: Erythema, rash, dyspnea, hyperventilation, glycosuria, ***lactic acidosis***

META: Hyperglycemia, hypokalemia

CNS: Headache, restlessness, anxiety, nervousness, sweating, chills, drowsiness, tremor

GI: Nausea, vomiting, anorexia, malaise, bloating, constipation, diarrhea

CV: Altered maternal, fetal heart rate, B/P, dysrhythmias, palpitations, chest pain, maternal pulmonary edema

Contraindications: Hypersensitivity, eclampsia, hypertension, dysrhythmias, thyrotoxicosis, before 20th wk of pregnancy, antepartum hemorrhage, intrauterine fetal death, maternal cardiac disease, pulmonary hypertension, uncontrolled diabetes, pheochromocytoma, bronchial asthma

Precautions: Migraine, sulfite sensitivity, pregnancy-induced hypertension, diabetes, pregnancy (B)

Pharmacokinetics:

IV: Immediate, distribution half-life 6 min, 2nd phase 1½-2½ hr, elimination phase >10 hr; metabolized in liver; 90% excreted in urine; crosses placenta

Interactions:

• Pulmonary edema: corticosteroids

• ↑ CV effects of ritodrine: magnesium sulfate, diazoxide, meperidine, potent general anesthetics

• ↑ effects of sympathomimetic amines

• Systemic hypertension: atropine

• ↓ action of ritodrine: β-blockers

Lab test interferences:

Increase: Blood glucose, free fatty acids, insulin, GTT

Decrease: Potassium

NURSING CONSIDERATIONS

Assess:

• Maternal, fetal heart tones during infusion; maternal ECG to determine CV disease

• Intensity, length of uterine contractions

• Fluid intake to prevent fluid overload; discontinue if this occurs

• Blood glucose in diabetics

Administer:

• Only clear sol

• After dilution: 150 mg/500 ml D_5W or NS, give at 0.3 mg/ml

• Using infusion pump

• Considered incompatible with any drug in sol or syringe

Perform/provide:

• Positioning of patient in left lateral recumbent position to decrease hypotension, increase renal blood flow

Evaluate:

• Therapeutic response: decreased intensity, length of contraction, absence of preterm labor, decreased B/P

Teach patient/family:

• To remain in bed during infusion

ritonavir (℞)

(ri-toe′na-veer)

Norvir

Func. class.: Antiretroviral

Chem. class.: Protease inhibitor

Action: Inhibits human immunodeficiency virus (HIV) protease and prevents maturation of the infectious virus

Uses: HIV in combination with other antiretrovirals

Dosage and routes:

• *Adult:* **PO** 600 mg bid. If nausea occurs begin dose at ½ and gradually increase

• *Child:* **PO** 250 mg/m^2 bid, titrate upward to 400 mg/m^2 bid

Available forms: Caps 100 mg; oral sol 80 mg/ml

Side effects/adverse reactions:

GI: Diarrhea, buccal mucosa ulceration, abdominal pain, *nausea,* taste perversion, dry mouth, dizziness, insomnia, headache, vomiting

CNS: Paresthesia, *headache,* vomiting, ***seizures***

INTEG: Rash

MS: Pain

MISC: Asthenia, ***angioedema, anaphylaxis, Stevens-Johnson syndrome,*** increase lipids

Contraindications: Hypersensitivity

Precautions: Hepatic disease, pregnancy (B), lactation, children

Do not confuse:

ritonavir/retrovir

Pharmacokinetics: Well absorbed; 98% protein binding, hepatic metabolism

Interactions:

• ↑ ritonavir levels: fluconazole

• ↓ ritonavir levels: rifamycins, nevirapine, barbiturates, phenytoin

• ↑ level of both drugs: clarithromycin, ddI

Toxicity, do not use together: amiodarone, azole antifungals, benzodiazepines, bepridil, buPROPion, clozapine, desipramine, dihydroergotamine, encainide, ergotamine, flecainide, HMG-CoA reductase inhibitors, interleukins, meperidine, midazolam, pimozide, piroxicam, propafenone, propoxyphene, quinidine, saquinavir, terfenadine, triazolam, zolpidem

• ↓ levels of: anticoagulants, atovaquone, divalproex, ethinyl estradiol, lamotrigine, phenytoin, sulfamethoxazole, theophylline, zidovudine

↓ ritonavir levels: St. John's wort; avoid concurrent use

Lab test interferences:

Increase: AST, ALT, CPK, cholesterol, GGT, triglycerides, uric acid

Decrease: Hct, RBC, Hgb, neutrophils, WBC

NURSING CONSIDERATIONS

Assess:

• Signs of infection, anemia

• Hepatic studies: ALT, AST

• Viral load and CD4 baseline and throughout therapy

• C&S before drug therapy; drug may be taken as soon as culture is taken; repeat C&S after treatment; determine the presence of other sexually transmitted diseases

• Bowel pattern before, during treatment; if severe abdominal pain with bleeding occurs, drug should be discontinued; monitor hydration

R

- Skin eruptions; rash
- Allergies before treatment, reaction to each medication

Administer:

- With food; mix oral powder with high-calorie drink such as Ensure
- Store caps in refrigerator

Teach patient/family:

- To take as prescribed; if dose is missed, take as soon as remembered up to 1 hr before next dose; do not double dose
- That drug must be taken in equal intervals around the clock to maintain blood levels for duration of therapy
- To take with food; mix liquid formulation with chocolate milk or liquid nutritional supplement
- That drug is not a cure for HIV; opportunistic infections may continue to be acquired
- That redistribution of body fat or accumulation of body fat may occur
- That others may continue to contract HIV from the patient
- Not to use St. John's wort; that it decreases this drug's effect

rituximab

(rih-tuks′ih-mab)

Rituxan

Func. class.: Misc. antineoplastic

Chem. class.: Murine/human monoclonal antibody

Action: Directed against the CD20 antigen that is found on malignant B lymphocytes; CD20 regulates a portion of cell-cycle initiation/differentiation

Uses: Non-Hodgkin's lymphoma (CD20 positive, B-cell), bulky disease (tumors >10 cm)

Dosage and routes:

- *Adult:* **IV INF** 375 mg/m^2 qwk × 4 doses; give at 50 mg/hr for 1st inf; if hypersensitivity does not occur, increase rate by 50 mg/hr q½h, max 400 mg/hr; slow/interrupt inf if hypersensitivity occurs; other inf can be given at 100 mg/hr and increased by 100 mg/hr, max 400 mg/hr

Available forms: Inj 10 mg/ml

Side effects/adverse reactions:

CV: ***Cardiac dysrhythmias***

GU: ***Renal failure***

SYST: ***Stevens-Johnson syndrome***

GI: Nausea, vomiting, anorexia

INTEG: Irritation at site, rash, ***fatal mucocutaneous infections (rare)***

HEMA: ***Leukopenia, neutropenia, thrombocytopenia***

OTHER: Fever, chills, asthenia, headache, ***angioedema,*** hypotension, myalgia, ***bronchospasm***

Contraindications: Hypersensitivity, murine proteins

Precautions: Lactation, children, elderly, pregnancy (C), cardiac conditions

Pharmacokinetics: Half-life 42-79 min

NURSING CONSIDERATIONS

Assess:

- ⬥ For signs of fatal infusion reaction: hypoxia, pulmonary infiltrates, acute respiratory distress syndrome, MI, ventricular fibrillation, cardiogenic shock; most fatal infusion reactions occur with first infusion; potentially fatal
- ⬥ For signs of severe mucocutaneous reactions: Stevens-Johnson syndrome, lichenoid dermatitis, toxic epidermal lysis; occur 1-13 wk after drug was given
- ⬥ Tumor lysis syndrome: acute renal failure requiring hemodialysis, hyperkalemia, hypocalcemia, hyperuricemia, hyperphosphatemia
- CBC, differential, platelet count weekly; withhold drug if WBC is <3500/mm^3, or platelet count <100,000/mm^3; notify prescriber

of these results; drug should be discontinued
• Food preferences: list likes, dislikes
• GI symptoms: frequency of stools
• Signs of dehydration: rapid respirations, poor skin turgor, decreased urine output, dry skin, restlessness, weakness

Administer:

IV INF route

• After diluting to a final conc. of 1-4 mg/ml; use 0.9% NaCl, D_5W, gently invert bag to mix; do not mix with other drugs

Perform/provide:

• Increased fluid intake to 2-3 L/day to prevent dehydration, unless contraindicated
• Changing of IV site q48h
• Nutritious diet with iron, vitamin supplement, low fiber, few dairy products
• Storage of vials at 36°-40° F, protect vials from direct sunlight, inf sol is stable at 36°-46° F × 24 hr and room temperature for another 12 hr

Evaluate:

• Therapeutic response: decrease in tumor size, decrease in spread of cancer

Teach patient/family:

• To report adverse reactions

rivastigmine (℞)

(riv-as-tig′mine)
Exelon
Func. class.: Anti-Alzheimer agent
Chem. class.: Cholinesterase inhibitor

Action: May enhance cholinergic functioning by increasing acetylcholine

Uses: Alzheimer's dementia

Dosage and routes:

• *Adult:* **PO** 1.5 mg bid, after 2 wk or more, may increase to 3 mg bid after 2 wk or more; may increase to 4.5 mg bid and thereafter 6 mg bid

Available forms: Caps 1.5, 3, 4.5, 6 mg; solution 2 mg/ml

Side effects/adverse reactions:

CNS: Tremors, confusion, insomnia, psychosis, hallucination, depression, dizziness, headache, anxiety, somnolence, fatigue, syncope

GI: Nausea, vomiting, anorexia, abdominal distress, flatulence, diarrhea, constipation

MISC: Urinary tract infection, asthenia, increased sweating, hypertension, flulike symptoms, weight change

Contraindications: Hypersensitivity to this drug, other carbamates; narrow-angle glaucoma, undiagnosed skin lesions

Precautions: Renal disease, hepatic disease, respiratory disease, seizure disorder, peptic ulcer, cardiac disease, urinary obstruction, asthma, pregnancy (B), asthma, lactation, children

Pharmacokinetics:

Rapidly and completely absorbed, metabolized to decarbamylated metabolite, half-life is 1.5 hr, excreted via kidneys (metabolites), clearance is lowered in the elderly, hepatic disease, and increased in nicotine use

Interactions:

• Synergistic effect: cholinomimetics, other cholinesterase inhibitors
↑ effect: pill-bearing spurge

NURSING CONSIDERATIONS

Assess:

• Hepatic studies: AST, ALT, alk phosphatase, LDH, bilirubin, CBC
• For severe GI effects: nausea, vomiting, anorexia, weight loss

• B/P, respiration during initial treatment; hypo/hypertension should be reported
• Mental status: affect, mood, behavioral changes, depression; complete suicide assessment

Administer:
• With meals; take with morning and evening meal even though absorption may be decreased

Perform/provide:
• Assistance with ambulation during beginning therapy

Evaluate:
• Therapeutic response: decreased dementia

Teach patient/family:
• The procedure for giving oral solution; use instruction sheet provided
• To notify prescriber of severe GI effects

rizatriptan (℞)

(rye-zah-trip′tan)
Maxalt, Maxalt-MLT
Func. class.: Migraine agent
Chem. class.: 5-HT_1 receptor agonist

Action: Binds selectively to the vascular 5-HT_1 receptor subtype, exerts antimigraine effect; causes vasoconstriction in cranial arteries

Uses: Acute treatment of migraine

Dosage and routes;
• *Adult:* **PO** 5-10 mg single dose, redosing separate by 2 hr or more; max 30 mg/24 hr

Available forms: Maxalt: tabs 5, 10 mg; Maxalt-MLT: tabs, orally disintegrating 5, 10 mg

Side effects/adverse reactions:
CNS: Dizziness, headache, fatigue, warm/cold sensations, flushing, hot flashes
RESP: Chest tightness, pressure, dyspnea
GI: Nausea, dry mouth, diarrhea
CV: ***MI, ventricular fibrillation, ventricular tachycardia, coronary artery vasospasm***

Contraindications: Angina pectoris, history of MI, documented silent ischemia, Prinzmetal's angina, ischemic heart disease, concurrent ergotamine-containing preparations, uncontrolled hypertension, hypersensitivity, basilar or hemiplegic migraine

Precautions: Postmenopausal women, men >40 yr, risk factors for CAD, hypercholesterolemia, obesity, diabetes, impaired hepatic or renal function, pregnancy (C), lactation, children, elderly

Pharmacokinetics: Onset of pain relief 10 min-2 hr, 14% plasma protein binding, metabolized in the liver (metabolite), excreted in urine, feces, half-life 2-3 hr

Interactions:
• Extended vasospastic effects: ergot, ergot derivatives, other 5-HT receptor agonists
• ↑ rizatriptan action: cimetidine, oral contraceptives, MAOIs, nonselective MAOI (type A and B), isocarboxazide, pargyline, phenelzine, propranolol, tranylcypromine
• Weakness, hyperreflexia, incoordination: SSRIs
Serotonin syndrome: SAM-e, St. John's wort
↑ effect: butterbur

NURSING CONSIDERATIONS

Assess:
• For stress level, activity, recreation, coping mechanisms
• Neurologic status: LOC, blurring vision, nausea, vomiting, tingling in extremities preceding headache
• Ingestion of tyramine foods (pickled products, beer, wine, aged cheese), food additives, preserva-

tives, colorings, artificial sweeteners, chocolate, caffeine, which may precipitate these types of headaches

Perform/provide:

• Quiet, calm environment with decreased stimulation for noise, bright light, excessive talking

Evaluate:

• Therapeutic response: decrease in frequency, severity of headache

Teach patient/family:

• Use of orally disintegrating tab: instruct patient not to open blister until use, to peel blister open with dry hands, to place tab on tongue, where it will dissolve, and to swallow with saliva (contains phenylalanine)

• To report any side effects to prescriber

• To use alternative contraception while taking drug if oral contraceptives are being used

HIGH ALERT

rocuronium (℞)

(ro-kyur-oh'nium)

Zemuron

Func. class.: Neuromuscular blocker (nondepolarizing)

Chem. class.: Biquaternary ammonium ester

Action: Inhibits transmission of nerve impulses by binding with cholinergic receptor sites, antagonizing action of acetylcholine

Uses: Facilitation of endotracheal intubation, skeletal muscle relaxation during mechanical ventilation, surgery, or general anesthesia

Dosage and routes:

Intubation

• *Adult and child:* **IV** 0.6 mg/kg

Available forms: Inj 10 mg/ml

Side effects/adverse reactions:

CV: Bradycardia, tachycardia, change in B/P

RESP: ***Prolonged apnea, bronchospasm, cyanosis, respiratory depression***

GI: Nausea, vomiting

INTEG: Rash, flushing, pruritus, urticaria

Contraindications: Hypersensitivity

Precautions: Pregnancy (C), cardiac disease, lactation, child <2 yr, electrolyte imbalances, dehydration, neuromuscular disease, respiratory disease, renal disease

Pharmacokinetics: Half-life 71-203 min, duration ½ hr

Interactions:

• Blocked action of rocuronium: phenylephrine

• ↑ effect of rocuronium: anesthetics

NURSING CONSIDERATIONS

Assess:

• For electrolyte imbalances (K, Mg), before drug is used; electrolyte imbalances may lead to increased action of this drug

• VS (B/P, pulse, respirations, airway) until fully recovered; rate, depth, pattern of respirations, strength of hand grip; patient should be intubated before use

• Recovery: decreased paralysis of face, diaphragm, leg, arm, rest of body; residual weakness and respiratory problems may occur during recovery

• Allergic reactions: rash, fever, respiratory distress, pruritus; drug should be discontinued

Administer:

• Using peripheral nerve stimulator by anesthesiologist to determine neuromuscular blockade; deep tendon reflexes should be monitored during extended use

R

• Undiluted direct IV over 2 min (only by qualified person, usually anesthesiologist); do not administer IM
• Maintenance q20-45min after 1st dose; titrate to response

Perform/provide:
• Storage in light-resistant area
• Reassurance if communication is difficult during recovery from neuromuscular blockade

Evaluate:
• Therapeutic response: paralysis of jaw, eyelid, head, neck, rest of body as evaluated by peripheral nerve stimulator

Teach patient/family:
• About all procedures or treatments; patient will remain conscious if anesthesia is not given also

Treatment of overdose: Edrophonium or neostigmine, atropine, monitor VS; may require mechanical ventilation

rofecoxib (℞)

(roh-fih-kox′ib)
Vioxx
Func. class.: Nonsteroidal antiinflammatory
Chem. class.: COX-2 inhibitor

Action: May inhibit prostaglandin synthesis by decreasing enzyme needed for biosynthesis; analgesic, antiinflammatory, antipyretic properties

Uses: Acute, chronic osteoarthritis pain, primary dysmenorrhea, relief of rheumatoid arthritis

Dosage and routes:

Osteoarthritis
• *Adult:* **PO** 12.5 mg/day as a single dose; may increase to 25 mg if needed

Primary dysmenorrhea
• *Adult:* **PO** 50 mg qd, use for <5 days

Rheumatoid arthritis
• *Adult:* **PO** 25 mg qd, max 25 mg qd

Available forms: Tabs 12.5, 25, 50 mg; susp 12.5, 25 mg/5 ml

Side effects/adverse reactions:
CNS: Fatigue, anxiety, depression, nervousness, paresthesia
CV: ***Tachycardia,*** angina, ***MI,*** *palpitations,* ***dysrhythmias,*** *hypertension, fluid retention*
EENT: Tinnitus, hearing loss, blurred vision, glaucoma, cataract, conjunctivitis, eye pain
GI: Nausea, anorexia, vomiting, constipation, dry mouth, diverticulitis, gastritis, gastroenteritis, hemorrhoids, hiatal hernia, stomatitis, ***GI bleeding***
GU: ***Nephrotoxicity: dysuria, hematuria, oliguria, azotemia,*** *cystitis, UTI*
HEMA: ***Blood dyscrasias,*** *epistaxis, bruising, anemia*
INTEG: Purpura, *rash, pruritus, sweating, erythema, petechiae, photosensitivity, alopecia*
RESP: Pharyngitis, shortness of breath, pneumonia, coughing

Contraindications: Hypersensitivity to aspirin, iodides, other NSAIDs, asthma

Precautions: Pregnancy (C), avoid in late pregnancy, lactation, children, bleeding disorders, GI disorders, cardiac disorders, hypersensitivity to other antiinflammatory agents

Pharmacokinetics: Well absorbed, crosses placenta, bound to plasma proteins

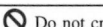

Interactions:
• ↓ effect, ↑ adverse reactions: aspirin, ACE inhibitors
• ↑ bleeding: aspirin, other NSAIDs, anticoagulants

• ↓ effect of: diuretics
• ↑ toxicity: lithium, antineoplastics
• ↑ adverse reaction: glucocorticosteroids
🌿 ↑ gastric irritation: arginine, gossypol
🌿 ↑ NSAIDs effect: bearberry, bilberry
🌿 ↑ bleeding risk: bogbean, chondroitin

NURSING CONSIDERATIONS

Assess:

◆ For patients with asthma, aspirin allergy, or nasal polyps; they may be hypersensitive

• For pain of rheumatoid arthritis, osteoarthritis; check ROM, inflammation of joints, characteristics of pain

◆ Blood counts during therapy; watch for decreasing platelets; if low, therapy may need to be discontinued, restarted after hematologic recovery; and for blood dyscrasias (thrombocytopenia): bruising, fatigue, bleeding, poor healing

Administer:

PO route

• With food or milk to decrease gastric symptoms

⊘ Do not crush, dissolve, or chew

Evaluate:

• Therapeutic response: decreased pain in arthritic conditions; decreased inflammation in arthritic conditions

Teach patient/family:

• That drug must be continued for prescribed time to be effective; to avoid other NSAIDs, aspirin, alcohol

• To report bleeding, bruising, fatigue, malaise, since blood dyscrasias do occur

• To take with a full glass of water to enhance absorption

ropinirole (℞)

(roh-pin′ih-role)

Requip

Func. class.: Antiparkinson agent

Chem. class.: Dopamine-receptor agonist, non-ergot

Action: Selective agonist for D_2 receptors (presynaptic/postsynaptic sites); binding at D_3 receptor contributes to antiparkinson effects

Uses: Parkinsonism

Dosage and routes:

• *Adult:* **PO** 0.25 mg tid, titrate weekly to a max of 24 mg/day

Available forms: Tabs 0.25, 0.5, 1, 2, 4, 5 mg

Side effects/adverse reactions:

HEMA: ***Hemolytic anemia, leukopenia, agranulocytosis***

CNS: Agitation, insomnia, psychosis, hallucination, dystonia, depression, dizziness, somnolence, ***sleep attacks***

GI: Nausea, vomiting, anorexia, dry mouth, constipation, dyspepsia, flatulence

INTEG: Rash, sweating

CV: Orthostatic hypotension, tachycardia, hypertension, hypotension, syncope, palpitations

EENT: Blurred vision

GU: Impotence, urinary frequency

RESP: Pharyngitis, rhinitis, sinusitis, bronchitis, dyspnea

Contraindications: Hypersensitivity

Precautions: Renal disease, cardiac disease, dysrhythmias, affective disorder, psychosis, pregnancy (C), hepatic disease

Pharmacokinetics:

PO: Half-life 6 hr; extensively metabolized by the liver by P450 CYP1A2 enzyme system

R

Interactions:

• ↑ ropinirole effect: cimetidine, ciprofloxacin, diltiazem, enoxacin, erythromycin, fluvoxamine, mexiletine, norfloxacin, tacrine, digoxin, theophylline, L-dopa

• ↓ ropinirole effects: butyrophenones, metoclopramide, phenothiazines, thioxanthenes

Herb: ↓ ropinirole action: chaste tree fruit, kava

NURSING CONSIDERATIONS

Assess:

• Involuntary movements in parkinsonism: akinesia, tremors, staggering gait, muscle rigidity, drooling

• B/P, respiration during initial treatment; hypo/hypertension should be reported

Alert: For sleep attacks, drowsiness, falling asleep without warning even during hazardous activities

• Mental status: affect, mood, behavioral changes, depression; complete suicide assessment

Administer:

• Drug until NPO before surgery

• Adjust dosage to patient response

• With meals

Perform/provide:

• Assistance with ambulation during beginning therapy

• Testing for diabetes mellitus, acromegaly if on long-term therapy

Evaluate:

• Therapeutic response: decrease in akathisia, increased mood

Teach patient/family:

• That therapeutic effects may take several wk to a few mo

• To change positions slowly to prevent orthostatic hypotension

• To use drug exactly as prescribed; if drug is discontinued abruptly, parkinsonian crisis may occur

ropivacaine (℞)

(roe-pi′va-kane)

Naropin

Func. class.: Local anesthetic

Chem. class.: Amide

Action: Competes with calcium for sites in nerve membrane that control sodium transport across cell membrane; decreases rise of depolarization phase of action potential

Uses: Peripheral nerve block, caudal anesthesia, central neural block, vaginal, epidural, spinal block

Dosage and routes:

• Varies with route of anesthesia

Available forms: Inj 2, 5, 7.5 mg/ml

Side effects/adverse reactions:

CNS: Anxiety, restlessness, ***convulsions, loss of consciousness,*** drowsiness, disorientation, tremors, shivering

CV: ***Myocardial depression, cardiac arrest, dysrhythmias,*** bradycardia, hypotension, hypertension, ***fetal bradycardia***

GI: Nausea, vomiting

EENT: Blurred vision, tinnitus, pupil constriction

INTEG: Rash, urticaria, allergic reactions, edema, burning, skin discoloration at inj site, tissue necrosis

RESP: ***Status asthmaticus, respiratory arrest, anaphylaxis***

Contraindications: Hypersensitivity, child <12 yr, elderly, severe liver disease

Precautions: Severe drug allergies, pregnancy (B), hyperthyroidism, cardiovascular disease

Pharmacokinetics: Onset varies with inj site 5-20 min, duration varies with inj site 2-8 hr; metabolized by liver, excreted in urine (metabolites)

Interactions:
• Dysrhythmias: epINEPHrine, halothane, enflurane
• Hypertension: MAOIs, tricyclics, phenothiazines
• ↓ action of ropivacaine: chloroprocaine

NURSING CONSIDERATIONS

Assess:
• B/P, pulse, respiration during treatment
• Fetal heart tones during labor
• Allergic reactions: rash, urticaria, itching
• Cardiac status: ECG for dysrhythmias, pulse, B/P during anesthesia

Administer:
• Only with crash cart, resuscitative equipment nearby
• Only drugs without preservatives for epidural or caudal anesthesia

Perform/provide:
• Use of new sol; discard unused portions

Evaluate:
• Therapeutic response: anesthesia necessary for procedure

Treatment of overdose: Airway, O_2, vasopressor, IV fluids, anticonvulsants for seizures

rosiglitazone (℞)

(ros-ih-glit'ah-zone)
Avandia
Func. class.: Antidiabetic, oral
Chem. class.: Thiazolidinedione

Action: Improves insulin resistance by hepatic glucose metabolism, insulin receptor kinase activity, insulin receptor phosphorylation

Uses: Stable adult-onset diabetes mellitus (type 2) NIDDM, alone or in combination with sulfonylureas, metformin, or insulin

Dosage and routes:

Monotherapy
• *Adult:* **PO** 4 mg qd or in 2 divided doses, may increase to 8 mg qd or in 2 divided doses after 12 wk

Combination therapy
• *Adult:* **PO** This drug should be added to metformin, sulfonylurea at the adult dose

Available forms: Tabs 2, 4, 8 mg

Side effects/adverse reactions:
MISC: Accidental injury, URI, sinusitis, anemia, back pain, diarrhea, edema
CNS: Fatigue, headache
ENDO: Hyper/hypoglycemia

Contraindications: Hypersensitivity to thiazolidinediones, children, lactation, diabetic ketoacidosis

Precautions: Pregnancy (C), elderly, thyroid disease, hepatic, renal disease

Pharmacokinetics: Maximal reductions in FBS after 6-12 wk, protein binding 99.8%, excreted in urine, feces, elimination half-life 3-4 hr, may be excreted in breast milk

Interactions:
• ↓ effect of: oral contraceptives, alternative method advised
Hypoglycemia: chromium, coenzyme Q10, fenugreek
Poor glucose control: glucosamine
↓ antidiabetic effect: bee pollen, blue cohosh, broom, chromium, elecampane, eucalyptus, gotu kola
↑ antidiabetic effect: alfalfa, aloe, basil, bay, bilberry, bitter melon, black catechu, buchu, burdock, coriander, dandelion, eyebright (po), fenugreek, garlic, ginseng, glucomannan, glucosamine, goat's rue, gymnema, horehound, horse chestnut, jambul, myrrh, myrtle

NURSING CONSIDERATIONS

Assess:

- For hypoglycemic reactions (sweating, weakness, dizziness, anxiety, tremors, hunger), hyperglycemic reactions soon after meals
- CBC (baseline, q3mo) during treatment; check liver function tests periodically AST, ALT (if ALT >2.5 × ULN, do not use), LDH, renal tests: BUN, creatinine, urinary glucose
- FBS, HbA_{1C}, fasting plasma insulin, plasma lipids/lipoproteins, B/P, body weight during treatment

Administer:

- Once or in 2 divided doses
- Tabs crushed and mixed with food or fluids for patients with difficulty swallowing

Perform/provide:

- Conversion from other oral hypoglycemic agents if needed; change may be made without gradual dosage change; monitor serum or urine glucose and ketones tid during conversion
- Storage in tight container in cool environment

Teach patient/family:

- To use capillary blood glucose test or Chemstrip tid; that periodic LFTs mandatory
- The symptoms of hypo/hyperglycemia, what to do about each
- That the drug must be continued on daily basis: explain consequence of discontinuing drug abruptly
- To avoid OTC medications or herbal preparations unless approved by prescriber
- That diabetes is lifelong illness; that this drug is not a cure; only controls symptoms
- That all food included in diet plan must be eaten to prevent hypoglycemia
- To carry emergency ID and glucagon emergency kit for emergencies
- To notify prescriber if oral contraceptives are used
- Not to use if breast-feeding, may be secreted in breast milk

Evaluate:

- Therapeutic response: Decrease in polyuria, polydipsia, polyphagia; clear sensorium; absence of dizziness; stable gait, blood glucose at normal level

salmeterol (℞)

(sal-met′er-ole)

Serevent

Func. class.: β_2-Adrenergic agonist, bronchodilator

Action: Causes bronchodilation by action on β_2 (pulmonary) receptors by increasing levels of cAMP, which relaxes smooth muscle; with very little effect on heart rate, maintains improvement in FEV from 3 to 12 hr; prevents nocturnal asthma symptoms

Uses: Prevention of exercise-induced asthma, bronchospasm, COPD

Dosage and routes:

- *Adult:* **INH** 2 puffs bid (AM and PM); exercise-induced bronchospasm: 50 mcg (2 inh) ½-1 hr prior to exercise
- *Child 4-12 yr:* **INH** 50 mcg as dry powder bid; exercise-induced bronchospasm 50 mcg as dry powder ½-1 hr prior to exercise

Available forms: Aerosol 25 mcg/actuation; inhalation pwd 50 mcg/blister

Side effects/adverse reactions:

CNS: Tremors, anxiety, insomnia, headache, dizziness, stimulation, restlessness, hallucinations, flushing, irritability

CV: Palpitations, tachycardia, hypertension, angina, hypotension, dysrhythmias

EENT: Dry nose, irritation of nose and throat
GI: Heartburn, nausea, vomiting
MS: Muscle cramps
RESP: ***Bronchospasm***

Contraindications: Hypersensitivity to sympathomimetics, tachydysrhythmias, severe cardiac disease

Precautions: Lactation, pregnancy (C), cardiac disorders, hyperthyroidism, diabetes mellitus, hypertension, prostatic hypertrophy, narrow-angle glaucoma, seizures, acute asthma, as a substitute to corticosteroids

Pharmacokinetics:
INH: Onset 5-15 min, peak 4 hr, duration 12 hr, metabolized in liver, excreted in urine, breast milk; crosses placenta; blood-brain barrier

Interactions:
- ↑ action of aerosol bronchodilators
- ↑ action of salmeterol: tricyclics, MAOIs
- ↓ salmeterol action: other β-blockers

↑ stimulation: betel palm, butterbur, coffee, cola nut, figwort, fumitory, guarana, hawthorn, lily of the valley, motherwort, plantain, tea (black/green), yerba maté

NURSING CONSIDERATIONS

Assess:
- Respiratory function: vital capacity, forced expiratory volume, ABGs, lung sounds, heart rate and rhythm

Administer:
- After shaking; exhale, place mouthpiece in mouth, inhale slowly, hold breath, remove, exhale slowly
- Gum, sips of water for dry mouth
- Using spacing device for pediatric/geriatric patients

Perform/provide:
- Storage in light-resistant container; do not expose to temperatures over 86° F (30° C)

Evaluate:
- Therapeutic response: absence of dyspnea, wheezing

Teach patient/family:
- Not to use OTC medications; extra stimulation may occur
- Use of inhaler; review package insert with patient
- To avoid getting aerosol in eyes
- To wash inhaler in warm water qd and dry
- To avoid smoking, smoke-filled rooms, persons with respiratory infections

Treatment of overdose: β_2-Adrenergic blocker

salsalate (℞)

(sal'sah-late)

Amigesic, Anaflex, Disalcid, Marthritic, Mono-Gesic, Salflex, salsalate, Salgesic, Salsitab

Func. class.: Nonopioid analgesic, nonsteroidal antiinflammatory

Chem. class.: Salicylate

Action: Blocks formation of peripheral prostaglandins, which cause pain and inflammation; antipyretic action results from inhibition of hypothalamic heat-regulating center; does not inhibit platelet aggregation

Uses: Mild to moderate pain or fever, including arthritis, juvenile rheumatoid arthritis

Dosage and routes:
- *Adult:* **PO** 3 g/day in divided doses

Available forms: Caps 500 mg; tabs 500, 750 mg

Side effects/adverse reactions:
HEMA: ***Thrombocytopenia, agran-***

ulocytosis, leukopenia, neutropenia, hemolytic anemia, increased pro-time
CNS: Stimulation, drowsiness, dizziness, confusion, ***convulsions,*** headache, flushing, hallucinations, ***coma***
GI: Nausea, vomiting, GI bleeding, diarrhea, heartburn, anorexia, ***hepatotoxicity***
INTEG: Rash, urticaria, bruising
EENT: Tinnitus, hearing loss
CV: Rapid pulse, ***pulmonary edema***
RESP: Wheezing, hyperpnea
ENDO: Hypoglycemia, hyponatremia, hypokalemia, alteration in acid-base balance

Contraindications: Hypersensitivity to salicylates, NSAIDs, GI bleeding, bleeding disorders, children <3 yr, vit K deficiency

Precautions: Anemia, hepatic disease, renal disease, Hodgkin's disease, pregnancy (C) 1st trimester, lactation, elderly

Pharmacokinetics: Metabolized by liver; excreted by kidneys; half-life 1 hr; highly protein bound; crosses blood-brain barrier and placenta slowly

Interactions:
- ↓ effects of salsalate: antacids, steroids, urinary alkalizers
- ↑ blood loss: alcohol, heparin, ibuprofen, warfarin
- ↑ effects of anticoagulants, insulin, methotrexate, probenecid, penicillins, phenytoin
- ↓ effects of spironolactone, sulfinpyrazone, sulfonamides, loop diuretics
- Toxic effects: PABA
- ↓ blood glucose levels: salicylates
- Drug/food: foods that cause acidic urine, may ↑ salsalate levels

Lab test interferences:
Increase: Coagulation studies, hepatic studies, serum uric acid, amylase, CO_2, urinary protein
Decrease: Serum potassium, PBI, cholesterol, blood glucose
Interference: Urine catecholamines, pregnancy test

NURSING CONSIDERATIONS

Assess:
- Pain: frequency, intensity, characteristics; relief of pain after medication

For asthma, aspirin hypersensitivity, nasal polyps; may develop hypersensitivity to this product
- Hepatic studies: AST, ALT, bilirubin (long-term therapy)
- Renal studies: BUN, urine creatinine (long-term therapy)
- Blood studies: CBC, Hct, Hgb, PT (long-term therapy)
- I&O ratio; decreasing output may indicate renal failure (long-term therapy)
- Hepatotoxicity: dark urine, clay-colored stools; jaundiced skin, sclera; itching, abdominal pain, fever, diarrhea (long-term therapy)
- Allergic reactions: rash, urticaria; drug may have to be discontinued
- Ototoxicity: tinnitus, ringing, roaring in ears; audiometric testing is needed before, after long-term therapy
- Visual changes: blurring, halos, corneal and retinal damage
- Edema in feet, ankles, legs
- Drug history; many interactions

Administer:
- To patient crushed or whole; chewable tablets may be chewed
- With food or milk to decrease gastric symptoms; give 30 min before or 2 hr after meals

Evaluate:
- Therapeutic response: decreased pain, fever

Teach patient/family:
- To report any symptoms of hepatotoxicity, renal toxicity, visual changes, ototoxicity, allergic reactions (long-term therapy)

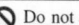

• Not to exceed recommended dosage; acute poisoning may result
• To read label on other OTC drugs; many contain aspirin
• That therapeutic response takes 2 wk (arthritis)
• To avoid alcohol ingestion; GI bleeding may occur
• To watch for signs of bleeding: dark stools

Treatment of overdose: Lavage, activated charcoal, monitor electrolytes, VS

saquinavir (℞)

(sa-quen'ah-veer)
Fortovase, Invirase
Func. class.: Antiretroviral
Chem. class.: Protease inhibitor

Action: Inhibits human immunodeficiency virus (HIV) protease, which prevents maturation of the infectious virus

Uses: HIV in combination with other antiretrovirals

Dosage and routes:
• *Adult:* **PO** 600 mg (hard cap-Invirase) or 1200 mg (soft cap-Fortovase) tid within 2 hr after a full meal

Available forms: Caps 200 mg (soft); 200 mg (hard)

Side effects/adverse reactions:
GI: Diarrhea, buccal mucosa ulceration, *abdominal pain, nausea*
CNS: Paresthesia, headache
INTEG: Rash
MS: Pain
MISC.: Asthenia, hyperglycemia

Contraindications: Hypersensitivity

Precautions: Hepatic disease, pregnancy (B), lactation, children

Pharmacokinetics: Absorption increased with food, protein binding 98%, extensive first-pass metabolism

Interactions:
• Toxicity: ergots, midazolam, triazolam, dapsone, quinidine, calcium channel blockers, clindamycin
• ↑ saquinavir levels: ketoconazole, indinavir, delaviridine, nelfinavir, ritonavir, clarithromycin
• ↓ saquinavir levels: rifamycins, carbamazepine, phenobarbital, phenytoin, nevirapine, dexamethasone
• Avoid use with HmG-CoA reductase inhibitors
↑ vasoconstriction: ergots, do not use concurrently
↑ CNS depression: midazolam, triazolam, do not use concurrently
• Drug/food: ↑ bioavailability after high-fat meal; grapefruit juice ↑ levels
St. John's wort may ↓ saquinavir levels, avoid concurrent use

Lab test interferences:
CPK, glucose (low)

NURSING CONSIDERATIONS

Assess:
• Signs of infection, anemia
• Hepatic studies: ALT, AST
• C&S before drug therapy; drug may be taken as soon as culture is taken; repeat C&S after treatment; determine the presence of other sexually transmitted diseases
• Bowel pattern before, during treatment; if severe abdominal pain with bleeding occurs, drug should be discontinued; monitor hydration
• Skin eruptions, rash, urticaria, itching
• Allergies before treatment, reaction of each medication

Teach patient/family:
• To take as prescribed within 2 hr of a full meal; if dose is missed, take as soon as remembered up to 1 hr before next dose; do not double dose
• That drug must be taken in equal intervals around the clock to maintain blood levels for duration of therapy

S

• That Invirase and Fortovase are not interchangeable

sargramostim (℞)

(sar-gram'oh-stim)

Leukine, rhu GM-CSF

Func. class.: Biologic modifier: cytokine

Chem. class.: Granulocyte macrophage colony-stimulating factor (GM-CSF)

Action: Stimulates proliferation and differentiation of hematopoietic progenitor cells (granulocytes, macrophages)

Uses: Acceleration of myeloid recovery in patients with non-Hodgkin's lymphoma, acute lymphoblastic leukemia, autologous bone marrow transplantation in Hodgkin's disease; bone marrow transplantation failure or engraftment delay, mobilization and transplant of peripheral blood progenitor cells (PBPCs)

Dosage and routes:

Myeloid reconstitution after autologous bone marrow transplantation

• *Adult:* **IV** 250 mcg/m^2/day × 3 wk; give over 2 hr, 2-4 hr after autologous bone marrow infusion, not less than 24 hr after last dose of antineoplastics and 12 hr after last dose of radiotherapy, bone marrow transplantation failure, or engraftment delay

Acceleration of myeloid recovery

• *Adult:* **IV** 250 mcg/m^2/day × 14 days; give over 2 hr; may repeat in 7 days, may repeat 500 mcg/m^2/day × 14 days after another 7 days if no improvement

Mobilization of PBPCs

• *Adult:* **IV/SC** 250 mcg/m^2/day during collection of PBPCs

After PBPC transplantation

• *Adult:* **IV/SC** 250 mcg/m^2/day until ANC >1500 cells/mm^3 × 3 days

Available forms: Powder for inj lyophilized 250, 500 mcg

Side effects/adverse reactions:

CNS: Fever, malaise, CNS disorder, weakness, chills

GI: Nausea, vomiting, diarrhea, anorexia, ***GI hemorrhage,*** stomatitis, ***liver damage***

HEMA: ***Blood dyscrasias, hemorrhage***

INTEG: Alopecia, rash, peripheral edema

GU: Urinary tract disorder, abnormal kidney function

RESP: Dyspnea

CV: ***Transient supraventricular tachycardia,*** peripheral edema, ***pericardial effusion***

Contraindications: Hypersensitivity to GM-CSF, yeast products; excessive leukemic myeloid blast in bone marrow, peripheral blood

Precautions: Pregnancy (C), lactation, child; renal, hepatic, lung disease; cardiac disease; pleural, pericardial effusions

Do not confuse:

Leukine/leucovorin

Leukine/Leukeran

Pharmacokinetics: Half-life 2 hr, detected within 5 min after administration, peak 2 hr

Interactions:

• Do not use this drug concomitantly with antineoplastics

• ↑ myeloproliferation: lithium, corticosteroids

NURSING CONSIDERATIONS

Assess:

◆ Blood studies: CBC, differential count before treatment and twice weekly; leukocytosis may occur (WBC >50,000 cells/mm^3, ANC >20,000 cells/mm^3), platelets; if ANC >20,000/mm^3 or 10,000/mm^3 after nadir has occurred, or platelets

>500,000/mm^3 reduce dose by ½ or discontinue; if blast cells occur, discontinue

- Renal, hepatic studies before treatment: BUN, creatinine, urinalysis; AST, ALT, alk phosphatase; twice weekly monitoring is needed in renal, hepatic disease
- For hypersensitivity, rashes, local inj site reactions; usually transient
- For increased fluid retention in cardiac disease
- For myalgia, arthralgia in legs, feet, use analgesics

Administer:

SC route

- Use reconstituted sol

IV route

- After reconstituting with 1 ml sterile water for inj without preservative; do not reenter vial; discard unused portion; direct reconstitution sol at side of vial; rotate contents; do not shake
- Dilute in 0.9% NaCl inj to prepare IV inf; if final concentration is <10 mcg/ml, add human albumin to make a final concentration of 0.1% to NaCl before adding sargramostim to prevent adsorption; for a final concentration of 0.1% albumin, add 1 mg human albumin/1 ml 0.9% NaCl inj run over 2 hr (bone marrow transplant or failure of graft); over 4 hr (chemotherapy for AML); over 24 hr as cont inf (PBPCs); give within 6 hr after reconstitution

Y-site compatibilities: Amikacin, aminophylline, aztreonam, bleomycin, butorphanol, calcium gluconate, carboplatin, carmustine, cefazolin, cefepime, cefotaxime, cefotetan, ceftizoxime, ceftriaxone, cefuroxime, cimetidine, cisplatin, clindamycin, cyclophosphamide, cycloSPORINE, cytarabine, dacarbazine, dactinomycin, dexamethasone, diphenhydrAMINE, DOPamine, DOXOrubicin, doxycycline, droperidol, etoposide, famotidine, fentanyl, floxuridine, fluconazole, fluorouracil, furosemide, gentamicin, granisetron, heparin, idarubicin, ifosfamide, immune globulin, magnesium sulfate, mannitol, mechlorethamine, meperidine, mesna, methotrexate, metoclopramide, metronidazole, mezlocillin, miconazole, minocycline, mitoxantrone, netilmicin, pentostatin, piperacillin/tazobactam, potassium chloride, prochlorperazine, promethazine, ranitidine, teniposide, ticarcillin, ticarcillin/clavulanate, trimethoprim-sulfamethoxazole, vinBLAStine, vinCRIStine, zidovudine

Perform/provide:

- Storage in refrigerator; do not freeze

Evaluate:

- Therapeutic response: WBC and differential recovery

scopolamine (℞)

(skoe-pol'a-meen)

Scopolamine Hydrobromide Injection

Func. class.: Cholinergic blocker

Chem. class.: Belladonna alkaloid

Action: Inhibits acetylcholine at receptor sites in autonomic nervous system, which controls secretions, free acids in stomach; blocks central muscarinic receptors, which decreases involuntary movements

Uses: Reduction of secretions before surgery, calm delirium, motion sickness, parkinsonian symptoms

Dosage and routes:

Parkinsonian symptoms

- *Adult:* **IM/SC/IV** 0.3-0.6 mg tid-qid using dilution provided

Preoperatively

- *Adult:* **SC** 0.4-0.6 mg

Nausea and vomiting

• *Child:* **SC** 0.006 mg/kg or 0.2 mg/m^2

Available forms: Inj 0.3, 0.4, 0.86, 1 mg/ml

Side effects/adverse reactions:

CNS: Confusion, anxiety, restlessness, irritability, delusions, hallucinations, headache, sedation, depression, incoherence, dizziness, excitement, delirium, flushing, weakness
INTEG: Urticaria
MISC: Suppression of lactation, nasal congestion, decreased sweating
EENT: Blurred vision, photophobia, dilated pupils, difficulty swallowing, mydriasis, cycloplegia
CV: Palpitations, tachycardia, postural hypotension, paradoxic bradycardia
GI: Dryness of mouth, constipation, nausea, vomiting, abdominal distress, ***paralytic ileus***
GU: Urinary hesitancy, retention

Contraindications: Hypersensitivity, narrow-angle glaucoma, myasthenia gravis, GI/GU obstruction, hypersensitivity to belladonna, barbiturates

Precautions: Pregnancy (C), elderly, lactation, prostatic hypertrophy, CHF, hypertension, dysrhythmia, children, gastric ulcer

Pharmacokinetics:

SC/IM: Peak 30-45 min, duration 7 hr
IV: Peak 10-15 min, duration 4 hr
Excreted in urine, bile, feces (unchanged)

Interactions:

• ↑ anticholinergic effect: alcohol, opioids, antihistamines, phenothiazines, tricyclics

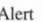

↑ anticholinergic effects: henbane, jimsonweed, scopolia

NURSING CONSIDERATIONS

Assess:

• I&O ratio; retention commonly causes decreased urinary output
• Parkinsonism, EPS: shuffling gait, muscle rigidity, involuntary movements
• Urinary hesitancy, retention; palpate bladder if retention occurs
• Constipation; increase fluids, bulk, exercise if this occurs
• For tolerance over long-term therapy; dose may have to be increased or changed
• Mental status: affect, mood, CNS depression, worsening of mental symptoms during early therapy

Administer:

• Parenteral dose with patient recumbent to prevent postural hypotension
• Parenteral dose slowly; keep in bed for at least 1 hr after dose
• With or after meals for GI upset; may give with fluids other than H_2O
• At hs to avoid daytime drowsiness in patient with parkinsonism
• With analgesic to avoid behavioral changes when given as a preop

Additive compatibilities: Floxacillin, furosemide, meperidine, succinylcholine

Syringe compatibilities: Atropine, benzquinamide, butorphanol, chlorproMAZINE, cimetidine, diamorphine, dimenhyDRINATE, diphenhydrAMINE, droperidol, fentanyl, glycopyrrolate, hydromorphone, hydrOXYzine, meperidine, metoclopramide, midazolam, morphine, nalbuphine, pentazocine, pentobarbital, perphenazine, prochlorperazine, promazine, promethazine, ranitidine, sufentanil, thiopental

Y-site compatibilities: Heparin, hydrocortisone, potassium chloride, propofol, sufentanil, vit B/C

Perform/provide:

• Storage at room temperature in light-resistant container
• Hard candy, frequent drinks, sugarless gum to relieve dry mouth

Evaluate:
• Therapeutic response: decreased secretions
Teach patient/family:
• Not to discontinue this drug abruptly; to taper off over 1 wk
• To avoid driving, other hazardous activities; drowsiness may occur
• To avoid OTC medication: cough, cold preparations with alcohol, antihistamines unless directed by prescriber

scopolamine ophthalmic

See appendix c

scopolamine (℞) (transdermal)

(skoe-pol'-a-meen)
Transderm-Scop, Transderm-V
Func. class.: Antiemetic, anticholinergic
Chem. class.: Belladonna alkaloid

Action: Competitive antagonism of acetylcholine at receptor site in eye, smooth muscle, cardiac muscle, glandular cells; inhibition of vestibular input to the CNS, resulting in inhibition of vomiting reflex
Uses: Prevention of motion sickness
Investigational uses: Drooling
Dosage and routes:
• *Adult:* **PATCH** 1 placed behind ear 4-5 hr before travel, reapply q3d, alternate ears
Not recommended for children
Drooling (off-label)
• *Adult:* **TD** 1.5 mg patch q3d
Available forms: Patch, 0.5, 1 mg delivered in 72 hr

Side effects/adverse reactions:
INTEG: Rash, erythema
GU: Difficult urination
CNS: Dizziness, drowsiness, confusion, disorientation, memory disturbances, hallucinations
EENT: Blurred vision, altered depth perception, *dilated pupils,* photophobia, *dry mouth;* dry, itchy, red eyes; acute narrow-angle glaucoma
Contraindications: Hypersensitivity, glaucoma
Precautions: Children, elderly, pregnancy (C); pyloric, urinary, bladder neck, intestinal obstruction; liver, kidney disease
Pharmacokinetics:
Patch: Onset 4-5 hr, duration 72 hr
Interactions:
• ↑ anticholinergic effects: antihistamines, antidepressants

NURSING CONSIDERATIONS
Teach patient/family:
• To avoid hazardous activities, activities requiring alertness; dizziness may occur
• To wash, dry hands before and after applying to surface behind ear
• To change patch q72h
• To apply at least 4 hr before traveling
• If blurred vision, severe dizziness, drowsiness occurs, to discontinue use, use another type of antiemetic or rotate the patch to other ear
• To read label of all OTC medications; if any scopolamine is found in product, avoid use
• To keep out of children's reach

S

RARELY USED

secobarbital (℞)

(see-koe-bar'bi-tal)

Secogen Sodium♣, Seconal Sodium Pulvules, Seral♣

Func. class.: Sedative/hypnotic-barbiturate

Controlled Substance Schedule II (USA), Schedule G (Canada)

Uses: Insomnia, sedation, preoperative medication, status epilepticus, acute tetanus convulsions

Dosage and routes:

Insomnia

- *Adult:* **PO/IM** 100-200 mg hs
- *Child:* **IM** 3-5 mg/kg, not to exceed 100 mg, not to inject >5 ml in one site

Sedation/preoperatively

- *Adult:* **PO** 200-300 mg 1-2 hr preoperatively
- *Child:* **PO** 50-100 mg 1-2 hr preoperatively

Status epilepticus

- *Adult and child:* **IM/IV** 250-350 mg

Acute psychotic agitation

- *Adult and child:* **IM/IV** 5.5 mg/kg q3-4h

Contraindications: Hypersensitivity to barbiturates, pregnancy (D), respiratory depression, addiction to barbiturates, severe liver impairment, porphyria, uncontrolled severe pain

selegiline (℞)

(se-le'ji-leen)

Apo-Selegiline, Carbex, Eldepryl, Gen-Selegiline, Novo-Selegiline♣, Nu-Selegiline, SD-Deprenyl

Func. class.: Antiparkinson agent

Chem. class.: MAOI, type B

Action: Increased dopaminergic activity by inhibition of MAO type B activity; not fully understood

Uses: Adjunct management of Parkinson's disease in patients being treated with levodopa/carbidopa who had poor response to therapy

Investigational uses: Alzheimer's disease

Dosage and routes:

- *Adult:* **PO** 10 mg/day given with levodopa/carbidopa in divided doses 5 mg at breakfast and lunch; after 2-3 days begin to reduce dose of levodopa/carbidopa 10%-30%

Available forms: Tabs 5 mg, caps 5 mg

Side effects/adverse reactions:

CNS: Increased tremors, chorea, restlessness, blepharospasm, increased bradykinesia, grimacing, tardive dyskinesia, dystonic symptoms, involuntary movements, increased apraxia, hallucinations, *dizziness,* mood changes, nightmares, delusions, lethargy, apathy, overstimulation, sleep disturbances, headache, migraine, numbness, muscle cramps, confusion, anxiety, tiredness, vertigo, personality change, back/leg pain

CV: Orthostatic hypotension, hypertension, dysrhythmia, palpitations, angina pectoris, hypotension, ***tachycardia,*** edema, ***sinus bradycardia,*** syncope

GI: Nausea, vomiting, constipation,

weight loss, anorexia, diarrhea, heartburn, rectal bleeding, poor appetite, dysphagia, xerostomia
GU: Slow urination, nocturia, prostatic hypertrophy, urinary hesitation, retention, frequency, sexual dysfunction
INTEG: Increased sweating, alopecia, hematoma, rash, photosensitivity, facial hair
RESP: Asthma, shortness of breath
EENT: Diplopia, dry mouth, blurred vision, tinnitus
Contraindications: Hypersensitivity
Precautions: Pregnancy (C), lactation, children
Do not confuse:
Eldepryl/enalapril
Pharmacokinetics: Rapidly absorbed, peak ½-2 hr; rapidly metabolized (active metabolites: *N*-desmethyldeprenyl, amphetamine, methamphetamine), metabolites excreted in urine, half-life 9 min
Interactions:
Fatal interaction: Opioids (especially meperidine); do not administer together
• ↑ side effects of: levodopa/carbidopa
Serotonin syndrome (confusion, seizures, fever, hypertension, agitation): fluoxetine, paroxetine, sertraline, fluvoxamine (discontinue 5 wk prior to selegiline); do not use together
Fatal interaction: Do not use with tricyclics
↓ selegiline action: chaste tree fruit, kava
Lab test interferences:
False positive: Urine ketones, urine glucose
False negative: Urine glucose (glucose oxidase)
False increase: Uric acid, urine protein
Decrease: VMA

NURSING CONSIDERATIONS
Assess:
• Decreased parkinsonian symptoms: rigidity, unsteady gait, weakness, tremors
• B/P, respiration throughout treatment
• Mental status: affect, mood behavioral changes, depression; perform suicide assessment
Administer:
• Drug until NPO before surgery
• Adjusting dosage to response
• With meals; limit protein taken with drug
• At doses <10 mg/day, because of risks associated with nonselective inhibition of MAO
Perform/provide:
• Assistance with ambulation during beginning therapy
Evaluate:
• Therapeutic response: decrease in akathisia, improved mood
Teach patient/family:
• To change positions slowly to prevent orthostatic hypotension
• To report side effects: twitching, eye spasms; indicate overdose
• To use drug exactly as prescribed; if discontinued abruptly, parkinsonian crisis may occur
• To avoid foods high in tyramine: cheese, pickled products, wine, beer, large amounts of caffeine
• Not to exceed recommended dose of 10 mg; might precipitate hypertensive crisis; report severe headache, other unusual symptoms
Treatment of overdose: IV fluids for hypertension, IV dilute pressure agent for B/P titration

selenium topical
See appendix c

S

senna, sennosides (OTC)

(sen'na)

Black Draught, Dr. Caldwell Dosalax, Ex-Lax Gentle, Fletcher's Castoria, Gentlax, Senexon, Senna-Gen, Senokot, Senokotxtra, Senolax

Func. class.: Laxative-stimulant

Chem. class.: Anthraquinone

Action: Stimulates peristalsis by action on Auerbach's plexus; softens feces by increasing water, electrolytes in large intestine

Uses: Acute constipation; bowel preparation for surgery or examination

Dosage and routes:

• *Adult:* **PO** 1-8 tabs (Senokot)/day or ½ to 4 tsp of granules (1 tsp-4 ml) added to water or juice; **RECT SUPP** 1-2 hs; **SYR** 1-4 tsp hs, 7.5-15 ml (Black Draught) ¾ oz dissolved in 2.5 oz liquid given between 2-4 PM the day before procedure (X-Prep)

• *Child >27 kg:* **PO** ½ adult dose; do not use Black Draught for children

• *Child 1 mo-1 yr:* **SYR** 1.25-2.5 ml (Senokot) hs

Available forms: Supp 625 mg, 30 mg sennosides; powder 662 mg/g, 6, 15 mg sennosides/3 g; tabs 8.6 mg sennosides, 180 mg; oral sol 3 mg sennosides/ml

Side effects/adverse reactions:

GI: Nausea, vomiting, anorexia, cramps, diarrhea, flatulence

META: Hypocalcemia, enteropathy, alkalosis, hypokalemia, ***tetany***

GU: Pink, red or brown, black urine

Contraindications: Hypersensitivity, GI bleeding, obstruction, CHF, lactation, abdominal pain, nausea/vomiting, appendicitis, acute surgical abdomen

Precautions: Pregnancy (C)

Pharmacokinetics:

PO: Onset 6-24 hr; metabolized by liver, excreted in feces

Interactions:

• Do not use with disulfiram (Antabuse)

↑ laxative effect: Flax, senna

NURSING CONSIDERATIONS

Assess:

• Stool: color, consistency, amount

• Blood, urine electrolytes if drug is used often

• I&O ratio to identify fluid loss

• Cause of constipation; fluids, bulk, exercise missing

• Cramping, rectal bleeding, nausea, vomiting; drug should be discontinued

Administer:

• In morning or evening (oral dose) with full glass of water

• Dissolve granules in water or juice before administration

• On empty stomach for more rapid results

• Shake oral sol before giving

Evaluate:

• Therapeutic response: decrease in constipation

Teach patient/family:

• That urine, feces may turn yellow-brown to red

• Not to use laxatives for long-term therapy; bowel tone will be lost

• That normal bowel movements do not always occur daily

• Not to use in presence of abdominal pain, nausea, vomiting

• To notify prescriber if constipation unrelieved or of symptoms of electrolyte imbalance: muscle cramps, pain, weakness, dizziness, excessive thirst

sertraline (℞)

(ser′tra-leen)

Zoloft

Func. class.: Antidepressant

Chem. class.: SSRI

Action: Inhibits serotonin reuptake in CNS; increases action of serotonin; does not affect dopamine, norepinephrine

Uses: Major depression, obsessive-compulsive disorder (OCD), post-traumatic stress disorder (PTSD), panic disorder

Investigational uses: Extended-interval dosing, premenstrual disorders, premenstrual disphoric disorder (PMDD)

Dosage and routes:

- *Adult:* **PO** 50 mg qd; may increase to max of 200 mg/day; do not change dose at intervals of <1 wk; administer qd in AM or PM; or 100 mg 3 ×/wk (off-label)
- *Geriatric:* **PO** 25 mg qd, increase by 25 mg q3 days to desired dose
- *Child 6-12 yr:* **PO** 25 mg qd
- *Child 13-17 yr:* **PO** 50 mg qd

Premenstrual disorders (off-label)

- *Adult:* **PO** 50-150 mg qhs

Available forms: Tabs 25, 50, 100 mg; liq 20 mg/ml

Side effects/adverse reactions:

CNS: Insomnia, agitation, somnolence, dizziness, headache, tremor, fatigue, paresthesia, twitching, confusion, ataxia, gait abnormality (elderly)

GU: Male sexual dysfunction, micturition disorder

GI: Diarrhea, nausea, constipation, anorexia, dry mouth, dyspepsia, *vomiting, flatulence*

CV: Palpitations, chest pain

EENT: Vision abnormalities

INTEG: Increased sweating, rash, hot flashes

ENDO: SIADH (elderly)

Contraindications: Hypersensitivity to this drug or SSRIs

Precautions: Pregnancy (B), lactation, elderly, hepatic, renal disease, epilepsy, recent MI

Do not confuse:

Zoloft/Zocor

Pharmacokinetics:

PO: Peak 4.5-8.4 hr; steady state 1 wk; plasma protein binding 99%, elimination half-life 1-4 days, extensively metabolized, metabolite excreted in urine, bile

Interactions:

- ↑ effects of: antidepressants (tricyclics), diazepam, TOLBUTamide, warfarin, benzodiazepines, sumatriptan

Fatal reactions: MAOIs

- ↑ sertraline levels: cimetidine, warfarin, other highly protein-bound drugs
- Altered lithium levels: lithium
- Sertraline is contraindicated with pimozide

↑ of SSRI, serotonin syndrome: St. John's wort, SAM-e; do not use together

↑ anticholinergic effect: corkwood, jimsonweed

Hypertensive crisis: ephedra

↑ CNS effect: Hops, lavender

Lab test interferences:

Increase: AST, ALT

NURSING CONSIDERATIONS

Assess:

- Mental status: mood, sensorium, affect, suicidal tendencies, increase in psychiatric symptoms, depression, panic
- B/P (lying/standing), pulse q4h; if systolic B/P drops 20 mm Hg, hold drug, notify prescriber; VS q4h in patients with cardiovascular disease
- Weight qwk; appetite may decrease with drug

S

• Urinary retention, constipation, especially in elderly
• Alcohol consumption; hold dose until morning
Administer:
• Increased fluids, bulk in diet for constipation, urinary retention
• With food, milk for GI symptoms
• Crushed if patient is unable to swallow medication whole
• Sugarless gum, hard candy, frequent sips of water for dry mouth
Perform/provide:
• Storage at room temperature; do not freeze
• Assistance with ambulation during therapy, since drowsiness, dizziness occur
• Safety measures, including side rails, primarily for elderly
• Checking to see that PO medication is swallowed
Evaluate:
• Therapeutic response: significant improvement in depression, OCS
Teach patient/family:
• That therapeutic effect may take 1 wk or longer
• To use caution in driving, other activities requiring alertness; drowsiness, dizziness, blurred vision may occur
• Not to discontinue medication quickly after long-term use; may cause nausea, headache, malaise
• To avoid alcohol, other CNS depressants
• To notify prescriber if pregnant or plan to become pregnant or breastfeed

RARELY USED

sevelamer (℞)

(seh-vel'ah-mer)
Renagel
Func. class.: Polymeric phosphate binder

Uses: End-stage renal disease (ESRD)
Dosage and routes:
Reduction of serum phosphorus in adults not taking phosphate binders
• *Adult:* **PO** initially 800-1600 mg tid with meals based on serum phosphorus level (see below); adjust dose gradually at 2-wk intervals until serum phosphorus 6 mg/dl
• *Adult, serum phosphorus 9 mg/dl:* 1600 mg tid with meals
• *Adult, serum phosphorus 7.5 and <9 mg/dl:* 1200-1600 mg tid with meals
• *Adult, serum phosphorus >6 and <7.5 mg/dl:* 800 mg tid with meals
Contraindications: Hypophosphatemia, bowel obstruction, hypersensitivity

RARELY USED

sibutramine (℞)

(si-byoo'tra-meen)
Meridia
Func. class.: Appetite suppressant

Controlled Substance Schedule IV
Uses: Obesity in conjunction with other treatments
Dosage and routes:
• *Adult:* **PO** 10 mg qd; may be increased to 15 mg qd after 4 wk, or lowered to 5 mg qd depending on response
Contraindications: Hypersensitiv-

ity, hypothyroidism, anorexia nervosa, severe hepatic/renal disease, uncontrolled hypertension, history of CAD, CHF, dysrhythmias, lactation, CVA

sildenafil (℞)

(sil-den'a-fill)

Viagra

Func. class.: Erectile agent

Chem. class.: Selective inhibitor of cGMP-PDE5

Action: Enhances the effect of nitric oxide (NO) by inhibiting phosphodiesterase type 5 (PDE5), which is necessary for degrading cGMP in the corpus cavernosum

Uses: Treatment of erectile dysfunction

Dosage and routes:

• *Adult:* **PO** 50 mg 1 hr before sexual activity, may be taken ½-4 hr before sexual activity; may be increased to 100 mg or decreased to 25 mg; max once/day

Renal/hepatic dose

• *Adult:* **PO** 25 mg, take 1 hr before sexual activity; do not use more than 1 ×/day

Available forms: Tabs 25, 50, 100 mg

Side effects/adverse reactions:

CV: ***MI, sudden death, CV collapse***

CNS: Headache, flushing, dizziness

MISC.: Dyspepsia, nasal congestion, UTI, abnormal vision, diarrhea, rash

Contraindication: Hypersensitivity

Precautions: Anatomical penile deformities, sickle cell anemia, leukemia, multiple myeloma, pregnancy (B)

Pharmacokinetics: Rapidly absorbed; bioavailability 40%; metabolized by liver (active metabolites); terminal half-life 4 hr, peak ½-1½ hr; reduced absorption with high-fat meal; excreted feces, urine

Interactions:

• ↑ sildenafil levels: cimetidine, erythromycin, ketoconazole, itraconazole

• ↓ sildenafil levels: rifampin

• ↓ B/P: amlodipine

⬥Do not use with nitrates; fatal fall in B/P

NURSING CONSIDERATIONS

Assess:

• Use of organic nitrates that should not be used with this drug

Administer:

PO route

• Approximately 1 hr before sexual activity, do not use more than once a day

Teach patient/family:

• That drug does not protect against sexually transmitted diseases, including HIV

• That drug absorption is reduced with a high-fat meal

• That drug should not be used with nitrates in any form

• That tabs may be split

silver nitrate (℞)

Func. class.: Keratolytic

Action: Antiinfective, astringent, caustic

Uses: Cauterization of lesions, warts, burns (low concentrations)

Dosage and routes:

• *Adult and child:* **TOP** apply to area to be treated

Available forms: Sticks, sol 10%, 25%, 50%

Side effects/adverse reactions:

INTEG: Skin discoloration

Contraindications: Hypersensitivity

Interactions:

• Not to be used with alkalies, phosphates, thimerosal, benzalkonium chloride, halogenated acids

NURSING CONSIDERATIONS

Administer:

• After moistening stick with water

• To burns using a wet dressing (low concentrations 0.125%)

Perform/provide:

• Storage in cool area

Evaluate:

• Therapeutic response: absence of lesions, healing of burned areas

Teach patient/family:

• To avoid contact with clothing, unaffected areas; discoloration may occur

silver nitrate 1% sulfacetamide sodium ophthalmic

See appendix c

silver protein, mild (℞, OTC)

Argyrol S.S. 10%, Argyrol S.S. 20%

Func. class.: Disinfectant

Chem. class.: Silver colloidal compound

Action: Destroys gram-positive, gram-negative organisms

Uses: Eye, nose, throat, swelling, infection

Dosage and routes:

• *Adult and child:* **TOP** sol use as needed

Available forms: Top sol 5%, 10%, 25%; eyedrops 20%

Side effects/adverse reactions:

INTEG: Irritation, discolored tissue

Contraindications: Hypersensitivity

Precautions: Pregnancy (C)

NURSING CONSIDERATIONS

Administer:

• To area to be treated only; do not apply to healthy skin

Perform/provide:

• Storage in tight container

Evaluate:

• Area of body involved: irritation, rash, breaks, dryness, scales

silver sulfadiazine topical

See appendix c

simethicone (OTC, ℞)

(si-meth'i-kone)

Extra Strength Gas-X, Extra Strength Maalox Anti-Gas, Extra Stength Maalox GRFGas Relief Formula✤, Flatulex, Gas-Relief, Gas-X, Genasyme, Maalox Anti-Gas, Maalox GRF Gas Relief Formula✤, Maximum Strength Gas Relief, Maximum Strength Mylanta Gas Relief, Maximum Strength Phazyme, Mylanta Gas, Mylicon, Ovol✤, Phazyme, Phazyme 95, Phazyme 125

Func. class.: Antiflatulent

Action: Disperses, prevents gas pockets in GI system; does not decrease gas production

Uses: Flatulence

Dosage and routes:

• *Adult and child >12 yr:* **PO** 40-100 mg pc, hs

• *Child <2 yr:* **PO** 20 mg qid

Available forms: Chew tabs 40, 80, 125 mg; tabs 60, 80, 95 mg; drops 40 mg/0.6 ml, 40 mg/ml, 95 mg/1.425 ml; caps 95, 125 mg; caps, soft gel 125 mg

Side effects/adverse reactions:
GI: Belching, rectal flatus
Contraindications: Hypersensitivity
Precautions: Pregnancy (C)
Do not confuse:
Mylicone/Mylanta Gas
NURSING CONSIDERATIONS
Assess:
- Reason for excess gas production, decreased bowel sounds, recent surgery, other GI conditions

Administer:
- After meals, hs; shake susp well before giving; chew tabs should be chewed

Evaluate:
- Therapeutic response: absence of flatulence

Teach patient/family:
- That tablets must be chewed
- To shake suspension well before pouring

simvastatin (℞)

(sim-va-sta′tin)
Zocor
Func. class.: Antilipidemic
Chem. class.: HMG-CoA reductase inhibitor

Action: Inhibits HMG-CoA reductase enzyme, which reduces cholesterol synthesis
Uses: As an adjunct in primary hypercholesterolemia (types IIa, IIb), isolated hypertriglyceridemia (Frederickson type IV) and type III hyperlipoproteinemia, coronary artery disease
Dosage and routes:
- *Adult:* **PO** 20 mg qd in PM initially; usual range 5-40 mg/day qd in PM, not to exceed 80 mg/day; dosage adjustments may be made in 4-wk intervals or more; those taking verapamil max 20 mg/day
- *Elderly/renal disease/those taking cycloSPORINE:* **PO** 5 mg/day, initially

Available forms: Tabs 5, 10, 20, 40, 80 mg
Side effects/adverse reactions:
INTEG: Rash, pruritus, photosensitivity
GI: Nausea, constipation, diarrhea, dyspepsia, flatus, abdominal pain, ***liver dysfunction,*** pancreatitis
EENT: Lens opacities
MS: Muscle cramps, myalgia, ***myositis, rhabdomyolysis***
CNS: Headache
RESP: Upper respiratory tract infection
Contraindications: Hypersensitivity, pregnancy (X), lactation, active hepatic disease
Precautions: Past hepatic disease, alcoholism, severe acute infections, trauma, severe metabolic disorders, electrolyte imbalances
Do not confuse:
Zocor/Cozaar
Zocor/Zoloft
Pharmacokinetics: Metabolized in liver (active metabolites), highly protein bound, excreted primarily in bile, feces (60%)
Interactions:
- ↑ effects of warfarin
- ↑ myalgia, myositis: cycloSPORINE, gemfibrozil, niacin, erythromycin, clofibrate, clarithromycin, ketoconazole, itraconazole, protease inhibitors
- ↑ serum level of digoxin

↑ effect: glucomannan
↓ effect: gotu kola
Lab test interferences:
Increase: CPK, LFTs
NURSING CONSIDERATIONS
Assess:
- 12-hr fasting lipid profile: LDL, ADL, TG, cholesterol at 6-8 wk, and q6mo

• Hepatic studies q1-2mo during the first 1½ yr of treatment; AST, ALT, LFTs may increase

⬥For rhabdomyolysis: muscle tenderness, increased CPK levels; therapy should be discontinued

• Renal studies in patients with compromised renal system: BUN, I&O ratio, creatinine

• Eyes with slit lamp before, 1 mo after treatment begins, annually; lens opacities may occur

Administer:

• Total daily dose in evening

Perform/provide:

• Storage in cool environment in tight container protected from light

Evaluate:

• Therapeutic response: decrease in cholesterol to desired level after 8 wk

Teach patient/family:

• That blood work and eye exam will be necessary during treatment

• To report blurred vision, severe GI symptoms, dizziness, headache

• That previously prescribed regimen will continue: low-cholesterol diet, exercise program

sirolimus (℞)

(seer-oh-lie'mus)

Rapamune

Func. class.: Immunosuppressant

Chem. class.: Macrolide

Action: Produces immunosuppression by inhibiting T-lymphocyte activation and proliferation

Uses: Organ transplants to prevent rejection, recommended use is with cycloSPORINE and corticosteroids

Investigational uses: Psoriasis

Dosage and routes:

• *Adult:* **PO** 2 mg qd with a 6 mg loading dose, may use 5 mg qd with a 15 mg loading dose

• *Child >13 yr weighing <40 kg (88 lb):* to 1 mg/m^2/day, 3 mg/m^2 loading dose

Hepatic dose

• *Adult/child ≥13 yr/<40 kg:* **PO** Reduce by 33% in maintenance dose

Available forms: Oral sol 1 mg/ml

Side effects/adverse reactions:

HEMA: ***Anemia, leukopenia, thrombocytopenia, purpura***

GI: Nausea, vomiting, diarrhea, constipation

CV: Hypertension, *atrial fibrillation, CHF, hypotension, palpitation, tachycardia*

CNS: Tremors, headache, insomnia, paresthesia, chills, fever

GU: UTIs, ***albuminuria, hematuria, proteinuria, renal failure***

META: Hyperglycemia, increased creatinine, edema, hypercholesterolemia, *hyperlipemia,* hypophosphatemia, weight gain, hyperkalemia, hyperuricemia, hypokalemia, hypomagnesemia

RESP: ***Pleural effusion, atelectasis,*** *dyspnea*

INTEG: Rash, acne, photosensitivity

EENT: Blurred vision, photophobia

SYST: ***Lymphoma***

Contraindications: Hypersensitivity to this drug or to components of the drug

Precautions: Severe renal, hepatic disease; pregnancy (C), diabetes mellitus, hyperkalemia, hyperuricemia, lymphomas, infection, other malignancies, lactation, children <13 yr, hypertension

Pharmacokinetics: Rapidly absorbed, peak 1 hr single dose, 2 hr multiple dosing, protein binding 92%; extensively metabolized by CYP3A4 enzyme system

Interactions:

• ↑ blood levels: antifungals, calcium channel blockers, cimetidine, danazol, erythromycin, cycloSPORINE, metoclopramide, bromocriptine, HIV-protease inhibitors

• ↓ blood levels: carbamazepine, phenobarbital, phenytoin, rifamycin, rifapentine

• ↓ effect of: vaccines

• Drug/food: alters bioavailability; use consistently with or without food; do not use with grapefruit juice

↓ immunosuppression: astragalus, echinacea, melatonin

St. John's wort: may ↓ the effect of sirolimus

↑ effect: ginseng, maitake, mistletoe

NURSING CONSIDERATIONS

Assess:

• Blood levels in those that may have altered metabolism, trough level ≥15 ng/ml are associated with increased adverse reactions

• Lipid profile: cholesterol, triglycerides, a lipid-lowering agent may be needed

For infection and development of lymphoma

Blood studies: Hgb, WBC, platelets during treatment qmo; if leukocytes <3000/mm^3 or platelets <100,000/mm^3, drug should be discontinued or reduced; decreased hemoglobulin level may indicate bone marrow suppression

• Hepatic studies: alk phosphatase, AST, ALT, amylase, bilirubin, and for hepatotoxicity: dark urine, jaundice, itching, light-colored stools; drug should be discontinued

Administer:

• Prophylaxis for *Pneumocystis carinii* pneumonia for 1 yr after transplantation; prophylaxis for cytomegalovirus (CMV) is recommended for 90 days after transplantation in those at increased risk for CMV

• All medications PO if possible, avoiding IM inj; bleeding may occur

• For 3 days before transplant surgery; patients should be placed in protective isolation

• Use amber oral dose syringe and withdraw amount needed oral sol from the bottle, empty correct dose into plastic/glass container holding 60 ml of water/orange juice, stir vigorously and have patient drink at once, refill container with additional 120 ml water/orange juice, stir vigorously and drink at once, if using a pouch squeeze entire contents into container and follow above directions

• Store protected from light, refrigerate, stable for 24 mo

Evaluate:

• Therapeutic response: absence of graft rejection; immunosuppression in autoimmune disorders

Teach patient/family:

• To report fever, rash, severe diarrhea, chills, sore throat, fatigue; serious infections may occur; clay-colored stools, cramping (hepatotoxicity)

• To avoid crowds, persons with known infections to reduce risk of infection

• To use contraception before, during and 12 wk after drug has been discontinued, avoid breastfeeding

• Use sunscreen, protective clothing to prevent burns

S

sodium bicarbonate (℞, OTC)

Baking Soda, Bellans, Citrocarbonate, Neut, Soda Mint

Func. class.: Alkalinizer

Chem. class.: $NaHCO_3$

Action: Orally neutralizes gastric

acid, which forms water, NaCl, CO_2; increases plasma bicarbonate, which buffers H^+-ion concentration; reverses acidosis IV

Uses: Acidosis (metabolic), cardiac arrest, alkalinization (systemic/urinary) antacid

Dosage and routes:

Acidosis, metabolic

• *Adult and child:* **IV INF** 2-5 mEq/kg over 4-8 hr depending on CO_2, pH

Cardiac arrest

• *Adult and child:* **IV BOL** 1 mEq/kg of 7.5% or 8.4% sol, then 0.5 mEq/kg q10 min, then doses based on ABGs

• *Infant:* **IV INF** not to exceed 8 mEq/kg/day based on ABGs (4.2% sol)

Alkalinization of urine

• *Adult:* **PO** 325 mg-2 g qid or 48 mEq (4g), then 12-24 mEq q4h

• *Child:* **PO** 12-120 mg/kg/day (1-10 mEq/kg)

Antacid

• *Adult:* **PO** 300 mg-2 g chewed, taken with H_2O qd-qid

Available forms: Tabs 300, 325, 600, 650 mg; inj 4.2%, 5%, 7.5%, 8.4%

Side effects/adverse reactions:

CNS: Irritability, headache, confusion, stimulation, tremors, *twitching, hyperreflexia,* ***tetany,*** weakness, ***seizures*** of alkalosis

CV: Irregular pulse, ***cardiac arrest,*** water retention, edema, weight gain

GI: Flatulence, *belching, distention,* ***paralytic ileus,*** acid rebound

META: Alkalosis

GU: Calculi

RESP: Shallow, slow respirations; cyanosis, ***apnea***

Contraindications: Hypertension, peptic ulcer, renal disease, hypocalcemia

Precautions: CHF, cirrhosis, toxemia, renal disease, pregnancy (C)

Pharmacokinetics:

PO: Onset 2 min, duration 10 min

IV: Onset 15 min, duration 1-2 hr, excreted in urine

Interactions:

• ↑ effects: amphetamines, mecamylamine, quinine, quinidine, pseudoephedrine, flecainide, anorexiants

• ↓ effects: lithium, chlorpropamide, barbiturates, salicylates, benzodiazepines

• ↑ sodium and ↓ potassium: corticosteroids

↓ action of sodium bicarbonate: oak bark

Lab test interferences:

Increase: Urinary urobilinogen

False positive: Urinary protein, blood lactate

NURSING CONSIDERATIONS

Assess:

• Respiratory and pulse rate, rhythm, depth, lung sounds; notify prescriber of abnormalities

• Fluid balance (I&O, weight qd, edema); notify prescriber of fluid overload

• Electrolytes, blood pH, PO_2, HCO_3^-, during treatment; ABGs frequently during emergencies

• Urine pH, urinary output, during beginning treatment

• Extravasation with IV administration (tissue sloughing, ulceration, and necrosis)

• Weight qd with initial therapy

• Alkalosis: irritability, confusion, twitching, hyperreflexia stimulation, slow respirations, cyanosis, irregular pulse

• Milk-alkali syndrome: confusion, headache, nausea, vomiting, anorexia, urinary stones, hypercalcemia

• For GI perforation secondary to CO_2 in GI tract; may lead to perforation if ulcer is severe enough

Administer:

IV route

• In prepared sol or diluted in an equal amount of compatible sol given 2-5 mEq/kg over 4-8 hr, not to exceed 50 mEq/hr; slower rate in children

Additive compatibilities: Amikacin, aminophylline, amobarbital, amphotericin B, atropine, bretylium, calcium gluceptate, cefoxitin, ceftazidime, cephalothin, cephapirin, chloramphenicol, chlorothiazide, cimetidine, clindamycin, cytarabine, droperidol/fentanyl, ergonovine, erythromycin, esmolol, floxacillin, furosemide, heparin, hyaluronidase, hydrocortisone, kanamycin, lidocaine, mannitol, metaraminol, methotrexate, methyldopate, multivitamins, nafcillin, nalmefene, netilmicin, nizatidine, ofloxacin, oxacillin, oxytocin, phenobarbital, phenylephrine, phenytoin, phytonadione, potassium chloride, prochlorperazine, thiopental, verapamil

Syringe compatibilities: Milrinone, pentobarbital

Y-site compatibilities: Acyclovir, amifostine, asparaginase, aztreonam, cefepime, cefmetazole, ceftriaxone, cladribine, cyclophosphamide, cytarabine, DAUNOrubicin, dexamethasone, dexchlorpheniramine, DOXOrubicin, etoposide, famotidine, filgrastim, fludarabine, gallium, granisetron, heparin, ifosfamide, indomethacin sodium trihydrate, insulin, melphalan, mesna, methylPREDNISolone, morphine, paclitaxel, piperacillin/tazobactam, potassium chloride, propofol, remifentanil, tacrolimus, teniposide, thiotepa, tolazoline, vancomycin, vit B/C

Evaluate:

• Therapeutic response: ABGs, electrolytes, blood pH, HCO_3^- WNL

Teach patient/family:

• To chew antacid tablets and drink 8 oz water

• Not to take antacid with milk, or milk-alkali syndrome may result

• Not to use antacid for more than 2 wk

• To notify prescriber if indigestion is accompanied by chest pain, dyspnea, diarrhea, dark, tarry stools

• About sodium-restricted diet; to avoid use of baking soda for indigestion

sodium biphosphate/ sodium phosphate (OTC)

Fleet Enema, Phospho-Soda

Func. class.: Laxative, saline

Action: Increases water absorption in the small intestine by osmotic action, laxative effect occurs by increased peristalsis and water retention

Uses: Constipation, bowel or rectal preparation for surgery, exam

Dosage and routes:

• *Adult:* **PO** 20-30 ml (Phospho-Soda)

• *Child:* **PO** 5-15 ml (Phospho-Soda)

• *Adult and child >12 yr:* **RECT** 1 enema (118 ml)

• *Child 2-12 yr:* **RECT** ½ enema (59 ml)

Available forms: Enema 7 g phosphate/19 g biphosphate/118 ml; oral sol 18 g phosphate/48 g biphosphate/100 ml

Side effects/adverse reactions:

GI: Nausea, cramps, diarrhea

META: Electrolyte, fluid imbalances

CV: ***Dysrhythmias, cardiac arrest,*** hypotension, widening QRS complex

S

Contraindications: Hypersensitivity, rectal fissures, abdominal pain, nausea/vomiting, appendicitis, acute surgical abdomen, ulcerated hemorrhoids, sodium-restricted diets, renal failure, hyperphosphatemia, hypocalcemia, hypokalemia, hypernatremia, Addison's disease, CHF, ascites, bowel perforation
Precautions: Pregnancy (C)
Pharmacokinetics: Excreted in feces

NURSING CONSIDERATIONS
Assess:
- Stools: color, amount, consistency
- Bowel pattern, bowel sounds, flatulence, distention, fever, dietary patterns, exercise
- Blood, urine electrolytes if drug is used often by patient
- Cramping, rectal bleeding, nausea, vomiting; if these symptoms occur, drug should be discontinued

Administer:
- Alone for better absorption; do not take within 1 hr of other drugs

Evaluate:
- Therapeutic response: decrease in constipation

Teach patient/family:
- Not to use laxatives for long-term therapy; bowel tone will be lost
- That normal bowel movements do not always occur daily
- Not to use in presence of abdominal pain, nausea, vomiting
- To notify prescriber if constipation unrelieved or if symptoms of electrolyte imbalance occur: muscle cramps, pain, weakness, dizziness, excessive thirst
- To maintain fluid consumption

sodium polystyrene sulfonate (℞)
(po-lee-stye'reen)
Kayexalate, K-Exit✦, Kionex, PMS Sodium Polystyrene Sulfonate✦, SPS
Func. class.: Potassium-removing resin
Chem. class.: Cation exchange resin

Action: Removes potassium by exchanging sodium for potassium in body primarily in large intestine
Uses: Hyperkalemia in conjunction with other measures
Dosage and routes:
- *Adult:* **PO** 15 g qd-qid; **RECT** enema 30-50 g/100 ml of sorbitol warmed to body temp q6h
- *Child:* **PO/RECT** 1 mEq of potassium exchanged/g of resin, approximate dose 1 g/kg q6h

Available forms: Susp 15 g polystyrene sulfonate, 21.5 ml sorbitol, 15 g (65 mEq) Na/60 ml; powder 15 g/4 level tsp
Side effects/adverse reactions:
GI: Constipation, anorexia, nausea, vomiting, diarrhea (sorbitol), fecal impaction, gastric irritation
META: Hypocalcemia, hypokalemia, hypomagnesemia, sodium retention
Precautions: Pregnancy (C), renal failure, CHF, severe edema, severe hypertension
Interactions:
- ↓ effect of sodium polystyrene: antacids, laxatives

NURSING CONSIDERATIONS
Assess:
- Hyperkalemia: confusion, dyspnea, weakness, dysrhythmias
- ECG for spiked T waves, depressed ST segments, prolonged QT and widening QRS complex

• Bowel function qd, note consistency of stools, times/day
• Hypotension: confusion, irritability, muscular pain, weakness
• Serum K, Ca, Mg, Na, acid-base balance
• I&O ratio, weight qd

Administer:
• Oral dose as susp mixed with H_2O or syr (20-100 ml)
• Mild laxative as ordered to prevent constipation, fecal impaction
• Sorbitol as ordered to prevent constipation
• Retention enema after mixing with warm water; introduce by gravity, continue stirring, flush with 100 ml of fluid, clamp, and leave in place

Perform/provide:
• Retention of enema for at least ½-1 hr
• Irrigation of colon after enema with 1-2 qt nonsodium sol, drain
• Storage of freshly prepared sol 24 hr at room temperature

Evaluate:
• Therapeutic response: potassium level 3.5-5 mg/dl

Teach patient/family:
• Reason for medication and expected results

sodium sulfacetamide lotion 10% topical

See appendix c

somatropin (℞)

(soe-ma-troe′pin)

Genotropin, Humatrope, Norditropin, Nutropin, Nutropin Depot, Nutropin AQ, Saizen, Serostim

Func. class.: Pituitary hormone
Chem. class.: Growth hormone

Action: Stimulates growth; somatropin similar to natural growth hormone; both preparations developed by recombinant DNA

Uses: Pituitary growth hormone deficiency (hypopituitary dwarfism), children with human growth hormone deficiency, AIDS wasting syndrome, cachexia, adults with somatropin deficiency syndrome (SDS)

Dosage and routes:

Genotropin
SC 0.16-0.24 mg/kg/wk divided into 6 or 7 inj, give in abdomen, thigh, buttocks

Humatrope
SC/IM 0.18 mg/kg divided into equal doses either on 3 alternate days or 6 ×/wk, max wk dose is 0.3 mg/kg

Nutropin/Nutropin AQ (growth hormone deficiency)
SC 0.3 mg/kg/wk

Serostim
SC at hs >55 kg, 6 mg; 45-55 kg, 5 mg; 35-45 kg, 4 mg

Norditropin
SC 0.024-0.034 mg/kg 6-7 ×/wk

Available forms: Powder for inj (lyophilized) 1.5 mg (4 international units/ml), 4 mg (12 international units/vial), 5 mg (13 international units/vial), 5 mg (15 international units/vial), 5 mg (15 international units/vial) rDNA origin, 5.8 mg (15 international units/ml), 6 mg (18 international units/ml), 8 mg (24 international units/vial), 10 mg (26 international units/vial); inj 10 mg (30 international units/vial), 5 mg/1.5 ml, 10 mg/1.5 ml, 15 mg/1.5 ml

Side effects/adverse reactions:
GU: Hypercalciuria
INTEG: Rash, urticaria, pain; inflammation at inj site
CNS: Headache, growth of intracranial tumor
ENDO: ***Hyperglycemia, ketosis, hypothyroidism***

S

SYST: ***Antibodies to growth hormone***
MS: Tissue swelling, joint and muscle pain
Contraindications: Hypersensitivity to benzyl alcohol, closed epiphyses, intracranial lesions
Precautions: Diabetes mellitus, hypothyroidism, pregnancy (C)
Pharmacokinetics: Half-life 15-60 min, duration 7 days; metabolized in liver
Interactions:
- ↓ growth: glucocorticosteroids
- Epiphyseal closure: androgens, thyroid hormones

NURSING CONSIDERATIONS
Assess:
- Growth hormone antibodies if patient fails to respond to therapy
- Thyroid function tests: T_3, T_4, T_7, TSH to identify hypothyroidism
- Allergic reaction: rash, itching, fever, nausea, wheezing
- Hypercalciuria: urinary stones; groin, flank pain; nausea, vomiting, urinary frequency, hematuria, chills
- Growth rate of child at intervals during treatment

Administer:
IM route
- Rotate inj site
- Norditropin: after reconstituting 4 or 8 mg/2 ml diluent
- Humatrope: 5 mg/1.5-5 ml diluent, do not shake
- Nutropin/Nutropin AQ: reconstitute 5 mg/1-5 ml or 10 mg/1-10 ml bacteriostatic water for inj (benzyl alcohol preserved)

Perform/provide:
- Storage in refrigerator for <1 mo, if reconstituted <1 wk; do not use discolored or cloudy sol

Evaluate:
- Therapeutic response: growth in children

Teach patient/family:
- That treatment may continue for years; regular assessments are required

sotalol (℞)
(sot′ah-lahl)
Betapace, Betapace AF, Sotacar✦
Func. class.: Antidysrhythmic group III
Chem. class.: Nonselective β-blocker

Action: Blockade of β_1- and β_2-receptors leads to antidysrhythmic effect, prolongs action potential in myocardial fibers without affecting conduction, prolongs QT interval, no effect on QRS duration
Uses: Life-threatening ventricular dysrhythmias; Betapace AF: to maintain sinus rhythm in symptomatic atrial fibrillation/flutter
Dosage and routes:
- *Adult:* **PO** initial 80 mg bid, may increase to 240-320 mg/day

Renal dose
- *Adult:* **PO** *CCr 30-60 ml/min:* Give q24h; *CCr 10-29 ml/min:* give q36-48h; *CCr <10 ml/min:* individualize dose

Betapace AF
- *Adult:* **PO** initial 80 mg bid, titrate upward to 120 mg bid during initial hospitalization

Renal dose (Betapace AF)
- *Adult:* **PO** *CCr >60 ml/min:* Give q12h; *CCr 40-60 ml/min:* give q24h; *CCr <40 ml/min:* do not use

Available forms: Tabs 80, 120, 160, 240 mg; Betapace AF 80, 120, 160 mg
Side effects/adverse reactions:
CV: ***Prodysrhythmia,*** orthostatic hypotension, bradycardia, ***CHF,*** chest pain, ventricular dysrhythmias, AV block, peripheral vascular insufficiency, palpitations, torsades de

pointes; ***life-threatening ventricular dysrhythmias (Betapace AF)***
CNS: Dizziness, mental changes, drowsiness, fatigue, headache, catatonia, depression, anxiety, nightmares, paresthesia, lethargy, insomnia, decreased concentration
GI: Nausea, vomiting, diarrhea, dry mouth, flatulence, constipation, anorexia
INTEG: Rash, alopecia, urticaria, pruritus, fever
HEMA: ***Agranulocytosis, thrombocytopenic purpura*** (rare), ***thrombocytopenia, leukopenia***
EENT: Tinnitus, visual changes, sore throat, double vision; dry, burning eyes
GU: Impotence, dysuria, ejaculatory failure, urinary retention
RESP: ***Bronchospasm,*** dyspnea, wheezing, nasal stuffiness, pharyngitis
MS: Joint pain, arthralgia, muscle cramps, pain
MISC.: Facial swelling, decreased exercise tolerance, weight change, Raynaud's disease

Contraindications: Hypersensitivity to β-blockers, cardiogenic shock, heart block (2nd or 3rd degree), sinus bradycardia, CHF, bronchial asthma, congenital or acquired long QT syndrome

Precautions: Major surgery, pregnancy (B), lactation, diabetes mellitus, renal disease, thyroid disease, COPD, well-compensated heart failure, CAD, nonallergic bronchospasm, electrolyte disturbances, bradycardia, cardiac dysrhythmias, peripheral vascular disease

Pharmacokinetics:
PO: Onset 1-2 hr, peak 2-4 hr, duration 8-12 hr, half-life 12 hr; excreted unchanged in urine, crosses placenta, excreted in breast milk, protein binding 0%

Interactions:
- ↑ hypotension: diuretics, other antihypertensives, nitroglycerin
- ↓ β-blocker effects: sympathomimetics
- ↑ hypoglycemia effect: insulin
- ↑ effects of lidocaine
- ↓ bronchodilating effects of theophylline, β_2-agonists
- ↓ hypoglycemic effects of sulfonylureas

Hypokalemia, ↑ antidysrhythmic effect: aloe, buckthorn, cascara sagrada, senna
↑ toxicity, death: aconite
↑ effect: aloe, broom, chronic buckthorn use, cascara sagrada (chronic use), Chinese rhubarb, figwort, fumitory, goldenseal, kudzu, licorice
↓ effect: coltsfoot
↑ serotonin effect: horehound

Lab test interferences:
- *False increase:* Urinary catecholamines
- *Interference:* Glucose, insulin tolerance tests

NURSING CONSIDERATIONS

Assess:
- I&O, weight qd; edema in feet, legs qd
- B/P, pulse q4h; note rate, rhythm, quality

Apical/radial pulse before administration: notify prescriber of any significant changes; monitor ECG continuously (Betapace AF); use QT interval to determine patient eligibility; baseline QT must be ≤450 msec
- Baselines in renal studies before therapy begins
- Skin turgor, dryness of mucous membranes for hydration status

Administer:
- PO: ac, hs; tablet may be crushed or swallowed whole
- Reduced dosage in renal dysfunction

S

• Betapace and Betapace AF are not interchangeable

Perform/provide:

• Storage in dry area at room temperature; do not freeze

Evaluate:

• Therapeutic response: absence of life-threatening dysrhythmias

Teach patient/family:

• Not to discontinue drug abruptly; taper over 2 wk or may precipitate angina

• Not to use OTC products containing α-adrenergic stimulants (nasal decongestants, OTC cold preparations) unless directed by prescriber

• To report bradycardia, dizziness, confusion, depression, fever

• To take pulse at home; advise when to notify prescriber

• To avoid alcohol, smoking, sodium intake

• To carry emergency ID to identify drug being taken, allergies

• To avoid hazardous activities if dizziness is present

• To report symptoms of CHF including: difficulty in breathing, especially on exertion or when lying down; night cough, swelling of extremities

• To wear support hose to minimize effects of orthostatic hypotension

Treatment of overdose: Lavage, IV atropine for bradycardia, IV theophylline for bronchospasm, digitalis, O_2, diuretic for cardiac failure; hemodialysis is useful for removal; administer vasopressor (norepinephrine) for hypotension, isoproterenol for heart block

sparfloxacin

(spar-floks'a-sin)

Zagam

Func. class.: Antiinfective

Chem. class.: Fluoroquinolone

Action: Interferes with conversion of intermediate DNA fragments into high-molecular-weight DNA in bacteria; DNA-gyrase inhibitor

Uses: Community-acquired pneumonia; chronic bronchitis caused by *Klebsiella pneumoniae, Haemophilus influenzae, Haemophilus parainfluenzae, Moraxella catarrhalis*

Dosage and routes:

• *Adult:* **PO** 400 mg loading dose, then 200 mg q24h × 10 days

Renal dose

• *Adult:* CCr <50 ml/min day 400 mg on 1st day then 200 mg qod day 2-10

Available forms: Tabs 200 mg

Side effects/adverse reactions:

HEMA: ***Leukopenia,*** eosinophilia, anemia

CNS: Headache, dizziness, insomnia

GI: Nausea, flatulence, *vomiting,* diarrhea, *abdominal pain,* ***pseudomembranous colitis***

CV: QT interval prolongation, vasodilation

INTEG: Rash, pruritus, photosensitivity

SYST: ***Anaphylaxis, Stevens-Johnson syndrome***

Contraindications: Hypersensitivity to quinolones, photosensitivity

Precautions: Pregnancy (C), lactation, children, renal disease, seizure disorders

Pharmacokinetics: Slow, erratic absorption, widely distributed; metabolized by liver, excreted in urine, feces; half-life 20 hr

Interactions:
• ↓ absorption of sparfloxacin: antacids with aluminum, magnesium, iron products, zinc, sucralfate, give 4 hr apart
• Torsades de pointes: amiodarone, bepridil, disopyramide, erythromycin, pentamidine, phenothiazines, tricyclics, class Ia antidysrhythmics, class III antidysrhythmics
• ↑ theophylline level, lead to toxicity
• ↑ warfarin level
• Nephrotoxicity may occur with cycloSPORINE
↑ effect: cola tree

Lab test interferences:
Increase: AST, ALT

NURSING CONSIDERATIONS

Assess:
• For previous sensitivity reaction
• For signs and symptoms of infection: characteristics of sputum, WBC >10,000/mm^3, fever; obtain baseline information before and during treatment
• C&S before beginning drug therapy to identify if correct treatment has been initiated
For allergic reactions, anaphylaxis: rash, urticaria, pruritus, chills, fever, joint pain; may occur a few days after therapy begins; epINEPHrine and resuscitation equipment should be available for anaphylactic reaction
• Blood studies: LFTs if patient is on long-term therapy
• Bowel pattern qd; if severe diarrhea occurs, drug should be discontinued
• For overgrowth of infection: perineal itching, fever, malaise, redness, pain, swelling, drainage, rash, diarrhea, change in cough, sputum

Administer:
• As directed only
• 4 hr before or 2 hr after antacids, zinc, calcium

Evaluate:
• Therapeutic response: absence of signs/symptoms of infection (WBC <10,000/mm^3, temp WNL, C&S negative for organism)

Teach patient/family:
• To avoid hazardous activities until response is known
• To contact prescriber if vaginal itching, loose, foul-smelling stools, furry tongue occur (may indicate superinfection); report itching, rash, pruritus, urticaria
• To take all medication prescribed for the length of time ordered; drug must be taken as directed to maintain blood levels; do not give medication to others
• To notify prescriber of diarrhea with blood or pus
• To increase fluid intake to 2 L/day to prevent crystalluria
• To take 4 hr before or 2 hr after antacids, dairy products, zinc products
• To avoid direct sunlight or use sunscreen to prevent phototoxicity
• Not to use theophylline with this product unless approved by prescriber
• To use frequent rinsing of mouth, sugarless candy, or gum for dry mouth

spironolactone (℞)

(speer′on-oh-lak′tone)
Aldactone, Novo-Spiroton ✦
Func. class.: Potassium-sparing diuretic
Chem. class.: Aldosterone antagonist

Action: Competes with aldosterone at receptor sites in distal tubule, resulting in excretion of sodium chloride, water, retention of potassium, phosphate

Uses: Edema of CHF, hypertension, diuretic-induced hypokalemia, primary hyperaldosteronism (diagnosis, short-term treatment, long-term treatment), edema of nephrotic syndrome, cirrhosis of the liver with ascites

Investigational uses: CHF

Edema/hypertension

• *Adult:* **PO** 25-400 mg/qd in single or divided doses

CHF

• *Adult:* **PO** 12.5-25 mg/day

Edema

• *Child:* **PO** 3.3 mg/kg/day in single or divided doses

Hypertension

• *Child:* **PO** 1-2 mg/kg bid

Hypokalemia

• *Adult:* **PO** 25-100 mg/day; if **PO,** potassium supplements must not be used

Primary hyperaldosteronism diagnosis

• *Adult:* **PO** 400 mg/day × 4 days or 4 wk depending on test, then 100-400 mg/day maintenance

Available forms: Tabs 25, 50, 100 mg

Side effects/adverse reactions:

CNS: Headache, confusion, drowsiness, lethargy, ataxia

GI: Diarrhea, cramps, ***bleeding,*** gastritis, *vomiting,* anorexia, nausea

INTEG: Rash, pruritus, urticaria

ENDO: Impotence, gynecomastia, irregular menses, amenorrhea, postmenopausal bleeding, hirsutism, deepening voice

HEMA: ***Agranulocytosis***

ELECT: Hyperchloremic metabolic acidosis, ***hyperkalemia,*** hyponatremia

Contraindications: Hypersensitivity, anuria, severe renal disease, hyperkalemia, pregnancy (D)

Precautions: Dehydration, hepatic disease, lactation, renal impairment

Pharmacokinetics:

PO: Onset 24-48 hr, peak 48-72 hr; metabolized in liver, excreted in urine, crosses placenta

Interactions:

• ↓ effect of anticoagulants

• ↑ action of antihypertensives, digitalis, lithium

• ↑ hyperkalemia: potassium-sparing diuretics, potassium products, ACE inhibitors, salt substitutes

• ↓ effect of spironolactone: ASA

Hypokalemia: bearberry, gossypol

↑ effect: cucumber, dandelion, horsetail, licorice, nettle, pumpkin, Queen Anne's lace

↑ hypotension: khella

Severe photosensitivity: St. John's wort

Fatal hypokalemia: arginine

Lab test interferences:

Interference: 17-OHCS, 17-KS, radioimmunoassay, digoxin assay

NURSING CONSIDERATIONS

Assess:

• Electrolytes: Na, Cl, K, BUN, serum creatinine, ABGs, CBC

• Weight, I&O qd to determine fluid loss; effect of drug may be decreased if used qd; ECG periodically (long-term therapy)

• Signs of metabolic acidosis: drowsiness, restlessness

• Rashes, temp qd

• Confusion, especially in elderly; take safety precautions if needed

• Hydration: skin turgor, thirst, dry mucous membranes

Administer:

• In AM to avoid interference with sleep

• With food; if nausea occurs, absorption may be decreased slightly

Evaluate:

• Therapeutic response: improvement in edema of feet, legs, sacral area qd if medication is being used in CHF

Teach patient/family:

- To avoid foods with high potassium content: oranges, bananas, salt substitutes, dried apricots, dates
- That drowsiness, ataxia, mental confusion may occur; observe caution in driving
- To notify prescriber of cramps, diarrhea, lethargy, thirst, headache, skin rash, menstrual abnormalities, deepening voice, breast enlargement

Treatment of overdose: Lavage if taken orally; monitor electrolytes, administer IV fluids, monitor hydration, renal, CV status

stavudine (℞)

(sta'vyoo-deen)

d4t, Zerit

Func. class.: Antiretroviral

Chem. class.: Nucleoside reverse transcriptase inihibitor

Action: Prevents replication of HIV by the inhibition of the enzyme reverse transcriptase, causes DNA chain termination

Uses: Treatment of HIV-1 in combination with other antiretrovirals

Dosage and routes:

- *Adult >60 kg:* **PO** 40 mg q12h
- *Adult <60 kg:* **PO** 30 mg q12h
- *Child <30 kg:* **PO** 1 mg/kg q12h
- *Child ≥30 kg ≤60 kg:* **PO** 30 mg q12h
- *Child >60 kg:* **PO** 40 mg q12h

Renal dose

- *Adult: >60 kg:* **PO** CCr 26-50 ml/min 20 mg q12h; CCr 10-25 ml/min 20 mg q24h
- *Adult: <60 kg:* **PO** CCr 26-50 ml/min 15 mg q12h; CCr 10-25 ml/min 15 mg q24h

Available forms: Caps 15, 20, 30, 40 mg; powder for oral sol 1 mg/ml

Side effects/adverse reactions:

HEMA: ***Bone marrow suppression***

CNS: Peripheral neuropathy, insomnia, anxiety, neuropathy, depression, dizziness, confusion, headache, chills/fever, malaise

GI: ***Hepatotoxicity,*** diarrhea, nausea, vomiting, anorexia, dyspepsia, constipation, stomatitis, ***pancreatitis***

MS: Myalgia, arthralgia

CV: Chest pain, vasodilation, hypertension

MISC: ***Lactic acidosis***

RESP: Dyspnea, pneumonia, asthma

INTEG: Rash, sweating, pruritus, benign neoplasms

EENT: Conjunctivitis, abnormal vision

Contraindications: Hypersensitivity to this drug or zidovudine, didanosine, zalcitabine; severe peripheral neuropathy

Precautions: Advanced HIV infection; pregnancy (C); lactation, bone marrow suppression; renal, hepatic disease; peripheral neuropathy

Interactions:

- ↑ myelosuppression: other myelosuppressants
- ↑ peripheral neuropathy: lithium, dapsone, chloramphenicol didanosine, ethambutol, hydrALAZINE, phenytoin, vinCRIStine, zalcitabine

Pharmacokinetics: Excreted in urine, breast milk; peak 1 hr; half-life: elimination: 1-1.6 hr, intracellular: 3-3.5 hr

NURSING CONSIDERATIONS

Assess:

⬍ For lactic acidosis and severe hepatomegaly with steatosis, death may result

- Blood studies: WBC, differential, RBC, Hct, Hgb, platelets
- Renal tests: urinalysis, protein, blood
- C&S before drug therapy; drug

may be given as soon as culture is taken
• Bowel pattern before, during treatment
• Weakness, tremors, confusion, dizziness; drug may have to be decreased or discontinued
• Viral load and CD4 counts baseline and throughout treatment
• For peripheral neuropathy: tingling, pain, in extremities; discontinue drug
◆ For pancreatitis: severe upper abdominal pain, nausea, vomiting throughout treatment, discontinue drug

Administer:
• With or without meals; absorption does not appear to be lowered when taken with food

Teach patient/family:
• The signs of peripheral neuropathy: burning, weakness, pain, prickling feeling in the extremities
• That drug should not be given with antineoplastics
• That drug is not a cure for AIDS, but will control symptoms
• To call prescriber if sore throat, swollen lymph nodes, malaise, fever occur; other drugs may be needed to prevent other infections
• That even with this drug, patient may pass AIDS virus to others
• That follow-up visits are necessary; serious toxicity may occur; blood counts must be done q2wk
• To take q12h around clock
• That serious drug interactions may occur if other medications are ingested; see prescriber before taking chloramphenicol, dapsone, cisplatin, didanosine, ethambutol, lithium, antifungals, antineoplastics
• That drug may cause fainting or dizziness

Evaluate:
• Therapeutic response: decreased symptoms of HIV

HIGH ALERT

streptokinase (℞)

(strep-toe-kye′nase)
Kabikinase, Streptase

Func. class.: Thrombolytic enzyme

Chem. class.: β-Hemolytic streptococcus filtrate (purified)

Action: Activates conversion of plasminogen to plasmin (fibrinolysin): plasmin breaks down clots (fibrin), fibrinogen, factors V, VII; occlusion of venous access lines

Uses: Deep-vein thrombosis, pulmonary embolism, arterial thrombosis, arterial embolism, arteriovenous cannula occlusion, lysis of coronary artery thrombi after MI, acute evolving transmural MI

Dosage and routes:

Lysis of coronary artery thrombi
• *Adult:* **IC** 20,000 international units, then 2000 international units/min over 1 hr as **IV INF**

Arteriovenous cannula occlusion
• *Adult:* **IV INF** 250,000 international units/2 ml sol into occluded limb of cannula run over ½ hr; clamp for 2 hr; aspirate contents; flush with NaCl sol and reconnect

Thrombosis/embolism/DVT/pulmonary embolism
• *Adult:* **IV INF** 250,000 international units over ½ hr, then 100,000 international units/hr for 72 hr for deep-vein thrombosis; 100,000 international units/hr over 24-72 hr for pulmonary embolism; 100,000 international units/hr × 24-72 hr for arterial thrombosis or embolism

Acute evolving transmural MI
• *Adult:* **IV INF** 1,500,000 international units diluted to a volume of 45 ml; give within 1 hr; intracoronary **INF** 20,000 international units

by **BOL,** then 2000 international units/min × 1 hr, total dose 140,000 international units

Available forms: Powder for inj, lyophilized, 250,000, 600,000, 750,000, 1,500,000 international units/vial

Side effects/adverse reactions:

CV: Dysrhythmias, hypotension, noncardiogenic pulmonary edema, ***pulmonary embolism***

CNS: Headache, fever

EENT: Periorbital edema

GI: Nausea

HEMA: Decreased Hct, ***bleeding***

INTEG: Rash, urticaria, phlebitis at IV inf site, itching, flushing

MS: Low back pain

RESP: Altered respirations, SOB, ***bronchospasm***

SYST: ***GI, GU, intracranial, retroperitoneal bleeding, surface bleeding, anaphylaxis***

Contraindications: Hypersensitivity, active internal bleeding, recent CVA, intracranial intrapleural surgery, intraspinal surgery, CNS neoplasms, uncontrolled severe hypertension

Precautions: Arterial emboli from left side of heart, pregnancy (C), ulcerative colitis, enteritis, severe renal disease, hepatic disease, hypocoagulation, COPD, subacute bacterial endocarditis, rheumatic valvular disease, cerebral embolism/thrombosis/hemorrhage, intraarterial diagnostic procedure or surgery (10 days), recent major surgery

Pharmacokinetics:

IV: Onset immediate, duration <12 hr; half-life <20 min; excreted in bile, urine

Interactions:

• Bleeding potential: aspirin, indomethacin, phenylbutazone, anticoagulants, other NSAIDs, abciximab, eptifibatide, tirofiban, clopidogrel, ticlopidine, some cephalosporins, plicamycin, valproic acid, dipyridamole, GP IIb, IIIa inhibitors

Lab test interferences:

Increase: PT, aPTT, TT

Decrease: Plasminogen, fibrinogen

NURSING CONSIDERATIONS

Assess:

• Allergy: fever, rash, itching, chills; mild reaction may be treated with antihistamines

⬥ For bleeding during 1st hr of treatment; hematuria, hematemesis, bleeding from mucous membranes, epistaxis, ecchymosis; may require tranfusion (rare), continue to assess for bleeding for 24 hr

• Blood studies (Hct, platelets, PTT, PT, TT, aPTT) before starting therapy; PT or aPTT must be less than 2× control before starting therapy; PTT or PT q3-4h during treatment

⬥ For hypersensitive reactions: fever, rash, dyspnea, facial swelling; drug should be discontinued; for streptokinase reactions previously; notify prescriber immediately, stop drug, keep resuscitative equipment nearby

• VS, B/P, pulse, respirations, neurologic signs, temp at least q4h; temp >104° F (40° C) indicates internal bleeding; systolic pressure increase >25 mm Hg should be reported to prescriber; assess neurologic status, neurologic change may indicate intracranial bleeding

⬥ For neurologic changes that may indicate intracranial bleeding

⬥ Retroperitoneal bleeding: back pain, leg weakness, diminished pulses

• For Guillain-Barré syndrome that may occur after treatment with this drug

• ECG continuously, cardiac enzymes, radionuclide myocardial scanning/coronary angiography

• For respiratory depression

S

Administer:

IV route

- As soon as thrombi identified; not useful for thrombi over 1 wk old
- Cryoprecipitate or fresh frozen plasma if bleeding occurs
- Loading dose at beginning of therapy; may require increased loading doses
- Heparin after fibrinogen level >100 mg/dl; heparin infusion to increase PTT to 1.5-2 × baseline for 3-7 days; IV heparin with loading dose is recommended after discontinuing streptokinase to prevent redevelopment of thrombi
- After reconstituting with 5 ml NS or D_5W; do not shake; further dilute to total volume of 45 ml; may be diluted to 500 ml in 45 ml increments; may dilute vial in 15 ml NS, further dilute 750,000 international units/50 ml NS or D_5W; further dilute 1,500,000 international units dose/100 ml or more
- About 10% patients have high streptococcal antibody titers requiring increased loading doses
- IV therapy using 0.8-μm filter

Y-site compatibilities: DOBUTamine, DOPamine, heparin, lidocaine, nitroglycerin

Perform/provide:

- Storage of reconstituted sol in refrigerator; discard after 24 hr
- Bed rest during entire course of treatment
- Avoidance of venous or arterial puncture, inj, rectal temp; any invasive treatment
- Treatment of fever with acetaminophen or aspirin
- Pressure for 30 sec to minor bleeding sites; inform prescriber if this does not attain hemostasis; apply pressure dressing

Evaluate:

- Therapeutic response: resolution of thrombosis, embolism

Teach patient/family:

- Reason for medication and expected results

streptomycin (℞)

(strep-toe-mye′sin)

Func. class.: Antiinfective/antitubercular

Chem. class.: Aminoglycoside

Action: Interferes with protein synthesis in bacterial cell by binding to ribosomal subunit, causing inaccurate peptide sequence to form in protein chain, causing bacterial death

Uses: Sensitive strains of *Mycobacterium tuberculosis,* nontuberculous infections caused by sensitive strains of *Yersinia pestis, Brucella, Haemophilus influenzae, Klebsiella pneumoniae, Escherichia coli, Enterobacter aerogenes, Streptococcus viridans, Francisella tularensis, Proteus*

Dosage and routes:

Tuberculosis

- *Adult:* **IM** 15 mg/kg (max 1 g) qd × 2-3 mo, then 1 g 2-3 ×/week with other antitubercular drugs
- *Child:* **IM** 20-40 mg/kg/day in divided doses with other antitubercular drugs; max 15 mg/kg/day

Streptococcal endocarditis

- *Adult:* **IM** 1 g q12h × 1 wk with penicillin, then 500 mg bid × 1 wk

Enterococcal endocarditis

- *Adult:* **IM** 1 g q12h × 2 wk, then 500 mg q12h × 4 wk with penicillin, max 15 mg/kg/day

Available forms: Inj 500 mg, 1 g/ml

Side effects/adverse reactions:

GU: ***Oliguria, hematuria, renal damage, azotemia, renal failure, nephrotoxicity***

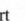

CNS: Confusion, depression, numb-

ness, tremors, ***convulsions,*** muscle twitching, ***neurotoxicity,*** dizziness
EENT: ***Ototoxicity,*** deafness, visual disturbances, tinnitus
HEMA: ***Agranulocytosis, thrombocytopenia, leukopenia, eosinophilia, anemia***
GI: Nausea, vomiting, anorexia, increased ALT, AST, bilirubin; hepatomegaly, ***hepatic necrosis,*** splenomegaly
CV: Hypotension, myocarditis, palpitations
INTEG: Rash, burning, urticaria, dermatitis, alopecia
Contraindications: Severe renal disease, hypersensitivity, pregnancy (D)
Precautions: Neonates, mild renal disease, myasthenia gravis, lactation, hearing deficit, elderly, Parkinson's disease
Pharmacokinetics:
IM: Onset rapid, peak 1-2 hr; plasma half-life 2-2½ hr; not metabolized, excreted unchanged in urine, crosses placental barrier, poor penetration into CSF, small amounts enter breast milk
Interactions:
- ↑ ototoxicity, neurotoxicity, nephrotoxicity: other aminoglycosides, amphotericin B, polymyxin, vancomycin, ethacrynic acid, furosemide, mannitol, methoxyflurane, cisplatin, cephalosporins, bacitracin
- ↑ effects: nondepolarizing muscle relaxants, succinylcholine, warfarin

↑ toxicity: lysine (large amounts)

NURSING CONSIDERATIONS

Assess:
- Weight before treatment; calculation of dosage is usually based on ideal body weight, but may be calculated on actual body weight
- I&O ratio, urinalysis qd for proteinuria, cells, casts; report sudden change in urine output
- Serum peak 20-30 min after IM inj, trough level drawn 8 hr; acceptable levels—peak 5-25 mcg/ml, trough should not be >5 mcg/ml
- Urine pH if drug is used for UTI; urine should be kept alkaline
- Renal impairment by collecting urine for CCr testing, BUN, serum creatinine; lower dosage should be given in renal impairment (CCr <80 ml/min), monitor electrolytes: K, Na, Cl, Mg
- Deafness by audiometric testing, ringing, roaring in ears, vertigo; assess hearing before, during, after treatment
- Dehydration: high specific gravity, decrease in skin turgor, dry mucous membranes, dark urine
- Overgrowth of infection: fever, malaise, redness, pain, swelling, perineal itching, diarrhea, stomatitis, change in cough, sputum
- C&S before starting treatment to identify infecting organism
- Vestibular dysfunction: nausea, vomiting, dizziness, headache; drug should be discontinued if severe
- Inj sites for redness, swelling, abscesses; use warm compresses at site

Administer:
- IM inj in large muscle mass; rotate inj sites
- Drug in evenly spaced doses to maintain blood level

Additive compatibilities: Bleomycin
Syringe compatibilities: Penicillin G sodium
Y-site compatibilities: Esmolol
Perform/provide:
- Adequate fluids of 2-3 L/day unless contraindicated to prevent irritation of tubules
- Supervised ambulation, other safety measures with vestibular dysfunction

Evaluate:

• Therapeutic effect: absence of fever, draining wounds, negative C&S after treatment

Teach patient/family:

• To report headache, dizziness, symptoms of overgrowth of infection, renal impairment

• To report loss of hearing, ringing, roaring in ears, fullness in head

Treatment of overdose: Hemodialysis; monitor serum levels of drug

succimer (℞)

(sux'i-mer)

Chemet

Func. class.: Heavy metal antagonist

Chem. class.: Chelating agent

Action: Binds with ions of lead to form a water-soluble complex excreted by kidneys

Uses: Lead poisoning in children with lead levels above 45 mcg/dl; may be beneficial in mercury, arsenic poisoning

Dosage and routes:

• *Child:* **PO** 10 mg/kg or 350 mg/m^2 q8h × 5 days, then 10 mg/kg or 350 mg/m^2 q12h × 2 wk; another course may be required depending on lead levels; allow 2 wk between courses

Available forms: Caps 100 mg

Side effects/adverse reactions:

SYST: Back, stomach, head, rib, flank pain; abdominal cramps, chills, fever, flulike symptoms, head cold, headache

HEMA: ***Increased platelets, intermittent eosinophilia***

GU: ***Proteinuria,*** decreased urination, voiding difficulties

INTEG: Rash, urticaria, pruritus

META: Increased AST, ALT, alk phosphatase, cholesterol

GI: Nausea, vomiting, diarrhea, metallic taste, anorexia

CNS: Drowsiness, dizziness, paresthesia, sensorimotor neuropathy

EENT: Otitis media, watery eyes, film in eyes, plugged ears

RESP: Sore throat, rhinorrhea, nasal congestion, cough

Contraindications: Hypersensitivity

Precautions: Pregnancy (C), lactation, children <1 yr

Pharmacokinetics:

PO: Peak 1-2 hr, 49% excreted (39% in feces, 9% urine, 1% as CO_2 from lungs)

Interactions:

• Not recommended concurrently with other chelating agents

NURSING CONSIDERATIONS

Assess:

• Renal, hepatic studies: ALT, AST, alk phosphatase, BUN, creatinine, serum lead level

• I&O

• For lead sources in home, school

• Allergic reactions: rash, pruritus, urticaria; drug should be discontinued if antihistamines fail to help

Administer:

PO route

• To children who cannot swallow capsule by separating the capsule and sprinkling content on food or in a spoon followed by a drink

Perform/provide:

• Adequate fluids; check hydration status qd

Evaluate:

• Therapeutic response: decrease in serum lead level

Teach patient/family:

• That therapeutic effect may take 1-3 mo

• To report urticaria, rash

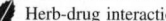

• To increase fluid intake

HIGH ALERT

succinylcholine (℞)

(suk-sin-ill-koe′leen)

Anectine, Anectine Flo-Pack, Quelicin, succinylcholine chloride, Sucostrin, Suxamethonium

Func. class.: Neuromuscular blocker (depolarizing–ultra short)

Action: Inhibits transmission of nerve impulses by binding with cholinergic receptor sites, antagonizing action of acetylcholine; causes release of histamine

Uses: Facilitation of endotracheal intubation, skeletal muscle relaxation during orthopedic manipulations

Dosage and routes:

- *Adult:* **IV** 0.6 mg/kg, then 2.5 mg/min as needed; **IM** 2.5 mg/kg, not to exceed 150 mg
- *Child:* **IV/IM** 1-2 mg/kg, not to exceed 150 mg **IM**

Available forms: Inj 20, 50, 100 mg/ml; powder for inj 100, 500 mg/vial, 1 g/vial

Side effects/adverse reactions:

CV: Bradycardia, tachycardia; increased, decreased B/P; ***sinus arrest, dysrhythmias***

RESP: ***Prolonged apnea, bronchospasm, cyanosis, respiratory depression***

EENT: Increased secretions, increased intraocular pressure

MS: Weakness, muscle pain, fasciculations, prolonged relaxation

HEMA: ***Myoglobulinemia***

INTEG: Rash, flushing, pruritus, urticaria

Contraindications: Hypersensitivity, malignant hyperthermia, decreased plasma pseudocholinesterase, penetrating eye injuries, acute narrow-angle glaucoma

Precautions: Pregnancy (C), cardiac disease, severe burns, fractures—fasciculations may increase damage—lactation, children <2 yr, electrolyte imbalances, dehydration, neuromuscular disease, respiratory disease, collagen diseases, glaucoma, eye surgery, elderly or debilitated patients

Pharmacokinetics:

IV: Onset 1 min, peak 2-3 min, duration 6-10 min

IM: Onset 2-3 min

Hydrolyzed in urine (active/inactive metabolites)

Interactions:

- ↑ neuromuscular blockade: aminoglycosides, clindamycin, lincomycin, quinidine, local anesthetics, polymyxin antibiotics, lithium, opioids, thiazides, enflurane, isoflurane, magnesium salts, oxytocin
- Dysrhythmias: theophylline

Blocks succinylcholine: melatonin

NURSING CONSIDERATIONS

Assess:

- For electrolyte imbalances (K, Mg); may lead to increased action of this drug
- VS (B/P, pulse, respirations, airway) until fully recovered; rate, depth, pattern of respirations, strength of hand grip
- I&O ratio; check for urinary retention, frequency, hesitancy
- Recovery: decreased paralysis of face, diaphragm, leg, arm, rest of body
- Allergic reactions: rash, fever, respiratory distress, pruritus; drug should be discontinued

Administer:

- Deep IM inj, preferably high in deltoid muscle

S

IV route
- Using nerve stimulator by anesthesiologist to determine neuromuscular blockade
- Anticholinesterase to reverse neuromuscular blockade
- IV inf; dilute 1-2 mg/ml in D_5, isotonic saline sol, give 0.5-10 mg/min, titrate to response; may be given directly over 1 min

Additive compatibilities: Amikacin, cephapirin, isoproterenol, meperidine, methyldopate, morphine, norepinephrine, scopolamine
Syringe compatibilities: Heparin
Y-site compatibilities: Etomidate, heparin, potassium chloride, propofol, vit B/C
Perform/provide:
- Storage in refrigerator, powder at room temperature; close tightly
- Reassurance if communication is difficult during recovery from neuromuscular blockade; postoperative stiffness is normal, soon subsides

Evaluate:
- Therapeutic response: paralysis of jaw, eyelid, head, neck, rest of body

Treatment of overdose: Edrophonium or neostigmine, atropine, monitor VS; may require mechanical ventilation

sucralfate (℞)

(soo-kral′fate)
Carafate, Sulcrate ♣
Func. class.: Protectant, antiulcer
Chem. class.: Aluminum hydroxide, sulfated sucrose

Action: Forms a complex that adheres to ulcer site, adsorbs pepsin
Uses: Duodenal ulcer, oral mucositis, stomatitis after radiation of head and neck
Investigational uses: Gastric ulcers, gastroesophageal reflux
Dosage and routes:
Ulcers
- *Adult:* **PO** 1 g qid 1 hr ac, hs
- *Child:* **PO** 40-80 mg/kg/day

Prevention of ulcers
- *Adult:* **PO** 1 g bid, 1 hr ac

GERD
- *Adult:* **PO** 1 g qid 1 hr ac and hs
- *Child:* **PO** 500 mg-1 g qid, 1 hr ac and hs

Available forms: Tabs 1 g; oral susp 500 mg/5 ml
Side effects/adverse reactions:
CNS: Drowsiness, dizziness
GI: Dry mouth, constipation, nausea, gastric pain, vomiting
INTEG: Urticaria, rash, pruritus
Contraindications: Hypersensitivity
Precautions: Pregnancy (B), lactation, children, renal failure
Do not confuse:
Carafate/Cafergot
Pharmacokinetics:
PO: Duration up to 6 hr
Interactions:
- ↓ action of tetracyclines, phenytoin, fat-soluble vitamins, cimetidine, digoxin, ketoconazole, ranitidine, theophylline
- ↓ absorption of fluoroquinolones
- ↓ absorption of sucralfate: antacids

NURSING CONSIDERATIONS
Assess:
- Gastric pH (>5 should be maintained); blood in stools

Administer:
PO route
- On an empty stomach, 1 hr before meals and hs
- ⊘ Do not crush, chew tabs

Perform/provide:
- Storage at room temperature

Evaluate:
- Therapeutic response: absence of pain, GI complaints

Teach patient/family:
- To take on empty stomach
- To take full course of therapy, not to use over 8 wk, to avoid smoking
- To avoid antacids within ½ hr of drug

* sulfADIAZINE (℞)

(sul-fa-dye'a-zeen)

Coptin, sulfADIAZINE

Func. class.: Antiinfective

Chem. class.: Sulfonamide, intermediate acting

Action: Interferes with bacterial biosynthesis of proteins by competitive antagonism of PABA

Uses: UTIs, rheumatic fever prophylaxis, with pyrimethamine for *Toxoplasma gondii* encephalitis, chancroid, inclusion conjunctivitis, malaria, meningitis, *Haemophilus influenzae,* meningococeal meningitis, nocardiosis, acute otitis media, trachoma, chloroquine-resistant malaria

Dosage and routes:

Meningococcal carriers (asymptomatic)
- *Adult:* **PO** 1 g q12h × 2 days
- *Child 1-12 yr:* **PO** 500 mg q12h × 2 days
- *Child 2-12 mo:* **PO** 500 mg qd × 2 days

Rheumatic fever prophylaxis
- *Child >30 kg:* **PO** 1 g qd
- *Child <30 kg:* **PO** 500 mg qd

Available forms: Tabs 500 mg

Side effects/adverse reactions:

SYST: ***Anaphylaxis***

GI: Nausea, vomiting, abdominal pain, stomatitis, ***hepatitis,*** glossitis, pancreatitis, diarrhea, ***enterocolitis,*** anorexia

CNS: Headache, insomnia, hallucinations, depression, vertigo, fatigue, anxiety, ***convulsions,*** drug fever, chills, drowsiness

HEMA: ***Leukopenia, thrombocytopenia, agranulocytosis, hemolytic anemia, aplastic anemia***

INTEG: Rash, dermatitis, urticaria, ***Stevens-Johnson syndrome,*** erythema, photosensitivity, alopecia

GU: ***Renal failure, toxic nephrosis,*** increased BUN, creatinine, crystalluria, hematuria, proteinuria

CV: ***Allergic myocarditis***

Contraindications: Hypersensitivity to sulfonamides, sulfonylureas, thiazide and loop diuretics, salicylates, sunscreens with PABA, lactation, infants <2 mo (except congenital toxoplasmosis), pregnancy at term, porphyria

Precautions: Pregnancy (B), impaired hepatic function, severe allergy, bronchial asthma, renal dysfunction

Do not confuse:

sulfADIAZINE/sulfiSOXAZOLE

Pharmacokinetics:

PO: Rapidly absorbed, onset ½ hr; peak 3-6 hr, 30%-50% bound to plasma proteins, half-life 8-10 hr; excreted in urine, breast milk; crosses placenta, metabolized in liver

Interactions:
- ↑ hypoglycemic response: sulfonylurea agents
- ↑ anticoagulant effects: warfarin
- ↓ renal excretion of: methotrexate
- ↓ hepatic clearance of: phenytoin
- ↑ effects of: barbiturates, TOLBUTamide, uricosurics
- ↑ free-drug concentrations: indomethacin, probenecid, salicylates
- ↑ thrombocytopenia: thiazide diuretics
- ↑ nephrotoxicity; cycloSPORINE

Lab test interferences:

False positive: Urinary glucose test (Benedict's method)

NURSING CONSIDERATIONS

Assess:

- I&O ratio; note color, character, pH of urine if drug administered for UTIs; output should be 800 ml less than intake; if urine is highly acidic, alkalization may be needed
- Renal studies: BUN, creatinine, urinalysis (long-term therapy)
- Blood dyscrasias: skin rash, fever, sore throat, bruising, bleeding, fatigue, joint pain, monitor CBC before and periodically
- Allergic reaction: rash, dermatitis, urticaria, pruritus, dyspnea, bronchospasm

Administer:

- On an empty stomach
- With full glass of H_2O to maintain adequate hydration; increase fluids to 2 L/day to decrease crystallization in kidneys
- Medication after C&S; repeat C&S after full course of medication

Perform/provide:

- Storage in tight, light-resistant container at room temperature

Evaluate:

- Therapeutic response: absence of pain, fever, C&S negative

Teach patient/family:

- To take each oral dose with full glass of water to prevent crystalluria
- To complete full course of treatment to prevent superinfection
- To avoid sunlight or use sunscreen to prevent burns
- To avoid OTC medication (aspirin, vit C) unless directed by prescriber
- To notify prescriber of skin rash, sore throat, fever, mouth sores, unusual bruising, bleeding

sulfamethoxazole (℞)

(sul-fa-meth-ox′a-zole)

Apo-Sulfamethoxazole✱, Gantanol, Urobak

Func. class.: Antiinfective

Chem. class.: Sulfonamide, intermediate acting

Action: Interferes with bacterial biosynthesis of proteins by competitive antagonism of PABA

Uses: UTIs, chancroid, inclusion conjunctivitis, malaria, meningococcal meningitis, nocardiosis, acute otitis media, toxoplasmosis, trachoma

Dosage and routes:

- *Adult:* **PO** 2 g, then 1 g bid or tid for 7-10 days
- *Child>2 mo:* **PO** 50-60 mg/kg × 1 dose then 25-30 mg/kg bid, not to exceed 75 mg/kg/day

Renal dose

- *Adult:* **PO** CCr <50 ml/min give 50% of dose

Available forms: Tabs 500 mg, oral susp 500 mg/5 ml

Side effects/adverse reactions:

SYST: ***Anaphylaxis***

GI: Nausea, vomiting, abdominal pain, stomatitis, ***hepatitis,*** glossitis, pancreatitis, diarrhea, ***enterocolitis,*** anorexia

CNS: Headache, insomnia, hallucinations, depression, vertigo, fatigue, anxiety, ***convulsions, drug fever,*** chills, drowsiness

HEMA: ***Leukopenia, thrombocytopenia, agranulocytosis, hemolytic anemia, aplastic anemia***

INTEG: Rash, dermatitis, urticaria, ***Stevens-Johnson syndrome,*** erythema, photosensitivity, alopecia

GU: ***Renal failure, toxic nephrosis,*** increased BUN, creatinine, crystalluria, hematuria, proteinuria

CV: ***Allergic myocarditis***

Contraindications: Hypersensitivity to sulfonamides, sulfonylureas, thiazide and loop diuretics, salicylates, sunscreens with PABA, infants <2 mo (except congenital toxoplasmosis), pregnancy at term, porphyria, lactation, G6PD deficiency
Precautions: Pregnancy (C), lactation, impaired hepatic/renal function, severe allergy, bronchial asthma
Pharmacokinetics:
PO: Poorly absorbed, peak 3-4 hr, 50%-70% bound to plasma proteins, half-life 7-12 hr; excreted in urine (unchanged 90%), breast milk; crosses placenta
Interactions:
• ↑ effects of: barbiturates, uricosurics
• ↑ drug-free concentrations: indomethacin, probenecid, salicylates
• ↑ thrombocytopenia: thiazide diuretics
• ↑ nephrotoxicity: cycloSPORINE
• ↑ hypoglycemic response: sulfonylurea agents
• ↑ anticoagulant effects: warfarin
• ↓ renal excretion of methotrexate
• ↓ hepatic clearance of phenytoin
Lab test interferences:
False positive: Urinary glucose test (Benedict's method)
NURSING CONSIDERATIONS
Assess:
• I&O ratio; note color, character, pH of urine if drug administered for UTIs; output should be 800 ml less than intake; if urine is highly acidic, alkalization may be needed
• Renal studies: BUN, creatinine, urinalysis (long-term therapy)
• Blood dyscrasias: skin rash, fever, sore throat, bruising, bleeding, fatigue, joint pain, monitor CBC before and periodically
⬥ Allergic reaction: rash, dermatitis, urticaria, pruritus, dyspnea, bronchospasm
Administer:
PO route
• On empty stomach
• With full glass of H_2O to maintain adequate hydration; increase fluids to 2 L/day to decrease crystallization in kidneys
• Medication after C&S; repeat C&S after full course of medication
Perform/provide:
• Storage in tight, light-resistant container at room temperature
Evaluate:
• Therapeutic response: absence of pain, fever, C&S negative
Teach patient/family:
• To take each oral dose with full glass of H_2O to prevent crystalluria
• To complete full course of treatment to prevent superinfection
• To avoid sunlight or use sunscreen to prevent burns
• To avoid OTC medication (aspirin, vit C) unless directed by prescriber
⬥ To notify prescriber of skin rash, sore throat, fever, mouth sores, unusual bruising, bleeding

sulfasalazine (℞)

(sul-fa-sal'a-zeen)
Azulfidine, Azulfidine EN-tabs, PMS-Sulfasalazine✤, S.A.S.✤, Salazopyrin✤, sulfasalazine
Func. class.: GI antiinflammatory, antirheumatic (DMARD)
Chem. class.: Sulfonamide

Action: Prodrug to deliver sulfapyridine and 5-aminosalicylic acid to colon; antiinflammatory in connective tissue also
Uses: Ulcerative colitis; rheumatoid arthritis in patients who inadequately respond to or are intolerant of analgesics/NSAIDs; juvenile,

S

rheumatoid arthritis (Azulfidine EN-tabs)

Investigational uses: Ankylosing spondylitis, Crohn's disease, psoriasis

Dosage and routes:

Bowel disease

• *Adult:* **PO** 3-4 g/day in divided doses; maintenance 2 g/day in divided doses q6h

• *Child >2 yr:* **PO** 40-60 mg/kg/day in 4-6 divided doses, then 30 mg/kg/day in 4 doses, max 2 g/day

Rheumatoid arthritis

• *Adult:* **PO** 2 g/day in evenly divided doses, initiate treatment with a lower dose of enteric-coated tab

• *Child ≥2 yr:* **PO** 30 mg/kg/24 hr, divided into 4 doses

Renal dose

• *Adult:* **PO** CCr 10-30 ml/min give bid; CCr <10 ml/min give qd

Available forms: Tabs 500 mg; oral susp 250 mg/5 ml; tabs, del rel 500 mg

Side effects/adverse reactions:

SYST: ***Anaphylaxis***

GI: Nausea, vomiting, abdominal pain, stomatitis, ***hepatitis,*** glossitis, pancreatitis, diarrhea

CNS: Headache, confusion, insomnia, hallucinations, depression, vertigo, fatigue, anxiety, ***convulsions,*** drug fever, chills

HEMA: ***Leukopenia, neutropenia, thrombocytopenia, agranulocytosis, hemolytic anemia***

INTEG: Rash, dermatitis, urticaria, ***Stevens-Johnson syndrome,*** erythema, photosensitivity

GU: ***Renal failure, toxic nephrosis,*** increased BUN, creatinine, crystalluria

CV: ***Allergic myocarditis***

Contraindications: Hypersensitivity to sulfonamides or salicylates, pregnancy at term, child <2 yr, intestinal, urinary obstruction

Precautions: Pregnancy (C), lactation, impaired hepatic function, severe allergy, bronchial asthma, impaired renal function

Do not confuse:

sulfasalazine/sulfiSOXAZOLE

Pharmacokinetics:

PO: Partially absorbed, peak 1½-6 hr, duration 6-12 hr, half-life 6 hr, excreted in urine as sulfasalazine (15%), sulfapyridine (60%), 5-aminosalicylic acid and metabolites (20%-33%), in breast milk; crosses placenta

Interactions:

• ↓ absorption of digoxin

• ↑ hypoglycemic response: oral hypoglycemics

• ↑ anticoagulant effects: oral anticoagulants

• ↓ renal excretion of methotrexate

• ↓ hepatic clearance of phenytoin

• Drug/food: ↓ iron/folic acid absorption

Lab test interferences:

False positive: Urinary glucose test

NURSING CONSIDERATIONS

Assess:

• Renal studies: BUN, creatinine, urinalysis (long-term therapy)

Blood dyscrasias: skin rash, fever, sore throat, bruising, bleeding, fatigue, joint pain; monitor CBC before and q3mo

Allergic reaction: rash, dermatitis, urticaria, pruritus, dyspnea, bronchospasm

Administer:

• With full glass of H_2O to maintain adequate hydration; increase fluids to 2 L/day to decrease crystallization in kidneys

• Total daily dose in evenly spaced doses and after meals to help minimize GI intolerance

Perform/provide:

• Storage in tight, light-resistant container at room temperature

Evaluate:
• Therapeutic response: absence of fever, mucus in stools, pain in joints
Teach patient/family:
• To take each oral dose with full glass of H_2O to prevent crystalluria
• That contact lens, urine/skin may be yellow-orange
• To avoid sunlight or use sunscreen to prevent burns
• To notify prescriber of skin rash, sore throat, fever, mouth sores, unusual bruising, bleeding

sulfinpyrazone (℞)

(sul-fin-peer'a-zone)
Anturan✤, Anturane, sulfinpyrazone
Func. class.: Uricosuric
Chem. class.: Pyrazolone

Action: Inhibits tubular reabsorption of urates, with increased excretion of uric acid; inhibits prostaglandin synthesis, which decreases platelet aggregation
Uses: Inhibition of platelet aggregation, gout
Dosage and routes:
Inhibition of platelet aggregation
• *Adult:* **PO** 200 mg qid
Gout/gouty arthritis
• *Adult:* **PO** 100-200 mg bid × 1 wk, then 200-400 mg bid, not to exceed 800 mg/day
Available forms: Tabs 100 mg; caps 200 mg
Side effects/adverse reactions:
CNS: Dizziness, ***convulsions, coma***
EENT: Tinnitus
GU: Renal calculi, hypoglycemia
GI: Gastric irritation, nausea, vomiting, anorexia, ***hepatic necrosis, GI bleeding***
INTEG: Rash, dermatitis, pruritus, fever, photosensitivity
HEMA: ***Agranulocytosis*** (rare)
RESP: ***Apnea,*** irregular respirations
Contraindications: Hypersensitivity to pyrazolone derivatives, blood dyscrasias, CCr <50 ml/min, active peptic ulcer, GI inflammation
Precautions: Pregnancy (C)
Pharmacokinetics:
PO: Peak 1-2 hr, duration 4-6 hr, half-life 4 hr; metabolized by liver, excreted in urine
Interactions:
• ↑ toxicity: acetaminophen
• ↑ effects of: warfarin, TOLBUTamide
• ↓ effects of: verapamil, theophylline
• ↓ effects of sulfinpyrazone: salicylates, niacin
Lab test interferences:
Increase: PSP, aminohippuric acid
False positive: Clinitest
NURSING CONSIDERATIONS
Assess:
• Uric acid levels (3-7 mg/dl); joint mobility, pain, swelling
• Respiratory rate, rhythm, depth; notify prescriber of abnormalities
• Renal function
• Bleeding tendencies, RBC, Hct
• I&O
• Electrolytes, CO_2 before, during treatment
• Urine pH, output, glucose during beginning treatment
Administer:
• With glass of milk
• With food for GI symptoms
• Increased fluids to prevent calculi; alkalinization of urine may be required
Evaluate:
• Therapeutic response: absence of pain, stiffness in joints
Teach patient/family:
• To avoid aspirin, alcohol, high-purine diet

*sulfiSOXAZOLE (℞)

(sul-fi-sox'a-zole)

Gantrisin, Novo-Soxazole♣, sulfiSOXAZOLE, Gantrisin Pediatric

Func. class.: Antiinfective

Chem. class.: Sulfonamide, short acting

Action: Interferes with bacterial biosynthesis of proteins by competitive antagonism of PABA

Uses: Urinary tract, systemic infections; chancroid; trachoma; toxoplasmosis; acute otitis media, malaria, *Haemophilus influenzae* meningitis, meningococcal meningitis, nocardiosis, eye infections

Dosage and routes:

UTIs, other systemic infections

• *Adult:* **PO** 2-4 g loading dose, then 1-2 g qid × 7-10 days

• *Child >2 mo:* **PO** 75 mg/kg or 2 g/m^2 loading dose, then 120-150 mg/kg/day or 4 g/m^2/day in divided doses q6h, not to exceed 6 g/day

Chlamydia trachomatis

• *Adult:* **PO** 500 mg-1 g qid × 3 wk

Renal dose

• *Adult:* **PO** CCr 10-50 ml/min give q8-12h; CCr <10 ml/min give q12-24h

Available forms: Tabs 500 mg; liquid 500 mg/5 ml

Side effects/adverse reactions:

SYST: ***Anaphylaxis***

GI: Nausea, vomiting, abdominal pain, stomatitis, ***hepatitis,*** glossitis, pancreatitis, diarrhea, ***enterocolitis,*** anorexia

CNS: Headache, insomnia, hallucinations, depression, vertigo, fatigue, anxiety, ***seizures,*** drug fever, chills, drowsiness

HEMA: ***Leukopenia, thrombocytopenia, agranulocytosis, hemolytic anemia, aplastic anemia***

INTEG: Rash, dermatitis, urticaria, ***Stevens-Johnson syndrome,*** erythema, photosensitivity, alopecia

GU: ***Renal failure, toxic nephrosis,*** increased BUN, creatinine, crystalluria, hematuria, proteinuria

CV: ***Allergic myocarditis***

Contraindications: Hypersensitivity to sulfonamides and sulfonylureas, thiazide and loop diuretics, salicylates; sunscreen with PABA, lactation, infants < 2 mo (except congenital toxoplasmosis), pregnancy at term, porphyria

Precautions: Pregnancy (B), lactation, impaired hepatic/renal function, severe allergy, bronchial asthma

Do not confuse:

sulfiSOXAZOLE/sulfasalazine

sulfiSOXAZOLE/sulfADIAZINE

Pharmacokinetics:

PO: Rapidly absorbed, peak 2-4 hr, 85% protein bound; half-life 4-7 hr, excreted in urine, crosses placenta

Interactions:

• ↑ effects of: barbiturates, TOLBUTamide, uricosurics

• ↑ free-drug concentrations: indomethacin, probenecid, salicylates

• ↑ thrombocytopenia: thiazides

• ↑ nephrotoxicity: cycloSPORINE

• ↑ hypoglycemic response: sulfonylurea agents

• ↑ anticoagulant effect: warfarin

• ↓ renal excretion of methotrexate

• ↓ hepatic clearance of phenytoin

Lab test interferences:

False positive: Urinary glucose test

NURSING CONSIDERATIONS

Assess:

• I&O ratio; note color, character, pH of urine if drug administered for UTIs; output should be 800 ml less than intake; if urine is highly acidic, alkalization may be needed

• Renal studies: BUN, creatinine, urinalysis (long-term therapy)

◆ Blood dyscrasias: skin rash, fever, sore throat, bruising, bleeding, fatigue, joint pain, monitor CBC before and periodically

◆ Allergic reaction: rash, dermatitis, urticaria, pruritus, dyspnea, bronchospasm

Administer:

- On an empty stomach
- With full glass of H_2O to maintain adequate hydration; increase fluids to 2 L/day to decrease crystallization in kidneys
- Medication after C&S; repeat C&S after full course of medication

Perform/provide:

- Storage in tight, light-resistant container at room temperature

Evaluate:

- Therapeutic response: absence of pain, fever, C&S negative

Teach patient/family:

- To take each oral dose with full glass of H_2O to prevent crystalluria
- To complete full course of treatment to prevent superinfection
- To avoid sunlight or use sunscreen to prevent burns; avoid hazardous activities if dizziness occurs
- To avoid OTC medication (aspirin, vit C) unless directed by prescriber
- To notify prescriber of skin rash, sore throat, fever, mouth sores, unusual bruising, bleeding

sulindac (℞)

(sul-in'dak)

Apo-Sulin✱, Clinoril, NovoSundac✱, sulindac

Func. class.: Nonsteroidal antiinflammatory, antirheumatic

Chem. class.: Indeneacetic acid derivative

Action: Inhibits prostaglandin synthesis by decreasing an enzyme needed for biosynthesis; analgesic, antiinflammatory, antipyretic

Uses: Mild to moderate pain, osteoarthritis; rheumatoid, gouty arthritis; ankylosing spondylitis

Dosage and routes:

Arthritis

- *Adult:* **PO** 150 mg bid, may increase to 200 mg bid

Bursitis/acute arthritis

- *Adult:* **PO** 200 mg bid × 1-2 wk, then reduce dose

Available forms: Tabs 150, 200 mg

Side effects/adverse reactions:

GI: Nausea, anorexia, vomiting, diarrhea, jaundice, ***cholestatic hepatitis,*** constipation, flatulence, cramps, dry mouth, peptic ulcer, ***bleeding, ulceration, perforation***

CNS: Dizziness, drowsiness, fatigue, tremors, confusion, insomnia, anxiety, depression, headache

CV: Tachycardia, peripheral edema, palpitations, dysrhythmias

INTEG: Purpura, *rash, pruritus,* sweating, photosensitivity

GU: ***Nephrotoxicity: dysuria, hematuria, oliguria, azotemia***

HEMA: ***Blood dyscrasias*** with prolonged use

EENT: Tinnitus, hearing loss, blurred vision

Contraindications: Hypersensitivity, asthma, severe renal disease, severe hepatic disease, active ulcers

Precautions: Pregnancy (C) 1st trimester, lactation, children, bleeding disorders, GI disorders, cardiac disorders, hypersensitivity to other antiinflammatory agents, renal disease

Do not confuse:

Clinoril/Clozaril

Clinoril/Oruvail

Pharmacokinetics:

PO: Peak 2 hr, half-life 3-3½ hr; metabolized in liver; excreted in urine (metabolites), breast milk; 93% protein binding

S

Interactions:
• ↑ bleeding risk: anticoagulants, thrombolytics, plicamycin, tirofiban, eptifibatide, clopidogrel, ticlopidine, valproic acid, some cephalosporins
• ↑ nephrotoxicity: cycloSPORINE
• ↓ sulindac effect: diflunisal, do not use together
• ↑ toxicity: methotrexate, sulfonamides, sulfonylureas, probenecid
• GI side effects: aspirin, corticosteroids, other NSAIDs
↑ gastric irritation: arginine, gossypol
↑ NSAIDs effect: bearberry, bilberry
↑ bleeding risk: bogbean, chondroitin

NURSING CONSIDERATIONS
Assess:
• Pain: frequency, intensity, characteristics, relief after med
Asthma, aspirin hypersensitivity, nasal polyps; increased hypersensitivity
• Renal, hepatic studies: BUN, creatinine, AST, ALT, Hgb, before treatment, periodically thereafter
• Have B/P checked qmo; drug causes sodium retention
• Audiometric, ophthalmic exam before, during, after treatment
• For eye, ear problems: blurred vision, tinnitus may indicate toxicity

Administer:
• With food to decrease GI symptoms; take on empty stomach to facilitate absorption; tablet may be crushed

Perform/provide:
• Storage at room temperature

Evaluate:
• Therapeutic response: decreased pain, stiffness, swelling in joints, ability to move more easily

Teach patient/family:
• To report blurred vision or ringing, roaring in ears (may indicate toxicity)
• To avoid driving, other hazardous activities if dizzy or drowsy
• To report change in urine pattern, weight increase, edema, pain increase in joints, fever, blood in urine (indicates nephrotoxicity)
• That therapeutic effects may take up to 1 mo
• To avoid alcohol and aspirin
• To take with full glass of water
• To use sunscreen

sumatriptan (℞)
(soo-ma-trip'tan)
Imitrex
Func. class.: Antimigraine agent
Chem. class.: 5-HT_1 receptor agonist

Action: Binds selectively to the vascular 5-HT_1 receptor subtype, exerts antimigraine effect; causes vasoconstriction in cranial arteries

Uses: Acute treatment of migraine with or without aura and cluster headache

Dosage and routes:
• *Adult:* **SC** 6 mg or less; may repeat in 1 hr; not to exceed 12 mg/24 hr; **PO** 25 mg with fluids, max 100 mg; **NASAL** one dose of 5, 10, or 20 mg in one nostril, may repeat in 2 hr, max 40 mg/24 hr

Hepatic dose
• *Adult:* **PO** 25 mg, if no response after 2 hr, give up to 50 mg

Available forms: Inj 12 mg/ml; tabs 25, 50, 100 mg, nasal spray 5 mg/100 mcl-U dose spray device, 20 mg/100 mcl-U

Side effects/adverse reactions:
CNS: Tingling, hot sensation, burning, feeling of pressure, tightness, numbness, dizziness, sedation, headache, anxiety, fatigue, cold sensation
*CV: Flushing, **MI***

RESP: Chest tightness, pressure
EENT: Throat, mouth, nasal discomfort; vision changes
GI: Abdominal discomfort
MS: *Weakness, neck stiffness,* myalgia
INTEG: Inj site reaction, sweating

Contraindications: Angina pectoris, history of MI, documented silent ischemia, Prinzmetal's angina, ischemic heart disease, IV use, concurrent ergotamine-containing preparations, uncontrolled hypertension, hypersensitivity, basilar or hemiplegic migraine

Precautions: Postmenopausal women, men >40 yr, risk factors for CAD, hypercholesterolemia, obesity, diabetes, impaired hepatic or renal function, pregnancy (C), lactation, children, elderly

Pharmacokinetics: Onset of pain relief 10 min-2 hr, peak 10-20 min, 10%-20% plasma protein binding, metabolized in the liver (metabolite), excreted in urine, feces

Interactions:
- Extended vasospastic effects: ergot, ergot derivatives
- ↑ sumatriptan effect: MAOIs, SSRIs

Serotonin syndrome: SAM-e, St. John's wort
↑ effect: butterbur

NURSING CONSIDERATIONS

Assess:
- B/P; signs/symptoms of coronary vasospasms
- Tingling, hot sensation, burning, feeling of pressure, numbness, flushing, inj site reaction
- For stress level, activity, recreation, coping mechanisms
- Neurologic status: LOC, blurring vision, nausea, vomiting, tingling in extremities preceding headache
- Ingestion of tyramine foods (pickled products, beer, wine, aged cheese), food additives, preservatives, colorings, artificial sweeteners, chocolate, caffeine, which may precipitate these types of headaches

Administer:
- SC only just below the skin; avoid IM or IV administration, use only for actual migraine attack

⊘ PO, swallow whole; take with fluids as soon as symptoms appear; may take a second dose >4 hr; max 200 mg/24 hr

Perform/provide:
- Quiet, calm environment with decreased stimulation for noise, bright light, excessive talking

Evaluate:
- Therapeutic response: decrease in frequency, severity of migraine

Teach patient/family:
- To report chest pain, tightness; sudden, severe abdominal pain to prescriber immediately
- To use contraception while taking drug
- To use nasal spray: one spray in one nostril, may repeat if headache returns, do not repeat if pain continues after 1st dose
- To have dark, quiet environment

suprofen ophthalmic
See appendix c

tacrine (℞)
(tack′rin)
Cognex
Func. class.: Anti-Alzheimer agent
Chem. class.: Reversible cholinesterase inhibitor

Action: Elevates acetylcholine concentrations (cerebral cortex) by slowing degradation of acetylcholine released in cholinergic neurons; does not alter underlying dementia

Uses: Treatment of mild to moderate dementia in Alzheimer's disease

Dosage and routes:

• *Adult:* **PO** 10 mg qid × 6 wk, then 20 mg qid × 6 wk, increase at 6-wk intervals if patient tolerating drug well and if transaminase is WNL

Available forms: Caps 10, 20, 30, 40 mg

Side effects/adverse reactions:

CNS: Dizziness, confusion, insomnia, tremor, *ataxia, somnolence, anxiety, agitation, depression, hallucinations, hostility, abnormal thinking,* chills, fever

CV: Hypotension or hypertension

GI: Nausea, vomiting, anorexia, abdominal pain, constipation, dyspepsia, flatulence, ***hepatotoxicity, GI bleeding***

GU: Urinary frequency, UTI, incontinence

INTEG: Rash, flushing

RESP: Rhinitis, URI, cough, pharyngitis

Contraindications: Hypersensitivity to this drug or acridine derivatives, patients treated with this drug who developed jaundice with a total bilirubin of >3 mg/dl

Precautions: Sick sinus syndrome, history of ulcers, GI bleeding, hepatic disease, bladder obstruction, asthma, pregnancy (C), lactation, children, seizure disorders

Do not confuse:

Cognex/Corgard

Pharmacokinetics: Rapidly absorbed PO, 55% bound to plasma proteins, extensively metabolized to metabolites by CYP450 enzyme system, elimination half-life 2-4 hr

Interactions:

• ↓ activity of anticholinergics
• ↑ tacrine levels: cimetidine
• ↑ elimination half-life of theophylline
• Synergistic effect: succinylcholine, cholinesterase inhibitors, cholinergic agonists

NURSING CONSIDERATIONS

Assess:

• B/P: hypotension, hypertension
• Mental status: affect, mood, behavioral changes, depression; complete suicide assessment; hallucinations, confusion
• GI status: nausea, vomiting, anorexia, constipation, abdominal pain; add bulk, increase fluids for constipation
• GU status: urinary frequency, incontinence
• Serum ALT qo wk × 4-16 wk, then q3mo

Administer:

• Between meals; may be given with meals for GI symptoms
• Dosage adjusted to response no more than q6wk

Perform/provide:

• Assistance with ambulation during beginning therapy; dizziness, ataxia may occur

Evaluate:

• Therapeutic response: decrease in confusion, improved mood

Teach patient/family:

• To report side effects: twitching, eye spasms; indicate overdose
• To use drug exactly as prescribed: at regular intervals, preferably between meals; may be taken with meals for GI upset; drug is not a cure
• To notify prescriber of nausea, vomiting, diarrhea (dose increase or beginning treatment), or rash; very dark or very light stools, jaundice (delayed onset)
• Not to increase or abruptly decrease dose; serious consequences may result

Treatment of overdose: Withdraw drug, administer tertiary anticholinergics, provide supportive care

tacrolimus (℞)

(tak-roe-li'mus)
Prograf

tacrolimus topical

Protopic
Func. class.: Immunosuppressant
Chem. class.: Macrolide

Action: Produces immunosuppression by inhibiting T-lymphocytes
Uses: Organ transplants to prevent rejection; topical: atopic dermatitis
Investigational uses: Autoimmune diseases, severe recalcitrant psoriasis
Dosage and routes:
• *Adult and child:* **IV** 0.03-0.05 mg/kg/day × 3 days then **PO** 0.15 mg/kg bid; adjust dose in renal impairment
• *Adult:* **TOP** apply ointment bid × 7 days
• *Child ≥2-15 yr:* apply ointment bid × 7 days
Available forms: Inj 5 mg/ml; caps 0.5, 1, 5 mg; ointment 0.03%, 0.1%
Side effects/adverse reactions:
HEMA: ***Anemia, leukocytosis, thrombocytopenia, purpura***
GI: Nausea, vomiting, diarrhea, constipation, ***GI bleeding***
CV: Hypertension
CNS: Tremors, headache, insomnia, paresthesia, chills, fever, ***seizures***
GU: UTIs, ***albuminuria, hematuria, proteinuria, renal failure***
META: Hirsutism, hyperglycemia, hyperkalemia, hyperuricemia, hypokalemia, hypomagnesemia
RESP: ***Pleural effusion, atelectasis,*** dyspnea
INTEG: Rash, flushing, itching, alopecia
EENT: Blurred vision, photophobia
SYST: ***Anaphylaxis***

Contraindications: Hypersensitivity to this drug or to some kinds of castor oil
Precautions: Severe renal, hepatic disease; pregnancy (C), diabetes mellitus, hyperkalemia, hyperuricemia, lymphomas, lactation, children <12, hypertension
Pharmacokinetics: Extensively metabolized, half-life 10 hr, 75% protein binding
Interactions:
• ↑ toxicity: aminoglycosides, cisplatin, cycloSPORINE
• ↑ blood levels: antifungals, calcium channel blockers, cimetidine, danazol, erythromycin, mycophenolate, mofetil
• ↓ blood levels: carbamazepine, phenobarbital, phenytoin, rifamycin
• ↓ effect of: vaccines
↓ immunosuppression: astragalus, echinacea, melatonin
↓ effect: ginseng, maitake, mistletoe

NURSING CONSIDERATIONS
Assess:
• Blood studies: Hgb, WBC, platelets during treatment qmo; if leukocytes <3000/mm^3 or platelets <100,000/mm^3, drug should be discontinued or reduced; decreased hemoglobulin level may indicate bone marrow suppression
• Hepatic studies: alk phosphatase, AST, ALT, amylase, bilirubin, and for hepatotoxicity: dark urine, jaundice, itching, light-colored stools; drug should be discontinued
Administer:
• All medications PO if possible, avoiding IM inj; bleeding may occur
• With meals to reduce GI upset; nausea is common
• For several days before transplant surgery; patients should be placed in protective isolation

◆ Anaphylaxis: rash, pruritus, wheezing, laryngeal edema; stop infusion, initiate emergency procedures

IV route

• After diluting in 0.9% NaCl or D_5W to 0.004 to 0.02 mg/ml as a continuous infusion

Additive compatibilities: Cimetidine

Y-site compatibilities: Acyclovir, aminophylline, amphotericin B, ampicillin, ampicillin/sulbactam, benztropine, calcium gluconate, cefazolin, cefotetan, ceftazidime, ceftriaxone, cefuroxime, chloramphenicol, cimetidine, ciprofloxacin, clindamycin, dexamethasone, digoxin, diphenhydrAMINE, DOBUTamine, DOPamine, doxycycline, erythromycin, esmolol, fluconazole, furosemide, ganciclovir, gentamicin, haloperidol, heparin, hydrocortisone, imipenem/cilastatin, insulin (regular), isoproterenol, leucovorin, lorazepam, methylPREDNISolone, metoclopramide, metronidazole, mezlocillin, multivitamins, nitroglycerin, oxacillin, penicillin G potassium, perphenazine, phenytoin, piperacillin, potassium chloride, propranolol, ranitidine, sodium bicarbonate, sodium nitroprusside, trimethoprim - sulfamethoxazole, vancomycin

Evaluate:

• Therapeutic response: absence of graft rejection; immunosuppression in autoimmune disorders

Teach patient/family:

• To report fever, rash, severe diarrhea, chills, sore throat, fatigue; serious infections may occur; clay-colored stools, cramping (hepatotoxicity)

• To avoid crowds, persons with known infections to reduce risk of infection

tamoxifen (℞)

(ta-mox′i-fen)

Alpha-Tamoxifen✤, Med Tamoxifen✤, Nolvadex, Nolvadex-D✤, Novo-Tamoxifen✤, Tamofen✤, Tamone✤, Tamoplex✤

Func. class.: Antineoplastic

Chem. class.: Antiestrogen hormone

Action: Inhibits cell division by binding to cytoplasmic estrogen receptors; resembles normal cell complex but inhibits DNA synthesis and estrogen response of target tissue

Uses: Advanced breast carcinoma not responsive to other therapy in estrogen-receptor-positive patients (usually postmenopausal), prevention of breast cancer, following breast surgery/radiation in ductal carcinoma in situ

Investigational uses: Mastalgia, to reduce pain/size of gynecomastia, ovulation stimulation, malignant carcinoid tumor, carcinoid syndrome

Dosage and routes:

Breast cancer

• *Adult:* **PO** 20-40 mg qd; doses >20 mg/day, divide AM/PM

High risk for breast cancer

• *Adult:* **PO** 20 mg qd × 5 yr

DCIS

• *Adult:* **PO** 20 mg qd × 5 yr

Available forms: Tabs 10, 20 mg

Side effects/adverse reactions:

HEMA: ***Thrombocytopenia, leukopenia,*** DVT, PE

GI: Nausea, vomiting, altered taste (anorexia)

GU: Vaginal bleeding, pruritus vulvae

INTEG: Rash, alopecia

CV: Chest pain

CNS: Hot flashes, headache, lightheadedness, depression

META: Hypercalcemia
EENT: Ocular lesions, retinopathy, corneal opacity, blurred vision (high doses)
Contraindications: Hypersensitivity, pregnancy (D)
Precautions: Leukopenia, thrombocytopenia, lactation, cataracts
Pharmacokinetics:
PO: Peak 4-7 hr, half-life 7 days (1 wk terminal), excreted primarily in feces
Interactions:
- ↑ chance of bleeding: anticoagulants
- ↑ tamoxifen levels: bromocriptine
- ↑ thromboembolic events: cytotoxics
- ↓ tamoxifen levels: aminoglutethimide, medroxyprogesterone, rifamycin
- ↓ letrozole levels: letrozole

Lab test interferences:
Increase: Serum calcium

NURSING CONSIDERATIONS
Assess:
- CBC, differential, platelet count qwk; withhold drug if WBC is <3500 or platelet count is <100,000; notify prescriber
- Bleeding q8h: hematuria, guaiac, bruising, petechiae, mucosa or orifices
- Effects of alopecia on body image; discuss feelings about body changes
- ⬥ For uterine malignancies, symptoms of stroke, pulmonary embolism that may occur in women with ductal carcinoma in situ (DCIS) and women at high risk for breast cancer
- ⬥ Symptoms indicating severe allergic reactions: rash, pruritus, urticaria, purpuric skin lesions, itching, flushing

Administer:
- Antacid before oral agent; give drug after evening meal, before bedtime
- Antiemetic 30-60 min before giving drug to prevent vomiting
- ⊘ Do not crush, break, chew tabs

Perform/provide:
- Liquid diet, if needed, including cola, Jell-O; dry toast or crackers may be added if patient is not nauseated or vomiting
- Increase fluid intake to 2-3 L/day to prevent dehydration
- Nutritious diet with iron, vitamin supplements as ordered
- Storage in light-resistant container at room temperature

Evaluate:
- Therapeutic response: decreased tumor size, spread of malignancy

Teach patient/family:
- To report any complaints, side effects to prescriber
- To increase fluids to 2 L/day unless contraindicated
- To wear sun screen, protective clothing, sunglasses
- That vaginal bleeding, pruritus, hot flashes are reversible after discontinuing treatment
- To report immediately decreased visual acuity, which may be irreversible; stress need for routine eye exams; care providers should be told about tamoxifen therapy
- To report vaginal bleeding immediately
- That tumor flare—increase in size of tumor, increased bone pain—may occur and will subside rapidly; may take analgesics for pain
- That premenopausal women must use mechanical birth control because ovulation may be induced
- That hair may be lost during treatment; a wig or hairpiece may make patient feel better; new hair may be different in color, texture

tamsulosin (℞)

(tam-sue-lo′sen)

Flomax

Func. class.: Selective α_1-adrenergic blocker

Chem. class.: Sulfamoylphenethylamine derivative

Action: Binds preferentially to α_{1A}-adrenoceptor subtype located mainly in the prostate

Uses: Symptoms of benign prostatic hyperplasia

Dosage and routes:

• *Adult:* **PO** 0.4 mg qd, increasing up to 0.8 mg qd if required

Available forms: Caps 0.4 mg

Side effects/adverse reactions:

CV: Chest pain

CNS: Dizziness, headache, asthenia

GI: Nausea, diarrhea

GU: Decreased libido, abnormal ejaculation

EENT: Amblyopia

MS: Back pain

RESP: Rhinitis, pharyngitis, cough

Contraindications: Hypersensitivity

Precautions: Pregnancy (C), children, lactation, hepatic disease, coronary artery disease, severe renal disease

Pharmacokinetics:

PO: Onset 2 hr, peak 2-6 hr, duration 6-12 hr; half-life 9-15 hr; metabolized in liver; excreted via urine; extensively protein bound (98%)

Interactions:

• Not to be taken with: prazosin, terazosin, doxazosin

NURSING CONSIDERATIONS

Assess:

• Prostatic hyperplasia: change in urinary patterns, baseline and throughout treatment

• CBC with diff and LFTs; B/P and heart rate

• BUN, uric acid, urodynamic studies (urinary flow rates, residual volume)

• I&O ratios, weight qd, edema, report weight gain or edema

Administer:

PO route

• Whole; do not chew or crush tablets; may be given with food ½ hr after same meal each day

Perform/provide:

• Storage in tight container in cool environment

Evaluate:

• Therapeutic response: decreased symptoms of benign prostatic hyperplasia

Teach patient/family:

• Not to drive or operate machinery for 4 hr after first dose or after dosage increase

tegaserod (℞)

(teg-as′er-odd)

Zelnorm

Func. class.: 5-HT_4 receptor partial agonist, misc. GI agent

Action: A 5-HT_4 receptor partial agonist that binds 5-HT_4 receptors, stimulating peristalsis and intestinal secretion

Uses: Irritable bowel symdrome (IBS) where primary bowel symptom is constipation

Dosage and routes:

• *Adult:* **PO** 6 mg bid before meals × 4-6 wk, another 4-6 wk course may be used

Available forms: Tabs 2, 6 mg

Side effects/adverse reactions:

SYST: ***Anaphylaxis***

GI: Nausea, abdominal pain, increased appetite, eructation, increased AST, increased ALT, diar-

rhea, irritable colon, tenesmus, flatulence

CNS: Headache, dizziness, depression, vertigo, fatigue, suicide attempt, poor concentration

MISC: Pain, facial edema, increased CPK, asthma, breast carcinoma

MS: Back pain, arthralgia

GU: Polyuria, renal pain, ovarian cyst, miscarriage, albuminuria

CV: Hypotension, angina, ***dysrrhythmias, bundle branch block, supraventricular tachycardia***

Contraindications: Hypersensitivity, severe renal disease, moderate to severe hepatic disease, history of bowel obstruction, gallbladder disease, abdominal adhesions, sphincter of Oddi dysfunction

Precautions: Pregnancy (B), lactation, children, diarrhea

Pharmacokinetics: Peak 1 hr, 98% protein binding, terminal half-life 11 hr, ⅔ excreted unchanged in feces, remainder in urine as metabolite

Interactions:

- ↓ effect of: digoxin, oral contraceptives
- Drug/food: Food ↓ absorption, but is minimized when taken ½ hr before meal

NURSING CONSIDERATIONS

Assess:

- GI symptoms: nausea, abdominal pain
- CV status: B/P, pulse, chest pain

Administer:

- Before meals, bid

Perform/provide:

- Store at room temperature

Evaluate:

- Therapeutic response: Decreased constipation in IBS

Teach patient/family:

- To notify prescriber of GI symptoms, hypersensitivity reactions

telmisartan (℞)

(tel-mih-sar′tan)

Micardis

Func. class.: Antihypertensive

Chem. class.: Angiotensin II receptor (Type AT_1)

Action: blocks the vasoconstrictor and aldosterone-secreting effects of angiotensin II; selectively blocks the binding of angiotensin II to the AT_1 receptor found in tissues

Uses: Hypertension, alone or in combination

Investigational uses: Heart failure

Research note: Telmisartan administered with digoxin resulted in an increased digoxin level[37]

Dosage and routes:

- *Adult:* **PO** 40 mg qd; range 20-80 mg

Available forms: Tabs 20, 40, 80 mg

Side effects/adverse reactions:

CNS: Dizziness, insomnia, *anxiety,* headache, fatigue

GI: Diarrhea, dyspepsia, *anorexia, vomiting*

MS: Myalgia, pain

RESP: Cough, *upper respiratory infection,* sinusitis, pharyngitis

Contraindications: Hypersensitivity, pregnancy (D) 2nd/3rd trimesters

Precautions: Hypersensitivity to ACE inhibitors: pregnancy (C) 1st trimester, lactation, children, elderly

Pharmacokinetics: Extensively metabolized, terminal half-life 24 hr, highly bound to plasma proteins, excreted feces >97%

Interactions:

- ↑ digoxin peak/trough concentrations: digoxin
- ↑ antihypertensive action: diuretics, other antihypertensives
- ↑ toxicity, death: aconite

T

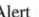

↑ or ↓ antihypertensive effect: astragalus, cola tree

↑ antihypertensive effect: barberry, betony, black catechu, black cohosh, bloodroot, broom, burdock, cat's claw, dandelion, goldenseal, Irish moss, Jamaican dogwood, kelp, khella, mistletoe, parsley

↓ antihypertensive effect: coltsfoot, guarana, khat, licorice

NURSING CONSIDERATIONS

Assess:

- B/P, pulse q4h; note rate, rhythm, quality
- Electrolytes: K, Na, Cl
- Baselines in renal, hepatic studies before therapy begins
- Edema in feet, legs qd
- Skin turgor, dryness of mucous membranes for hydration status

Administer:

- Without regard to meals
- Increased dose to black patients, B/P response may be reduced

Evaluate:

- Therapeutic response: decreased B/P

Teach patient/family:

- To comply with dosage schedule, even if feeling better
- To notify prescriber of mouth sores, fever, swelling of hands or feet, irregular heartbeat, chest pain
- That excessive perspiration, dehydration, vomiting, diarrhea may lead to fall in blood pressure; consult prescriber if these occur
- That drug may cause dizziness, fainting; light-headedness may occur
- To use contraception while taking this drug
- To notify prescriber of all prescriptions, OTC, and supplements taken

temazepam (℞)

(te-maz′e-pam)

Razepam, Restoril, temazepam

Func. class.: Sedative-hypnotic

Chem. class.: Benzodiazepine

Controlled Substance Schedule IV (USA), Schedule F (Canada)

Action: Produces CNS depression at limbic, thalamic, hypothalamic levels of the CNS; may be mediated by neurotransmitter γ-aminobutyric acid (GABA); results are sedation, hypnosis, skeletal muscle relaxation, anticonvulsant activity, anxiolytic action

Uses: Insomnia

Dosage and routes:

- *Adult:* **PO** 15-30 mg hs
- *Geriatric:* **PO** 7.5 mg hs

Available forms: Caps 7.5, 15, 30 mg

Side effects/adverse reactions:

HEMA: ***Leukopenia, granulocytopenia*** (rare)

CNS: Lethargy, drowsiness, daytime sedation, dizziness, confusion, lightheadedness, headache, anxiety, irritability

GI: Nausea, vomiting, diarrhea, heartburn, abdominal pain, constipation, anorexia

CV: Chest pain, pulse changes

Contraindications: Hypersensitivity to benzodiazepines, pregnancy (X), lactation, intermittent porphyria

Precautions: Anemia, hepatic disease, renal disease, suicidal individuals, drug abuse, elderly, psychosis, children <15 yr, acute narrow-angle glaucoma, seizure disorders

Pharmacokinetics:

PO: Onset 30-45 min, duration 6-8 hr, half-life 10-20 hr; metabolized by liver, excreted by kidneys, crosses placenta, excreted in breast milk

Interactions:

- ↑ effects of cimetidine, disulfiram, oral contraceptives
- ↑ action of both drugs: alcohol, CNS depressants
- ↓ effect of antacids, theophylline, rifampin

↑ CNS depression: catnip, chamomile, clary, cowslip, hops, kava, lavender, mistletoe, nettle, pokeweed, poppy, Queen Anne's lace, senega, skullcap, valerian

↑ hypotension: black cohosh

Lab test interferences:

Increase: ALT, AST, serum bilirubin

Decrease: RAI uptake

False increase: Urinary 17-OHCS

NURSING CONSIDERATIONS

Assess:

- Blood studies: Hct, Hgb, RBCs (long-term therapy)
- Hepatic studies: AST, ALT, bilirubin (long-term therapy)
- Mental status: mood, sensorium, affect, memory (long, short)

Blood dyscrasias: fever, sore throat, bruising, rash, jaundice, epistaxis (rare)

- Type of sleep problem: falling asleep, staying asleep

Administer:

- After removal of cigarettes to prevent fires
- After trying conservative measures for insomnia
- ½-1 hr before hs for sleeplessness
- On empty stomach for fast onset, but may be taken with food if GI symptoms occur

Perform/provide:

- Assistance with ambulation after receiving dose
- Safety measures: night-light, call bell within easy reach
- Checking to see if PO medication has been swallowed
- Storage in tight container in cool environment

Evaluate:

- Therapeutic response: ability to sleep at night, decreased early morning awakening if taking drug for insomnia

Teach patient/family:

- To avoid driving, other activities requiring alertness until stabilized
- To avoid alcohol ingestion, CNS depressants; serious CNS depression may result
- That effects may take 2 nights for benefits to be noticed
- Alternative measures to improve sleep: reading, exercise several hours before hs, warm bath, warm milk, TV, self-hypnosis, deep breathing
- That hangover, memory impairment are common in elderly but less common than with barbiturates
- To use contraception while taking this product

Treatment of overdose: Lavage, activated charcoal; monitor electrolytes, VS

temozolomide (℞)

(tem-oh-zole′oh-mide)

Temodar

Func. class.: Antineoplastic-alkylating agent

Chem. class.: Imidazotetrazine derivative

Action: A prodrug that undergoes conversion to MTIC. MTIC action prevents DNA transcription

Uses: Anaplastic astrocytoma with relapse

Dosage and routes:

- *Adult:* **PO** Adjust dose based on nadir neutrophil and platelet counts 150 mg/m^2/day × 5 days during a 28-day cycle

Available forms: Caps 5, 20, 100, 250 mg

Side effects/adverse reactions:
HEMA: ***Thrombocytopenia, leukopenia,*** anemia
GI: Nausea, anorexia, vomiting
CNS: ***Seizures,*** *hemiparesis, dizziness, poor coordination, amnesia, insomnia, paresthesia, somnolence, paresis, ataxia, anxiety, dysphagia, depression, confusion*
INTEG: Rash, pruritus
GU: Urinary incontinence, UTI, frequency
RESP: URI, pharyngitis, sinusitis, coughing
MISC: Headache, fatigue, asthenia, fever, edema, back pain, weight increase, diplopia

Contraindications: Hypersensitivity to this drug or carbazine, pregnancy (D), lactation

Precautions: Radiation therapy, renal, hepatic disease

Pharmacokinetics: Absorption complete, rapid; crosses blood-brain barrier, excreted urine/feces, half-life 1.8 hr, peak 1 hr

Interactions:
- ↑ myelosuppression: radiation, other antineoplastics
- ↓ antibody reaction: live virus vaccines

NURSING CONSIDERATIONS

Assess:
- CBC on day 22 (21 days after 1st dose), CBC weekly until recovery if ANC is $<1.5 \times 10^9$/L and platelets $<100 \times 10^9$/L, do not administer to patients that do not tolerate 100 mg/m^2, myelosuppression usually occurs late in the treatment cycle
- For seizures throughout treatment
- Monitor temp q4h (may indicate beginning infection)
- Hepatic studies before, during therapy (bilirubin, AST, ALT, LDH), as needed or monthly
- Bleeding: hematuria, guaiac, bruising or petechiae, mucosa or orifices q8h

Administer:
- Antiemetic 30-60 min before giving drug to prevent vomiting

⊘ Caps one at a time with 8 oz of water at same time of day; do not open, break, chew

- Fluids IV or PO before chemotherapy to hydrate patient
- Caps should not be opened; if accidentally damaged, do not allow contact with skin, or inhale
- Give on empty stomach to prevent nausea/vomiting

Perform/provide:
- Storage in light-resistant container, dry area

Evaluate:
- Therapeutic response: decreased tumor size, spread of malignancy

Teach patient/family:
- To report signs of infection: fever, sore throat, flulike symptoms
- To report signs of anemia: fatigue, headache, faintness, shortness of breath, irritability
- To report bleeding; avoid use of razors, commercial mouthwash
- To avoid use of aspirin products or ibuprofen

HIGH ALERT

tenecteplase (℞)

(ten-ek'ta-place)

TNKase

Func. class.: Thrombolytic enzyme

Chem. class.: Tissue Plasminogen Activator

Action: Activates conversion of plasminogen to plasmin (fibrinolysin): plasmin breaks down clots (fibrin), fibrinogen, factors V, VII; occlusion of venous access lines

Uses: Acute myocardial infarction

Dosage and routes:
- *Adult <60 kg:* **IV BOL** 30 mg, give over 5 sec
- *Adult ≥60-<70 kg:* **IV BOL** 35 mg, give over 5 sec
- *Adult ≥70-<80 kg:* **IV BOL** 40 mg, give over 5 sec
- *Adult ≥80-<90 kg:* **IV BOL** 45 mg, give over 5 sec
- *Adult ≥90 kg:* **IV BOL** 50 mg, give over 5 sec

Available forms: Powder for inj, lyophilized 50 mg

Side effects/adverse reactions:

CV: Dysrhythmias, hypotension, pulmonary edema, ***pulmonary embolism, cardiogenic shock, cardiac arrest, heart failure, myocardial reinfarction, myocardial rupture, tamponade, pericarditis, pericardial effusion, thrombosis***

HEMA: Decreased Hct, ***bleeding***

INTEG: Rash, urticaria, phlebitis at IV inf site, itching, flushing

SYST: ***GI, GU, intracranial, retroperitoneal bleeding, surface bleeding, anaphylaxis***

Contraindications: Hypersensitivity, arteriovenous malformation, aneurysm, active bleeding, intracranial, intraspinal surgery, CNS neoplasms, severe hypertension, severe renal disease, hepatic disease

Precautions: Arterial emboli from left side of heart, pregnancy (C), lactation, children, hypocoagulation, COPD, subacute bacterial endocarditis, rheumatic valvular disease, cerebral embolism/thrombosis/hemorrhage, intraarterial diagnostic procedure or surgery (10 days), recent major surgery, ulcerative colitis, enteritis

Pharmacokinetics:

IV: Onset immediate, half-life 20-24 min; metabolized by the liver

Interactions:
- Bleeding potential: aspirin, indomethacin, phenylbutazone, anticoagulants, antithrombolytics, glycoprotein IIb, IIIa inhibitors, dipyridamole

↑ risk of bleeding: agrimony, alfalfa, angelica, anise, basil, bay, bilberry, black haw, bogbean, bromelain, buchu, chondroitin, cinchona bark, dong quai, fenugreek, feverfew, garlic, ginger, ginkgo, ginseng, horse chestnut, Irish moss, kelp, kelpware, khella, lovage, lungwort, meadowsweet, motherwort, mugwort, nettle, papaya, parsley (large amts), pau d'arco, pineapple, poplar, prickly ash, safflower, saw palmetto, tonka bean, turmeric, wintergreen, yarrow

↓ anticoagulant effect: chamomile, coenzyme Q10, flax, glucomannan, goldenseal, guar gum

Lab test interferences:

Increase: PT, aPTT, TT

Decrease: Plasminogen, fibrinogen

NURSING CONSIDERATIONS

Assess:
- Allergy: fever, rash, itching, chills; mild reaction may be treated with antihistamines

For bleeding during 1st hr of treatment; hematuria, hematemesis, bleeding from mucous membranes, epistaxis, ecchymosis; may require tranfusion (rare), continue to assess for bleeding for 24 hr
- Blood studies (Hct, platelets, PTT, PT, TT, aPTT) before starting therapy; PT or aPTT must be less than 2× control before starting therapy; PTT or PT q3-4h during treatment
- For hypersensitive reactions: fever, rash, dyspnea; drug should be discontinued
- VS, B/P, pulse, respirations, neurologic signs, temp at least q4h; temp >104° F (40° C) indicates internal bleeding; systolic pressure increase >25 mm Hg should be reported to prescriber

T

For neurologic changes that may indicate intracranial bleeding

Retroperitoneal bleeding: back pain, leg weakness, diminished pulses

Administer:

IV route

- As soon as thrombi identified; not useful for thrombi over 1 wk old
- Cryoprecipitate or fresh frozen plasma if bleeding occurs
- Heparin after fibrinogen level >100 mg/dl; heparin infusion to increase PTT to 1.5-2 × baseline for 3-7 days; IV heparin with loading dose is recommended
- Aseptically withdraw 10 ml of sterile H_2O for inj from diluent vial, use red cannula syringe-filling device, inject all contents of syringe into drug vial, direct into powder, swirl, withdraw correct dose, discard any unused solution; stand the shield with dose vertically on flat surface and passively recap the red cannula, remove entire shield assembly by twisting counter-clockwise, give by IV BOL
- IV therapy: use upper extremity vessel that is accessible to manual compression

Perform/provide:

- Bed rest during entire course of treatment
- Avoidance of venous or arterial puncture, inj, rectal temp; any invasive treatment
- Treatment of fever with acetaminophen or aspirin
- Pressure for 30 sec to minor bleeding sites; inform prescriber if this does not attain hemostasis; apply pressure dressing

Evaluate:

- Therapeutic response: resolution of myocardial infarction

RARELY USED

teniposide (℞)

(ten-i-poe'side)

Vumon, VM 26

Func. class.: Antineoplastic

Uses: Childhood acute lymphoblastic leukemia (ALL), refractory childhood acute lymphocytic leukemia

Dosage and routes:

- *Child:* **IV INF** combo teniposide 165 mg/m^2 and cytarabine 300 mg/m^2 2×/wk × 8-9 doses or combo teniposide 250 mg/m^2 and vinCRIStine 1.5 mg/m^2 qwk × 4-8 wk and predniSONE 40 mg/m^2 **PO** × 28 days

Contraindications: Hypersensitivity, bone marrow depression, severe hepatic disease, severe renal disease, bacterial infection, pregnancy (D)

tenofovir (℞)

(ten-oh-foh'veer)

Viread

Func. class.: Antiretroviral

Chem. class.: Nucleoside analog reverse transcriptase inhibitor

Action: Inhibits replication of HIV virus by competing with the natural substrate and then incorporating into cellular DNA by viral reverse transcriptase, thereby terminating cellular DNA chain

Uses: HIV-1 infection with other antiretrovirals

Dosage and routes:

- *Adult:* **PO** 300 mg with meal; if used with didanosine, give tenofovir 2 hr before or 1 hr after didanosine

Available form: Tabs 300 mg (300

mg of fumarate salt equivalent to 245 mg tenofovir disoproxil)
Side effects/adverse reactions:
CNS: Headache
GI: Nausea, vomiting, diarrhea, anorexia, *flatulence, abdominal pain*
SYST: Change in body fat distribution
Contraindications: Hypersensitivity, CCr <60 ml/min
Precautions: Pregnancy (B), lactation, children, elderly, renal disease, hepatic insufficiency
Pharmacokinetics: Rapidly absorbed, distributed to extravascular space, excreted unchanged in urine
Interactions:
• ↑ tenofovir level: cidofovir, acyclovir, valacyclovir, ganciclovir, valganciclovir
• ↑ level of didanosine when given with tenofovir
• ↑ tenofovir level: any drug that decreases renal function
NURSING CONSIDERATIONS
Assess:
• Hepatic studies: AST, ALT, bilirubin; amylase, lipase, triglycerides periodically during treatment
• For bone, renal toxicity: if bone abnormalities are suspected, obtain tests; serum phosphorus, creatinine
⬦ For lactic acidosis, severe hepatomegaly with steatosis
Administer:
• PO qd with meal
Perform/provide:
• Storage at 25° C (77° F)
Evaluate:
• Therapeutic response: Decrease in signs/symptoms of HIV
Teach patient/family:
• To take this drug 2 hr before or 1 hr after taking didanosine (if used)
• To take with meal
• That GI complaints resolve after 3-4 wk of treatment
• Not to breastfeed while taking this drug
• That drug must be taken qd even if patient feels better
• That follow-up visits must be continued because serious toxicity may occur; blood counts must be done q2wk
• That drug will control symptoms but is not a cure for HIV; patient is still infectious, may pass HIV virus on to others
• That other drugs may be necessary to prevent other infections
• That changes in body fat distribution may occur

terazosin (℞)
(ter-ay′zoe-sin)
Hytrin
Func. class.: Antihypertensive
Chem. class.: α-Adrenergic blocker

Action: Decreases total vascular resistance, which is responsible for a decrease in B/P; this occurs by blockade of α_1-adrenoreceptors
Uses: Hypertension, as a single agent or in combination with diuretics or β-blockers, BPH
Dosage and routes:
Hypertension
• *Adult:* **PO** 1 mg hs, may increase dose slowly to desired response; not to exceed 20 mg/day
Benign prostatic hyperplasia
• *Adult:* **PO** 1 mg hs, gradually increase up to 5-10 mg
Available forms: Tabs 1, 2, 5, 10 mg
Side effects/adverse reactions:
CV: Palpitations, orthostatic hypotension, tachycardia, edema, rebound hypertension
CNS: Dizziness, headache, drowsiness, anxiety, depression, vertigo, weakness, fatigue
GI: Nausea, vomiting, diarrhea, constipation, abdominal pain

T

GU: Urinary frequency, incontinence, impotence, priapism
EENT: Blurred vision, epistaxis, tinnitus, dry mouth, red sclera, nasal congestion, sinusitis
RESP: Dyspnea, cough, pharyngitis
Contraindications: Hypersensitivity
Precautions: Pregnancy (C), children, lactation
Pharmacokinetics: Peak 1 hr, half-life 9-12 hr, highly bound to plasma proteins; metabolized in liver, excreted in urine, feces
Interactions:
- ↑ hypotensive effects: β-blockers, nitroglycerin, verapamil, other antihypertensives, alcohol
- ↓ hypotensive effects: estrogens, NSAIDs, sympathomimetics

NURSING CONSIDERATIONS
Assess:
- Urinary symptoms associated with BPH
- Orthostatic B/P, pulse, jugular venous distention q4h
- BUN, uric acid if on long-term therapy
- Weight qd, I&O
- Skin turgor, dryness of mucous membranes for hydration status
- Rales, dyspnea, orthopnea q30min

Perform/provide:
- Cool storage in tight container

Evaluate:
- Therapeutic response: decreased B/P, edema in feet, legs, decreased symptoms of BPH

Teach patient/family:
- That fainting occasionally occurs after first dose; not to drive or operate machinery for 4 hr after first dose or after an increase in dose; or take first dose hs
- To rise slowly from sitting/lying position

terbinafine (℞)

(ter-bin'a-feen)
Lamisil
Func. class.: Antifungal
Chem. class.: Synthetic allylamine derivative

Action: Interferes with cell membrane permeability in fungi such as *Trichophyton rubrum, Trichophyton mentagrophytes, Trichophyton tonsurans, Epidermophyton floccosum, Microsporum canis, Microsporum audouinii, Microsporum gypseum, Candida,* broad-spectrum antifungal
Uses: (TOP) Tinea cruris, tinea corporis, tinea pedis; (oral) onychomycosis of the toenail or fingernail due to dermatophytes
Investigational uses: Cutaneous candidiasis, tinea versicolor
Dosage and routes:
Topical
- Massage into affected area, surrounding area qd or bid, continue for 7-14 days, not to exceed 4 wk

Oral
- *Fingernail:* 250 mg/day × 6 wk
- *Toenail:* 250 mg/day × 12 wk

Available forms: Cream 1%, tabs 250 mg
Side effects/adverse reactions:
Topical
INTEG: Burning, stinging, dryness, itching, local irritation
Oral
HEME: ***Neutropenia***
GI: Diarrhea, dyspepsia, abdominal pain, nausea
INTEG: Rash, pruritus, urticaria, ***Stevens-Johnson syndrome***
MISC: Headache, hepatic enzyme changes, taste, visual disturbance
Contraindications: Hypersensitivity, chronic/active liver disease

Precautions: Pregnancy (B), lactation, children, renal disease
Interactions:
• ↑ levels of: dextromethorphan
• ↓ terbinafine clearance: cimetidine
• ↑ terbinafine clearance: rifampin
• ↑ clearance of: cycloSPORINE
Side effects: cola nut, guarana, yerba maté, tea (black, green) coffee

NURSING CONSIDERATIONS
Assess:
• Hepatic studies (ALT, AST) prior to beginning treatment; do not use in presence of liver disease
• CBC in treatment >6 wk
• For continuing infection: increased size, number of lesions
Administer:
• To affected area, surrounding area; do not cover with occlusive dressings
Perform/provide:
• Storage below 30° C (86° F)
Evaluate:
• Therapeutic response: decrease in size, number of lesions
Teach patient/family:
Topical
• To wear cotton clothing
• To use clean towel, dry well
• To avoid contact with mucous membranes
• Not to cover areas unless directed by prescriber
• To report excessive itching, burning
• How to apply; massage cream into affected area and surrounding skin in AM, PM; effects observed within 1 wk, continue 1-2 wk after symptoms decrease
Oral
• To notify prescriber of nausea, vomiting, fatigue, jaundice, dark urine, clay-colored stool, RUQ pain, that may indicate liver dysfunction

terbinafine topical
See appendix c

terbutaline (℞)
(ter-byoo'te-leen)
Brethine, Bricanyl
Func. class.: Selective β_2-agonist; bronchodilator
Chem. class.: Catecholamine

Action: Relaxes bronchial smooth muscle by direct action on β_2-adrenergic receptors through accumulation of cAMP at β-adrenergic receptor sites; bronchodilation, diuresis, CNS, cardiac stimulation occur; relaxes uterine smooth muscle
Uses: Bronchospasm, hyperkalemia
Investigational uses: Premature labor
Dosage and routes:
Bronchodilation
• *Adult and child >15 yr:* 2.5-5 mg q6h during the day, max 15 mg/24 hr
• *Child 12-15 yr:* **PO** 2.5 mg tid q6h
Bronchospasm
• *Adult and child >12 yr:* **INH** 2 puffs q1min, then q4-6h; **PO** 2.5-5 mg q8h; **SC** 0.25 mg q15-30 min, max 0.5 mg in 4 hr
Renal dose
• *Adult:* **PO** GFR 10-50 ml/min 50% of dose severe renal failure; avoid GFR if <10 ml/min
Available forms: Tabs 2.5, 5 mg; aerosol 0.2 mg/actuation; inj 1 mg/ml
Side effects/adverse reactions:
CNS: Tremors, anxiety, insomnia, headache, dizziness, stimulation
CV: Palpitations, tachycardia, hypertension, dysrhythmias, ***cardiac arrest***
GI: Nausea, vomiting

T

Contraindications: Hypersensitivity to sympathomimetics, narrow-angle glaucoma, tachydysrhythmias
Precautions: Pregnancy (B), cardiac disorders, hyperthyroidism, diabetes mellitus, prostatic hypertension, lactation, elderly, hypertension, glaucoma
Pharmacokinetics:
PO: Onset ½ hr, peak 1-2 hr, duration 4-8 hr
SC: Onset 6-15 min, peak ½-1 hr, duration 1½-4 hr
INH: Onset 5-30 min, peak 1-2 hr, duration 3-6 hr
Interactions:
- ↑ effects of both drugs: other sympathomimetics
- ↓ action: β-blockers
- Hypertensive crisis: MAOIs
- Incompatible with bleomycin

↑ effect: green tea (large amounts), guarana

NURSING CONSIDERATIONS
Assess:
- Respiratory function: vital capacity, forced expiratory volume, ABGs, B/P, pulse, respiratory pattern, lung sounds, sputum before and after treatment
- Tolerance over long-term therapy; dose may have to be changed; monitor for rebound bronchospasm

Paradoxical bronchospasm: dyspnea, wheezing, keep emergency equipment nearby
- Labor: maternal heart rate, B/P, contraction, fetal heart rate

Administer:
- With food; may be crushed
- 2 hr before hs to avoid sleeplessness

IV route
- IV after diluting each 5 mg/1 L D_5W for inf
- IV, run 5 mcg/min; may increase 5 mcg q10min, titrate to response; after ½-1 hr taper dose by 5 mcg; switch to PO as soon as possible

Additive compatibilities: Aminophylline
Syringe compatibilities: Doxapram
Y-site compatibilities: Insulin (regular)
Perform/provide:
- Storage at room temperature; do not use discolored sol

Evaluate:
- Therapeutic response: absence of dyspnea, wheezing

Teach patient/family:
- Not to use OTC medications; extra stimulation may occur
- The use of inhaler; review package insert with patient
- To avoid getting aerosol in eyes; burning, stinging will occur
- To wash inhaler in warm water and dry qd, rinse mouth after use
- All aspects of drug; avoid smoking, smoke-filled rooms, persons with respiratory infections
- To increase fluids >2 L/day; allow 15 min between inhalation of this drug and inhaler containing steroid
- To take on time; if missed, do not make up after 1 hr; wait until next dose

Treatment of overdose: Administer an α-blocker, then norepinephrine for severe hypotension

terconazole vaginal antifungal
See appendix c

teriparatide (℞)
(tah-ree-par′ah-tide)
Forteo
Func. class.: Parathyroid hormone (rDNA)

Action: Contains human recombinant parathyroid hormone, to stimulate new bone growth

Uses: Postmenopausal women with osteoporosis, men with primary or hypogonadal osteoporosis who are at high risk for fracture

Dosage and routes:

• *Adult:* **SC** 20 mcg qd

Available forms: Inj 250 mcg/ml

Side effects/adverse reactions:

CNS: Dizziness, headache, insomnia, depression, vertigo

GI: Nausea, diarrhea, dyspepsia, vomiting, constipation

RESP: Rhinitis, cough, pharyngitis, pneumonia, dyspnea

MS: Arthralgia, leg cramps

CV: Hypertension, angina, syncope

MISC: Pain, asthenia

INTEG: Rash, sweating

Contraindications: Hypersensitivity, increased baseline risk of osteosarcoma (Paget's disease, open epiphyses; previous bone radiation), bone metastases, history of skeletal malignancies, other metabolic bone diseases, pre-existing hypercalcemia

Precautions: Pregnancy (C), lactation, urolithiasis, hypotension, use >2 yrs, bone metastasis, or history of skeletal malignancies

Pharmacokinetics:

SC: Extensively and rapidly absorbed, metabolized by liver, excreted by kidneys

Interactions:

• ↑ digoxin toxicity: digoxin

Lab test interferences:

Increase: Calcium

NURSING CONSIDERATIONS

Assess:

• Uric acid, chloride, magnesium, electrolytes, urine pH, vit D, phosphate for normal serum levels. Serum calcium may be transiently increased after dosing (max at 4-6 hrs post-dose)

• For bone pain, headache, fatigue, changes in LOC, leg cramps

• For signs of persistent hypercalcemia: nausea, vomiting, constipation, lethargy, muscle weakness

• Nutritional status: diet for sources of vit D (milk, some seafood); calcium (dairy products, dark green vegetables), phosphates (dairy products)

Administer:

SC route

• Give by SC only, rotate inj sites

Perform/provide:

• Store refrigerated, do not freeze

Evaluate:

• Therapeutic response: increased bone mineral density

Teach patient/family:

• The symptoms of hypercalcemia

• About foods rich in calcium

• How to use delivery device, dispose of needles, not to share pen with others

• To sit or lie down if dizziness or fast heartbeat occurs after the first few doses

testolactone (℞)

(tess-toe-lak'tone)

Teslac

Func. class.: Antineoplastic

Chem. class.: Androgen hormone

Controlled Substance Schedule III

Action: Acts on adrenal cortex to suppress activity; reduces estrone synthesis

Uses: Advanced breast carcinoma in postmenopausal women; prostatic cancer

Dosage and routes:

• *Adult:* **PO** 250 mg qid

Available forms: Tabs 50 mg

Side effects/adverse reactions:

GI: Nausea, vomiting, anorexia, glossitis

GU: Urinary retention, ***renal failure***

INTEG: Rash, nail changes, facial hair growth
CV: Orthostatic hypertension, edema
CNS: Paresthesias, dizziness
EENT: Deepening voice
META: Hypercalcemia
Contraindications: Hypersensitivity, premenopausal women, carcinoma of male breast, lactation
Precautions: Renal disease, hypercalcemia, cardiac disease, pregnancy (C)
Pharmacokinetics: None known
Interactions:
• Enhanced effects of oral anticoagulants
Lab test interferences:
Increase: Urinary 17-OHCS
Decrease: Estradiol

NURSING CONSIDERATIONS
Assess:
• Calcium levels
• B/P q4h; tell patient to rise slowly from sitting or lying down
• Food preferences; list likes, dislikes
• Edema in feet; joint, stomach pain; shaking
Symptoms indicating severe allergic reaction: rash, pruritus, urticaria, purpuric skin lesions, itching, flushing
• Anorexia, nausea, vomiting, constipation, weakness, loss of muscle tone (indicating hypercalcemia)
Administer:
PO route
• For 1 mo or longer for desired response
Evaluate:
• Therapeutic response: decreased tumor size, spread of malignancy
Teach patient/family:
• To recognize and report signs of hepatotoxicity, hypercalcemia, virilization (in females), bleeding if on anticoagulants

testosterone cypionate (℞)
Andro-Cyp, Andronate, depAndro, Depotest, Depo-Testosterone, Dura-test, T-Cypionate, Testa-C, Testred, Testoject-LA, Virilon IM

testosterone enanthate (℞)
Andro LA, Andropository, Andryl, Delatest, Delatestryl, Everone, Malog-x✱, Testone LA, Testrin-PA

testosterone gel (℞)
AndroGel 1%

testosterone, long-acting (℞)

testosterone pellets (℞)
Testopel

testosterone transdermal (℞)
Androderm, Testoderm, Testoderm TTS, Testoderm with Adhesive

Func. class.: Androgenic anabolic steroid
Chem. class.: Halogenated testosterone derivative

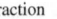

Controlled Substance Schedule III
Action: Increases weight by building body tissue, increases potassium, phosphorus, chloride, nitrogen levels, bone development
Uses: Female breast cancer, eunuchoidism, male climacteric, oligospermia, impotence, osteoporosis, weight loss in AIDS patients, vulvar dystrophies, low testosterone levels
Dosage and routes:
Replacement
• *Adult:* **IM** 25-50 mg 2-3 ×/wk

(base or propionate) or 50-400 mg q2-4wk (enanthate or cypionate)
• *Adult:* **Trans Testoderm** 4-6 mg applied q24h; **Androderm, AndroGel** 5 mg applied q24h; once qd (gel)

Breast cancer
• *Adult:* **IM** 50-100 mg 3 ×/wk (propionate) or 200-400 mg q2-4wk (cypionate or enanthate)

Delayed male puberty
• *Child>12 yr:* **IM** up to 100 mg/mo for up to 6 mo

Available forms: Enanthate: inj 200 mg/ml; ***cypionate:*** inj 100, 200 mg/ml; pellets 75 mg; transdermal 2.5, 4, 5, 6 mg/24 hr; gel 1%

Side effects/adverse reactions:
INTEG: Rash, acneiform lesions, oily hair and skin, flushing, sweating, acne vulgaris, alopecia, hirsutism
CNS: Dizziness, headache, fatigue, tremors, paresthesias, flushing, sweating, anxiety, lability, insomnia, carpal tunnel syndrome
MS: Cramps, spasms
CV: Increased B/P
GU: Hematuria, amenorrhea, vaginitis, decreased libido, decreased breast size, clitoral hypertrophy, testicular atrophy
GI: Nausea, vomiting, constipation, weight gain, ***cholestatic jaundice***
EENT: Conjunctival edema, nasal congestion
ENDO: Abnormal GTT

Contraindications: Severe renal, severe cardiac, severe hepatic disease, hypersensitivity, pregnancy (X), lactation, genital bleeding (rare)

Precautions: Diabetes mellitus, CV disease, MI

Pharmacokinetics:
PO: Metabolized in liver, excreted in urine, breast milk; crosses placenta

Interactions:
• ↑ effects of oxyphenbutazone
• ↑ PT: anticoagulants
• Edema: ACTH, adrenal steroids
• ↓ glucose levels may alter need for: oral antidiabetics, insulin

Lab test interferences:
Increase: Serum cholesterol, blood glucose, urine glucose
Decrease: Serum calcium, serum potassium, T_4, T_3, thyroid ^{131}I uptake test, urine 17-OHCS, 17-KS, PBI

NURSING CONSIDERATIONS

Assess:
• Weight qd; notify prescriber if weekly weight gain is >5 lb
• B/P q4h
• I&O ratio; be alert for decreasing urinary output, increasing edema
• Growth rate in children; growth rate may be uneven (linear/bone growth) with extended use
• Electrolytes: K, Na, Cl, Ca; cholesterol
• Hepatic studies: ALT, AST, bilirubin
• Edema, hypertension, cardiac symptoms, jaundice
• Mental status: affect, mood, behavioral changes, aggression
• Signs of masculinization in female: increased libido, deepening of voice, decreased breast tissue, enlarged clitoris, menstrual irregularities; male: gynecomastia, impotence, testicular atrophy
• Hypercalcemia: lethargy, polyuria, polydipsia, nausea, vomiting, constipation; drug may have to be decreased
• Hypoglycemia in diabetics; oral antidiabetic action is increased

Administer:
• Titrated dose; use lowest effective dose
• IM inj deep into upper outer quadrant of gluteal muscle
• Transdermal patches: Testoderm to skin of scrotum; Androderm to skin of back, upper arms, thighs,

T

abdomen; area must be dry-shaved; may be reapplied after bathing, swimming

• Gel: apply qd to clean, dry area on shoulders, upper arms or abdomen

Perform/provide:

• Diet with increased calories, protein; decrease sodium if edema occurs

Evaluate:

• Therapeutic response: 4-6 wk in osteoporosis

Teach patient/family:

• That drug must be combined with complete health plan: diet, rest, exercise

• To notify prescriber if therapeutic response decreases; if edema occurs

• Not to discontinue abruptly

• About changes in sex characteristics

• That women should report menstrual irregularities, voice changes, acne, facial hair growth, if pregnancy is planned or suspected

• That 1-3-mo course is necessary for response in breast cancer

• The proper application of patches

tetracaine (℞)

(tet′ra-kane)

Pontocaine

Func. class.: Local anesthetic

Chem. class.: Ester

Action: Competes with calcium for sites in nerve membrane that control sodium transport across cell membrane; decreases rise of depolarization phase of action potential

Uses: Spinal anesthesia, epidural and peripheral nerve block, perineum, lower extremities

Dosage and routes:
Varies with route of anesthesia

Available forms: Inj 0.2%, 0.3%, 1%; powder

Side effects/adverse reactions:

CNS: Anxiety, restlessness, ***convulsions, LOC,*** drowsiness, disorientation, tremors, shivering

CV: ***Myocardial depression, cardiac arrest, dysrhythmias,*** bradycardia, hypo/hypertension, fetal bradycardia

GI: Nausea, vomiting

EENT: Blurred vision, tinnitus, pupil constriction

INTEG: Rash, urticaria, allergic reactions, edema, burning, skin discoloration at inj site, tissue necrosis

RESP: ***Status asthmaticus, respiratory arrest, anaphylaxis***

Contraindications: Hypersensitivity, severe liver disease, heart block

Precautions: Elderly, severe drug allergies, pregnancy (C), lactation, children

Pharmacokinetics: Onset, ophthalmic: 1 min; MS 3 min; spinal 3-8 min; duration 1.5-3 hr; metabolized by liver, excreted in urine (metabolites)

Interactions:

• Dysrhythmias: epINEPHrine, halothane, enflurane

• Hypertension: MAOIs, tricyclics, phenothiazines

• ↓ action of tetracaine: chloroprocaine

• ↓ action of sulfonamides

NURSING CONSIDERATIONS

Assess:

• B/P, pulse, respiration during treatment

• Fetal heart tones during labor

• Allergic reactions: rash, urticaria, itching

• Cardiac status: ECG for dysrhythmias, pulse, B/P, during anesthesia

Administer:

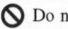

• Only if not cloudy, does not contain precipitate

• Only with crash cart, resuscitative equipment nearby
• Only without preservatives for epidural or caudal anesthesia

Perform/provide:

• Use of new sol, discard unused portions, store in refrigerator

Evaluate:

• Therapeutic response: anesthesia necessary for procedure

Treatment of overdose: Airway, O_2, vasopressor, IV fluids, anticonvulsants for seizures

tetracaine ophthalmic

See appendix c

tetracaine topical

See appendix c

tetracycline (℞)

(tet-ra-sye'kleen)

Achromycin V, Actisite (dental product), Alatel, Apo-Tetra✤, Novotetra✤, Nu-Tetra✤, Panmycin, Robitet, Sumycin, Teline, Tetracap, tetracycline HCl, Tetracyn, Tetralan, Tetram

Func. class.: Broad-spectrum antiinfective

Chem. class.: Tetracycline

Action: Inhibits protein synthesis and phosphorylation in microorganisms; bacteriostatic

Uses: Syphilis, *Chlamydia trachomatis,* gonorrhea, lymphogranuloma venereum; uncommon gram-positive, gram-negative organisms; rickettsial infections

Dosage and routes:

• *Adult:* **PO** 250-500 mg q6h
• *Child >8 yr:* **PO** 25-50 mg/kg/day in divided doses q6h

Gonorrhea

• *Adult:* **PO** 1.5 g, then 500 mg qid for a total of 9 g over 7 days

Chlamydia trachomatis

• *Adult:* **PO** 500 mg qid × 7 days

Syphilis

• *Adult:* **PO** 2-3 g in divided doses × 10-15 days; if syphilis duration >1 yr, must treat 30 days

Brucellosis

• *Adult:* **PO** 500 mg qid × 3 wk with 1 g streptomycin **IM** 2 × /day × 1 wk, and 1 × /day the second wk

Urethral syndrome in women

• *Adult:* **PO** 500 mg qid × 7 days

Acne

• *Adult:* 1 g/day in divided doses; maintenance 125-500 mg/day

Available forms: Oral susp 125 mg/5 ml; caps 100, 250, 500 mg; tabs 250, 500 mg

Side effects/adverse reactions:

CNS: Fever, headache, paresthesia

HEMA: ***Eosinophilia, neutropenia, thrombocytopenia, leukocytosis, hemolytic anemia***

EENT: Dysphagia, glossitis, decreased calcification, discoloration of deciduous teeth, oral candidiasis, oral ulcers

GI: Nausea, abdominal pain, *vomiting, diarrhea,* anorexia, enterocolitis, ***hepatotoxicity,*** flatulence, abdominal cramps, epigastric burning, stomatitis

CV: Pericarditis

GU: Increased BUN

INTEG: Rash, urticaria, photosensitivity, increased pigmentation, ***exfoliative dermatitis,*** pruritus, ***angioedema***

Contraindications: Hypersensitivity to tetracyclines, children <8 yr, pregnancy (D), lactation

Precautions: Renal disease, hepatic disease

Pharmacokinetics:

PO: Peak 2-3 hr, duration 6 hr, half-life 6-10 hr; excreted in urine, breast milk; crosses placenta; 20%-60% protein bound

Interactions:

• ↓ effect of tetracycline: antacids, $NaHCO_3$, dairy products, alkali products, iron, kaolin/pectin, cimetidine

• ↑ effect: warfarin, digoxin

• ↓ effect of penicillins, oral contraceptives

• Nephrotoxicity: methoxyflurane

Photosensitivity: dong quai

Lab test interferences:

False negative: Urine glucose with Clinistix or Tes-Tape

False increase: Urinary catecholamines

NURSING CONSIDERATIONS

Assess:

• Signs of anemia: Hct, Hgb, fatigue

• I&O ratio

• Blood studies: PT, CBC, AST, ALT, BUN, creatinine

• Allergic reactions: rash, itching, pruritus, angioedema

• Nausea, vomiting, diarrhea; administer antiemetic, antacids as ordered

• Overgrowth of infection: fever, malaise, redness, pain, swelling, drainage, perineal itching, diarrhea, changes in cough or sputum

Administer:

• After C&S obtained

• 2 hr before or after iron products; 3 hr after antacid or kaolin/pectin products

• Should be given on an empty stomach

Perform/provide:

• Storage in tight, light-resistant container at room temperature

Evaluate:

• Therapeutic response: decreased temp, absence of lesions, negative C&S

Teach patient/family:

• To avoid sun exposure; sunscreen does not seem to decrease photosensitivity

• That diabetic should avoid use of Clinistix, Diastix, or Tes-Tape for urine glucose testing

• That all prescribed medication must be taken to prevent superinfection

• To avoid milk products, antacids, or separate by 2 hr; take with a full glass of water

tetracycline ophthalmic

See appendix c

tetracycline topical

See appendix c

tetrahydrozoline nasal agent

See appendix c

tetrahydrozoline ophthalmic

See appendix c

theophylline (℞)

(thee-off'i-lin)

Accurbron, Aquaphyllin, Asmalix, Bronkodyl, Elixomin, Elixophyllin, Lanophyllin, Quibron-T Dividose, Quibron-T/SR Dividose, Respbid, Slo-bid Gyrocaps, Slo-Phyllin, Sustaire, Theo-24, Theobid Duracaps, Theochron, Theoclear-80, Theoclear L.A., Theo-Dur, Theolair-SR, Theo-Sav, Theospan-SR, Theostat 80, Theovent, Theo-X, T-Phyl, Uni-Dur, Uniphyl

Func. class.: Spasmolytic

Chem. class.: Xanthine, ethylenediamide

Action: Relaxes smooth muscle of respiratory system by blocking phosphodiesterase, which increases cAMP

Uses: Bronchial asthma, bronchospasm of COPD, chronic bronchitis

Dosage and routes:

Hepatic dose

• *Adult:* **PO** 6 mg/kg loading dose, then 2 mg/kg q8h × 2 doses, then 1-2 mg/kg q12h; **IV** 4.7 mg/kg, then 0.39 mg/kg/hr for 12 hr, then 0.08-0.16 mg/kg/hr maintenance

Bronchospasm, bronchial asthma

• *Adult:* **PO** 100-200 mg q6h; dosage must be individualized; **RECT** 250-500 mg q8-12h

• *Child:* **PO** 50-100 mg q6h, not to exceed 12 mg/kg/24 hr

COPD, chronic bronchitis

• *Adult:* **PO** 330-660 mg q6-8h pc

• *Child 1-9 yr:* **PO** 5 mg/kg loading dose, then 4 mg/kg q6h

• *Child 9-16 yr:* **PO** 5 mg/kg loading dose, then 3 mg/kg q6h

Apnea of prematurity

• *Neonate:* 2-10 mg/kg/day divided q8-12h (usual loading dose is 4 mg/kg **PO**)

Available forms: Caps 50, 100, 200, 250 mg; tabs 100, 125, 200, 225, 250, 300 mg; tabs, time rel 100, 200, 250, 300, 400, 500 mg; caps, time rel 50, 65, 100, 125, 130, 200, 250, 260, 300, 400, 500 mg; elix 80, 11.25 mg/15 ml; sol 80 mg/15 ml; liquid 80, 150, 160 mg/15 ml; susp 300 mg/15 ml

Side effects/adverse reactions:

CNS: Anxiety, restlessness, insomnia, dizziness, ***seizures,*** headache, light-headedness, muscle twitching, tremors

CV: Palpitations, sinus tachycardia, hypotension, ***dysrhythmias,*** fluid retention with tachycardia

ENDO: Hyperglycemia

GI: Nausea, vomiting, anorexia, diarrhea, bitter taste, dyspepsia, gastric distress

RESP: Increased rate

INTEG: Flushing, urticaria

Contraindications: Hypersensitivity to xanthines, tachydysrhythmias

Precautions: Elderly, CHF, cor pulmonale, hepatic disease, active peptic ulcer disease, diabetes mellitus, hyperthyroidism, hypertension, children, pregnancy (C)

Pharmacokinetics:

PO: Peak 2 hr

SOL: Peak 1 hr

Metabolized in liver, excreted in urine and breast milk, crosses placenta

Interactions:

• ↓ theophylline level: phenytoin, phenobarbital, carbamazepine, rifampin, smoking

• ↑ theophylline action: cimetidine, propranolol, erythromycin, ciprofloxacin, oral contraceptives, influenza vaccine, fluoroquinones, mexiletine, corticosteroids, disulfiram, fluvoxamine, interferons

• ↑ effects of anticoagulants

T

• Cardiotoxicity: β-blockers
• ↓ effect of lithium
↓ theophylline levels: St. John's wort
Toxicity: ephedra (ma huang), cola nut, guarana, yerba maté, tea (black, green) coffee

NURSING CONSIDERATIONS

Assess:

Theophylline blood levels (therapeutic level is 5-15 mcg/ml); toxicity may occur with small increase above 20 mcg/ml
• Monitor I&O; diuresis occurs; elderly or child may be dehydrated
• Signs of toxicity: irritability, insomnia, restlessness, tremors, nausea, vomiting
• Respiratory rate, rhythm, depth; auscultate lung fields bilaterally; notify prescriber of abnormalities
• Allergic reactions: rash, urticaria; drug should be discontinued

Administer:

• PO after meals for GI symptoms; absorption may be affected

IV route

• Loading dose over 20-30 min, max 20-25 mg/min; do not give by rapid IV, use only cont inf

Additive compatibilities: Cefepime, chlorproMAZINE, fluconazole, furosemide, hydrocortisone, lidocaine, methylprednisolone, verapamil

Y-site compatibilities: Acyclovir, ampicillin, ampicillin/sulbactam, aztreonam, cefazolin, cefotetan, ceftazidime, ceftriaxone, cimetidine, cisatracurium, clindamycin, dexamethasone, diltiazem, DOBUTamine, DOPamine, doxycycline, erythromycin, famotidine, fluconazole, gentamicin, haloperidol, heparin, hydrocortisone, lidocaine, methyldopate, methylPREDNISolone, metronidazole, midazolam, nafcillin, nitroglycerin, penicillin G potassium, piperacillin, potassium chloride, ranitidine, remifentanil, sodium nitroprusside, ticarcillin, ticarcillin/clavulanate, tobramycin, vancomycin

Evaluate:

• Therapeutic response: ability to breathe more easily

Teach patient/family:

• To check OTC medications, current prescription medications for ephedrine, which will increase stimulation; to avoid alcohol, caffeine
• To avoid hazardous activities; dizziness may occur
• That if GI upset occurs, to take drug with 8 oz H_2O; avoid food; absorption may be decreased
Not to break, crush, chew, or dissolve slow-release products
• That contents of bead-filled capsule may be sprinkled over food for children's use
• To notify prescriber of toxicity: nausea, vomiting, anxiety, insomnia, convulsions
• To notify prescriber of change in smoking habit; dosage may have to be changed

thiamine (vit B_1)

(PO-OTC, IV, IM-℞)

Betalin S, Betaxin♣, Biamine, Revitonus, Thiamilate, thiamine HCl

Func. class.: Vit B_1

Chem. class.: Water soluble

Action: Needed for pyruvate metabolism, carbohydrate metabolism

Uses: Vit B_1 deficiency or polyneuritis, cheilosis adjunct with thiamine beriberi, Wernicke-Korsakoff syndrome, pellagra, metabolic disorders

Dosage and routes:

RDA

• *Adult:* Male 1.2-1.5 mg; females

1.1 mg; pregnancy 1.5 mg; lactation 1.6 mg
Child 7-10 yr: 1.3 mg
Child 4-6 yr: 0.9 mg
Child 1-3 yr: 0.7 mg
Infants 6 mo-1 yr: 0.4 mg
Neonates and infants to 6 mo: 0.3 mg
Beriberi
• *Adult:* **IM** 10-20 mg tid × 2 wk, then 5-10 mg qd × 1 mo
Beriberi with cardiac failure
• *Adult and child:* **IV** 10-30 mg tid
Available forms: Tabs 50, 100, 250, 500 mg; inj 100 mg/ml; enteric coated tabs 20 mg
Side effects/adverse reactions:
CNS: Weakness, restlessness
GI: Hemorrhage, *nausea, diarrhea*
CV: ***Collapse, pulmonary edema,*** hypotension
INTEG: ***Angioneurotic edema,*** cyanosis, sweating, warmth
SYST: ***Anaphylaxis***
EENT: Tightness of throat
Contraindications: Hypersensitivity
Precautions: Pregnancy (A)
Do not confuse:
thiamine/Tenormin
Pharmacokinetics:
PO/INJ: Unused amounts excreted in urine (unchanged)
NURSING CONSIDERATIONS
Assess:
• Thiamine levels throughout treatment
• Nutritional status: yeast, beef, liver, whole or enriched grains, legumes
Administer:
IM route
• By IM inj; rotate sites if pain and inflammation occur; do not mix with alkaline sols; Z-track to minimize pain
IV route
• Undiluted over 5 min or diluted with IV sol and given as an inf at 100 mg or less/5 min or more
Syringe compatibilities: Doxapram
Y-site compatibilities: Famotidine
Perform/provide:
• Storage in tight, light-resistant container
• Application of cold to help decrease pain
Evaluate:
• Therapeutic response: absence of nausea, vomiting, anorexia, insomnia, tachycardia, paresthesias, depression, muscle weakness
Teach patient/family:
• The necessary foods to be included in diet: yeast, beef, liver, legumes, whole grain

thiethylperazine (℞)
(thye-eth-il-per′a-zeen)
Norzine, Torecan
Func. class.: Antiemetic
Chem. class.: Phenothiazine, piperazine derivative

Action: Acts centrally by blocking chemoreceptor trigger zone, which in turn acts on vomiting center
Uses: Nausea, vomiting
Dosage and routes:
• *Adult:* **PO/IM** 10 mg/qd-tid
Available forms: Tabs 10 mg; inj 5 mg/ml
Side effects/adverse reactions:
HEMA: ***Agranulocytosis, leukopenia***
GU: Urinary retention, dark urine
CNS: Euphoria, depression, restlessness, tremor, EPS, ***seizures,*** drowsiness, confusion, ***neuroleptic malignant syndrome***
GI: Nausea, vomiting, anorexia, dry mouth, diarrhea, constipation, weight loss, metallic taste, cramps
CV: ***Circulatory failure, tachycardia,*** postural hypotension, ECG changes
RESP: ***Respiratory depression***

T

Contraindications: Hypersensitivity to phenothiazines, coma, seizure, encephalopathy, bone marrow depression, pregnancy (X)
Precautions: Children <2 yr, elderly, lactation
Do not confuse:
Torecan/Toradol
Pharmacokinetics:
PO: Onset 45-60 min
RECT: Onset 45-60 min, metabolized by liver, crosses placenta, excreted in urine, breast milk
Interactions:
- ↓ effect of thiethylperazine: barbiturates, antacids
- ↑ anticholinergic action: anticholinergics, antiparkinson drugs, antidepressants

NURSING CONSIDERATIONS
Assess:
- VS, B/P; check patients with cardiac disease more often

◆ For neuroleptic malignant syndrome: dyspnea, fever, seizures, diaphoresis, fatigue, loss of urinary control, tachycardia; have emergency equipment nearby
- Respiratory status before, during, after administration of emetic; check rate, rhythm, character; respiratory depression can occur rapidly with elderly or debilitated patients

Administer:
- IM inj in large muscle mass; aspirate to avoid IV administration; patient should remain recumbent 1 hr after inj

Syringe compatibilities: Butorphanol, hydromorphone, midazolam, ranitidine
Y-site compatibilities: Aldesleukin
Evaluate:
- Therapeutic response: absence of nausea, vomiting

Teach patient/family:
- To avoid hazardous activities, activities requiring alertness; dizziness may occur

---

RARELY USED

thioguanine (6-TG) (℞)
(thye-oh-gwah'neen)
thioguanine, Lanvis🍁
Func. class.: Antineoplastic-antimetabolite

Uses: Acute leukemias, chronic granulocytic leukemia, lymphomas, multiple myeloma, solid tumors
Dosage and routes:
- *Adult and child:* **PO** 2 mg/kg/day, then increase slowly to 3 mg/kg/day after 4 wk

Contraindications: Prior drug resistance, leukopenia (<2500/mm^3), thrombocytopenia (<100,000/mm^3), anemia, pregnancy (D)

HIGH ALERT

thiopental (℞)
(thye-oh-pen'tal)
Pentothal, thiopental sodium
Func. class.: General anesthetic
Chem. class.: Barbiturate

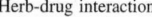

Controlled Substance Schedule III
Action: Acts in reticular-activating system to produce anesthesia, raises seizure threshold
Uses: Short, general anesthesia; narcoanalysis, induction anesthesia before other anesthetics
Investigational uses: Increased intracranial pressure
Dosage and routes:
Test dose
- *Adult:* **IV** 25-75 mg

Induction
- *Adult:* **IV** 210-280 mg or 3-5 mg/kg

General anesthetic
- *Child:* **IV** 3-5 mg/kg then 1 mg/kg as needed
- *Adult:* **IV** 50-75 mg given at 20-40 sec intervals

Narcoanalysis
- *Adult:* **IV** 100 mg/min, not to exceed 50 ml/min

Sedation or narcosis
- *Adult:* **RECT** 12-20 mg/lb

Available forms: Powder for inj 2%, 2.5% (20 mg/ml, 25 mg/ml)

Side effects/adverse reactions:

RESP: ***Respiratory depression, bronchospasm***

CNS: Retrograde amnesia, prolonged somnolence

CV: Tachycardia, hypotension, ***myocardial depression, dysrhythmias***

EENT: Sneezing, coughing

INTEG: Chills, *shivering,* necrosis, pain at inj site

MS: Muscle irritability

Contraindications: Hypersensitivity, status asthmaticus, hepatic/intermittent porphyrias

Precautions: Severe cardiovascular disease, renal disease, hypotension, liver disease, myxedema, myasthenia gravis, asthma, increased intracranial pressure, pregnancy (C)

Pharmacokinetics:

IV: Onset 30-60 sec; duration 4-15 min; half-life 11½ hr; crosses placenta

Interactions:
- ↑ action: CNS depressants
- ↑ CNS depression: kava

NURSING CONSIDERATIONS

Assess:
- VS q3-5min during IV administration, after dose, q4h postoperatively
- Extravasation; if it occurs, use nitroprusside or chloroprocaine to decrease pain, increase circulation
- Dysrhythmias or myocardial depression

Administer:
- Only with crash cart, resuscitative equipment nearby

IV route
- After diluting 500 mg/20 ml sterile H_2O for inj; give each 25 mg or less/min, titrate to response

Additive compatibilities: Chloramphenicol, hydrocortisone sodium succinate, oxytocin, pentobarbital, phenobarbital, potassium chloride, sodium bicarbonate

Solution compatibilities: D_5/0.45% NaCl, D_5W, multiple electrolyte sol, 0.45% NaCl, 0.9% NaCl, 1/6 M sodium lactate

Syringe compatibilities: Aminophylline, hyaluronidase, hydrocortisone sodium succinate, neostigmine, pentobarbital, propofol, scopolamine, tubocurarine

Y-site compatibilities: Doxacurium, fentanyl, heparin, milrinone, mivacurium, nitroglycerin, ranitidine, remifentanil

Evaluate:
- Therapeutic response: maintenance of anesthesia

thioridazine (℞)

(thye-or-rid′a-zeen)

Apo-Thioridazine♣, Mellaril, Mellaril Concentrate, Mellaril-5, Novo-Ridazine♣, PMS-Thioridazine♣, thioridazine HCl

Func. class.: Antipsychotic, neuroleptic

Chem. class.: Phenothiazine piperidine

Action: Depresses cerebral cortex, hypothalamus, limbic system, which control activity, aggression; blocks neurotransmission produced by dopamine at synapse; exhibits strong α-adrenergic, anticholinergic blocking action; mechanism for antipsychotic effects is unclear

Uses: Psychotic disorders, schizophrenia, behavioral problems in children, anxiety, major depressive disorders, organic brain syndrome, dementia in elderly

Dosage and routes:

Psychosis

• *Adult:* **PO** 25-100 mg tid, max dose 800 mg/day; dose is gradually increased to desired response, then reduced to minimum maintenance

Depression/behavioral problems/ organic brain syndrome

• *Adult:* **PO** 25 mg tid, range from 10 mg bid-qid to 50 mg tid-qid

• *Geriatric:* **PO** 10-25 mg qd-bid, increase 4-7 days by 10-25 mg to desired dose

• *Child 2-12 yr:* **PO** 0.5-3 mg/kg/ day in divided doses

Available forms: Tabs 10, 15, 25, 50, 100, 150, 200 mg; conc 30, 100 mg/ml; susp 25, 100 mg/5 ml; syr 10 mg/15 ml

Side effects/adverse reactions:

RESP: ***Laryngospasm,*** dyspnea, ***respiratory depression***

CNS: EPS (rare): pseudoparkinsonism, akathisia, dystonia, tardive dyskinesia, ***seizures,*** *headache,* confusion, ***neuroleptic malignant syndrome,*** dizziness

HEMA: Anemia, ***leukopenia, leukocytosis, agranulocytosis***

INTEG: Rash, photosensitivity, dermatitis

EENT: Blurred vision, glaucoma, dry eyes

GI: Dry mouth, nausea, vomiting, anorexia, constipation, diarrhea, jaundice, weight gain

GU: Urinary retention, urinary frequency, enuresis, impotence, amenorrhea, gynecomastia

CV: Orthostatic hypotension, ***cardiac arrest,*** ECG changes, ***tachycardia***

Contraindications: Hypersensitivity, blood dyscrasias, coma, children <2 yr, brain damage, bone marrow depression

Precautions: Pregnancy (C), lactation, seizure disorders, hypertension, hepatic disease, cardiac disease

Do not confuse:

Mellaril/Elavil

Pharmacokinetics:

PO: Onset erratic, peak 2-4 hr; metabolized by liver, excreted in urine, breast milk; crosses placenta, half-life 26-36 hr

Interactions:

• Oversedation: other CNS depressants, alcohol, barbiturate anesthetics

• ↓ thioridazine effect: lithium, barbiturates

• ↓ antihypertensive effect: centrally acting antihypertensives

• ↓ absorption: aluminum hydroxide, magnesium hydroxide antacids

• ↑ anticholinergic effects: anticholinergics

↑ CNS depression: kava

↑ EPS: betel palm, kava

↑ effect: cola tree, hops, nettle, nutmeg

Lab test interferences:

Increase: LFTs, cardiac enzymes, cholesterol, blood glucose, prolactin, bilirubin, PBI, cholinesterase, ^{131}I

Decrease: Hormones (blood, urine)

False positive: Pregnancy test, PKU

False negative: Urinary steroid, pregnancy test

NURSING CONSIDERATIONS

Assess:

• Mental status before first dose

• Swallowing of PO medication; check for hoarding or giving of medication to other patients

• I&O ratio; palpate bladder if low urinary output occurs, urinary retention may be the cause
• Bilirubin, CBC, LFTs qmo
• Urinalysis is recommended before and during prolonged therapy
• Affect, orientation, LOC, reflexes, gait, coordination, sleep pattern disturbances
• B/P standing and lying; also include pulse and respirations q4h during initial treatment; establish baseline before starting treatment; report drops of 30 mm Hg
• Dizziness, faintness, palpitations, tachycardia on rising
• EPS including akathisia (inability to sit still, no pattern to movements), tardive dyskinesia (bizarre movements of jaw, mouth, tongue, extremities), pseudoparkinsonism (rigidity, tremors, pill rolling, shuffling gait)
◆ For neuroleptic malignant syndrome: altered mental status, muscle rigidity, increased CPK, hyperthermia, dyspnea, fatigue
• Skin turgor qd
• Constipation, urinary retention qd; increase bulk, water in diet

Administer:
• Antiparkinsonian agent on order from prescriber for EPS
• Concentrate mixed in citrus juices or distilled or acidified tap water
• Decreased dose in elderly

Perform/provide:
• Decreased sensory input by dimming lights, avoiding loud noises
• Supervised ambulation until stabilized on medication if needed; do not involve in strenuous exercise program because fainting is possible; patient should not stand still for long periods
• Increased fluids to prevent constipation
• Sips of water, candy, gum for dry mouth
• Storage in tight, light-resistant container; avoid contact with skin

Evaluate:
• Therapeutic response: decrease in emotional excitement, hallucinations, delusions, paranoia, reorganization of patterns of thought, speech

Teach patient/family:
• That orthostatic hypotension occurs frequently, to rise from sitting or lying position gradually; to avoid hazardous activities until stabilized on medication
• To remain lying down after IM inj for at least 30 min
• To avoid hot tubs, hot showers, tub baths; hypotension may occur
• To avoid abrupt withdrawal of thioridazine, or EPS may result; drug should be withdrawn slowly
• To avoid OTC preparations (cough, hay fever, cold) unless approved by prescriber; serious drug interactions may occur; avoid use with alcohol, CNS depressants; increased drowsiness may occur
• To use a sunscreen
• About compliance with drug regimen
• About the necessity for meticulous oral hygiene, since oral candidiasis may occur
• To report sore throat, malaise, fever, bleeding, mouth sores; if these occur, CBC should be drawn and drug discontinued
• That in hot weather, heat stroke may occur; take extra precautions to stay cool

Treatment of overdose: Lavage if orally ingested, provide an airway; do not induce vomiting, CV monitoring, continuous EKG

T

RARELY USED

thiotepa (℞)

(thye-oh-tep'a)
Thioplex
Func. class.: Antineoplastic

Uses: Hodgkin's disease, lymphomas; breast, ovarian, lung, bladder cancer; neoplastic effusions

Dosage and routes:
• *Adult:* **IV** 0.3-0.4 mg/kg at 1-4 wk intervals

Neoplastic effusions
• *Adult:* **INTRACAVITY** 0.6-0.8 mg/kg

Bladder cancer
• *Adult:* **INSTILL** 60 mg/30-60 ml water for inj instilled in bladder for 2 hr once weekly × 4 wk

Contraindications: Hypersensitivity, pregnancy (D)

RARELY USED

thiothixene (℞)

(thye-oh-thix'een)
Navane, thiothixene
Func. class.: Antipsychotic, neuroleptic

Uses: Psychotic disorders, schizophrenia, acute agitation

Dosage and routes:
• *Adult:* **PO** 2-5 mg bid-qid depending on severity of condition; dose gradually increased to 15-30 mg if needed; **IM** 4 mg bid-qid; max dose 30 mg qd; administer **PO** dose as soon as possible
• *Geriatric:* **PO** 1-2 mg qd-bid, increase by 1-2 mg q4-7 days to desired dose

Contraindications: Hypersensitivity, blood dyscrasias, child <12 yr, bone marrow depression, circulatory collapse, CNS depression, coma, alcoholism, CV disease, hepatic disease, Reye's syndrome, narrow-angle glaucoma

Do not confuse:
Navane/Norvasc

thyroid USP (desiccated) (℞)

(thye'roid)
Armour Thyroid, Thyrar, Thyroid Strong, Westhroid
Func. class.: Thyroid hormone
Chem. class.: Active thyroid hormone in natural state and ratio

Action: Increases metabolic rates, increases cardiac output, O_2 consumption, body temp, blood volume, growth, development at cellular level

Uses: Hypothyroidism, cretinism (juvenile hypothyroidism), myxedema

Dosage and routes:

Hypothyroidism
• *Adult:* **PO** 65 mg qd, increased by 65 mg q30d until desired response; maintenance dose 65-195 mg qd
• *Elderly:* **PO** 7.5-15 mg qd, double dose q6-8wk until desired response

Cretinism/juvenile hypothyroidism
• *Child over 1 yr:* **PO** up to 180 mg qd titrated to response
• *Child 4-12 mo:* **PO** 30-60 mg qd
• *Child 1-4 mo:* **PO** 15-30 mg qd; may increase q2wk; titrated to response; maintenance dose 30-45 mg qd

Myxedema
• *Adult:* **PO** 16 mg qd, double dose q2wk, maintenance 65-195 mg/day

Available forms: Tabs 16, 32, 65, 98, 130, 195, 260, 325 mg; tabs enteric coated 32, 65, 130 mg; sugar-coated tabs 32, 65, 130, 195 mg; caps 65, 130, 195, 325 mg

Side effects/adverse reactions:
CNS: Insomnia, tremors, headache, ***thyroid storm***
CV: Tachycardia, palpitations, angina, dysrhythmias, hypertension, ***cardiac arrest***
GI: Nausea, diarrhea, increased or decreased appetite, cramps
MISC: Menstrual irregularities, weight loss, sweating, heat intolerance, fever

Contraindications: Adrenal insufficiency, MI, thyrotoxicosis

Precautions: Elderly, angina pectoris, hypertension, ischemia, cardiac disease, pregnancy (A), lactation

Do not confuse:
Thyrar/Thyrolar

Pharmacokinetics:
PO: Peak 12-48 hr, half-life 6-7 days

Interactions:
- ↓ thyroid absorption: bile acid sequestrants
- ↑ effects of: anticoagulants, sympathomimetics, tricyclics, catecholamines
- ↓ effects of: digoxin, insulin, hypoglycemics
- ↓ thyroid effects: estrogens
- ↓ thyroid effect: agar, bugleweed, carnitine, kelpware, soy, spirulina

Lab test interferences:
Increase: CPK, LDH, AST, PBI, blood glucose
Decrease: Thyroid function tests

NURSING CONSIDERATIONS

Assess:
- B/P, pulse before each dose
- I&O ratio
- Weight qd in same clothing, using same scale, at same time of day
- Height, growth rate of child
- T_3, T_4, which are decreased; radioimmunoassay of TSH, which is increased; radio uptake, which is decreased if dosage is too low
- PT may require decreased anticoagulant; check for bleeding, bruising
- Increased nervousness, excitability, irritability; may indicate too high dose of medication, usually after 1-3 wk of treatment
- Cardiac status: angina, palpitation, chest pain, change in VS

Administer:
- In AM if possible as a single dose to decrease sleeplessness
- At same time each day to maintain drug level
- Only for hormone imbalances; not to be used for obesity, male infertility, menstrual disorders, lethargy
- Lowest dose that relieves symptoms

Perform/provide:
- Removal of medication 4 wk before RAIU test

Evaluate:
- Therapeutic response: absence of depression; increased weight loss, diuresis, pulse, appetite; absence of constipation, peripheral edema, cold intolerance; pale, cool, dry skin; brittle nails, alopecia, coarse hair, menorrhagia, night blindness, paresthesias, syncope, stupor, coma, rosy cheeks

Teach patient/family:
- That hair loss will occur in child, is temporary
- To report excitability, irritability, anxiety; indicates overdose
- Not to switch brands unless directed by prescriber
- That hypothyroid child will show almost immediate behavior/personality change
- That treatment drug is not to be taken to reduce weight
- To avoid OTC preparations with iodine; read labels

T

• To avoid iodine food, iodized salt, soybeans, tofu, turnips, some seafood, some bread

tiagabine (℞)

(tie-ah-ga'been)

Gabitril

Func. class.: Anticonvulsant

Action: Mechanism unknown; may increase seizure threshold; structurally similar to GABA; tiagabine binding sites in neocortex, hippocampus

Uses: Adjunct treatment of partial seizures

Dosage and routes:

• *Adult:* **PO** 4 mg qd, may increase by 4-8 mg qwk until desired response, max 56 mg/day

• *Child 12-18 yr:* **PO** 4 mg qd, may increase by 4 mg at beginning of wk 2; may increase by 4-8 mg qwk until desired response; max 32 mg/day

Available forms: Tabs 4, 12, 16, 20 mg

Side effects/adverse reactions:

CNS: Dizziness, anxiety, somnolence, ataxia, confusion, asthenia, unsteady gait, depression

CV: Vasodilation

GI: Nausea, vomiting, diarrhea

INTEG: Pruritus, rash

RESP: Pharyngitis, coughing

Contraindications: Hypersensitivity to this drug

Precautions: Hepatic disease, renal disease, pregnancy (C), lactation, children <12 yr, elderly

Pharmacokinetics: Absorption >95%, half-life 7-9 hr

Interactions:

• Lower doses may be needed when used with valproate

• ↑ CNS depression: CNS depressants

NURSING CONSIDERATIONS

Assess:

• Renal studies: urinalysis, BUN, urine creatinine q3mo

• Hepatic studies: ALT, AST, bilirubin

• Description of seizures: location, duration, presence of aura

• Mental status: mood, sensorium, affect, behavioral changes; if mental status changes, notify prescriber

Perform/provide:

• Storage at room temperature away from heat and light

• Assistance with ambulation during early part of treatment; dizziness occurs

• Seizure precautions: padded side rails; move objects that may harm patient

Evaluate:

• Therapeutic response: decreased seizure activity; document on patient's chart

Teach patient/family:

• To carry emergency ID stating patient's name, drugs taken, condition, prescriber's name and phone number

• To avoid driving, other activities that require alertness

• Not to discontinue medication quickly after long-term use

• To take with food

Treatment of overdose: Lavage, VS

ticarcillin (℞)

(tye-kar-sill'in)

Ticar

Func. class.: Broad-spectrum antiinfective

Chem. class.: Extended-spectrum penicillin

Action: Interferes with cell wall replication of susceptible organisms; osmotically unstable cell wall swells, bursts from osmotic pressure

Uses: Respiratory, soft tissue, urinary tract infections, bacterial septicemia; effective for gram-positive cocci *(Staphylococcus aureus, Streptococcus faecalis, Streptococcus pneumoniae)*, gram-negative cocci *(Neisseria gonorrhoeae)*, gram-positive bacilli *(Clostridium perfringens, Clostridium tetani)*, gram-negative bacilli *(Bacteroides, Fusobacterium nucleatum, Escherichia coli, Proteus mirabilis, Salmonella, Morganella morganii, Proteus rettgeri, Enterobacter, Pseudomonas aeruginosa, Serratia); and Peptococcus, Peptostreptococcus, Eubacterium*

Dosage and routes:

Bacterial septicemia, respiratory, skin, soft tissue, intra-abdominal, reproductive infections

• *Adult:* **IV INF** 200-300 mg/kg/day in divided doses q4-6h

• *Child <40 kg:* **IV INF** 200-300 mg/kg/day in divided doses q4-6h

Urinary tract complicated infections

• *Adult/child:* **IV INF** 150-200 mg/kg/day in divided doses q4-6h

Uncomplicated urinary infections

• *Adult:* **IV Direct/IM** 1 g q6h

• *Child <40 kg:* **IV Direct/IM** 50-100 mg/kg/day q6-8h

Severe infections (Pseudomonas, Proteus, E. coli)

• *Neonates:* **IM/IV** <2 kg: 75 mg/kg q8-12h; **IM/IV** >2 kg: 75-100 mg/kg q8h

Renal dose/hepatic dose

• CCr >60 ml/min 3 g q4h; CCr 30-60 ml/min 2 g q4h; CCr 10-30 ml/min 2 g q8h; CCr <10 ml/min 2 g q12h or 1 g q6h; CCr <10 ml/min and hepatic dysfunction 2 g q24h or 1 g q12h

Available forms: Inj 1, 3, 6, 20, 30 g

Side effects/adverse reactions:

HEMA: Anemia, increased bleeding time, ***bone marrow depression, granulocytopenia***

GI: Nausea, vomiting, diarrhea; increased AST, ALT; abdominal pain, glossitis, colitis

GU: Oliguria, proteinuria, hematuria, *vaginitis, moniliasis,* ***glomerulonephritis***

CNS: Lethargy, hallucinations, anxiety, depression, twitching, ***coma, seizures***

INTEG: Rash

META: Hypokalemia

SYST: ***Anaphylaxis***

Contraindications: Hypersensitivity to penicillins

Precautions: Hypersensitivity to cephalosporins, pregnancy (B), lactation, renal disease

Pharmacokinetics:

IM: Peak 1 hr, duration 4-6 hr

IV: Peak 30-45 min, duration 4 hr, half-life 70 min; small amount metabolized in liver; excreted in urine, breast milk

Interactions:

• ↓ antimicrobial effect of ticarcillin: tetracyclines, aminoglycosides IV

• ↑ effect of: neuromuscular blockers, heparin

• ↑ ticarcillin concentrations: aspirin, probenecid

• ↓ effect: oral contraceptives, erythromycins

Delayed absorption: khat

Lab test interferences:

False positive: Urine glucose, urine protein

NURSING CONSIDERATIONS

Assess:

• I&O ratio; report hematuria, oliguria, since penicillin in high doses is nephrotoxic

Any patient with compromised renal system, since drug is excreted slowly in poor renal system function; toxicity may occur rapidly

For anaphylaxis: wheezing, rash, pruritus, laryngeal edema, keep emergency equipment nearby
• Hepatic studies: AST, ALT
• Blood studies: WBC, RBC, Hgb, Hct, bleeding time
• Renal tests: urinalysis, protein, blood, BUN, creatinine
• C&S before drug therapy; drug may be given as soon as culture is taken
• Bowel pattern before, during treatment
• Skin eruptions after administration of penicillin to 1 wk after discontinuing drug
• Allergies before initiation of treatment, reaction of each medication

Administer:
• Drug after C&S has been completed

IM route
• Inject into well-developed muscle
• Reconstitute ticarcillin 1 g/2 ml sterile water for inj, NaCl inj, 1% lidocaine HCl without epINEPHrine (385 mg/ml)

IV route
• After diluting 1 g or less/4 ml sterile H_2O for inj; dilute further with 10-20 ml or more D_5W, NS, or sterile H_2O for inj sol; give 1 g or less/5 min or more or by intermittent inf over ½-2 hr or by continuous inf at prescribed rate

Additive compatibilities: Ranitidine, verapamil

Y-site compatibilities: Acyclovir, allopurinol, amifostine, aztreonam, cisatracurium, cyclophosphamide, diltiazem, DOXOrubicin, famotidine, filgrastim, fludarabine, granisetron, heparin, hydromorphone, IL-2, insulin (regular), magnesium sulfate, melphalan, meperidine, morphine, ondansetron, perphenazine, propofol, remifentanil, sargramostim, teniposide, theophylline, thiotepa, verapamil, vinorelbine

Perform/provide:
• Adrenalin, suction, tracheostomy set, endotracheal intubation equipment
• Adequate fluid intake (2 L) during diarrhea episodes
• Scratch test to assess allergy on order from prescriber; done when penicillin is only drug of choice
• Storage at room temperature, reconstituted sol 72 hr at room temperature

Evaluate:
• Therapeutic response: absence of fever, purulent drainage, redness, inflammation

Teach patient/family:
• That culture may be taken after completed course of medication
• To report sore throat, fever, fatigue (may indicate superinfection)
• To wear or carry emergency ID if allergic to penicillins
• To notify nurse of diarrhea

Treatment of overdose: Withdraw drug, maintain airway, administer epINEPHrine, aminophylline, O_2, IV corticosteroids for anaphylaxis

ticarcillin/ clavulanate (℞)

Timentin

Func. class.: Broad-spectrum antiinfective

Chem. class.: Extended-spectrum penicillin

Action: Interferes with cell wall replication of susceptible organisms; osmotically unstable cell wall swells, bursts from osmotic pressure

Uses: Respiratory, soft tissue, and urinary tract infections, bacterial septicemia; effective for gram-positive cocci (*Staphylococcus aureus, Strep-*

tococcus faecalis, Streptococcus pneumoniae), gram-negative cocci *(Neisseria gonorrhoeae),* gram-positive bacilli *(Clostridium perfringens, Clostridium tetani),* gram-negative bacilli *(Bacteroides, Fusobacterium nucleatum, Escherichia coli, Proteus mirabilis, Salmonella, Morganella morganii, Proteus rettgeri, Enterobacter, Pseudomonas aeruginosa, Serratia);* and *Peptococcus, Peptostreptococcus, Eubacterium*

Dosage and routes:

Renal dose

- CCr 60 ml/min 3.1 g q4h; CCr 30-60 ml/min 2 g q4h; CCr 10-30 ml/min 2 g q8h; CCr <10 ml/min 2 g q12h; CCr <10 ml/min with hepatic dysfunction 2 g q24h

Systemic/urinary tract infections, serious infections

- *Adult ≥60 kg:* **IV INF** 3.1 g q4-6h
- *Adult <60 kg:* **IV INF** 200-300 mg/kg/day q4-6h
- *Child >60 kg:* **IV INF** 3.1 g q4h
- *Child <60 kg:* **IV INF** 300 mg/kg/day q4h

Mild/moderate infections

- *Child ≥60 kg:* **IV INF** 3.1 g q6h
- *Child <60 kg:* **IV INF** 200 mg/kg/day q6h

Available forms: Inj 3 g ticarcillin, 0.1 g clavulanate; IV inf 3 g ticarcillin, 0.1 g clavulanate; powder for inj 3 g ticarcillin, 0.1 g clavulanate; 30 g ticarcillin, 1 g clavulanate

Side effects/adverse reactions:

HEMA: Anemia, increased bleeding time, ***bone marrow depression, granulocytopenia***

GI: Nausea, vomiting, diarrhea; increased AST, ALT; abdominal pain, glossitis, colitis

GU: Oliguria, proteinuria, hematuria, *vaginitis, moniliasis,* ***glomerulonephritis***

CNS: Lethargy, hallucinations, anxiety, depression, twitching, ***coma, seizures***

META: Hyperkalemia, hypokalemia, alkalosis, hypernatremia

SYST: ***Anaphylaxis***

Contraindications: Hypersensitivity to penicillins; neonates

Precautions: Hypersensitivity to cephalosporins, pregnancy (B), renal disease

Pharmacokinetics:

IV: Peak 30-45 min, duration 4 hr, half-life 64-68 min; excreted in urine

Interactions:

- ↓ antimicrobial effect of ticarcillin: tetracyclines, aminoglycosides IV
- ↓ effect: oral contraceptives, erythromycin
- ↑ effect of: neuromuscular blockers, heparin
- ↑ ticarcillin concentrations: aspirin, probenecid

↓ absorption: khat

Lab test interferences:

False positive: Urine glucose, urine protein, Coombs' test

NURSING CONSIDERATIONS

Assess:

- I&O ratio; report hematuria, oliguria, since penicillin in high doses is nephrotoxic

Any patient with compromised renal system, since drug is excreted slowly in poor renal system function; toxicity may occur rapidly

For anaphylaxis: wheezing, rash, laryngeal edema; have emergency equipment nearby

- Hepatic studies: AST, ALT
- Blood studies: WBC, RBC, Hct, Hgb, bleeding time
- Renal studies: urinalysis, protein, blood, BUN, creatinine
- C&S before drug therapy; drug may be given as soon as culture is taken
- Bowel pattern before, during treatment

T

• Skin eruptions after administration of penicillin to 1 wk after discontinuing drug
• Allergies before initiation of treatment, reaction of each medication

Administer:

• Drug after C&S

IV route

• After diluting 3.1 g or less/13 ml of sterile H_2O or NaCl (200 mg/ml), shake; may further dilute in 50-100 ml or more NS, D_5W, or LR sol and run over ½ hr

Y-site compatibilities: Allopurinol, amifostine, aztreonam, cefepime, cyclophosphamide, diltiazem, DOXOrubicin liposome, famotidine, filgrastim, fluconazole, fludarabine, foscarnet, gallium, granisetron, heparin, insulin (regular), melphalan, meperidine, morphine, ondansetron, perphenazine, propofol, remifentanil, sargramostim, teniposide, theophylline, thiotepa, vinorelbine

Perform/provide:

• Adrenaline, suction, tracheostomy set, endotracheal intubation equipment
• Adequate fluid intake (2 L) during diarrhea episodes
• Scratch test to assess allergy on order from prescriber; usually done when penicillin is only drug of choice
• Storage of reconstituted sol 12-24 hr at room temperature, or 3-7 days refrigerated

Evaluate:

• Therapeutic response: absence of fever, purulent drainage, redness, inflammation

Teach patient/family:

• To report persistent diarrhea
• That culture may be taken after completed course of medication
• To report sore throat, fever, fatigue (may indicate superinfection)
• To wear or carry emergency ID if allergic to penicillins

Treatment of overdose: Withdraw drug, maintain airway, administer epinephrine, O_2, IV corticosteroids for anaphylaxis

ticlopidine (℞)

(tye-cloe'pi-deen)

Ticlid

Func. class.: Platelet aggregation inhibitor

Action: Inhibits first and second phases of ADP-induced effects in platelet aggregation

Uses: Reducing the risk of stroke in high-risk patients

Investigational uses: Intermittent claudication, chronic arterial occlusion, subarachnoid hemorrhage, uremic patients with AV shunts/fistulas, open heart surgery, coronary artery bypass grafts, primary glomerulonephritis, sickle cell disease

Dosage and routes:

• *Adult:* **PO** 250 mg bid with food

Available forms: Tabs 250 mg

Side effects/adverse reactions:

INTEG: *Rash,* pruritus

GI: Nausea, vomiting, *diarrhea,* GI discomfort, ***cholestatic jaundice, hepatitis,*** increased cholesterol, LDL, VLDL, TG

HEMA: ***Bleeding (epistaxis, hematuria, conjunctival hemorrhage, GI bleeding), agranulocytosis, neutropenia, thrombocytopenia, thrombotic thombocytopenic purpura***

CNS: Dizziness

Contraindications: Hypersensitivity, severe hepatic disease, blood dyscrasias, active bleeding

Precautions: Past hepatic disease, renal disease, elderly, pregnancy (B), lactation, children, increased bleeding risk

Pharmacokinetics: Peak 1-3 hr, metabolized by liver, excreted in urine, feces; half-life increases with repeated dosing

Interactions:

• ↑ levels of: phenytoin

• ↑ bleeding tendencies: anticoagulants, salicylates, thrombolytics

• ↓ plasma levels of ticlopidine: antacids

• ↓ plasma levels of digoxin

• ↑ effects of ticlopidine: cimetidine

• ↑ effects of theophylline

NURSING CONSIDERATIONS

Assess:

• Hepatic studies: AST, ALT, bilirubin, creatinine (long-term therapy)

◆ Blood studies: CBC; CBC q2 wk × 3 mo, Hct, Hgb, PT (long-term therapy)

◆ Bleed time baseline and throughout, levels may be 2-5 × normal limit

Administer:

• With food to decrease gastric symptoms

Evaluate:

• Therapeutic response: absence of stroke

Teach patient/family:

• That blood work will be necessary during treatment

• To report any unusual bleeding to prescriber

• To report side effects such as diarrhea, skin rashes, subcutaneous bleeding, signs of cholestasis (jaundiced skin and sclera, dark urine, light-colored stools)

tiludronate (℞)

(till-oo'droe-nate)

Skelid

Func. class.: Bone resorption inhibitor

Chem. class.: Bisphosphonate

Action: Decreases bone resorption and new bone development

Uses: Paget's disease

Dosage and routes:

• *Adult:* **PO** 400 mg qd, with 8 oz water × 3 mo

Available forms: Tabs 240 mg (equivalent to 200 mg tiludronic acid)

Side effects/adverse reactions:

GI: Nausea, diarrhea, dry mouth, gastritis, vomiting, flatulence, gastric ulcers, gastritis, dyspepsia

RESP: Rhinitis, rales, sinusitis, URI

CNS: Headache, somnolence, dizziness, anxiety, vertigo, nervousness, involuntary movements

ENDO: Hyperparathyroidism

INTEG: Rash, epidermal necrosis, pruritus, sweating

GU: ***Nephrotoxicity,*** UTI

MS: Bone pain, decreased mineralization of nonaffected bones, pathological fractures

Contraindications: Hypersensitivity to bisphosphonates, severe renal disease with creatinine >5 mg/dl

Precautions: Pregnancy (C), renal disease, lactation, restricted vit D/calcium, GI disease

Pharmacokinetics:

Protein binding 90%, excreted by kidneys

Half-life 150 hr

Interactions:

• ↓ tiludronate absorption: antacids, mineral supplements with magnesium, calcium, aluminum, aspirin

• ↑ tiludronate effect: indomethacin

NURSING CONSIDERATIONS

Assess:

• GI symptoms, polyuria, flushing, head swelling, tingling, headache—may indicate hypercalcemia; nervousness, irritability, twitching, seizures, spasm, paresthesia indicates hypocalcemia at start of treatment

• Nutritional status; evaluate diet for sources of vit D (milk, some seafood), calcium (dairy products, dark green vegetables), phosphates

• BUN, creatinine, uric acid, chloride, electrolytes, urine pH, urinary calcium, magnesium, phosphate, urinalysis (calcium should be kept at 9-10 mg/dl), albumin, alk phosphatase baseline and q3-6 mo; check urine sediment for casts throughout treatment

• For increased drug level—toxic reactions occur rapidly; have calcium chloride or gluconate on hand if calcium level drops too low; check for tetany

Administer:

• On empty stomach to improve absorption (2 hr ac), with 6-8 oz water

• Take calcium or mineral supplements 2 hr before or 2 hr after tiludronate

• Take aluminum or magnesium antacids ≥2 hr after tiludronate

• Do not take indomethacin within 2 hr

Evaluate:

• Therapeutic response: calcium levels 9-10 mg/dl; decreasing symptoms of Paget's disease

Teach patient/family:

• To notify prescriber of hypercalcemic relapse: renal calculi, nausea, vomiting, thirst, lethargy, deep bone or flank pain

• To follow a low-calcium diet as prescribed (Paget's disease, hypercalcemia)

• To notify prescriber of diarrhea, nausea; dose may be divided to lessen these symptoms

timolol (℞)

(tye'moe-lole)

Apo-Timol✤, Blocadren, Novo-Timol✤, timolol maleate

Func. class.: Antihypertensive

Chem. class.: Nonselective β-blocker

Action: Competitively blocks stimulation of β-adrenergic receptor within vascular smooth muscle (decreases rate of SA node discharge, increases recovery time), slows conduction of AV node, decreases heart rate, which decreases O_2 consumption in myocardium; also decreases renin-aldosterone-angiotensin system, at high doses inhibits β_2-receptors in bronchial system

Uses: Mild to moderate hypertension

Investigational uses: Mitral valve prolapse, hypertrophic cardiomyopathy, thyrotoxicosis, tremors, anxiety, pheochromocytoma, tachydysrhythmias, angina pectoris

Dosage and routes:

Hypertension

• *Adult:* **PO** 10 mg bid, or 20 mg qd, may increase by 10 mg q7d, not to exceed 60 mg/day

Myocardial infarction

• *Adult:* **PO** 10 mg bid beginning 1-4 wks after MI

Migraine headache prevention

• *Adult:* **PO** 10 mg bid or 20 mg qd; may increase to 30 mg/day, 20 mg in AM, 10 mg in PM

Available forms: Tabs 5, 10, 20 mg

Side effects/adverse reactions:

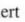

CV: Hypotension, bradycardia, ***CHF***, edema, chest pain, claudication, an-

gina, AV block, ventricular dysrhythmias
CNS: Insomnia, dizziness, hallucinations, anxiety, fatigue, depression
GI: Nausea, vomiting, ***ischemic colitis,*** diarrhea, *abdominal pain,* ***mesenteric arterial thrombosis,*** flatulence, constipation
INTEG: Rash, alopecia, pruritus, fever
HEMA: ***Agranulocytosis, thrombocytopenia, purpura***
EENT: Visual changes, sore throat, *double vision,* dry burning eyes
GU: Impotence, urinary frequency
RESP: ***Bronchospasm,*** *dyspnea,* cough, rales, nasal stuffiness
META: Hypoglycemia
MUSC: Joint pain, muscle pain

Contraindications: Hypersensitivity to β-blockers, cardiogenic shock, heart block (2nd or 3rd degree), sinus bradycardia, CHF, cardiac failure, severe COPD

Precautions: Major surgery, pregnancy (C), lactation, diabetes mellitus, renal disease, thyroid disease, COPD, well-compensated heart failure, CAD, nonallergic bronchospasm, peripheral vascular disease, hepatic disease

Do not confuse:
Timoptic/Viroptic

Pharmacokinetics:
PO: Peak 1-2 hr; half-life 4 hr; metabolized by liver; excreted in urine, breast milk, protein binding <10%

Interactions:
- ↑ hypotension, bradycardia: reserpine, hydrALAZINE, methyldopa, prazosin, anticholinergics, alcohol, reserpine, nitrates
- ↑ effects of: β-blockers, calcium channel blockers
- ↓ antihypertensive effects: NSAIDs, sympathomimetics, thyroid
- ↓ hypoglycemic effects: insulin, sulfonylureas
- ↓ bronchodilation: theophyllines

↑ toxicity, death: aconite
↑ or ↓ antihypertensive effect: astragalus, cola tree
↑ antihypertensive effect: barberry, betony, black catechu, black cohosh, bloodroot, broom, burdock, cat's claw, dandelion, goldenseal, Irish moss, Jamaican dogwood, kelp, khella, mistletoe, parsley
↓ antihypertensive effect: coltsfoot, guarana, khat, licorice

Lab test interferences:
Increase: Renal, hepatic studies, potassium, uric acid
Decrease: Hct, Hgb, HDL
Interference: Glucose, insulin tolerance test

NURSING CONSIDERATIONS

Assess:
- Headaches: location, severity, duration, frequency baseline and throughout treatment
- I&O, weight qd
- B/P during initial treatment, periodically thereafter, pulse q4h; note rate, rhythm, quality
- Apical/radial pulse before administration; notify prescriber of any significant changes
- Baselines in renal, hepatic studies before therapy begins
- Edema in feet, legs qd
- Skin turgor, dryness of mucous membranes for hydration status

Administer:
- PO ac, hs, tablet may be crushed or swallowed whole
- Reduced dosage in renal dysfunction

Perform/provide:
- Dry storage at room temperature; do not freeze

Evaluate:
- Therapeutic response: decreased B/P after 1-2 wk

Teach patient/family:
- To take with or immediately after meals

• Not to discontinue drug abruptly; taper over 2 wk; may cause precipitate angina
• Not to use OTC products containing α-adrenergic stimulants (nasal decongestants, cold preparations) unless directed by prescriber
• To report bradycardia, dizziness, confusion, depression, fever, sore throat, shortness of breath to prescriber
• To take pulse at home; advise when to notify prescriber
• To avoid alcohol, smoking, sodium intake
• To comply with weight control, dietary adjustments, modified exercise program
• To carry emergency ID to identify drug, allergies
• To avoid hazardous activities if dizziness is present
• To report symptoms of CHF: difficulty breathing, especially on exertion or when lying down; night cough; swelling of extremities
• To take medication hs to minimize effect of orthostatic hypotension
• To wear support hose to minimize effects of orthostatic hypotension

Treatment of overdose: Lavage, IV atropine for bradycardia, IV theophylline for bronchospasm, digitalis, O_2, diuretic for cardiac failure, hemodialysis; administer vasopressor (norepinephrine)

timolol ophthalmic

See appendix c

HIGH ALERT

tinzaparin (℞)

(tin-zay-par′in)

Innohep

Func. class.: Anticoagulant

Chem. class.: Unfractionated porcine heparin

Action: Prevents conversion of fibrinogen to fibrin and prothrombin to thrombin by enhancing inhibitory effects of antithrombin III; produces higher ratio of antifactor Xa to antifactor IIa

Uses: Treatment of deep-vein thrombosis, pulmonary emboli when given with warfarin

Dosage and routes:
• *Adult:* **SC** 175 anti-Xa international units/kg qd ≥6 days and until adequate anticoagulation with warfarin (INR ≥2 for 2 consecutive days)

Available forms: Inj 40,000 international units/2 ml

Side effects/adverse reactions:

CV: Angina, dysrhythmias, peripheral edema

CNS: Fever, confusion, dizziness, insomnia

GI: Nausea, constipation, flatulence, dyspepsia, ***hepatitis***

GU: UTI, hematuria, urinary retention, dysuria

HEMA: Hemorrhage, ***hypochromic anemia, thrombocytopenia,*** bleeding

INTEG: Ecchymosis

MISC: Headache, chest pain

Contraindications: Hypersensitivity to this drug, heparin, pork or benzyl alcohol; hemophilia, leukemia with bleeding, peptic ulcer disease, thrombocytopenic purpura, heparin-induced thrombocytopenia

Precautions: Alcoholism, elderly, pregnancy (C), hepatic disease (severe), renal disease (severe), blood dyscrasias, severe, uncontrolled hypertension, subacute bacterial endocarditis, acute nephritis, lactation, children

Pharmacokinetics:

Maximum antithrombin activity (3-5 hr), elimination half-life 4.5 hr

Interactions:

- ↑ action of tinzaparin: oral anticoagulants, salicylates, thrombolytics, NSAIDs, platelet inhibitors, ticlopidine
- Do not mix with other drugs or infusion fluids

↑ risk of bleeding: agrimony, alfalfa, angelica, anise, basil, bay, bilberry, black haw, bogbean, bromelain, buchu, chondroitin, cinchona bark, Dong quai, fenugreek, feverfew, garlic, ginger, ginkgo, ginseng, horse chestnut, Irish moss, kelp, kelpware, khella, lovage, lungwort, meadowsweet, motherwort, mugwort, nettle, papaya, parsley (large amts), pau d' arco, pineapple, poplar, prickly ash, safflower, saw palmetto, tonka bean, turmeric, wintergreen, yarrow

↓ anticoagulant effect: chamomile, coenzyme Q10, flax, glucomannan, goldenseal, guar gum

NURSING CONSIDERATIONS

Assess:

- Blood studies (Hct, platelets, occult blood in stools), anti-Xa; thrombocytopenia may occur
- Bleeding gums, petechiae, ecchymosis, black tarry stools, hematuria

Administer:

- Only after screening patient for bleeding disorders
- SC only; do not give IM
- To recumbent patient; give SC; rotate inj sites (left/right anterolateral, left-right posterolateral abdominal wall)
- Insert whole length of needle into skin fold held with thumb and forefinger

Only this drug when ordered; not interchangeable with heparin or LMWHs

- At same time each day to maintain steady blood levels
- Do not massage area or aspirate when giving SC inj
- Avoiding all IM inj that may cause bleeding

Perform/provide:

- Storage at 77° F (25° C); do not freeze

Evaluate:

- Therapeutic response: resolution of deep vein thrombosis

Teach patient/family:

- To use soft-bristle toothbrush to avoid bleeding gums, to use electric razor
- To report any signs of bleeding: gums, under skin, urine, stools

Treatment of overdose: Protamine 1 mg/100 anti-Xa international units of tinzaparin

tioconazole vaginal antifungal

See appendix c

HIGH ALERT

tirofiban (℞)

(tie-roh-fee′ban)

Aggrastat

Func. class.: Antiplatelet

Chem. class.: Glycoprotein IIb/IIIa inhibitor

Action: Antagonist of platelet glycoprotein (GP) IIb/IIIa receptor that leads to binding of fibrinogen and von Willebrand's factor, which inhibits platelet aggregation

Uses: Acute coronary syndrome in combination with heparin

Dosage and routes:

• *Adult:* **IV** 0.4 mcg/kg/min × 30 min, then 0.1 mcg/kg/min

Renal dose

• *Adult:* **IV** CCr <30 ml/min 0.2 mcg/kg/min × 30 min, then 0.05 mcg/kg/min, during angiography and for up to 24 hr after angioplasty

Available forms: Inj for sol 250 mcg/ml, inj 50 mcg/ml

Side effects/adverse reactions:

CV: Bradycardia

CNS: Dizziness

INTEG: Rash

HEMA: ***Bleeding, thrombocytopenia***

OTHER: Dissection, coronary artery edema, pain in legs/pelvis, sweating

Contraindications: Hypersensitivity, active internal bleeding, stroke, major surgery, severe trauma, intracranial neoplasm, aneurysm, hemorrhage, acute pericarditis, platelets $<100,000/mm^3$, history of thrombocytopenia

Precautions: Pregnancy (B), lactation, elderly, renal disease, bleeding tendencies

Pharmocokinetics: Half-life 2 hr, excretion via urine/feces; plasma clearance 20%-25% lower in elderly with coronary artery disease; renal insufficiency decreases plasma clearance

Interactions:

• ↑ bleeding: aspirin, heparin, NSAIDs, abciximab, eptifibatide, clopidogrel, ticlopidine, dipyridamole, cefamandole, cefotetan, cefoperazone, plicamycin, valproic acid

↑ risk of bleeding: agrimony, alfalfa, angelica, anise, basil, bay, bilberry, black haw, bogbean, bromelain, buchu, chondroitin, cinchona bark, Dong quai, fenugreek, feverfew, garlic, ginger, ginkgo, ginseng, horse chestnut, Irish moss, kelp, kelpware, khella, lovage, lungwort, meadowsweet, motherwort, mugwort, nettle, papaya, parsley (large amts), pau d' arco, pineapple, poplar, prickly ash, safflower, saw palmetto, tonka bean, turmeric, wintergreen, yarrow

↓ anticoagulant effect: chamomile, coenzyme Q10, flax, glucomannan, goldenseal, guar gum

NURSING CONSIDERATIONS

Assess:

Platelet counts, Hct, Hgb, prior to treatment, within 6 hr of loading dose and at least qd thereafter; watch for bleeding from puncture sites, catheters or in stools, urine

Administer:

IV route

• IV: Give ½ dose in renal disease

• Dilute inj: withdraw and discard 100 ml from a 500 ml bag of sterile 0.9% NaCl or D_5W and replace this vol with 50 ml of tirofiban inj from one vial

• Tirofiban inj for sol is premixed in containers of 500 ml 0.9% NaCl (50 mg/ml)

• Minimize other arterial/venous punctures; IM inj, catheter use, intubation, to reduce bleeding risks

Y-site compatibility: Heparin

Evaluate:
• Therapeutic response: treatment of acute coronary syndrome

Teach patient/family:
• That it is necessary to quit smoking to prevent excessive vasoconstriction

tizanidine

(ti-za′nih-deen)

Zanaflex

Func. class.: Skeletal muscle relaxant, α_2-adrenergic agonist

Chem. class.: Imidazoline

Action: Increases presynaptic inhibition of motor neurons and reduces spasticity by α_2-adrenergic agonism

Uses: Acute/intermittent management of increased muscle tone associated with spasticity

Dosage and routes:
• *Adult:* **PO** 4-8 mg, increase gradually by 2-4 mg increments, may repeat dose q6-8h, not to exceed 36 mg/24 hr

Available forms: Tabs 2, 4 mg

Side effects/adverse reactions:

GI: Dry mouth, vomiting, increased ALT, abnormal LFTs, constipation

CNS: Somnolence, dizziness, speech disorder, dyskinesia, nervousness, hallucination, psychosis

OTHER: UTI, infection, blurred vision, urinary frequency, flulike symptoms, pharyngitis, rhinitis

Contraindications: Hypersensitivity

Precautions: Hypotension, liver disease, pregnancy (C), lactation, elderly, children, renal disease

Pharmacokinetics: Completely absorbed, widely distributed; half-life 2.5 hr, peak 1½ hr; protein binding 30%; metabolized by liver, excreted in urine, feces

Interactions:
• ↑ CNS depression: alcohol
• ↓ clearance of tizanidine: oral contraceptives

NURSING CONSIDERATIONS

Assess:
• For muscle spasticity baseline and throughout treatment
• For hypotension, gradual dosage increase should lessen hypotensive effects; have patient rise slowly from supine to upright; watch those patients receiving antihypertensives for increased effects
• For increased sedation, dizziness, hallucinations, psychosis; drug may need to be discontinued
• Vision by ophthalmic exam, corneal opacities may occur
• Hepatic studies: 1, 3, 6 mo during treatment and periodically thereafter

Teach patient/family:
• To rise slowly from lying or sitting to upright position
• To ask for assistance if dizziness, sedation occur; to avoid drinking alcohol, to avoid operating machinery or driving until effects are known

tobramycin (℞)

(toe-bra-mye′sin)

Nebcin, TOBI, tobramycin sulfate

Func. class.: Antiinfective

Chem. class.: Aminoglycoside

Action: Interferes with protein synthesis in bacterial cell by binding to ribosomal subunit, causing inaccurate peptide sequence to form in protein chain, causing bacterial death

Uses: Severe systemic infections of CNS, respiratory, GI, urinary tract, bone, skin, soft tissues caused by *Pseudomonas aeruginosa, Escherichia coli, Enterobacter, Providen-*

T

cia, Citrobacter, Staphylococcus, Proteus, Klebsiella, Serratia; cystic fibrosis (nebulizer) for *Pseudomonas aeruginosa*

Dosage and routes:

- *Adult:* **IM/IV** 3 mg/kg/day in divided doses q8h; may give up to 5 mg/kg/day in divided doses q6-8h; once qd dosing is an option
- *Child:* **IM/IV** 6-7.5 mg/kg/day in 3-4 equal divided doses
- *Child ≥6 yr:* **NEB** 300 mg bid in repeating cycles of 28 days on/28 days off of drug; give **INH** over 10-15 min using a handheld PARI LC PLUS reusable nebulizer with a DeVilbiss Pulmo-Aid compressor
- *Neonate <1 wk:* **IM** up to 4 mg/kg/day in divided doses q12h; **IV** up to 4 mg/kg/day in divided doses q12h diluted in 50-100 mg NS or D_5W; give over 30-60 min

Renal dose

- *Adult:* **IM/IV** 1 mg/kg, then dose determined by blood levels

Available forms: Inj 10, 40 mg/ml; powder for inj 1.2 g; inj 20 mg/2 ml; neb sol 300 mg/5 ml

Side effects/adverse reactions:

GU: ***Oliguria, hematuria, renal damage, azotemia, renal failure, nephrotoxicity***

CNS: Confusion, depression, numbness, tremors, ***convulsions,*** muscle twitching, ***neurotoxicity,*** dizziness, vertigo

EENT: ***Ototoxicity,*** deafness, visual disturbances, tinnitus

HEMA: ***Agranulocytosis, thrombocytopenia, leukopenia, eosinophilia,*** anemia

GI: Nausea, vomiting, anorexia; increased ALT, AST, bilirubin, hepatomegaly, ***hepatic necrosis,*** splenomegaly

CV: Hypo/hypertension, palpitation

INTEG: Rash, burning, urticaria, dermatitis, alopecia

Contraindications: Severe renal disease, hypersensitivity to aminoglycosides, pregnancy (D)

Precautions: Neonates, mild renal disease, myasthenia gravis, lactation, hearing deficits, Parkinson's disease, elderly

Pharmacokinetics:

IM: Onset rapid, peak 1 hr

IV: Onset immediate, peak 1 hr

Plasma half-life 2-3 hr prolonged in neonates; not metabolized, excreted unchanged in urine, crosses placental barrier, poor penetration into CSF

Interactions:

- ↑ ototoxicity, neurotoxicity, nephrotoxicity: other aminoglycosides, amphotericin B, polymyxin, vancomycin, ethacrynic acid, furosemide, mannitol, methoxyflurane, cisplatin, cephalosporins, bacitracin, acyclovir, penicillins

Toxicity: Lysine (large amounts)

NURSING CONSIDERATIONS

Assess:

- Weight before treatment; dosage is usually based on ideal body weight, but may be calculated on actual body weight
- I&O ratio, urinalysis qd for proteinuria, cells, casts; report sudden change in urine output
- VS during infusion; watch for hypotension, change in pulse
- IV site for thrombophlebitis, including pain, redness, swelling q30min; change site if needed; apply warm compresses to discontinued site
- Serum peak, drawn at 30-60 min after IV infusion or 60 min after IM inj, trough drawn just before next dose, peak 4-12 mcg/ml, trough 1-2 mcg/ml
- Urine pH if drug is used for UTI; urine should be kept alkaline
- Renal impairment by securing urine for CCr testing, BUN, serum creatinine; lower dosage should be given in renal impairment (CCr <80

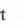

ml/min); monitor electrolytes: potassium, sodium, chloride, magnesium monthly, if patient is on long-term therapy
• Deafness by audiometric testing; ringing, roaring in ears; vertigo; assess hearing before, during, after treatment
• Dehydration: high specific gravity, decrease in skin turgor, dry mucous membranes, dark urine
• Overgrowth of infection: fever, malaise, redness, pain, swelling, perineal itching, diarrhea, stomatitis, change in cough, sputum
• C&S before starting treatment to identify infecting organism
• Vestibular dysfunction: nausea, vomiting, dizziness, headache; drug should be discontinued if severe
• Inj sites for redness, swelling, abscesses; use warm compresses at site

Administer:
• Bicarbonate to alkalinize urine if ordered in treating UTI, as drug is most active in an alkaline environment
• Drug in evenly spaced doses to maintain blood level; separate aminoglycosides and penicillins by ≥1 hr

IM route
• IM inj in large muscle mass; rotate inj sites

IV route
• Diluted in 50-100 ml 0.9% NaCl or D_5W (adult), infuse over 20-60 min

Additive compatibilities: Aztreonam, bleomycin, calcium gluconate, cefoxitin, ciprofloxacin, clindamycin, furosemide, metronidazole, ofloxacin, ranitidine, verapamil

Syringe compatibilities: Doxapram

Y-site compatibilities: Acyclovir, amifostine, amiodarone, amsacrine, aztreonam, ciprofloxacin, cisatracurium, cyclophosphamide, diltiazem, doxorubicin liposome, enalaprilat, esmolol, filgrastim, fluconazole, fludarabine, foscarnet, furosemide, granisetron, hydromorphone, IL-2, insulin (regular), labetalol, magnesium sulfate, melphalan, meperidine, midazolam, morphine, perphenazine, remifentanil, tacrolimus, teniposide, theophylline, thiotepa, tolazoline, vinorelbine, zidovudine

Nebulizer
• Give as close to q12hr apart as possible; do not use <6 hr apart
• Do not mix with dornase alfa in the nebulizer

Perform/provide:
• Adequate fluids of 2-3 L/day unless contraindicated to prevent irritation of tubules
• Flush of IV line with NS or D_5W after infusion
• Supervised ambulation, other safety measures with vestibular dysfunction

Evaluate:
• Therapeutic response: absence of fever, draining wounds, negative C&S after treatment

Teach patient/family:
• To report headache, dizziness, symptoms of overgrowth of infection, renal impairment
• To report loss of hearing; ringing, roaring in ears; feeling of fullness in head

Nebulizer
• Have patient inhale sitting or standing, breathe normally through the mouthpiece; may use noseclips
• To use multiple therapies first, then tobramycin

Treatment of overdose: Hemodialysis; monitor serum levels of drug

tobramycin ophthalmic

See appendix c

tocainide (℞)

(toe-kay′nide)

Tonocard

Func. class.: Antidysrhythmic (Class Ib)

Chem. class.: Lidocaine analog

Action: Produces dose-dependent decreases in sodium and potassium conduction, thereby decreasing the excitability of myocardial cells; does not affect heart rate or B/P

Uses: Life-threatening ventricular dysrhythmias (multifocal/unifocal PVCs), ventricular tachycardia

Dosage and routes:

• *Adult:* **PO** 400 mg q8h, may increase to 1.2-1.8 g/day in divided doses q8-12h

Available forms: Tabs 400, 600 mg

Side effects/adverse reactions:

CNS: Headache, dizziness, involuntary movement, confusion, psychosis, restlessness, irritability, paresthesias, tremors, ***seizures***

EENT: Tinnitus, blurred vision, hearing loss

GI: Nausea, vomiting, anorexia, diarrhea, hepatitis

CV: Hypotension, bradycardia, angina, PVCs, ***heart block, cardiovascular collapse, sinus arrest, CHF,*** chest pain, tachycardia, prodysrhythmia

RESP: Dyspnea, ***respiratory depression, pulmonary fibrosis,*** pulmonary edema, interstitial pneumonitis pneumonia

INTEG: Rash, urticaria, lupus, alopecia, sweating

HEMA: ***Blood dyscrasias: leukopenia, agranulocytosis, hypoplastic anemia, thrombocytopenia, bone marrow depression***

Contraindications: Hypersensitivity to amides, severe heart block

Precautions: Pregnancy (C), lactation, children, renal disease, liver disease, CHF, pulmonary depression, myasthenia gravis, blood dyscrasias, hypokalemia, atrial flutter/fibrillation

Pharmacokinetics:

PO: Peak 0.5-3 hr; half-life 10-17 hr; metabolized by liver, excreted in urine, 40% unchanged

Interactions:

• ↑ tocainide effects: metoprolol

• ↓ tocainide effects: cimetidine, rifampin

↑ toxicity, death: aconite

↑ effect: aloe, broom, chronic buckthorn use, cascara sagrada (chronic use), Chinese rhubarb, figwort, fumitory, goldenseal, kudzu, licorice

↓ effect: coltsfoot

↑ serotonin effect: horehound

Lab test interferences:

Increase: CPK

False positive: ANA titer

NURSING CONSIDERATIONS

Assess:

Chest x-ray film, pulmonary function tests, hepatic enzymes during treatment, monitor for lung sounds, sputum, SOB after 3-18 wk

• CBC, with differential and platelet count during beginning treatment and q3mo

• I&O ratio; check for decreasing output

• Blood levels (therapeutic level 4-10 mcg/ml)

• B/P continuously for fluctuations

• Lung fields; bilateral rales may occur in CHF patient

• Increased respiration, increased pulse; drug should be discontinued

• Toxicity: fine tremors, dizziness

• Blood dyscrasias: fatigue, sore throat, fever, bruising

• Cardiac status, respiration: rate, rhythm, character

Administer:

• With meals to decrease GI symptoms

Evaluate:

• Therapeutic response: decreased dysrhythmia

Teach patient/family:

• Of reason for medication and expected results

• Method for taking pulse at home and what to report to prescriber

• To avoid hazardous activities until drug response is known; dizziness, confusion, sedation may occur

• To use a bracelet or other emergency ID indicating medications taken, condition, and prescriber's name and phone number

• To report bleeding, bruising, respiratory symptoms, chills, fever, sore throat to prescriber

Treatment of overdose: O_2, artificial ventilation, ECG; administer dopamine for circulatory depression, diazepam or thiopental for convulsions

tolcapone (℞)

(toll'cah'pone)

Tasmar

Func. class.: Antiparkinson agent

Chem. class.: Catecholamine inhibitor (comt)

Action: Selective, reversible inhibitor of catecholamine; used as adjunct to levodopa/carbidopa therapy

Uses: Parkinsonism

Dosage and routes:

• *Adult:* **PO** 100-200 mg tid, with levodopa/carbidopa therapy; max 600 mg/day, discontinue if no benefit in 3 wk

Renal dose

• *Adult:* **PO** Use 100 mg tid or less

Available forms: Tabs 100, 200 mg

Side effects/adverse reactions:

CNS: Dystonia, dyskinesia, dreaming, *fatigue, headache, confusion,* psychosis, hallucination, dizziness

CV: Orthostatic hypotension, chest pain, hypotension

EENT: Cataract, eye inflammation

GI: Nausea, vomiting, anorexia, abdominal distress, diarrhea, constipation, ***fatal liver failure,*** increased LFTs

GU: UTI, urine discoloration, uterine tumor, micturition disorder, hematuria

HEMA: ***Hemolytic anemia, leukopenia, agranulocytosis***

INTEG: Sweating, alopecia

Contraindications: Hypersensitivity

Precautions: Renal disease, cardiac disease, hepatic disease, hypertension, pregnancy (C), asthma, lactation

Pharmacokinetics: Rapidly absorbed, peak 2 hr, protein binding 99%, extensively metabolized, half-life 2-3 hr, excreted in urine (60%), feces (40%)

Interactions:

• Inhibition of normal catecholamine metabolism: MAOIs, MAO-B inhibitor may be used

• May influence pharmacokinetics of: α-methyldopa, DOBUTamine, apomorphine, isoproterenol

↓ effect: kava

NURSING CONSIDERATIONS

Assess:

• Hepatic studies: AST, ALT, alk phosphatase, LDH, bilirubin, CBC, monitor ALT, AST q2wk × 1 yr, then q4wk × 6 mo, and q8wk thereafter; if LFTs are elevated, this drug should not be used

• Involuntary movements in parkinsonism: akinesia, tremors, staggering gait, muscle rigidity, drooling

• B/P, respiration during initial treat-

ment; hypo/hypertension should be reported
• Mental status: affect, mood, behavioral changes
Administer:
• PO tid with levodopa/carbidopa therapy, only to be used if levodopa/carbidopa does not provide satisfactory result
Perform/provide:
• Assistance with ambulation during beginning therapy
Evaluate:
• Therapeutic response: decrease in akathisia, increased mood
Teach patient/family:
• To change positions slowly to prevent orthostatic hypotension
• That urine, sweat may change color
• That food taken within 1 hr ac or 2 hr pc decreases action of drug by 20%
• To report signs of liver injury: clay-colored stools, jaundice, fatigue, appetite loss, lethargy
• To report nausea, vomiting, anorexia

tolnaftate topical

See appendix c

tolterodine (℞)

(toll-tehr′oh-deen)
Detrol, Detrol LA
Func. class.: Overactive bladder product
Chem. class.: Muscarinic receptor antagonist

Action: Relaxes smooth muscles in urinary tract by inhibiting acetylcholine at postganglionic sites
Uses: Overactive bladder (urinary frequency, urgency)
Dosage and routes:
• *Adult:* **PO** 2 mg bid, hepatic disease 1 mg bid; 4 mg qd, may decrease to 2 mg if needed
Available forms: Tabs 1, 2 mg; cap, ext rel 2, 4 mg
Side effects/adverse reactions:
CNS: Anxiety, paresthesia, fatigue, *dizziness,* headache
CV: Chest pain, hypertension
EENT: Vision abnormalities, xerophthalmia
GI: Nausea, vomiting, anorexia, abdominal pain, constipation, dry mouth, dyspepsia
GU: Dysuria, urinary retention, frequency, UTI
INTEG: Rash, pruritus
RESP: Bronchitis, cough, pharyngitis, URI
Contraindications: Hypersensitivity, uncontrolled narrow-angle glaucoma, urinary retention, gastric retention
Precautions: Pregnancy (C), lactation, children, renal/hepatic disease, controlled narrow-angle glaucoma
Pharmacokinetics: Rapidly absorbed, highly protein bound, extensively metabolized, excreted in urine/feces
Interactions:
• ↑ action of tolterodine: macrolide antiinfectives, antifungals
• Drug/food: food ↑ the bioavailability of tolterodine
NURSING CONSIDERATIONS
Assess:
• Urinary patterns: distention, nocturia, frequency, urgency, incontinence
• Allergic reactions: rash; if this occurs, drug should be discontinued
Evaluate:
• Urinary status: dysuria, frequency, nocturia, incontinence

Teach patient/family:
• To avoid hazardous activities; dizziness may occur

topiramate (℞)
(toh-pire′ah-mate)
Topamax
Func. class.: Anticonvulsant, miscellaneous
Chem. class.: Monosaccharide derivative

Action: Mechanism of action unknown; may prevent seizure spread as opposed to an elevation of seizure threshold
Uses: Partial seizures, in adults and children 2-16 yr old; tonic-clonic seizures; seizures in Lennox-Gastaut syndrome
Investigational uses: Bipolar disorder, cluster headache, infantile spasms
Dosage and routes:
Renal dose
• CCr <70 ml/min give ½ dose
Adjunctive therapy
• *Adult:* **PO** 25-50 mg/day initially, titrate by 25-50 mg/wk, up to 400 mg/day in 2 divided doses
Bipolar disorder (off-label)
• *Adult:* **PO** 50-200 mg/day, max 400 mg/day
Available forms: Tabs 25, 100, 200 mg; sprinkle cap 15, 25 mg
Side effects/adverse reactions:
RESP: URI, pharyngitis
EENT: Diplopia, vision abnormality
INTEG: Rash
MISC: Weight loss, leukopenia
CNS: Dizziness, fatigue, cognitive disorder, insomnia, anxiety, depression, paresthesia
GI: Diarrhea, anorexia, nausea, dyspepsia, abdominal pain, constipation, dry mouth
GU: Breast pain, dysmenorrhea, menstrual disorder

Contraindications: Hypersensitivity
Precautions: Hepatic, renal disease, acute myopia, secondary angle closure glaucoma, lactation, children, pregnancy (C)
Pharmacokinetics: Well absorbed, terminal half-life 21 hr; excreted in urine (55%-97% unchanged), crosses placenta, excreted in breast milk, protein binding (9%-17%); steady state 4 days
Interactions:
• ↓ levels of: oral contraceptives, digoxin
• ↑ CNS depression: alcohol, CNS depressants
• ↓ topiramate levels: phenytoin, carbamazepine, valproic acid
• Kidney stones: carbonic anhydrase inhibitors
↑ effect: gingko
↓ effect: ginseng, santonica

NURSING CONSIDERATIONS
Assess:
• Renal studies: urinalysis, BUN, urine creatinine q3mo
• Hepatic studies: ALT, AST, bilirubin if on long-term treatment
• CBC during long-term therapy
• Description of seizures: location, type, duration, aura
• Mental status: mood, sensorium, affect, behavioral changes; if mental status changes, notify prescriber
• Body weight, evidence of cognitive disorder
Administer:
⊘ Whole; do not break, crush, or chew tabs, very bitter
• May take without regard to meals
• Sprinkle cap can be given whole or opened and sprinkled on soft food; do not chew
Perform/provide:
• Storage at room temperature away from heat and light
• Assistance with ambulation dur-

T

ing early part of treatment; dizziness occurs
• Seizure precautions: padded side rails, move objects that may harm patient
Evaluate:
• Therapeutic response: decreased seizure activity
Teach patient/family:
• To carry emergency ID stating patient's name, drugs taken, condition, prescriber's name, phone number
• To avoid driving, other activities that require alertness
• Not to discontinue medication quickly after long-term use
Treatment of overdose: Lavage, VS

HIGH ALERT

topotecan

(toh-poh-tee′kan)
Hycamtin
Func. class.: Antineoplastic hormone
Chem. class.: Semisynthetic derivative of camptothecin (topoisomerase inhibitor)

Action: Antitumor drug with topoisomerase I–inhibitory activity topoisomerase I relieves torsional strain in DNA by causing single-strand breaks; causes double-strand DNA damage
Uses: Metastatic carcinoma of the ovary after failure of traditional chemotherapy
Dosage and routes:
• *Adult:* **IV INF** 1.5 mg/m^2 over 30 min qd × 5 days starting on day 1 of a 21-day course × 4 courses; may be reduced to 0.25 mg/m^2 for subsequent courses if severe neutropenia occurs
Renal dose
• *Adult:* **IV** CCr 20-39 ml/min 0.75 mg/m^2/day × 5 days starting on day 1 of a 21 day course
Available forms: Lyophilized powder for inj 4 mg
Side effects/adverse reactions:
HEMA: ***Neutropenia, leukopenia, thrombocytopenia, anemia, sepsis***
GI: Abdominal pain, constipation, diarrhea, obstruction, nausea, stomatitis, vomiting; increased ALT, AST; anorexia
CNS: Arthralgia, asthenia, headache, myalgia, pain
RESP: Dyspnea
INTEG: Total alopecia
Contraindications: Hypersensitivity, lactation, severe bone marrow depression, pregnancy (D)
Precautions: Children
Pharmacokinetics: Rapidly and completely absorbed; excreted in urine and feces as metabolites; half-life 6 hr, geriatric half-life 8 hr; 94% bound to plasma proteins
Interactions:
• ↑ duration of neutropenia when used with: G-CSF
• ↑ myelosuppression when used with: cisplatin

NURSING CONSIDERATIONS
Assess:
• Hepatic studies: AST, ALT, alk phosphatase, which may be elevated
• For CNS symptoms: drowsiness, confusion, depression, anxiety
• CBC, differential, platelet count weekly; withhold drug if WBC is <3500/mm^3 or platelet count is <100,000/mm^3; notify prescriber of these results; drug should be discontinued
• Buccal cavity q8h for dryness, sores or ulceration, white patches, oral pain, bleeding, dysphagia
• GI symptoms: frequency of stools, cramping

• Signs of dehydration: rapid respiration, poor skin turgor, decreased urine output, dry skin, restlessness, weakness

Perform/provide:

• Increased fluid intake to 2-3 L/day to prevent dehydration, unless contraindicated

• Changing of IV site q48h

• Rinsing of mouth tid-qid with water, club soda; brushing of teeth bid-tid with soft brush or cotton-tipped applicator for stomatitis; use unwaxed dental floss

• Nutritious diet with iron, vit K supplements, low fiber, few dairy products

Evaluate:

• Therapeutic response: decreased tumor size, spread of malignancy

Teach patient/family:

• To avoid foods with citric acid or hot or rough texture if stomatitis is present; to drink adequate fluids

• To report stomatitis; any bleeding, white spots, ulcerations in mouth; tell patient to examine mouth qd; report symptoms

• To report signs of anemia: fatigue, headache, faintness, shortness of breath, irritability

• To use contraception during therapy

toremifene (℞)

(tor-em'ih-feen)

Fareston

Func. class.: Antineoplastic

Chem. class.: Antiestrogen hormone

Action: Inhibits cell division by binding to cytoplasmic estrogen receptors; resembles normal cell complex but inhibits DNA synthesis and estrogen response of target tissue

Uses: Advanced breast carcinoma not responsive to other therapy in estrogen-receptor-positive patients (usually postmenopausal)

Dosage and routes:

• *Adult:* **PO** 60 mg qd

Available forms: Tabs 60 mg

Side effects/adverse reactions:

HEMA: ***Thrombocytopenia, leukopenia***

CV: ***CHF, MI, pulmonary embolism***

GI: Nausea, vomiting, altered taste (anorexia)

GU: Vaginal bleeding, pruritus vulvae

INTEG: Rash, alopecia

CV: Chest pain

CNS: Hot flashes, headache, lightheadedness, depression

META: Hypercalcemia

EENT: Ocular lesions, retinopathy, corneal opacity, blurred vision (high doses)

Contraindications: Hypersensitivity, pregnancy (D), history of thromboembolism

Precautions: Leukopenia, thrombocytopenia, lactation, cataracts

Pharmacokinetics:

PO: Peak 3 hr, excreted primarily in feces

Interactions:

• May ↑ the effect of: warfarin

Lab test interferences:

Increase: Serum calcium

NURSING CONSIDERATIONS

Assess:

• CBC, differential, platelet count qwk; withhold drug if WBC is $<3500/mm^3$ or platelet count is $<100,000/mm^3$; notify prescriber

• Bleeding: hematuria, guaiac, bruising, petechiae, mucosa or orifices q8h

• Effects of alopecia on body image; discuss feelings about body changes

◆ Symptoms indicating severe allergic reactions: rash, pruritus, ur-

T

ticaria, purpuric skin lesions, itching, flushing

Administer:

- Antacid before oral agent; give drug after evening meal, before bedtime
- Antiemetic 30-60 min before giving drug to prevent vomiting

Perform/provide:

- Liquid diet, if needed, including cola, Jell-O; dry toast or crackers may be added if patient is not nauseated or vomiting
- Increase fluid intake to 2-3 L/day to prevent dehydration
- Nutritious diet with iron, vitamin supplements as ordered
- Storage in light-resistant container at room temperature

Evaluate:

- Therapeutic response: decreased tumor size, spread of malignancy

Teach patient/family:

- To report any complaints, side effects to prescriber
- That vaginal bleeding, pruritus, hot flashes are reversible after discontinuing treatment
- To report immediately decreased visual acuity, which may be irreversible; stress need for routine eye exams; care providers should be told about tamoxifen therapy
- To report vaginal bleeding immediately
- That tumor flare—increase in size of tumor, increased bone pain—may occur and will subside rapidly; may take analgesics for pain
- That premenopausal women must use mechanical birth control because ovulation may be induced
- That hair may be lost during treatment; a wig or hairpiece may make patient feel better; new hair may be different in color, texture

torsemide (℞)

(tor'suh-mide)

Demadex

Func. class.: Loop diuretic

Chem. class.: Sulfonamide derivative

Action: Acts on loop of Henle, proximal, distal tubule by inhibiting absorption of chloride, sodium, water

Uses: Treatment of hypertension and edema in CHF, hepatic disease, renal disease

Dosage and routes:

CHF

- *Adult:* **PO/IV** 10-20 mg/day, may increase as needed up to 200 mg/day

Chronic renal failure

- *Adult:* **PO/IV** 20 mg/day, may increase up to 200 mg/day

Hepatic cirrhosis

- *Adult:* **PO/IV** 5-10 mg/day may increase as needed up to 40 mg/day

Hypertension

- *Adult:* **PO** 5 mg/day may increase to 10 mg/day

Available forms: Tabs 5, 10, 20, 100 mg; inj 10 mg/ml

Side effects/adverse reactions:

CNS: Headache, dizziness, asthenia, insomnia, nervousness

CV: Orthostatic hypotension, chest pain, ECG changes, ***circulatory collapse,*** ventricular tachycardia

EENT: Loss of hearing, ear pain, tinnitus, blurred vision

ENDO: Hyperglycemia, hyperuricemia

ELECT: Hypokalemia, hypochloremic alkalosis, hypomagnesemia, hypocalcemia, hyponatremia, metabolic alkalosis

GI: Nausea, diarrhea, dyspepsia, GI hemorrhage, rectal bleeding, cramps

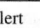

GU: Polyuria, ***renal failure,*** glycosuria

INTEG: Rash, photosensitivity
MS: Cramps, stiffness
RESP: Rhinitis, cough increase
Contraindications: Hypersensitivity to sulfonamides, anuria, hypovolemia, infants, lactation, electrolyte depletion
Precautions: Diabetes mellitus, dehydration, severe renal disease, pregnancy (C)
Pharmacokinetics:
PO: Rapidly absorbed; duration 6 hr; excreted in urine, feces, breast milk; crosses placenta; half-life 2-4 hr, plasma protein binding 97%-99%
Interactions:
- ↑ toxicity: lithium, non-depolarizing skeletal muscle relaxants, digitalis
- ↑ action of antihypertensives, oral anticoagulants, nitrates
- ↑ ototoxicity: aminoglycosides, cisplatin, vancomycin
- ↓ antihypertensive effect of torsemide: indomethacin, metolazone
- Incompatible with acidic sol, vit C, corticosteroids, diphenhydrAMINE, DOBUTamine, esmolol, epINEPHrine, gentamicin, meperidine, milrinone, netilmicin, norepinephrine, reserpine, spironolactone, tetracyclines in sol
- Incompatible with any drug in syringe

🍃 ↑ effect: aloe, cucumber, dandelion, horsetail, pumpkin, Queen Anne's lace
🍃 ↑ hypotension khella
🍃 Severe photosensitivity: St. John's wort

Lab test interferences:
Interference: GTT
NURSING CONSIDERATIONS
Assess:
- Hearing when giving high doses
- Weight, I&O daily to determine fluid loss; effect of drug may be decreased if used qd
- Rate, depth, rhythm of respiration, effect of exertion
- B/P lying, standing; postural hypotension may occur
- Electrolytes: K, Na, Cl; include BUN, blood glucose, CBC, serum creatinine, blood pH, ABGs, uric acid, Ca, Mg
- Glucose in urine of diabetic
- Signs and symptoms of metabolic alkalosis: drowsiness, restlessness
- Signs and symptoms of hypokalemia: postural hypotension, malaise, fatigue, tachycardia, leg cramps, weakness
- Rashes, temp elevation qd
- Confusion, especially in elderly; take safety precautions if needed

Administer:
- In AM to avoid interference with sleep if using drug as a diuretic
- Potassium replacement if potassium <3 mg/dl
- With food if nausea occurs; absorption may be decreased slightly

Evaluate:
- Therapeutic response: improvement in edema of feet, legs, sacral area qd if medication is being used in CHF

Teach patient/family:
- To rise slowly from lying, sitting position
- To recognize adverse reactions: muscle cramps, weakness, nausea, dizziness
- To take with food or milk for GI symptoms
- To take early in day to prevent nocturia

Treatment of overdose: Lavage if taken orally; monitor electrolytes, administer dextrose in saline; monitor hydration, CV, renal status

T

trace elements (℞)

Concentrated Multiple Trace Elements, ConTE-PAK-4, M.T.E.-4, M.T.E.-4 Concentrated, M.T.E.-5, M.T.E.-5 Concentrated, M.T.E.-6, M.T.E.-6 Concentrated, M.T.E.-7, MulTE-PAK-4, MulTE-PAK-5, Multiple Trace Element, Multiple Trace Element Neonatal, Multiple Trace Element Pediatric, Neotrace 4, PedTE-PAK-4, Pedtrace-4, P.T.E.-4, P.T.E.-5

Func. class.: Mineral supplements

Action: Needed for adequate absorption and synthesis of amino acids

Uses: Prevention of trace element deficiency

Dosage and routes:

Usual dosage may be given in TPN sol

Chromium

- *Adult:* **IV** 10-15 mcg qd
- *Child:* **IV** 0.14-0.20 mcg/kg/day

Copper

- *Adult:* **IV** 0.5-1.5 mg/day
- *Child:* **IV** 0.05-0.2 mg/kg/day

Iodine

- *Adult:* **IV** 1 mcg/kg/day

Manganese

- *Adult:* **IV** 1-3 mg/day

Selenium

- *Adult:* 40-120 mcg/day
- *Child:* 3 mcg/kg/day

Zinc

- *Adult:* **IV** 2-4 mg/day
- *Child:* **IV** 0.05 mg/kg/day

Available forms: Many forms available—see particular elements

Side effects/adverse reactions:

CHROMIUM: Seizures, coma, nausea, vomiting, ulcers, renal/hepatic toxicity

COPPER: Personality changes, diarrhea, weakness, photophobia, muscle weakness

IODINE: Headache, edema of eyelids, acne, metallic taste, sore mouth, running nose

MANGANESE: Incoordination, headache, irritability, lability, slurred speech, impotence

SELENIUM: Alopecia, depression, vomiting, GI cramping, nervousness, garlic smell

ZINC: Vomiting, oliguria, hypothermia, vision changes, tachycardia, jaundice, coma

Precautions: Hepatic, biliary disease, pregnancy (C), lactation, vomiting, diarrhea

NURSING CONSIDERATIONS

Assess:

- Trace element levels; notify prescriber if low; copper 0.07-0.15 mg/ml, zinc 0.05-0.15 mg/100 ml, manganese 4-20 mcg/100 ml, selenium 0.1-0.19 mcg/ml
- Trace element deficiency of patient receiving TPN for extended period

Administer:

- By IV infusion, often mixed with TPN solution

Evaluate:

- Therapeutic response: absence of element deficiency

tramadol (℞)

(tram′a-dole)

Ultram

Func. class.: Central analgesic

Action: Not completely understood, binds to opioid receptors, inhibits reuptake of norepinephrine, serotonin; does not cause histamine release or affect heart rate

Uses: Management of moderate to severe pain

Dosage and routes:
Renal dose
- CCr <30 ml/min give q12h, max 200 mg/day
- *Adult:* **PO** 50-100 mg prn q4-6h; not to exceed 400 mg/day
- *Elderly (>75 years):* **PO** <300 mg/day in divided doses

Hepatic impairment
- **PO** 50 mg q12h

Available forms: Tabs 50 mg

Side effects/adverse reactions:

CNS: Dizziness, CNS stimulation, somnolence, headache, anxiety, confusion, euphoria, ***seizures,*** hallucinations

GI: Nausea, constipation, vomiting, dry mouth, diarrhea, abdominal pain, anorexia, flatulence, *GI bleeding*

CV: Vasodilation, orthostatic hypotension, tachycardia, hypertension, abnormal ECG

INTEG: Pruritus, rash, urticaria, vesicles

GU: Urinary retention/frequency, menopausal symptoms, dysuria, menstrual disorder

Contraindications: Hypersensitivity, acute intoxication with any CNS depressant

Precautions: Seizure disorder, pregnancy (C), lactation, children, elderly, renal or hepatic disease, respiratory depression, head trauma, increased intracranial pressure, acute abdominal condition, drug abuse

Do not confuse:
tramadol/Toradol

Pharmacokinetics: Rapidly and almost completely absorbed, steady state 2 days, may cross blood-brain barrier, extensively metabolized, 30% excreted in the urine as unchanged drug

Interactions:
- ↓ levels of tramadol: carbamazepine
- Inhibition of norepinephrine and serotonin reuptake: MAO inhibitors, use together with caution
- ↑ CNS depression: alcohol, sedatives, hypnotics, opiates
- ↑ CNS depression: chamomile, hops, kava, skullcap, valerian

Lab test interferences:
Increase: Creatinine, hepatic enzymes
Decrease: Hgb

NURSING CONSIDERATIONS

Assess:
- Pain: location, type, character, give before pain becomes extreme
- I&O ratio: check for decreasing output; may indicate urinary retention
- Need for drug
- Bowel pattern; for constipation increase fluids, bulk in diet
- CNS changes: dizziness, drowsiness, hallucinations, euphoria, LOC, pupil reaction
- Allergic reactions: rash, urticaria

Administer:

PO route
- With antiemetic for nausea, vomiting
- When pain is beginning to return; determine dosage interval by patient response

Perform/provide:
- Storage in cool environment, protected from sunlight
- Assistance with ambulation
- Safety measures: side rails, nightlight, call bell within easy reach

Evaluate:
- Therapeutic response: decrease in pain

Teach patient/family:
- To report any symptoms of CNS changes, allergic reactions
- That drowsiness, dizziness, and confusion may occur, to call for assistance
- To make position changes slowly, orthostatic hypotension may occur

T

- To avoid OTC medications and alcohol unless approved by prescriber

trandolapril (℞)

(tran-doe′la-prill)

Mavik

Func. class.: Antihypertensive

Chem. class.: Angiotensin-converting enzyme inhibitor

Action: Selectively suppresses renin-angiotensin-aldosterone system; inhibits ACE; prevents conversion of angiotensin I to angiotensin II, dilates arterial and venous vessels, lowers B/P

Uses: Hypertension, heart failure, post-MI/left ventricular dysfunction post MI

Dosage and routes:

Hypertension

- *Adult:* **PO** 1 mg/day, 2 mg/day in African-Americans, make dosage adjustment ≥wk; up to 8 mg/day

Heart failure post-MI/left ventricular dysfunction post MI

- *Adult:* **PO** 1 mg/day, titrate upward to 4 mg/day if tolerated

Renal/hepatic dose

- CCr <30 ml/min give 0.5 mg/day, may increase gradually up to 4 mg/day

Available forms: Tabs 1, 2, 4 mg

Side effects/adverse reactions:

CV: Hypotension, ***MI,*** palpitations, angina, TIAs, ***stroke,*** bradycardia, dysrhythmias

CNS: Dizziness, paresthesias, headache, fatigue, drowsiness, depression, sleep disturbances, anxiety

GI: Nausea, vomiting, cramps, diarrhea, constipation, pancreatitis, *dyspepsia*

INTEG: Rash, purpura, pruritus

HEMA: ***Agranulocytosis, neutropenia, leukopenia, anemia***

GU: ***Proteinuria, renal failure***

RESP: Dyspnea, *cough*

MISC: Hyperkalemia, hyponatremia, impotence, *myalgia,* ***angioedema,*** muscle cramps, asthenia, hypocalcemia, gout

Contraindications: Hypersensitivity, history of angioedema, pregnancy (D) (2nd/3rd trimester)

Precautions: Hyperkalemia, hepatic disease, bilateral renal stenosis, post kidney transplant, aorta/mitral valve stenosis, cirrhosis, severe renal disease, untreated CHF, autoimmune disease, severe hypertension

Pharmacokinetics:

PO: Peak 4-10 hr; half-life 0.6-1.1 hr, 16-24 hr; metabolized by liver, excreted in urine

Interactions:

- Severe hypotension: diuretics, other antihypertensives
- ↓ effects of trandolapril: antacids
- ↑ potassium levels: salt substitutes, potassium-sparing diuretics, potassium supplements
- ↑ effects of ergots, neuromuscular blocking agents, antihypertensives, hypoglycemics, barbiturates, reserpine, levodopa
- Effects ↑: phenothiazines, diuretics

↑ toxicity, death: aconite

↑ or ↓ antihypertensive effect: astragalus, cola tree

↑ antihypertensive effect: barberry, betony, black catechu, black cohosh, bloodroot, broom, burdock, cat's claw, dandelion, goldenseal, Irish moss, Jamaican dogwood, kelp, khella, mistletoe, parsley

↓ antihypertensive effect: coltsfoot, guarana, khat, licorice

NURSING CONSIDERATIONS

Assess:

- B/P, pulse q4h; note rate, rhythm, quality
- Electrolytes: K, Na, Cl
- Baselines in renal, hepatic studies before therapy begins

• Edema in feet, legs daily
• Skin turgor, dryness of mucous membranes for hydration status
• Symptoms of CHF: edema, dyspnea, wet rales

Evaluate:

• Therapeutic response: decreased B/P

Teach patient/family:

• Not to use OTC (cough, cold, orallergy) products unless directed by prescriber
• To avoid sunlight or wear sunscreen for photosensitivity
• To comply with dosage schedule, even if feeling better
• To notify prescriber of mouth sores, sore throat, fever, swelling of hands or feet, irregular heartbeat, chest pain, signs of angioedema
• That excessive perspiration, dehydration, vomiting, diarrhea may lead to fall in blood pressure; consult prescriber if these occur
• That drug may cause dizziness, fainting; light-headedness may occur during 1st few days of therapy
• That drug may cause skin rash or impaired perspiration
• Not to discontinue drug abruptly
• Not to use OTC products unless directed by prescriber
• To rise slowly to sitting or standing position to minimize orthostatic hypotension

tranylcypromine (℞)

(tran-ill-sip′roe-meen)
Parnate

Func. class.: Antidepressant-MAOI
Chem. class.: Nonhydrazine

Action: Increases concentrations of endogenous epinephrine, norepinephrine, serotonin, dopamine in storage sites in CNS by inhibition of MAO; increased concentration reduces depression

Uses: Depression, when uncontrolled by other means

Investigational uses: Bulimia, cocaine addiction, migraines, seasonal affective disorder, panic disorder

Dosage and routes:

• *Adult:* **PO** 10 mg bid; may increase to 30 mg/day after 2 wk; up to 60 mg/day

Available forms: Tabs 10 mg

Side effects/adverse reactions:

HEMA: Anemia
CNS: Dizziness, drowsiness, confusion, headache, anxiety, tremors, stimulation, weakness, hyperreflexia, mania, insomnia, fatigue
GI: Constipation, dry mouth, nausea, vomiting, *anorexia,* diarrhea, weight gain
GU: Change in libido, urinary frequency
INTEG: Rash, flushing, increased perspiration
CV: Orthostatic hypotension, hypertension, dysrhythmias, ***hypertensive crisis***
EENT: Blurred vision
ENDO: ***SIADH-like syndrome***

Contraindications: Hypersensitivity to MAOIs, elderly, uncontrolled hypertension, CHF, severe hepatic disease, pheochromocytoma, severe renal disease, severe cardiac disease

Precautions: Suicidal patients, convulsive disorders, severe depression, schizophrenia, hyperactivity, diabetes mellitus, pregnancy (C), lactation, child <16 yr

Pharmacokinetics: Metabolized by liver, excreted by kidneys, crosses placenta, excreted in breast milk

Interactions:

• ↑ pressor effects: guanethidine, clonidine, indirect-acting sympathomimetics (epHEDrine), busPIRone

T

• ↑ effects of: direct-acting sympathomimetics (epINEPHrine), alcohol, barbiturates, benzodiazepines, CNS depressants, levodopa, β-blockers, antidiabetics, sulfonamide, rauwolfia alkaloids, methyldopa, thiazide diuretics, sumatriptan

Serotonin-syndrome: fluoxetine, fluvoxamine, sertraline, paroxetine

Hypertensive crisis: tricyclics, meperidine, dibenzazepine agents, methylphenidate, dextromethorphan, nasal decongestants, sinus medications, appetite suppressants, asthma inhalants

• Drug/food: tyramine foods; avoid all

Hypertensive crisis: betel palm, butcher's broom, capsicum peppers, galanthamine, green tea (large amounts), guarana (large amounts), night-blooming cereus

Mania: ginseng

Serotonin syndrome: parsley

NURSING CONSIDERATIONS

Assess:

• B/P (lying, standing), pulse; if systolic B/P drops 20 mm Hg, stop drug, notify prescriber

• Blood studies: CBC, leukocytes, cardiac enzymes (long-term therapy)

• Hepatic studies: ALT, AST, bilirubin; hepatotoxicity may occur

Toxicity: increased headache, palpitation; discontinue drug immediately; prodromal signs of hypertensive crisis

• Mental status changes: mood, sensorium, affect, memory (long, short), increase in psychiatric symptoms

• Urinary retention, constipation, edema: take weight weekly

• Withdrawal symptoms: headache, nausea, vomiting, muscle pain, weakness

Administer:

• Increased fluids, bulk in diet if constipation occurs

• With food or milk for GI symptoms

• Crushed if patient is unable to swallow medication whole

• Dosage hs if oversedation occurs during day

• Gum, hard candy, frequent sips of water for dry mouth

• Phentolamine for severe hypertension

Perform/provide:

• Cool storage in tight container

• Assistance with ambulation during beginning therapy for drowsiness/dizziness

• Safety measures including side rails

• Checking to see if PO medication swallowed

Evaluate:

• Therapeutic response: decreased depression

Teach patient/family:

• That therapeutic effects may take 48 hr-3 wks

• To avoid driving, other activities requiring alertness

• To avoid alcohol ingestion, CNS depressants, OTC medications: cold, weight loss, hay fever, cough syrup

• Not to discontinue medication quickly after long-term use

To avoid high-tyramine foods: cheese (aged), sour cream, yogurt, beer, wine, pickled products, liver, raisins, bananas, figs, avocados, meat tenderizers, chocolate, increased caffeine, ginseng; give complete list of tyramine foods

• To report headache, palpitation, neck stiffness

• To rise slowly to prevent postural hypotension

Treatment of overdose: Lavage, activated charcoal; monitor electrolytes, vital signs; diazepam IV, $NaHCO_3$

HIGH ALERT

trastuzumab (℞)

(tras-tuz'uh-mab)

Herceptin

Func. class.: Miscellaneous antineoplastic

Chem. class.: Humanized monoclonal antibody

Action: DNA-derived monoclonal antibody selectively binds to extracellular portion of human epidermal growth factor receptor 2; it inhibits proliferation of cancer cells

Uses: Breast cancer; metastatic with overexpression of HER2

Dosage and routes:

• *Adult:* **IV** 4 mg/kg given over 90 min, then maintenance 2 mg/kg given over 30 min; do not give as IV push or BOL

Available forms: Lyophilized powder 440 mg

Side effects/adverse reactions:

CNS: Dizziness, numbness, paresthesias, depression, insomnia, neuropathy, peripheral neuritis

*CV: **Tachycardia, CHF***

INTEG: Rash, acne, herpes simplex

GI: Nausea, vomiting, anorexia, diarrhea

MISC: Flulike symptoms; fever, headache, chills

HEMA: Anemia, ***leukopenia***

MS: Arthralgia, bone pain

META: Edema, peripheral edema

RESP: Cough, dyspnea, pharyngitis, rhinitis, sinusitis

*SYST: **Anaphylaxis, angioedema***

Contraindications: Hypersensitivity to this drug, Chinese hamster ovary cell protein

Precautions: Pregnancy (B), lactation, children, elderly, cardiac disease, anemia, leukopenia

Pharmacokinetics: Half-life 1.7-12 days

Interactions:

• ↑ chance of cardiomyopathy: anthracyclines, cyclophosphamide, avoid use

NURSING CONSIDERATIONS

Assess:

◆ CHF and other cardiac symptoms: dyspnea, coughing; gallop; obtain a full cardiac workup including ECG, echo, MUGA

• For symptoms of infection; may be masked by drug

• CNS reaction: LOC, mental status, dizziness, confusion

◆ For hypersensitive reactions, anaphylaxis

◆ For infusion reactions that may be fatal: fever, chills, nausea, vomiting, pain, headache, dizziness, hypotension, discontinue drug

Administer:

• Acetaminophen as ordered to alleviate fever and headache

IV route

• After reconstituting vial with 20 ml bacteriostatic water for inj, 1.1% benzyl alcohol preserved (supplied) to yield 21 mg/ml, mark date on vial 28 days from reconstitution date, if patient is allergic to benzyl alcohol, reconstitute with sterile water for inj—use immediately

• Do not mix or dilute with other drugs or dextrose sol

Perform/provide:

• Increased fluid intake to 2-3 L/day

Evaluate:

• Therapeutic response: decrease in size of tumors

Teach patient/family:

• To take acetaminophen for fever

• To avoid hazardous tasks, since confusion, dizziness may occur

• To report signs of infection: sore throat, fever, diarrhea, vomiting

• Emotional lability is common; notify prescriber if severe or incapacitating

travoprost ophthalmic

See appendix c

trazodone (℞)

(tray'zoe-done)

Desyrel, Desyrel Dividose, trazodone HCl, Trazon, Trialodine

Func. class.: Antidepressant, miscellaneous

Chem. class.: Triazolopyridine

Action: Selectively inhibits serotonin, norepinephrine uptake by brain, potentiates behavorial changes

Uses: Depression

Investigational uses: Chronic pain

Dosage and routes:

• *Adult:* **PO** 150 mg/day in divided doses; may increase by 50 mg/day q3-4d, not to exceed 600 mg/day

• *Child 6-18 yr:* **PO** 1.5-2 mg/kg/day in divided dose, may increase q3-4d, up to 6 mg/kg/day

• *Geriatric:* **PO** 25-50 mg hs, increase by 25-50 mg q3-7d to desired dose, usual 75-150 mg/day

Available forms: Tabs 50, 100, 150, 300 mg

Side effects/adverse reactions:

HEMA: ***Agranulocytosis, thrombocytopenia, eosinophilia, leukopenia***

CNS: Dizziness, drowsiness, confusion, headache, anxiety, tremors, stimulation, weakness, insomnia, nightmares, EPS (elderly), increase in psychiatric symptoms

GI: Diarrhea, dry mouth, nausea, vomiting, ***paralytic ileus,*** increased appetite, cramps, epigastric distress, jaundice, ***hepatitis,*** stomatitis, constipation

GU: Urinary retention, ***acute renal failure,*** priapism

INTEG: Rash, urticaria, sweating, pruritus, photosensitivity

CV: Orthostatic hypotension, ECG changes, tachycardia, ***hypertension,*** palpitations

EENT: Blurred vision, tinnitus, mydriasis

Contraindications: Hypersensitivity to tricyclics, recovery phase of MI, convulsive disorders, prostatic hypertrophy

Precautions: Suicidal patients, severe depression, increased intraocular pressure, narrow-angle glaucoma, urinary retention, cardiac disease, hepatic disease, hyperthyroidism, electroshock therapy, elective surgery, pregnancy (C)

Pharmacokinetics: Metabolized by liver, excreted by kidneys, feces; half-life 4.4-7.5 hr

Interactions:

• ↓ effects of guanethidine, clonidine, indirect-acting sympathomimetics (epHEDrine)

• ↑ toxicity: fluoxetine

• ↑ effects of direct-acting sympathomimetics (epINEPHrine), alcohol, barbiturates, benzodiazepines, CNS depressants

◆ Hyperpyretic crisis, convulsions, hypertensive episode: MAOI (pargyline [Eutonyl])

🍃 ↑ CNS depression: chamomile, hops, kava, lavender, skullcap, valerian

🍃 Serotonin syndrome: SAM-e, St. John's wort

🍃 ↑ anticholinergic effect: corkwood, jimsonweed

Lab test interferences:

Increase: Serum bilirubin, blood glucose, alk phosphatase

False increase: Urinary catecholamines
Decrease: VMA, 5-HIAA

NURSING CONSIDERATIONS

Assess:

• Pain: location, duration, intensity before and 1-2 hr after medication
• B/P (lying, standing), pulse q4h; if systolic B/P drops 20 mm Hg, hold drug, notify prescriber; take vital signs q4h in patients with cardiovascular disease
• Blood studies: CBC, leukocytes, differential, cardiac enzymes if patient is receiving long-term therapy
• Hepatic studies: AST, ALT, bilirubin
• Weight qwk; appetite may increase with drug
• ECG for flattening of T wave, bundle branch block, AV block, dysrhythmias in cardiac patients
• EPS, primarily in elderly: rigidity, dystonia, akathisia
• Mental status changes: mood, sensorium, affect, suicidal tendencies, increase in psychiatric symptoms, depression, panic
• Urinary retention, constipation; constipation most likely in children
• Withdrawal symptoms: headache, nausea, vomiting, muscle pain, weakness; not usual unless drug discontinued abruptly
• Alcohol consumption; hold dose until morning

Administer:

• Increased fluids, bulk in diet if constipation occurs, especially in elderly
• With food, milk for GI symptoms
• Dosage hs for oversedation during day; may take entire dose hs; elderly may not tolerate qd dosing
• Gum, hard candy, frequent sips of water for dry mouth

Perform/provide:

• Storage in tight, light-resistant container at room temperature
• Assistance with ambulation during beginning therapy for drowsiness/dizziness
• Safety measures, including side rails, primarily for elderly
• Checking to see if PO medication swallowed

Evaluate:

• Therapeutic response: decreased depression

Teach patient/family:

• That therapeutic effects may take 2-3 wk
• To use caution in driving, other activities requiring alertness because of drowsiness, dizziness, blurred vision
• To avoid alcohol ingestion, other CNS depressants
• Not to discontinue medication quickly after long-term use; may cause nausea, headache, malaise
• To report urinary retention immediately
• To wear sunscreen or large hat, since photosensitivity occurs
• Signs of suicidal ideation

Treatment of overdose: ECG monitoring; induce emesis; lavage, activated charcoal; administer anticonvulsant

treprostinil (℞)

(treh-prah'stin-ill)
Remodulin
Func. class.: Antiplatelet agent

Action: Direct vasodilation of pulmonary, systemic arterial vascular beds, inhibition of platelet aggregation

Uses: Pulmonary arterial hypertension (PAH) NYHA class II through IV

Dosage and routes:

• *Adult:* **SC INF** 1.25 ng/kg/min by **CONT INF,** may reduce to 0.625 mg if not tolerated

Hepatic dose

• *Adult:* **SC INF** 0.625 ng/kg/min and increase cautiously

Available forms: Inj 1, 2.5, 5, 10 mg/ml

Side effects/adverse reactions:

INTEG: Rash, pruritus

GI: Nausea, *diarrhea*

CV: Vasodilation, hypotension, edema

CNS: Dizziness, headache

SYST: Infusion site reactions, infusion site pain

OTHER: Jaw pain

Contraindications: Hypersensitivity

Precautions: Past liver disease, renal disease, elderly, pregnancy (B), lactation, children

Pharmacokinetics: Metabolized by liver, excreted in urine, feces; terminal half-life 2-4 hr

Interactions:

• ↑ bleeding tendencies: anticoagulants, aspirin

• Excessive hypotension: diuretics, antihypertensives, vasodilators

NURSING CONSIDERATIONS

Assess:

• Hepatic studies: AST, ALT, bilirubin, creatinine (long-term therapy)

Blood studies: CBC; CBC q2wk × 3 mo, Hct, Hgb, PT (long-term therapy)

Bleed time baseline and throughout; levels may be 2-5 × normal limit

Administer:

• SC infusion continuous

Evaluate:

• Therapeutic response: decreased pulmonary arterial hypertension (PAH)

Teach patient/family:

• That blood work will be necessary during treatment

• To report side effects such as diarrhea, skin rashes

tretinoin (vit A acid, retinoic acid) (℞)

(tret′i-noyn)

Retin-A, Stievaa✦, Tretinoin LF, IV, Vesanoid

Func. class.: Vit A acid, acne product; antineoplastic (misc.)

Chem. class.: Tretinoin derivative

Action: Decreases cohesiveness of follicular epithelium, decreases microcomedone formation (TOP); induces maturation of acute promyelocytic leukemia, exact action is unknown (PO)

Uses: Acne vulgaris (grades 1-3) (top); (PO) acute promyelocytic leukemia

Investigational uses: Skin cancer

Dosage and routes:

• *Adult and child:* **TOP** cleanse area, apply hs; cover lightly

Promyelocytic leukemia

• *Adult:* **PO** 45 mg/m^2/day given as 2 evenly divided doses until remission, discontinue treatment 30 days after remission or 90 days of treatment, whichever is first

Available forms: Cream 0.01%, 0.05%; gel 0.01%, 0.025%; liquid 0.05%; caps 10 mg

Side effects/adverse reactions:

INTEG: (top) Rash, stinging, warmth, redness, erythema, blistering, crusting, peeling, contact dermatitis, hypopigmentation, hyperpigmentation

Oral

CNS: Headache, fever, sweating

GI: Nausea, vomiting, ***hemorrhage,*** *abdominal pain, diarrhea, consti-*

pation, dyspepsia, distention, hepatitis

Contraindications: Hypersensitivity to retinoids or sensitivity to parabens, pregnancy (D) (PO)

Precautions: Lactation, eczema, sunburn, pregnancy (C) (top)

Pharmacokinetics:

TOP: Poor systemic absorption

Interactions:

• ↑ peeling: medication containing agents such as sulfur, benzoyl peroxide, resorcinol, salicylic acid (top)

• Use with caution: medicated, abrasive soaps, cleansers that have drying effect, products with high concentrations of alcohol astringents (top)

• ↑ plasma concentrations of tretinoin: ketoconazole (oral)

NURSING CONSIDERATIONS

Assess:

Topical

• Area of body involved, what helps or aggravates condition; cysts, dryness, itching; lesions may worsen at beginning of treatment

Oral

• Hepatic function, coagulation, hematologic parameters, also cholesterol, triglyceride

Administer:

Topical

• Once daily before hs; cover area lightly using gauze; use gloves to apply

Perform/provide:

Topical

• Storage at room temperature

• Hand washing after application

Evaluate:

• Therapeutic response: decrease in size and number of lesions

Teach patient/family:

Topical

• To avoid application on normal skin, getting cream in eyes, nose, other mucous membranes

• To avoid sunlight, sunlamps, or use protective clothing, sunscreen

• That treatment may cause warmth, stinging, dryness, peeling will occur

• That cosmetics may be used over drug; not to use shaving lotions

• That rash may occur during first 1-3 wk of therapy

• That drug does not cure condition; only relieves symptoms

• That therapeutic results may be seen in 2-3 wk but may not be optimal until after 6 wk

triamcinolone (℞)

(trye-am-sin'oh-lone)

Amcort, Aristocort, Aristocort Forte, Aristocort Intralesional, Aristospan Intra-Articular, Aristospan Intralesional, Articulose L.A., Atolone, Azmacort, Cenocort A-40, Cenocort Forte, Kenacort, Kenaject-40, Kenalog, Kenalog-10, Kenalog-40, Tac-3, Tac-40, Triam-A, triamcinolone, triamcinolone acetonide, Triam Forte, Triamolone 40, Triamonide 40, Tri-Kort, Trilog, Trilone, Trisoject

Func. class.: Corticosteroid

Chem. class.: Glucocorticoid, intermediate-acting

Action: Decreases inflammation by suppression of migration of polymorphonuclear leukocytes, fibroblasts, reversal to increase capillary permeability and lysosomal stabilization

Uses: Severe inflammation, immunosuppression, neoplasms, asthma (steroid dependent), collagen, respiratory, dermatologic disorders

T

Dosage and routes:

• *Adult:* **PO** 4-12 mg/day in divided doses qd-qid; **IM** 40 mg qwk (acetonide, or diacetate), 5-48 mg into neoplasms (diacetate, acetonide), 2-40 mg into joint or soft tissue (diacetate, acetonide), 0.5 mg/in^2 of affected intralesional skin (hexacetonide), 2-20 mg into joint or soft tissue (hexacetonide)

• *Child:* **PO** 117 mcg/kg/day as a single or divided dose

Asthma

• *Adult:* **INH** 2 tid-qid, not to exceed 16 **INH**/day

• *Child 6-12 yr:* **INH** 1-2 tid-qid, not to exceed 12 **INH**/day

Available forms: Tabs 1, 2, 4, 8 mg; syr 2 mg/5 ml, 4.85 mg/5 ml; inj 25, 40 mg/ml diacetate; inj 3, 10, 40 mg/ml acetonide; inj 20, 5 mg/ml hexacetonide; aerosol actuation/100 mcg (acetonide)

Side effects/adverse reactions:

INTEG: Acne, poor wound healing, ecchymosis, petechiae

CNS: Depression, flushing, sweating, headache, mood changes

CV: Hypertension, ***circulatory collapse, thrombophlebitis, embolism,*** tachycardia, edema

HEMA: ***Thrombocytopenia***

MS: Fractures, osteoporosis, weakness

GI: Diarrhea, nausea, abdominal distention, ***GI hemorrhage,*** *increased appetite,* ***pancreatitis***

EENT: Fungal infections, increased intraocular pressure, blurred vision

Contraindications: Psychosis, hypersensitivity, idiopathic thrombocytopenia, acute glomerulonephritis, amebiasis, fungal infections, nonasthmatic bronchial disease, child <2 yr, AIDS, TB, adrenal insufficiency

Precautions: Pregnancy (C), diabetes mellitus, glaucoma, osteoporosis, seizure disorders, ulcerative colitis, CHF, myasthenia gravis, renal disease, esophagitis, peptic ulcer, lactation

Pharmacokinetics:

PO/IM: Peak 1-2 hr, half-life 2-5 hr

Interactions:

• ↓ action of triamcinolone: cholestyramine, colestipol, barbiturates, rifampin, epHEDrine, phenytoin, theophylline

• ↓ effects of anticoagulants, anticonvulsants, antidiabetics, ambenonium, neostigmine, isoniazid, toxoids, vaccines, anticho-linesterases, salicylates, somatrem

• ↑ side effects: alcohol, salicylates, indomethacin, amphotericin B, digitalis, cycloSPORINE, diuretics

• ↑ action of triamcinolone: salicylates, estrogens, indomethacin, oral contraceptives, ketoconazole, macrolide antiinfectives

Hypokalemia: aloe, buckthorn, cascara, Chinese rhubarb, senna

Lab test interferences:

Increase: Cholesterol, sodium, blood glucose, uric acid, calcium, urine glucose

Decrease: Ca, K, T_4, T_3, thyroid ^{131}I uptake test, urine 17-OHCS, 17-KS, PBI

False negative: Skin allergy tests

NURSING CONSIDERATIONS

Assess:

• Potassium, blood glucose, urine glucose while on long-term therapy; hypokalemia and hyperglycemia

• Weight qd; notify prescriber if weekly gain >5 lb

• B/P q4h, pulse; notify prescriber if chest pain occurs

• I&O ratio; be alert for decreasing urinary output, increasing edema

• Plasma cortisol levels during long-term therapy (normal level: 138-635 nmol/L SI units when drawn at 8 AM)

• Infection: increased temp, WBC, even after withdrawal of medication; drug masks infection
• Potassium depletion: paresthesias, fatigue, nausea, vomiting, depression, polyuria, dysrhythmias, weakness
• Edema, hypertension, cardiac symptoms
• Mental status: affect, mood, behavioral changes, aggression

Administer:
• After shaking susp (parenteral)
• Titrated dose; use lowest effective dose
• IM inj deep in large muscle mass; rotate sites; avoid deltoid; use 21G needle
• In one dose in AM to prevent adrenal suppression; avoid SC administration; may damage tissue
• With food or milk to decrease GI symptoms, tablet may be crushed

Perform/provide:
• Assistance with ambulation for patient with bone tissue disease to prevent fractures
• Use of spacer device for elderly patients with inhaler

Evaluate:
• Therapeutic response: ease of respirations, decreased inflammation

Teach patient/family:
• That emergency ID as steroid user should be carried
• To notify prescriber if therapeutic response decreases; dosage adjustment may be needed
• Not to discontinue abruptly; adrenal crisis can result
• To avoid OTC products: salicylates, alcohol in cough products, cold preparations unless directed by prescriber
• About cushingoid symptoms
• The symptoms of adrenal insufficiency: nausea, anorexia, fatigue, dizziness, dyspnea, weakness, joint pain

triamcinolone topical

See appendix c

triamcinolone (topical-oral) (OTC)

(trye-am-sin'oh-lone)

Kenalog in Orabase, Oralone Dental

Func. class.: Topical anesthetic

Chem. class.: Synthetic fluorinated adrenal corticosteroid

Action: Inhibits nerve impulses from sensory nerves

Uses: Oral pain

Dosage and routes:
• *Adult and child:* **TOP** press ¼ inch into affected area until film appears, repeat bid-tid

Available forms: Paste 0.1%

Side effects/adverse reactions:

INTEG: Rash, irritation, sensitization

Contraindications: Hypersensitivity, infants <1 yr, application to large areas, presence of fungal, viral, or bacterial infections of mouth or throat

Precautions: Child <6 yr, sepsis, pregnancy (C), denuded skin

NURSING CONSIDERATIONS

Assess:
• Allergy: rash, irritation, reddening, swelling
• Infection: if affected area is infected, do not apply

Administer:
• After cleansing oral cavity

Evaluate:
• Therapeutic response: absence of pain in affected area

Teach patient/family:
• To report rash, irritation, redness, swelling
• How to apply paste

triamterene (℞)

(trye-am′ter-een)

Dyrenium

Func. class.: Potassium-sparing diuretic

Chem. class.: Pteridine derivative

Action: Acts on distal tubule to inhibit reabsorption of sodium, chloride; increase potassium retention

Uses: Edema, may be used with other diuretics; hypertension

Dosage and routes:

• *Adult:* **PO** 100 mg bid pc, not to exceed 300 mg/day

• *Geriatric:* **PO** 50 mg qd, max 100 mg/day

Available forms: Caps 50, 100 mg

Side effects/adverse reactions:

GI: Nausea, diarrhea, vomiting, dry mouth, jaundice, ***liver disease***

ELECT: Hyperkalemia, hyponatremia, hypochloremia

CNS: Weakness, headache, dizziness, fatigue

INTEG: Photosensitivity, rash

HEMA: ***Thrombocytopenia, megaloblastic anemia,*** low folic acid levels

GU: ***Azotemia, interstitial nephritis,*** increased BUN, creatinine, renal stones, bluish discoloration of urine

Contraindications: Hypersensitivity, anuria, severe renal disease, severe hepatic disease, hyperkalemia, lactation

Precautions: Dehydration, hepatic disease, CHF, renal disease, pregnancy (B), cirrhosis

Pharmacokinetics:

PO: Onset 2 hr, peak 6-8 hr, duration 12-16 hr; half-life 3 hr; metabolized in liver, excreted in bile and urine

Interactions:

• Nephrotoxicity: indomethacin

• ↑ antihypertensives, amantadine

• ↑ hyperkalemia: other potassium-sparing diuretics, potassium products, ACE inhibitors, salt substitutes

• ↓ renal clearance of triamterene: cimetidine

Fatal hypokalemia: arginine

Hypokalemia: bearberry, gossypol

↑ diuretic: cucumber, dandelion, horsetail, licorice, nettle, pumpkin, Queen Anne's lace

Severe photosensitivity: St. John's wort

Lab test interferences:

Interference: Quinidine serum levels, LDH

NURSING CONSIDERATIONS

Assess:

• Weight, I&O qd to determine fluid loss; effect of drug may be decreased if used qd

• Electrolytes: K, Na, Cl; include BUN, blood glucose, CBC, serum creatinine, blood pH, ABGs, LFTs

• Improvement in CVP q8h

• Signs of metabolic acidosis: drowsiness, restlessness

• Rashes, temp qd

• Confusion, especially in elderly; take safety precautions if needed

• Hydration: skin turgor, thirst, dry mucous membranes

Administer:

• In AM to avoid interference with sleep

• With food if nausea occurs; absorption may be decreased slightly

Evaluate:

• Therapeutic response: improvement in edema of feet, legs, sacral area qd if medication is being used in CHF

Teach patient/family:

• To take medication after meals for GI upset

• To avoid prolonged exposure to sunlight; photosensitivity may occur; may turn urine blue
• To avoid foods high in potassium: oranges, bananas, salt substitutes, dried apricots, dates
• To notify prescriber of weakness, headache, nausea, vomiting, dry mouth, fever, sore throat, mouth sores, unusual bleeding or bruising

Treatment of overdose: Lavage if taken orally; monitor electrolytes; administer IV fluids, dialysis; monitor hydration, CV, renal status

triazolam (℞)

(trye-ay′zoe-lam)

Apo-Triazo♣, Gen-Triazolam♣, Halcion, Novo-Triolam♣, Nu-Triazol♣

Func. class.: Sedative-hypnotic, antianxiety

Chem. class.: Benzodiazepine

Controlled Substance Schedule IV (USA), Schedule F (Canada)

Action: Produces CNS depression at limbic, thalamic, hypothalamic levels of CNS; may be mediated by neurotransmitter γ-aminobutyric acid (GABA); results are sedation, hypnosis, skeletal muscle relaxation, anticonvulsant activity, anxiolytic action

Uses: Insomnia, sedative, hypnotic

Dosage and routes:
• *Adult:* **PO** 0.125-0.5 mg hs
• *Elderly:* **PO** 0.625-0.125 mg hs

Available forms: Tabs 0.125, 0.25 mg

Side effects/adverse reactions:

HEMA: ***Leukopenia, granulocytopenia*** (rare)

CNS: Headache, lethargy, drowsiness, daytime sedation, dizziness, confusion, light-headedness, anxiety, irritability, amnesia, poor coordination

GI: Nausea, vomiting, diarrhea, heartburn, abdominal pain, constipation

CV: Chest pain, pulse changes

Contraindications: Hypersensitivity to benzodiazepines, pregnancy (X), lactation, intermittent porphyria

Precautions: Anemia, hepatic disease, renal disease, suicidal individuals, drug abuse, elderly, psychosis, child <15 yr, acute narrow-angle glaucoma, seizure disorders

Pharmacokinetics:

PO: Onset 30-45 min, duration 6-8 hr; metabolized by liver, excreted by kidneys (inactive metabolites), crosses placenta, excreted in breast milk; half-life 2-3 hr

Interactions:

↑ effects of cimetidine, disulfiram, erythromycin, macrolides, probenecid, isoniazid, oral contraceptives; do not use concurrently
• ↑ action of both drugs: alcohol, CNS depressants
• ↓ effect of antacids, theophylline, rifampin, smoking

↑ CNS depression: catnip, chamomile, clary, cowslip, hops, kava, lavender, mistletoe, nettle, pokeweed, poppy, Queen Anne's lace, senega, skullcap, valerian

↑ hypotension: black cohosh

Lab test interferences:

Increase: ALT, AST, serum bilirubin

Decrease: RAI uptake

False increase: Urinary 17-OHCS

NURSING CONSIDERATIONS

Assess:
• Blood studies: Hct, Hgb, RBC if blood dyscrasias suspected (rare)
• Hepatic studies: AST, ALT, bilirubin if liver damage has occurred
• Mental status: mood, sensorium, affect, memory (long, short)

T

- Blood dyscrasias: fever, sore throat, bruising, rash, jaundice, epistaxis (rare)
- Type of sleep problem: falling asleep, staying asleep

Administer:

- After removal of cigarettes to prevent fires
- After trying conservative measures for insomnia
- ½ hr before hs for sleeplessness
- On empty stomach for fast onset, but may be taken with food if GI symptoms occur

Perform/provide:

- Assistance with ambulation after receiving dose
- Safety measures: side rails, nightlight, call bell within easy reach
- Checking to see if PO medication has been swallowed
- Cool storage in tight container

Evaluate:

- Therapeutic response: ability to sleep at night, decreased amount of early morning awakening if taking drug for insomnia

Teach patient/family:

- That dependence is possible after long-term use
- To avoid driving, other activities requiring alertness until drug is stabilized
- To avoid alcohol ingestion, CNS depressants; serious CNS depression may result
- That effects may take 2 nights for benefits to be noticed; for short-term use only
- Alternative measures to improve sleep: reading, exercise several hours before hs, warm bath, warm milk, TV, self-hypnosis, deep breathing
- That hangover is common in elderly but less common than with barbiturates; rebound insomnia may occur for 1-2 nights after discontinuing drug

Treatment of overdose: Lavage, activated charcoal; monitor electrolytes, VS

trifluoperazine (℞)

(trye-floo-oh-per′a-zeen)
Apo-Trifluoperazine🍁, Novoflurazine🍁, Solazine🍁, Stelazine, Suprazine, Terfluzine, trifluoperazine HCl, Triflurin

Func. class.: Antipsychotic, neuroleptic

Chem. class.: Phenothiazine, piperazine

Action: Depresses cerebral cortex, hypothalamus, limbic system, which control activity, aggression; blocks neurotransmission produced by dopamine at synapse; exhibits strong α-adrenergic, anticholinergic blocking action; mechanism for antipsychotic effects is unclear

Uses: Psychotic disorders, nonpsychotic anxiety, schizophrenia

Dosage and routes:

Psychotic disorders

- *Adult:* **PO** 2-5 mg bid, usual range 15-20 mg/day, may require 40 mg/day or more; **IM** 1-2 mg q4-6h
- *Geriatric:* **PO** 0.5-1 mg qd-bid, increase q4-7d by 0.5-1 mg/day to desired dose
- *Child >6 yr:* **PO** 1 mg qd or bid; **IM** not recommended for children, but 1 mg may be given qd or bid

Nonpsychotic anxiety

- *Adult:* **PO** 1-2 mg bid, not to exceed 6 mg/day; do not give longer than 12 wk

Available forms: Tabs 1, 2, 5, 10 mg; conc 10 mg/ml; inj 2 mg/ml

Side effects/adverse reactions:

RESP: ***Laryngospasm,*** dyspnea, ***respiratory depression***

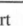

CNS: EPS: pseudoparkinsonism, akathisia, dystonia, tardive dyski-

nesia, ***seizures,*** *headache,* ***neuroleptic malignant syndrome,*** dizziness
HEMA: Anemia, ***leukopenia, leukocytosis, agranulocytosis***
INTEG: Rash, photosensitivity, dermatitis
EENT: Blurred vision, glaucoma, dry eyes
GI: Dry mouth, nausea, vomiting, anorexia, constipation, diarrhea, jaundice, weight gain
GU: Urinary retention, urinary frequency, enuresis, impotence, amenorrhea, gynecomastia
CV: Orthostatic hypotension, hypertension, ***cardiac arrest,*** ECG changes, ***tachycardia***

Contraindications: Hypersensitivity, cardiovascular disease, coma, blood dyscrasias, severe hepatic disease, child <6 yr, narrow-angle glaucoma

Precautions: Breast cancer, seizure disorders, pregnancy (C), lactation, diabetes mellitus, respiratory conditions, prostatic hypertrophy, elderly

Do not confuse:
trifluoperazine/trihexyphenidyl

Pharmacokinetics:
PO: Onset rapid, peak 2-3 hr, duration 12 hr
IM: Onset immediate, peak 1 hr, duration 12 hr
Metabolized by liver, excreted in urine, breast milk; crosses placenta

Interactions:
- Oversedation: other CNS depressants, alcohol, barbiturate anesthetics
- ↓ absorption: aluminum hydroxide, magnesium hydroxide antacids
- ↓ effects of lithium, levodopa, anticonvulsants
- ↑ effects of both drugs: β-adrenergic blockers, alcohol
- ↑ anticholinergic effects: anticholinergics

↑ EPS: betel palm, kava
↑ action: cola tree, hops, nettle, nutmeg
↑ CNS depression: chamomile, hops, kava, skullcap, valerian

Lab test interferences:
Increase: LFTs, cardiac enzymes, cholesterol, blood glucose, prolactin, bilirubin, PBI, cholinesterase, ^{131}I
Decrease: Hormones (blood, urine)
False positive: Pregnancy tests, PKU
False negative: Urinary steroids, 17-OHCS, pregnancy tests

NURSING CONSIDERATIONS

Assess:

For neuroleptic malignant syndrome: seizures, hyper/hypotension, dyspnea, diaphoresis, fatigue, muscle stiffness; notify prescriber immediately
- Mental status before initial administration
- Swallowing of PO medication; check for hoarding or giving of medication to other patients
- I&O ratio; palpate bladder if low urinary output occurs, urinary retention may be the cause
- Bilirubin, CBC, LFTs qmo
- Urinalysis is recommended before and during prolonged therapy
- Affect, orientation, LOC, reflexes, gait, coordination, sleep pattern disturbances
- For hypo/hyperglycemia; appetite patterns
- B/P standing and lying; also include pulse, respirations q4h during initial treatment; establish baseline before starting treatment; report drops of 30 mm Hg
- Dizziness, faintness, palpitations, tachycardia on rising
- EPS including akathisia (inability to sit still, no pattern to movements), tardive dyskinesia (bizarre movements of jaw, mouth, tongue, extremities), pseudoparkinsonism (ri-

T

gidity, tremors, pill rolling, shuffling gait)

- Skin turgor qd
- Constipation, urinary retention qd; if these occur increase bulk, water in diet

Administer:

- Reduced dose in elderly
- Antiparkinsonian agent on order from prescriber for EPS

PO route

- Conc in 60 ml of tomato or fruit juice, milk, carbonated beverage, coffee, tea, water, or semisolid foods (soup, pudding)

Perform/provide:

- Decreased stimulus by dimming lights, avoiding loud noises
- Supervised ambulation until stabilized on medication if needed; do not involve in strenuous exercise program because fainting is possible; patient should not stand still for long periods
- Increased fluids and bulk in diet to prevent constipation
- Sips of water, candy, gum for dry mouth
- Storage in tight, light-resistant container, oral sol in amber bottles; slight yellowing of inj or conc is common, does not affect potency

Evaluate:

- Therapeutic response: decrease in emotional excitement, hallucinations, delusions, paranoia, reorganization of patterns of thought, speech

Teach patient/family:

- That orthostatic hypotension occurs frequently, and to rise from sitting or lying position gradually; avoid hazardous activities until stabilized on medication
- To remain lying down after IM injection for at least 30 min
- To avoid hot tubs, hot showers, tub baths; hypotension may occur
- To avoid abrupt withdrawal of this drug, or EPS may result; drug should be withdrawn slowly
- To avoid OTC preparations (cough, hay fever, cold) unless approved by prescriber, since serious drug interactions may occur; avoid use with alcohol, CNS depressants; increased drowsiness may occur
- To use a sunscreen
- About compliance with drug regimen
- About the necessity for meticulous oral hygiene; oral candidiasis may occur
- To report sore throat, malaise, fever, bleeding, mouth sores; CBC should be drawn and drug discontinued
- That in hot weather, heat stroke may occur; take extra precautions to stay cool

Treatment of overdose: Lavage if orally ingested; provide an airway; do not induce vomiting

trifluridine ophthalmic

See appendix c

trihexyphenidyl (℞)

(trye-hex-ee-fen′i-dill)

Apo-Trihex ✤, Artane, Artane Sequels, Novohexidyl ✤, PMS-Trihexyphenidyl ✤, Trihexane, Trihexy-2, Trihexy-5, trihexyphenidyl HCl

Func. class.: Cholinergic blocker

Chem. class.: Synthetic tertiary amine

Action: Blocks central muscarinic receptors, which decreases involuntary movements, sweating, salivation

Uses: Parkinson symptoms, drug-induced EPS

Dosage and routes:

Parkinson symptoms

• *Adult:* **PO** 1 mg, increased by 2 mg q3-5d to a total of 6-10 mg/day, given in 3-4 divided doses; give ext rel q12h

Drug-induced EPS

• *Adult:* **PO** 1 mg/day; usual dose 5-15 mg/day, in 3-4 divided doses; give ext rel q12h

Available forms: Tabs 2, 5 mg; caps ext rel 5 mg; elix 2 mg/5 ml

Side effects/adverse reactions:

CNS: Confusion, anxiety, restlessness, irritability, delusions, hallucinations, headache, sedation, depression, incoherence, dizziness, flushing, weakness

EENT: Blurred vision, photophobia, dilated pupils, difficulty swallowing, dry eyes, increased intraocular tension, angle-closure glaucoma

CV: Palpitations, tachycardia, postural hypotension

INTEG: Urticaria, rash

MISC: Suppression of lactation, nasal congestion, decreased sweating, increased temp, hyperthermia, heat stroke, numbness of fingers

MS: Weakness, cramping

GI: Dryness of mouth, constipation, nausea, vomiting, abdominal distress, ***paralytic ileus***

GU: Urinary hesitancy, retention, dysuria

Contraindications: Hypersensitivity, narrow-angle glaucoma, myasthenia gravis, GI/GU obstruction, myocardial ischemia, unstable CV disease, prostatic hypertrophy

Precautions: Pregnancy (C), elderly, lactation, tachycardia, abdominal obstruction, infection, children, gastric ulcer

Do not confuse:

tryhexyphenidyl/trifluoperazine

Artane/Altace

Pharmacokinetics:

PO: Onset 1 hr, peak 2-3 hr, duration 6-12 hr, excreted in urine, half-life 5-10 hr

Interactions:

• ↑ anticholinergic effects: antihistamines, phenothiazines, amantadine

• ↓ action of haloperidol

• ↑ CNS depression: analgesics, alcohol, sedatives/hypnotics, antihistamines, opioids

• ↑ levels of: digoxin

NURSING CONSIDERATIONS

Assess:

• For Parkinson's and EPS baseline and throughout treatment

• I&O ratio; retention commonly causes decreased urinary output

• B/P, pulse frequently while dose is being determined

• Urinary hesitancy, retention; palpate bladder if retention occurs

• Constipation; increase fluids, bulk, exercise

• For tolerance over long-term therapy; dosage may have to be increased or medication changed

• Mental status: affect, mood, CNS depression, worsening of mental symptoms during early therapy

Administer:

• With or after meals for GI upset; may give with fluids other than water

• At hs to avoid daytime drowsiness in patient with parkinsonism

Perform/provide:

• Storage at room temperature in light-resistant container

• Hard candy, frequent drinks, sugarless gum to relieve dry mouth

Evaluate:

• Therapeutic response: parkinsonism: shuffling gait, muscle rigidity, involuntary movements

Teach patient/family:

• Not to discontinue this drug abruptly; to taper off over 1 wk

• To avoid driving, other hazardous activities; drowsiness may occur

• To avoid OTC medications: cough, cold preparations with alcohol, antihistamines unless directed by prescriber
• To avoid sudden position changes
• To avoid hot climates; overheating may occur

trimethobenzamide (℞)

(trye-meth-oh-ben'za-mide)
Arrestin, Benzacot, Brogan, Stemetic, T-Gen, Tebamide, Ticon, Tigan, Tiject-20, Triban, Trimazide, Trimethobenzamide, trimethobenzamide HCl

Func. class.: Antiemetic, anticholinergic

Chem. class.: Ethanolamine derivative

Action: Acts centrally by blocking chemoreceptor trigger zone, which in turn acts on vomiting center
Uses: Nausea, vomiting, prevention of postoperative vomiting
Dosage and routes:
Postoperative vomiting
• *Adult:* **IM/RECT** 200 mg before or during surgery; may repeat 3 hr after
Discontinuing anesthesia
• *Child 13-40 kg:* **PO/RECT** 100-200 mg tid-qid
• *Child <13 kg:* **PO/RECT** 100 mg tid-qid
Nausea/vomiting
• *Adult:* **PO** 250-300 mg tid-qid; **IM/RECT** 200 mg tid-qid
Available forms: Caps 100, 250, 300 mg; supp 100, 200 mg; inj 100 mg/ml
Side effects/adverse reactions:
CNS: Drowsiness, restlessness, headache, dizziness, insomnia, confusion, nervousness, tingling, *vertigo,* EPS
GI: Nausea, anorexia, diarrhea, vomiting, constipation
CV: Hypertension, hypotension, palpitation
INTEG: Rash, urticaria, fever, chills, flushing
EENT: Dry mouth, blurred vision, diplopia, nasal congestion, photosensitivity
Contraindications: Hypersensitivity to opioids, shock, children (parenterally)
Precautions: Children, cardiac dysrhythmias, elderly, asthma, pregnancy (C), prostatic hypertrophy, bladder-neck obstruction, narrow-angle glaucoma, stenosing peptic ulcer, pyloroduodenal obstruction
Pharmacokinetics:
PO: Onset 20-40 min, duration 3-4 hr
IM: Onset 15 min, duration 2-3 hr
Metabolized by liver, excreted by kidneys
Interactions:
• ↑ effect: CNS depressants
• May mask ototoxic symptoms associated with antibiotics

NURSING CONSIDERATIONS
Assess:
• For nausea, vomiting before, after treatment
• VS, B/P; check patients with cardiac disease more often
• Signs of toxicity of other drugs or masking of symptoms of disease: brain tumor, intestinal obstruction
• Observe for drowsiness, dizziness
Administer:
• IM inj in large muscle mass; aspirate to avoid IV administration
• Tablets may be swallowed whole, chewed, allowed to dissolve
Syringe compatibilities: Glycopyrrolate, hydromorphone, midazolam, nalbuphine
Y-site compatibilities: Heparin, hydrocortisone, potassium chloride, vit B/C

Evaluate:
• Therapeutic response: decreased nausea, vomiting
Teach patient/family:
• To avoid hazardous activities, activities requiring alertness; dizziness may occur; to request assistance with ambulation
• To avoid alcohol, other depressants
• To keep out of children's reach

trimethoprim (℞)

(trye-meth'oh-prim)
Primsol, Proloprim, trimethoprim, Trimpex
Func. class.: Urinary antiinfective
Chem. class.: Folate antagonist

Action: Prevents bacterial synthesis by blocking enzyme reduction of dihydrofolic acid
Uses: *Escherichia coli, Proteus mirabilis, Klebsiella, Enterobacter* UTIs
Dosage and routes:
Urinary tract infection
• *Adult:* **PO** 100 mg q12h × 10 days
• *Child:* 4 mg/kg/day divided q12h
Otitis media
• *Child >6 mo:* **PO** 5 mg/kg q12h
Pneumocystis carinii pneumonia
• *Adult:* **PO** 20 mg/kg/day with 100 mg dapsone × 21 days
Renal dose
• *Adult:* **PO** CCr 15-30 ml/min 50 mg q12h; CCr <15 ml/min avoid use
Available forms: Tabs 100, 200 mg
Side effects/adverse reactions:
INTEG: ***Exfoliative dermatitis,*** pruritus, rash
HEMA: ***Thrombocytopenia, leukopenia, neutropenia, megaloblastic anemia*** (rare)
GI: Nausea, vomiting, abdominal pain, abnormal taste, increased AST, ALT, bilirubin, creatinine
CNS: Fever
Contraindications: Hypersensitivity, CCr <15 ml/min, megaloblastic anemia
Precautions: Folate deficiency, pregnancy (C), lactation, fragile X chromosome, child <12 yr old, renal disease, hepatic disease
Pharmacokinetics:
PO: Peak 1-4 hr, half-life 8-11 hr; metabolized in liver, excreted in urine (unchanged 60%), breast milk; crosses placenta
Interactions:
• ↑ action of phenytoin
NURSING CONSIDERATIONS
Assess:
• For symptoms of UTI: fever, frequency, burning or pain when urinating; baseline and throughout
• Nocturia; may indicate drug resistance
• Signs of infection, anemia
• AST, ALT, BUN, bilirubin, creatinine, urine cultures
• C&S; drug may be given as soon as culture is obtained
• Skin eruptions
Administer:
• With full glass of water
Perform/provide:
• Storage in tight, light-resistant container
• Adequate intake of fluids (2 L) to decrease bacteria in bladder
Evaluate:
• Therapeutic response: absence of pain in bladder area, negative C&S
Teach patient/family:
• All aspects of drug therapy: need to complete entire course of medication to ensure organism death (10-14 days); culture may be taken after completed course of medication

• That drug must be taken in equal intervals around clock to maintain blood levels
• To notify nurse of nausea, vomiting, rash, severe fatigue, sore throat

trimethoprim-sulfamethoxazole (℞)

(trye-meth'oh-prim–sul-fa-meth-ox'a-zole)
Apo-Sulfatrim♣, Apo-Sulfatrim DS♣, Bactrim, Bactrim IV, Bethaprim, Comoxol, Cotrim, Novo-Trimel♣, Novo-Trimel DS♣, Nu-Cotrimox♣, Nu-Cotrimox DS♣, Roubac♣, Septra, Septra DS, SMZ/TMP, Sulfatrim

Func. class.: Antiinfective
Chem. class.: Miscellaneous sulfonamide

Action: Sulfamethoxazole (SMZ) interferes with bacterial biosynthesis of proteins by competitive antagonism of PABA when adequate levels are maintained; trimethoprim (TMP) blocks synthesis of tetrahydrofolic acid; combination blocks 2 consecutive steps in bacterial synthesis of essential nucleic acids, protein

Uses: UTI, otitis media, acute and chronic prostatitis, shigellosis, *Pneumocystis carinii* pneumonitis, chronic bronchitis, chancroid, traveler's diarrhea

Dosage and routes: Based on TMP content

UTI
• *Adult:* **PO** 160 mg TMP q12h × 10-14 days
• *Child:* **PO** 8 mg/kg TMP qd in 2 divided doses q12h

Otitis media
• *Child:* **PO** 8 mg/kg TMP qd in 2 divided doses q12h × 10 days

Chronic bronchitis
• *Adult:* **PO** 160 mg TMP q12h × 14 days

Pneumocystis carinii *pneumonitis*
• *Adult and child:* **PO** 20 mg/kg TMP qd in 4 divided doses q6h × 14 days; **IV** 15-20 mg/kg/day (based on TMP) in 3-4 divided doses for up to 14 days
• Dosage reduction necessary in moderate to severe renal impairment (CCr <30 ml/min)

Available forms: Tabs 80 mg trimethoprim/400 mg sulfamethoxazole, 160 mg trimethoprim/800 mg sulfamethoxazole; susp 40 mg/200 mg/5 ml; IV 16 mg/80 mg/ml

Side effects/adverse reactions:
CNS: Headache, insomnia, hallucinations, depression, vertigo, fatigue, anxiety, ***convulsions, drug fever,*** chills, ***aseptic meningitis***
CV: ***Allergic myocarditis***
GI: Nausea, vomiting, abdominal pain, stomatitis, ***hepatitis,*** glossitis, pancreatitis, diarrhea, ***enterocolitis,*** anorexia
GU: ***Renal failure, toxic nephrosis;*** increased BUN, creatinine; crystalluria
HEMA: ***Leukopenia, neutropenia, thrombocytopenia, agranulocytosis, hemolytic anemia, hypoprothrombinemia, Henoch-Schönlein purpura, methemoglobinemia, eosinophilia I***
INTEG: Rash, dermatitis, urticaria, ***Stevens-Johnson syndrome,*** erythema, photosensitivity, pain, inflammation at inj site, ***toxic epidermal necrolysis, erythema multiforme***
RESP: Cough, shortness of breath
SYST: ***Anaphylaxis, SLE***

Contraindications: Hypersensitivity to trimethoprim or sulfonamides, pregnancy at term, megaloblastic anemia, infants <2 mo, CCr <15 ml/min, lactation, porphyria

Precautions: Pregnancy (C), renal disease, elderly, G6PD deficiency, impaired hepatic/renal function, possible folate deficiency, severe allergy, bronchial asthma

Pharmacokinetics:

PO: Rapidly absorbed, peak 1-4 hr; half-life 8-13 hr, excreted in urine (metabolites and unchanged), breast milk; crosses placenta; 68% bound to plasma proteins; TMP achieves high levels in prostatic tissue and fluid

Interactions:

• ↑ hypoglycemic response: sulfonylurea agents
• ↑ anticoagulant effects: oral anticoagulants
• ↓ hepatic clearance of phenytoin
• ↓ response: cycloSPORINE
• ↑ bone marrow depressant effects: methotrexate
• Thrombocytopenia: thiazide diuretics

Lab test interferences:

Increase: Alk phosphatase, creatinine, bilirubin
False positive: Urinary glucose test

NURSING CONSIDERATIONS

Assess:

• Allergic reactions: rash, fever (AIDS patients more susceptible)
• I&O ratio; note color, character, pH of urine if drug administered for UTI; output should be 800 ml less than intake; if urine is highly acidic, alkalization may be needed
• Renal studies: BUN, creatinine, urinalysis (long-term therapy)
• Type of infection; obtain C&S before starting therapy
• Blood dyscrasias, skin rash, fever, sore throat, bruising, bleeding, fatigue, joint pain
• Allergic reaction: rash, dermatitis, urticaria, pruritus, dyspnea, bronchospasm

Administer:

PO route

• Medication after C&S; repeat C&S after full course of medication
• With resuscitative equipment, epINEPHrine available; severe allergic reactions may occur
• With full glass of water to maintain adequate hydration; increase fluids to 2 L/day to decrease crystallization in kidneys

IV route

• After diluting 5 ml of drug/125 ml D_5W, run over 1-1½ hr

Syringe compatibilities: Heparin

Y-site compatibilities: Acyclovir, aldesleukin, allopurinol, amifostine, amphotericin B cholesteryl, atracurium, aztreonam, cefepime, cyclophosphamide, diltiazem, DOXOrubicin liposome, enalaprilat, esmolol, filgrastim, fludarabine, gallium, granisetron, hydromorphone, labetalol, lorazepam, magnesium sulfate, melphalan, meperidine, morphine, pancuronium, perphenazine, piperacillin/tazobactam, remifentanil, sargramostim, tacrolimus, teniposide, thiotepa, vecuronium, zidovudine

Perform/provide:

• Storage in tight, light-resistant container at room temperature

Evaluate:

• Therapeutic response: absence of pain, fever, C&S negative

Teach patient/family:

• To take each oral dose with full glass of water to prevent crystalluria; drink 8-10 glasses of water/day; to take on an empty stomach 1 hr ac, 2 hr pc
• To complete full course of treatment to prevent superinfection
• To avoid sunlight or use sunscreen to prevent burns
• To avoid OTC medications (aspirin, vit C) unless directed by prescriber

T

• If diabetic, to use Clinistix or Tes-Tape
• To use alternative contraceptive measures; decreased effectiveness of oral contraceptives may result
• To notify prescriber if skin rash, sore throat, fever, mouth sores, unusual bruising, bleeding occur

trimipramine (℞)

(tri-mip′ra-meen)

Apo-Trimip, Novo-Tripramine, Rhotrimine, Surmontil

Func. class.: Antidepressant—tricyclic

Chem. class.: Tertiary amine

Action: Selectively inhibits serotonin uptake by brain; potentiates behavioral changes

Uses: Depression, enuresis in children

Dosage and routes:

• *Adult:* **PO** 50-150 mg/day in divided doses, may be increased to 200 mg/day
• *Geriatric:* **PO** 25 mg hs, increase by 25 mg q3-7 days, max 100 mg/day
• *Child >6 yr:* 25 mg hs, may increase to 50 mg in child <12 yr or 75 mg in child >12 yr

Available forms: Caps 25, 50, 100 mg

Side effects/adverse reactions:

HEMA: ***Agranulocytosis, thrombocytopenia, eosinophilia, leukopenia***

CNS: Dizziness, drowsiness, confusion, headache, anxiety, tremors, stimulation, weakness, insomnia, nightmares, EPS (elderly), increase in psychiatric symptoms

GI: Diarrhea, *dry mouth,* nausea, vomiting, ***paralytic ileus,*** increased appetite, cramps, epigastric distress, jaundice, ***hepatitis,*** stomatitis, *constipation,* taste change

GU: Urinary retention, ***acute renal failure***

INTEG: Rash, urticaria, sweating, pruritus, photosensitivity

CV: Orthostatic hypotension, ECG changes, tachycardia, ***hypertension,*** palpitations

EENT: Blurred vision, tinnitus, mydriasis

Contraindications: Hypersensitivity to tricyclics, recovery phase of MI, convulsive disorders, prostatic hypertrophy

Precautions: Suicidal patients, severe depression, increased intraocular pressure, narrow-angle glaucoma, urinary retention, cardiac disease, hepatic disease, renal disorders, hyperthyroidism, electroshock therapy, elective surgery, pregnancy (C), elderly

Pharmacokinetics: Metabolized by liver, excreted by kidneys, steady state 2-6 days; half-life 20-26 hr

Interactions:

• ↓ effects of: guanethidine, clonidine, indirect-acting sympathomimetics (epHEDrine)
• ↑ effects of direct-acting sympathomimetics (epINEPHrine), alcohol, barbiturates, benzodiazepines, CNS depressants, cimetidine, methylphenidate

Hyperpyretic crisis, convulsions, hypertensive episode: MAOIs

↑ anticholinergic effect: belladonna, corkwood, henbane, jimsonweed

Serotonin syndrome: SAM-e, St. John's wort

↑ hypertension: yohimbe

↑ antidepressant action: scopolia

Lab test interferences:

Increase: Serum bilirubin, blood glucose, alk phosphatase

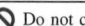

False increase: Urinary catecholamines
Decrease: VMA, 5-HIAA

NURSING CONSIDERATIONS

Assess:

• B/P (lying, standing), pulse q4h; if systolic B/P drops 20 mm Hg, hold drug, notify prescriber; take VS q4h in patients with cardiovascular disease
• Blood studies: CBC, leukocytes, differential, cardiac enzymes if patient is receiving long-term therapy
• Hepatic studies: AST, ALT, bilirubin, creatinine
• Weight qwk; appetite may increase with drug
• ECG for flattening of T wave, bundle branch block, AV block, dysrhythmias in cardiac patients
• EPS primarily in elderly: rigidity, dystonia, akathisia
• Mental status changes: mood, sensorium, affect, suicidal tendencies, increase in psychiatric symptoms, depression, panic
• Urinary retention, constipation; constipation is more likely to occur in children, elderly
• Withdrawal symptoms: headache, nausea, vomiting, muscle pain, weakness; not usual unless drug is discontinued abruptly
• Alcohol consumption; hold dose until morning

Administer:

• Increased fluids, bulk in diet for constipation, urinary retention
• With food, milk for GI symptoms
• Dosage hs for oversedation during day; may take entire dose hs; elderly may not tolerate once/day dosing
• Gum, hard candy, or frequent sips of water for dry mouth

Perform/provide:

• Storage in tight, light-resistant container at room temperature
• Assistance with ambulation during beginning therapy for drowsiness/dizziness
• Safety measures, including side rails, primarily for elderly
• Checking to see if PO medication swallowed

Evaluate:

• Therapeutic response: decreased depression or enuresis

Teach patient/family:

• That therapeutic effects may take 2-3 wk
• To use caution in driving, other activities requiring alertness because of drowsiness, dizziness, blurred vision
• That appetite and weight may increase
• That urine may turn blue-green; to report urinary retention
• To avoid alcohol ingestion, other CNS depressants
• Not to discontinue medication quickly after long-term use; may cause nausea, headache, malaise
• To wear sunscreen or large hat, since photosensitivity occurs

Treatment of overdose: ECG monitoring; induce emesis; lavage, activated charcoal; administer anticonvulsant

triptorelin (℞)

(trip-toe'rel-in)
Trelstar Depot
Func. class.: Gonadotropin-releasing hormone
Chem. class.: Synthetic decapeptide analog of LHRH

Action: Inhibitor of pituitary gonadotropin secretion; initially increases LH and FSH, with increases in testosterone, reduction in sex steroid levels
Uses: Advanced prostate cancer

Dosage and routes:
• *Adult:* **IM** 3.75 mg qmo
Available forms: Microgranules, depot inj 3.75 mg
Side effects/adverse reactions:
CNS: Headache, insomnia, dizziness, lability, fatigue
CV: Hypertension
ENDO: Gynecomastia, breast tenderness, hot flashes
GI: Nausea, vomiting, diarrhea
GU: Impotence, urinary retention, UTI
INTEG: Rash, pain on inj, pruritus, hypersensitivity
MS: Osteoneuralgia
MISC: ***Anaphylaxis, angioedema***
Contraindications: Hypersensitivity to this product or other LHRH agonists or LHRH, pregnancy (X), lactation
Pharmacokinetics: Metabolism may be by CYP 450, eliminated by liver, kidneys; terminal half-life is 3 hr in healthy males
Lab test interferences:
Increase: Alk phosphatase, estradiol, FSH, LH, testosterone levels
Decrease: Testosterone levels, progesterone

NURSING CONSIDERATIONS
Assess:
• Severe hypersensitivity: discontinue drug and give antihistamines, have emergency equipment nearby
• I&O ratios; palpate bladder for distention in urinary obstruction
• For relief of bone pain (back pain)
• Assess levels of testosterone and PSA
Administer:
• IM using implant, inserted by qualified person
• Using syringe with 20G needle, withdraw 2 ml sterile water for inj, inject into vial, shake well, withdraw vial contents, inject immediately
Evaluate:
• Therapeutic response: more normal levels of prostate-specific antigen, acid phosphatase, alk phosphatase; testosterone level of <25 ng/dl
Teach patient/family:
• That postmenopausal symptoms may occur but will decrease after treatment is discontinued
• That disease flare may occur at beginning of therapy

tromethamine (℞)
(troe-meth'a-meen)
Tham
Func. class.: Alkalinizer
Chem. class.: Amine

Action: Proton acceptor that corrects acidosis by combining with hydrogen ions to form bicarbonate and buffer; acts as diuretic (osmotic)
Uses: Acidosis (metabolic) associated with cardiac disease, COPD
Dosage and routes:
• *Adult:* **IV** 0.3 M required = kg of weight × HCO_3^- deficit (mEq/L)
• *Child:* **IV** same as above given over 3-6 hr, not to exceed 40 ml/kg
Available forms: Inj 18 g/500 ml
Side effects/adverse reactions:
CV: Irregular pulse, ***cardiac arrest***
META: Alkalosis, hypoglycemia, ***hyperkalemia with oliguria***
RESP: Shallow, slow respirations, cyanosis, ***apnea***
GI: ***Hepatic necrosis***
INTEG: Infection at inj site, extravasation, phlebitis
Contraindications: Hypersensitivity, anuria, uremia
Precautions: Severe respiratory disease/respiratory depression, pregnancy (C), cardiac edema, renal disease, infants

Pharmacokinetics:
IV: Excreted in urine
Interactions:
↓ alkaline effect: oak bark
NURSING CONSIDERATIONS
Assess:
• Respiratory rate, rhythm, depth; notify prescriber of abnormalities that may indicate acidosis
• Electrolytes, blood glucose, chloride; CO_2, before, during treatment
• Urine pH, urinary output, urine glucose during beginning treatment
• I&O ratio, report large increase or decrease
• IV site for extravasation, phlebitis, thrombosis
• For signs of potassium depletion
Administer:
• IV slowly to avoid pain at infusion site and toxicity
• IV undiluted as inf or added to priming fluid or ACD blood; give 5 ml or less/min
Evaluate:
• Therapeutic response: decreased metabolic acidosis
Teach patient/family:
• To increase potassium in diet: bananas, oranges, cantaloupe, honeydew, spinach, potatoes, dried fruit

tropicamide ophthalmic
See appendix c

HIGH ALERT

tubocurarine (℞)
(too-boe-kyoor-ar′een)
Tubarine✤, Tubocuraine
Func. class.: Neuromuscular blocker
Chem. class.: Curare alkaloid

Action: Inhibits transmission of nerve impulses by binding with cholinergic receptor sites, antagonizing action of acetylcholine
Uses: Facilitation of endotracheal intubation, skeletal muscle relaxation during mechanical ventilation, surgery, or general anesthesia
Dosage and routes:
• *Adult:* **IV BOL** 0.4-0.5 mg/kg, then 0.08-0.10 mg/kg 20-45 min after 1st dose if needed for long procedures
Available forms: Inj 3 mg/ml, 20 units/ml
Side effects/adverse reactions:
CV: Bradycardia, tachycardia, increased, decreased B/P
RESP: ***Prolonged apnea, bronchospasm, cyanosis, respiratory depression***
EENT: Increased secretions
INTEG: Rash, flushing, pruritus, urticaria
Contraindications: Hypersensitivity
Precautions: Pregnancy (C), cardiac disease, lactation, children <2 yr, electrolyte imbalances, dehydration, neuromuscular disease, respiratory disease
Pharmacokinetics:
IV: Onset 3-5 min, dose dependent, peak 2-3 min, duration ½-1½ hr; half-life 1-3 hr; degraded in liver, kidney (minimally); excreted in urine (unchanged) crosses placenta
Interactions:
• ↑ neuromuscular blockade: aminoglycosides, clindamycin, lincomycin, quinidine, local anesthetics, polymyxin antiinfectives, lithium, opioid analgesics, thiazides, enflurane, isoflurane, trimethaphan, magnesium salts
• Dysrhythmias: theophylline

T

NURSING CONSIDERATIONS
Assess:
- For electrolyte imbalances (K, Mg); may lead to increased action of this drug
- VS (B/P, pulse, respirations, airway) q15min until fully recovered; rate, depth, pattern of respirations, strength of hand grip
- I&O ratio; check for urinary retention, frequency, hesitancy
- Recovery: decreased paralysis of face, diaphragm, leg, arm, rest of body; allow to recover fully before completing neurologic assessment
- Allergic reactions: rash, fever, respiratory distress, pruritus; drug should be discontinued

Administer:
- With diazepam or morphine when used for therapeutic paralysis; provides no sedation alone
- Using nerve stimulator by anesthesiologist to determine neuromuscular blockade
- Anticholinesterase to reverse neuromuscular blockade
- IV undiluted 3 mg/ml; give single dose over 1-1½ sec by qualified person; diluted to 4 ml in NS given 0.5 ml/2 min for myasthenia testing

Solution compatibilities: D_5, $D_{10}W$, 0.9% NaCl, 0.45% NaCl, Ringer's, LR, dextrose/Ringer's or dextrose/LR combinations
Syringe compatibilities: Pentobarbital, thiopental
Perform/provide:
- Storage in light-resistant area; use only fresh sol
- Reassurance if communication is difficult during recovery from neuromuscular blockade

Evaluate:
- Therapeutic response: paralysis of jaw, eyelid, head, neck, rest of body

Treatment of overdose: Edrophonium or neostigmine, atropine, monitor VS; may require mechanical ventilation

undecylenic acid topical

See appendix c

unoprostone ophthalmic

See appendix c

urea (℞)

(yoor-ee'a)
Ureaphil
Func. class.: Diuretic, osmotic
Chem. class.: Carbonic acid diamide salt

Action: Elevates plasma osmolality, increasing flow of water into plasma from ocular and cranial fluids
Uses: To decrease intracranial pressure, intraocular pressure
Dosage and routes:
- *Adult:* **IV** 1-1.5 g/kg of 30% sol over 1-3 hr, not to exceed 4 ml/min; do not exceed 120 g/day
- *Child >2 yr:* **IV** 0.5-1.5 g/kg, not to exceed 4 ml/min
- *Child <2 yr:* **IV** 0.1 g/kg, not to exceed 4 ml/min

Available forms: Inj 40 g/150 ml
Side effects/adverse reactions:
CNS: Dizziness, disorientation, fever, syncope, *headache*
GI: Nausea, vomiting
INTEG: Venous thrombosis, phlebitis, extravasation
Contraindications: Severe renal disease, active intracranial bleeding, marked dehydration, liver fail-

ure, sickle cell disease with CNS involvement
Precautions: Hepatic disease, renal disease, pregnancy (C), electrolyte imbalances, lactation
Pharmacokinetics:
IV: Onset ½-1 hr, peak 1 hr, duration 3-10 hr (diuresis), 5-6 hr (intraocular pressure); half-life 1 hr; excreted in urine, breast milk; crosses placenta
Interactions:
- Incompatible with whole blood, alkalies in sol or syringe
- ↑ renal excretion of lithium

NURSING CONSIDERATIONS
Assess:
- Weight, I&O qd to determine fluid loss; effect of drug may be decreased if used qd; for hourly urinary output
- Rate, depth, rhythm of respiration, effect of exertion
- B/P lying, standing, postural hypotension may occur
- Electrolytes: K, Na, Cl; include BUN, blood glucose, CBC, serum creatinine, blood pH, ABGs, LFTs
- Fever, signs of extravasation
- Confusion, especially in elderly; take safety precautions if needed
- Hydration: skin turgor, thirst, dry mucous membranes

Administer:
- IV after diluting 30 g/100 ml diluent with D_5, D_{10}; run 30% sol over 1-2 hr; check for extravasation; do not exceed 4 ml/min; may cause bleeding; use IV filter
- Within minutes of reconstitution; sol becomes ammonia on standing

Evaluate:
- Therapeutic response: improvement in edema of feet, legs, sacral area daily in CHF

Teach patient/family:
- That drug will cause diuresis in ½ hr

Treatment of overdose: Lavage if taken orally; monitor electrolytes, administer IV fluids, monitor BUN, hydration, CV status

HIGH ALERT

urokinase (℞)

(yoor-oh-kin′ase)
Abbokinase, Abbokinase Open-Cath
Func. class.: Thrombolytic enzyme
Chem. class.: β-Hemolytic streptococcus filtrate (purified)

Action: Promotes thrombolysis by directly converting plasminogen to plasmin
Uses: Venous thrombosis, pulmonary embolism, arterial thrombosis, arterial embolism, arteriovenous cannula occlusion, lysis of coronary artery thrombi after MI
Dosage and routes:
Lysis of pulmonary emboli
- *Adult and child:* **IV** 4400 international units/kg/hr × 12-24 hr, not to exceed 200 ml; then **IV** heparin, then anticoagulants

Coronary artery thrombosis
- *Adult:* **INSTILL** 6000 international units/min into occluded artery for 1-2 hr after giving **IV BOL** of heparin 2500-10,000 units
- May also give as **IV INF** 2 million-3 million units over 45-90 min

Venous catheter occlusion
- *Adult and child:* **INSTILL** 5000 international units into line, wait 5 min, then aspirate, repeat aspiration attempts q5min × ½ hr; if occlusion has not been removed, cap line and wait ½-1 hr, then aspirate; may need 2nd dose if still occluded

Available forms: Powder for inj, lyophilized: 250,000 international units/vial; powder for catheter clearance

Side effects/adverse reactions:

HEMA: Decreased Hct, ***bleeding***

INTEG: Rash, urticaria, phlebitis at IV inf site, itching, flushing

CNS: Headache, fever

GI: Nausea, vomiting

RESP: Altered respirations, SOB, ***bronchospasm,*** cyanosis

MS: Low back pain

CV: Hypotension, dysrhythmias

SYST: ***GI, GU, intracranial, retroperitoneal bleeding,*** surface bleeding, ***anaphylaxis*** (rare)

Contraindications: Hypersensitivity, internal active bleeding, intraspinal surgery, neoplasms of CNS, ulcerative colitis/enteritis, severe uncontrolled hypertension, renal disease, hepatic disease, hypocoagulation, COPD, subacute bacterial endocarditis, rheumatic valvular disease, cerebral embolism/thrombosis/hemorrhage, intraarterial diagnostic procedure or surgery (10 days), recent major surgery/trauma, aneurysm AV malformation

Precautions: Arterial emboli from left side of heart, pregnancy (B), hepatic disease

Pharmacokinetics:

IV: Half-life 10-20 min; small amounts excreted in urine

Interactions:

- Bleeding potential: aspirin, indomethacin, phenylbutazone, anticoagulants, other NSAIDs, abciximab, eptifibatide, tirofiban, clopidogrel, ticlopidine, some cephalosporins, plicamycin, valproic acid, dipyridamole, glycoprotein IIb, IIIa inhibitors

Lab test interferences:

Increase: PT, APTT, TT

NURSING CONSIDERATIONS

Assess:

- VS, B/P, pulse, resp, neurologic signs, temp at least q4h; temp >104° F (40° C) is an indicator of internal bleeding; cardiac rhythm following intracoronary administration
- For neurologic changes that may indicate intracranial bleeding
- Retroperitoneal bleeding: back pain, leg weakness, diminished pulses
- Peripheral pulses, lung sounds, respiratory function
- Hypersensitivity: fever, rash, itching, chills, facial swelling, dyspnea; mild reaction may be treated with antihistamines; notify prescriber of severe reactions, stop drug, keep resuscitative equipment nearby
- Bleeding during 1st hr of treatment (hematuria, hematemesis, bleeding from mucous membranes, epistaxis, ecchymosis)
- Blood studies (Hct, platelets, PTT, PT, TT, APTT) before starting therapy; PT or APTT must be less than 2 × control before starting therapy TT; or PT q3-4h during treatment
- ECG continuously, cardiac enzymes, radionuclide myocardial scanning/coronary angiography

Administer:

IV route

- Using infusion pump, terminal filter (0.45 μm or smaller)
- Reconstituting only with 5.2 ml sterile water for inj (not bacteriostatic water), and roll (not shake) to enhance reconstitution; further dilute with 190 ml; give as intermittent inf or give to clear cannula by using 1 ml of diluted drug; inject into cannula slowly, clamp 5 min, aspirate clot; avoid excessive pressure when urokinase is injected into catheter; force could rupture catheter or expel clot into circulation
- As soon as thrombi identified; not useful for thrombi over 1 wk old
- Cryoprecipitate or fresh frozen plasma if bleeding occurs

• Loading dose at beginning of therapy; may require increased loading doses
• Heparin therapy after thrombolytic therapy is discontinued, TT or APTT less than 2 × control (about 3-4 hr)

Y-site compatibilities: TPN 55, 56

Perform/provide:
• Storage in refrigerator; use immediately after reconstitution
• Bed rest during entire course of treatment; use caution in handling patients
• Avoidance of venous, arterial puncture procedures, inj, rectal temp
• Treatment of fever with acetaminophen or aspirin
• Placement of sign above patient's bed stating urokinase therapy
• Pressure for 30 sec to minor bleeding sites; 30 min to sites of arterial puncture followed by pressure dressing; inform prescriber if hemostasis not attained, apply pressure dressing

Evaluate:
• Therapeutic response: decreased clotting, thrombosis, embolism

ursodiol (℞)

(ur-soh-die′-ohl)

Actigall

Func. class.: Gallstone solubilizing agent

Chem. class.: Ursodeoxycholic acid

Action: Suppresses hepatic synthesis, secretion of cholesterol; inhibits intestinal absorption of cholesterol

Uses: Dissolution of radiolucent, noncalcified gallbladder stones (less than 20 mm in diameter) in which surgery is not indicated

Investigational uses: Severe pruritus

Dosage and routes:
• *Adult:* **PO** 8-10 mg/kg/day in 2-3 divided doses using gallbladder ultrasound q6mo; determine if stones have dissolved; if so, continue therapy, repeat ultrasound within 1-3 mo

Available forms: Caps 300 mg

Side effects/adverse reactions:

GI: Diarrhea, nausea, vomiting, abdominal pain, constipation, stomatitis, flatulence, dyspepsia, biliary pain

INTEG: Pruritus, rash, urticaria, dry skin, sweating, alopecia

CNS: Headache, anxiety, depression, insomnia, fatigue

MS: Arthralgia, myalgia, back pain

OTHER: Cough, rhinitis

Contraindications: Calcified cholesterol stones, radiopaque stones, radiolucent bile pigment stones, chronic hepatic disease, hypersensitivity

Precautions: Pregnancy (B), lactation, children

Pharmacokinetics: 80% excreted in feces, 20% metabolized, excreted into bile, lost in feces

Interactions:
• ↓ action of ursodiol: cholestyramine, colestipol, aluminum-based antacids
• ↑ risk of stone formation: clofibrate, gemfibrozil, estrogens, oral contraceptives

NURSING CONSIDERATIONS

Assess:
• GI status: diarrhea, abdominal pain, nausea, vomiting; drug may have to be discontinued if side effects are severe
• Skin for pruritus, rash, urticaria, dry skin; provide soothing lotion to lesions
• Musculoskeletal status: aches or stiffness in joints

Administer:
• For up to 9-12 mo; if no improvement is seen, discontinue drug

Evaluate:

• Therapeutic response: decreasing size of stones on ultrasound

Teach patient/family:

• That anxiety, depression, insomnia are side effects and are reversible after discontinuing drug

valacyclovir (℞)

(val-a-sye'kloh-vir)

Valtrex

Func. class.: Antiviral

Chem. class.: Acyclic purine nucleoside analog

Action: Interferes with DNA synthesis by conversion to acyclovir, causing decreased viral replication, time of lesional healing

Uses: Treatment or suppression of herpes zoster, genital herpes, herpes labialis

Investigational uses: Prevention of CMV in advanced HIV, posttransplant patients

Dosage and routes:

Genital herpes

• *Adult:* **PO** 1 g bid × 10 days initially; 1 g qd or 500 mg bid in those with <10 recurrences/yr

Recurrent episodes

• *Adult:* **PO** 500 mg bid × 3 days

Suppressive therapy

• *Adult:* **PO** 1 g qd if those ≤ recurrences/yr

Herpes zoster

• *Adult:* **PO** 1 g tid × 1 wk

Herpes labialis

• *Adult:* **PO** 2 g bid × 1 day

Renal dose

• *Adult:* **PO** CCr 30-49 ml/min 1 g q12h (herpes zoster); CCr 10-29 ml/min 1 g q24h (genital herpes); 500 mg q24h (recurrent genital herpes); CCr <10 ml/min 500 mg q24h (genital herpes), 500 mg q24h (recurrent genital herpes)

Available forms: Tabs 500 mg, 1 g

Side effects/adverse reactions:

CNS: Tremors, lethargy, *dizziness, headache,* weakness

GI: Nausea, vomiting, diarrhea, abdominal pain, constipation

INTEG: Rash

HEMA: Thrombocytopenic purpura, hemolytic uremic syndrome

Contraindications: Hypersensitivity to this drug or acyclovir

Precautions: Lactation, hepatic disease, renal disease, electrolyte imbalance, dehydration, pregnancy (B)

Pharmacokinetics:

PO: Onset unknown, terminal half-life 2½-3½ hr; converted to acyclovir that crosses placenta and enters breast milk

Interactions:

• ↑ blood levels of valacyclovir: cimetidine, probenecid

NURSING CONSIDERATIONS

Assess:

• Signs of infection; characteristics of lesions

◆ For thrombocytopenic purpura, hemolytic uremic syndrome; may be fatal

• C&S before drug therapy; drug may be taken as soon as culture is taken; repeat C&S after treatement; determine the presence of other sexually transmitted diseases

• Bowel pattern before, during treatment

• Skin eruptions: rash

• Allergies before treatment, reaction of each medication

Evaluate:

• Therapeutic response: absence of itching, painful lesions; crusting and healed lesions

Teach patient/family:

• To take as prescribed; if dose is missed, take as soon as remembered up to 1 hr before next dose; do not double dose

• That drug may be taken orally before infection occurs; drug should be taken when itching or pain occurs, usually before eruptions
• That partners need to be told that patient has herpes; they can become infected; condoms must be worn to prevent reinfections
• That drug does not cure infection, just controls symptoms and does not prevent infection of others
• Women must use a reliable form of contraception during treatment and for 90 days following; men should use barrier contraceptive during treatment and for 90 days following

Treatment of overdose: Discontinue drug, hemodialysis, resuscitate if needed

valdecoxib (℞)

(val-deh-cock'sib)
Bextra
Func. class.: Nonsteroidal antiinflammatory
Chem. class.: COX-2 inhibitor

Action: Inhibits prostaglandin synthesis by decreasing COX-2 enzyme needed for biosynthesis; analgesic, antiinflammatory, antipyretic properties

Uses: Acute, chronic rheumatoid arthritis, osteoarthritis, primary dysmenorrhea

Dosage and routes:

Osteoarthritis/adult rheumatoid arthritis
• *Adult:* **PO** 10 mg qd

Primary dysmenorrhea
• *Adult:* **PO** 20 mg bid, prn

Available forms: Tabs 10, 20 mg

Side effects/adverse reactions:

CNS: Fatigue, anxiety, depression, nervousness, paresthesia, dizziness, insomnia

CV: ***Tachycardia,*** angina, ***MI,*** palpitations, dysrhythmias, hypertension, fluid retention

EENT: Tinnitus, hearing loss, blurred vision, glaucoma, cataract, conjunctivitis, eye pain

GI: Nausea, anorexia, vomiting, constipation, dry mouth, diverticulitis, gastritis, gastroenteritis, hemorrhoids, hiatal hernia, stomatitis, ***GI bleeding***

GU: ***Nephrotoxicity:*** *dysuria,* ***hematuria, oliguria, azotemia,*** cystitis, UTI

HEMA: ***Blood dyscrasias,*** epistaxis, bruising, anemia

INTEG: Purpura, rash, pruritus, sweating, erythema, petechiae, photosensitivity, alopecia

RESP: Pharyngitis, shortness of breath, pneumonia, coughing

SYST: ***Stevens-Johnson syndrome, anaphylaxis***

Contraindications: Hypersensitivity to this drug, aspirin, iodides, other NSAIDs, sulfonamides; asthma triad, asthma, pregnancy 3rd trimester (D)

Precautions: Pregnancy 1st, 2nd trimester (C), lactation; bleeding; GI, cardiac, renal, hepatic disorders; hypersensitivity to other antiinflammatory agents, glucocorticoids, anticoagulants; hypertension, severe dehydration, elderly, children <18 yr

Pharmacokinetics: Well absorbed; peak 3 hr, delayed 1-2 hr by high-fat meal; 98% bound to plasma proteins; half-life 8-11 hr; metabolized in liver by CYP450 and non-CYP450 systems, excreted in urine (metabolites, 70%)

Interactions:
• ↑ effect of: anticoagulants
• ↓ effect of: aspirin, ACE inhibitors, thiazide diuretics, furosemide
• ↑ adverse reactions: glucocorticoids, NSAIDs, aspirin

V

- ↑ toxicity: lithium, antineoplastics
- ↑ valdecoxib blood level: fluconazole, ketoconazole

↑ gastric irritation: arginine, gossypol

↑ NSAIDs effect: bearberry, bilberry

↑ bleeding risk: bogbean, chondroitin

NURSING CONSIDERATIONS

Assess:

- For pain of rheumatoid arthritis, osteoarthritis; check ROM, inflammation of joints, characteristics of pain
- Blood counts during therapy; watch for decreasing platelets; if low, therapy may need to be discontinued, restarted after hematologic recovery

◆ For blood dyscrasias (thrombocytopenia): bruising, fatigue, bleeding, poor healing

Administer:

PO route

- With food or milk to decrease gastric symptoms, do not increase dose

Evaluate:

- Therapeutic response: decreased pain, inflammation in arthritic conditions, decreased dysmenorrhea

Teach patient/family:

- To check with prescriber to determine when drug should be discontinued before surgery
- That drug must be continued for prescribed time to be effective; to avoid other NSAIDs, aspirin, sulfonamides
- To notify prescriber if pregnancy is planned or suspected
- To notify prescriber of GI symptoms: black, tarry stools; cramping or rash; edema of extremities, weight gain
- To report bleeding, bruising, fatigue, malaise because blood dyscrasias do occur
- To take with a full glass of water to enhance absorption

valganciclovir (℞)

(val-gan-sy'kloh-veer)

Valcyte

Func. class.: Antiviral

Chem. class.: Synthetic nucleoside analog

Action: Valganciclovir is metabolized to ganciclovir; inhibits replication of human cytomegalovirus in vivo and in vitro by selective inhibition of viral DNA synthesis

Uses: Cytomegalovirus (CMV) retinitis in immunocompromised persons, including those with AIDS, after indirect ophthalmoscopy confirms diagnosis

Dosage and routes:

- *Adult:* **PO** induction 900 mg bid × 21 days with food; maintenance 900 mg qd with food

Renal dose

- *Adult:* **PO** reduce dose; CCr ≥60 ml/min same as above; CCr 40-59 ml/min 450 mg bid, then 450 mg qd; CCr 25-39 ml/min 450 mg qd, then 450 mg q2 days; CCr 10-24 ml/min 450 mg q2 days, then 450 mg 2×/ week

Available form: Tab 450 mg

Side effects/adverse reactions:

CNS: Fever, chills, ***coma***, *confusion*, abnormal thoughts, dizziness, bizarre dreams, *headache*, psychosis, tremors, somnolence, *paresthesia, weakness,* ***seizures***

EENT: Retinal detachment in CMV retinitis

GI: Abnormal LFTs, nausea, vomiting, anorexia, diarrhea, abdominal pain, ***hemorrhage***

GU: ***Hematuria***, increased creatinine, BUN

HEMA: ***Granulocytopenia, throm-***

bocytopenia, irreversible neutropenia, anemia, eosinophilia
INTEG: Rash, alopecia, *pruritus*, urticaria, pain at site, phlebitis
MISC: Local and systemic infections and sepsis
Contraindications: Hypersensitivity to acyclovir or ganciclovir, absolute neutrophil count <500, platelet count <25,000, hemodialysis
Precautions: Preexisting cytopenias, renal function impairment, pregnancy (C), lactation, children <6 mo, elderly
Pharmacokinetics: Metabolized to ganciclovir, which has a half-life of 3-4½ hr, excreted by kidneys (unchanged); crosses blood-brain barrier, CSF
Interactions:
- ↓ renal clearance of valganciclovir: probenecid
- ↑ toxicity: dapsone, pentamidine, flucytosine, vinCRIStine, vinBLAStine, adriamycin, DOXOrubicin, amphotericin B, trimethoprim-sulfamethoxazole combinations or other nucleoside analogs, cycloSPORINE
- Severe granulocytopenia: zidovudine, antineoplastics, radiation; do not give together
- ↑ seizures: imipenem/cilastatin

NURSING CONSIDERATIONS
Assess:
- For leukopenia/neutropenia/thrombocytopenia: WBCs, platelets q2d during 2×/day dosing and then q1wk
- For leukopenia with qd WBC count in patients with prior leukopenia with other nucleoside analogs or for whom leukopenia counts are <1000 cells/mm^3 at start of treatment
- Serum creatinine or CCr ≥q2wk

Administer:
PO route
- With food

Evaluate:
- Therapeutic response: decreased symptoms of CMV

Teach patient/family:
- That drug does not cure condition, that regular ophthalmologic exams are necessary
- That major toxicities may necessitate discontinuing drug
- To use contraception during treatment and that infertility may occur; men should use barrier contraception for 90 days after treatment
- To take with food
- ◆ To report infection: fever, chills, sore throat; blood dyscrasias: bruising, bleeding, petechiae
- To avoid crowds, persons with respiratory infections
- To use sunscreen to prevent burns

valproate
(val′proh-ate)
Depacon
valproic acid
(val′proh-ik)
Depakene, Myproic acid
divalproex sodium
(dye-val′proh-ex)
Depakote, Depakote ER, Epival✤
Func. class.: Anticonvulsant
Chem. class.: Carboxylic acid derivative

Action: Increases levels of γ-aminobutyric acid (GABA) in brain, which decreases seizure activity

Uses: Simple (petit mal), complex (petit mal) absence, mixed, manic episodes associated with bipolar disorder, prophylaxis of migraine, adjunct in schizophrenia, tardive dyskensia, aggression in children with ADHD, organic brain syndrome

Investigational uses: Tonic-clonic (grand mal), myoclonic seizures, migraines; rectal (valproic acid)

Dosage and routes:

Epilepsy

• *Adult and child:* **PO** 10-15 mg/kg/day divided in 2-3 doses, may increase by 5-10 mg/kg/day qwk, not to exceed 60 mg/kg/day in 2-3 divided doses; **IV** ≤20 mg/min over 1 hr

Mania (divalproex sodium)

• *Adult:* **PO** 750 mg qd in divided doses, max 60 mg/kg/day

Migraine (divalproex sodium)

• *Adult:* **PO** 250 mg bid, may increase to 1000 mg/day if needed or 500 mg (Depakote ER) qd × 7 days, then 1000 mg qd

Available forms: Valproic acid: caps 250 mg; divalproex: tabs delayed rel 125, 250, 500 mg; 125 mg; ext rel tabs 250, 500 mg sprinkle cap; valproate: inj 100 mg/ml; syr 250 mg/5 ml

Side effects/adverse reactions:

HEMA: ***Thrombocytopenia, leukopenia, lymphocytosis,*** increased PT, bruising, epistaxis

CNS: Sedation, drowsiness, dizziness, headache, incoordination, depression, hallucinations, behavioral changes, tremors, aggression, weakness

GI: Nausea, vomiting, constipation, diarrhea, dyspepsia, anorexia, cramps, ***hepatic failure, pancreatitis, toxic hepatitis,*** stomatitis

INTEG: Rash, alopecia, photosensitivity, dry skin

GU: Enuresis, irregular menses

EENT: Visual disturbances, taste perversion

Contraindications: Hypersensitivity, pregnancy (D), hepatic disease

Precautions: Lactation, child <2 yr, elderly

Pharmacokinetics:

PO: Onset 15-30 min, peak 1-4 hr, duration 4-6 hr

Metabolized by liver; excreted by kidneys, breast milk; crosses placenta; half-life 9-16 hr

Interactions:

• ↑ CNS depression: alcohol, opioids, barbiturates, antihistamines, MAOIs

• ↑ toxicity of valproic acid: salicylates

• ↑ action of: phenytoin

• ↑ bleeding: antiplatelets, NSAIDs, tirofiban, eptifibatide, abciximab, cefamandole, cefoperazone, cefotetan, heparin, thrombolytics

• ↓ metabolism of valproic acid: cimetidine

Lab test interferences:

False positive: Ketones

Interference: Thyroid function tests

NURSING CONSIDERATIONS

Assess:

• Blood studies: Hct, Hgb, RBC, serum folate, PT, platelets, vit D if on long-term therapy

• Hepatic studies: AST, ALT, bilirubin, hepatic failure

• Blood levels: therapeutic level 50-100 mcg/ml

• Mental status: mood, sensorium, affect, memory (long, short)

• Respiratory dysfunction: respiratory depression, character, rate, rhythm; hold drug if respirations are <12/min or if pupils are dilated

Administer:

PO route

Tablets or capsules whole; do not break, crush, or chew

• Elixir alone; do not dilute with carbonated beverage; do not give syrup to patients on sodium restriction

• Give with food or milk to decrease GI symptoms

Evaluate:

• Therapeutic response: decreased seizures

Teach patient/family:

• That physical dependency may result from extended use

• To avoid driving, other activities that require alertness

• Not to discontinue medication quickly after long-term use; convulsions may result

• To report visual disturbances, rash, diarrhea, light-colored stools, jaundice, protracted vomiting to prescriber

valrubicin (℞)

(val-roo'bih-sin)

Valstar

Func. class.: Antineoplastic, antibiotic

Chem. class.: Anthracycline glycoside

Action: A semisynthetic analog of DOXOrubicin that inhibits DNA synthesis primarily; replication is decreased by binding to DNA, which causes strand splitting; active throughout entire cell cycle; a vesicant

Uses: Bladder cancer

Dosage and routes:

• *Adult:* Intravesically 800 mg qwk × 6 wk, delay administration ≥2 wk after transurethral resection or fulguration

Available forms: Sol for intravesical instillation: 40 mg/ml

Side effects/adverse reactions:

HEMA: ***Thrombocytopenia, leukopenia,*** *anemia*

GI: Nausea, vomiting, anorexia, diarrhea

GU: UTI, urinary retention, hematuria

INTEG: Rash

CV: Chest pain

Contraindications: Hypersensitivity to anthracyclines or *Cremophor El,* urinary tract infection, small bladder

Precautions: Pregnancy (C), lactation, children

Pharmacokinetics: Penetrates into bladder wall, not metabolized

NURSING CONSIDERATIONS

Assess:

• I&O ratio; report fall in urine output to <30 ml/hr

• Monitor temp q4h; fever may indicate beginning infection

• Local irritation, pain, burning at inj site

Administer:

• After urinary catheter is inserted under aseptic conditions, drain bladder and instill the diluted 75 ml valrubicin by gravity for several min, withdraw catheter, drug should be retained for 2 hr, then void

• Use procedure for handling and disposal of cytotoxic agents

• Do not use polyvinyl chloride (PVC) or IV tubing

• Prepare/store valrubicin sol in glass, polypropylene, or polyolefin tubing/containers

• For instillation, 5 ml vials (200 mg valrubicin/5 ml/vial) should be warmed to room temperature, withdraw 20 ml for the 4 vials and dilute with 55 ml 0.9% NaCl inj to 75 ml of diluted valrubicin sol

• Valrubicin sol is clear red, at lower temps a waxy precipitate may form, warm in hand until sol is clear

Perform/provide:

• Strict hand-washing technique, gloves, protective clothing

• Increased fluid intake to 2-3 L/day to prevent urate, calculi formation

• Storage at room temperature for 12 hr after reconstituting

Evaluate:

• Therapeutic response: decreased tumor size, spread of malignancy

Teach patient/family:

• To consume fluids 2 L/day unless contraindicated

• To report any complaints, side effects to nurse or prescriber

• That urine and other body fluids may be red-orange for 48 hr

• That contraceptive measures are recommended during therapy

valsartan (℞)

(val'sahr-tan)

Diovan

Func. class.: Antihypertensive

Chem. class.: Angiotensin II receptor antagonist (Type AT_1)

Action: Blocks the vasoconstrictor and aldosterone-secreting effects of angiotensin II; selectively blocks the binding of angiotensin II to the AT_1 receptor found in tissues

Uses: Hypertension, alone or in combination

Dosage and routes:

• *Adult:* **PO** 80-160 mg qd alone or in combination with other antihypertensives, may increase to 320 mg

Available forms: Tabs 80, 160, 320 mg

Side effects/adverse reactions:

CNS: Dizziness, insomnia, drowsiness, vertigo, headache, fatigue

CV: Angina pectoris, 2nd-degree AV block, ***cerebrovascular accident,*** hypotension, ***myocardial infarction,*** *dysrhythmias*

EENT: Conjunctivitis

GI: Diarrhea, abdominal pain, nausea, ***hepatotoxicity***

GU: Impotence, ***nephrotoxicity***

HEMA: Anemia, neutropenia

MS: Cramps, myalgia, pain, stiffness

RESP: Cough

Contraindications: Hypersensitivity, severe hepatic disease, bilateral renal artery stenosis, pregnancy (D) 2nd/3rd trimester

Precautions: Hypersensitivity to ACE inhibitors: congestive heart failure, hypertrophic cardiomyopathy aortic/mitral valve stenosis, CAD; lactation, children, elderly

Pharmacokinetics:

Peak 2 hr, duration >24 hr, extensively metabolized, half-life 6 hr; excreted in feces, urine, breast milk

Interactions:

↑ toxicity, death: aconite

↑ or ↓ antihypertensive effect: astragalus, cola tree

↑ antihypertensive effect: barberry, betony, black catechu, black cohosh, bloodroot, broom, burdock, cat's claw, dandelion, goldenseal, Irish moss, Jamaican dogwood, kelp, khella, mistletoe, parsley

↓ antihypertensive effect: coltsfoot, guarana, khat, licorice

NURSING CONSIDERATIONS

Assess:

• B/P, pulse q4h; note rate, rhythm, quality

• Blood studies; BUN, creatinine, LFTs before treatment

• Electrolytes: K, Na, Cl, total CO_2

• Baselines in renal, hepatic studies before therapy begins

• Edema in feet, legs qd

• Skin turgor, dryness of mucous membranes for hydration status

Administer:

PO route

• Without regard to meals

Evaluate:

• Therapeutic response: decreased B/P

Teach patient/family:

• To comply with dosage schedule, even if feeling better

- To notify prescriber of fever, swelling of hands or feet, irregular heartbeat, chest pain
- That excessive perspiration, dehydration, diarrhea may lead to fall in blood pressure; consult prescriber if these occur
- That drug may cause dizziness, fainting; light-headedness may occur
- To rise slowly to sitting or standing position to minimize orthostatic hypotension
- Not to take this medication if pregnant or breastfeeding, or have had an allergic reaction to this drug
- That if a dose is missed, to take it as soon as possible, unless it is within an hour before next dose

vancomycin (℞)

(van-koe-mye′sin)
Lyphocin, Vancocin, Vancoled, vancomycin HCl

Func. class.: Antiinfective, misc.

Chem. class.: Tricyclic glycopeptide

Action: Inhibits bacterial cell wall synthesis

Uses: Resistant staphylococcal infections, pseudomembranous colitis, staphylococcal enterocolitis, endocarditis prophylaxis for dental procedures, diphtheroid endocarditis

Dosage and routes:

Serious staphylococcal infections

- *Adult:* **IV** 500 mg q6-8h or 1 g q12h
- *Child:* **IV** 40 mg/kg/day divided q6-8h
- *Neonate:* **IV** 15 mg/kg initially followed by 10 mg/kg q8-24h

Pseudomembranous/staphylococcal enterocolitis

- *Adult:* **PO** 500 mg/day in divided doses for 7-10 days
- *Child:* **PO** 40 mg/kg/day divided q6h, not to exceed 2 g/day

Endocarditis prophylaxis for dental procedures

- *Adult:* **IV** 1 g over 1 hr, 1 hr before procedure
- *Child:* **IV** 20 mg/kg over 1 hr, 1 hr prior to procedure

Available forms: Pulvules 125, 250 mg; powder for oral sol 1, 10 g; powder for inj 500 mg, 1, 5, 10 g

Side effects/adverse reactions:

CV: ***Cardiac arrest, vascular collapse*** (rare)

EENT: ***Ototoxicity, permanent deafness,*** tinnitus

HEMA: ***Leukopenia, eosinophilia, neutropenia***

GI: ***Nausea, pseudomembranous colitis***

RESP: Wheezing, dyspnea

SYST: ***Anaphylaxis***

GU: ***Nephrotoxicity,*** *increased BUN, creatinine, albumin,* ***fatal uremia***

INTEG: Chills, fever, rash, thrombophlebitis at inj site, urticaria, pruritus, necrosis (red man's syndrome)

Contraindications: Hypersensitivity, previous hearing loss

Precautions: Renal disease, pregnancy (C), lactation, elderly, neonates

Pharmacokinetics:

IV: Peak 5 min; half-life 4-8 hr; excreted in urine (active form)

PO: Absorption: poor

Interactions:

- Ototoxicity or nephrotoxicity: aminoglycosides, cephalosporins, colistin, polymyxin, bacitracin, cisplatin, amphotericin B, nondepolarizing muscle relaxants

V

NURSING CONSIDERATIONS

Assess:

- I&O ratio; report hematuria, oliguria; nephrotoxicity may occur

➡ Any patient with compromised renal system; drug is excreted slowly in poor renal system function; toxicity may occur rapidly; BUN, creatinine

- Blood studies: WBC
- Serum levels: peak 1 hr after 1 hr inf 25-40 mg/ml, trough prior to next dose 5-10 mg/ml
- C&S; drug may be given as soon as culture is taken
- Auditory function during, after treatment
- B/P during administration; sudden drop may indicate red man syndrome
- Signs of infection
- Hearing loss, ringing, roaring in ears; drug should be discontinued
- Skin eruptions
- Respiratory status: rate, character, wheezing, tightness in chest
- Allergies before treatment, reaction of each medication

Administer:

- Antihistamine if red man's syndrome occurs: decreased B/P, flushing of neck, face
- Dose based on serum concentration

IV route

- After reconstitution with 10 ml sterile water for injection (500 mg/10 ml); further dilution is needed for IV, 500 mg/100 ml 0.9%NaCl, D_5W given as int inf over 1 hr; decrease rate of infusion if red man syndrome occurs

Additive compatibilities: Amikacin, atracurium, calcium gluconate, cefepime, cimetidine, corticotropin, dimenhydrinate, famotidine, hydrocortisone, meropenem, ofloxacin, potassium chloride, ranitidine, verapamil, vit B/C

Y-site compatibilities: Acyclovir, allopurinol, amifostine, amiodarone, amsacrine, atracurium, cisatracurium, cyclophosphamide, diltiazem, DOXOrubicin liposome, enalaprilat, esmolol, filgrastim, fluconazole, fludarabine, gallium, granisetron, hydromorphone, insulin (regular), labetalol, lorazepam, magnesium sulfate, melphalan, meperidine, meropenem, midazolam, morphine, ondansetron, paclitaxel, pancuronium, perphenazine, propofol, remifentanil, sodium bicarbonate, tacrolimus, teniposide, theophylline, thiotepa, tolazoline, vecuronium, vinorelbine, warfarin, zidovudine

Perform/provide:

- Storage at room temperature for up to 2 wk after reconstitution
- Adrenaline, suction, tracheostomy set, endotracheal intubation equipment on unit; anaphylaxis may occur
- Adequate intake of fluids (2 L/day) to prevent nephrotoxicity

Evaluate:

- Therapeutic response: absence of fever, sore throat; negative culture

Teach patient/family:

- All aspects of drug therapy: need to complete entire course of medication to ensure organism death (7-10 days); culture may be taken after completed course of medication
- To report sore throat, fever, fatigue; could indicate superinfection
- That drug must be taken in equal intervals around clock to maintain blood levels

vasopressin (℞)

(vay-soe-press'in)

Pitressin Synthetic

Func. class.: Pituitary hormone

Chem. class.: Lysine vasopressin

Action: Promotes reabsorption of water by action on renal tubular epithelium; causes vasoconstriction

Uses: Diabetes insipidus (nonnephrogenic/nonpsychogenic), abdominal distention postoperatively, bleeding esophageal varices

Dosage and routes:
Diabetes insipidus
• *Adult:* **IM/SC** 5-10 units bid-qid as needed; **IM/SC** 2.5-5 units q2-3 days (Pitressin Tannate) for chronic therapy
• *Child:* **IM/SC** 2.5-10 units bid-qid as needed; **IM/SC** 1.25-2.5 units q2-3 days (Pitressin Tannate) for chronic therapy
Abdominal distention
• *Adult:* **IM** 5 units, then q3-4h, increasing to 10 units if needed (aqueous)
Available forms: Inj 20, 5 units/ml (tannate), spray, cotton pledgets
Side effects/adverse reactions:
EENT: Nasal irritation, congestion, rhinitis
CNS: Drowsiness, headache, lethargy, flushing
GU: Vulval pain, uterine cramping
GI: Nausea, heartburn, cramps
CV: Increased B/P
MISC: Tremor, sweating, vertigo, urticaria, bronchial constriction
Contraindications: Hypersensitivity, chronic nephritis
Precautions: CAD, pregnancy (C)
Pharmacokinetics:
Nasal: Onset 1 hr, duration 3-8 hr, half-life 15 min; metabolized in liver, kidneys; excreted in urine

NURSING CONSIDERATIONS
Assess:
• Nasal mucosa if given by intranasal spray; for irritation
• Pulse, B/P, when giving drug IV or IM
• I&O ratio, weight daily; check for edema in extremities; if water retention is severe, diuretic may be prescribed
• H_2O intoxication: lethargy, behavioral changes, disorientation, neuromuscular excitability
Evaluate:
• Therapeutic response: absence of severe thirst, decreased urine output, osmolality

---

HIGH ALERT

vecuronium (℞)
(vek-yoo-roe′nee-um)
Norcuron
Func. class.: Neuromuscular blocker
Chem. class.: Monoquaternary analog of pancuronium

Action: Inhibits transmission of nerve impulses by binding with cholinergic receptor sites, antagonizing action of acetylcholine
Uses: Facilitation of endotracheal intubation, skeletal muscle relaxation during mechanical ventilation, surgery, general anesthesia
Dosage and routes:
• *Adult and child >9 yr:* **IV BOL** 0.08-0.10 mg/kg, then 0.01-0.015 mg/kg for prolonged procedures
Available forms: 10 mg/5 ml vial
Side effects/adverse reactions:
CNS: Skeletal muscle weakness or paralysis (rare)
RESP: ***Prolonged apnea, possible respiratory paralysis***
Contraindications: Hypersensitivity
Precautions: Pregnancy (C), cardiac disease, lactation, children <2 yr, electrolyte imbalances, dehydration, neuromuscular disease, respiratory disease, hepatic disease
Do not confuse:
Nocuron/Narcan
Pharmacokinetics:
IV: Onset 2-3 min, peak 3-5 min, duration 15-25 (recovery index) min; half-life 65-75 min; not metabolized; excreted in feces; crosses placenta

V

Interactions:
• ↑ neuromuscular blockade: aminoglycosides, clindamycin, lincomycin, quinidine, local anesthetics, polymyxin antibiotics, lithium, opioid analgesics, thiazides, enflurane, isoflurane, succinylcholine
• Dysrhythmias: theophylline

NURSING CONSIDERATIONS

Assess:
• For electrolyte imbalances (K, Mg); may lead to increased action of this drug
• VS (B/P, pulse, respirations, airway) q15min until fully recovered; rate, depth, pattern of respirations, strength of hand grip
• I&O ratio; check for urinary retention, frequency, hesitancy
• Recovery: decreased paralysis of face, diaphragm, leg, arm, rest of body; allow to recover fully before completing neurologic assessment
• Allergic reactions: rash, fever, respiratory distress, pruritus; drug should be discontinued

Administer:
• With diazepam or morphine when used for therapeutic paralysis; provides no sedation alone
• Using nerve stimulator by anesthesiologist to determine neuromuscular blockade
• Anticholinesterase to reverse neuromuscular blockade
• IV after diluting with diluent provided; give by direct IV over 1 min; may give as continuous inf 10-20 mg/100 ml; titrate to patient response (only by qualified person)

Y-site compatibilities: Aminophylline, cefazolin, cefuroxime, cimetidine, diltiazem, DOBUTamine, DOPamine, epINEPHrine, esmolol, fentanyl, fluconazole, gentamicin, heparin, hydrocortisone, hydromorphone, isoproterenol, labetalol, lorazepam, midazolam, milrinone, morphine, niCARdipine, nitroglycerin, norepinephrine, propofol, ranitidine, sodium nitroprusside, trimethoprim-sulfamethoxazole, vancomycin

Perform/provide:
• Storage in refrigerator; discard in 24 hr
• Reassurance if communication is difficult during recovery from neuromuscular blockade

Evaluate:
• Therapeutic response: paralysis of jaw, eyelid, head, neck, rest of body

Treatment of overdose: Edrophonium or neostigmine, atropine, monitor VS; may require mechanical ventilation

venlafaxine (℞)

(ven-la-fax′een)

Effexor, Effexor-XR

Func. class.: Antidepressant (misc)

Action: Potent inhibitor of neuronal serotonin and norepinephrine uptake, weak inhibitor of DOPamine; no muscarinic, histaminergic, or α-adrenergic receptors in vitro

Uses: Prevention/treatment of depression, to treat depression at end of life, long-term treatment of general anxiety disorder (Effexor-XR)

Investigational uses: Hot flashes, obsessive-compulsive disorder (OCD)

Dosage and routes:

Renal dose
• Mild-moderate impairment, 75% of dose

Hepatic dose
• Moderate impairment, 50% of dose

Depression
• *Adult:* **PO** 75 mg/day in 2 or 3 divided doses; taken with food, may be increased to 150 mg/day; if needed, may be further increased to

225 mg/day; increments of 75 mg/day at intervals of no less than 4 days; some hospitalized patients may require up to 375 mg/day in 3 divided doses; ext rel 37.5-75 mg PO qd, max 225 mg/day; give XR qd

Hot flashes (Investigational)

• *Adult:* **PO** 12.5 mg bid × 4 wk or ext rel 37.5 mg × 4 wk

Available forms: Tabs scored 25, 37.5, 50, 75, 100 mg; cap ext rel 37.5, 75, 150 mg

Side effects/adverse reactions:

CNS: Emotional lability, vertigo, apathy, ataxia, CNS stimulation, euphoria, hallucinations, hostility, increased libido, hypertonia, hypotonia, psychosis, insomnia, anxiety

CV: Migraine, angina pectoris, hypertension, extrasystoles, postural hypotension, syncope, thrombophlebitis

EENT: Abnormal vision, taste, *ear pain,* cataract, conjunctivitis, corneal lesions, dry eyes, otitis media, photophobia

GI: Dysphagia, eructation, nausea, anorexia, dry mouth, colitis, gastritis, gingivitis, ***rectal hemorrhage,*** stomatitis, stomach and mouth ulceration

GU: Anorgasmia, abnormal ejaculation, *dysuria, hematuria, metrorrhagia, vaginitis, impaired urination,* albuminuria, amenorrhea, kidney calculus, cystitis, nocturia, breast and bladder pain, polyuria, ***uterine hemorrhage, vaginal hemorrhage,*** moniliasis

INTEG: Ecchymosis, acne, alopecia, brittle nails, dry skin, photosensitivity

META: Peripheral edema, weight loss or gain, diabetes mellitus, edema, glycosuria, hyperlipemia, hypokalemia

MS: Arthritis, bone pain, bursitis, myasthenia tenosynovitis, arthralgia

RESP: Bronchitis, dyspnea, asthma, chest congestion, epistaxis, hyperventilation, laryngitis

SYST: Malaise, neck pain, enlarged abdomen, cyst, facial edema, hangover, hernia

Contraindications: Hypersensitivity

Precautions: Mania, pregnancy (C), lactation, children, elderly, hypertension, seizure disorder, recent MI, cardiac disease

Pharmacokinetics: Well absorbed, extensively metabolized in the liver to an active metabolite; 87% of drug recovered in urine; 27% protein binding; half-life 5-7, 11-13 hr (active metabolite) respectively

Interactions:

⬍ Hyperthermia, rigidity, rapid fluctuations of vital signs, mental status changes, neuroleptic malignant syndrome: MAOIs

• ↑ CNS depression: alcohol, opioids, antihistamines, sedative/hypnotics

• ↑ serotonin effect: lithium

• ↑ toxicity: cimetidine, fluoxetine, sertraline, phenothiazine

↑ CNS depression: chamomile, hops, kava, lavender, skullcap, valerian

↑ anticholinergic effect: corkwood, jimsonweed

Serotonin syndrome: SAM-e, St. John's wort

↑ hypertension: yohimbe

NURSING CONSIDERATIONS

Assess:

• B/P lying, standing; pulse q/4 h; if systolic B/P drops 20 mm Hg, hold drug, notify prescriber; take VS q4h in patients with cardiovascular disease

• Blood studies: CBC, leukocytes, differential cardiac enzymes if patient is receiving long-term therapy

V

• Hepatic studies: AST, ALT, bilirubin
• Weight qwk; weight loss or gain; appetite may increase; peripherae edema may occur
• With food, milk for GI symptoms
• Sugarless gum, hard candy, frequent sips of water for dry mouth
• Mental status: mood, sensorium, affect, suicidal tendencies, increase in psychiatric symptoms; depression, panic
• Withdrawal symptoms: headache, nausea, vomiting, muscle pain, weakness; not usual unless drug is discontinued abruptly

Perform/provide:
• Storage in tight container at room temperature; do not freeze
• Assistance with ambulation during beginning therapy, since drowsiness, dizziness occur
• Checking to see if PO medication swallowed

Evaluate:
• Therapeutic response; decreased depression

Teach patient/family:
• To dispense in small amounts because of suicide potential, especially in the beginning of therapy
• To use with caution when driving or other activities requiring alertness because of drowsiness, dizziness, blurred vision
• To avoid alcohol ingestion, other CNS depressants
• Not to discontinue medication quickly after long-term use; may cause nausea, headache, malaise
• To wear sunscreen or large hat, since photosensitivity occurs

Treatment of overdose: ECG monitoring; induce emesis; lavage, activated charcoal; administer anticonvulsant

verapamil (℞)

(ver-ap′a-mill)

Apo-Verap✤, Calan, Calan SR, Covera-HS, Isoptin, Isoptin SR, verapamil HCl, verapamil HCl SR, Verelan

Func. class.: Calcium channel blocker; antihypertensive; antianginal

Chem. class.: Diphenylalkylamine

Action: Inhibits calcium ion influx across cell membrane during cardiac depolarization; produces relaxation of coronary vascular smooth muscle; dilates coronary arteries; decreases SA/AV node conduction; dilates peripheral arteries

Uses: Chronic stable, vasospastic, unstable angina; dysrhythmias, hypertension, supraventricular tachycardia, atrial flutter or fibrillation

Investigational uses: Prevention of migraine headaches, ventricular outflow obstruction in hypertrophic cardiomyopathy

Dosage and routes:

Angina
• *Adult:* **PO** 80-120 mg tid, increase qwk

Dysrhythmias
• *Adult:* **PO** 240-320 mg/day in 3-4 divided doses in digitalized patients

Hypertension
• *Adult:* **PO** 80 mg tid, may titrate upward; ext rel 120-240 mg/day as a single dose, may increase to 240-480 mg/day

IV route
• *Adult:* **IV BOL** 5-10 mg (0.075-0.15 mg/kg) over 2 min, may repeat 10 mg (0.15 mg/kg) ½ hr after 1st dose
• *Child 1-15 yr:* **IV BOL** 0.1-0.3 mg/kg >2 min, repeat in 30 min, not to exceed 5 mg in a single dose

• *Child 0-1 yr:* **IV BOL** 0.1-0.2 mg/kg over ≥2 min

Available forms: Tabs 40, 80, 120 mg; ext rel tabs 120, 180, 240 mg; inj 2.5 mg/ml; sus rel caps 120, 180, 240, 360 mg; sus rel tabs 120, 180, 240 mg; caps, ext rel 100, 120, 180, 200, 240, 300 mg

Side effects/adverse reactions:

CV: Edema, ***CHF,*** bradycardia, hypotension, palpitations, AV block

GI: Nausea, diarrhea, gastric upset, *constipation,* increased liver function tests

GU: Impotence, nocturia, polyuria

CNS: Headache, drowsiness, dizziness, anxiety, depression, weakness, insomnia, confusion, light-headedness, asthenia, fatigue

SYST: ***Stevens-Johnson syndrome***

INTEG: Rash

Contraindications: Sick sinus syndrome, 2nd- or 3rd-degree heart block, hypotension <90 mm Hg systolic, cardiogenic shock, severe CHF

Precautions: CHF, hypotension, hepatic injury, pregnancy (C), lactation, children, renal disease, concomitant β-blocker therapy, elderly

Pharmacokinetics:

IV: Onset 3 min, peak 3-5 min, duration 10-20 min

PO: Onset variable, peak 3-4 hr, duration 17-24 hr, half-life (biphasic) 4 min, 3-7 hr (terminal)

• Metabolized by liver, excreted in urine (70% as metabolites)

Interactions:

• ↑ hypotension: prazosin, quinidine

• ↑ effects of verapamil: β-blockers, antihypertensives, cimetidine

• ↓ effects of lithium

• ↑ levels of digoxin, theophylline, cycloSPORINE, carbamazepine, nondepolarizing muscle relaxants

• Food/drug: ↑ hypotensive effects: grapefruit juice

↑ effect: barberry, betel palm, burdock, goldenseal, khat, lily of the valley, plantain

↓ effect: yohimbe

Lab test interferences:

Increase: LFTs

NURSING CONSIDERATIONS

Assess:

• Cardiac status: B/P, pulse, respiration, ECG intervals (PR, QRS, QT)

I&O ratios, weight qd; CHF: rales, weight gain, dyspnea, jugular vein distention

Administer:

PO route

• Before meals, hs; sus rel give with food

Do not crush, break, or chew ext rel, sus rel products

IV route

• Undiluted through Y-tube or 3-way stopcock of compatible sol; give over 2 min, or 3 min elderly, discard unused solution

Additive compatibilities: Amikacin, amiodarone, ascorbic acid, atropine, bretylium, calcium chloride, calcium gluconate, cefamandole, cefazolin, cefotaxime, cefoxitin, cephapirin, chloramphenicol, cimetidine, clindamycin, dexamethasone, diazepam, digoxin, DOPamine, epINEPHrine, erythromycin, gentamicin, heparin, hydrocortisone sodium phosphate, hydrocortisone, hydromorphone, insulin (regular), isoproterenol, lidocaine, magnesium sulfate, mannitol, meperidine, metaraminol, methicillin, methyldopate, methylPREDNISolone, metoclopramide, mezlocillin, morphine, moxalactam, multivitamins, naloxone, nitroglycerin, norepinephrine, oxytocin, pancuronium, penicillin G potassium, penicillin G sodium, pentobarbital, phenobarbital, phentolamine, phenytoin, piperacillin, potassium chloride, potassium phosphates, procainamide, propranolol, protamine, quinidine, sodium bicar-

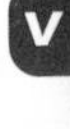

bonate, sodium nitroprusside, theophylline, ticarcillin, tobramycin, tolazoline, vancomycin, vasopressin, vit B/C

Syringe compatibilities: Amrinone, heparin, milrinone

Y-site compatibilities: Amrinone, ciprofloxacin, DOBUTamine, DOPamine, famotidine, hydrALAZINE, meperidine, methicillin, milrinone, penicillin G potassium, piperacillin, propofol, ticarcillin

Evaluate:

- Therapeutic response: decreased anginal pain, decreased B/P, dysrhythmias

Teach patient/family:

- To increase fluids/fiber to counteract constipation
- How to take pulse before taking drug; to keep record or graph
- To avoid hazardous activities until stabilized on drug, dizziness no longer a problem
- To limit caffeine consumption; no alcohol products
- To avoid OTC drugs unless directed by prescriber
- To comply with all areas of medical regimen: diet, exercise, stress reduction, drug therapy
- To change positions slowly to prevent syncope

Treatment of overdose: Defibrillation, atropine for AV block, vasopressor for hypotension

vidarabine ophthalmic

See appendix c

HIGH ALERT

*vinBLAStine (VLB) (℞)

(vin-blast′een)

Velban, Velbe, vinblastine sulfate

Func. class.: Antineoplastic

Chem. class.: Vinca rosea alkaloid

Action: Inhibits mitotic activity, arrests cell cycle at metaphase; inhibits RNA synthesis, blocks cellular use of glutamic acid needed for purine synthesis; a vesicant

Uses: Breast, testicular cancer, lymphomas, neuroblastoma; Hodgkin's, non-Hodgkin's lymphomas; mycosis fungoides, histiocytosis, Kaposi's sarcoma

Dosage and routes:

- *Adult:* **IV** 0.1 mg/kg or 3.7 mg/m^2 qwk or q2wk, not to exceed 0.5 mg/kg or 18.5 mg/m^2 qwk
- *Child:* 2.5 mg/m^2 then 3.75, 5, 6.25, 7.5 at 7-day intervals

Available forms: Inj, powder 10 mg for 10 ml IV

Side effects/adverse reactions:

HEMA: ***Thrombocytopenia, leukopenia, myelosuppression***

GI: Nausea, vomiting, ileus, *anorexia, stomatitis,* constipation, abdominal pain, ***GI, rectal bleeding, hepatotoxicity,*** pharyngitis

GU: Urinary retention, ***renal failure***

INTEG: Rash, alopecia, photosensitivity

RESP: ***Fibrosis, pulmonary infiltrate, bronchospasm***

CV: Tachycardia, orthostatic hypotension

CNS: Paresthesias, peripheral neuropathy, depression, headache, ***convulsions***

META: SIADH

Contraindications: Hypersensitiv-

ity, infants, pregnancy (D), leukopenia, granulocytopenia, lactation
Precautions: Renal disease, hepatic disease
Do not confuse:
vinBLAStine/vinCRIStine
Pharmacokinetics: Half-life (triphasic) 35 min, 53 min, 19 hr; metabolized in liver, excreted in urine, feces; crosses blood-brain barrier
Interactions:
- ↑ action of methotrexate
- Do not use with radiation
- Synergism: bleomycin
- ↓ phenytoin level: phenytoin
- Bronchospasm: mitomycin
- ↑ toxicity, bone marrow suppression: antineoplastics
- ↑ adverse reactions: live virus vaccines

NURSING CONSIDERATIONS
Assess:
- CBC, differential, platelet count qwk; withhold drug if WBC is <2000/mm^3 or platelet count is <75,000/mm^3; notify prescriber
- Pulmonary function tests, chest x-ray studies before, during therapy; chest x-ray film should be obtained q2wk during treatment
- Neurologic status: sensory-vibratory evaluation if side effects occur
- Renal studies: BUN, serum uric acid, urine CCr, electrolytes before, during therapy
- I&O ratio; report fall in urine output of 30 ml/hr
- Monitor temp q4h; may indicate beginning infection
- Hepatic studies before, during therapy (bilirubin, AST, ALT, LDH) as needed or qmo
- RBC, Hct, Hgb, since these may be decreased
- Bleeding: hematuria, guaiac, bruising or petechiae, mucosa of orifices q8h
- Dyspnea, rales, unproductive cough, chest pain, tachypnea, fatigue, increased pulse, pallor, lethargy
- Effects of alopecia on body image; discuss feelings about body changes
- Sensitivity of feet/hands, which precedes neuropathy
- Jaundiced skin, sclera; dark urine, clay-colored stools, itchy skin, abdominal pain, fever, diarrhea
- Buccal cavity q8h for dryness, sores or ulceration, white patches, oral pain, bleeding, dysphagia
- Local irritation, pain, burning, discoloration at inj site
- Symptoms indicating severe allergic reaction: rash, pruritus, urticaria, purpuric skin lesions, itching, flushing
- Frequency of stools and characteristics: cramping; acidosis; signs of dehydration: rapid respirations, poor skin turgor, decreased urine output, dry skin, restlessness, weakness

Administer:
- Antiemetic 30-60 min before giving drug and prn to prevent vomiting
- Transfusion for anemia

IV route
- After diluting 10 mg/10 ml NaCl; give through Y-tube or 3-way stopcock or directly over 1 min
- Hyaluronidase 150 units/ml in 1 ml NaCl, warm compress for extravasation for vesicant activity treatment

Additive compatibilities: Bleomycin
Syringe compatibilities: Bleomycin, cisplatin, cyclophosphamide, droperidol, fluorouracil, leucovorin, methotrexate, metoclopramide, mitomycin, vinCRIStine
Y-site compatibilities: Allopurinol, amifostine, amphotericin B cholesteryl, aztreonam, bleomycin, cisplatin, cyclophosphamide, DOXO-

rubicin, DOXOrubicin liposome, droperidol, filgrastim, fludarabine, fluorouracil, granisetron, heparin, leucovorin, melphalan, methotrexate, metoclopramide, mitomycin, ondansetron, paclitaxel, piperacillin/tazobactam, sargramostim, teniposide, thiotepa, vinCRIStine, vinorelbine

Perform/provide:

- Deep-breathing exercises with patient 3-4 ×/day; place in semi-Fowler's position
- Liquid diet: cola, Jell-O; dry toast or crackers may be added if patient is not nauseated or vomiting
- Increase fluid intake to 2-3 L/day to prevent urate deposits, calculi formation
- Rinsing of mouth tid-qid with water
- Brushing of teeth bid-tid with soft brush or cotton-tipped applicators for stomatitis; use unwaxed dental floss
- Nutritious diet with iron, vitamin supplements
- HOB raised to facilitate breathing

Evaluate:

- Therapeutic response: decreased tumor size, spread of malignancy

Teach patient/family:

- To report any complaints or side effects to nurse or prescriber
- To report any changes in breathing or coughing; to avoid exposure to persons with infection
- That hair may be lost during treatment, a wig or hairpiece may make patient feel better; tell patient that new hair may be different in color, texture
- To report change in gait or numbness in extremities; may indicate neuropathy
- To avoid foods with citric acid, hot or rough texture
- To report any bleeding, white spots or ulcerations in mouth to prescriber; to examine mouth qd
- To wear sunscreen, protective clothing, sunglasses
- To avoid receiving vaccinations

HIGH ALERT

*vinCRIStine (VCR) (℞)

(vin-kris'teen)

Oncovin, Vincasar PFS, vincristine sulfate

Func. class.: Antineoplastic-misc

Chem. class.: Vinca alkaloid

Action: Inhibits mitotic activity, arrests cell cycle at metaphase; inhibits RNA synthesis, blocks cellular use of glutamic acid needed for purine synthesis; a vesicant

Uses: Breast, lung cancer, lymphomas, neuroblastoma, Hodgkin's disease, acute lymphoblastic and other leukemias, rhabdomyosarcoma, Wilms' tumor, osteogenic and other sarcomas

Dosage and routes:

- *Adult:* **IV** 1-2 mg/m^2/wk, not to exceed 2 mg
- *Child:* **IV** 1.5-2 mg/m^2/wk, not to exceed 2 mg

Available forms: Inj 1 mg/ml; powder for inj 5 mg/vial

Side effects/adverse reactions:

INTEG: Alopecia

HEMA: ***Thrombocytopenia, leukopenia, myelosuppression, anemia***

GI: Nausea, vomiting, anorexia, stomatitis, constipation, ***paralytic ileus,*** *abdominal pain,* ***hepatotoxicity***

CV: Orthostatic hypotension

CNS: Decreased reflexes, numbness, weakness, motor difficulties, CNS depression, cranial nerve paralysis, ***seizures***

Contraindications: Hypersensitivity, infants, pregnancy (D), radiation therapy, lactation

Precautions: Renal disease, hepatic disease, hypertension, neuromuscular disease

Do not confuse:
vinCRIStine/vinBLAStine

Pharmacokinetics: Half-life (triphasic) 0.85 min, 7.4 min, 164 min; metabolized in liver; excreted in bile, feces; crosses placental barrier, blood-brain barrier

Interactions:

- ↑ action of methotrexate, anticoagulants
- Do not use with radiation
- Neurotoxicity: peripheral nervous system drugs
- ↓ digoxin level: digoxin
- ↓ action of vinCRIStine: L-asparaginase
- Acute pulmonary reactions: mitomycin-c

NURSING CONSIDERATIONS

Assess:

- CBC, differential, platelet count qwk; withhold drug if WBC is <4000/mm^3 or platelet count is <75,000/mm^3; notify prescriber
- Renal studies: BUN, serum uric acid, urine CCr, electrolytes before, during therapy
- I&O ratio, report fall in urine output of 30 ml/hr
- Monitor temp q4h; may indicate beginning infection
- Hepatic studies before, during therapy (bilirubin, AST, ALT, LDH) as needed or monthly
- RBC, Hct, Hgb; may be decreased
- Deep tendon reflexes; drug is neurotoxic
- Sensitivity of feet/hands, which precedes neuropathy
- Bleeding: hematuria, guaiac, bruising or petechiae, mucosa of orifices q8h
- Effects of alopecia on body image, discuss feelings about body changes
- Jaundiced skin, sclera; dark urine, clay-colored stools, itchy skin, abdominal pain, fever, diarrhea
- Buccal cavity q8h for dryness, sores or ulceration, white patches, oral pain, bleeding, dysphagia
- Symptoms indicating severe allergic reaction: rash, pruritus, urticaria, purpuric skin lesions, itching, flushing
- Frequency of stools, characteristics: cramping, acidosis; signs of dehydration: rapid respirations, poor skin turgor, decreased urine output, dry skin, restlessness, weakness

Administer:

- Agents to prevent constipation
- Antiemetic 30-60 min before giving drug and prn
- Transfusion for anemia
- Antispasmodic for GI symptoms

IV route

- After diluting with diluent provided or 1 mg/10 ml of sterile H_2O or NaCl; give through Y-tube or 3-way stopcock or directly over 1 min
- Hyaluronidase 150 units/ml in 1 ml NaCl; apply warm compress for extravasation

Additive compatibilities: Bleomycin, cytarabine, fluorouracil, methotrexate

Syringe compatibilities: Bleomycin, cisplatin, cyclophosphamide, doxapram, DOXOrubicin, droperidol, fluorouracil, heparin, leucovorin, methotrexate, metoclopramide, mitomycin, vinBLAStine

Y-site compatibilities: Allopurinol, amifostine, amphotericin B cholesteryl, aztreonam, bleomycin, cisplatin, cladribine, cyclophos-

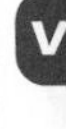

phamide, DOXOrubicin, DOXOrubicin liposome, droperidol, filgrastim, fludarabine, fluorouracil, granisetron, heparin, leucovorin, melphalan, methotrexate, metoclopramide, mitomycin, ondansetron, paclitaxel, piperacillin/tazobactam, sargramostim, teniposide, thiotepa, vinBLAStine, vinorelbine

Perform/provide:

- Liquid diet: cola, Jell-O; dry toast or crackers may be added if patient is not nauseated or vomiting
- Rinsing of mouth tid-qid with water
- Brushing of teeth bid-tid with soft brush or cotton-tipped applicators for stomatitis; use unwaxed dental floss
- Nutritious diet with iron, vitamin supplements

Evaluate:

- Therapeutic response: decreased tumor size, spread of malignancy

Teach patient/family:

- To report change in gait or numbness in extremities; may indicate neuropathy
- To report any complaints or side effects to nurse or prescriber
- To report any bleeding, white spots or ulcerations in mouth to prescriber; to examine mouth qd
- To increase bulk, fluids, exercise to prevent constipation
- To avoid persons with infections
- To avoid vaccinations

HIGH ALERT

vinorelbine (℞)

(vi-nor′el-bine)

Navelbine

Func. class.: Antineoplastic-misc

Chem. class.: Semisynthetic vinca alkaloid

Action: Inhibits mitotic activity, arrests cell cycle at metaphase; inhibits RNA synthesis, blocks cellular use of glutamic acid needed for purine synthesis; a vesicant

Uses: Unresectable advanced non-small cell lung cancer (NSCLC) stage IV; may be used alone or in combination with cisplatin for stage III or IV NSCLC breast cancer

Dosage and routes:

- *Adult:* **IV** 30 mg/m^2 qwk

Hepatic dose

- *Adult:* **IV** total bilirubin 2.1-3 mg/dl 15 mg/m^2 qwk; total bilirubin ≥3 mg/dl 7.5 mg/m^2 qd

Available forms: Inj 10 mg/ml

Side effects/adverse reactions:

CV: Chest pain

RESP: Shortness of breath

HEMA: ***Neutropenia, anemia, thrombocytopenia, granulocytopenia***

GI: Nausea, vomiting, ileus, *anorexia, stomatitis,* constipation, abdominal pain, diarrhea, ***hepatotoxicity***

INTEG: Rash, alopecia, photosensitivity

CNS: Paresthesias, peripheral neuropathy, depression, headache, ***convulsions,*** weakness, jaw pain

META: SIADH

MS: Myalgia

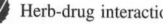

Contraindications: Hypersensitivity, infants, pregnancy (D), granu-

locyte count <1000 cells/mm^3 pretreatment
Precautions: Renal, hepatic disease, elderly, lactation, children
Pharmacokinetics: Half-life 27-43 hr, peak 1-2 hr
Interactions:
• Possible ↑ toxicity: fluorouracil

NURSING CONSIDERATIONS

Assess:
• B/P (baseline and q15min) during administration
• CBC, differential, platelet count weekly; withhold drug if WBC is <4000/mm^3 or platelet count is <75,000/mm^3; notify prescriber of results, recovery will take 3 wk
• For dyspnea, rales, unproductive cough, chest pain, tachypnea
• Renal studies: BUN, serum uric acid, urine CCr before, during therapy; I&O ratio; report fall in urine output to <30 ml/hr; for decreased hyperuricemia
• For cold, fever, sore throat (may indicate beginning infection); notify prescriber if these occur
• For bleeding: hematuria, guaiac, bruising or petechiae, mucosa or orifices q8h, no rectal temps; avoid IM inj; use pressure to venipuncture sites
• Nutritional status: an antiemetic may be needed
⬘ For symptoms of severe allergic reactions: rash, pruritus, urticaria, itching, flushing, bronchospasm, hypotension, epINEPHrine and crash cart should be nearby

Administer:
• Antiemetic 30-60 min before giving drug and prn to prevent vomiting

IV route
• Hyaluronidase 150 units/ml in 1 ml NaCl, warm compress for extravasation for vesicant activity treatment
• By cont inf: 40 mg/m^2 q3wk after an IV bol of 8 mg/m^2; may be given in combination with DOXOrubicin, fluorouracil, cisplatin

Y-site compatibilities: Amikacin, aztreonam, bleomycin, bumetanide, buprenorphine, butorphanol, calcium gluconate, carboplatin, carmustine, cefotaxime, ceftazidime, ceftizoxime, chlorproMAZINE, cimetidine, cisplatin, clindamycin, cyclophosphamide, cytarabine, dacarbazine, dactinomycin, DAUNOrubicin, dexamethasone, diphenhydrAMINE, DOXOrubicin, DOXOrubicin liposome, doxycycline, droperidol, enalaprilat, etoposide, famotidine, filgrastim, floxuridine, fluconazole, fludarabine, gallium, gentamicin, granisetron, haloperidol, heparin, hydrocortisone, hydromorphone, hydrOXYzine, idarubicin, ifosfamide, imipenem-cilastatin, lorazepam, mannitol, mechlorethamine, melphalan, meperidine, mesna, methotrexate, metoclopramide, metronidazole, minocycline, mitoxantrone, morphine, nalbuphine, netilmicin, ondansetron, plicamycin, streptozocin, teniposide, ticarcillin, ticarcillin/clavulanate, tobramycin, vancomycin, vinBLAStine, vinCRIStine, zidovudine

Perform/provide:
• Liquid diet: cola, Jell-O; dry toast or crackers if patient not nauseated or vomiting
• Brushing of teeth bid-tid with soft brush or cotton-tipped applicators for stomatitis; unwaxed dental floss
• Nutritious diet with iron, vitamin supplements

Evaluate:
• Therapeutic response: decreased tumor size, spread of malignancy

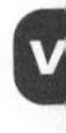

Teach patient/family:
• To report change in gait or numbness in extremities; may indicate neuropathy
• To report any complaints or side effects to nurse or prescriber
• To examine mouth qd for bleeding, white spots, ulcerations; notify prescriber
• To avoid crowds, people with infections, vaccinations

vitamin A (℞, OTC)

Aquasol A, Del-Vi-A, Vitamin A

Func. class.: Vitamin, fat soluble

Chem. class.: Retinol

Action: Needed for normal bone, tooth development, visual dark adaptation, skin disease, mucosa tissue repair, assists in production of adrenal steroids, cholesterol, RNA

Uses: Vit A deficiency

Dosage and routes:
• *Adult and child >8 yr:* **PO** 100,000-500,000 international units qd × 3 days, then 50,000 qd × 2 wk; dose based on severity of deficiency; maintenance 10,000-20,000 international units for 2 mo
• *Child 1-8 yr:* **IM** 5000-15,000 international units qd × 10 days
• *Infant <1 yr:* **IM** 5000-15,000 international units × 10 days

Maintenance
• *Child 4-8 yr:* **IM** 15,000 international units qd × 2 mo
• *Child <4 yr:* **IM** 10,000 international units qd × 2 mo

Available forms: Caps 10,000, 25,000, 50,000 international units; drops 5000 international units; inj 50,000 international units/ml; tabs 10,000, 25,000, 50,000 international units

Side effects/adverse reactions:
GI: Nausea, vomiting, anorexia, abdominal pain, ***jaundice***
CNS: Headache, ***increased intracranial pressure, intracranial hypertension,*** lethargy, malaise
EENT: Gingivitis, papilledema, exophthalmos, inflammation of tongue and lips
INTEG: Drying of skin, pruritus, increased pigmentation, night sweats, alopecia
MS: Arthralgia, retarded growth, hard areas on bone
META: Hypomenorrhea, hypercalcemia

Contraindications: Hypersensitivity to vit A, malabsorption syndrome (PO)

Precautions: Lactation, impaired renal function, pregnancy (C)

Pharmacokinetics: Stored in liver, kidneys, fat; excreted (metabolites) in urine, feces

Interactions:
• ↓ absorption of vit A: mineral oil, cholestyramine, colestipol
• ↑ levels of vit A: corticosteroids, oral contraceptives

Lab test interferences:
False increase: Bilirubin, serum cholesterol

NURSING CONSIDERATIONS

Assess:
• Nutritional status: yellow and dark green vegetables, yellow/orange fruits, vit A–fortified foods, liver, egg yolks
• Vit A deficiency: decreased growth, night blindness, dry, brittle nails; hair loss; urinary stones; increased infection, hyperkeratosis of skin; drying of cornea

Administer:

PO route
• With food (PO) for better absorption
• Do not administer IV because of risk of anaphylactic shock, IM only

• Oral preparations are not indicated for vitamin A deficiency in those with malabsorption syndrome

Perform/provide:

• Storage in tight, light-resistant container

Evaluate:

• Therapeutic response: increased growth rate, weight; absence of dry skin and mucous membranes, night blindness

Teach patient/family:

• That if dose is missed, it should be omitted

• That ophthalmic exams may be required periodically throughout therapy

• Not to use mineral oil while taking this drug

• To notify prescriber of nausea, vomiting, lip cracking, loss of hair, headache

• Not to take more than the prescribed amount

Treatment of overdose: Discontinue drug

vitamin D (cholecalciferol, vitamin D_3 or ergocalciferol, vitamin D_2) (℞, OTC)

Calciferol, Delta-D, Drisdol, Radiostol✤, Radiostol Forte✤, Vitamin D, Vitamin D_3

Func. class.: Vit D

Chem. class.: Fat soluble

Action: Needed for regulation of calcium, phosphate levels, normal bone development, parathyroid activity, neuromuscular functioning

Uses: Vit D deficiency, rickets, renal osteodystrophy, hypoparathyroidism, hypophosphatemia, psoriasis, rheumatoid arthritis

Dosage and routes:

Deficiency

• *Adult:* **PO/IM** 12,000 international units qd, then increased to 500,000 international units/day

• *Child:* **PO/IM** 1500-5000 international units qd × 2-4 wk, may repeat after 2 wk or 600,000 international units as single dose

Hypoparathyroidism

• *Adult and child:* **PO/IM** 200,000 international units given with 4 g calcium tab

Available forms: Tabs 400, 1000, 50,000 international units; caps 25,000, 50,000 international units; liq 8000 international units/ml; inj 500,000 international units/ml, 500,000 international units/5 ml

Side effects/adverse reactions:

GI: Nausea, vomiting, anorexia, cramps, diarrhea, constipation, metallic taste, dry mouth

CNS: Fatigue, weakness, drowsiness, ***convulsions,*** headache, psychosis

GU: Polyuria, nocturia, ***hematuria, albuminuria, renal failure,*** decreased libido

CV: Hypertension, dysrhythmias

MS: Decreased bone growth, early joint pain, early muscle pain

INTEG: Pruritus, photophobia

Contraindications: Hypersensitivity, hypercalcemia, renal dysfunction, hyperphosphatemia

Precautions: Cardiovascular disease, renal calculi, pregnancy (C)

Do not confuse:

Calciferol/calcitriol

Pharmacokinetics: Half-life 7-12 hr; stored in liver, duration 2 mo; excreted in bile (metabolites) and urine

Interactions:

• ↓ effects of vit D: cholestyramine, colestipol, phenobarbital, phenytoin

• ↑ toxicity: diuretics (thiazides), antacids, verapamil

NURSING CONSIDERATIONS

Assess:

• Vit D levels q2wk during treatment

• Calcium, PO_4, magnesium, BUN, alk phosphatase, urine Ca, creatinine

• In children, monitor height and weight

• Nutritional status: egg yolk, fortified dairy products, cod, halibut, salmon, sardines

Administer:

• IM inj deep in large muscle mass; administer slowly; aspirate carefully; rotate inj sites; avoid IV administration

Evaluate:

• Therapeutic response: absence of rickets/osteomalacia, adequate calcium/phosphate levels, decrease in bone pain

Teach patient/family:

• That if dose is missed, to omit

• The necessary foods in diet

• To avoid vitamin supplements unless directed by prescriber

• To keep appointments with health care providers; line between therapeutic and toxic doses is narrow

• To report weakness, lethargy, headache, anorexia, loss of weight

• To report nausea, vomiting, abdominal cramps, diarrhea, constipation, excessive thirst, polyuria, muscle and bone pain

• To decrease intake of antacids and laxatives containing magnesium

vitamin E (OTC)

Amino-Opti-E, Aquasol E, Daltose✦, E-Complex-600, E-Ferol, E-Vitamin Succinate, E-200 I.U. Softgels, Gordo-Vite E, Tocopherol, Vitamin E, Vita-Plus E Softgells, Vitec

Func. class.: Vit E

Chem. class.: Fat soluble

Action: Needed for digestion and metabolism of polyunsaturated fats, decreases platelet aggregation, decreases blood clot formation, promotes normal growth and development of muscle tissue, prostaglandin synthesis

Uses: Vit E deficiency, impaired fat absorption, hemolytic anemia in premature neonates, prevention of retrolental fibroplasia, sickle cell anemia, supplement in malabsorption syndrome

Dosage and routes:

Deficiency

• *Adult:* **PO** 60-75 international units qd

• *Child:* **PO** 1 mg/0.6 g of dietary fat

Prevention of deficiency

• *Adult:* **PO** 30 international units/day; **TOP** apply to affected areas

• *Infants:* **PO** 5 international units/day

Available forms: Caps 100, 200, 400, 500, 600, 1000 international units; tabs 100, 200, 400 international units; drops 50 mg/ml; chew tabs 400 units; ointment, cream, lotion, oil

Side effects/adverse reactions:

META: Altered metabolism of hormones: thyroid, pituitary, adrenal; altered immunity

MS: Weakness

CNS: Headache, fatigue

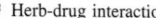

GI: Nausea, cramps, diarrhea

GU: Gonadal dysfunction
CV: Increased risk of thrombophlebitis
EENT: Blurred vision
INTEG: Sterile abscess, contact dermatitis
Contraindications: IV use in infants
Precautions: Pregnancy (A)
Pharmacokinetics:
PO: Metabolized in liver, excreted in bile
Interactions:
- ↑ action of oral anticoagulants
- ↓ absorption: cholestyramine, colestipol, mineral oil, sucralfate

NURSING CONSIDERATIONS
Assess:
- Vit E levels during treatment
- Nutritional status: wheat germ, dark green leafy vegetables, nuts, eggs, liver, vegetable oils, dairy products, cereals

Administer:
PO route
- Administer with or after meals
- *Chewable tabs:* Chew well
- *Sol:* May be dropped in mouth or mixed with food

TOP route
- To moisturize dry skin

Perform/provide:
- Storage in tight, light-resistant container

Evaluate:
- Therapeutic response: absence of hemolytic anemia, adequate vit E levels, improvement in skin lesions, decreased edema

Teach patient/family:
- The necessary foods in diet
- To omit if dose is missed
- To avoid vitamin supplements unless directed by prescriber

voriconazole (℞)
(vohr-i-kahn′a-zol)
Vfend
Func. class.: Antifungal
Chem. class.: Triazole

Action: Inhibits fungal CYP 450-mediation demethylation, needed for biosynthesis
Uses: Invasive aspergillosis, serious fungal infections (*Scedosporium apiospermum, Fusarium* sp.)
Dosage and routes:
- *Adult:* **PO** Give 1 hr ac or pc; ≥40 kg: 200 mg q12h; <40 kg: 100 mg q12h
- *Adult:* **IV** Loading dose 6 mg/kg q12h × 2 dose, then 4 mg/kg q12h; may switch to oral dosing

Available forms: Tabs 50, 200 mg; powder for inj, lyophilized 200 mg voriconazole, 3200 mg sulfobutyl ester β-cyclodextrin sodium (SBECD)
Side effects/adverse reactions:
CV: ***Tachycardia,*** hyper/hypotension, vasodilation, ***atrial arrhythmias, atrial fibrillation, AV block, bradycardia, CHF, MI***
EENT: Blurred vision, eye hemorrhage
INTEG: Burning, irritation, pain, necrosis at inj site with extravasation, dermatitis, rash, photosensitivity
CNS: Headache, paresthesias, peripheral neuropathy, hallucinations, psychosis, EPS, depression, Guillain-Barré syndrome, insomnia, suicidal ideation, dizziness
GU: Hypokalemia, azotemia, ***renal tubular necrosis, permanent renal impairment, anuria, oliguria***
GI: Nausea, vomiting, anorexia, diarrhea, cramps, ***hemorrhagic gastroenteritis, acute hepatic failure, hepatitis, intestinal perforation, pancreatitis***

V

HEMA: Anemia, ***eosinophilia,*** hypomagnesemia, ***thrombocytopenia, leucopenia, pancytopenia***
SYST: ***Stevens-Johnson syndrome, toxic epidermal necrolysis, sepsis***
MISC: Respiratory disorder
Contraindications: Hypersensitivity, severe bone marrow depression, pregnancy (D), lactation, children
Precautions: Renal disease
Pharmacokinetics: By P45 enzymes, protein binding 58%; max serum conc 1-2 hr after dosing; eliminated via hepatic metabolism
Interactions:
• ↑ effects of: benzodiazepines, calcium channel blockers, cycloSPORINE, ergots, HMG-CoA reductase inhibitors, pimozide, quinidine, prednisoLONE, sirolimus, sulfonylureas, tacrolimus, vinca alkaloids, warfarin, rifabutin, proton pump inhibitors, NNRTIs, protease inhibitors, phenytoin
• ↑ nephrotoxicity: other nephrotoxic antibiotics (aminoglycosides, cisplatin, vancomycin, cycloSPORINE, polymyxin B)
• ↑ hypokalemia: corticosteroids, digitalis, skeletal muscle relaxants, thiazides
• Drug/food: Avoid use with high-fat meals
↑ possibility of nephrotoxicity: gossypol

NURSING CONSIDERATIONS
Assess:
• VS q15-30min during first infusion; note changes in pulse, B/P
• I&O ratio; watch for decreasing urinary output, change in specific gravity; discontinue drug to prevent permanent damage to renal tubules
• Blood studies: CBC, K, Na, Ca, Mg q2wk, BUN, creatinine weekly
• Weight weekly; if weight increases over 2 lb/wk, edema is present; renal damage should be considered
For renal toxicity: increasing BUN, serum creatinine; if BUN is >40 mg/dl or if serum creatinine >3 mg/dl, drug may be discontinued or dosage reduced
For hepatotoxicity: increasing AST, ALT, alk phosphatase, bilirubin
• For allergic reaction: dermatitis, rash; drug should be discontinued, antihistamines (mild reaction) or epINEPHrine (severe reaction) administered
• For hypokalemia: anorexia, drowsiness, weakness, decreased reflexes, dizziness, increased urinary output, increased thirst, paresthesias
• For ototoxicity: tinnitus (ringing, roaring in ears), vertigo, loss of hearing (rare)
Administer:
IV route
• Drug only after C&S confirms organism, drug needed to treat condition; make sure drug is used in life-threatening infections
• Reconstitute powder with 19 ml water for inj to 10 mg/ml, shake until dissolved; infuse over 1-2 hr at a conc of 5 mg/ml or less; do not admix with other drugs, 4.2% sodium bicarbonate inf
• Store at room temp (powder, tabs)
Evaluate:
• Therapeutic response: decreased fever, malaise, rash, negative C&S for infecting organism
Teach patient/family:
• That long-term therapy may be needed to clear infection (2 wk–3 mo depending on type of infection)
• To notify prescriber of bleeding, bruising, or soft tissue swelling
• Take 1 hr before or after meal
• Do not drive at night because of vision changes
• Avoid strong, direct sunlight
• Women of childbearing age should use effective contraceptive

HIGH ALERT

warfarin (℞)

(war'far-in)

Coumadin, warfarin sodium, Warfilone♣

Func. class.: Anticoagulant

Action: Interferes with blood clotting by indirect means; depresses hepatic synthesis of vit K–dependent coagulation factors (II, VII, IX, X)

Uses: Pulmonary emboli, deep-vein thrombosis; prevention or treatment of venous thrombosis, pulmonary embolism, thromboembolic complications associated with atrial fibrillation, or cardiac valve replacement; after MI to reduce risk of death

Research note: Nevirapine given with warfarin resulted in decreased warfarin action[39]

Dosage and routes:

- *Adult:* **PO/IV** 2.5-10 mg/day × 3 days, then titrated to prothrombin time or INR qd
- *Geriatric:* **PO/IV** 2-10 mg/day
- *Child:* 0.1 mg/kg/day titrated to INR

Available forms: Tabs 1, 2, 2.5, 3, 4, 5, 6, 7.5, 10 mg; inj 5.4 mg powder for inj

Side effects/adverse reactions:

GI: Diarrhea, nausea, vomiting, anorexia, stomatitis, cramps, ***hepatitis***

GU: ***Hematuria***

INTEG: Rash, dermatitis, urticaria, alopecia, pruritus

CNS: Fever

HEMA: ***Hemorrhage, agranulocytosis, leukopenia, eosinophilia***

Contraindications: Hypersensitivity, hemophilia, leukemia with bleeding, peptic ulcer disease, thrombocytopenic purpura, hepatic disease (severe), malignant hypertension, subacute bacterial endocarditis, acute nephritis, blood dyscrasias, pregnancy (X), eclampsia, preeclampsia, lactation

Precautions: Alcoholism, elderly, CHF

Do not confuse:

Coumadin/Cardura

Coumadin/Compazine

Pharmacokinetics:

PO: Onset 12-24 hr, peak 1½-4 days, duration 3-5 days, effective half-life 1½-2½ days; metabolized in liver, excreted in urine/feces (active/inactive metabolites), crosses placenta, 99% bound to plasma proteins

Interactions:

- ↑ warfarin action: allopurinol, chloramphenicol, furosemide, HMG-CO reductase inhibitors, SSRIs, amiodarone, diflunisal, heparin, steroids, cimetidine, disulfiram, thyroid, glucagon, metronidazole, quinidine, sulindac, sulfinpyrazone, sulfonamides, clofibrate, salicylates, ethacrynic acids, indomethacin, mefenamic acid, oxyphenbutazones, phenylbutazone, penicillins, cefamandole, chloral hydrate, cotrimoxazole, erythromycin, quinolone antiinfectives, isoniazid, thrombolytic agents, tricyclics, NSAIDs, COX-2 selective inhibitors
- ↓ warfarin action: barbiturates, griseofulvin, ethchlorvynol, carbamazepine, rifampin, oral contraceptives, dicloxacillin, nafcillin, phenytoin, estrogens, vit K, sucralfate, vit K foods
- ↑ toxicity: oral sulfonylureas, phenytoin

↑ risk of bleeding: agrimony, alfalfa, angelica, anise, basil, bay, bilberry, black haw, bogbean, bromelain, buchu, chondroitin, cinchona bark, Dong quai, fenugreek, feverfew, garlic, ginger, ginkgo, ginseng, horse chestnut, Irish moss, kelp, kelpware, khella, lovage, lungwort, meadowsweet, motherwort, mug-

W

wort, nettle, papaya, parsley (large amts), pau d' arco, pineapple, poplar, prickly ash, safflower, saw palmetto, tonka bean, turmeric, wintergreen, yarrow

↓ anticoagulant effect: chamomile, coenzyme Q10, flax, glucomannan, goldenseal, guar gum, St. John's wort

Lab test interferences:

Increase: T_3 uptake

Decrease: Uric acid

NURSING CONSIDERATIONS

Assess:

- Blood studies (Hct, platelets, occult blood in stools) q3mo
- PT, which should be 1½-2 × control; PT often done qd initially or INR
- Bleeding gums, petechiae, ecchymosis, black tarry stools, hematuria
- Fever, skin rash, urticaria
- Needed dosage change q1-2wk; when stable, PT q3wk

Administer:

- At same time each day to maintain steady blood levels
- Tabs whole or crushed
- Avoiding all IM inj that may cause bleeding

IV route

- Reconstitute with 2.7 ml of sterile water for inj; do not use solution that is discolored or has particulates
- Give over 1-2 min into peripheral vein

Y-site compatibilities: Cefazolin, ceftriaxone, DOPamine, heparin, lidocaine, morphine, nitroglycerin, potassium chloride, ranitidine

Perform/provide:

- Storage in tight container

Evaluate:

- Therapeutic response: decrease of deep-vein thrombosis

Teach patient/family:

- To avoid OTC preparations that may cause serious drug interactions unless directed by prescriber
- To use soft-bristle toothbrush to avoid bleeding gums, and to use electric razor
- To carry emergency ID identifying drug taken
- The importance of compliance
- To report any signs of bleeding: gums, under skin, urine, stools
- To avoid hazardous activities (football, hockey, skiing), dangerous work
- The importance of avoiding unusual changes in vitamin intake, diet, or lifestyle
- To inform dentists and other physicians of anticoagulant intake
- To limit foods high in vit K (green leafy vegetables) may impair anticoagulation

Treatment of overdose: Administer vit K

xylometazoline nasal agent

See appendix c

zafirlukast (℞)

(za-feer'loo-cast)

Accolate

Func. class.: Bronchodilator

Chem class.: Leukotriene receptor antagonist

Action: Antagonizes the contractile action of leukotrienes (LTC_4, LTD_4, LTE_4) in airway smooth muscle; inhibits bronchoconstriction caused by antigens

Uses: Prophylaxis and chronic treatment of asthma in adults/children >5 yr

Investigational uses: Chronic urticaria

Dosage and routes:
• *Adult/child ≥12 yr:* **PO** 20 mg bid, take 1 hr ac or 2 hr pc
• *Child 5-11 yr:* **PO** 10 mg bid
Available forms: Tabs 10, 20 mg
Side effects/adverse reactions:
CNS: Headache, dizziness
GI: Nausea, diarrhea, abdominal pain, vomiting, dyspepsia
OTHER: Infections, pain, asthenia, myalgia, fever, increased ALT, urticaria, rash, ***angioedema***
Contraindications: Hypersensitivity
Precautions: Pregnancy (B), elderly, lactation, children, hepatic disease
Pharmacokinetics: Rapidly absorbed, peak 3 hr, 99% protein binding (albumin), extensively metabolized; inhibits P450 2C9 and 3A4 enzyme systems; excreted in feces, clearance is reduced in the elderly, hepatic impairment, half-life 10 hr
Interactions:
• ↑ plasma levels of zafirlukast: aspirin
• ↓ plasma levels of zafirlukast: erythromycin, theophylline
• ↑ PT: warfarin
• Drug/food: ↓ bioavailability
↑ effect: green tea (large amounts), guarana
NURSING CONSIDERATIONS
Assess:
Adult patients carefully for symptoms of Churg-Strauss syndrome (rare), including eosinophilia, vasculitic rash, worsening pulmonary symptoms, cardiac complications, and/or neuropathy
• Respiratory rate, rhythm, depth; auscultate lung fields bilaterally; notify prescriber of abnormalities
Administer:
• PO 1 hr ac or 2 hr pc; absorption may be decreased if given with food
Evaluate:
• Therapeutic response: ability to breathe more easily
Teach patient/family:
• To check OTC medications, current prescription medications, which will increase stimulation
• To avoid hazardous activities; dizziness may occur
• That if GI upset occurs, to take drug with 8 oz water; avoid food if possible, absorption may be decreased
• To notify prescriber of nausea, vomiting, diarrhea, abdominal pain, fatigue, jaundice, anorexia, flulike symptoms (hepatic dysfunction)
• Not to use for acute asthma episodes
• Not to take if breastfeeding
• To take even if symptom free

zalcitabine (℞)

(zal-sit′a-bin)
ddC, dideoxycytidine, HIVID
Func. class.: Antiretroviral
Chem. class.: (NRTI) Nucleoside reverse transcriptase inhibitor

Action: Inhibits HIV replication by the conversion of this drug by cellular enzymes to an active antiviral metabolite, a chain terminator
Uses: HIV infections in combination in adults, children >13 yr
Dosage and routes:
• *Adult:* **PO** 0.75 mg q8h in combination with other antiretrovirals, in presence of peripheral neuropathy initiate dose at 0.375 mg q8h of zalcitabine
Renal dose
• *Adult:* **PO** CCr 10-40 ml/min 0.75 mg q12h; CCr <10 ml/min 0.75 mg q24h

Available forms: Tabs 0.375, 0.75 mg

Side effects/adverse reactions:

GI: ***Pancreatitis,*** *diarrhea, nausea, vomiting,* abdominal pain, constipation, stomatitis, dysplasia, hepatic abnormalities, *oral ulcers,* flatulence, taste perversion, dry mouth, oral thrush, melena, *increased ALT, AST, alk phosphatase, amylase*

GU: Uric acid, ***toxic nephropathy,*** polyuria

CNS: Headache, peripheral neuropathy, ***seizures,*** confusion, anxiety, hypertonia, abnormal thinking, asthenia, insomnia, CNS depression, pain, *dizziness,* chills, *fever*

RESP: Cough, pneumonia, dyspnea, asthma, hypoventilation

ENDO: Hypoglycemia, hyponatremia, hyperbilirubinemia, hyperglycemia

INTEG: Rash, pruritus, alopecia, sweating, acne

MS: Myalgia, arthritis, myopathy, muscular atrophy

CV: Hypertension, vasodilation, dysrhythmia, syncope, palpitation, tachycardia, ***cardiomyopathy, CHF***

EENT: Ear pain, otitis, photophobia, visual impairment

HEMA: ***Leukopenia, granulocytopenia, thrombocytopenia,*** anemia

SYST: ***Lactic acidosis***

Contraindications: Hypersensitivity

Precautions: Renal, hepatic disease, pregnancy (C), lactation, child <13 yr, peripheral neuropathy, heart failure

Pharmacokinetics:

PO: Elimination half-life 1-3 hr; elimination via kidneys

Interactions:

- ↑ risk of pancreatitis with agents that can cause pancreatitis (ddI, d4T)
- ↑ risk of peripheral neuropathy with other agents that can cause peripheral neuropathy: aminoglycosides, amphotericin B, chloramphenicol, cimetidine, cisplatin, dapsone, disulfiram, ethionamide, foscarnet, glutethimide, gold, hydralazine, iodoquinol, isoniazid, metronidazole, nitrofurantoin, phenytoin, probenecid, ribavirin, vinCRIStine, other nucleoside analogs
- ↓ absorption: ketoconazole, dapsone, food, antacids, metoclopramide

NURSING CONSIDERATIONS

Assess:

- Neuropathy: tingling or pain in hands and feet, distal numbness
- Pancreatitis: abdominal pain, nausea, vomiting, elevated hepatic enzymes; drug should be discontinued, since condition can be fatal
- For lactic acidosis, severe hepatomegaly with steatosis that can be fatal, drug should be discontinued
- Children by dilated retinal exam q6mo to rule out retinal depigmentation
- Viral load CD4 baseline and throughout treatment
- CBC, differential, platelet count qwk; withhold drug if WBC is <4000/mm^3 or platelet count is <75,000/mm^3; notify prescriber
- Renal studies: BUN, serum uric acid, urine CCr before, during therapy
- Temp q4h; may indicate beginning infection
- Hepatic studies before, during therapy (bilirubin, AST, ALT), triglycerides, amylase prn or qmo

Perform/provide:

- Strict medical asepsis, protective isolation if WBC levels are low

Evaluate:

- Therapeutic response: absence of infection; symptoms of HIV

Teach patient/family:

- To report signs of infection: fever, sore throat, flulike symptoms

• To report signs of anemia: fatigue, headache, faintness, shortness of breath, irritability
• To report bleeding; avoid use of razors, commercial mouthwash
• That hair may be lost during therapy; a wig or hairpiece may make patient feel better

zaleplon (℞)

(zal'eh-plon)
Sonata
Func. class.: Sedative/hypnotic, antianxiety
Chem. class.: Pyrazolopyrimidine

Controlled Substance Schedule IV
Action: Binds selectively to omega-1 receptor of the $GABA_A$ receptor complex; results are sedation, hypnosis, skeletal muscle relaxation, anticonvulsant activity, anxiolytic action
Uses: Insomnia
Dosage and routes:
• *Adult:* **PO** 10 mg hs; may increase dose to 20 mg hs if needed; 5 mg may be used in low-weight persons
• *Elderly:* **PO** 15 mg hs; may increase if needed
Available forms: Caps 5, 10 mg
Side effects/adverse reactions:
CNS: Lethargy, drowsiness, daytime sedation, dizziness, confusion, anxiety, amnesia, depersonalization, hallucinations, hypesthesia, paresthesia, somnolence, tremor, vertigo
GI: Nausea, abdominal pain, constipation, anorexia, colitis, dyspepsia, dry mouth
EENT: Vision change, ear/eye pain, hyperacusis, parosmia
MISC: Asthenia, fever, headache, myalgia, dysmenorrhea
Contraindications: Hypersensitivity
Precautions: Hepatic disease, renal disease, elderly, psychosis, child <15 yr, pregnancy (C), lactation
Pharmacokinetics:
PO: Rapid onset, metabolized by liver extensively; excreted by kidneys (inactive metabolites); half-life 1 hr
Interactions:
• ↑ effects of zaleplon: cimetidine
• ↓ effect of zaleplon: rifampin
• Food: prolonged absorption, sleep onset reduced: high-fat/heavy meal
↑ CNS depression: catnip, chamomile, clary, cowslip, hops, kava, lavender, mistletoe, nettle, pokeweed, poppy, Queen Anne's lace, senega, skullcap, valerian
↑ hypotension: black cohosh

NURSING CONSIDERATIONS
Assess:
• Mental status: mood, sensorium, affect, memory (long, short)
• Type of sleep problem: falling asleep, staying asleep
Administer:
• After removal of cigarettes to prevent fires
• After trying conservative measures for insomnia
• Immediately before hs for sleeplessness
• On empty stomach for fast onset
Perform/provide:
• Assistance with ambulation after receiving dose
• Safety measure: nightlight, call bell within easy reach
• Checking to see if PO medication has been swallowed
• Storage in tight container in cool environment
Evaluate:
• Therapeutic response: ability to sleep at night, decreased amount of early morning awakening

Z

Teach patient/family:
- To avoid driving or other activities requiring alertness until drug is stabilized
- To avoid alcohol ingestion or CNS depressants
- Alternative measures to improve sleep: reading, exercise several hr before hs, warm bath, warm milk, TV, self-hypnosis, deep breathing
- That drug may cause memory problems, dependence (if used for longer periods of time), changes in behavior/thinking
- That drug is for short-term use only
- To take immediately before going to bed
- Not to ingest a high-fat/heavy meal before taking

zanamivir (℞)

(zan′ah-mih-veer)
Relenza
Func. class.: Antiviral
Chem. class.: Neuramidase inhibitor

Action: Inhibits the enzyme needed for influenza virus replication
Uses: Treatment of influenza type A for those that have been symptomatic for no more than 2 days
Dosage and routes:
- *Adult and child >12 yr:* **INH** 2 inhalations (two 5 mg blisters) q12h × 5 days, on the 1st day 2 doses should be taken with at least 2 hr between doses

Available forms: Blisters of powder for inhalation: 5 mg
Side effects/adverse reactions:
CNS: Headache, dizziness, fatigue
EENT: Ear, nose, throat infections
GI: Nausea, vomiting, diarrhea
RESP: Nasal symptoms, cough, sinusitis, bronchitis

Contraindications: Hypersensitivity
Precautions: Lactation, children <12 yr, respiratory disease, elderly, pregnancy (B)
Pharmacokinetics: Half-life 2½-5 hr, not metabolized, excreted in urine unchanged
Interactions:
- None known

NURSING CONSIDERATIONS
Assess:
- Bowel pattern before, during treatment
- Skin eruptions, photosensitivity after administration of drug
- Respiratory status: rate, character, wheezing, tightness in chest
- Allergies before initiation of treatment, reaction of each medication
- Signs of infection

Administer:
- Within 2 days of symptoms of influenza; continue for 5 days
- Give patient "Patient's Instruction for Use" and review all points before using delivery system

Perform/provide:
- Storage in tight, dry container

Evaluate:
- Therapeutic response: absence of fever, malaise, cough, dyspnea in infection

Teach patient/family:
- That this drug does not reduce transmission risk of influenza to others
- Patients with asthma or COPD to carry a fast-acting inhaled bronchodilator since bronchospasm may occur; to use scheduled inhaled bronchodilators before using this drug
- To avoid hazardous activities if dizziness occurs
- To take drug exactly as prescribed

zidovudine (℞)

(zye-doe′-vue-deen)

Apo-Zidovudine♣, Azidothymidine, AZT, Novo-AZT♣, Retrovir

Func. class.: Antiretroviral

Chem. class.: Nucleoside reverse transcriptase inhibitor (NRTI)

Action: Inhibits replication of HIV virus by incorporating into cellular DNA by viral reverse transcriptase, thereby terminating the cellular DNA chain

Uses: Used in combination with other antiretrovirals for HIV infection

Dosage and routes:

• *Adult:* **PO** 600 mg qd in divided doses, either 200 mg tid or 300 mg bid in combination with other antiretrovirals; **IV** 1-2 mg/kg q4h, initiate **PO** as soon as possible

• *Child 6 wk-12 yr:* **PO** 160 mg/m^2 q8h (480 mg/m^2/day, max 200 mg q8h) in combination with other antiretrovirals; **IV** same as adult

• *Neonates:* **PO** 2-3 mg/kg/dose q6h; **IV** 1.5 mg/kg infused over 30 min q6h

Prevention of maternal-fetal HIV transmission

• *Neonatal:* **PO** 2 mg/kg/dose q6h × 6 wk beginning 8-12 hr after birth; **IV** 1.5 mg/kg/dose over 30 min q6h until able to take **PO**

• *Maternal (>14 wk gestation):* **PO** 100 mg 5×/day until start of labor, then during labor/delivery **IV** 2 mg/kg over 1 hr followed by **IV INF** 1 mg/kg/hr until umbilical cord clamped

Symptomatic HIV infection

• *Adult:* **PO** 100 mg q4h; **IV** 1-2 mg/kg over 1 hr q4h

• *Child 3 mo to 12 yr:* **PO** 90-180 mg/m^2 q6h (max 200 mg q6h); **IV** 1-2 mg/kg over 1 hr q4h

Prevention of HIV following needlestick

• *Adult:* **PO** 200 mg tid plus lamivudine 150 mg bid, plus a protease inhibitor for high-risk exposure; begin within 2 hr of exposure

Available forms: Caps 100; tabs 300 mg; inj 200 mg/20 ml; oral syr 50 mg/5 ml

Side effects/adverse reactions:

HEMA: ***Granulocytopenia, anemia***

CNS: Fever, headache, malaise, diaphoresis, *dizziness, insomnia,* paresthesia, somnolence, chills, tremor, twitching, anxiety, confusion, depression, lability, vertigo, loss of mental acuity, ***seizures***

GI: Nausea, vomiting, diarrhea, anorexia, cramps, *dyspepsia,* constipation, dysphagia, *flatulence,* rectal bleeding, mouth ulcer

RESP: Dyspnea

EENT: Taste change, hearing loss, photophobia

INTEG: Rash, acne, pruritus, urticaria

MS: Myalgia, arthralgia, muscle spasm

GU: Dysuria, polyuria, urinary frequency, hesitancy

Contraindications: Hypersensitivity

Precautions: Granulocyte count <1000/mm^3 or Hgb <9.5 g/dl, pregnancy (C), lactation, child, severe renal disease, impaired hepatic disease

Pharmacokinetics:

PO: Rapidly absorbed from GI tract, peak ½-1½ hr, metabolized in liver (inactive metabolites), excreted by kidneys

Interactions:

• Toxicity: probenecid, fluconazole

• ↑ bone marrow depression: antineoplastics, radiation, ganciclovir

NURSING CONSIDERATIONS
Assess:

• Blood counts q2wk; watch for decreasing granulocytes, Hgb; if low, therapy may have to be discontinued and restarted after hematologic recovery; blood transfusions may be required; viral load, CD4 counts baseline and throughout

Administer:

• By mouth; capsules should be swallowed whole
• Trimethoprim-sulfamethoxazole, pyrimethamine, or acyclovir as ordered to prevent opportunistic infections; if these drugs are given, watch for neurotoxicity

IV route

• After diluting each 1 mg/0.25 ml or more D_5W to 4 mg/ml or less; give over 1 hr

Y-site compatibilities: Acyclovir, allopurinol, amifostine, amikacin, amphotericin B, amphotericin B cholesteryl, aztreonam, cefepime, ceftazidime, ceftriaxone, cimetidine, cisatracurium, clindamycin, dexamethasone, DOBUTamine, DOPamine, DOXOrubicin liposome, erythromycin, filgrastim, fluconazole, fludarabine, gentamicin, granisetron, heparin, imipenem/cilastatin, lorazepam, melphalan, metoclopramide, morphine, nafcillin, ondansetron, oxacillin, paclitaxel, pentamidine, phenylephrine, piperacillin, piperacillin/tazobactam, potassium chloride, ranitidine, remifentanil, sargramostim, teniposide, thiotepa, tobramycin, trimethoprim-sulfamethoxazole, trimetrexate, vancomycin, vinorelbine

Perform/provide:

• Storage in cool environment; protect from light

Evaluate:

• Blood dyscrasias (anemia, granulocytopenia): bruising, fatigue, bleeding, poor healing

Teach patient/family:

• That GI complaints and insomnia resolve after 3-4 wk of treatment
• That drug is not cure for AIDS but will control symptoms
• To notify prescriber of sore throat, swollen lymph nodes, malaise, fever; other infections may occur
• That patient is still infective, may pass AIDS virus on to others
• That follow-up visits must be continued since serious toxicity may occur; blood counts must be done q2wk
• That drug must be taken bid or tid
• That serious drug interactions may occur if OTC products are ingested; check with prescriber before taking aspirin, acetaminophen, indomethacin
• That other drugs may be necessary to prevent other infections
• That drug may cause fainting or dizziness

zileuton (℞)

(zye'loo-tahn)
Zyflo
Func. class.: Bronchodilator, leukotriene pathway inhibitor
Chem. class.: 5-Lipoxygenase inhibitor

Action: Inhibits leukotriene (LT) formation; leukotrienes exert their effects by increasing neutrophil, eosinophil migration; aggregation of neutrophils, monocytes; smooth muscle contraction, capillary permeability; these actions further lead to bronchoconstriction, inflammation, edema

Uses: Asthma

Investigational uses: Ulcerative colitis, rheumatoid arthritis

Dosage and routes:
Asthma
• *Adult and child:* 12 yr: **PO** 600 mg qid, may be given with meal and hs
Ulcerative colitis (off-label)
• *Adult:* **PO** 600 mg bid
Available forms: Tabs 600 mg
Side effects/adverse reactions:
CNS: Dizziness, insomnia, fatigue, paresthesias, headache
GI: Nausea, abdominal pain, dyspepsia, diarrhea, LFT abnormalities
INTEG: Hives
MS: Myalgia, asthenia
Contraindications: Active hepatic disease, elevations in LFTs 3× upper limits, hypersensitivity
Precautions: Acute attacks of asthma, alcohol consumption, pregnancy (C), lactation, history of hepatic disease
Pharmacokinetics:
PO: Rapidly absorbed, peak 1-3 hr, half-life 2.1-2.5 hr, protein binding 93% (albumin); metabolized by liver, excretion in urine
Interactions:
• ↑ effects of: theophylline, propranolol, warfarin
↑ effect: green tea (large amounts), guarana
NURSING CONSIDERATIONS
Assess:
• CBC, blood chemistry during treatment
• Hepatic studies before and qmo × 3 mo, then q2-3mo during first year treatment
• Respiratory rate, rhythm, depth; auscultate lung fields bilaterally; notify prescriber of abnormalities
• Allergic reactions: rash, urticaria; drug should be discontinued
Administer:
PO route
• After meals for GI symptoms
Evaluate:
• Therapeutic response: ability to breathe more easily
Teach patient/family:
• To check OTC medications, current prescription medications for epHEDrine, which will increase stimulation; to avoid alcohol
• To avoid hazardous activities; dizziness may occur
• That if GI upset occurs to take drug with 8 oz water or food
• To notify prescriber of nausea, vomiting, anxiety, insomnia
• Not to use for acute asthma attack
• To take even if without symptoms

zinc (℞, OTC)

Orazinc, PMS Egozine♣, Verazinc, Zinca-Pak, Zincate, Zinc 15, Zinc-220, zinc sulfate
Func. class.: Trace element; nutritional supplement

Action: Needed for adequate healing, bone and joint development (23% zinc)
Uses: Prevention of zinc deficiency, adjunct to vit A therapy
Investigational uses: Wound healing
Dosage and routes:
Dietary supplement
• *Adult:* **PO** 25-50 mg/day
Nutritional supplement (IV)
• *Adult:* **IV** 2.5-4 mg/day; may increase by 2 mg/day if needed
• *Child 1-5 yr:* **IV** 100 mcg/kg/day
• *Infant <1.5-3 kg:* **IV** 300 mcg/kg/day
Available forms: Tabs 66, 110 mg; caps 220 mg; inj 1 mg, 5 mg/ml
Side effects/adverse reactions:
GI: Nausea, vomiting, cramps, heartburn, ulcer formation
Overdose: Diarrhea, rash, dehydration, restlessness

Precautions: Pregnancy (A)
Interactions:
• ↓ absorption of other covalent cations
NURSING CONSIDERATIONS
Assess:
• Zinc levels during treatment
Administer:
• With meals to decrease gastric upset; avoid dairy products
Evaluate:
• Therapeutic response: absence of zinc deficiency
Teach patient/family:
• That element must be taken for 2 mo to be effective
• To report immediately nausea, diarrhea, rash, severe vomiting, restlessness, abdominal pain, tarry stools

ziprasidone (℞)

(zi-praz'ih-dohn)
Geodon
Func. class.: Antipsychotic/neuroleptic
Chem. class.: Benzisoxazole derivative

Action: Unknown; may be mediated through both DOPamine type 2 (D_2) and serotonin type 2 ($5\text{-}HT_2$) antagonism
Uses: Schizophrenia, acute agitation
Dosage and routes:
• *Adult:* **PO** 20 mg bid with food, adjust dosage every 2 days upward to max of 80 mg bid; **IM** 10-20 mg; may give 10 mg q2h; doses of 20 mg may be given q4h; max 40 mg/day
Available forms: Tabs 20, 40, 60, 80 mg; inj 20 mg/ml
Side effects/adverse reactions:
CNS: EPS, pseudoparkinsonism, akathisia, dystonia, tardive dyskinesia; drowsiness, insomnia, agitation, anxiety, headache, ***seizures, neuroleptic malignant syndrome,*** dizziness, tremor
CV: Orthostatic hypotension, ***tachycardia, prolonged QT/QTc, sudden death,*** hypertension
EENT: Blurred vision
GI: Nausea, vomiting, *anorexia, constipation,* jaundice, weight gain, diarrhea, dry mouth, abdominal pain
RESP: Rhinitis, dyspnea
Contraindications: Hypersensitivity, lactation, seizure disorders
Precautions: Children, renal disease, pregnancy (C), hepatic disease, elderly, breast cancer
Pharmacokinetics:
PO: Extensively metabolized by liver to a major active metabolite, plasma protein binding 90%
Interactions:
• ↑ sedation: other CNS depressants, alcohol
• ↑ EPS: other antipsychotics, lithium
• ↑ ziprasidone excretion: carbamazepine
• ↑ ziprasidone level: ketoconazole
• ↑ hypotension: antihypertensives
↑ CNS depression: chamomile, hops, kava, skullcap, valerian
↑ EPS: betel palm, kava
↑ action: cola tree, hops, nettle, nutmeg
Lab test interferences:
Not known
NURSING CONSIDERATIONS
Assess:
• Mental status before initial administration
• Swallowing of PO medication; check for hoarding or giving of medication to other patients
• I&O ratio; palpate bladder if urinary output is low
• Bilirubin, CBC, LFTs qmo
• Urinalysis before, during prolonged therapy

• Affect, orientation, LOC, reflexes, gait, coordination, sleep pattern disturbances
• B/P standing and lying; also pulse, respirations; take these q4h during initial treatment; establish baseline before starting treatment; report drops of 30 mm Hg; watch for ECG changes
• Dizziness, faintness, palpitations, tachycardia on rising
• EPS, including akathisia (inability to sit still, no pattern to movements), tardive dyskinesia (bizarre movements of the jaw, mouth, tongue, extremities), pseudoparkinsonism (rigidity, tremors, pill rolling, shuffling gait)
◆ For neuroleptic malignant syndrome: hyperthermia, increased CPK, altered mental status, muscle rigidity
• Skin turgor qd
• Constipation, urinary retention qd; if these occur, increase bulk and water in diet

Administer:

PO route
• Reduced dose in elderly
• Antiparkinsonian agent on order from prescriber, to be used for EPS

IM route
• Add 1.2 ml sterile water for inj to vial, shake vigorously until drug is dissolved, do not admix

Perform/provide:
• Decreased stimulus by dimming lights, avoiding loud noises
• Supervised ambulation until patient is stabilized on medication; do not involve in strenuous exercise program because fainting is possible; patient should not stand still for a long time
• Increased fluids to prevent constipation
• Sips of water, candy, gum for dry mouth
• Storage in tight, light-resistant container

Evaluate:
• Therapeutic response: decrease in emotional excitement, hallucinations, delusions, paranoia; reorganization of patterns of thought, speech

Teach patient/family:
• That orthostatic hypotension may occur and to rise from sitting or lying position gradually
• To avoid hot tubs, hot showers, tub baths; hypotension may occur
• To avoid abrupt withdrawal of this drug; EPS may result; drug should be withdrawn slowly
• To avoid OTC preparations (cough, hay fever, cold) unless approved by prescriber, since serious drug interactions may occur; avoid use with alcohol, CNS depressants; increased drowsiness may occur
• To avoid hazardous activities if drowsy or dizzy
• Compliance with drug regimen
• To report impaired vision, tremors, muscle twitching
• In hot weather, that heat stroke may occur; take extra precautions to stay cool

Treatment of overdose: Lavage if orally ingested; provide airway; *do not induce vomiting*

zoledronic acid (℞)

(zoh'leh-drah'nick ass'id)

Zometa

Func. class.: Bone-resorption inhibitor

Chem. class.: Bisphosphonate

Action: Inhibits normal and abnormal bone resorption, potent inhibitor of osteoclastic bone resorption; inhibits osteoclastic activity, inhibits skeletal calcium release caused by stimulating factors released by tumors; reduction of abnormal bone resorption is responsible for therapeutic effect in hypercalcemia; may directly block dissolution of hydroxyapatite bone crystals

Uses: Moderate to severe hypercalcemia associated with malignancy; multiple myeloma; bone metastases from solid tumors (used with antineoplastics)

Dosage and routes:

Hypercalcemia of malignancy

• *Adult:* **IV INF** 4 mg, given as a single infusion over ≥15 min; may re-treat with 4 mg if serum calcium does not return to normal within 1 wk

Multiple myeloma/metastatic bone lesions

• *Adult:* **IV INF** 4 mg, give over 15 min q3-4wk; may continue treatment for 9-15 months, depending on condition

Available form: Powder for inj 4 mg

Side effects/adverse reactions:

CV: Hypotension

GI: Abdominal pain, anorexia, constipation, nausea, diarrhea, vomiting

GU: UTI, possible reduced renal function

META: Anemia, hypokalemia, hypomagnesemia, hypophosphatemia

MISC: Fever, chills, flulike symptoms

MS: Bone pain, *arthralgias, myalgias*

Contraindications: Hypersensitivity to bisphosphonates, pregnancy (D)

Precautions: Children, nursing mothers, renal dysfunction, asthma-sensitive asthmatic patients

Pharmacokinetics: Rapidly cleared from circulation and taken up mainly by bones, not metabolized, eliminated primarily by kidneys; approximately 50% is eliminated in urine within 24 hr of administration

Interactions:

• Hypomagnesemia, hypokalemia: digoxin

• ↓ effect of zoledronic acid: calcium, vit D

• ↓ serum calcium, aminoglycosides, loop diuretics

• Do not mix with calcium-containing infusion sol such as lactated Ringer's sol

NURSING CONSIDERATIONS

Assess:

• Renal tests and Ca, P, Mg, K; creatinine, if creatinine is elevated hold treatment

• For hypercalcemia: paresthesia, twitching, laryngospasm; Chvostek's, Trousseau's signs

Administer:

• Saline hydration must be performed before administration; urine output should be 2 L/day during treatment, do not overhydrate

IV route

• Administer after reconstituting by adding 5 ml of sterile water for inj to each vial, then add to ≥100 ml of sterile 0.9% NaCl, D_5; run over ≥5 min

• Administer in separate IV line from all other drugs

Perform/provide:

• Sol reconstituted with sterile water may be stored under refrigeration for up to 24 hr

Evaluate:

• Therapeutic response: decreased calcium levels

Teach patient/family:

• To report hypercalcemic relapse: nausea, vomiting, bone pain, thirst

• To continue with dietary recommendations including calcium and vit D; take a multiple vitamin daily, 500 mg of calcium, 400 international units vit D in multiple myeloma

zolmitriptan (℞)

(zole-mih-trip'tan)

Zomig, Zomig-ZMT

Func. class.: Migraine agent

Chem. class.: 5-HT_1 receptor agonist

Action: Binds selectively to the vascular 5-HT_1 receptor subtype, exerts antimigraine effect; causes vasoconstriction in cranial arteries

Uses: Acute treatment of migraine with or without aura

Dosage and routes:

• *Adult:* **PO** Start on 2.5 mg or lower (tab may be broken), may repeat after 2 hr, max 10 mg/24 hr

Available forms: Tabs 2.5, 5 mg; orally disintegrating tab 2.5 mg

Side effects/adverse reactions:

CV: Palpitations

GI: Abdominal discomfort, nausea

MS: Weakness, neck stiffness, myalgia

CNS: Tingling, hot sensation, burning, feeling of pressure, tightness, numbness, dizziness, sedation

RESP: Chest tightness, pressure

Contraindications: Angina pectoris, history of MI, documented silent ischemia, ischemic heart disease, concurrent ergotamine-containing preparations, uncontrolled hypertension, hypersensitivity, basilar or hemiplegic migraine, risk of CV events

Precautions: Postmenopausal women, men >40 yr, risk factors for CAD, hypercholesterolemia, obesity, diabetes, impaired hepatic or renal function, pregnancy (C), lactation, children, elderly

Pharmacokinetics: Duration 2-3½ hr, 25% plasma protein binding, half-life 3-3½ hr, metabolized in the liver (metabolite), excreted in urine, feces

Interactions:

◆ Extended vasospastic effects: ergot, ergot derivatives

◆ Do not use within 2 wk of MAOIs

• ↑ half-life of zolmitriptan: cimetidine, oral contraceptives

◆ Weakness, hyperreflexia, incoordination: SSRIs (fluoxetine, fluvoxamine, paroxetine, sertraline)

Serotonin syndrome: SAM-e, St. John's wort

↑ effect: butterbur

NURSING CONSIDERATIONS

Assess:

• Tingling, hot sensation, burning, feeling of pressure, numbness, flushing

• For stress level, activity, recreation, coping mechanisms

• Neurologic status: LOC, blurring vision, nausea, vomiting, tingling in extremities preceding headache

• Ingestion of tyramine foods (pickled products, beer, wine, aged cheese), food additives, preservatives, colorings, artifical sweeteners, chocolate, caffeine, which may precipitate these types of headaches

• For serotonin syndrome, if also taking an SSRI

Administer:

• Take with fluids as soon as symptoms of migraine occur

Perform/provide:

• Quiet, calm environment with decreased stimulation for noise, bright light, excessive talking

Evaluate:

• Therapeutic response: decrease in frequency, severity of headache

Teach patient/family:

• To report any side effects to prescriber

• To use contraception while taking drug

zolpidem (℞)

(zole′pih-dem)
Ambien
Func. class.: Sedative-hypnotic
Chem. class.: Nonbenzodiazepine of imidazopyridine class

Controlled Substance Schedule IV
Action: Produces CNS depression at limbic, thalamic, hypothalamic levels of CNS; may be mediated by neurotransmitter γ-aminobutyric acid (GABA); results are sedation, hypnosis, skeletal muscle relaxation, anticonvulsant activity, anxiolytic action
Uses: Insomnia, short-term treatment
Dosage and routes:
• *Adult:* **PO** 10 mg hs × 7-10 days only; total dose should not exceed 10 mg
• *Geriatric:* **PO** 5 mg hs
Available forms: Tabs 5, 10 mg
Side effects/adverse reactions:
HEMA: ***Leukopenia, granulocytopenia*** (rare)
CNS: Headache, lethargy, drowsiness, daytime sedation, dizziness, confusion, light-headedness, anxiety, irritability, amnesia, poor coordination
GI: Nausea, vomiting, diarrhea, heartburn, abdominal pain, constipation
CV: Chest pain, palpitation
Contraindications: Hypersensitivity to benzodiazepines
Precautions: Anemia, hepatic disease, renal disease, suicidal individuals, drug abuse, elderly, psychosis, child <18 yr, seizure disorders, pregnancy (B), lactation
Pharmacokinetics:
PO: Onset 1.5 hr, metabolized by liver, excreted by kidneys (inactive metabolites), crosses placenta, excreted in breast milk; half-life 2-3 hr
Interactions:
• ↑ action of both drugs: alcohol, CNS depressants
↑ CNS depression: chamomile, hops, kava, skullcap, valerian
Lab test interferences:
Increase: ALT, AST, serum bilirubin
Decrease: RAI uptake
False increase: Urinary 17-OHCS
NURSING CONSIDERATIONS
Assess:
• Blood studies: Hct, Hgb, RBC, if blood dyscrasias are suspected (rare)
• Hepatic studies: AST, ALT, bilirubin if liver damage has occurred
• Mental status: mood, sensorium, affect, memory (long, short)
• Blood dyscrasias: fever, sore throat, bruising, rash, jaundice, epistaxis (rare)
• Type of sleep problem: falling asleep, staying asleep
Administer:
• After removal of cigarettes to prevent fires
• After trying conservative measures for insomnia
• ½-1 hr before hs for sleeplessness
• On empty stomach for fast onset but may be taken with food if GI symptoms occur
Perform/provide:
• Assistance with ambulation after receiving dose
• Safety measures: side rails, nightlight, call bell within easy reach
• Checking to see if PO medication has been swallowed
• Storage in tight container in cool environment
Evaluate:
• Therapeutic response: ability to sleep at night, decreased amount of early morning awakening if taking drug for insomnia

Teach patient/family:
• That dependence is possible after long-term use
• To avoid driving or other activities requiring alertness until drug is stabilized
• To avoid alcohol ingestion, CNS depressants; serious CNS depression may result
• That effects may take 2 nights for benefits to be noticed
• Alternative measures to improve sleep: reading, exercise several hours before hs, warm bath, warm milk, TV, self-hypnosis, deep breathing
• That hangover is common in elderly but less common than with barbiturates; rebound insomnia may occur for 1-2 nights after discontinuing drug

Treatment of overdose: Lavage, activated charcoal; monitor electrolytes, vital signs

zonisamide (℞)
(zone-is'a-mide)
Zonegran
Func. class.: Anticonvulsant
Chem. class.: Sulfonamides

Action: May act through action at sodium and calcium channels, but exact action is unknown

Uses: Epilepsy, adjunctive therapy of partial seizures

Dosage and routes:
• *Adults and child >16 yr:* 100 mg qd, may increase after 2 wk to 200 mg/day, may increase q2 wk, maximum dose 600 mg/day

Available forms: Caps 100 mg

Side effects/adverse reactions:
CNS: Dizziness, insomnia, paresthesias, depression, fatigue, headache, confusion, somnolence, agitation, irritability
EENT: Diplopia, verbal difficulty, speech abnormalities, taste perversion
GI: Nausea, constipation, anorexia, weight loss, diarrhea, dyspepsia
INTEG: Rash

Contraindications: Hypersensitivity to this drug or sulfonamides, psychiatric condition, hepatic failure

Precautions: Allergies, hepatic disease, renal disease, elderly, pregnancy (C), lactation, child <16 yr

Pharmacokinetics: Peak 2-6 hr, half-life 63 hr
Metabolized by liver, excreted by kidneys

Interactions:
• ↑ half-life of zonisamide: drugs inducing CYP 450 enzymes (carbamazepine, phenytoin, phenobarbital)

NURSING CONSIDERATIONS

Assess:
• For seizures: duration, type, intensity precipitating factors
• Renal function: albumin conc
• Mental status: mood, sensorium, affect, memory (long, short)

Evaluate:
• Therapeutic response; decrease in severity of seizures

Teach patient/family:
• Not to discontinue drug abruptly; seizures may occur
• To avoid hazardous activities until stabilized on drug
• To carry emergency ID stating drug use

Bibliography

Blumenthal M: *The complete German Commission E monographs: therapeutic guide to herbal medicines,* Austin, 2002, American Botanical Council.

Drug information: Bethesda, American Hospital Formulary Service.

Facts and comparisons: St Louis, updated monthly.

Gahart BL: *Intravenous medications,* ed 18, St Louis, 2004, Mosby.

Goodman A and others: *Goodman and Gilman's the pharmacological basis of therapeutics,* ed 11, New York, 2002, Pergamon Press.

McKenry LM, Salerno E: *Mosby's pharmacology in nursing,* ed 21, St Louis, 2003, Mosby.

Mediphor Editorial Group: *Drug interaction facts,* Philadelphia, updated quarterly, JB Lippincott.

Review of natural products: Philadelphia, updated monthly, *Facts and Comparisons.*

Appendixes

Appendix a

Selected new drugs

RARELY USED

agalsidase beta (℞)

(a-gal'sih-daze bay'tah)
Fabrazyme
Func. class.: Misc drug

Uses: Fabry disease
Dosage and routes:
• *Adult:* **IV INF** 1 mg/kg q2wks, run at ≤0.25 mg/min (15 mg/hr), slow if infusion-associated reaction occurs
Contraindications: Hypersensitivity

RARELY USED

alefacept (℞)

(ah-leh'fa-cept)
Amevive
Func. class.: Immunosuppressive

Uses: Adults with moderate to severe plaque psoriasis
Dosage and routes
• *Adult:* **IV BOL** 7.5 mg qwk or IM 15 mg qwk, for 12 wks
Contraindications: Hypersensitivity

alfuzosin (℞)

(al-fyoo'zoe-sin)
Uroxatral
Func. class.: Antiadrenergics
Chem. class.: Quinazolone

Action: Binds preferentially to α_{1A}-adrenoceptor subtype located mainly in the prostate
Uses: Symptoms of benign prostatic hyperplasia; has not been studied for and is not indicated for the treatment of high blood pressure
Dosage and routes:
• *Adult:* **PO** ext rel 10 mg qd, taken after same meal each day
Available forms: Tabs, ext rel 10 mg
Side effects/adverse reactions:
CV: Postural hypotension (dizziness, lightheadedness, fainting) within a few hours of administration, chest pain, tachycardia
CNS: Dizziness, headache, fatigue
GI: Nausea, abdominal pain, dyspepsia, constipation
GU: Impotence, priaprism
MISC: Body pain in general, rash
RESP: Upper respiratory infection, pharyngitis, bronchitis, sinusitis
Contraindications: Hypersensitivity, moderate to severe hepatic impairment
Precautions: Not indicated for use in women or children, pregnancy (C), lactation, coronary artery disease, coronary insufficiency, mild hepatic disease, mild/moderate/severe renal disease, history of QT prolongation or co-administration

with meds known to prolong QT interval

Pharmacokinetics:

PO: Elimination half-life: 10 hrs; metabolized in liver by CYP3A4 enzyme; excreted via urine; moderately protein binding (82-90%)

Interactions:

- Possible ↑ effects of alfuzosin: alcohol
- Not to be taken with: prazosin, terazosin, doxazosin
- Not to be taken with: CYP3A4 inhibitors (ketoconazole, itraconazole, and ritonavir)

NURSING CONSIDERATIONS

Assess:

- Prostatic hyperplasia: change in urinary patterns, baseline and throughout treatment
- CBC with diff and LFTs; B/P and heart rate
- BUN, uric acid, urodynamic studies (urinary flow rates, residual volume)
- I&O ratios, weight qd, edema, report weight gain or edema

Administer:

PO route

- Whole; do not chew or crush tablets

Perform/provide:

- Storage in tight container in cool environment

Evaluate:

- Therapeutic response: decreased symptoms of benign prostatic hyperplasia

Teach patient/family:

- Not to drive or operate machinery for 4 hr after first dose or after dosage increase

aprepitant (℞)

(ap-re′pi-tant)

Emend

Func. class.: Antiemetic

Chem. class.: Misc.

Action: A selective antagonist of human substance P/neurokinin 1 (NK_1) receptors

Uses: Prevention of nausea, vomiting associated with cancer chemotherapy including high-dose cisplatin, used in combination with other antiemetics

Dosage and routes:

- *Adult:* **PO** Day 1 (1 hour prior to chemotherapy) aprepitant 125 mg with 12 mg dexamethasone PO, with 32 mg ondansetron IV; Day 2 aprepitant 80 mg with 8 mg dexamethasone PO; Day 3 aprepitant 80 mg with 8 mg dexamethasone PO; Day 4 only dexamethasone 8 mg PO

Available forms: Caps 80, 125 mg

Side effects/adverse reactions:

CNS: Headache, dizziness, insomnia, anxiety, depression, confusion, peripheral neuropathy

CV: Bradycardia, DVT, hypertension

GI: Diarrhea, constipation, abdominal pain, anorexia, gastritis, ↑ AST, ALT, *nausea,* vomiting, heartburn

GU: Increased BUN, serum creatine, proteinuria, dysuria

HEMA: Anemia, ***thrombocytopenia, neutropenia***

MISC: Asthenia, fatigue, dehydration, fever, hiccups, tinnitus

Contraindications: Hypersensitivity

Precautions: Pregnancy (B), lactation, children

Pharmacokinetics: Metabolized in liver by CYP3A4 enzymes to an active metabolite; half-life 10-12 hr;

95% protein bound; not excreted in kidneys

Interactions:

- ↑ aprepitant action: CYP3A4 inhibitors (ketoconazole, itraconazole, nefazodone, troleandomycin, clarithromycin, ritonavir, nelfinavir, diltiazem)
- ↓ aprepitant action: CYP3A4 inducers (rifampin, carbamazepine, phenytoin)
- ↓ action of: CYP2C9 substrates (warfarin, tolbutamide, phenytoin), oral contraceptives
- ↑ action of: CYP3A4 substrates (pimozide, cisapride, dexamethasone, methylPREDNISolone, midazolam, alprazolam, triazolam, docetaxel, paclitaxel, etoposide, irinotecan, imatinib, ifosfamide, vinorelbine, vinBLAStine, vinCRIStine)
- ↓ action of both drugs: paroxetine

NURSING CONSIDERATIONS

Assess:

- For absence of nausea, vomiting during chemotherapy

Administer:

- PO on 3 day schedule

Perform/provide:

- Storage at room temperature

Evaluate:

- Therapeutic response: absence of nausea, vomiting during cancer chemotherapy

Teach patient/family:

- To report diarrhea, constipation
- To take only as prescribed, take 1st dose 1 hr prior to chemotherapy
- To report all medication to prescriber prior to taking this medication
- Advise to use nonhormonal form of contraception while taking this agent
- Advise those on warfarin to have clotting monitored closely during 2 wk period following administration of aprepitant

atazanavir (℞)

(at-a-za-na'veer)

Reyataz

Func. class.: Antiretroviral

Chem. class.: Protease inhibitor

Action: Inhibits human immunodeficiency virus (HIV-1) protease, which prevents maturation of the infectious virus

Uses: HIV-1 infection in combination with other antiretroviral agents

Dosage and routes:

- *Adult:* **PO** 400 mg qd

Hepatic dose

- *Adult:* **PO** (Child-Pugh B) 300 mg qd; (Child-Pugh C) do not use

Available forms: Caps 100, 150, 200 mg

Side effects/adverse reactions:

GI: Diarrhea, abdominal pain, nausea, ***hepatotoxicity***

CNS: Headache, depression, dizziness, insomnia, peripheral neurologic symptoms

INTEG: Rash, ***Stevens-Johnson syndrome,*** *photosensitivity*

MISC: Fatigue, fever, arthralgia, back pain, cough, lipodystrophy, pain

Contraindications: Hypersensitivity

Precautions: Liver disease, pregnancy (B), lactation, children, elderly

Pharmacokinetics: Rapidly absorbed, absorption increased with food, peak 2½ hr, 86% protein bound, extensively metabolized in liver, 27% excreted unchanged in urine/feces (minimal), half life 7 hr

Interactions:

- ↑ levels resulting in ↑ toxicity of immunosupressants (cycloSPORINE, sirolimus, tacrolimus, sildenafil), tricylic antidepressants, warfarin, calcium channel blockers, irinotecan, HMG CoA reductase inhibitors, antidysrhythmics, midazolam, triazolam, ergots, pimozide

- ↓ atazanavir levels: rifampin, antacids, didanosine, efavirenz, proton pump inhibitors, H_2-receptor antagonists
- ↑ effects of: oral contraceptives
- ↑ hyperbilirubinemia indinavir

↓ atazanavir levels: St. John's wort

Lab test interferences:

Increase: AST, ALT, total bilirubin, amylase, lipase

NURSING CONSIDERATIONS

Assess:

For hepatic failure

- Signs of infection, anemia
- Liver function studies: ALT, AST, bilirubin
- Bowel pattern before, during treatment; if severe abdominal pain with bleeding occurs, drug should be discontinued; monitor hydration
- Viral load, CD4 count throughout treatment
- Skin eruptions, rash, urticaria, itching
- Allergies before treatment, reaction of each medication; place allergies on chart

Administer:

- With food

Evaluate:

- Therapeutic response: Increasing CD4 counts; decreased viral load, resolution of symptoms of HIV-1 infection

Teach patient/family:

- To take as prescribed with other antiretrovirals as prescribed, if dose is missed, take as soon as remembered up to 1 hr before next dose; do not double dose, do not share with others
- That drug must be taken daily to maintain blood levels for duration of therapy
- May cause photosensitivity, use protective clothing, or stay out of the sun
- To notify prescriber if diarrhea, nausea, vomiting, rash occurs; dizziness, light-headedness, ECG may be altered
- That drug interacts with many drugs and St. John's wort, advise prescriber of all drugs, herbal products used
- That redistribution of body fat may occur, the effect is not known
- That drug does not cure HIV-1 infection or prevent transmission to others, only controls symptoms
- That if taking sildenafil with atazanavir, there may be at increased risk of sildenafil-associated adverse events, including hypotension and prolonged penile erection; notify physician promptly of these symptoms

bortezomib (℞)

(bor-tez'oh-mib)

Velcade

Func. class.: Antineoplastic, misc

Chem. class.: Proteasome inhibitor

Action: A reversible inhibitor of chymotrysin-like activity in mammalian cells. Causes a delay in tumor growth.

Uses: Multiple myeloma when at least two other treatments have failed.

Dosage and routes:

- *Adult:* **IV** BOL 1.3 mg/m^2/dose 2×/wk for 2 weeks (days 1, 4, 8, 11) followed by 10-day rest period (days 12 to 21)

• Grade 1 with pain or Grade 2: Reduce to 1 mg/m^2
• Onset of Grade 3 Nonhematological or Grade 4 Hematological toxicities, withhold use

Available forms: Lyophilized powder for inj 3.5 mg

Side effects/adverse reactions:

CV: Hypotension, edema

HEMA: Anemia, ***neutropenia, thrombocytopenia***

MS: Fatigue, malaise, weakness, arthralgia, bone pain, muscle cramps, myalgia, back pain

GI: Abdominal pain, constipation, diarrhea, dyspepsia, nausea, vomiting, anorexia

CNS: Anxiety, insomnia, dizziness, headache, peripheral neuropathy, rigors, paresthesia

RESP: Cough, pneumonia, dyspnea, URI

MISC: Dehydration, weight loss, herpes zoster, rash, pruritus, blurred vision

Contraindications: Hypersensitivity to this drug, boron, or Mannitol, pregnancy (D)

Precautions: Peripheral neuropathy, elderly, hepatic, renal disease, hypotension, lactation, children

Pharmacokinetics: Half-life 9-15 hrs, protein binding 83%, metabolized by P450 enzymes (3A4, 2D6, 2C19, 2C9, 1A2)

Interactions:

• Oral hypoglycemics: may result in hypo-, hyperglycemia
• ↑ exposure to CYP450 2C19 substrates when used with bortezomib
• ↑ toxicity or ↓ efficacy when administered with drugs that induce or inhibit cytochrome P450 3A4

NURSING CONSIDERATIONS

Assess:

• Hematological status: platelets, CBC throughout treatment
• For extravasation at inj site

Administer:

• Reconstitute each vial with 3.5 ml 0.9% NaCl
• Use protective clothing during handling, preparation, avoid contact with skin

Evaluate:

• Therapeutic response: improvement of multiple myeloma symptoms

Teach patient/family:

• To use contraception while on this drug, pregnancy (D), avoid breastfeeding
• To monitor blood glucose levels if diabetic
• To contact prescriber of new or worsening peripheral neuropathy, severe vomiting, diarrhea
• To avoid driving, operating machinery until effect is known
• To avoid using other medications unless approved by prescriber

daptomycin (℞)

(dap'toe-mye-sin)

Cubicin

Func. class.: Antiinfective, misc

Chem. class.: Lipopeptides

Action: A new class of antiinfective. It binds to the bacterial membrane and results in a rapid depolarization of the membrane potential, thus leading to inhibition of DNA, RNA and protein synthesis.

Uses: Complicated skin, skin structure infections caused by Staphylococcus aureus including methicillin-resistant strains, Streptococcus pyogenes, S. agalactiae, S. dysgalactiae, Enterococcus faecalis (vancomycin-susceptible strains only).

Dosage and routes:

• *Adult:* IV INF 4 mg/kg over ½ hr diluted in 0.9% NaCl, give q24h X7-14 days

Renal Dose
• *Adult:* IV INF CCr ≥30 ml/min 4 mg/kg q24h; CCr < 30 ml/min, hemodialysis, CAPD 4 mg/kg q48h
Available forms: Lyophilized powder for inj 250, 500 mg
Side effects/adverse reactions:
CV: Hypotension, hypertension, ↑ CPK
GI: Nausea, constipation, diarrhea, vomiting, dyspepsia, ***pseudomembraneous colitis***
CNS: Headache, insomnia, dizziness
MS: Muscle pain or weakness, arthralgia, pain
MISC: Fungal infections, UTI, anemia
GU: Nephrotoxicity: ↑ BUN, creatinine, albumin
INTEG: Rash, pruritus
Contraindications: Hypersensitivity
Precautions: Renal disease, pregnancy (B), children, lactation, elderly
Pharmacokinetics: Site of metabolism unknown, protein binding 92%
Interactions:
• Myopathy: HMG-CoA reductase inhibitors

NURSING CONSIDERATIONS
Assess:
• I&O ratio: report hematuria, oliguria; nephrotoxicity may occur
◆ Any patient with compromised renal system, toxicity may occur; BUN, creatinine
• Blood studies: CBC
• C&S, drug may be given as soon as culture is taken
• B/P during administration; hypo-, hypertension may occur
• Signs of infection
• Respiratory status: rate, character, wheezing
• Allergies before treatment, reaction of each medication

Administer:
IV route
• After reconstitution with 5 ml 0.9% NaCl (250 mg/5 ml) or 10 ml 0.9% NaCl (500 mg/10 ml), further dilution is needed with 0.9 NaCl, infuse over ½ hr.
Solution compatibilities: 0.9% NaCl, LR
Evaluate:
• Therapeutic response: Negative culture
Teach patient/family:
• Allergies before treatment, reaction of each medication
• All aspects of drug therapy
• To report sore throat, fever, fatigue, could indicate superinfection

desirudin (℞)
(des-i-rude'in)
Iprivask
Func. class.: Anticoagulant
Chem. class.: Thrombin inhibitor

Action: Inhibits thrombin resulting in prolongation of clotting time
Uses: Prophylaxis for deep vein thrombosis in those undergoing hip replacement
Dosage and routes:
• *Adult:* **SC** 15 mg, 1st dose 5-15 min before surgery, but after regional block anesthesia, then 15 mg q12h, up to 12 days
Available forms: Lyophilized powder 15 mg
Side effects/adverse reactions:
SYST: ***Bleeding, hemorrhage***
MISC: Inj site mass, nausea, deep thrombophelibitis, anemia, hypersensivity
Contraindications: Hypersensitivity to natural or synthetic hirudins, active bleeding, irreversible coagulation disorders

Precautions: Pregnancy (C), lactation, children, elderly, hepatic and renal impairment, patients with ↑ risks of hemorrhage

Pharmacokinetics: Metabolized and eliminated by the kidney (40-50% unchanged)

Interactions:

- ↑ anticoagulant effect: thrombolytics, anticoagulants, antiplatelets (salicylates, NSAIDS, ketorolac, triclopidine, sulfinpyrazone, clopidogrel, abciximab)

NURSING CONSIDERATIONS

Assess:

- APTT qd in those with increased risk for bleeding
- ◆ For neurologic changes that may indicate intracranial bleeding
- ◆ Retroperitoneal bleeding: back pain, leg weakness, diminished pulses
- For bleeding: gums, petechiae, ecchymosis, black tarry stool, hematuria; notify prescriber

Administer:

- Alone, do not mix with other drugs or solutions
- For 9-12 days
- Only after screening patient for bleeding disorders
- SC only, do not give IM
- Give to patient recumbent, rotate inj sites (left/right anterolateral, left/right posterolateral abdominal wall)
- Insert whole length of needle into skin fold held with thumb and forefinger
- Give at same time of day to maintain blood level
- Administer only this drug when ordered, not interchangeable with heparin

Perform/provide:

- Bed rest during entire course of treatment
- Avoidance of venous or arterial puncture, inj, rectal temp
- Treatment of fever with acetaminophen

Evaluate:

- Therapeutic response: absence of deep vein thrombosis

Teach patient/family:

- About drug use and expected results; to report adverse reactions; bleeding, bruising
- To avoid all OTC drugs unless prescribed
- To use soft-bristle toothbrush to avoid bleeding gums, to use electric razor

RARELY USED

efalizumab (℞)

(eh-fah-lih′zyoo-mab)

Raptiva

Func. class.: Immunosuppressive

Uses: Adults 18 years of age and older with moderate to severe plaque psoriasis

Dosage and routes:

- *Adult:* **SC** 0.7 mg/kg as a conditioning dose, then **SC** 1 mg/kg qwk, max single dose 200 mg

Contraindications: Hypersensitivity

emtricitabine (℞)

(em-tri-sit′uh-bean)

Emtriva

Func. class.: Antiretroviral

Chem. class.: Nucleoside reverse transcriptase inhibitor (NRTI)

Action: A synthetic nucleoside analog of cytosine. Inhibits replication of HIV virus by competing with the natural substrate and then becoming incorporated into cellular DNA by viral reverse transcriptase, thereby terminating cellular DNA chain.

Uses: HIV-1 infection with other antiretrovirals.

Dosage and routes:

• *Adult:* **PO** 200 mg qd

Renal dose

• *Adult:* **PO** CCr 30-49 ml/min 200 mg q48h; 15-29 ml/min 200 mg q72h; <15 ml/min 200 mg q96h

Available forms: cap 200 mg

Side effects/adverse reactions:

CNS: Headache, abnormal dreams, depression, dizziness, insomnia, neuropathy, paresthesia

GI: Nausea, vomiting, diarrhea, anorexia, abdominal pain, dyspepsia

MS: Arthralgia, myalgia

RESP: Cough

SYST: Change in body fat distribution

INTEG: Rash, skin discolorization

Contraindications: Hypersensitivity

Precautions: Pregnancy (B), lactation, children, elderly, renal disease, hepatic insufficiency, chronic hepatitis B

Pharmacokinetics: Rapidly, extensively absorbed, peak 1-2 hr, protein binding <4%, excreted unchanged in urine (86%), feces (14%); half-life 10 hrs.

Interactions:

None known

NURSING CONSIDERATIONS

Assess:

• Liver, renal function tests: AST, ALT, bilirubin, amylase, lipase, triglycerides periodically during treatment

◆ For lactic acidosis, severe hepatomegaly with steatosis; if lab reports confirm these conditions, discontinue treatment

Administer:

PO route

• Give without regard to meals

Perform/provide:

• Storage at 25° C (77° F)

Evaluate:

• Therapeutic response: ↓ in signs/symptoms of HIV

Teach patient/family:

• That GI complaints resolve after 3-4 wk of treatment

• Not to breastfeed while taking this drug

• That drug must be taken at same time of day to maintain blood level

• That drug will control symptoms, but is not a cure for HIV; patient is still infectious, may pass HIV virus on to others

• That other drugs may be necessary to prevent other infections

• That changes in body fat distribution may occur

enfuvirtide (℞)

(en-fyoo′vir-tide)

Fuzeon

Func. class.: Antiretroviral

Chem. class.: Fusion Inhibitor

Action: Inhibitor of the fusion of HIV-1 with CD4+ cells

Uses: Treatment of HIV-1 infection in combination with other antiretrovirals

Dosage and routes:

• *Adult:* **SC** 90 mg (1 ml) bid

• *6-16 yrs:* **SC** 2 mg/kg bid, max 90 mg bid

Available forms: Powder for inj, lyophilized 108 mg (90 mg/ml when reconstituted)

Side effects/adverse reactions:

GU: ***Glomerulonephritis, renal failure***

CNS: Anxiety, peripheral neuropathy, taste disturbance, ***Gullain-Barré Syndrome,*** insomnia, depression

APPENDIX

HEMA: ***Thrombocytopenia, neutropenia***
GI: Abdominal pain, anorexia, constipation, pancreatitis
INTEG: Inj site reactions
MISC: Influenza, cough, conjunctivitis, lymphadenopathy, myalgis, hyperglycemia, pneumonia
Contraindications: Hypersensitivity
Precautions: Liver disease, pregnancy (B), lactation, children <6 yr, myelosuppression, infections
Pharmacokinetics: Well absorbed, undergoes catabolism, 92% protein binding
Interactions:
• None known
NURSING CONSIDERATIONS
Assess:
• Signs of infection, inj site reactions
• Renal studies: BUN, creatitine, renal failure may occur
• Bowel pattern before, during treatment; if severe abdominal pain or constipation occurs, notify prescriber; monitor hydration
• Skin eruptions, rash, urticaria, itching
• Allergies before treatment, reaction to each medication
• CBC, blood chemistry, plasma HIV RNA, absolute CD4+/CD8+ cell counts/%, serum β_2 microglobulin, serum ICD+24 antigen levels, cholesterol
Administer:
• SC, give bid, rotate sites
Evaluate:
• Therapeutic response: increased CD4 cell counts; decreased viral load; slowing progression of HIV-1 infection
Teach patient/family:
• To notify prescriber if pregnancy is suspected, or if breastfeeding
• That pneumonia may occur, to contact prescriber if cough, fever occur
• That hypersensitive reactions may occur, rash, pruritus; stop drug, contact prescriber
• That this drug is not a cure for HIV-1 infection but controls symptoms, HIV-1 can still be transmitted to others
• This drug is to be used in combination only with other antiretrovirals

epinastine (Elestat)

See Appendix C

fosamprenavir (℞)

(fos-am-pren′a-veer)
Lexiva
Func. class.: Antiretroviral
Chem. class.: Protease inhibitor

Action: A prodrug of amprenavir. Inhibits human immunodeficiency virus (HIV) protease, which prevents maturation of the infectious virus
Uses: HIV-1 infection in combination with antiretrovirals
Dosage and routes:
Therapy-naïve patients
• *Adult:* **PO** 1400 mg bid without ritonavir or fosamprenavir 1400 mg qd and ritonavir 200 mg qd or fosamprenavir 700 mg bid and ritonavir 100 mg bid
Protease experienced patients (PI)
• *Adult:* **PO** 700 mg bid and ritonavir 100 mg bid
Combination with efavirenz
• *Adult:* **PO** Add another 100 mg/day of ritonavir for a total of 300 mg/day when all three drugs are given
Hepatic dose
• *Adult* (Child-Pugh 5-8): **PO** 700 mg bid, do not use in Child-Pugh 9-12

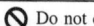

Available forms: Tabs 700 mg (equivalent to 600 mg amprenavir)
Side effects/adverse reactions:
GI: Nausea, diarrhea, vomiting, abdominal pain
INTEG: Rash, pruritus
CNS: Headache, fatigue, depression, oral paresthesia
MISC: Redistribution or accumulation of body fat
Contraindications: Hypersensitivity to protease inhibitors
Precautions: Liver disease, hemolytic anemia, diabetes, sulfa sensitivity, pregnancy (C), lactation, elderly
Pharmacokinetics: A prodrug of amprenavir, peak 1½-4 hrs., 90% protein binding, metabolized in the liver by Cytochrome P450 3AY (CYP3A4), excretion of unchanged drug is minimal
Interactions:
◆ Serious dysrhythmias: amiodarone, calcium channel blockers, lidocaine
• ↓ effect of: oral contraceptives, methadone
• ↑ effect: rifbutin, ketoconazole, itraconazole, sildenafil, vardenafil
• ↓ fosamprenavir levels: nevirapine, antacids, efavirenz, saquinavir, ranitidine
• ↑ toxicity: HMG-CoA reductase inhibitors
• Do not use with pimozide, ergots, midazolam, triazolam, flecainide, propafenone
• May affect coagulation: warfarin
• Avoid use with St. John's wort, rifampin, delavirdine, H2 receptor antagonists, proton-pump inhibitors, carbamazepine, phenobarbital, phenytoin because may lose virologic response and possibly lead to resistance to fosamprenavir

NURSING CONSIDERATIONS
Assess:
• Bowel pattern before, during treatment, monitor hydration
• Skin eruptions, rash, urticaria, itching
• Viral load, CD4 cell counts baseline and throughout treatment
Administer:
• Without regard to food
Teach patient/family:
• To avoid taking with other medications unless directed by provider
• That drug does not cure, but does manage symptoms and does not prevent transmission of HIV to others
• To use nonhormonal form of birth control while taking this drug
• If dose is missed, take as soon as remembered up to 1 hr before next dose, do not double dose
• Not to alter dose or stop therapy without talking to physician
• Advise physician if they have sulfa allergy
• To report all medications including herbal supplements to physician
• That patients receiving phosphodiesterase type 5 inhibitors may be at ↑ risk for PDE5 inhibitor adverse effects

gefitinib (℞)
(ge-fi'tye-nib)
Iressa
Func. class.: Antineoplastic, misc
Chem. class.: Epidermal growth factor receptor inhibitor

Action: Not fully understood. Inhibits intracellular phosphorylation of cell surface receptors associated with epidermal growth factor receptors.
Uses: Nonsmall cell lung cancer (NSCLC)

Dosage and routes:
• *Adult:* **PO** 250 mg qd
CYP3A4 inducers concurrently (such as rifampin or phenytoin)
• *Adult:* **PO** 500 mg qd
Available forms: Tabs 250 mg
Side effects/adverse reactions:
GI: Nausea, diarrhea, vomiting, anorexia, ***pancreatitis,*** mouth ulceration
INTEG: Rash, pruritus, acne, dry skin, ***toxic epidermal neurolysis, angioedema***
RESP: ***Interstitial lung disease,*** cough, dyspnea
MISC: Peripheral edema, amblyopia, conjunctivitis, eye pain, corneal erosion/ulcer
Contraindications: Hypersensitivity, pregnancy (D)
Precautions: Renal, hepatic, ocular, pulmonary disorders, lactation, children, elderly
Pharmacokinetics:
Slowly absorbed, peak 3-7 hrs, excreted in feces (86%), urine (<4%)
Interactions:
• ↑ Gefitinib concentrations: ketoconazole, itraconazole, erythromycin, clarithromycin
• ↓ Gefitinib levels: phenytoin, rifampin, cimetidine, rantidine, sodium bicarbonate
• ↑ plasma concentration of warfarin, metoprolol

NURSING CONSIDERATIONS
Assess:
⬥ Pulmonary changes: lung sounds, cough, dyspnea; interstitial lung disease may occur, my be fatal; discontinue therapy if confirmed
• Ocular changes: eye irritation, corneal erosion/ulcer, aberrant eyelash growth
⬥ Pancreatitis: abdominal pain, levels of amylase, lipase
⬥ Toxic epidermal necrosis, angioedema
• GI symptoms: frequency of stools, if diarrhea is poorly tolerated, therapy may be discontinued for up to 14 days
Administer:
• PO, without regard to food
Evaluate:
• Therapeutic response: ↓ Non-small cell lung cancer cells
Teach patient/family:
• To report adverse reactions immediately: SOB, severe abdominal pain, ocular changes, skin eruptions
• Reason for treatment, expected results
• Use contraception during treatment, pregnancy (D)

gemifloxacin (℞)
(gem-ah-flox'a-sin)
Factive
Func. class.: Antiinfective
Chem. class.: Fluoroquinolone

Action: Inhibits DNA gyrase which is an enzyme involved in replication, transcription and repair of bacterial DNA
Uses: Acute bacterial exacerbation of chronic bronchitis caused by *Streptococcus pneumoniae, Haemophilus influenzae, H. parainfluenzae, Moraxella catarrhalis*; community acquired pneumonia caused by *Streptococcus pneumoniae* including multi-drug resistant strains, *H. influenzae, M. catarrhalis, Mycoplasma pneumoniae, Chlamydia pneumoniae, Klebsiella pneumoniae*
Dosage and routes:
• *Adult:* **PO** 320 mg/day × 5-7 days depending on type of infection
Renal **dose**
• *Adult:* **PO** CCr ≤40 ml/min 160 mg q 24hr
Available forms: Tabs 320 mg

Side effects/adverse reactions:
CNS: Dizziness, headache, somnolence, depression, insomnia, nervousness, confusion, agitation, ***seizures***
GI: Diarrhea, *nausea,* vomiting, anorexia, flatulence, heartburn, dry mouth; increased AST, ALT; constipation, abdominal pain, oral thrush, glossitis, stomatitis, ***pseudomembranous colitis***
INTEG: Rash, pruritus, urticaria, *photosensitivity*
EENT: Visual disturbances
SYST: ***Anaphylaxis, Stevens-Johnson syndrome***
Contraindications: Hypersensitivity to quinolones
Precautions: Hypokalemia, hypomagnesium, pregnancy (C), lactation, children, elderly, renal disease, seizure disorders, excessive exposure to sunlight, psychosis, increased intracranial pressure, history of arrhythmias, history of QT interval prolongation, dysrhythmias
Pharmacokinetics:
PO: Peak 1-2 hr, half-life 6-8 hr; excreted in urine as active drug, metabolites
Interactions:
- ↓ absorption antacids containing aluminum, magnesium, sucralfate, zinc, iron, give 4 hr ac or 2 hr pc
- May ↑ CNS stimulation, seizures: NSAIDs
- May ↑ toxicity of gemifloxacin: cimetidine, probenecid
- ↑ levels: cycloSPORINE, warfarin, watch for toxicity
- May ↓ clearance of theophylline, toxicity may result
- May ↓ effect of antidysrhythmias (amiodarone, bretylusion, procainamide, quinidine, sotalol, disopyramide) result in life-threatening arrhythmias

NURSING CONSIDERATIONS
Assess:
- Kidney, liver function tests: BUN, creatinine, AST, ALT
- I&O ratio; urine pH, <5.5 is ideal
- CNS symptoms: insomnia, vertigo, headache, agitation, confusion

◆ Allergic reactions and anaphylaxis: rash, flushing, urticaria, pruritus, chills, fever, joint pain; may occur a few days after therapy begins; epINEPHrine and resuscitation equipment should be available for anaphylactic reaction
- Bowel pattern qd, if severe diarrhea occurs, drug should be discontinued
- For overgrowth of infection: perineal itching, fever, malaise, redness, pain, swelling, drainage, rash, diarrhea, change in cough, sputum

Administer:
- 4 hr before or 2 hrs after antacids, iron, calcium, zinc products

Evaluate
- Therapeutic response: negative C&S, absence of signs/symptoms of infection

Teach patient/family:
- May take with or without food
- That fluids must be increased to 2 L/day to avoid crystallization in kidneys
- That if dizziness or lightheadedness occurs, to ambulate, perform activities with assistance
- To complete full course of drug therapy
- To contact prescriber if adverse reactions occur
- To avoid iron- or mineral-containing supplements or antacids within 4 hr before and 2 hr after dosing
- That photosensitivity may occur and sunscreen should be used
- To use frequent rinsing of mouth, sugarless candy or gum for dry mouth

• To avoid other medication unless approved by prescriber
• Not to use theophylline with this product, toxicity may result; contact prescriber if taking theophylline

RARELY USED

laronidase (℞)

(lah-rah'nih-daze)
Aldurazyme
Func. class.: Misc. drug

Uses: Mucopolysaccharidosis I (MPSI), patients with Hurler and Hurler-Scheie forms of MPSI
Dosage and routes:
• *Adult:* **IV INF** 0.58 mg/kg qwk. Pretreat with antipyretic and/or antihistamines 1 hr prior to **IV INF**
Contraindications: Hypersensitivity

memantine (℞)

(me-man'teen)
Namenda
Func. class.: Anti-Alzheimer agent
Chem. class.: NMDA receptor antagonist

Action: Antagonist action of CNS NMDA receptors that may contribute to the symptoms of Alzheimer's disease
Uses: Treatment of moderate to severe dementia in Alzheimer's disease
Investigational uses: Vascular dementia
Dosage and routes:
• *Adult:* **PO** 5 mg qd, may increase dose in 5 mg increments ≥1 wk intervals
Available forms: Tabs 5, 10 mg
Side effects/adverse reactions:
CNS: Dizziness, confusion, somnolence, headache, hallucinations
CV: Hypertension
GI: Vomiting, constipation
INTEG: Rash
RESP: Coughing, dyspnea
MISC: Back pain, fatigue, pain
Contraindications: Hypersensitivity
Precautions: Renal disease, GU conditions which raises urine pH, pregnancy (B), lactation, children
Pharmacokinetics: Rapidly absorbed PO, 44% protein binding, very little metabolism, 57%-82% excreted unchanged in urine, terminal elimination half-life 60-80 hr
Interactions:
• May alter levels of both drugs: hydrochlorothiazide, triamterene, cimetidine, quinidine, ranitidine, nicotine
• ↓ clearance of memantine: drugs which makes the urine alkaline (sodium bicarbonate, carbonic anhydrase inhibitors)

NURSING CONSIDERATIONS
Assess:
• B/P: hypertension
• Mental status: affect, mood, behavioral changes; hallucinations, confusion
• GI status: vomiting, constipation, add bulk, increase fluids for constipation
• GU status: urinary frequency
Administer:
• Twice a day if dose >5 mg
• Dosage adjusted to response no more than q1wk
Perform/provide:
• Assistance with ambulation during beginning therapy; dizziness may occur
Evaluate:
• Therapeutic response: decrease in confusion, improved mood

Teach patient/family:
• To report side effects: restlessness, psychosis, visual hallucinations, stupor, loss of consciousness; indicate overdose
• To use drug exactly as prescribed; drug is not a cure

RARELY USED

miglustat (℞)

(mih'glue-stat)
Zavesca
Func. class.: Misc agent

Uses: Adults with mild to moderate type 1 Gaucher disease
Dosage and routes:
• *Adult:* **PO** 100 mg tid, without regard to food
Contraindications: Hypersensitivity, pregnancy (X)

omalizumab (℞)

(oh-mah-lye-zoo'mab)
Xolair
Func. class.: Monoclonal antibody

Action: Recombinant DNA-derived humanized IgG murine monoclonal antibody that selectively binds to IgE to limit the release of mediators in the allergic response
Uses: Moderate to severe persistent asthma
Investigational uses: Seasonal allergic rhinitis
Dosage and routes:
• Adult: **SC** 150-375 mg × 2-4 wks, divide injection into 2 sites, if dose is >150 mg
Available forms: Powder for inj, lyophilized 202.5 mg (150 mg/1.2 ml after reconstitution)

Side effects/adverse reactions:
MISC: Earache, dizziness, fatigue, pain, ***malignancies***, viral infections
RESP: Sinusitis, upper respiratory infections, pharyngitis
INTEG: Pruritus, dermatitis, inj site reactions
MS: Arthralgia, fracture, leg, arm pain
Contraindications: Hypersensitivity
Precautions: Acute attacks of asthma, lactation, children <12 yrs, pregnancy (B)
Pharmacokinetics: Slowly absorbed, peak 7-8 days, half-life 26 days, degradation by liver, excretion in bile
Interactions: None known

NURSING CONSIDERATIONS
Assess:
• Respiratory rate, rhythm, depth; auscultate lung fields bilaterally; notify prescriber of abnormalities
• Allergic reactions: rash, urticaria; drug should be discontinued
Administer:
SC route
• Given q 2-4 wks, product is viscous, if >150 mg is given divide into two sites, the inj may take 5-10 seconds to administer
Evaluate:
• Therapeutic response: ability to breathe more easily
Teach patient/family:
• That improvement will not be immediate
• Not to stop taking or decrease current asthma medications unless instructed by prescriber

APPENDIX

palonosetron (℞)

(pa-lone-o'se-tron)

Aloxi

Func. class.: Antiemetic

Chem. class.: 5-HT_3 receptor antagonist

Action: Prevents nausea, vomiting by blocking serotonin peripherally, centrally, and in the small intestine at the 5-HT_3 receptor

Uses: Prevention of nausea, vomiting associated with cancer chemotherapy

Dosage and routes:

• *Adult:* **IV** 0.25 mg as a single dose over 30 secs, ½ hr prior to chemotherapy

Available forms: Inj 0.25 mg/5 ml

Side effects/adverse reactions:

GI: Diarrhea, constipation, abdominal pain

CNS: Headache, dizziness, drowsiness, fatigue, insomnia

MISC: Weakness, hyperkalemia, anxiety, rash, ***bronchospasm*** (rare), arthralgia, *fever, urinary retention*

Contraindications: Hypersensitivity

Precautions: Pregnancy (B), lactation, children, elderly, prolongation of QT interval or other cardiac conduction intervals (patients with hypokalemia, hypomagnesium, taking diuretics, congenital QT syndrome and those taking antidysrhythmics or other drugs which many prolong QT interval and cumulative high dose antithramycline therapy)

Pharmacokinetics: 62% protein bound; metabolized by liver; unchanged drug and metabolites excreted by kidney; terminal elimination half life: 40 hrs

NURSING CONSIDERATIONS

Assess:

• For absence of nausea, vomiting during chemotherapy

• Hypersensitivity reaction: rash, bronchospasm

Administer:

IV route

• Give as a single dose over 30 secs

• Do not mix with other drugs, flush IV line before and after administration

Perform/provide:

• Storage at room temperature

Evaluate:

• Therapeutic response: absence of nausea, vomiting during cancer chemotherapy

Teach patient/family:

• To report diarrhea, constipation, rash, or changes in respirations or discomfort at insertion site

RARELY USED

pegvisomant (℞)

(peg-vi'soe-mant)

Somavert

Func. class.: Misc agent

Uses: Acromegaly, in those patients who have an inadequate response to other treatment.

Dosage and routes:

• *Adult:* **SC** Loading dose of 40 mg, under supervision of prescriber, then **SC** 10 mg qd, measure IGF-I levels q4-6 wks

Contraindications: Hypersensitivity, latex allergy

rosuvastatin (℞)

(roe-soo'va-sta-tin)
Crestor
Func. class.: Antilipemic
Chem. class.: HMG-CoA reductase inhibitor

Action: Inhibits HMG-CoA reductase enzyme, which reduces cholesterol synthesis
Uses: As an adjunct in primary hypercholesterolemia (types IIa, IIb), and mixed dyslipidemia elevated serum triglycerides, homozygous familial hypercholesterolemia (FH)
Dosage and routes:
(Patient should first be placed on a cholesterol-lowering diet)
Hypercholesterolemia
• *Adult:* **PO** 5-40 mg qd; initial dose 10 mg Q day, reanalyze lipid levels at 2-4 wks and adjust dosage accordingly
Homozygous FH
• *Adult:* **PO** 20 mg qd, max 40 mg
Dose in patients taking cyclosporine
• *Adult:* 5 mg qd
Dose when taken with gemfibrosil:
• *Adult:* 10 mg qd
Available forms: Tabs 5, 10, 20, 40 mg
Side effects/adverse reactions:
GI: Nausea, constipation, abdominal pain, flatus, diarrhea, dyspepsia, heartburn, ***liver dysfunction,*** vomiting
MS: Asthenia, muscle cramps, arthritis, arthralgia, myalgia, ***myositis, rhabdomyolysis,*** leg, shoulder or localized pain
CNS: Headache, dizziness, insomnia, paresthesia
INTEG: Rash, pruritus, photosensitivity
HEMA: ***Thrombocytopenia, hemolytic anemia, leucopenia***
RESP: Rhinitus, sinusitis, *pharygitis,* bronchitis, increased cough
Contraindications: Hypersensitivity, pregnancy (X), lactation, active liver disease
Precautions: Past liver disease, alcoholism, severe acute infections, trauma, hypotension, uncontrolled seizure disorders, severe metabolic disorders, electrolyte imbalances, children, severe renal impairment, elderly, hypothyroidism
Pharmacokinetics:
PO: Peak 3-5 hr, minimal live metabolism (about 10%), 88% protein bound; excreted primarily in feces (90%); crosses placenta; half life 19 hr
Interactions:
• ↑ effects of rosuvastatin: bile acid sequestrants
• ↑ myalgia, myositis: cycloSPORINE, gemfibrozil, niacin, clofibrate, azole antifungals
• ↑ bleeding: warfarin
• Drug/food: Possible toxicity: grapefruit juice
Lab test interferences:
Increase: CPK, LFTs

NURSING CONSIDERATIONS
Assess:
• Diet, obtain diet history including fat, cholesterol in diet
• Fasting cholesterol, LDL, HDL, triglycerides periodically during treatment
• Liver function tests q1-2mo during the first 1½ yr of treatment; AST, ALT, LFTs may increase (AST and ALT are types of LFTs)
• Renal function in patients with compromised renal system: BUN, creatinine, I&O ratio
• Ophthalmic exam before, 1 mo after treatment begins, annually; lens opacities may occur
• For muscle pain, tenderness, obtain CPK; if these occur, drug may need to be discontinued

Administer:
• May be taken at any time of day, with or without food
Perform/provide:
• Storage in cool environment in airtight, light-resistant container
Evaluate:
• Therapeutic response: cholesterol at desired level after 8 wk
Teach patient/family:
• To report suspected pregnancy
• That blood work and ophthalmic exam will be necessary during treatment
• To report blurred vision, severe GI symptoms, dizziness, headache, muscle pain, weakness
• To use sunscreen or stay out of the sun to prevent photosensitivity
• That previously prescribed regimen will continue: low-cholesterol diet, exercise program, smoking cessation

tadalafil (℞)
(tah-dal'a-fil)
Cialis
Func. class.: Impotence agent
Chem. class.: Phosphodiesterase type 5 inhibitor

Action: Inhibits phosphodiesterase type 5 (PDE5); enhances erectile function by increasing the amount of cGMP which causes smooth muscle relaxation and increased blood flow into the corpus cavernosum; improves erectile function for up to 36 hr
Uses: Treatment of erectile dysfunction
Dosage and routes:
• *Adult:* **PO** 10 mg, taken prior to sexual activity, dose may be reduced to 5 mg or increased to a max of 20 mg; usual max dosing frequency is once per day
Renal dose
• *Adult (CCr 31-50 ml/min):* **PO** 5 mg/qd, max 10 mg q 48 hr; CCr <30 ml/min, max 5 mg
Hepatic dose
• *Adult (Child-Pugh class A, B):* **PO** max 10 mg qd; (Child-Pugh class C), not recommended
Concomitant medications
• Ketoconazole, Ritonavir, max 10 mg q 72 hr
Available forms: Tabs 5, 10, 20 mg
Side effects/adverse reactions:
CV: ***MI, sudden death, CV collapse***
CNS: Headache, flushing, dizziness
MISC: Back pain/myalgia, *dyspepsia, nasal congestion, UTI,* blurred vision, changes in color vision, *diarrhea,* pruritus
Contraindications: Hypersensitivity, patients taking organic nitrates either regularly and/or intermittently, patients taking any alpha-adrenergic antagonist other than 0.4 mg once daily tamsulosin
Precautions: Anatomical penile deformities, sickle cell anemia, leukemia, multiple myeloma. Tadalafil is not indicated for use in newborns, children, or women.
Pharmacokinetics: Rapidly absorbed; metabolized by liver; terminal half-life 17.5 hr, peak ½-6 hr; excreted primarily as metabolites feces, urine; plasma concentration 61% in feces, 36% in urine; 94% protein bound; rate and extent of absorption of tadalafil are not influenced by food.
Interactions:
• ↑ tadalafil levels: ketoconazole, ritonavir (although not studied, may also include other HIV protease inhibitors)
◆ Do not use with nitrates because of unsafe drop in B/P which could result in MI or stroke
• ↓ B/P: antihypertensives

NURSING CONSIDERATIONS

Assess:

• Use of organic nitrates that should not be used with this drug

Administer:

PO route

• Give prior to sexual activity; do not use more than once a day

Teach patient/family:

• That drug does not protect against sexually transmitted diseases, including HIV

• To tell physician if patient has a bleeding problem

• That drug should not be used with nitrates in any form

• That drug has no effect in the absence of sexual stimulation

• To seek medical help if an erection lasts more than 4 hours

• To tell physician of all medicines, vitamins, and herbs patient is taking, especially ritonavir, indinavir, ketoconozole, itraconazole, erythromycin, nitrates, alpha-blockers

• That tadalafil is contraindicated for use with alpha-blockers except 0.4 mg/daily tamsulosin

vardenafil (℞)

(var-den′a-fil)

Levitra

Func. class.: Impotence agent

Chem. class.: Phosphodiesterase type 5 inhibitor

Action: Inhibits phosphodiesterase type 5 (PDE5), enhances erectile function by increasing the amount of cGMP which in turn causes smooth muscle relaxation and increased blood flow into the corpus cavernosum

Uses: Treatment of erectile dysfunction

Dosage and routes:

• *Adult:* **PO** 10 mg, taken 1 hr before sexual activity, dose may be reduced to 5 mg or increased to a max of 20 mg; max dosing frequency is once daily

• *Elderly >65 yr:* **PO** 5 mg initially

Hepatic dose (child-Pugh B)

• *Adult:* **PO** 5 mg, max 10 mg

Concomitant medications

• Ritonavir, max 2.5 mg q 72 hr; for indinavir, ketoconazole 400 mg/day and itraconazole 400 mg/day, max 2.5 mg/day; for ketoconazole 200 mg/day, itraconazole 200 mg/day and erythromycin max 5 mg/day

Available forms: Tabs 2.5, 5, 10, 20 mg

Side effects/adverse reactions:

CV: Hypertension, ***MI, CV collapse***

CNS: Headache, flushing, dizziness, insomnia

EENT: Conjunctivitis, tinnitus, photophobia, diminished vision, glaucoma

GU: Abnormal ejaculation, priapism

MS: Myalgia, arthralgia, neck pain

RESP: Rhinitis, sinusitis, dyspnea, pharyngitis, epistaxis

MISC: Rash, GERD, GGTP increased

Contraindications: Hypersensitivity, co-administration of alpha-blockers or nitrates

Precautions: Hepatic impairment, retinis pigmentosa, cardiovascular disease including congenital or acquired QT prolongation, anatomical penile deformities, sickle cell anemia, leukemia, multiple myeloma, pregnancy (B), not indicated for women, children, or newborns

Pharmacokinetics: Rapidly absorbed; bioavailability 15%; protein binding 95%; metabolized by liver; terminal half-life 4-5 hrs, onset 20 min, peak ½-1½ hr, duration <5 hrs, reduced absorption with high-fat meal; primarily excreted in feces (91-95%)

Interactions:

• ↑ vardenafil levels: erythromycin, ketoconazole, intraconazole, cimetadine

• ↓ B/P: NIFEdipine

• Hypotension: alpha-blockers, protease inhibitors, do not use concurrently

Do not use with nitrates because of unsafe ↓ in B/P which could result in MI or stroke

NURSING CONSIDERATIONS

Assess:

• Use of organic nitrates that should not be used with this drug

Administer:

PO route

• Approximately 1 hr before sexual activity, do not use more than once a day

Teach patient/family:

• That drug does not protect against sexually transmitted diseases, including HIV

• That drug absorption is reduced with a high-fat meal

• That drug should not be used with nitrates in any form

• That drug has no effect in the absence of sexual stimulation

• That patient should seek immediate medical attention if erections last for more than 4 hrs

• To inform physician of all medications being taken

Appendix b

Recent FDA drug approvals

Generic name	Trade name	Use
abarelix	Plenaxis	Prostate cancer
bevacizumab	Avastin	Metastatic colorectal carcinoma
botulism immune globulin IV (Human) (BIG-IV)	BabyBIG	Infant botulism
cetuximab	Erbitux	Metastatic colorectal cancer
cinacalet	Sensipar	Parathyroid carcinoma
pemetrexed	Alimta	Mesothelioma
sertaconazole	Ertaczo	*Tinea pedis*
tiotropium	Spiriva	COPD

Appendix c

Ophthalmic, otic, nasal, and topical products

OPHTHALMIC PRODUCTS

α-ADRENERGIC BLOCKER

dapiprazole (℞)
(da-pip′ra-zole)
Rev-Eyes

ANESTHETICS

proparacaine (℞)
(proe-par′a-kane)
Alcaine, Diocane✦, Ophthaine, Ophthestic

tetracaine (℞)
(tet′ra-kane)
Pontocaine, Tetracaine

ANTIHISTAMINES

azelastine (℞)
(ay-zell′ah-steen)
Optivar

emedastine (℞)
(ee-med′ah-steen)
Emadine

epinastine (℞)
(ep-een′as-teen)
Elestat

ketotifen (℞)
(kee-toh-tif′en)
Zaditor

olopatadine (℞)
(oh-loh-pat′ah-deen)
Patanol

ANTIINFECTIVES

bacitracin (℞)
(bass-i-tray′sin)
AK-Tracin, Bacitracin Ophthalmic

chloramphenicol (℞)
(klor-am-fen′i-kole)
AK-Chlor, Chloramphenicol, Chloromycetin Ophthalmic, Chloroptic, Chloroptic S.O.P., Fenicol✦, Isopto Fenical✦, Pentamycin✦

ciprofloxacin (℞)
(sip-ro-floks′a-sin)
Ciloxan

erythromycin (℞)
(er-ith-roe-mye′sin)
Erythromycin, Ilotycin

fomivirsen (℞)
(foh-muh-vir′sun)
Vitravene

ganciclovir (℞)
(gan-sye′kloe-vir)
Vitrasert

gatifloxacin (℞)
(gat-i-flox′a-sin)
Zymar

gentamicin (℞)
(jen-ta-mye′sin)
Garamycin Ophthalmic, Genoptic Ophthalmic, Genoptic S.O.P., Gentacidin, Gentamicin Ophthalmic, Gentak

idoxuridine-IDU (℞)
(eye-dox-yoor'i-deen)
Herplex

levofloxacin (℞)
(lee-voh-floks'a-sin)
Quixin

moxifloxacin (℞)
(mox-i-flox'a-sin)
Vigamox

natamycin (℞)
(nat-a-mye'sin)
Natacyn

norfloxacin (℞)
(nor-floks'a-sin)
Chibroxin

ofloxacin (℞)
(oh-flox'a-sin)
Ocuflox

polymyxin B (℞)
(pol-ee-mix'in)
Polymyxin B Sulfate Sterile

silver nitrate 1% (℞)
silver nitrate

sulfacetamide sodium (℞)
(sul-fa-seet'a-mide)
AK-Sulf, Bleph-10, Bleph-10 S.O.P., Cetamide, Isopto Cetamide, Ocusulf-10, Sodium Sulamyd, Sodium Sulfacetamide, Storzsulf, Sulf-10, Sulster

* **sulfiSOXAZOLE diolamine (℞)**
(sul-fih-sox'ah-zohl)
Gantrisin

tobramycin (℞)
(toe-bra-mye'sin)
AKTob, Defy, Tobrex

trifluridine (℞)
(trye-floor'i-deen)
Viroptic

vidarabine (℞)
(vye-dare'a-been)
Vira-A

β-ADRENERGIC BLOCKERS

betaxolol (℞)
(beh-tax'oh-lole)
Betoptic, Betoptic 5

carteolol (℞)
(kar-tee'oh-lole)
Carteolol HCl, Ocupress

levobetaxolol (℞)
(lee-voh-beh-tax'oh-lole)
Betaxon

levobunolol
(lee-voe-byoo'no-lole)
AKBeta, Betagen

metipranolol (℞)
(met-ee-pran'oh-lole)
OptiPranolol

timolol (℞)
(tye'moe-lole)
Apo-Timop♣, Betimol, Timoptic, Timoptic-XE[3]

CARBONIC ANHYDRASE INHIBITORS

brinzolamide (℞)
(brin-zoh'la-mide)
Azopt

dorzolamide (℞)
(dor-zol'a-mide)
Trusopt

CHOLINERGICS

(Direct-acting)

acetylcholine (℞)
(ah-see-til-koe'leen)
Miochol-E

carbachol (℞)
(kar'ba-kole)
Carbastat, Carboptic, Iosopto Carbachol, Miostat

pilocarpine (℞)
(pye-loe-kar′peen)
Adsorbocarpine, Akarpine, Isopto Carpine, Ocu-Carpine, Ocusert Pilo-20, Ocusert Pilo-40, Pilagan, Pilocar, pilocarpine, Pilopine HS, Piloptic-Y_2, Piloptic-1, Piloptic-2, Piloptic-3, Piloptic-4, Piloptic-6, Pilostat, Pilopto-Carpine

CHOLINESTERASE INHIBITORS

demecarium (℞)
(dem-e-kare′ee-um)
Humorsol

ecothiophate (℞)
(ek-oh-thye′eh-fate)
Phospholine Iodide

CORTICOSTEROIDS

dexamethasone (℞)
(dex-a-meth′a-sone)
AK-Dex, Decadron Phosphate, Dexamethasone Ophthalmic Suspension, Maxidex

fluorometholone (℞)
(flure-oh-meth′oh-lone)
Flarex, Fluor-Op, FML, FML Forte, FML S.O.P.

loteprednol (℞)
(loe-tee-pred′nole)
Alrex, Lotemax

medrysone (℞)
(me′dri-sone)
HMS

***prednisoLONE (℞)**
(pred-niss′oh-lone)
Econopred, Econopred Plus, AK-Pred, Inflamase Forte, Inflamase Mild, Pred-Forte

rimexolone (℞)
(ri-mex′a-lone)
Vexol

MYDRIATICS

atropine (℞)
(a′troe-peen)
Atropine-1, Atropine Care, Atropine Sulfate Ophthalmic, Atropisol, Isopto Atropine

cyclopentolate (℞)
(sye-kloe-pen′toe-late)
AK-Pentolate, Cyclogly, Cyclopentolate HC1

homatropine (℞)
(home-a′troe-peen)
Homatrine HBr, Isopto Homatropine, Minims Homatropine🍁

hydroxyamphetamine HBr (℞)
(hy-drox-ee-am-fet′a-meen)
Paredrine

phenylephrine (OTC)
(fen-ill-ef′rin)
AK-Dilate, AK-Nefrin, Isopto Frin, Neo-Synephrine 2.5%, Neo-Synephrine 10%, phenylephrine HCl, 2.5% Mydfrin, Phenoptic Relief, Prefrin

scopolamine (℞)
(skoe-pol′a-meen)
Isopto Hyoscine

tropicamide
(troe-pik′a-mide)
Mydriacyl, Opticyl, Tropicacyl, Tropicamide

NONSTEROIDAL ANTIINFLAMMATORIES

diclofenac (℞)
(dye-kloe′fen-ak)
Voltaren

flurbiprofen (℞)
(flure-bih-proh'fen)
Ocufen

ketorolac (℞)
(kee-toe'role-ak)
Acular

suprofen (℞)
(soo-proe'fen)
Profenal

SYMPATHOMIMETICS

apraclonidine (℞)
(a-pra-klon'i-deen)
Lopidine

brimonidine (℞)
(brih-moh'nih-deen)
Alphagan, Alphagan P

dipivefrin (℞)
(dye-pi'vef-rin)
Propine, AKPro

* **epINEPHrine/ epinephryl borate (℞)**
(ep-i-nef'rin)
Epifrin, Glaucon/Epinal, Eppy✦

OPHTHALMIC DECONGESTANTS/ VASOCONSTRICTORS

levocabastine (℞)
(lee-voh-cab'ah-steen)
Livostin

lodoxamide
(loe-dox'a-mide)
Alomide

naphazoline (OTC, ℞)
(naf-az'oh-leen)
20/20 Eye Drops Allergy Drops, AK-Con, Albalon, Allerest Eye Drops, Clear Eyes, Clear Eyes ACR, Comfort Eye Drops, Degest 2, Maximum Strength Allergy Drops, Nafazair, naphazoline HCl, Naphcon, Naphcon Forte, Opcon, Vasoclear, Vasocon Regular

oxymetazoline (℞)
(ox-i-meth'oh-lone)
OcuClear, Visine L.R.

tetrahydrozoline (OTC)
(tet-ra-hye-dro'zoe-leen)
Collyrium Fresh, Eyesine, Geneye, Geneye Extra, Mallazine Eye Drops, Murine Plus, Optigene 3, tetrahydrozoline HCl, Tetrasine, Tetrasine Extra, Visine Moisturizing

MISCELLANEOUS OPHTHALMICS

bimatoprost
(by-mat'oh-prahst)
Lumigan

brinzolamide (℞)
(brin-zole'a-mide)
Azopt

dorzolamide (℞)
(dor-zol'a-mide)
Trusopt

ketotifen
(ke-toe-tie'fen)
Zaditor

latanoprost
(la-tan'oh-proest)
Xalatan

travoprost
(trav'oh-prahst)
Travatan

unoprostone (℞)
(un-oh-proe'stone)
Rescula

Pregnancy categories: Demecarium, isoflurophate (X); apraclonidine, cyclopentolate, ecothiophate, glucocorticoids, levobunalol, metipranolol, pilocarpine, proparacaine, suprofen, tetracaine (C); dapiprazole, dipivefrin (B)

β-Adrenergic blockers

Action: Reduces production of aqueous humor by unknown mechanism

Uses: Ocular hypertension, chronic open-angle glaucoma

Anesthetics

Action: Decreases ion permeability by stabilizing neuronal membrane

Uses: Cataract extraction, tonometry, gonioscopy, removal of foreign objects, corneal suture removal, glaucoma surgery (ophth); pruritus, sunburn, toothache, sore throat, cold sores, oral pain, rectal pain and irritation, control of gagging (top)

Antiinfectives

Action: Inhibits folic acid synthesis by preventing PABA use, which is necessary for bacterial growth

Uses: Conjunctivitis, superficial eye infections, corneal ulcers, prophylaxis against infection after removal of foreign matter from the eye

Antiinflammatories

Action: Decreases inflammation, resulting in decreased pain, photophobia, hyperemia, cellular infiltration

Uses: Inflammation of eye, eyelids, conjunctiva, cornea; uveitis, iridocyclitis, allergic conditions, burns, foreign bodies, postoperatively in cataract

Carbonic anhydrase inhibitor

Action: Converted to epINEPHrine, which decreases aqueous production and increases outflow

Uses: Open-angle glaucoma, ocular hypertension

Direct-acting miotic

Action: Acts directly on cholinergic receptor sites; induces miosis, spasm of accommodation, fall in intraocular pressure, caused by stimulation of ciliary, pupillary sphincter muscles, which leads to pulling away of iris from filtration angle, resulting in increased outflow of aqueous humor

Uses: Primary glaucoma, early stages of wide-angle glaucoma (less useful in advanced stages), chronic open-angle glaucoma, acute narrow-angle glaucoma before emergency surgery; also neutralizes mydriatics used during eye exam; may be used alternately with mydriatics to break adhesions between iris and lens

Side effects/adverse reactions:

CNS: Headache

CV: Hypertension, tachycardia, dysrhythmias

EENT: Burning, stinging

GI: Bitter taste

Contraindications: Hypersensitivity

Precautions: Pregnancy, lactation, children, aphakia, hypersensitivity to carbonic anhydrase inhibitors, sulfonamides, thiazide diuretics, ocular inhibitors, hepatic and renal insufficiency

NURSING CONSIDERATIONS

Assess:

- Ophth exams and intraocular pressure readings
- Blood counts; liver, renal function tests and serum electrolytes during long-term treatment

Perform/provide:

- Storage at room temperature away from light

Evaluate:

- Positive therapeutic response
- Absence of increased intraocular pressure

Teach patient/family:

- How to instill drops
- That drug may cause burning, itching, blurring, dryness of eye area

NASAL AGENTS

NASAL DECONGESTANTS

azelastine (℞)
(ay-zell'ah-steen)
Astelin

desoxyephedrine (OTC)
(des-oxy-e-fed'rin)
Vicks Inhaler

* **epHEDrine** (OTC)
(e-fed'rin)
Pretz-D

* **epINEPHrine** (OTC)
(ep-i-neff'rin)
Adrenalin

naphazoline (OTC)
(naff-a-zoe'leen)
Privine

oxymetazoline (OTC)
(ox-i-met-az'oh-leen)
12-Hour Nasal, Afrin 12-Hour Original, Afrin 12-Hour Original Pump Mist, Afrin Severe Congestion with Menthol, Afrin Sinus with Vapornase, Afrin No-Drip 12-Hour, Afrin No-Drip 12-Hour Extra Moisturizing, Dristan, Duramist Plus, Duration, Genasal, Nafrine♣, Nasal Relief, Neo-Synephrine 12 Hour, Nostrilla, oxymetazoline HCl, Nasal Decongestant, Maximum Strength, Vicks Sinex 12-Hour Long-Acting, Vicks Sinex 12-Hour Ultra Fine Mist for Sinus Relief

phenylephrine (OTC)
(fen-ill-eff'rin)
Alconefrin 12, Children's Nostril, Neo-Synephrine, Sinex

propylhexadrine (OTC)
(proe-pil-hex'a-dreen)
Benzedrex Inhaler

tetrahydrozoline (OTC)
(tet-ra-hye-dro'zoe-leen)
Tyzine, Tyzine Pediatric

xylometazoline (OTC)
(zye-loh-meh-tazz'oh-leen)
Natru-vent, Otrivin, Otrivin Pediatric Nasal

NASAL STEROIDS

beclomethasone (℞)
(be-kloe-meth'a-sone)
Beconase AQ Nasal, Beconase Inhalation, Vancenase AQ Nasal, Vancenase Pocket Inhaler

budesonide (℞)
(byoo-des'oh-nide)
Rhinocort, Rhinocort Aqua

flunisolide (℞)
(floo-niss'oh-lide)
Nasalide, Nasarel

fluticasone (℞)
(floo-tic'a-son)
Flonase

mometasone (℞)
(mo-met'a-sone)
Nasonex

triamcinolonex (℞)
(trye-am-sin'oh-lone)
Nasacort, Nasacort AQ

Pregnancy category: C
Action: Produces vasoconstriction (rapid, long acting) of arterioles, thereby decreasing fluid exudation, mucosal engorgement by stimulation of α-adrenergic receptors in vascular smooth muscle
Uses: Nasal congestion
Dosage and routes:
Desoxyephedrine
• *Adult and child >6 yr:* 1-2 **INH** in each nostril q2h or less
EpHEDrine
• *Adult:* Fill dropper to the level

marked, then use in each nostril q4h or less

EpINEPHrine

• *Adult and child >6 yr:* Apply with swab, drops, spray prn

Naphazoline

• *Adult and child >6 yr:* 1-2 drops/spray q6h or less

Oxymetazoline

• *Adult and child >6 yr:* **INSTILL** 2-3 gtt or sprays to each nostril bid

• *Child 2-6 yr:* **INSTILL** 2-3 gtt or sprays 0.025 sol bid, not to exceed 3 days

Phenylephrine

• *Adult and child >12 yr:* 2-3 drops/spray (0.25-0.5) in each nostril q3-4h or less; or 2-3 drops/spray (1%) in each nostril q4h or less

• *Child 6-12 yr:* 2-3 drops/spray (0.25%) in each nostril q3-4h

• *Infant >6 mo:* 1-2 drops (0.16%) in each nostril q3h

Propylhexadrine

• *Adult and child >6 yr:* 1-2 **INH** in each nostril q2h or less

Tetrahydrozoline

• *Adult and child >6 yr:* 2-4 drops (0.1%) q3-4h prn or 3-4 sprays in each nostril q4h prn

• *Child 2-6 yr:* 2-3 drops (0.05%) in each nostril q4-6h prn

Xylometazoline

• *Adult and child >12 yr:* 2-3 drops/spray (0.1%) in each nostril q8-10h

• *Child 2-12 yr:* 2-3 drops (0.05%) in each nostril q8-10h

Available forms: Nasal sol 0.025%, 0.05%

Side effects/adverse reactions:

CNS: Anxiety, restlessness, tremors, weakness, insomnia, dizziness, fever, headache

EENT: Irritation, burning, sneezing, stinging, dryness, rebound congestion

GI: Nausea, vomiting, anorexia

INTEG: Contact dermatitis

Contraindications: Hypersensitivity to sympathomimetic amines

Precautions: Children <6 yr, elderly, diabetes, cardiovascular disease, hypertension, hyperthyroidism, increased intracranial pressure, prostatic hypertrophy, pregnancy (C), glaucoma

NURSING CONSIDERATIONS

Assess:

• For redness, swelling, pain in nasal passages before and during treatment

• For syst absorption; hypertension, tachycardia; notify prescriber; syst absorption occurs at high doses or after prolonged use

Administer:

• Having patient tilt head back, squeeze bulb to create a vacuum, and draw correct amount of sol into dropper; insert 2 gtt of sol into nostril; repeat in other nostril

• Store in light-resistant container; do not expose to high temp or let sol come into contact with aluminum

• For <4 consecutive days

• Environmental humidification to decrease nasal congestion, dryness

Evaluate:

• Therapeutic response: decreased nasal congestion

Teach patient/family:

• That stinging may occur for several applications; drying of mucosa may be decreased by environmental humidification

• To notify prescriber if irregular pulse, insomnia, dizziness, or tremors occur

• Proper administration to avoid syst absorption

• To rinse dropper with very hot water to prevent contamination

TOPICAL GLUCOCORTICOIDS

alclometasone (℞)
(al-kloe-met′a-sone)
Adovate

amcinonide (℞)
(am-sin′oh-nide)
Cyclocort

augmented betamethasone (℞)
(bay-ta-meth′a-sone)
Diprolene, Diprolene AF

betamethasone (℞)
(bay-ta-meth′a-sone)
Alphatrex, Beben♣, Betacort♣, Betatrex, Beta-Val, Bethovate♣, Celestoderm♣, Diprosone, Ectosonel♣, Luxiq, Maxivate, Metaderm♣, Psorion, Valisone

clobetasol (℞)
(kloe-bay′ta-sol)
Cormax, Dermovate♣, Embeline E 0.05%, Temovate

clocortolone (℞)
(kloe-kore′toe-lone)
Cloderm

desonide (℞)
(dess′oh-nide)
Desonide, DesOwen, Tridesilon

desoximetasone (℞)
(dess-ox-i-met′a-sone)
Topicort, Topicort LP

dexamethasone (℞)
(dex-a-meth′a-sone)
Aeroseb-Dex, Decaspray

diflorasone (℞)
(dye-flor′a-sone)
Florone, Maxiflor, Psorcon

fluocinolone (℞)
(floo-oh-sin′oh-lone)
Fluocin, Licon, Lidemol♣, Lidex, Lyderm♣, Topsyn♣, Vasoderm

flurandrenolide (℞)
(flure-an-dren′oh-lide)
Cordran, Cordran SP, Drenison 1/4♣, Drenison Tape♣

fluticasone (℞)
(floo-tik′a-sone)
Cutivate

halcinonide (℞)
(hal-sin′oh-nide)
Halog, Halog-E

halobetasol (℞)
(hal-oh-bay′ta-sol)
Ultravate

hydrocortisone (℞)
(hye-droe-kor′ti-sone)
Actiocort, Aeroseb-HC, Ala-Cort, Allercort, Alphaderm, Anusol HC, Bactine, Barriere-HC♣, Calde-CORT Anti-Itch, Carmol HC, Cetacort, Cortacet♣, Cortaid, Cortate♣, Cort-Dome, Cortef♣, Corticaine, Corticreme♣, Cortifair, Cortizone, Cortoderm♣, Cortril, Delcort, Dermacort, DemiCort, Dermtex HC, Emo-Cort, Epifoam, FoilleCort, Gly-Cort, Gynecort, Hi-Cor, Hycort, Hyderm♣, Hydro-Tex, Hytone, Lacti-Care-HC, Lanacort, Lemoderm, Locoid, My Cort, Novoehydrocort♣, Nutracort Pharm, Pharmacort, Pentacort, Rederm, Rhulicort S-T Cort, Synacort, Sarna HC♣, Texa-Cort, Unicort♣, Westcort

mometasone (℞)
(moe-met′a-sone)
Elocon

prednicarbate (℞)
(pred-ni-kar′bate)
Dermatop

APPENDIX

triamcinolone
(trye-am-sin'oh-lone)
Aristocort, Delta-Tritex, Flutex, Kenac, Kenalog, Kenonel, Triaderm, Trianide✤, Triderm, Trymex

Pregnancy category: C
Action: Antipruritic, antiinflammatory
Uses: Psoriasis, eczema, contact dermatitis, pruritus; usually reserved for severe dermatoses that have not responded to less potent formulation
Dosage and routes:
- *Adult and child:* Apply to affected area

Side effects/adverse reactions:
INTEG: Acne, atrophy, epidermal thinning, purpura, striae
Contraindications: Hypersensitivity, viral infections, fungal infections
Precautions: Pregnancy (C)
NURSING CONSIDERATIONS
Assess:
- Temp; if fever develops, drug should be discontinued
- For systemic absorption, increased temp, inflammation, irritation

Administer:
- Only to affected areas; do not get in eyes
- Leaving site uncovered or lightly covered; occlusive dressing is not recommended—systemic absorption may occur
- Use only on dermatoses; do not use on weeping, denuded, or infected area
- Cleansing before application of drug
- Continuing treatment for a few days after area has cleared
- Store at room temperature

Evaluate:
- Therapeutic response: absence of severe itching, patches on skin, flaking

Teach patient/family:
- To avoid sunlight on affected area, burns may occur
- To limit treatment to 14 days

TOPICAL ANTIFUNGALS

amphotericin B (OTC)
(am-foe-ter'i-sin)
Fungizone
butenafine (℞)
(byoo-tin'a-feen)
Lotrimin Ultra, Mentex
ciclopirox (OTC)
(sye-kloe-peer'ox)
Loprox, Penlac Nail Lacquer
clioquinol (OTC)
(klye-oh-kwin'ole)
Vioforim
clotrimazole (OTC)
(kloe-trye'ma-zole)
Canestew✤, Clotrimaderm✤, Clotrimazole, Cruex, Desenex, Lotrimin AF, Myclo✤, Neozol✤
econazole (OTC)
(ee-kon'a-zole)
Spectazole
haloprogin (OTC)
(hal-oh-proe'jin)
Halotex
ketoconazole (OTC)
(kee-toe-kon'a-zole)
Nizoral
miconazole (OTC)
(mye-kon'a-zole)
Absorbine Antifungal Foot Powder, Breeze Mist Antifungal, Fungoid Tincture, Lotrimin AF, Maximum Strength Desenex Antifungal, Micatin, Monistat-Derm, Onyclear, Tetterine, Zeasorb-AF

naftifine (OTC)
(naff′ti-feen)
Naftin

nystatin (OTC)
(nye-stat′in)
Mycostatin, Nodostine✦, Nilstat, Nyoderm✦, Nystex

oxiconazole (OTC)
(ox-i-kon′a-zole)
Oxistat

selenium (OTC)
(see-leen′ee-um)
Exsel, Head and Shoulders Intensive Treatment, Selenium Sulfide, Selsun, Selsun Blue

terbinafine (OTC)
(ter-bin′a-feen)
Lamisil

tolnaftate (OTC)
(tole-naf′tate)
Absorbine Athlete's Foot Cream, Aftate for Athlete's Foot, Aftate for Jock Itch, Genaspor, Quinsana Plus, Tinactin, Ting, tolnaftate

undecylenic acid (OTC)
(un-deh-sih-len′ik)
Blis-To-Sol, Breeze Mist, Caldesene, Cruex, Decylenes, Desenex, Desenex Maximum Strength, Pedi-Pro, Phicon F, Protectol

Pregnancy category: B
Action: Interferes with fungal cell membrane permeability
Uses: Tinea cruris, tinea pedis, diaper rash, minor skin irritations; amphotericin B is used for *Candida* infections
Dosage and routes:
• Massage into affected area, surrounding area qd or bid, continue for 7-14 days, not to exceed 4 wk

Side effects/adverse reactions:
INTEG: Burning, stinging, dryness, itching, local irritation
Contraindications: Hypersensitivity
Precautions: Pregnancy (B), lactation, children
Interactions: None

NURSING CONSIDERATIONS
Assess:
• Skin for fungal infections; peeling, dryness, itching before and throughout treatment
• For continuing infection; increased size, number of lesions

Administer:
Topical route
• To affected area, surrounding area; do not cover with occlusive dressings
• Store below 30° C (86° F)

Evaluate:
• Therapeutic response: decrease in size, number of lesions

Teach patient/family:
• To apply with glove to prevent further infection; not to cover with occlusive dressings
• That long-term therapy may be needed to clear infection (2 wk-6 mo depending on organism); compliance is needed even after feeling better
• Proper hygiene; hand-washing technique, nail care, use of concomitant top agents if prescribed
• To avoid use of OTC creams, ointments, lotions unless directed by prescriber
• To use medical asepsis (hand washing) before, after each application; to change socks and shoes once a day during treatment of tinea pedis
• To report to health care prescriber if infection persists or recurs; if blisters, burning, oozing, swelling occur
• To avoid alcohol because nausea, vomiting, hypertension may occur

• To use sunscreen or avoid direct sunlight to prevent photosensitivity
• To notify health-care prescriber of sore throat, fever, skin rash, which may indicate overgrowth of organisms

TOPICAL ANTIINFECTIVES

azelaic acid (℞)
(a-zuh-lay′ic)
Azelex, Finacen

bacitracin (OTC)
(bass-i-tray′sin)
Bacitin♣, Bacitracin

clindamycin (℞)
(klin-da-my′sin)
Cleocin T, Clindagel, ClindaMax, Clindets

erythromycin (OTC)
(er-ith-roe-mye′sin)
A/T/S, Akne-Mycin, Eryderm, Erygel, Erythromycin, Staticin, T-Statd

gentamicin (℞)
(jen-ta-mye′sin)
Gentamicin

mafenide (℞)
(ma′fe-nide)
Sulfamylon

metronidazole (℞)
(met-roh-nye′da-zole)
MetroGel, MetroCream, MetroLotion, Noritate

mupirocin (℞)
(myoo-peer′oh-sin)
Bactroban

neomycin (OTC)
(nee-oh-mye′sin)
Neomycin Sulfate

nitrofurazone (℞)
(nye-troe-fyoor′a-zone)
Furacin, Nitrofurazone

***silver sulfADIAZINE** (℞)
(sul-fa-dye′a-zeen)
Flamazine♣, Silvadene, SSD, SSD AF, Thermazene

Pregnancy category: C
Action: Interferes with bacterial protein synthesis
Uses: Skin infections, minor burns, wounds, skin grafts, primary pyodermas, otitis externa
Side effects/adverse reactions:
INTEG: Rash, urticaria, scaling, redness
Contraindications: Hypersensitivity, large areas, burns, ulcerations
Precautions: Pregnancy (C), lactation, impaired renal function, external ear or perforated eardrum

NURSING CONSIDERATIONS
Assess:
• Allergic reaction: burning, stinging, swelling, redness
• For signs of nephrotoxicity or ototoxicity

Administer:
• Enough medication to cover lesions completely
• After cleansing with soap, water before each application; dry well
• To less than 20% of body surface area when patient has impaired renal function

Perform/provide:
• Storage at room temperature in dry place

Evaluate:
• Therapeutic response: decrease in size, number of lesions

TOPICAL ANTIVIRALS

acyclovir (℞)
(ay-sye'kloe-ver)
Zovirax
penciclovir (℞)
(pen-sye'kloe-ver)
Denavir

Pregnancy category: C
Action: Interferes with viral DNA replication
Uses: Simple mucocutaneous herpes simplex, in immunocompromised clients with initial herpes genitalis
Side effects/adverse reactions:
INTEG: Rash, urticaria, stinging, burning, pruritus, vulvitis
Contraindications: Hypersensitivity
Precautions: Pregnancy (C), lactation
NURSING CONSIDERATIONS
Assess:
• Allergic reaction: burning, stinging, swelling, redness, rash, vulvitis, pruritus
Administer:
• Using finger cot or rubber glove to prevent further infection
• Enough medication to cover lesions completely
• After cleansing with soap, water before each application; dry well
Perform/provide:
• Storage at room temperature in dry place
Evaluate:
• Therapeutic response: decrease in size, number of lesions
Teach patient/family:
• Not to use in eyes or when there is no evidence of infection
• To apply with glove to prevent further infection
• To avoid use of OTC creams, ointments, lotions unless directed by prescriber
• To use medical asepsis (hand washing) before, after each application and avoid contact with eyes
• To adhere strictly to prescribed regimen to maximize successful treatment outcome
• To begin taking drug when symptoms arise

TOPICAL ANESTHETICS

benzocaine (OTC)
(ben'zoe-kane)
Americaine Anesthetic, Anbesol Maximum Strength, Baby Anbesol, Biozene, Boil-Ease, Children's Chloraseptic, Dermoplast, Foille, Foille Plus, Hurraccaine, Lanacaine, Medamint, Orabase, Oracin, Ora-Jel
dibucaine (OTC)
(dye'byoo-kane)
Dibucaine, Nupercainal
lidocaine (OTC, ℞)
(lye'doe-kane)
Anestacon, Burn-O-Jel, Derma Flex, Dentipatch, ELA-Max, Lidocaine HCl Topical, Lidocaine Viscous, Numby Stuff, Solarcaine Aloe Extra Burn Relief, Xylocaine, Xylocaine 10% oral, Xylocaine Viscous, Zilactin-L
pramoxine (OTC)
(pra-mox'een)
Itch-X, PrameGel, Prax, Tronothane
tetracaine (OTC, ℞)
(tet'ra-cane)
Pontocaine, Viractin

Pregnancy category: C
Action: Inhibits conduction of nerve impulses from sensory nerves

Uses: Oral irritation, sore throat, toothache, cold sore, canker sore, sunburn, minor cuts, insect bites, pain, itching

Dosage and routes:

• *Adult and child:* **TOP** apply qid as needed; **RECT** insert tid and after each BM

Side effects/adverse reactions:

INTEG: Rash, irritation, sensitization

Contraindications: Hypersensitivity, infants <1 yr, application to large areas

Precautions: Child <6 yr, sepsis, pregnancy (C), denuded skin

NURSING CONSIDERATIONS

Assess:

• Pain: location, duration, characteristics before and after administration

• For infection: redness, drainage, inflammation; this drug should not be used until infection is treated

Perform/provide:

• Storage in tight, light-resistant container; do not freeze, puncture, or incinerate aerosol container

Evaluate:

• Therapeutic response: decreased redness, swelling, pain

Teach patient/family:

• To avoid contact with eyes

• Not to use for prolonged periods: use for <1 wk; if condition remains, prescriber should be contacted

TOPICAL MISCELLANEOUS

docosanol (OTC)
(doe-koe'san-ole)
Abreva

pimecrolimus (℞)
(pim-eh-croh'lim-us)
Elidel

VAGINAL ANTIFUNGALS

butoconazole (OTC)
(byoo-toh-kone'ah-zole)
Femstat-3, Gynazol-1, Mycelex-3

clotrimazole (OTC)
(kloe-trye'ma-zole)
Canesten♣, Clotrimazole, Gyne-Lotrimin 3, Gyne-Lotrimin 7, Mycelex 7, Myclo♣

miconazole (OTC)
(mye-kon'a-zole)
Femizole-M, Monistat, Monistat 3, Monistat 7, Monistat Dual Pak, M-Zole 7 Dual Pack

nystatin (OTC)
(nye-stat'in)
Nystatin

terconazole (OTC)
(ter-kone'ah-zole)
Terazol 7, Terazol 3

tioconazole (OTC)
(tye-oh-kone'ah-zole)
Gyne-Trosyd♣, Monistat 1, Vagistat-1

Pregnancy category: Nystatin (A); clotrimazole (B); butoconazole, terconazole, tioconazole (C)

Action: Interferes with fungal DNA replication; binds sterols in fungal cell membranes, which increases permeability, leaking of nutrients

Uses: Vaginal, vulval, vulvovaginal candidiasis (moniliasis)

Dosage and routes:

Butoconazole

• *Adult:* **VAG** 5 g (1 applicator) hs × 3-6 days

Clotrimazole

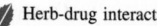

• *Adult:* 100 mg (1 vag tab, 100 mg) hs × 1 wk, or 200 mg (2 vag tab, 100 mg) hs × 3 nights, or 500 mg (1 vag tab, 500 mg); or 5 g (1 applicator) hs × 1-2 wk

Miconazole

• *Adult:* 200 mg supp hs × 3 days or 100 mg supp × 1 wk

Nystatin

• *Adult:* 100,000 units qd × 2 wk

Terconazole

• *Adult:* **VAG** 5 g (1 applicator) hs × 7 days

Tioconazole

• *Adult:* 1 applicator hs × 1 wk

Side effects/adverse reactions:
GU: Vulvovaginal burning, itching, pelvic cramps
INTEG: Rash, urticaria, stinging, burning
MISC: Headache, body pain

Contraindications: Hypersensitivity

Precautions: Children <2 yr, pregnancy, lactation

Interactions: None

NURSING CONSIDERATIONS

Assess:

• For allergic reaction: burning, stinging, itching, discharge, soreness

Administer:

Topical route

• One full applicator every night high into the vagina

• Store at room temperature in dry place

Evaluate:

• Therapeutic outcome: decrease in itching or white discharge (vaginal)

Teach patient/family:

• About asepsis (hand washing) before, after each application

• To apply with applicator only; to avoid use of any other vaginal product unless directed by prescriber; sanitary napkin may prevent soiling of undergarments

• To abstain from sexual intercourse until treatment is completed; reinfection and irritation may occur

• To notify prescriber if symptoms persist

OTIC ANTIINFECTIVES

ofloxacin (℞)

(o-flox'a-sin)

Floxin

Pregnancy category: C

Action: Interferes with conversion of intermediate DNA fragments into high-molecular-weight DNA in bacteria, inhibits DNA gyrase

Uses: Treatment of lower respiratory tract infections (pneumonia, bronchitis), genitourinary infections (prostatitis, UTIs) caused by *Escherichia coli, Klebsiella pneumoniae, Chlamydia trachomatis, Neisseria gonorrhoeae;* skin and skin structure infections; conjunctivitis (ophthalmic)

Dosage and routes:

Renal dose

• *Adult:* **PO** CCr 10-50 ml/min give q24h; CCr <10 ml/min give × of dose q24h

Lower respiratory tract infections/skin and skin structure infections

• *Adult:* **PO, IV** 400 mg q12h × 10 days

Cervicitis, urethritis

• *Adult:* **PO, IV** 300 mg q12h × 7 days

Prostatitis

• *Adult:* **PO, IV** 300 mg q12h × 6 wk

Acute, uncomplicated gonorrhea

• *Adult:* **PO, IV** 400 mg as a single dose

Urinary tract infection

• *Adult:* **PO, IV** 200-400 mg q12h × 3-10 days

Side effects/adverse reactions:
CNS: Dizziness, headache, fatigue, somnolence, depression, insomnia, lethargy, malaise, ***seizures***

EENT: Visual disturbances
GI: Diarrhea, nausea, vomiting, anorexia, flatulence, heartburn, dry mouth, increased AST, ALT, abdominal pain, constipation, ***pseudomembranous colitis***
INTEG: Rash, pruritus
SYST: ***Anaphylaxis, Stevens-Johnson syndrome***

Contraindications: Hypersensitivity to quinolones

Precautions: Pregnancy (C), lactation, children, elderly, renal disease, seizure disorders, excessive sunlight

NURSING CONSIDERATIONS

Assess:

• Renal, hepatic studies: BUN, creatinine, AST, ALT
• I&O ratio; urine pH <5.5 is ideal
• CNS symptoms: insomnia, vertigo, headache, agitation, confusion
• Allergic reactions: rash, flushing, urticaria, pruritus

Administer:

PO route

• 2 hr before or 2 hr after antacids, calcium, iron, zinc products
• After clean-catch urine for C&S

IV route

• Dilute to 4 mg/ml with 0.9% NaCl, D_5W, D_5/LR, D_5/0.9% NaCl, 5% $NaCO_3$, D_5 plasmalyte 56, sodium lactate; give over 1 hr or more

Perform/provide:

• Storage for 2 wk refrigerated or 6 mo frozen after reconstitution

Evaluate:

• Therapeutic response: urine culture, absence of symptoms of infection

Teach patient/family:

• That fluid intake must be 3 L/day to avoid crystallization in kidneys
• That if dizziness or lightheadedness occurs, ambulate, perform activities with assistance
• To complete full course of therapy
• To notify prescriber of adverse reactions or tendon pain
• To avoid iron- or mineral-containing supplements within 2 hr before or after dose
• To prevent sun exposure, photosensitivity can occur

Appendix d

Commonly used antiinfectives in adults and children

amoxicillin

Adult: **PO** 750 mg-1.5 g qd in divided doses q8h
Child: **PO** 20-40 mg/kg/day in divided doses q8h

ampicillin

Adult: **PO** 1-2 g qd in divided doses q6h
IM/IV 2-8 g qd in divided doses q4-6h
Child: **PO** 50-100 mg/kg/day in divided doses q6h
IM/IV 100-200 mg/kg/day in divided doses q6h

cefaclor

Adult: **PO** 250-500 mg q8h
Child: **PO** 24-40 mg/kg/day in divided doses q8h

cephalexin

Adult: **PO** 250-500 mg q6h
Child: **PO** 25-50 mg/kg/day in 4 equal doses

chloramphenicol

Adult and child >3 mo: 50-100 mg/kg/day in divided doses q6h

clindamycin

Adult: **PO** 150-450 mg q6h
IM/IV 300 mg q6-12h
Child >1 mo: **PO** 8-25 mg/kg/day in divided doses q6-8h
IM/IV 15-40 mg/kg/day in divided doses q6-8h

erythromycin

Adult: 250-500 mg q6h
Child: 30-50 mg/kg/day in divided doses q6h

gentamicin

Adult: **IV INF** 3-5 mg/kg/day in divided doses q8h
Child: **IV/IM** 2-2.5 mg/kg q8h
Neonate and infant: **IV/IM** 2.5 mg/kg q8h

kanamycin

Adult and child: **IV INF/IM** 15 mg/kg/day in divided doses q8-12h

methicillin

Adult: **IM/IV** 4-12 g/day in divided doses q4-6h
Child: **IM/IV** 50-300 mg/kg/day in divided doses q4-12h
PO 25-50 mg/kg/day in divided doses q6h
Neonate: **IM** 10 mg/kg q12h

nafcillin

Adult: **PO/IM/IV** 2-6 g/day in divided doses q4-6h

Child: **IM** 25 mg/kg q12h

nitrofurantoin

Adult and child >12 yr: **PO** 50-100 mg qid pc

oxacillin

Adult: **PO** 2-6 g/day in divided doses q4-6h
IM/IV 2-12 g/day in divided doses q4-6h

Child: **PO/IM/IV** 50-100 mg/kg/day in divided doses q6h

penicillin G benzathine

Adult: **IM** 1.2 million units

penicillin G potassium

Adult: **PO** 400,000-500,000 units q6-8h

Child <12 yr: **PO** 25,000-90,000 units/kg/day in 3-6 divided doses

penicillin G procaine

Adult and child: **IM** 600,000-1.2 million units in 1-2 doses/day

Neonate: **IM** 50,000 units/kg qd

sulfisoxazole

Adult: **PO** 2-4 g loading dose, then 1-2 g qid

Child >2 mo: **PO** 75 mg/kg or 2 g/m^2 loading dose, then 150 mg/kg/day or 4 g/m^2/day in divided doses q6h

ticarcillin

Adult: **IV/IM** 12-24 g/day in divided doses q3-6h

Child: **IV/IM** 50-300 mg/kg/day in divided doses q4-8h

Neonate: **IV INF** 75-100 mg/kg q8-12h

Appendix e Vaccines and toxoids

GENERIC NAME	TRADE NAME	USES	DOSAGE AND ROUTES	CONTRAINDICATIONS
BCG vaccine	TICE BCG	TB exposure	Adult/child >1 mo: 0.2-0.3 ml Child <1 mo: Reduce dose by 50% using 2 ml of sterile water after reconstituting	Hypersensitivity, hypogammaglobulinemia, positive TB test, burns
cholera vaccine	No trade name	Immunization for cholera in other countries	Adult/child >10 yr: IM/SC 2× of 0.5 ml, 7-30 days before traveling to cholera areas Booster is used q6mo 0.5 ml prn	Hypersensitivity, acute febrile illness
diphtheria and tetanus toxoids, adsorbed	No trade name	Induces antitoxins to provide immunity to diphtheria and tetanus	Adult/child ≥7 yr: IM (adult strength) 0.5 ml q4-8 wk × 2 doses, then 3rd dose 6-12 mo after 2nd dose, booster IM 0.5 ml q10yr Child 1-6 yr: IM (pediatric strength) 0.5 ml q4wk × 2 doses, booster 6-12 mo after 2nd dose Infant 6 wk-1 yr: IM (pediatric strength) 0.5 ml q4wk × 3 doses, booster 6-12 mo after 3rd dose	Hypersensitivity to mercury, thimerosal; immunocompromised patients; radiation; corticosteroids; acute illness
diphtheria and tetanus toxoids and whole-cell pertussis vaccine (DPT, DTP) diphtheria and tetanus toxoids and acellular pertussis vaccine	DTwP, Tr-Immunol Acel-Imune, DTaP, Tripedia	Prevention of diphtheria, tetanus, pertussis	Adult: booster dose q10yr Child >6 wk-6 yr: IM 0.5 ml at 2, 4, 6 mo, 1½ yr; booster needed 0.5 ml at age 6	Hypersensitivity, active infection, poliomyelitis outbreak, immunosuppression, febrile illness
haemophilus b conjugate vaccine, diphtheria CRM_{197} protein conjugate (HbOC)	HibTITER	Polysaccharide immunization of children 2-6 yr against *H. influenzae* b, conjugate	**HibTITER (IM only)** Child: IM 0.5 ml Child 2-6 mo: 0.5 ml q2mo × 3 inj	Hypersensitivity, febrile illness, active infection

Continued

Appendix e *Vaccines and toxoids—cont'd*

GENERIC NAME	TRADE NAME	USES	DOSAGE AND ROUTES	CONTRAINDICATIONS
haemophilus b conjugate vaccine, meningococcal protein conjugate (PRP-OMP)	PedvaxHIB	Immunization of child 2, 4, 6 mo	Child 7-11 mo: Previously unvaccinated 0.5 ml q2mo inj Child 12-14 mo: Previously unvaccinated 0.5 ml × 1 inj **PedvaxHIB (IM only)** Child 2-14 mo: 0.5 ml × 2 inj at 2, 4 mo of age (6 mo dose not needed), then booster at 12-18 mo against invasive disease Child ≥15 mo: Previously unvaccinated 0.5 ml inj	
hepatitis A vaccine, inactivated	Havrix, Vaqta	Active immunization against hepatitis A virus	Adults: IM 1440 EL units (Havrix) or 50 units (Vagta) as a single dose; booster dose is the same given at 6, 12 mo) Child 2-18 yr: IM 720 EL units (Havrix) or 25 units (Vagta) as a single dose, booster dose is the same given at 6, 12 mo	Hypersensitivity
hepatitis B vaccine, recombinant	Engerix-B, Recombivax HB	Immunization against all subtypes of hepatitis B virus	Varies widely	Hypersensitivity to this vaccine or yeast
influenza virus vaccine, trivalent A and B (whole virus/split virus)	Fluogen, FluShield, Fluviral*, Fluvirin, Fluzone, influenza virus vaccine, trivalent	Prevention of Russian, Chilean, Philippine influenza	Adult/child >12 yr: IM 0.5 ml in 1 dose Child 3-12 yr: IM 0.5 ml, repeat in 1 mo (split) unless 1978-1985 vaccine was given Child 6 mo to 3 yr: IM 0.25 ml, repeat in 1 mo (split) unless 1978-1985 vaccine was given	Hypersensitivity, active infection, chicken egg allergy, Guillain-Barré syndrome, active neurologic disorders
Japanese encephalitis virus vaccine, inactivated	JE-VAX	Active immunity against Japanese encephalitis (JE)	Adult/child ≥3 yr: SC 1 ml, days 0, 7, 30; booster SC 1 ml 2 yr after last dose Child 1-3 yr: SC 0.5 ml, days 0, 7, 30; booster SC 0.5 ml 2 yr after last dose	Hypersensitivity to murine, thimerosal; allergic reactions to previous dose
Lyme disease vaccine (recombinant OspA)	LYMErix	Immunization against Lyme disease	Adult and adolescent 15-70: IM 30 mcg in deltoid, repeat at 1, 12 mo after first dose	Hypersensitivity, antibiotic refractory Lyme arthritis

measles and rubella virus vaccine, live attenuated	M-R-Vax II	Immunity to measles and rubella by antibody production	Adult/child ≥15 mo: SC 0.5 ml (1000 units)	Hypersensitivity, immunocompromised patients, active untreated TB, cancer, blood dyscrasias, radiation, corticosteroids, pregnancy; allergic reactions to neomycin, eggs
measles, mumps, and rubella vaccine, live	M-M-R-II	Prevention of measles, mumps, rubella	Adult: SC 1 vial; 2 vials separated by 1 mo, in person born after 1957 Child >15 mo and adult: SC 0.5 ml	Hypersensitivity, blood dyscrasias, anemia, active infection, immunosuppression; egg, chicken allergy; pregnancy, febrile illness, neomycin allergy, neoplasms
measles virus vaccine, live attenuated	Attenuvax	Immunity to measles by antibody production	Adult/child ≥15 mo: SC 0.5 ml (1000 units), 1 dose 15 mo, 2nd dose age 4-6 or 11, or 12	Hypersensitivity to eggs, neomycin; cancer, radiation, corticosteroids, pregnancy, immunocompromised patients, blood dyscrasias, active untreated TB
meningococcal polysaccharide vaccine	Menomune-A/C/Y/W-135	Prophylaxis to meningococcal meningitis	Adult/child >2 yr: SC 0.5 ml	Hypersensitivity to thimerosal, pregnancy, acute illness
mumps virus vaccine, live	Mumpsvax	Active immunity to mumps	Adult/child ≥1 yr: SC 0.5 ml (20,000 units)	Hypersensitivity to eggs, neomycin; cancer, radiation, corticosteroids, pregnancy, immunocompromised patients, blood dyscrasias, active untreated TB
plague vaccine	No trade name	Active immunity to *Yersinia pestis* plague	Adult: IM 1 ml, then 0.2 ml in 4-12 wk, then 0.2 ml 5-6 mo after 2nd dose; booster 0.1-0.2 ml q6mo when in plague area	Hypersensitivity to phenol, sulfites, formaldehyde, beef, soy, casein; pregnancy, coagulation disorders

*Canada only.

Continued

Appendix e Vaccines and toxoids—cont'd

GENERIC NAME	TRADE NAME	USES	DOSAGE AND ROUTES	CONTRAINDICATIONS
pneumococcal 7-valent conjugate vaccine	Prevnar	Immunity against *Streptococcus pneumoniae*	Child: IM 0.5 ml × 3 doses (7-11 mo); × 2 doses (12-23 mo); × 1 dose >2-9 yr	Hypersensitivity to diphtheria toxoid or this product
pneumococcal vaccine, polyvalent	Pneumovax 23, Pnu-Imune 23	Pneumococcal immunization	Adult/child >2 yr: IM/SC 0.5 ml	Hypersensitivity, Hodgkin's disease, ARDS
poliovirus vaccine, live, oral, trivalent (TOPV) poliovirus vaccine (IPV)	Orimune, IPOL	Prevention of polio	Adult/child >2 yr: PO 0.5 ml, given q8wk × 2 doses, then 0.5 ml ½-1 yr after dose 2 Infant: PO 0.5 ml at 2, 4, 18 mo; booster at 4-6 yr; may also be given: IPV at 2, 4 mo, then TOPV at 12-18 mo, booster at 4-6 yr	Hypersensitivity, active infection, allergy to neomycin/streptomycin, immunosuppression, vomiting, diarrhea
rabies vaccine, adsorbed	No trade name	Active immunity to rabies	**Preexposure** Adult/child: IM 1 ml day 0, 7, 21, or 28 days (total 3 doses); booster IM 1 ml prn q2-5 yr **Postexposure** Adult/child not vaccinated: IM 20 international units/kg of human rabies immune globulin (HRIG), give 5 total doses of 1-ml inj of rabies vaccine on days 0, 3, 7, 14, 28	Severe hypersensitivity to previous inj of vaccine, thimerosol
rabies vaccine, human diploid cell (HDCV)	Imovax Rabies, Imovax Rabies I.D.	Active immunity to rabies	**Preexposure** Adult/child: IM 1 ml day 0, 7, 21 or 28 (total 4 doses) **Postexposure** Adult/child: IM 1 ml on day 0, 3, 7, 14, 28 (total 5 doses)	No contraindications
rubella and mumps virus vaccine, live	Biavax II	Immunity to rubella and mumps by antibody production	Adult/child ≥1 yr: SC 0.5 ml	Hypersensitivity to eggs, neomycin; cancer, radiation, corticosteroids, pregnancy, immunocompromised patients, blood dyscrasias, active untreated TB

rubella virus vaccine, live attenuated (RA 27/3)	Meruvax II	Immunity to rubella by antibody production	Adult/child ≥1 yr: SC 0.5 ml (1000 units)	Hypersensitivity to eggs, neomycin; cancer, radiation, corticosteroids
tetanus toxoid, adsorbed/ tetanus toxoid	No trade name	Tetanus toxoid: used for prophylactic treatment of wounds	Adult/child: IM 0.5 ml q4-6wk × 2 doses, then 0.5 ml 1 yr after dose 2 (adsorbed); SC/IM 0.5 ml q4-8wk × 3 doses, then 0.5 ml ½-1 yr after dose 3, booster dose 0.5 ml q10yr	Hypersensitivity, active infection, poliomyelitis outbreak, immunosuppression
typhoid vaccine, parenteral	No trade name	Active immunity to typhoid fever	Adult: PO 1 cap 1 hr before meals × 4 doses, booster q5yr	Parenteral: systemic or allergic reaction, acute respiratory or other acute infection, intensive physical exercise in high temperatures Oral: hypersensitivity, acute febrile illness, suppressive or antibiotic drugs
typhoid vaccine, oral	Vivotif Berna Vaccine		Adult/child >10 yr: SC 0.5 ml, repeat in 4 wk, booster q3yr Child 6 mo-10 yr: SC 0.25 ml, repeat in 4 wk, booster q3yr	
typhoid Vi polysaccharide vaccine	Typhim Vi	Active immunity to typhoid fever	Adult/child ≥2 yr: IM 0.5 ml as a single dose, reimmunize q2yr 0.5 ml IM, if needed	Hypersensitivity, chronic typhoid carriers
varicella virus vaccine	Varivax	Prevention of varicella-zoster (chickenpox)	Adult/child ≥13 yr: SC 0.5 ml, 2nd dose SC 0.5 ml 4-8 wk later	Hypersensitivity to neomycin; blood dyscrasias, immunosuppression, active untreated TB, acute illness, prenancy, diseases of lymphatic system
yellow fever vaccine	YF-Vax	Active immunity to yellow fever	Adult/child ≥9 mo: SC 0.5 ml deeply, booster q10yr Child 6-9 mo: same as above if exposed	Hypersensitivity to egg or chicken embryo protein, pregnancy, child <6 mo, immunodeficiency

*Canada only.

Appendix f *Antitoxins and antivenins*

GENERIC NAME	TRADE NAME	USE	DOSAGE AND ROUTES	CONTRAINDICATIONS
Black widow spider antivenin *(Lactrodectus mactans)*	No trade name	Black widow spider bite	Adult/child: IM 2.5 ml, 2nd dose may be given if severe; give in anterolateral thigh, obtain test for sensitivity before inj	Hypersensitivity to this product or horse serum
Crotalidae antivenom, polyvalent	No trade name	Rattlesnake bite	Adult/child: IV 20-150 ml depending on seriousness of bite, may give additional doses based on response	Hypersensitivity
Diphtheria antitoxin, equine	No trade name	Diphtheria	Adult/child: IM/slow IV 20,000-120,000 units, may give additional doses after 24 hr	Hypersensitivity
Micrurus fulvius antivenin	No trade name	East/Texas coral snake bite	Adult/child: IV 30-50 ml, give through running IV line of normal saline, give 1st 1-2 ml over 4-5 min, watch for allergic reaction	Hypersensitivity

Appendix g Less frequently used antihistamines

GENERIC NAME	TRADE NAME(S)	USES	DOSAGES AND ROUTES	AVAILABLE FORMS	INTERACTIONS	CONTRAINDICATIONS
acrivastine/ pseudoephedrine (℞)	Semprex-D	• Rhinitis • Allergy symptoms • Chronic idiopathic urticaria	• Adult, child >12 yr: PO 8 mg q4-6h	• Caps 8 mg/60 mg	• Increased CNS depression: alcohol, narcotics, sedatives, hypnotics • Hypertensive crisis: MAOIs (herb) May increase CNS depression: kava (herb) May increase anticholinergic effect: henbane leaf	• Hypersensitivity to this drug or triprolidine • Severe hypertension • Cardiac disease
azatadine (℞)	Optimine	• Allergy symptoms • Rhinitis • Chronic urticaria	• Adult: PO 1-2 mg bid, not to exceed 4 mg/day • Geriatric: PO 1 mg qd-bid	• Tabs 1 mg	• Increased CNS depression: barbiturates, narcotics, hypnotics, tricyclics, alcohol • Decreased effect of: oral anticoagulants • Increased effect of azatadine: MAOIs (herb) Increased CNS depression: kava (herb) Increased anticholinergic effect: henbane leaf	• Hypersensitivity to H_1-receptor antagonists • Acute asthma attack • Lower respiratory tract disease • Child <12 yr
buclizine (℞)	Bucladin-S, Softabs	• Motion sickness • Dizziness • Nausea • Vomiting • Antihistamine	• Adult: PO 25-50 mg prn ½ hr before travel; may be repeated q4-6h prn	• Tabs 50 mg	• Increased anticholinergic effect: henbane leaf (herb) Increased CNS depression: kava	• Hypersensitivity to cyclizines • Shock

KEY: * = Canada only; (herb) = herb/drug interaction

Continued

Appendix g Less frequently used antihistamines—cont'd

GENERIC NAME	TRADE NAME(S)	USES	DOSAGES AND ROUTES	AVAILABLE FORMS	INTERACTIONS	CONTRAINDICATIONS
clemastine (℞)	Contac Allergy 12 Hour, Tavist, Antihist-1	• Allergy symptoms • Rhinitis • Angioedema • Urticaria • Common cold	• Adult and child >12 yr: PO 1.34-2.68 mg bid-tid, not to exceed 8.04 mg/day	• Tabs 1.34, 2.68 mg; Syr 0.67 mg/ml	• Increased CNS depression: barbiturates, opioids, hypnotics, tricyclics, alcohol • Increased effect of clemastine: MAOIs Increased CNS depression: kava Increased anticholinergic effect: henbane leaf	• Hypersensitivity to H_1-receptor antagonists • Acute asthma attack • Lower respiratory tract disease
cyclizine (OTC, ℞)	Marezine	• Motion sickness • Prevention of postoperative vomiting • Antihistamine	*Vomiting* • Adult: IM 25-50 mg ½ hr before termination of surgery, then q4-6h prn (lactate) • Child: IM 3 mg/kg divided in 3 equal doses *Motion sickness* • Adult: PO 50 mg then q4-6h prn, not to exceed 200 mg/day (HCl) • Child: PO 25 mg q4-6h prn	• Tabs 50 mg • Inj 50 mg/ml	• May increase CNS effect: alcohol, tranquilizers, opioids Increased CNS depression: kava	• Hypersensitivity to cyclizines • Shock
dexchlorpheniramine (℞)	Dexchlor, dexclorpheniramine maleate, Poladex, Polaramine	• Allergy symptoms • Rhinitis • Pruritus • Contact dermatitis	• Adult: PO 1-2 mg tid-qid; repeat action 4-6 mg bid-tid • Child 6-11 yr: PO 1 mg q4-6h, or time rel 4 mg hs	• Tabs 2 mg • Repeat action tabs 4, 6 mg • Syr 2 mg/5 ml	• Increased CNS depression: barbiturates, opioids, hypnotics, tricyclics, alcohol • Decreased effect: oral	• Hypersensitivity to H_1-receptor antagonists • Acute asthma attack • Lower respiratory tract disease

			• Child 2-5 yr: PO 0.5 mg q4-6h; do not use repeat action form		anticoagulants, heparin • Increased effect of dexchlorpheniramine: MAOIs (herb) Increased anticholinergic effect: henbane leaf	
trimeprazine (℞)	Panectyl*, Temaril	• Pruritus	• Adult: PO 2.5 mg qid; time-rel 5 mg bid • Geriatric: PO 2.5 mg bid • Child 3-12 yr: PO 2.5 mg tid or hs • Child 6 mo-1 yr: PO 1.25 mg tid or hs	• Tabs 2.5 mg • Time-rel spanules 5 mg • Syr 2.5 mg/5 ml	• Increased CNS depression: barbiturates, opioids, hypnotics, tricyclics, alcohol • Decreased effect of oral anticoagulants, heparin • Increased effect of trimeprazine: MAOIs (herb) Increased anticholinergic effect: henbane leaf	• Hypersensitivity to H_1-receptor antagonists • Acute asthma attack • Lower respiratory tract disease
tripelennamine (℞)	PBZ, PBZ-SR, Pelamine, tripelennamine HC1	• Rhinitis • Allergy symptoms	• Adults: PO 25-50 mg q4-6h, not to exceed 600 mg/day; time-rel 100 mg bid-tid, not to exceed 600 mg/day • Child >5 yr: PO time-rel 50 mg q8-12h, not to exceed 300 mg/day • Child <5 yr: PO 5 mg/kg/day in 4-6 divided doses, not to exceed 300 mg/day	• Tabs 25, 50 mg • Time-rel tabs 100 mg • Elix 37.5 mg/5 ml	• Increased CNS depression: barbiturates, opioids, hypnotics, tricyclics, alcohol • Decreased effect of oral anticoagulants, heparin • Increased effect of tripelennamine: MAOIs (herb) Increased anticholinergic effect: henbane leaf	• Hypersensitivity to H_1-receptor antagonists • Acute asthma attack • Lower respiratory tract disease

KEY: * = Canada only; (herb) = herb/drug interaction

Appendix h

Herbal products

agrimony

Uses: Mild diarrhea, gastroenteritis, intestinal mucous secretion, inflammation of the mouth and throat, cuts and scrapes, amenorrhea

alfalfa

Uses: Poor appetite, hay fever and asthma, high cholesterol, nutrient source

aloe

Uses of aloe vera gel:
- *External:* Minor burns, skin irritations, minor wounds, frostbite, radiation-caused injuries
- *Internal:* To heal intestinal inflammation and ulcers, as a digestive aid to stimulate bile secretion

angelica

Uses: Heartburn, indigestion, gas, colic, poor blood flow to the extremities, bronchitis, poor appetite, psoriasis, vitiligo, as an antiseptic

arnica

Uses: Topical application for muscle and joint inflammation and swelling; in homeopathic preparations as a remedy for shock, injury, pain

astragalus

Uses: Immune stimulant, viral infections, HIV/AIDS, cancer, vascular disorders, improve circulation, lower blood pressure, possible efficacy in myasthenia gravis

bilberry

Uses: Diabetic retinopathy, macular degeneration, glaucoma, cataract, capillary fragility, varicose veins, hemorrhoids, mild diarrhea

black cohosh

Uses:
- *Menopause:* Hot flashes, nervous conditions associated with menopause
- *Dysmenorrhea:* Menstrual cramps, pain, inflammation

Adapted from: Debusk, Ruth, and Treadwell, Phillip. *Serious Drug/Herb Interactions.* Skidmore-Roth Publishing, Inc. 1999.

black haw (cramp bark)

Uses: Dysmenorrhea, menstrual cramps and pain, menopausal metrorrhagia, hysteria, asthma, lower blood pressure, heart palpitations

blessed thistle

Uses: Loss of appetite, indigestion, intestinal gas

blue cohosh

Uses: Menopausal symptoms, uterine and ovarian pain, improve flow of menstrual blood, antiinflammatory, antirheumatic, popular remedy in black ethnic medicine

borage

Uses: Antiinflammatory for premenstrual syndrome, rheumatoid arthritis, Raynaud's disease, other inflammatory conditions, atopic dermatitis, infant cradle cap, cystic fibrosis, high blood pressure, diabetes

burdock root

Uses: Skin diseases, inflammation, rashes, cold and fever, cancer, gout, arthritis

calendula

Uses:
- *External:* Minor skin ailments
- *Internal:* Inflammation throughout the gastrointestinal tract, toxic liver and gallbladder, menstrual bleeding and pain, yeast infections

capsicum (cayenne)

Uses: Muscle spasms, pain of inflammation, neuromas, psoriasis, dry mouth, as an antioxidant food, as a food seasoning

cascara

Uses: Chronic constipation, hepatitis, gallstones

cat's claw

Uses: Cancer, herpes, HIV/AIDS, rheumatoid arthritis, gastritis, gout, wounds, gastric ulcers

chamomile

Uses:
- *External:* As an antiseptic and soothing agent for inflamed skin and minor wounds
- *Internal:* As an antispasmodic, gas-relieving, and antiinflammatory agent for the treatment of digestive problems; light sleep aid and sedative for adults and children; possible anticancer agent

chaparral

Uses: Not recommended—potentially toxic to the liver and kidneys

chicory

Uses: Coffee substitute, source of fructo-oligosaccharides, mild laxative for children, gout, rheumatism, loss of appetite, digestive distress

comfrey

Uses: Bruises, sprains, broken bones, acne, boils

cranberry

Uses: Urinary tract infections (UTIs); susceptibility to kidney stones

dong quai

Uses: To restore vitality to tired women; for a variety of gynecologic, menstrual, and menopausal symptoms; cirrhosis of the liver

echinacea

Uses: Low immune status, hard-to-heal superficial wounds, sun protection

elder (elderberry)

Uses: Susceptibility to colds, flu, yeast infections; nasal and chest congestion; earache associated with chronic congestion; hay fever

eleuthero (See siberian ginseng)

evening primrose

Uses: Premenstrual syndrome, arthritis and inflammatory disorders in general, dry skin, eczema, asthma, diabetes, migraines, chronic fatigue syndrome, heart disease and stroke, circulatory disorders, Raynaud's disease, NSAID use, multiple sclerosis

fenugreek

Uses: Loss of appetite, inflamed areas of the skin, water retention, cancer, constipation, diarrhea, high cholesterol, high blood sugar, calcium oxalate stones

feverfew

Uses: Migraines, cluster headaches, fever, psoriasis, inflammation

flaxseed

Uses: Constipation, as a source of omega-3 fatty acids

fo-ti

Uses: Tiredness, constipation, elevated cholesterol

garcinia cambogia

Uses: Appetite control, weight loss, high cholesterol

garlic

Uses: Vascular disease, elevated LDL, elevated triglycerides, low HDL, high blood pressure, poor circulation, risk of cancer, inflammatory disorders, childhood ear infection, yeast infection

ginger

Uses: Nausea, motion sickness, indigestion, inflammation

ginkgo

Uses: Poor circulation; age-related decline in cognition, memory; diabetes; vascular disease; cancer; inflammatory disorders; impotence; degenerative nerve conditions

ginseng

Uses: Physical and mental exhaustion, stress, viral infections, diabetes, sluggishness, fatigue, weak immunity, convalescence

goldenseal

Uses: High blood pressure, poor appetite, infections, menstrual problems, minor sciatic pain, muscle spasms, eye washes

gotu kola

Uses: Chronic wounds, psoriasis

grape seed

Uses: Antioxidant, chronic disease prevention, inflammation

green tea

Uses: Cancer prevention, heart disease prevention, hypercholesterolemia, diarrhea

guggul

Uses: High LDL cholesterol, elevated triglycerides, weight loss

gymnema sylvestre

Uses: High blood sugar levels

hawthorn

Uses: Poor circulation, chest pain, irregular heartbeat, high blood fats, high blood pressure

hops

Uses: Mild sedative, diuretic, weak antibiotic, insomnia, hyperactivity, pain, fever, jaundice, improve appetite

horse chestnut

Uses: Fever, fluid retention, frostbite, hemorrhoids, inflammation, lower extremity swelling, phlebitis, varicose veins, wounds

horsetail

Uses: Diuretic, genitourinary astringent, antihemorrhagic, Bell's palsy, healing broken bones

kava

Uses: Nervous anxiety, restlessness, sleep disturbances, stress

khat

Uses: Obesity, gastric ulcers, stimulant

kombucha

Uses: Numerous claims for a wide variety of ills; none has been substantiated to date

konjac

Uses: Blood sugar control, constipation, high blood fats, high blood pressure, excessive appetite

kudzu

Uses: Alcohol cravings, menopausal symptoms

lapacho (pau d'arco)

Uses: Cancer, inflammation, infection

lemon balm (melissa)

Uses: Abdominal gas and cramping, cold sores

licorice

Uses: Allergies, arthritis, asthma, constipation, esophagitis, gastritis, hepatitis, inflammatory conditions, peptic ulcers, poor adrenal function, poor appetite

maitake

Uses: Immunostimulant activity, diabetes, hypertension, high cholesterol, obesity

maté

Uses: Diuretic, depurative

melatonin

Uses: Jet lag, insomnia, cancer protection, oral contraceptive

milk thistle

Uses: Protection for alcoholic cirrhosis and hepatitis, antiinflammatory

monascus

Uses: Maintaining acceptable cholesterol levels

morinda

Uses: Headache, digestive, heart and liver conditions, arthritis

nettle

Uses: Diuretic, hay fever

octacosanol

Uses: Herpes, inflammation of the skin, physical endurance

passionflower

Uses: Antifungal, hypertension, sedative, group A hemolytic streptococcus

peppermint

Uses: GI disorders

pygeum

Uses: Benign prostate hypertrophy, antiinflammatory

raspberry leaves

Uses: Facilitation of childbirth, dysmenorrhea, uterine tonic, fever, vomiting

red clover

Uses: Antispasmodic, expectorant, sedative, psoriasis, eczema, amenorrhea

rose hips

Uses: Source of vit C, cold, fever, mild infections

st. john's wort

Uses: Depression, antiviral

sarsaparilla

Uses: Antiinflammatory, antiseptic, syphilis, skin diseases, rheumatism, necrosis, mercury poisoning

sassafras

Uses: Banned in the United States

saw palmetto

Uses: Benign prostatic hypertrophy

schisandra

Uses: GI disorders, liver protection, tonic

scull cap

Uses: Antibacterial, sedative

senna

Uses: Laxative

siberian ginseng (eleuthero)

Uses: Improve appetite, memory loss, hypertension, insomnia, rheumatism, improve circulation, heart ailments, diabetes, headache

tea tree oil

Uses: Topical use for infections; inhaled for respiratory disorders

uva ursi

Uses: Diuretic, urinary tract infections, contact dermatitis, arthritis

valerian

Uses: Sedative

vitex

Uses: Premenstrual and menstrual disorders, spasms, estrogen gestagen imbalance

yarrow

Uses: To decrease bleeding, GI disorders, hypertension, thrombi, to improve circulation

yohimbe

Uses: Male organic impotence

APPENDIX

Appendix i

Combination products

A-200 Shampoo:
0.33% pyrethrins
4% piperonyl butoxide
Uses: Scabicide, pediculicide

Accuretic 10/12.5:
quinapril 10 mg
hydrochlorthiazide 12.5 mg
Uses: Antihypertensive

Accuretic 20/12.5:
quinapril 20 mg
hydrochlorthiazide 12.5 mg
Uses: Antihypertensive

Accuretic 20/25:
quinapril 20 mg
hydrochlorthiazide 25 mg
Uses: Antihypertensive

Aceta w/Codeine:
acetaminophen 300 mg
codeine 30 mg
Uses: Opioid analgesic

Acid-X:
acetaminophen 500 mg
calcium carbonate 250 mg
Uses: Analgesic, antacid

Actagen C Cough Syrup:
Per 5 ml:
triprolidine 1.25 mg
pseudoephrine 30 mg
codeine 10 mg
Uses: Antihistamine, adrenergic, antitussive

Actagen Tablets:
triprolidine 2.5 mg
pseudoephedrine 60 mg
Uses: Antihistamine, adrenergic

Actifed:
pseudoephedrine 60 mg
triprolidine 2.5 mg
Uses: Decongestant

Actifed Allergy, Daytime:
pseudoephedrine 30 mg
Uses: Adrenergic

Actifed Allergy, Nighttime:
pseudoephedrine 30 mg
diphenhydrAMINE 25 mg
Uses: Decongestant, antihistamine

Actifed with Codeine:
pseudoephedrine 30 mg
triprolidine 1.25 mg
codeine 10 mg
Uses: Adrenergic, antihistamine, antitussive

Actifed with Codeine Cough Syrup:
Per 3 ml:
pseudoephedrine 30 mg
triprolidine 1.25 mg
codeine 10 mg
Uses: Adrenergic, antihistamine, antitussive

Actifed Cold and Allergy:
pseudoephedrine 60 mg
triprolidine 2.5 mg
Uses: Adrenergic, antihistamine

Actifed Cold and Sinus:
chlorpheniramine 2 mg
pseudoephedrine 30 mg
acetaminophen 500 mg
Uses: antihistamine, adrenergic, analgesic

Actifed Plus:
pseudoephedrine 30 mg
triprolidine 1.25 mg
acetaminophen 500 mg
Uses: Decongestant, antihistamine

Actifed Plus ES Caplets:
pseudoephedrine 60 mg
triprolidine 2.5 mg

acetaminophen 500 mg
Uses: Adrenergic, antihistamine, analgesic

Actifed Sinus Daytime:
pseudoephedrine 30 mg
acetaminophen 500 mg
Uses: Decongestant

Actifed Sinus Nighttime:
pseudoephedrine 30 mg
diphenhydrAMINE 25 mg
acetaminophen 500 mg
Uses: Decongestant, antihistamine

Actifed Syrup:
Per 5 ml:
triprolidine 1.25 mg
pseudoephedrine 30 mg
Uses: Antihistamine, adrenergic

Activella Tablets:
estriol 1 mg
norethindrone 0.5 mg
Uses: Menopause

Adderall 5 mg:
dextroamphetamine sulfate 1.25 mg
dextroamphetamine saccharate 1.25 mg
amphetamine sulfate 1.25 mg
amphetamine aspartate 1.25 mg
Uses: CNS stimulant

Adderall 10 mg:
dextroamphetamine sulfate 5 mg
dextroamphetamine saccharate 2.5 mg
amphetamine sulfate 2.5 mg
amphetamine aspartate 2.5 mg
Uses: CNS stimulant

Adderall 20 mg:
dextroamphetamine sulfate 5 mg
dextroamphetamine saccharate 5 mg
amphetamine sulfate 5 mg
amphetamine aspartate 5 mg
Uses: CNS stimulant

Adderall 30 mg:
dextroamphetamine sulfate 7.5 mg
dextroamphetamine saccharate 7.5 mg
amphetamine sulfate 7.5 mg
amphetamine aspartate 7.5 mg
Uses: CNS stimulant

Adderall XR 10 mg:
dextroamphetamine sulfate 2.5 mg
dextroamphetamine saccharate 2.5 mg
amphetamine sulfate 2.5 mg
amphetamine aspartate 2.5 mg
Uses: CNS stimulant

Adderall XR 20 mg:
dextroamphetamine sulfate 5 mg
dextroamphetamine saccharate 5 mg
amphetamine sulfate 5 mg
amphetamine aspartate 5 mg
Uses: CNS stimulant

Adderall XR 30 mg:
dextroamphetamine sulfate 7.5 mg
dextroamphetamine saccharate 7.5 mg
amphetamine sulfate 7.5 mg
amphetamine aspartate 7.5 mg
Uses: CNS stimulant

Advair Diskus 100:
fluticasone 100 mcg
salmetrol 50 mcg
Uses: Corticosteroid, bronchodilator

Advair Diskus 250:
fluticasone 250 mcg
salmetrol 50 mcg
Uses: Corticosteroid, bronchodilator

Advair Diskus 500:
fluticasone 500 mcg
salmetrol 50 mcg
Uses: Corticosteroid, bronchodilator

Advicor 500:
niacin 500 mg
lovastatin 20 mg
Uses: Antilipidemic

Advicor 750:
niacin 750 mg
lovastatin 20 mg
Uses: Antilipidemic

Advicor 1000:
niacin 1000 mg

lovastatin 20 mg
Uses: Antilipidemic

Advil Cold & Sinus Caplets:
pseudoephedrine 30 mg
ibuprofen 200 mg
Uses: Decongestant

Aggrenox:
200 mg ext rel dipyridamole
25 mg aspirin
Uses: Antiplatelet

AK-Cide Ophthalmic Suspension/ Ointment:
10% sulfacetamide sodium
0.5% prednisoLONE acetate
Uses: Ophth antiinfective, antiinflammatory

Aldactazide 25/25:
spironolactone 25 mg
hydrochlorothiazide 25 mg
Uses: Diuretic

Aldactazide 50/50:
spironolactone 50 mg
hydrochlorothiazide 50 mg
Uses: Diuretic

Aldoclor-150:
methyldopa 250 mg
chlorothiazide 150 mg
Uses: Antihypertensive

Aldoclor-250:
methyldopa 250 mg
chlorothiazide 250 mg
Uses: Antihypertensive

Aldori 15:
methyldopa 250 mg
hydrochlorothiazide 15 mg
Uses: Antihypertensive

Aldoril 25:
methyldopa 250 mg
hydrochlorothiazide 25 mg
Uses: Antihypertensive

Aldoril D30
hydrochlorothiazide 30 mg
methyldopa 500 mg
Uses: Antihypertensive

Aldoril D50:
hydrochlorothiazide 50 mg
methyldopa 500 mg
Uses: Antihypertensive

Aleve Cold & Sinus:
naproxen 200 mg
ER pseudoephedrine 120 mg
Uses: Analgesic, adrenergic

Alka-Seltzer Effervescent, Original:
sodium bicarbonate 1916 mg
citric acid 1000 mg
aspirin 325 mg
Uses: Antacid, adsorbent, antiflatulent

Alka-Seltzer Cold:
sodium bicarbonate 958 mg
citric acid 832 mg
potassium bicarbonate 312 mg
Uses: Antacid, adsorbent

Alka-Seltzer Plus Cold & Cough Liqui-Gels:
pseudoephedrine 30 mg
chlorpheniramine 2 mg
dextromethorphan 10 mg
acetaminophen 250 mg
Uses: Antitussive, decongestant

Alka-Seltzer Plus Cold Liqui-Gels:
pseudoephedrine 30 mg
chlorpheniramine 2 mg
acetaminophen 250 mg
Uses: Decongestant, antihistamine

Alka-Seltzer Plus Night-Time Cold Liqui-Gels:
doxylamine 6.25 mg
dextromethorphan 10 mg
pseudoephedrine 30 mg
acetaminophen 250 mg
Uses: Antitussive, decongestant

Allegra-D:
fexofenadine 60 mg
pseudoephedrine 120 mg
Uses: Antihistamine, adrenergic

Allercon Tablets:
triprolidine 2.5 mg
pseudoephedrine 60 mg
Uses: Antihistamine, adrenergic

Allerest Headache Strength Advanced Formula:
pseudoephedrine 30 mg
chlorpheniramine 2 mg
acetaminophen 325 mg
Uses: Decongestant, antihistamine
Allerest Maximum Strength Tablets:
pseudoephedrine 30 mg
chlorpheniramine 2 mg
Uses: Decongestant, antihistamine
Allerest No-Drowsiness:
pseudoephedrine 30 mg
acetaminophen 325 mg
Uses: Decongestant, analgesic
Allerest Sinus Pain Formula:
pseudoephedrine 30 mg
chlorpheniramine 2 mg
acetaminophen 500 mg
Uses: Decongestant, antihistamine, analgesic
Allerfrim Syrup:
Per 5 ml:
triprolidine 1.25 mg
pseudoephrine 30 mg
Uses: Antihistamine, adrenergic
Allerfrim Tablets:
triprolidine 2.5 mg
pseudoephrine 60 mg
Uses: Antihistamine, adrenergic
All-Nite Cold Formula Liquid:
Per 5 ml:
pseudoephedrine 10 mg
doxylamine 1.25 mg
dextromethorphan 5 mg
acetaminophen 167 mg
Uses: Decongestant, antihistamine, analgesic
Alor 5/500:
hydrocodone 5 mg
aspirin 500 mg
Uses: Analgesic
Amaphen:
acetaminophen 325 mg
butalbital 50 mg
caffeine 40 mg
Uses: Analgesic, barbiturates
Ambenyl Cough Syrup:
Per 5 ml:
bromodiphenhydramine 12.5 mg
codeine 10 mg
5% alcohol
Uses: Antihistamine, opioid analgesic
Anacin:
aspirin 400 mg
caffeine 32 mg
Uses: Analgesic
Anacin Maximum Strength:
aspirin 500 mg
caffeine 32 mg
Uses: Analgesic
Anacin PM (Aspirin Free):
diphenhydrAMINE 25 mg
acetaminophen 500 mg
Uses: Analgesic
Anacin w/Codeine:
aspirin 325 mg
codeine 8 mg
caffeine 32 mg
Uses: Opioid analgesic
Anaplex HD Syrup:
Per 5 ml:
hydrocodone 1.7 mg
phenylephrine 5 mg
chlorpheniramine 2 mg
Uses: Analgesic, adrenergic, antihistamine
Anaplex Liquid:
Per 5 ml:
chlorpheniramine 2 mg
pseudoephedrine 30 mg
Uses: Antihistamine, decongestant
Anatuss LA:
pseudoephedrine 120 mg
guaifenesin 400 mg
Uses: Adrenergic, expectorant
Anexsia 5/500:
hydrocodone 5 mg
acetaminophen 500 mg
Uses: Analgesic

Anexsia 7.5/650:
hydrocodone 7.5 mg
acetaminophen 650 mg
Uses: Analgesic

Apresazide 25/25:
hydrALAZINE 25 mg
hydrochlorothiazide 25 mg
Uses: Antihypertensive

Apresazide 50/50:
hydrALAZINE 50 mg
hydrochlorothiazide 50 mg
Uses: Antihypertensive

Apri:
desorgestrel 0.15 mg
ethinyl estradiol 30 mcg
Uses: Estrogen, progestin

Arthritis Pain Formula:
aspirin 500 mg
aluminum hydroxide 27 mg
magnesium hydroxide 100 mg
Uses: Analgesic, antacid

Arthrotec:
diclofenac 50 or 75 mg
misoprostol 200 mcg
Uses: NSAID, gastric protectant

Ascriptin:
aspirin 325 mg
magnesium hydroxide 50 mg
aluminum hydroxide 50 mg
calcium carbonate 50 mg
Uses: Nonopioid analgesic, antipyretic

Ascriptin A/D:
aspirin 325 mg
aluminum hydroxide 75 mg
magnesium hydroxide 75 mg
calcium carbonate 75 mg
Uses: Analgesic

Aspirin-Free Bayer Select Allergy Sinus:
pseudoephedrine 30 mg
chlorpheniramine 2 mg
acetaminophen 500 mg
Uses: Adrenergic, antihistamine, analgesic

Aspirin Free Excedrin:
acetaminophen 500 mg
caffeine 65 mg
Uses: Analgesic

Aspirin Free Excedrin Dual:
acetaminophen 500 mg
calcium carbonate 111 mg
magnesium carbonate 64 mg
magnesium oxide 30 mg
Uses: Analgesic, antacid

Atacand HCT 16:
candesartan 16 mg
hydrochlorthiazide 12.5 mg
Uses: Antihypertensive

Atacand HCT 32:
candesartan 32 mg
hydrochlorthiazide 12.5 mg
Uses: Antihypertensive

Augmentin 250:
amoxicillin 250 mg
clavulanic acid 125 mg
Uses: Antiinfective

Augmentin 500:
amoxicillin 500 mg
clavulanic acid 125 mg
Uses: Antiinfective

Augmentin 875:
amoxicillin 875 mg
clavulanic acid 125 mg
Uses: Antiinfective

Augmentin 125 Chewable:
amoxicillin 125 mg
clavulanic acid 31.25 mg
Uses: Antiinfective

Augmentin 200 Chewable:
amoxicillin 200 mg
clavulanic acid 28.5 mg
Uses: Antiinfective

Augmentin 250 Chewable:
amoxicillin 250 mg
clavulanic acid 62.5 mg
Uses: Antiinfective

Augmentin 400 Chewable:
amoxicillin 400 mg
clavulanic acid 57 mg
Uses: Antiinfective

Augmentin 125 mg/5 ml Suspension:
Per 5 ml:
amoxicillin 125 mg
clavulanic acid 31.25 mg
Uses: Antiinfective
Augmentin 200 mg/5 ml Suspension:
Per 5 ml:
amoxicillin 200 mg
clavulanic acid 28.5 mg
Uses: Antiinfective
Augmentin 250 mg/5 ml Suspension:
Per 5 ml:
amoxicillin 250 mg
clavulanic acid 62.5 mg
Uses: Antiinfective
Augmentin 400 mg/5 ml Suspension:
Per 5 ml:
amoxicillin 400 mg
clavulanic acid 57 mg
Uses: Antiinfective
Auralgan Otic Solution:
5.4% antipyrine
1.4% benzocaine
Uses: Otic analgesic
Avalide:
hydrochlorthiazide 12.5 mg
irbesartan 150 mg
Uses: Antihypertensive
Avalide 300:
hydrochlorthiazide 12.5 mg
irbesartan 300 mg
Uses: Antihypertensive
Azo-Gantanol:
sulfamethoxazole 500 mg
phenazopyridine 100 mg
Uses: Sulfonamide
Azo-Gantrisin:
sulfiSOXAZOLE 500 mg
phenazopyridine 50 mg
Uses: Sulfonamide
Azo-Sulfamethoxazole:
sulfamethoxazole 500 mg
phenazopyridine 100 mg
Uses: Sulfonamide
Azo-SulfiSOXAZOLE:
sulfiSOXAZOLE 500 mg
phenazopyridine 50 mg
Uses: Sulfonamide
B&O Supprettes No. 15A Supps:
belladonna extract 15 mg
opium 30 mg
Uses: Anticholinergic, opioid analgesic
B&O Supprettes No. 16A Supps:
belladonna extract 16.2 mg
opium 60 mg
Uses: Anticholinergic, narcotic analgesic
Bactrim: trimethoprim 80 mg
sulfamethoxazole 400 mg
Uses: Antiinfective
Bactrim DS:
trimethoprim 160 mg
sulfamethoxazole 800 mg
Uses: Antiinfective
Bactrim I.V.:
Per 5 ml:
trimethoprim 80 mg
sulfamethoxazole 400 mg
Uses: Antiinfective
Bancap HC:
acetaminophen 500 mg
hydrocodone 5 mg
Uses: Analgesic
Bayer Plus, Extra Strength:
aspirin 500 mg
calcium carbonate 250 mg
Uses: Analgesic, antacid
Bayer Select Chest Cold:
dextromethorphan 15 mg
acetaminophen 500 mg
Uses: Antitussive, analgesic
Bayer Select Flu Relief:
acetaminophen 500 mg
pseudoephedrine 30 mg
dextromethorphan 15 mg

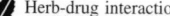

chlorpheniramine 2 mg
Uses: Analgesic, adrenergic, antitussive, antihistamine

Bayer Select Head Cold:
pseudoephedrine 30 mg
acetaminophen 500 mg
Uses: Adrenergic, analgesic

Bayer Select Maximum Strength Headache:
acetaminophen 500 mg
caffeine 65 mg
Uses: Nonopioid analgesic

Bayer Select Maximum Strength Menstrual:
acetaminophen 500 mg
pamabrom 25 mg
Uses: Nonopioid analgesic

Bayer Select Maximum Strength Night-Time Pain Relief:
acetaminophen 500 mg
diphenhydrAMINE 25 mg
Uses: Analgesic, antihistamine

Bayer Select Maximum Strength Sinus Pain Relief:
acetaminophen 500 mg
pseudoephedrine 30 mg
Uses: Analgesic, adrenergic

Bayer Select Night Time Cold:
acetaminophen 500 mg
pseudoephedrine 30 mg
dextromethorphan 15 mg
triprolidine 1.25 mg
Uses: Analgesic, adrenergic, antitussive, antihistamine

Bellatal:
phenobarbital 16.2 mg
hyoscyamine sulfate 0.1037 mg
atropine sulfate 0.0194 mg
scopolamine hydrobromide 0.0065 mg
Uses: Barbiturate, anticholinergic

Bellergal-S:
ergotamine 0.6 mg
belladonna alkaloids 0.2 mg
phenobarbital 40 mg
Uses: α-Adrenergic blocker, anticholinergic, barbiturate

Bel-Phen-Ergot-SR:
phenobarbital 40 mg
ergotamine tartrate 0.6 mg
belladonna alkaloids 0.2 mg
Uses: α-Adrenergic blocker, anticholinergic, barbiturate

Benadryl Allergy Decongestant Liquid:
Per 5 ml:
diphenhydrAMINE 12.5 mg
pseudoephedrine 30 mg
Uses: Antihistamine, adrenergic

Benadryl Allergy/Sinus Headache Caplets:
diphenhydrAMINE 12.5 mg
pseudoephedrine 30 mg
acetaminophen 500 mg
Uses: Antihistamine, adrenergic, analgesic

Benadryl Decongestant Allergy:
pseudoephedrine 60 mg
diphenhydrAMINE 25 mg
Uses: Adrenergic, antihistamine

Benylin Expectorant Liquid:
Per 5 ml:
dextromethorphan 5 mg
guaifenesin 100 mg
5% alcohol
Uses: Expectorant, antitussive

Benylin Multi-Symptom Liquid:
Per 5 ml:
dextromethorphan 5 mg
pseudoephedrine 15 mg
guaifenesin 100 mg
Uses: Antitussive, adrenergic, expectorant

Benzamycin:
benzoyl peroxide 5%
erythromycin 3%
Uses: Antiinfective

BenzaClin:
clindamycin 10%
benzoyl peroxide 5%
Uses: Antiinfective

Blephamide Ophthalmic Suspension/Ointment:
0.2% prednisoLONE
10% sodium sulfacetamide
Uses: Ophthalmic antiinfective, antiinflammatory

Bromfed Capsules:
pseudoephedrine 120 mg
brompheniramine 12 mg
Uses: Antihistamine, adrenergic

Bromfed-PD Capsules:
pseudoephedrine 60 mg
brompheniramine 6 mg
Uses: Adrenergic, antihistamine

Bromfed Tablets:
pseudoephedrine 60 mg
brompheniramine 4 mg
Uses: Antihistamine, adrenergic

Bromfenex:
brompheniramine 12 mg
pseudoephedrine 120 mg
Uses: Antihistamine, adrenergic

Bromfenex PD:
brompheniramine 6 mg
pseudoephedrine 60 mg
Uses: Antihistamine, adrenergic

Bromo-Seltzer:
sodium bicarbonate 2781 mg
acetaminophen 325 mg
citric acid 2224 mg
Uses: Antacid, analgesic

Bufferin:
aspirin 325 mg
calcium carbonate 158 mg
magnesium oxide 63 mg
magnesium carbonate 34 mg
Uses: Analgesic, antacid

Bufferin AF Nite-Time:
acetaminophen 500 mg
diphenhydrAMINE 38 mg
Uses: Analgesic, antihistamine

Butibel:
belladonna extract 15 mg
butabarbital 15 mg
Uses: Anticholinergic, barbiturate

Cafatine PB:
ergotamine 1 mg
caffeine 100 mg
belladonna alkaloids 0.125 mg
pentobarbital 30 mg
Uses: Migraine agent

Cafergot:
ergotamine 1 mg
caffeine 100 mg
Uses: Adrenergic blocker

Cafergot Suppositories:
ergotamine 2 mg
caffeine 100 mg
Uses: Adrenergic blocker

Caladryl:
8% calamine, camphor
2.2% alcohol
1% pramoxine
Uses: Top antihistamine

Calcet:
calcium 152.8 mg
vitamin D 100 international units
Uses: Supplement

Caltrate 600+D:
vitamin D 200 international units
calcium 600 mg
Uses: Supplement

Cama Arthritis Pain Reliever:
aspirin 500 mg
magnesium oxide 150 mg
aluminum hydroxide 125 mg
Uses: Nonopioid analgesic, antacid

Capital w/Codeine:
Per 5 ml:
acetaminophen 120 mg
codeine 12 mg
Uses: Opioid analgesic

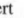

Capozide 25/15:
captopril 25 mg
hydrochlorothiazide 15 mg
Uses: Antihypertensive

Capozide 25/25:
captopril 25 mg
hydrochorothiazide 25 mg
Uses: Antihypertensive
Capozide 50/15:
captopril 50 mg
hydrochlorothiazide 15 mg
Uses: Antihypertensive
Capozide 50/25:
captopril 50 mg
hydrochlorothiazide 25 mg
Uses: Antihypertensive
Cardec DM Syrup:
Per 5 ml:
pseudoephedrine 60 mg
carbinoxamine 4 mg
dextromethorphan 15 mg
Uses: Adrenergic, antitussive
Cenafed Plus Tablets:
triprolidine 2.5 mg
pseudoephedrine 60 mg
Uses: Antihistamine, adrenergic
Cetapred Ophthalmic Ointment:
0.25% prednisoLONE
10% sodium sulfacetamide
Uses: Ophthalmic antiinfective, antiinflammatory
Cheracol Syrup:
Per 5 ml:
codeine 10 mg
guaifenesin 100 mg
Uses: Analgesic, expectorant
Children's Cepacol Liquid:
Per 5 ml:
acetaminophen 160 mg
pseudoephedrine 15 mg
Uses: Analgesic, adrenergic
Chlor-Trimeton Allergy 4 Hour Decongestant:
pseudoephedrine 60 mg
chlorpheniramine 4 mg
Uses: Antihistamine, adrenergic
Chlor-Trimeton 12 Hour Relief Tablets:
pseudoephedrine 120 mg
chlorpheniramine 8 mg
Uses: Antihistamine, adrenergic
Chromagen:
ferrous fumarate 66 mg
vitamin B_{12} 10 mcg
vitamin C 250 mg
intrinsic factor 100 mg
Uses: Supplement
Cipro HC Otic:
Per 1 ml:
ciprofloxacin 2 mg
hydrocortisone 10 mg
Uses: Antiinfective/antiinflammatory
Claritin-D 12 Hour:
loratidine 5 mg
pseudoephedrine 120 mg
Uses: Antihistamine, adrenergic
Claritin-D 24-Hour:
loratidine 10 mg
pseudoephedrine 240 mg
Uses: Antihistamine, adrenergic
Clindex:
chlordiazepoxide 5 mg
clidinium 2.5 mg
Uses: Antianxiety, anticholinergic
Clomycin Ointment:
bacitracin 500 units
neomycin sulfate 3.5 g
polymyxin B sulfate 500 units
lidocaine 40 mg
Uses: Antiinfective, local anesthetic
Co-Apap:
pseudoephedrine 30 mg
chlorpheniramine 2 mg
dextromethorphan 15 mg
acetaminophen 325 mg
Uses: Adrenergic, antihistamine, antitussive, analgesic
Co-Gesic:
acetaminophen 500 mg
hydrocodone 5 mg
Uses: Analgesic
Codiclear DH Syrup:
Per 5 ml:
hydrocodone 5 mg

guaifenesin 100 mg
Uses: Analgesic, expectorant

Codimal:
pseudoephedrine 30 mg
chlorpheniramine 2 mg
acetaminophen 500 mg
Uses: Adrenergic, antihistamine, analgesic

CombiPatch 0.05/0.14:
estradiol 0.05 mg
norethindone 0.14 mg
Uses: Menopause

CombiPatch 0.05/0.25:
estradiol 0.05 mg
norethindone 0.25 mg
Uses: Menopause

Codimal DH Syrup:
Per 5 ml:
hydrocodone 1.66 mg
phenylephrine 5 mg
pyrilamine 8.33 mg
Uses: Analgesic, adrenergic

Codimal DM Syrup:
Per 5 ml:
phenylephrine 5 mg
pyrilamine 8.33 mg
dextromethorphan 10 mg
Uses: Adrenergic, antitussive

Codimal-LA:
chlorpheniramine 8 mg
pseudoephedrine 120 mg
Uses: Antihistamine, adrenergic

Codimal PH Syrup:
Per 5 ml:
codeine 10 mg
phenylephrine 5 mg
pyrilamine 8.33 mg
Uses: Analgesic, adrenergic

Col-Probenecid:
probenecid 500 mg
colchicine 0.5 mg
Uses: Antigout agent

ColBenemid:
probenecid 500 mg
colchicine 0.5 mg
Uses: Antigout agent

Coldrine:
pseudoephedrine 30 mg
acetaminophen 500 mg
Uses: Decongestant, nonnarcotic analgesic

Col-Probenecid:
probenecid 500 mg
colchicine 0.5 mg
Uses: Antigout

Coly-Mycin S Otic Suspension:
1% hydrocortisone
neomycin base 3.3 mg/ml
colistin 3 mg/ml
0.05% thonzonium bromide
Uses: Otic antiinfective

CombiPatch 0.05/0.14:
estradiol 0.05 mg/day
norethindrone 0.14 mg/day
Uses: Estrogen, progestin

CombiPatch 0.05/0.25:
estradiol 0.05 mg/day
norethindrone 0.25 mg/day
Uses: Estrogen, progestin

Combipres 0.1:
chlorthalidone 15 mg
clonidine 0.1 mg
Uses: Antihypertensive

Combipres 0.2:
chlorthalidone 15 mg
clonidine 0.2 mg
Uses: Antihypertensive

Combipres 0.3:
chlorthalidone 15 mg
clonidine 0.3 mg
Uses: Antihypertensive

Combisor:
mometasone 0.1%
salicylic acid 5%
Uses: Corticosteroid

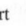

Combivent:
ipratropium bromide 18 mcg
albuterol 103 mcg/actuation
Uses: Bronchodilator

Combivir:
lamivudine 150 mg
zidovudine 300 mg
Uses: Antiviral

Comtrex Allergy-Sinus:
chlorpheniramine 2 mg
acetaminophen 500 mg
pseudoephedrine 30 mg
Uses: Antihistamine, analgesic, decongestant

Comtrex Liquid:
Per 5 ml:
chlorpheniramine 0.67 mg
acetaminophen 108.3 mg
dextromethorphan 3.3 mg
pseudoephedrine 10 mg
Uses: Antihistamine, analgesic, antitussive, decongestant

Comtrex Maximum Strength Caplets:
acetaminophen 500 mg
pseudoephedrine 30 mg
chlorpheniramine 2 mg
dextromethorphan 15 mg
Uses: Analgesic, decongestant, antihistamine, antitussive

Comtrex Maximum Strength Multi-Symptoms Cold, Flu Relief:
pseudoephedrine 30 mg
dextromethorphan 15 mg
chlorpheniramine 2 mg
acetaminophen 500 mg
Uses: Analgesic, decongestant, antihistamine, antitussive

Comtrex Maximum Strength Non-Drowsy Caplets:
acetaminophen 500 mg
pseudoephedrine 30 mg
dextromethorphan 15 mg
Uses: Analagesic, decongestant, antitussive

Congess SR:
guaifenesin 250 mg
pseudoephedrine 120 mg
Uses: Expectorant, decongestant

Congestac:
guaifenesin 400 mg
pseudoephedrine 60 mg
Uses: Expectorant, decongestant

Contac Cough & Chest Cold Liquid:
Per 5 ml:
pseudoephedrine 15 mg
dextromethorphan 5 mg
guaifenesin 50 mg
acetaminophen 125 mg
Uses: Decongestant, antitussive, expectorant, analgesic

Contac Cough & Sore Throat Liquid:
Per 5 ml:
dextromethorphan 5 mg
acetaminophen 125 mg
Uses: Antitussive, analgesic

Contac Day Allergy/Sinus:
pseudoephedrine 60 mg
acetaminophen 650 mg
Uses: Decongestant, analgesic

Contac Day Cold and Flu:
pseudoephedrine 60 mg
dextromethorphan 30 mg
acetaminophen 650 mg
Uses: Decongestant, antitussive, analgesic

Contac Night Allergy Sinus:
pseudoephedrine 60 mg
diphenhydrAMINE 50 mg
acetaminophen 650 mg
Uses: Decongestant, antihistamine, analgesic

Contac Night Cold and Flu Caplets:
pseudoephedrine 60 mg
diphenhydrAMINE 50 mg
acetaminophen 650 mg
Uses: Decongestant, antihistamine, antitussive, analgesic

Contac Non-Drowsy Maximum Strength 12 Hour:
pseudoephedrine 120 mg
Uses: Adrenergic

Contac Severe Cold & Flu Nighttime Liquid:
Per 5 ml:
pseudoephedrine 10 mg
chlorpheniramine 0.67 mg
dextromethorphan 5 mg
acetaminophen 167 mg
18.5% alcohol
Uses: Decongestant, antihistamine, antitussive, analgesic

Coricidin:
chlorpheniramine 2 mg
acetaminophen 325 mg
Uses: Antihistamine, analgesic

Coricidin D Tablets:
chlorpheniramine 2 mg
acetaminophen 325 mg
Uses: Antihistamine, analgesic

Coricidin D Cold, Flu & Sinus:
chlorpheniramine 2 mg
acetaminophen 325 mg
pseudoephedrine sulfate 30 mg
Uses: Antihistamine, analgesic, decongestant

Corcidin HBP Cold and Flu:
acetaminophen 325 mg
chlorpheniramine 2 mg
Uses: Analgesic, antihistamine

Corcidin HBP Cough and Cold:
chlorpheniramine 4 mg
dextromethorphan 30 mg
Uses: Antihistamine, expectorant

Corcidin HBP Nighttime Cold and Flu:
acetaminophen 325 mg
diphenhydrAMINE 25 mg
Uses: Analgesic, antihistamine

Corcidin HBP Maximum Strength Flu:
acetaminophen 500 mg
chlorpheniramine 2 mg
dextromethorphan 15 mg
Uses: Analgesic, antihistamine, expectorant

Cortisporin Ophthalmic/Otic Suspension:
0.35% neomycin polymyxin B 10,000 units/ml
1% hydrocortisone
Uses: Ophthalmic antiinfective, antiinflammatory

Cortisporin Ophthalmic Ointment:
0.35% neomycin base
bacitracin 400 units
polymyxin B 10,000 units
hydrocortisone 1%
Uses: Ophthalmic antiinfective

Cortisporin Topical Cream:
0.5% neomycin sulfate
polymyxin B 10,000 units
0.5% hydrocortisone
Uses: Topical antiinfective

Cortisporin Topical Ointment:
0.5% neomycin sulfate
bacitracin 400 units
polymyxin B 5000 units
1% hydrocortisone
Uses: Topical antiinfective

Corzide 40/5:
nadolol 40 mg
bendroflumethiazide 5 mg
Uses: Antihypertensive

Corzide 80/5:
nadolol 80 mg
bendroflumethiazide 5 mg
Uses: Antihypertensive

Cosopt:
dorzolamide 2%
timolol 0.5%
Uses: Antihypertensive

Cough-X:
dextromethorphan 5 mg
benzocaine 2 mg
Uses: Antitussive, local anesthetic

Creon:
lipase 8000 units
amylase 30,000 units

protease 13,000 units
pancreatin 300 mg
Uses: Digestive enzyme

Cyclomydril Ophthalmic Solution:
0.2% cyclopentolate
1% phenylephrine
Uses: Mydriatic

Dallergy Caplets:
chlorpheniramine 8 mg
phenylephrine 20 mg
methscopolamine 2.5 mg
Uses: Antihistamine, adrenergic

Dallergy Syrup:
Per 5 ml:
chlorpheniramine 2 mg
phenylephrine 10 mg
methscopolamine 0.625 mg
Uses: Antihistamine, adrenergic

Dallergy Tablets:
chlorpheniramine 4 mg
phenylephrine 10 mg
methscopolamine 1.25 mg
Uses: Antihistamine, adrenergic

Dallergy-D Syrup:
Per 5 ml:
phenylephrine 5 mg
chlorpheniramine 2 mg
Uses: Antihistamine, adrenergic

Damason-P:
hydrocodone 5 mg
aspirin 500 mg
Uses: Analgesic

Darvocet-N 100:
propoxyphene-N 100 mg
acetaminophen 650 mg
Uses: Analgesic

Darvon Compound-65:
propoxyphene 65 mg
aspirin 389 mg
caffeine 32.4 mg
Uses: Analgesic

✤Darvon-N Compound:
aspirin 375 mg
propoxyphene 100 mg
caffeine 30 mg
Uses: Analgesic

✤Darvon-N w/A.S.A.:
aspirin 325 mg
propoxyphene 100 mg
Uses: Analgesic

Deconamine:
pseudoephedrine 60 mg
chlorpheniramine 4 mg
Uses: Antihistamine, decongestant

Deconamine CX:
hydrocodone 5 mg
pseudoephedrine 30 mg
guaifenesin 300 mg
Uses: Analgesic, decongestant, expectorant

Deconamine SR:
pseudoephedrine 120 mg
chlorpheniramine 8 mg
Uses: Antihistamine, decongestant

Deconamine Syrup:
Per 5 ml:
pseudoephedrine 30 mg
chlorpheniramine 2 mg
Uses: Antihistamine, decongestant

Defen-LA:
pseudoephedrine 60 mg
guaifenesin 600 mg
Uses: Decongestant, expectorant

Demi-Regroton:
chlorthalidone 25 mg
reserpine 0.125 mg
Uses: Antihypertensive

Demulen 1/35:
ethinyl estradiol 35 mcg
ethynodiol diacetate 1 mg
Uses: Oral contraceptive

Demulen 1/50:
ethinyl estradiol 50 mcg
ethynodiol diacetate 1 mg
Uses: Oral contraceptive

Depo-Testadiol:
estradiol cypionate 2 mg
testosterone cypionate 50 mg
Uses: Menopause

Desogen:
ethinyl estradiol 30 mcg
desorgestrel 0.15 mg
Uses: Estrogen, progestin

Dexacidin Ophthalmic Ointment/ Suspension:
Per ml:
0.1% dexamethasone
0.35% neomycin
polymyxin B 10,000 units/g
Uses: Ophth, antiinfective/ antiinflammatory

Dexasporin Ophthalmic Ointment:
Per gram:
0.1% dexamethasone
0.35% neomycin
polymyxin B 10,000 units
Uses: Ophth, antiinfective/ antiinflammatory

DHC Plus:
dihydrocodeine 16 mg
acetaminophen 356.4 mg
caffeine 30 mg
Uses: Analgesic

Dialose Plus:
docusate sodium 100 mg
yellow phenolphthalein 65 mg
Uses: Laxative

Di-Gel Advanced Formula:
magnesium hydroxide 128 mg
calcium carbonate 280 mg
simethicone 20 mg
Uses: Antacid, adsorbent, antiflatulent

Di-Gel Liquid:
Per 5 ml:
aluminum hydroxide 200 mg
magnesium hydroxide 200 mg
simethicone 20 mg
Uses: Antacid, adsorbent, antiflatulent

Dihistine DH Liquid:
Per 5 ml:
pseudoephedrine 30 mg
chlorpheniramine 2 mg
codeine 10 mg
Uses: Decongestant, antihistamine, analgesic

Dilaudid Cough Syrup:
Per 5 ml:
guaifenesin 100 mg
hydromorphone 1 mg
5% alcohol
Uses: Expectorant, analgesic

Dilor-G:
dyphylline 200 mg
guaifenesin 200 mg
Uses: Bronchodilator, expectorant

Dimetane Decongestant:
brompheniramine 4 mg
phenylephrine 10 mg
Uses: Antihistamine, adrenergic

Dimetane-DX Cough Syrup:
Per 5 ml:
brompheniramine 2 mg
pseudoephedrine 30 mg
dextromethorphan 10 mg
Uses: Antihistamine, decongestant, antitussive

Dimetapp DM Elixir:
Per 5 ml:
pseudoephedrine 5 mg
brompheniramine 2 mg
dextromethorphan 10 mg
Uses: Antihistamine, adrenergic, expectorant

Dimetapp Sinus:
pseudoephedrine 30 mg
ibuprofen 200 mg
Uses: Decongestant, analgesic

Diovan 80 HCT:
valsartan 80 mg
hydrochlorthiazide 12.5 mg
Uses: Antihypertensive

Diovan 160 HCT:
valsartan 160 mg
hydrochlorthiazide 12.5 mg
Uses: Antihypertensive

Diurigen w/Reserpine:
chlorothiazide 250 mg
reserpine 0.125 mg
Uses: Antihypertensive

Diutensin-R:
methylclothiazide 2.5 mg
reserpine 0.1 mg
Uses: Antihypertensive

Doan's PM Extra Strength:
magnesium salicylate 500 mg
diphenhydrAMINE 25 mg
Uses: Analgesic, antihistamine

Dolacet:
hydrocodone 5 mg
acetaminophen 500 mg
Uses: Analgesic

Donnatal:
phenobarbital 16.2 mg
hyoscyamine 0.1037 mg
atropine 0.0194 mg
scopolamine 0.0065 mg
Uses: Anticholinergic, barbiturate

Donnatal Elixir:
Per 5 ml:
phenobarbital 16.2 mg
hyoscyamine 0.1037 mg
atropine 0.0194 mg
scopolamine 0.0065 mg
23% alcohol
Uses: Anticholinergic, barbiturate

Donnatal Extentabs:
phenobarbital 48.6 mg
hyoscyamine 0.3111 mg
atropine 0.0582 mg
scopolamine 0.0195 mg
Uses: Anticholinergic, barbiturate

Donnazyme:
pancreatin 500 mg
lipase 1000 units
protease 12,500 units
amylase 12,500 units
Uses: Pancreatic enzymes

Dorcol Children's Cold Formula Liquid:
Per 5 ml:
pseudoephedrine 15 mg
chlorpheniramine 1 mg
Uses: Decongestant, antihistamine

Doxidan:
docusate calcium 60 mg
phenolphthalein 65 mg
Uses: Stool softener

Dristan Cold:
pseudoephedrine 30 mg
acetaminophen 500 mg
Uses: Decongestant, analgesic

Dristan Cold Maximum Strength Caplets:
pseudoephedrine 30 mg
brompheniramine 2 mg
acetaminophen 500 mg
Uses: Decongestant, antihistamine, analgesic

Dristan Cold Multi-Symptom Formula:
acetaminophen 325 mg
phenylephrine 5 mg
chlorpheniramine 2 mg
Uses: Analgesic, adrenergic, antihistamine

Dristan Sinus:
pseudoephedrine 30 mg
ibuprofen 200 mg
Uses: Decongestant, analgesic

Drixoral Allergy Sinus:
pseudoephedrine 60 mg
dexbrompheniramine 3 mg
acetaminophen 500 mg
Uses: Decongestant, antihistamine, analgesic

Drixoral Cold & Allergy:
pseudoephedrine 120 mg
dexbrompheniramine 6 mg
Uses: Decongestant, antihistamine

Drixoral Cold & Flu:
pseudoephedrine 60 mg
dexbrompheniramine 3 mg
acetaminophen 500 mg
Uses: Decongestant, antihistamine, analgesic

Drixoral Nasal Decongestant:
pseudoephedrine 120 mg
Uses: Decongestant

DT:
Per 5 ml dose:
diphtheria toxoid 2LfU
tetanus toxoid 5LfU
Uses: Vaccine

DTP:
Per 0.5 ml dose:
diphtheria toxoid 6.5LfU
tetanus toxoid 5LfU
pertussis 4LfU
Uses: Vaccine

DuoNeb:
Per 3 ml:
albuterol 3 mg
ipratroprium 0.5 mg
Uses: Bronchodilator

Dura-Vent/DA:
phenylephrine 20 mg
chlorpheniramine 8 mg
methscopolamine 2.5 mg
Uses: Adrenergic, antihistamine

Dyazide:
hydrochlorothiazide 25 mg
triamterene 37.5 mg
Uses: Diuretic

Dylline-GG Tablets:
dyphylline 200 mg
quaifenesin 200 mg
Uses: Bronchodilator, expectorant

Dynafed Asthma Relief:
epHEDrine 25 mg
guaifenesin 200 mg
Uses: Adrenergic, expectorant

Dynafed Plus Maximum Strength:
pseudoephedrine 30 mg
acetaminophen 500 mg
Uses: Decongestant, analgesic

Dyphylline-GG Elixir:
Per 5 ml:
dyphylline 100 mg
guaifenesin 100 mg
Uses: Bronchodilator, expectorant

E-Lor:
acetaminophen 650 mg
propoxyphene 65 mg
Uses: Analgesic

E-Pilo-1 Ophthalmic Solution:
1% epINEPHrine
1% pilocarpine
Uses: Mydriatic, miotic

E-Pilo-2 Ophthalmic Solution:
1% epINEPHrine
2% pilocarpine
Uses: Mydriatic, miotic

E-Pilo-4 Ophthalmic Solution:
1% epINEPHrine
4% pilocarpine
Uses: Mydriatic, miotic

E-Pilo-6 Ophthalmic Solution:
1% epINEPHrine
6% pilocarpine
Uses: Mydriatic, miotic

Elase Ointment:
Per gram:
fibrinolysin 1 unit
desoxyribonuclease 666.6 units
Uses: Enzyme

Elixophyllin GG Liquid:
Per 5 ml:
theophylline 100 mg
guaifenesin 100 mg
Uses: Expectorant, bronchodilator

EMLA Cream:
lidocaine 2.5 mg
prilocaine 2.5 mg
Uses: Local anesthetic

Empirin w/Codeine #3:
aspirin 325 mg
codeine phosphate 30 mg
Uses: Analgesic

Empirin w/Codeine #4:
aspirin 325 mg
codeine phosphate 60 mg
Uses: Analgesic

✤Empracet-60:
acetaminophen 300 mg
codeine 60 mg
Uses: Analgesic

Endocet:
acetaminophen 325 mg
oxycodone 5 mg
Uses: Analgesic

✦Endodan:
aspirin 325 mg
oxycodone 5 mg
Uses: Analgesic

Enduronyl:
methyclothiazide 5 mg
deserpidine 0.25 mg
Uses: Antihypertensive

Enduronyl Forte:
methyclothiazide 5.0 mg
deserpidine 0.5 mg
Uses: Antihypertensive

Entex PSE:
pseudoephedrine 120 mg
guaifenesin 600 mg
Uses: Adrenergic, expectorant

Epifoam Aerosol Foam:
1% hydrocortisone
1% pramoxine
Uses: Topical corticosteroid

Equagesic:
meprobamate 200 mg
aspirin 325 mg
Uses: Antianxiety

Eryzole:
Per 5 ml:
erythromycin 200 mg
sulfisoxazole 600 mg
Uses: Macrolide antiinfective

Esgic-Plus:
butalbital 50 mg
acetaminophen 500 mg
caffeine 40 mg
Uses: Barbiturate, analgesic

Esimil:
guanethidine 10 mg
hydrochlorothiazide 25 mg
Uses: Antihypertensive

Estratest:
esterified estrogens 1.25 mg
methyltestosterone 2.5 mg
Uses: Menopause

Estratest HS:
esterified estrogens 1.25 mg
methyltestosterone 2.5 mg
Uses: Menopause

Etrafon:
perphenazine 2 mg
amitriptyline 25 mg
Uses: Antipsychotic, antidepressant

Etrafon 2-10:
perphenazine 2 mg
amitriptyline 10 mg
Uses: Antidepressant

Etrafon A:
perphenazine 4 mg
amitriptyline 10 mg
Uses: Antidepressant

Etrafon Forte:
perphenazine 4 mg
amitriptyline 25 mg
Uses: Antipsychotic, antidepressant

Excedrin Migraine:
aspirin 250 mg
acetaminophen 250 mg
caffeine 65 mg
Uses: Migraine agent

Excedrin P.M.:
acetaminophen 500 mg
diphenhydrAMINE citrate 38 mg
Uses: Analgesic, antihistamine

Excedrin P.M. Liquigels:
acetaminophen 500 mg
diphenhydrAMINE 25 mg
Uses: Analgesic, antihistamine

Excedrin Sinus Extra Strength:
pseudoephedrine 30 mg
acetaminophen 500 mg
Uses: Decongestant, analgesic

Fansidar:
sulfidoxine 500 mg
pyrimethamine 25 mg
Uses: Antimalarial

Fedahist:
pseudoephedrine 60 mg
chlorpheniramine 4 mg
Uses: Decongestant, antihistamine

Fedahist Expectorant Syrup:
Per 5 ml:
guaifenesin 200 mg
pseudoephedrine 20 mg
Uses: Expectorant, decongestant

Fedahist Gyrocaps:
pseudoephedrine 65 mg
chlorpheniramine 10 mg
Uses: Decongestant, antihistamine

Fedahist Timecaps:
pseudoephedrine 120 mg
chlorpheniramine 8 mg
Uses: Decongestant, antihistamine

Feen-A-Mint Pills:
docusate sodium 100 mg
phenolphthalein 65 mg
Uses: Laxative

Fem-1:
acetaminophen 500 mg
pamabrom 25 mg
Uses: Nonopioid analgesic

Fembrt 1/5:
norethindrone 1 mg
ethinyl estradiol 5 mcg
Uses: Menopause

Ferro-Sequels:
docusate sodium 100 mg
ferrous fumarate 150 mg
Uses: Laxative, hematinic

Fioricet:
acetaminophen 325 mg
caffeine 40 mg
butalbital 50 mg
Uses: Analgesic, barbiturate

Fioricet w/Codeine:
acetaminophen 325 mg
caffeine 40 mg
butalbital 50 mg
codeine 30 mg
Uses: Analgesic, barbiturate

Fiorinal:
aspirin 325 mg
caffeine 40 mg
butalbital 50 mg
Uses: Analgesic, barbiturate

Fiorinal w/Codeine:
aspirin 325 mg
caffeine 40 mg
butalbital 50 mg
codeine 30 mg
Uses: Analgesic, barbiturate

FML-S Ophthalmic Suspension:
0.1% flurometholone
10% sulfacetamide
Uses: Ophth, antiinfective/antiinflammatory

Gas-Ban:
calcium carbonate 500 mg
simethicone 40 mg
Uses: Antiflatulent, antacid

Gas-Ban DS Liquid:
Per 5 ml:
aluminum hydroxide 400 mg
magnesium hydroxide 400 mg
simethicone 40 mg
Uses: Antiflatulent, antacid

Gaviscon:
magnesium trisilicate 20 mg
aluminum hydroxide 80 mg
Uses: Antacid, adsorbent, antiflatulent

Gaviscon Liquid:
Per 5 ml:
aluminum hydroxide 31.7 mg
magnesium carbonate 119.3 mg
Uses: Antacid, adsorbent, antiflatulent

Gelprin:
acetaminophen 125 mg
aspirin 240 mg
caffeine 32 mg
Uses: Analgesic

Gelusil:
aluminum hydroxide 200 mg
magnesium hydroxide 200 mg
simethicone 25 mg
Uses: Antacid, adsorbent, antiflatulent

Genac Tablets:
triprolidine 2.5 mg
pseudoephedrine 60 mg
Uses: Antihistamine

Genatuss DM Syrup:
Per 5 ml:
guaifenesin 100 mg
dextromethorphan 10 mg
Uses: Expectorant, antitussive

Glucovance 1.25:
glyBURIDE: 1.25 mg
metformin: 250 mg
Uses: Antidiabetic

Glucovance 2.50:
glyBURIDE: 2.5 mg
metformin: 500 mg
Uses: Antidiabetic

Glucovance 5:
glyBURIDE: 5 mg
metformin: 500 mg
Uses: Antidiabetic

Granulex Aerosol:
Per 0.82 ml:
trypsin 0.1 mg
balsam peru 72.5 mg
castor oil 650 mg
Uses: Top enzyme

Guaifenex PSE 60:
pseudoephedrine 60 mg
guaifenesin 600 mg
Uses: Decongestant, expectorant

Guaifenex PSE 120:
pseudoephedrine 120 mg
guaifenesin 600 mg
Uses: Decongestant, expectorant

Guaituss AC:
Per 5 ml:
codeine 10 mg
guafenesin 100 mg
Uses: Analgesic, expectorant

Haley's M-O Liquid:
Per 15 ml:
magnesium hydroxide 900 mg
mineral oil 3.75 ml
Uses: Laxative

Halotussin-DM Sugar Free Liquid:
Per 5 ml:
guaifenesin 100 mg
dextromethorphan 10 mg
Uses: Expectorant, antitussive

Helidac:
In a compliance package:
bismuth subsalicylate 262.4 mg tabs
metronidazole 250 mg tabs
tetracycline 500 mg caps
Uses: Antiinfective

Humalog Mix 50/50:
insulin lispro protamine 50%
insulin lispro (rDNA) 50%
Uses: Antidiabetic

Humalog Mix 75/25:
insulin lispro protamine 75%
insulin lispro (rDNA) 25%
Uses: Antidiabetic

Humibid DM Sprinkle Caps:
dextromethorphan 15 mg
guaifenesin 300 mg
Uses: Expectorant, antitussive

Humibid DM Tablets:
dextromethorphan 30 mg
guaifenesin 600 mg
Uses: Expectorant, antitussive

HycoClear Tuss:
Per 5 ml:
hydrocodone 5 mg
guaifenesin 100 mg
Uses: Analgesic, expectorant

Hycodan:
hydrocodone 5 mg
homatropine 1.5 mg
Uses: Analgesic, mydriatic

Hycodan Syrup:
Per 5 ml:
hydrocodone 5 mg
homatropine 1.5 mg
Uses: Analgesic, mydriatic

Hycomine Compound:
chlorpheniramine 2 mg
acetaminophen 250 mg
phenylephrine 10 mg

hydrocodone 5 mg
caffeine 30 mg
Uses: Antihistamine, analgesic, adrenergic

Hycotuss Expectorant:
Per 5 ml:
guaifenesin 100 mg
hydrocodone 5 mg
10% alcohol
Uses: Expectorant

Hydergine:
dihydroergocornine 0.167 mg
dihydroergocristine 0.167 mg
dihydroergocryptine 0.167 mg
Uses: Adrenergic blocker

Hydrocet:
hydrocodone 5 mg
acetaminophen 500 mg
Uses: Opioid analgesic

Hydrogesic:
hydrocodone 5 mg
acetaminophen 500 mg
Uses: Opioid analgesic

Hydropres-50:
hydrochlorothiazide 50 mg
reserpine 0.125 mg
Uses: Antihypertensive

Hydroserpine:
hydrochlorothiazide 25 mg
reserpine 0.125 mg
Uses: Antihypertensive

Hydroserpine:
hydrochlorothiazide 50 mg
reserpine 0.125 mg
Uses: Antihypertensive

Hyzaar:
losartan potassium 50 mg
hydrochlorothiazide 12.5 mg
potassium 4.24 mg
Uses: Antihypertensive

Imodium Advanced:
loperamide 2 mg
simethicone 125 mg
Uses: Antidiarrheal, antiflatulent

Inderide 40/25:
propranolol 40 mg
hydrochlorothiazide 25 mg
Uses: Antihypertensive

Inderide 80/25:
propranolol 80 mg
hydrochlorothiazide 25 mg
Uses: Antihypertensive

Inderide LA 80/50:
propranolol 80 mg
hydrochlorothiazide 50 mg
Uses: Antihypertensive

Inderide LA 120/50:
propranolol 120 mg
hydrochlorothiazide 50 mg
Uses: Antihypertensive

Inderide LA 160/50:
propranolol 160 mg
hydrochlorothiazide 50 mg
Uses: Antihypertensive

Innovar:
Per ml:
droperidol 2.5 mg
fentanyl 0.05 mg
Uses: Opioid analgesic, general anesthetic

Iofed:
brompheniramine 12 mg
pseudoephedrine 120 mg
Uses: Antihistamine, adrenergic

Iofed PD:
brompheniramine 6 mg
pseudoephedrine 60 mg
Uses: Antihistamine, adrenergic

Isopap:
isometheptene 65 mg
APAP 325 mg
dicloral-phenazone 100 mg
Uses: Migraine agent

Kaletra Capsules:
lopinavir 133.3 mg
ritonavir 33.3 mg
Uses: HIV

Kaletra Solution:
Per 1 ml:
lopinavir 80 mg
ritonavir 20 mg
Uses: HIV

Lactinex:
Mixed culture of:
Lactobacillus acidophilus and
Lactobacillus bulgaricus
Uses: Supplement
Lenoltec w/Codeine No. 1:
acetaminophen 650 mg
hydrocodone 10 mg
Uses: Analgesic
Levlite:
levonorgestrel 0.100 mg
ethinyl estradiol 20 mcg
Uses: Estrogen, progestin
Levsin PB Drops:
Per ml:
hyoscyamine 0.125 mg
phenobarbital 15 mg
5% alcohol
Uses: Anticholinergic, barbiturate
Levsin w/Phenobarbital:
hyoscyamine 0.125 mg
phenobarbital 15 mg
Uses: Anticholinergic, barbiturate
Lexxel 1:
enalapril 5 mg
felodipine 5 mg
Uses: Antihypertensive
Lexxel 2:
enalapril 5 mg
felodipine 2.5 mg
Uses: Antihypertensive
Librax:
chlordiazepoxide 5 mg
clidinium 2.5 mg
Uses: Antianxiety, anticholinergic
Lida-Mantel-HC-Cream:
0.5% hydrocortisone
3% lidocaine
Uses: Antiinflammatory, analgesic
Limbitrol DS 10-25:
chlordiazepoxide 10 mg
amitriptyline 25 mg
Uses: Antidepressant, antianxiety
Lobac:
salicylamide 200 mg
phenyltoloxamine 20 mg
acetaminophen 300 mg
Uses: Skeletal muscle relaxant, analgesic
Loestrin Fe 1/20:
norethindrone acetate 1 mg/tablet
ethinyl estradiol 20 mcg/tablet
with 7 tablets of ferrous fumarate 75 mg/container
Uses: Oral contraceptive
Loestrin Fe 1.5/30:
norethindrone acetate 1.5 mg
ethinyl estradiol 30 mcg
Uses: Oral contraceptive
Lomotil:
diphenoxylate 2.5 mg
atropine 0.025 mg
Uses: Antidiarrheal, anticholinergic
Lomotil Liquid:
Per 5 ml:
diphenoxylate 2.5 mg
atropine 0.025 mg
Uses: Antidiarrheal, anticholinergic
Lo Ovral:
ethinyl estradiol 30 mcg
norgestrel 0.3 mg
Uses: Oral contraceptive
Lopressor HCT 50/25:
metoprolol 50 mg
hydrochlorothiazide 25 mg
Uses: Antihypertensive
Lopressor HCT 100/25:
metoprolol 100 mg
hydrochlorothiazide 25 mg
Uses: Antihypertensive
Lopressor HCT 100/50:
metoprolol 100 mg
hydrochlorothiazide 50 mg
Uses: Antihypertensive
Lorcet 10/650:
acetaminophen 650 mg
hydrocodone 10 mg
Uses: Analgesic
Lorcet-HD:
hydrocodone 10 mg
acetaminophen 300 mg
Uses: Analgesic

Lorcet Plus:
acetaminophen 650 mg
hydrocodone 7.5 mg
Uses: Analgesic

Lortab 2.5/500:
hydrocodone 2.5 mg
acetaminophen 500 mg
Uses: Analgesic

Lortab 5/500:
hydrocodone 5 mg
acetaminophen 500 mg
Uses: Analgesic

Lortab 7.5/500:
hydrocodone 7.5 mg
acetaminophen 500 mg
Uses: Analgesic

Lortab 10/500:
hydrocodone 10 mg
acetaminophen 500 mg
Uses: Analgesic

Lortab ASA:
aspirin 500 mg
hydrocodone 5 mg
Uses: Analgesic

Lortab Elixir:
Per 5 ml:
hydrocodone 2.5 mg
acetaminophen 167 mg
Uses: Analgesic

Losec 1-2-3A:
omeprazole 20 mg
clarithromycin 500 mg
amoxicillin 1 g
Uses: Antiinfective

Losec 1-2-3M:
omeprazole 20 mg
clarithromycin 250 mg
medtronidazole 500 mg
Uses: Antiinfective

Lotensin HCT 5/6.25:
benazepril 5 mg
hydrochlorothiazide 6.25 mg
Uses: Antihypertensive

Lotensin HCT 10/12.5:
benazepril 10 mg
hydrochlorothiazide 12.5 mg
Uses: Antihypertensive

Lotensin HCT 20/12.5:
benazepril 20 mg
hydrochlorothiazide 12.5 mg
Uses: Antihypertensive

Lotensin HCT 20/25:
benazepril 20 mg
hydrochlorothiazide 25 mg
Uses: Antihypertensive

Lotrel 2.5/10:
amlopidine 2.5 mg
benazepril 10 mg
Uses: Antihypertensive

Lotrel 5/10:
amlodipine 5 mg
benazepril 10 mg
Uses: Antihypertensive

Lotrel 5/20:
amlodipine 5 mg
benazepril 20 mg
Uses: Antihypertensive

Lotrisone Topical:
0.05% betamethasone
1% clotrimazole
Uses: Local antiinfective, antiinflammatory

Lufyllin-EPG Elixir:
Per 5 ml:
dyphylline 150 mg
epHEDrine 24 mg
guaifenesin 300 mg
phenobarbital 24 mg
Uses: Bronchodilator, expectorant

Lufyllin-GG:
dyphylline 200 mg
guaifenesin 200 mg
Uses: Bronchodilator, expectorant

Lunelle Monthly Contraceptive Injection:
25 mg medroxyprogesterone
5 mg estradiol/0.5 ml
Uses: Contraceptive

M-M-R-II:
measles
mumps
rubella
Uses: Vaccine, toxoid

Maalox:
aluminum hydroxide 200 mg
magnesium hydroxide 200 mg
Uses: Antacid, adsorbent, antiflatulent

Maalox Plus:
aluminum hydroxide 200 mg
magnesium hydroxide 200 mg
simethicone 25 mg
Uses: Antacid, adsorbent, antiflatulent

Maalox Plus Extra Strength Suspension:
Per 5 ml:
aluminum hydroxide 500 mg
magnesium hydroxide 450 mg
simethicone 40 mg
Uses: Antacid, adsorbent, antiflatulent

Maalox Suspension:
Per 5 ml:
aluminum hydroxide 225 mg
magnesium hydroxide 200 mg
Uses: Antacid, adsorbent, antiflatulent

Macrobid:
nitrofurantoin macrocrystals 25 mg
nitrofurantoin monohydrate 75 mg
Uses: Antiinfective

Magnaprin:
aspirin 325 mg
magnesium hydroxide 50 mg
aluminum hydroxide 50 mg
calcium carbonate 50 mg
Uses: Nonopioid analgesic

Magnaprin Arthritis Strength:
aspirin 325 mg
magnesium hydroxide 75 mg
aluminum hydroxide 75 mg
calcium carbonate 75 mg
Uses: Nonnarcotic analgesic

Malarone:
250 mg atovaquone
100 mg proguanil
Uses: Malaria

Malarone Pediatric:
62.5 mg atovaquone
25 mg proguanil
Uses: Malaria

Mapap Cold Formula:
acetaminophen 325 mg
chlorpheniramine 2 mg
pseudoephedrine 30 mg
dextromethorphan 15 mg
Uses: Bronchodilator, expectorant

Marax:
epHEDrine 25 mg
theophylline 130 mg
hydrOXYzine 10 mg
Uses: Bronchodilator, sedative/hypnotic

Maxitrol Ophthalmic Suspension/Ointment:
Per ml:
0.35% neomycin
0.1% dexamethasone
polymyxin B 10,000 units
Uses: Ophthalmic antiinfective, antiinflammatory

Maxzide:
hydrochlorothiazide 50 mg
triamterene 75 mg
Uses: Antihypertensive, diuretic

Maxzide-25 MG:
hydrochlorothiazide 25 mg
triamterene 37.5 mg
Uses: Diuretic

Medi-Flu Liquid:
Per 5 ml:
pseudoephedrine 10 mg
chlorpheniramine 0.67 mg
dextromethorphan 5 mg
acetaminophen 167 mg
18.5% alcohol
Uses: Decongestant, antihistamine, antitussive, analgesic

Medigesic:
acetaminophen 325 mg
caffeine 40 mg
butalbital 50 mg
Uses: Nonopioid analgesic

Mepergan Fortis:
meperidine 50 mg
promethazine 25 mg
Uses: Analgesic, antihistamine

Mepergan Injection:
meperidine 25 mg
promethazine 25 mg
Uses: Analgesic

Metimyd Ophthalmic Suspension/ Ointment:
0.5% prednisoLONE
10% sodium sulfacetamide
Uses: Ophthalmic antiinfective, antiinflammatory

Micardis HCT 40:
telmesartan 40 mg
hydrochlorthiazide 12.5 mg
Uses: Antihypertensive

Micardis HCT 80:
telmesartan 80 mg
hydrochlorthiazide 12.5 mg
Uses: Antihypertensive

Microgestin Fe 1/20:
norethindrone 1 mg
ethinyl estradiol 20 mcg
ferrous fumarate 75 mg in container
Uses: Estrogen, progestin

Microgestin Fe 1.5/30:
norethindrone 1.5 mg
ethinyl estradiol 30 mcg
ferrous fumarate 75 mg in container
Uses: Estrogen, progestin

Midol Maximum Strength Multi-Symptom Menstrual Gelcaps:
acetaminophen 500 mg
pyrilamine 15 mg
caffeine 60 mg
Uses: Analgesic

Midol PM:
acetaminophen 500 mg
diphenhydrAMINE 25 mg
Uses: Analgesic, antihistamine

Midol PMS Maximum Strength Caplets:
acetaminophen 500 mg
pyrilamine 15 mg
pamabrom 25 mg
Uses: Analgesic

Midol, Teen:
acetaminophen 400 mg
pamabrom 25 mg
Uses: Analgesic

Midrin:
isometheptene 65 mg
acetaminophen 325 mg
dichloralphenazone 100 mg
Uses: Analgesic

Minizide 1:
prazosin 1 mg
polythiazide 0.5 mg
Uses: Antihypertensive

Minizide 2:
prazosin 2 mg
polythiazide 0.5 mg
Uses: Antihypertensive

Minizide 5:
prazosin 5 mg
polythiazide 0.5 mg
Uses: Antihypertensive

Moduretic:
hydrochlorothiazide 50 mg
amiloride 5 mg
Uses: Diuretic

Monopril-HCT 10:
fosinopril 10 mg
hydrochlorthiazine 12.5 mg
Uses: Antihypertensive

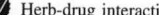

Monopril-HCT 20:
fosinopril 20 mg
hydrochlorthiazine 12.5 mg
Uses: Antihypertensive

Motrin Children's Cold Suspension:
Per 5 ml:
ibuprofen 100 mg
pseudoephedrine 15 mg
Uses: Nonopioid analgesic, decongestant

Motrin IB Sinus:
pseudoephedrine 30 mg
ibuprofen 200 mg
Uses: Adrenergic, analgesic

Murocoll-2 Ophthalmic Drops:
0.3% scopolamine
10% phenylephrine
Uses: Ophthalmic anticholinergic, mydriatic

Mycolog II Topical:
Per gram:
0.1% triamcinolone acetonide
nystatin 100,000 units
Uses: Local antiinfective, antiinflammatory

Mylanta:
aluminum hydroxide 200 mg
magnesium hydroxide 200 mg
simethicone 20 mg
Uses: Antacid, adsorbent, antiflatulent

Mylanta Double Strength Liquid:
Per 5 ml:
aluminum hydroxide 400 mg
magnesium hydroxide 400 mg
simethicone 40 mg
Uses: Antacid, adsorbent, antiflatulent

Mylanta Gelcaps:
calcium carbonate 311 mg
magnesium carbonate 232 mg
Uses: Antacid, adsorbent, antiflatulent

Naldecon Senior DX Liquid:
Per 5 ml:
dextromethorphan 10 mg
guaifenesin 200 mg
Uses: Expectorant, antitussive

Naphcon-A Ophthalmic
Solution:
0.25% naphazoline
0.3% pheniramine
Uses: Ophthalmic vasoconstrictor

Nasatab LA:
guaifenesin 500 mg
pseudoephedrine 120 mg
Uses: Expectorant, decongestant

NeoDecadron Ophthalmic Ointment:
0.35% neomycin
0.05% dexamethasone
Uses: Ophthalmic antiinfective, antiinflammatory

NeoDecadron Ophthalmic Solution:
0.35% neomycin
0.1% dexamethasone
Uses: Ophthalmic antiinfective, antiinflammatory

Neosporin Cream:
Per gram:
polymyxin B 10,000 units
neomycin 3.5 mg
Uses: Top antiinfective

Neosporin G.U. Irrigant:
Per ml:
neomycin 40 mg
polymyxin B 200,000 units
Uses: Antiinfective

Neosporin Ointment:
Per gram:
polymyxin B 5000 units
bacitracin zinc 400 units
neomycin 3.5 mg
Uses: Top antiinfective

Neosporin Ophthalmic Solution:
Per ml:
neomycin 1.75 mg
polymyxin B 10,000 units
gramicidin 0.025 mg
Uses: Ophthalmic antiinfective

Neosporin Ophthalmic Ointment:
Per gram:
neomycin 3.5 mg

polymyxin B 10,000 units
bacitracin zinc 400 units
Uses: Ophthalmic antiinfective

Neosporin Plus Cream:
polymyxin B 10,000 units
neomycin 3.5 mg
lidocaine 40 mg
Uses: Top antiinfective

Niferex-150 Forte:
ferrous sulfate 150 mg
vitamin B_{12} 25 mcg
folic acid 1 mg
Uses: Supplement

Norco 5/325:
hydrocodone 5 mg
acetaminophen 325 mg
Uses: Analgesic, opioid, nonopioid

Norco:
hydrocodone 10 mg
acetaminophen 325 mg
Uses: Analgesic, opioid, nonopioid

Norgesic:
orphenadrine 25 mg
aspirin 385 mg
caffeine 30 mg
Uses: Skeletal muscle relaxant, analgesic

Norgesic Forte:
orphenadrine 50 mg
aspirin 770 mg
caffeine 60 mg
Uses: Skeletal muscle relaxant, analgesic

Novacet Lotion:
sodium sulfacetamine 10%
sulfur 5%
Uses: Acne agent

Novafed A:
pseudoephedrine 120 mg
chlorpheniramine 8 mg
Uses: Adrenergic, antihistamine

Novahistone Elixir:
Per 5 ml:
phenylephrine 5 mg
chlorpheniramine 2 mg
alcohol 5%
Uses: Antihistamine

Novo-Gesic🍁 C8:
acetaminophen 300 mg
codeine 8 mg
caffeine 15 mg
Uses: Analgesic

NuLytely:
PEG 3350/420 g
sodium bicarbonate 5.72 g
sodium chloride 11.2 g
potassium chloride 1.48 g
Uses: Laxative

NyQuil Hot Therapy:
Per packet:
acetaminophen 1000 mg
pseudoephedrine 60 mg
dextromethorphan 30 mg
doxylamine 12.5 mg
Uses: Analgesic, adrenergic, antitussive

NyQuil Nightime Cold/Flu Medicine Liquid:
Per 5 ml:
pseudoephedrine 10 mg
doxylamine 1.25 mg
dextromethorphan 5 mg
acetaminophen 167 mg
25% alcohol
Uses: Adrenergic, antitussive, analgesic

Octicair Otic Suspension:
hydrocortisone 1%
neomycin 5 mg/ml
polymyxin B 10,000 units/ml
Uses: Otic antiinflammatory, antiinfective

Opcon-A Ophthalmic Solution:
0.027% naphazoline
0.315% pheniramine
Uses: Ophth vasoconstrictor

Ornade Spansules:
phenylpropanolamine 75 mg
chlorpheniramine 12 mg
Uses: Antihistamine, decongestant

Ornex:
pseudoephedrine 30 mg
acetaminophen 500 mg
Uses: Adrenergic, analgesic

Ornex No Drowsiness Caplets:
acetaminophen 325 mg
pseudoephedrine 30 mg
Uses: Adrenergic, analgesic

Orphengesic:
orphenadrine 25 mg
aspirin 385 mg
caffeine 30 mg
Uses: Analgesic

Orphengesic Forte:
orphenadrine 50 mg
aspirin 770 mg
caffeine 60 mg
Uses: Analgesic

Ortho-cept:
ethinyl estradiol 30 mcg
desogestrel 0.15 mg
Uses: Oral contraceptive

Ortho-cyclen:
ethinyl estradiol 35 mcg
norgestimate 0.25 mg
Uses: Oral contraceptive

Ortho-Novum 7/7/7:
Phase I:
0.5 mg norethindrone
35 mcg ethinyl estradiol
Phase II:
0.75 mg norethindrone
35 mcg ethinyl estradiol
Phase III:
1 mg norethinidrone
35 mcg estradiol
Uses: Oral contraceptive

Ortho-Prefest:
estradiol 1 mg (15)
norgestimate 0.09 mg (15)
Uses: Menopause

Ovcon-50:
ethinyl estradiol 50 mcg
norethindrone 1 mg
Uses: Oral contraceptive

✤Oxycocet:
acetaminophen 325 mg
oxycodone 5 mg
Uses: Analgesic

P-A-C Analgesic:
aspirin 400 mg
caffeine 32 mg
Uses: Nonnarcotic analgesic

Pain-X Topical:
0.05% capsaicin
5% menthol
4% camphor
Uses: Top analgesic

Pamprin Maximum Pain Relief:
acetaminophen 250 mg
pamabrom 25 mg
magnesium salicylate 250 mg
Uses: Analgesic

Pamprin Multi-Symptom:
acetaminophen 500 mg
pamabrom 25 mg
pyrilamine 15 mg
Uses: Analgesic

Panacet 5/500:
hydrocodone 5 mg
acetaminophen 500 mg
Uses: Analgesic

Panasal 5/500:
hydrocodone 5 mg
aspirin 500 mg
Uses: Analgesic

Pancrease Capsules:
amylase 20,000 units
protease 25,000 units
lipase 4500 units (microspheres)
Uses: Digestive enzyme

Pedia Care Cold-Allergy Chewable:
pseudoephedrine 15 mg
chlorpheniramine 1 mg
Uses: Adrenergic, antihistamine

Pedia Care Cough-Cold Liquid:
Per 5 ml:
pseudoephedrine 15 mg
chlorpheniramine 1 mg

dextromethorphan 5 mg
Uses: Adrenergic, antihistamine, antitussive

Pedia Care NightRest Cough-Cold Liquid:
Per 5 ml:
pseudoephedrine 15 mg
chlorpheniramine 1 mg
dextromethorphan 7.5 mg
Uses: Adrenergic, antihistamine, antitussive

Pediacof Syrup:
Per 5 ml:
codeine 5 mg
phenylephrine 2.5 mg
chlorpheniramine 0.75 mg
potassium iodide 75 mg
5% alcohol
Uses: Opioid, narcotic analgesic, antihistamine

Pediazole Suspension:
Per 5 ml:
erythromycin 200 mg
sulfiSOXAZOLE 600 mg
Uses: Antiinfective

Pepcid Complete:
calcium carbonate 800 mg
magnesium hydroxide 165 mg
famotidine 10 mg
Uses: Antiulcer agent

Percocet 2.5/325:
oxycodone 2.5 mg
acetaminophen 325 mg
Uses: Analgesic

Percocet 5/325:
oxycodone 5 mg
acetaminophen 325 mg
Uses: Analgesic

Percocet 7.5/500:
oxycodone 7.5 mg
acetaminophen 500 mg
Uses: Analgesic

Percocet 10/650:
oxycodone 10 mg
acetaminophen 650 mg
Uses: Analgesic

Percodan:
oxycodone 4.88 mg
aspirin 325 mg
Uses: Analgesic

Percodan-Demi:
aspirin 325 mg
oxycodone HCl 2.25 mg
oxycodone terephthalate 0.19 mg
Uses: Analgesic

Percodan-Demi:
aspirin 325 mg
oxycodone 2.5 mg
Uses: Analgesic

Percogesic:
phenyltoloxamine 30 mg
acetaminophen 325 mg
Uses: Analgesic

Perdiem Granules:
Per teaspoon:
senna 0.74 g
psyllium 3.25 g
sodium 1.8 mg
potassium 35.5 mg
Uses: Laxative

Peri-Colace:
docusate sodium 100 mg
casanthranol 30 mg
Uses: Laxative

Peri-Colace Syrup:
Per 15 ml:
docusate sodium 60 mg
casanthranol 30 mg
Uses: Laxative

Phenaphen w/Codeine No. 3:
aspirin 325 mg
codeine 30 mg
Uses: Analgesic

Phenaphen w/Codeine No. 4:
aspirin 325 mg
codeine 60 mg
Uses: Analgesic

Phenerbel-S:
ergotamine tartrate 0.6 mg
belladonna alkaloids 0.2 mg

phenobarbital 40 mg
Uses: α-Adrenergic blocker, anticholinergic

Phenergan VC Syrup:
Per 5 ml:
phenylephrine 5 mg
promethazine 6.25 mg
Uses: Adrenergic, antihistamine

Phenergan VC w/Codeine Syrup:
Per 5 ml:
phenylephrine 5 mg
promethazine 6.25 mg
codeine 10 mg
Uses: Adrenergic, antihistamine, opioid analgesic

Phenergan w/Codeine Syrup:
Per 5 ml:
promethazine 6.25 mg
codeine 10 mg
Uses: Antihistamine, analgesic

Pherazine DM Syrup:
Per 5 ml:
dextromethorphan 15 mg
promethazine 6.25 mg
7% alcohol
Uses: Antitussive, antihistamine

Phillips' Laxative Gelcaps:
docusate sodium 83 mg
phenolphthalein 90 mg
Uses: Laxative

PMB-400:
conjugated estrogens 0.45 mg
meprobamate 400 mg
Uses: Oral contraceptive

Polaramine Expectorant Liquid:
Per 5 ml:
guaifenesin 100 mg
dexchlorpheniramine 2 mg
pseudoephedrine 20 mg
7.5% alcohol
Uses: Expectorant

Polycillin-PRB Oral Suspension:
Per single dose:
ampicillin 3.5 g
probenecid 1 g
Uses: Antiinfective

Polycitra Syrup:
Per 5 ml:
potassium citrate 550 mg
sodium citrate 500 mg
citric acid 334 mg
Uses: Laxative

Poly-Histine Elixir:
Per 5 ml:
pheniramine 4 mg
pyrilamine 4 mg
phenyltoloxamine 4 mg
4% alcohol
Uses: Antihistamine

Polysporin Topical Ointment:
Per gram:
polymyxin B 10,000 units
bacitracin zinc 500 units
Uses: Top antiinfective

Polysporin Ophthalmic Ointment:
Per gram:
polymyxin B 10,000 units
bacitracin zinc 500 units
Uses: Ophthalmic antiinfective

Polytrim Ophthalmic Solution:
Per ml:
trimethoprim 1 mg
polymyxin B 10,000 units
Uses: Ophthalmic antiinfective

Premphase:
In a compliance package:
conjugated estrogens 0.625 mg
medroxyprogesterone 5 mg
Uses: Menopause

Prempro:
In a compliance package:
conjugated estrogens 0.625 mg
medroxyPROGESTERone 2.5 mg
Uses: Menopause

Premsyn PMS:
acetaminophen 500 mg
pamabrom 25 mg
pyrilamine 15 mg
Uses: Analgesic

Prevpac:
In a compliance package:
amoxicillin 500 mg caps

clarithromycin 500 mg tabs
lansoprazole 30 mg caps
Uses: Antiinfective

Primatene:
theophylline 130 mg
epHEDrine 24 mg
phenobarbital 7.5 mg
Uses: Bronchodilator, barbiturate

Primaxin 250 mg IV for Injection:
imipenem 250 mg
cilastatin sodium 250 mg
Uses: Antiinfective

Primaxin 500 mg IV for Injection:
imipenem 500 mg
cilastatin sodium 500 mg
Uses: Antiinfective

Prinzide 10-12.5:
lisinopril 10 mg
hydrochlorothiazide 12.5 mg
Uses: Antihypertensive

Prinzide 20-12.5:
lisinopril 20 mg
hydrochlorothiazide 12.5 mg
Uses: Antihypertensive

Prinzide 20-25:
lisinopril 20 mg
hydrochlorothiazide 25 mg
Uses: Antihypertensive

Probampacin Oral Suspension:
Per single dose:
ampicillin 3.5 g
probenecid 1 g
Uses: Antiinfective

Proben-C:
colchicine 0.5 mg
probenecid 500 mg
Uses: Antigout agent

Proctofoam-HC Aerosol Foam:
1% hydrocortisone
1% pramoxine
Uses: Topical corticosteroid

Propacet 100:
propoxyphene-N 100 mg
acetaminophen 650 mg
Uses: Analgesic

Pseudo-Chlor:
pseudoephedrine 120 mg
chlorpheniramine 8 mg
Uses: Antihistamine

Pseudo-Gest Plus:
pseudoephedrine 60 mg
chlorpheniramine 4 mg
Uses: Antihistamine

P-V-Tussin:
phenindamine 25 mg
guaifenesin 200 mg
hydrocodone 5 mg
Uses: Antihistamine, analgesic

P-V-Tussin Syrup:
Per 5 ml:
chlorpheniramine 2 mg
phenindamine 5 mg
phenylephrine 5 mg
pyrilamine 6 mg
Uses: Antihistamine, decongestant

Quadrinal:
epHEDrine 24 mg
theophylline 65 mg
potassium iodide 320 mg
phenobarbital 24 mg
Uses: Adrenergic, bronchodilator, barbiturate

Quelidrine Cough Syrup:
Per 5 ml:
dextromethorphan 10 mg
phenylephrine 5 mg
epHEDrine 5 mg
chlorpheniramine 2 mg
ammonium chloride 40 mg
ipecac 0.005 ml
Uses: Expectorant, adrenergic, antihistamine

Quibron-300:
theophylline 300 mg
guaifenesin 180 mg
Uses: Bronchodilator, expectorant

Quibron:
theophylline 150 mg
guaifenesin 90 mg
Uses: Bronchodilator, expectorant

R&C Shampoo:
0.3% pyrethrins
3% piperonyl butoxide
Uses: Scabicide, pediculicide

Rauzide:
bendroflumethiazide 4 mg
powdered *Rauwolfia serpentina* 50 mg
Uses: Diuretic, antihypertensive

Rebetron:
interferon alfa-2b/oral ribavarine 200 mg
Uses: Biologic response modifier, antiviral

Regroton:
chlorthalidone 50 mg
reserpine 0.25 mg
Uses: Diuretic, antihypertensive

Regulace:
docusate sodium 100 mg
casanthranol 30 mg
Uses: Laxative

Renese-R:
polythiazide 2 mg
reserpine 0.25 mg
Uses: Diuretic, antihypertensive

Repan:
acetaminophen 325 mg
caffeine 40 mg
butalbital 50 mg
Uses: Nonopioid analgesic

Respahist:
pseudoephedrine 60 mg
brompheniramine 6 mg
Uses: Adrenergic, antihistamine

Respaire-60:
guaifenesin 200 mg
pseudoephedrine 60 mg
Uses: Expectorant, adrenergic

RID Mousse:
pyrethrins 0.33%
piperonyl butoxide 4%
Uses: Scabicide, pediculicide

RID Shampoo:
0.3% pyrethrins
3% piperonyl butoxide
Uses: Scabicide, pediculicide

Rifamate:
isoniazid 150 mg
rifampin 300 mg
Uses: Antitubercular, antileprotic

Rifater:
rifampin 120 mg
isoniazid 50 mg
pyrazinamide 300 mg
Uses: Antitubercular

Rimactane/INH Dual Pack:
isoniazid 300 mg (30 tabs)
rifampin 300 mg (60 caps)
Uses: Antitubercular

Riopan Plus Suspension:
Per 5 ml:
magaldrate 540 mg
simethicone 40 mg
Uses: Antacid, adsorbent, antiflatulent

Robaxisal:
methocarbamol 400 mg
aspirin 325 mg
Uses: Skeletal muscle relaxant, analgesic

Robitussin A-C Syrup:
Per 5 ml:
codeine 10 mg
guaifenesin 100 mg
3.5% alcohol
Uses: Analgesic, expectorant

Robitussin Cold & Cough Liqui-Gels:
pseudoephedrine 30 mg
guaifenesin 200 mg
dextromethorphan 10 mg
Uses: Antitussive, expectorant

Robitussin-DAC Syrup:
Per 5 ml:
codeine 10 mg
guaifenesin 100 mg
pseudoephedrine 30 mg
1.4% alcohol
Uses: Analgesic, expectorant, adrenergic

Robitussin-DM Liquid:
Per 5 ml:
guaifenesin 100 mg
dextromethorphan 10 mg
Uses: Expectorant, antitussive

Robitussin Maximum Strength Cough and Cold Liquid:
dextromethorphan 15 mg
pseudoephedrine 30 mg
Uses: Antitussive, adrenergic

Robitussin Night Relief Liquid:
dextromethorphan 5 mg
pyrilamine 8.3 mg
pseudoephedrine 10 mg
acetaminophen 108.3 mg
Uses: Antitussive, adrenergic

Robitussin Pediatric Cough & Cold Liquid:
Per 5 ml:
pseudoephedrine 15 mg
dextromethorphan 7.5 mg
Uses: Antitussive, adrenergic

Robitussin-PE Syrup:
guaifenesin 100 mg
pseudoephedrine 30 mg
1.4% alcohol
Uses: Expectorant, adrenergic

Robitussin Severe Congestion Liqui-Gels:
guaifenesin 200 mg
pseudoephedrine 30 mg
Uses: Expectorant, adrenergic

Rolaids Calcium Rich:
magnesium hydroxide 80 mg
calcium carbonate 412 mg
Uses: Antacid, adsorbent, antiflatulent

Rondec:
pseudoephedrine 60 mg
carbinoxamine 4 mg
Uses: Adrenergic

Rondec DM Drops:
Per ml:
pseudoephedrine 25 mg
carbinoxamine 2 mg
dextromethorphan 4 mg
Uses: Adrenergic, antitussive

Rondec DM Syrup:
Per 5 ml:
pseudoephedrine 60 mg
carbinoxamine 4 mg
dextromethorphan 15 mg
Uses: Adrenergic, antitussive

Rondec Oral Drops:
Per 5 ml:
pseudoephedrine 25 mg
carbinoxamine 2 mg
Uses: Adrenergic

Roxicet:
Per 5 ml:
acetaminophen 325 mg
oxycodone 5 mg
Uses: Opioid analgesic

Roxicet 5/500:
oxycodone 5 mg
acetaminophen 500 mg
Uses: Opioid analgesic

Roxicet Oral Solution:
Per 5 ml:
acetaminophen 325 mg
oxycodone 5 mg
Uses: Analgesic

Roxiprin:
aspirin 325 mg
oxycodone HCl 4.5 mg
oxycodone terephthalate 0.38 mg
Uses: Analgesic

Ru-Tuss DE:
pseudoephedrine 120 mg
guaifenesin 600 mg
Uses: Adrenergic, expectorant

Ru-Tuss Expectorant Liquid:
Per 5 ml:
guaifenesin 100 mg
pseudoephedrine 30 mg
dextromethorphan 10 mg
10% alcohol
Uses: Adrenergic, expectorant, antitussive

Ru-Tuss with Hydrocodone Liquid:
Per 5 ml:
hydrocodone: 1.7 mg
phenylephrine 5 mg
pyrilamine 3.3 mg
pheniramine 3.3 mg
phenylpropanolamine 3.3 mg
alcohol 5%
Uses: Antihistamine, analgesic, decongestant

Ryna-C Liquid:
Per 5 ml:
pseudoephedrine 30 mg
chlorpheniramine 2 mg
codeine 10 mg
Uses: Adrenergic, antihistamine, analgesic

Ryna Liquid:
Per 5 ml:
pseudoephedrine 30 mg
chlorpheniramine 2 mg
Uses: Adrenergic, antihistamine

Rynatan:
phenylephrine 25 mg
chlorpheniramine 8 mg
pyrilamine 25 mg
Uses: Adrenergic, antihistamine

Rynatan Pediatric Suspension:
Per 5 ml:
phenylephrine 5 mg
chlorpheniramine 2 mg
pyrilamine 12.5 mg
Uses: Adrenergic, antihistamine

Rynatuss:
epHEDrine 10 mg
carbetapentane 60 mg
chlorpheniramine 5 mg
phenylephrine 10 mg
Uses: Adrenergic, antihistamine

Saleto Tablets:
115 mg acetaminophen
210 mg aspirin
65 mg salicylamide
16 mg caffeine
Uses: Nonopioid analgesic

Salutensin:
hydroflumethiazide 50 mg
reserpine 0.125 mg
Uses: Antihypertensive

Salutensin Demi:
hydroflumethiazide 25 mg
reserpine 0.125 mg
Uses: Antihypertensive

Scot-Tussin DM Liquid:
Per 5 ml:
chlorpheniramine 2 mg
dextromethorphan 15 mg
Uses: Antihistamine, antitussive

Scot-Tussin Original 5-Action Liquid:
phenylephrine 4.2 mg
pheniramine 13.3 mg
sodium citrate 83.3 mg
sodium salicylate 83.3 mg
caffeine citrate 25 mg
Uses: Adrenergic, analgesic

Scot-Tussin Senior Clear Liquid:
Per 5 ml:
guaifenesin 200 mg
dextromethorphan 15 mg
Uses: Antitussive, expectorant

Sedapap-10:
acetaminophen 650 mg
butalbital 50 mg
Uses: Analgesic, barbiturate

Semprex-D:
acrivastine 8 mg
pseudoephedrine 60 mg
Uses: Adrenergic, bronchodilator

Senokot-S:
docusate 50 mg
senna concentrate 187 mg
Uses: Laxative

Septra:
sulfamethoxazole 400 mg
trimethroprim 80 mg
Uses: Antiinfective

Septra DS:
sulfamethoxazole 800 mg
trimethroprim 160 mg
Uses: Antiinfective

Septra I.V. for Injection:
Per 5 ml:
trimethoprim 80 mg
sulfamethoxazole 400 mg
Uses: Antiinfective

Septra Suspension:
Per 5 ml:
trimethoprim 40 mg
sulfamethoxazole 200 mg
Uses: Antiinfective

Ser-A-Gen:
hydrochlorothiazide 15 mg
hydralazine 25 mg
reserpine 0.1 mg
Uses: Antihypertensive

Ser-Ap-Es:
hydrochlorothiazide 15 mg
reserpine 0.1 mg
hydrALAZINE 25 mg
Uses: Diuretic, antihypertensive

Silafed Syrup:
Per 5 ml:
pseudoephedrine 30 mg
triprolidine 1.25 mg
Uses: Adrenergic, antihistamine

Silaminic Cold Syrup:
Per 5 ml:
phenylpropanolamine 12.5 mg
chlorpheniramine 2 mg
Uses: Antihistamine, decongestant

Sinarest Extra Strength:
pseudoephedrine 30 mg
chlorpheniramine 2 mg
acetaminophen 500 mg
Uses: Adrenergic, antihistamine, analgesic

Sinarest No Drowsiness:
pseudoephedrine 30 mg
acetaminophen 500 mg
Uses: Adrenergic, analgesic

Sinarest Sinus:
pseudoephedrine 30 mg
chlorpheniramine 2 mg
acetaminophen 325 mg
Uses: Adrenergic, antihistamine, analgesic

Sine-Aid IB:
pseudoephedrine 30 mg
ibuprofen 200 mg
Uses: Adrenergic, analgesic

Sine-Aid Maximum Strength:
pseudoephedrine 30 mg
acetaminophen 500 mg
Uses: Adrenergic, analgesic

Sinemet 10/100:
carbidopa 10 mg
levodopa 100 mg
Uses: Antiparkinsonian

Sinemet 25/100:
carbidopa 25 mg
levodopa 100 mg
Uses: Antiparkinsonian

Sinemet 25/250:
carbidopa 25 mg
levodopa 250 mg
Uses: Antiparkinsonian

Sinemet CR 25-100:
carbidopa 25 mg
levodopa 100 mg
Uses: Antiparkinsonian

Sinemet CR 50-200:
carbidopa 50 mg
levodopa 200 mg
Uses: Antiparkinsonian

Sine-Off Maximum Strength No Drowsiness Formula Caplets:
pseudoephedrine 30 mg
acetaminophen 500 mg
Uses: Adrenergic, analgesic

Sine-Off Sinus Medicine:
pseudoephedrine 30 mg
chlorpheniramine 2 mg
acetaminophen 500 mg
Uses: Adrenergic, antihistamine, analgesic

Sinus-Relief:
acetaminophen 325 mg
pseudoephedrine 30 mg
Uses: Nonopioid analgesic

Sinutab:
acetaminophen 325 mg
chlorpheniramine 2 mg
pseudoephedrine 30 mg
Uses: Nonopioid analgesic

Sinutab Maximum Strength Sinus Allergy:
acetaminophen 500 mg
pseudoephedrine 30 mg
chlorpheniramine 2 mg
Uses: Analgesic, adrenergic, antihistamine

Sinutab Maximum Strength Without Drowsiness:
acetaminophen 500 mg
pseudoephedrine 30 mg
Uses: Analgesic, adrenergic

Sinutab Non-Drying:
pseudoepedrine 30 mg
guaifenesin 200 mg
Uses: Adrenergic, expectorant

Slo-Phyllin GG Syrup:
theophylline 150 mg
guaifenesin 90 mg
Uses: Bronchodilator, expectorant

Slow-Salt-K:
sodium chloride 410 mg
potassium chloride 15 mg
Uses: Potassium, sodium supplement

Solage:
mequinol 2%
tretinoin 0.01%
Uses: Antineoplastic

Soma Compound w/Codeine:
carisoprodol 200 mg
aspirin 325 mg
codeine 16 mg
Uses: Skeletal muscle relaxant

Synophylate-GG Syrup:
theophylline 150 mg
guaifenesin 100 mg
alcohol 15%
Uses: Bronchodilator, expectorant

Soma Compound:
carisoprodol 200 mg
aspirin 325 mg
Uses: Skeletal muscle relaxant, analgesic

Spec-T Lozenge:
dextromethorphan 10 mg
benzocaine 10 mg
Uses: Antitussive, topical anesthetic

Stalevo 50:
carbidopa 12.5 mg
levodopa 50 mg
entacapone 200 mg
Uses: Parkinsonism

Stalevo 100:
carbidopa 25 mg
levodopa 100 mg
entacapone 200 mg
Uses: Parkinsonism

Stalevo 150:
carbidopa 37.5 mg
levodopa 150 mg
entacapone 200 mg
Uses: Parkinsonism

Sudafed Cold & Allergy:
pseudoephedrine 60 mg
chlorpheniramine 4 mg
Uses: Adrenergic, antihistamine

Sudafed Cold & Cough Liquicaps:
pseudoephedrine 30 mg
dextromethorphan 10 mg
guaifenesin 100 mg
acetaminophen 250 mg
Uses: Adrenergic, antitussive, expectorant, analgesic

Sudafed Cold & Sinus:
pseudoephedrine 30 mg

acetaminophen 325 mg
Uses: Adrenergic, analgesic

Sudafed Plus:
pseudoephedrine 60 mg
chlorpheniramine 4 mg
Uses: Adrenergic, antihistamine

Sudafed Severe Cold:
pseudoephedrine 30 mg
dextromethorphan 15 mg
Uses: Adrenergic, antitussive

Sudafed Sinus Maximum Strength:
pseudoephedrine 30 mg
acetaminophen 500 mg
Uses: Adrenergic, analgesic

Sudal 60/500:
pseudoephedrine 60 mg
guaifenesin 500 mg
Uses: Adrenergic, expectorant

Sudal 120/600:
pseudoephedrine 120 mg
guaifenesin 600 mg
Uses: Adrenergic, expectorant

Sulfimycin Suspension:
Per 5 ml:
erythromycin 200 mg
sulfiSOXAZOLE 600 mg
Uses: Macrolide antiinfective

Sultrin Triple Sulfa Vaginal Cream:
3.42% sulfathiazole
2.86% sulfacetamine
3.7% sulfabenzamide
Uses: Antiinfective

Sultrin Triple Sulfa Vaginal Tablets:
sulfathiazole 172.5 mg
sulfacetamide 143.75
sulfabenzamide 184 mg
Uses: Antiinfective

Synalgos-DC:
aspirin 356.4 mg
caffeine 30 mg
dihydrocodeine 16 mg
Uses: Analgesic

Synercid:
quinupristin 150 mg
dalfopristin 350 mg
Uses: Antiinfective

Syntest D.S.:
esterified estrogens 1.25 mg
methylTESTOSTERone 2.5 mg
Uses: Menopause

Syntest H.S.:
esterified estrogens 0.625 mg
methylTESTOSTERone 1.25 mg
Uses: Menopause

Talacen:
acetaminophen 650 mg
pentazocine 25 mg
Uses: Analgesic

Talwin Compound:
aspirin 325 mg
pentazocine 12.5 mg
Uses: Analgesic

Talwin NX:
pentazocine 50 mg
naloxone 0.5 mg
Uses: Analgesic, opioid antagonist

Tarka 182:
trandolapril 2 mg (immed rel)
verapamil 180 mg (sus rel)
Uses: Antihypertensive, calcium channel blocker

Tarka 241:
trandolapril 1 mg (immed rel)
verapamil 240 mg (sus rel)
Uses: Antihypertensive, calcium channel blocker

Tarka 242:
trandolapril 2 mg (immed rel)
verapamil 240 mg (sus rel)
Uses: Antihypertensive, calcium channel blocker

Tarka 244:
trandolapril 4 mg (immed rel)
verapamil 240 mg (sus rel)
Uses: Antihypertensive, calcium channel blocker

Tavist Allergy / Sinus Headache:
clemastine 0.335 mg

pseudoephedrine 30 mg
acetaminophen 500 mg
Uses: Antihistamine, adrenergic, analgesic

Tavist Sinus:
acetaminophen 500 mg
pseudoephedrine 30 mg
Uses: Analgesic, adrenergic

✤Tecnal:
aspirin 330 mg
caffeine 40 mg
butalbital 50 mg
Uses: Nonopioid analgesic

Teczem:
enalapril 5 mg (extended release)
diltiazem 180 mg (extended release)
Uses: Antihypertensive, calcium channel blocker

Tedrigen:
epHEDrine 22.5 mg
theophylline 120 mg
phenobarbital 7.5 mg
Uses: Adrenergic, bronchodilator, barbiturate

Tegrin-LT Shampoo:
0.33% pyrethrins
3.15% piperonyl butoxide
Uses: Scabicide, pediculicide

Tenoretic 50:
atenolol 50 mg
chlorthalidone 25 mg
Uses: Antihypertensive

Tenoretic 100:
atenolol 100 mg
chlorthalidone 25 mg
Uses: Antihypertensive

Terra-Cortril Ophthalmic Suspension:
1.5% hydrocortisone acetate
0.5% oxytetracycline
Uses: Ophthalmic antiinflammatory, antiinfective

Terramycin w/Polymycin B Sulfate Ophthalmic Ointment:
Per gram:
polymyxin B 10,000 units
oxytetracycline 5 mg
Uses: Ophthalmic antiinfective

T-Gesic:
hydrocodone 5 mg
acetaminophen 500 mg
Uses: Analgesic

Theodrine:
epHEDrine 22.5 mg
theophylline 120 mg
Uses: Adrenergic, bronchodilator

Thera-Flu, Flu & Cold Medicine Powder:
Per packet:
pseudoephedrine 60 mg
chlorpheniramine 4 mg
acetaminophen 650 mg
Uses: Adrenergic, antihistamine, analgesic

Thera-Flu, Flu, Cold & Cough Powder:
Per packet:
pseudoephedrine 60 mg
chlorpheniramine 4 mg
dextromethorphan 20 mg
acetaminophen 650 mg
Uses: Adrenergic, antihistamine, antitussive, analgesic

Thera-Flu NightTime Powder:
Per packet:
pseudoephedrine 60 mg
chlorpheniramine 4 mg
dextromethorphan 30 mg
acetaminophen 1000 mg
Uses: Adrenergic, antihistamine, antitussive, analgesic

Thera-Flu Non-Drowsy Flu, Cold & Cough Maximum Strength Powder:
Per packet:
pseudoephedrine 60 mg
dextromethorphan 30 mg
acetaminophen 1000 mg
Uses: Adrenergic, antitussive, analgesic

Thera-Flu Non-Drowsy Formula Maximum Strength Caplets:
pseudoephedrine 30 mg
dextromethorphan 15 mg
acetaminophen 500 mg
Uses: Adrenergic, antitussive, analgesic

Timentin for Injection:
Per 3.1-g vial:
ticarcillin 3 g
clavulanic acid 0.1 g
Uses: Antiinfective

Timolide 10/25:
timolol 10 mg
hydrochlorothiazide 25 mg
Uses: Antihypertensive

Titralac Plus:
calcium carbonate 420 mg
simethicone 21 mg
Uses: Antacid, adsorbent, antiflatulent

Tobra Dex Ophthalmic Suspension/Ointment:
tobramycin 0.3%
dexamethasone 0.1%
Uses: Ophthalmic antiinfective, antiinflammatory

Triacin-C Cough Syrup:
Per 5 ml:
codeine 10 mg
pseudoephedrine 30 mg
triprolidine 1.25 mg
Uses: Analgesic, adrenergic, antihistamine

Triad:
acetaminophen 325 mg
caffeine 40 mg
butalbital 50 mg
Uses: Nonopioid analgesic

Tri-Hydroserpine:
hydrALAZINE 25 mg
hydrochlorothiazide 15 mg
reserpine 0.1 mg
Uses: Antihypertensive

Tri-Levlen:
Phase I:
levonorgestrel 0.05 mg
ethinyl estradiol 30 mcg
Phase II:
levonorgestrel 0.075 mg
ethinyl estradiol 40 mcg;
Phase III:
levonorgestrel 0.125 mg
ethinyl estradiol 30 mcg
Uses: Oral contraceptive

Triaminic AM Cough & Decongestant Formula Liquid:
Per 5 ml:
pseudoephedrine 15 mg
dextromethorphan 7.5 mg
Uses: Adrenergic, antitussive

Triaminic Nite Light Liquid:
Per 5 ml:
pseudoephedrine 15 mg
chlorpheniramine 1 mg
dextromethorphan 7.5 mg
Uses: Adrenergic, antihistamine, antitussive

Triaminic Sore Throat Formula Liquid:
Per 5 ml:
pseudoephedrine 15 mg
dextromethorphan 7.5 mg
acetaminophen 160 mg
Uses: Adrenergic, antitussive

Triavil 2-10:
perphenazine 2 mg
amitriptyline 10 mg
Uses: Antipsychotic, antidepressant

Triavil 2-25:
perphenazine 2 mg
amitriptyline 25 mg
Uses: Antipsychotic, antidepressant

Triavil 4-10:
perphenazine 4 mg
amitriptyline 10 mg

Triavil 4-25:
perphenazine 4 mg
amitriptyline 25 mg
Uses: Antipsychotic, antidepressant

Triavil 4-50:
perphenazine 4 mg
amitriptyline 50 mg
Uses: Antipsychotic, antidepressant

Trinalin Repetabs:
azatadine maleate 1 mg
pseudoephedrine 120 mg
Uses: Antihistamine

Triphasil:
Phase I:
levonorgestrel 0.05 mg
ethinyl estradiol 30 mcg
Phase II:
levonorgestrel 0.075 mg
ethinyl estradiol 40 mcg
Phase III:
levonorgestrel 0.125 mg
ethinyl estradiol 30 mcg
Uses: Oral contraceptive

Triple Antibiotic Ophthalmic Ointment:
Per gram:
polymyxin B 10,000 units
neomycin 3.5 mg
bacitracin 400 units
Uses: Antiinfective

Triprolidine/Pseudoephedrine Syrup (generic):
Per 5 ml
triprolidine 1.25 mg
pseudoephedrine 50 mg
Uses: Antihistamine, decongestant

Triprolidine/Pseudoephedrine Tablets (generic):
triprolidine 2.5 mg
pseudoephedrine 60 mg
Uses: Antihistamine, decongestant

Triposed Tablets:
triprolidine 150 mg
pseudoephedrine 60 mg
Uses: Decongestant, antihistamine

Trizivir:
300 mg abacavir
150 mg lamivudine
300 mg zidovudine
Uses: HIV

Tuinal 100 mg:
amobarbital 50 mg
secobarbital 50 mg
Uses: Sedative-hypnotic

Tuinal 200 mg:
amobarbital 100 mg
secobarbital 100 mg
Uses: Sedative-hypnotic

Tusibron-DM Syrup:
Per 5 ml:
guaifenesin 100 mg
dextromethorphan 15 mg
Uses: Expectorant, antitussive

Tussionex Pennkinetic Suspension:
Per 5 ml:
chlorpheniramine 8 mg
hydrocodone 10 mg
Uses: Antihistamine, analgesic

Tussi-Organidin NR Liquid:
Per 5 ml:
codeine 10 mg
guaifenesin 100 mg
Uses: Analgesic, expectorant

Tussi-Organidin DM NR Liquid:
Per 5 ml:
guaifenesin 100 mg
dextromethorphan 10 mg
Uses: Expectorant, antitussive

Twinrix:
hepatitis A vaccine
hepatitis B vaccine
Uses: Vaccine

Two-Dyne:
acetaminophen 325 mg
caffeine 40 mg
butalbital 50 mg
Uses: Nonopioid analgesic

Tylenol Allergy Sinus, Maximum Strength Gelcaps:
acetaminophen 500 mg
chlorpheniramine 2 mg
pseudoephedrine 30 mg
Uses: Antihistamine, adrenergic, analgesic

Tylenol Children's Cold:
acetaminophen 80 mg
chlorpheniramine 0.5 mg
pseudoephedrine 7.5 mg
Uses: Antihistamine, adrenergic, analgesic

Tylenol Children's Cold Liquid:
Per 5 ml:
acetaminophen 160 mg
chlorpheniramine 1 mg
pseudoephedrine 15 mg
Uses: Antihistamine, adrenergic, analgesic

Tylenol Children's Cold Multi-Symptom Plus Cough Liquid:
Per 5 ml:
acetaminophen 160 mg
dextromethorphan 5 mg
chlorpheniramine 1 mg
pseudoephedrine 15 mg
Uses: Antihistamine, adrenergic, analgesic

Tylenol Children's Cold Plus Cough Chewable:
acetaminophen 80 mg
pseudoephedrine 7.5 mg
dextromethorphan 2.5 mg
chlorpheniramine 0.5 mg
Uses: Antihistamine, adrenergic, analgesic

Tylenol Cold Multi-Symptom:
acetaminophen 325 mg
chlorpheniramine 2 mg
pseudoephedrine 30 mg
dextromethorphan 15 mg
Uses: Antihistamine, adrenergic, analgesic

Tylenol Cold No Drowsiness:
acetaminophen 325 mg
pseudoephedrine 30 mg
dextromethorphan 15 mg
Uses: Analgesic, adrenergic, antitussive

Tylenol Flu Maximum Strength Gelcaps:
dextromethorphan 15 mg
pseudoephedrine 30 mg
acetaminophen 500 mg
Uses: Analgesic, adrenergic, antitussive

Tylenol Flu NightTime Maximum Strength Gelcaps:
pseudoephedrine 30 mg
chlorpheniramine 2 mg
acetaminophen 500 mg
Uses: Adrenergic, antihistamine, analgesic

Tylenol Flu NightTime Maximum Strength Powder:
pseudoephedrine 60 mg
diphenhydramine 50 mg
acetaminophen 1000 mg
Uses: Adrenergic, antihistamine, analgesic

Tylenol Headache Plus, Extra Strength:
acetaminophen 500 mg
calcium carbonate 250 mg
Uses: Analgesic, antacid

Tylenol Multi-Symptom Cough Liquid:
Per 5 ml:
dextromethorphan 10 mg
acetaminophen 216.7 mg
5% alcohol
Uses: Antitussive, analgesic

Tylenol Multi-Symptom Cough w/Decongestant Liquid:
Per 5 ml:
dextromethorphan 10 mg
acetaminophen 200 mg
pseudoephedrine 20 mg
Uses: Antitussive, analgesic, adrenergic

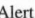

Tylenol Multi-Symptom Hot Medication:
Per packet:
acetaminophen 650 mg
chlorpheniramine 4 mg

pseudoephedrine 60 mg
dextromethorphan 30 mg
Uses: Analgesic, antihistamine, adrenergic, antitussive

Tylenol PM, Extra Strength:
acetaminophen 500 mg
diphenhydrAMINE 25 mg
Uses: Analgesic, antihistamine

Tylenol Severe Allergy:
diphenhydrAMINE 12.5 mg
acetaminophen 500 mg
Uses: Analgesic, antihistamine

Tylenol Sinus Maximum Strength:
pseudoephedrine 30 mg
acetaminophen 500 mg
Uses: Adrenergic, analgesic

Tylenol w/Codeine Elixir:
Per 5 ml:
acetaminophen 120 mg
codeine 12 mg
Uses: Analgesic

Tylenol w/Codeine No. 1:
acetaminophen 300 mg
codeine 7.5 mg
Uses: Analgesic

Tylenol w/Codeine No. 2:
acetaminophen 300 mg
codeine 15 mg
Uses: Analgesic

Tylenol w/Codeine No. 3:
acetaminophen 300 mg
codeine 30 mg
Uses: Analgesic

Tylenol w/Codeine No. 4:
acetaminophen 300 mg
codeine 60 mg
Uses: Analgesic

Tylox:
oxycodone 5 mg
acetaminophen 500 mg
Uses: Analgesic

Tyrodone Liquid:
Per 5 ml:
hydrocodone 5 mg
pseudoephedrine 60 mg
5% alcohol
Uses: Analgesic, adrenergic

Ultracet:
tramadol 37.5 mg
acetaminophen 325 mg
Uses: Analgesic

Unasyn for Injection 3 g:
ampicillin 2 g
sulbactam 1 g
Uses: Antiinfective

Uniretic:
moexipril 7.5 mg
hydrochlorothiazide 12.5 mg
or moexipril 15 mg
hydrochlorothiazide 25 mg
Uses: Antihypertensive, diuretic

Unituss HC Syrup:
hydrocodone 2.5 mg
phenylephrine 5 mg
chlorpheniramine 2 mg
Uses: Analgesic, adrenergic, antihistamine

Urised:
methenamine 40.8 mg
phenylsalicylate 18.1 mg
atropine 0.03 mg
hyoscyamine 0.03 mg
benzoic acid 4.5 mg
methylene blue 5.4 mg
Uses: Antiinfective

Urobiotic 250:
oxytetracycline 250 mg
sulfamethizole 250 mg
phenazopyridine 50 mg
Uses: Antiinfective

Vanquish:
aspirin 227 mg
acetaminophen 194 mg
caffeine 33 mg
aluminum hydroxide 25 mg
magnesium hydroxide 50 mg
Uses: Nonopioid analgesic

Vaseretic 5-12.5:
enalapril 5 mg
hydrochlorthiazide 12.5 mg
Uses: Antihypertensive diuretic

Vaseretic 10-25:
enalapril 10 mg
hydrochlorothiazide 25 mg
Uses: Antihypertensive, diuretic

Vasocidin Ophthalmic Ointment:
sulfacetamide 10%
prednisoLONE 0.5%
Uses: Ophthalmic antiinfective, antiinflammatory

Vasocidin Ophthalmic Solution:
sulfacetamide 10%
prednisoLONE 0.25%
Uses: Ophthalmic antiinfective, antiinflammatory

Vasocon-A Ophthalmic Solution:
naphazoline 0.05%
antazoline 0.5%
Uses: Ophthalmic vasoconstrictor

Vicks 44D Cough & Head Congestion Liquid:
Per 5 ml:
dextromethorphan 10 mg
pseudoephedrine 20 mg
Uses: Antitussive, adrenergic

Vicks 44E Liquid:
Per 5 ml:
dextromethorphan 6.7 mg
guaifenesin 66.7 mg
Uses: Antitussive, expectorant

Vicks 44M Cold, Flu, & Cough LiquiCaps:
dextromethorphan 10 mg
pseudoephedrine 30 mg
chlorpheniramine 2 mg
acetaminophen 250 mg
Uses: Antitussive, adrenergic, antihistamine, analgesic

Vicks 44 Non-Drowsy Cold & Cough LiquiCaps:
dextromethorphan 30 mg
pseudoephedrine 60 mg
Uses: Antitussive, adrenergic

Vicks Children's NyQuil Nighttime Cough/Cold Liquid:
Per 5 ml:
pseudoephedrine 10 mg
chlorpheniramine 0.67 mg
dextromethorphan 5 mg
Uses: Adrenergic, antihistamine, antitussive

Vicks Cough Silencers:
dextromethorphan 2.5 mg
benzocaine 1 mg
Uses: Antitussive, top anesthetic

Vicks DayQuil Liquid:
Per 5 ml:
dextromethorphan 3.3 mg
pseudoephedrine 10 mg
acetaminophen 108.3 mg
guaifenesin 33.3 mg
Uses: Antitussive, adrenergic, analgesic, expectorant

Vicks DayQuil Sinus Pressure & Pain Relief:
pseudoephedrine 30 mg
acetaminophen 500 mg
Uses: Adrenergic, analgesic

Vicks NyQuil Liquicaps:
pseudoephedrine 30 mg
doxylamine 6.25 mg
dextromethorphan 10 mg
acetaminophen 250 mg
Uses: Adrenergic, antihistamine, antitussive, analgesic

Vicks NyQuil Multi-Symptom Cold Flu Relief Liquid:
pseudoephedrine 10 mg
doxylamine 2.1 mg
dextromethorphan 5 mg
acetaminophen 167 mg
Uses: Adrenergic, antihistamine, antitussive, analgesic

Vicks Pediatric Formula 44e Liquid:
Per 5 ml:
dextromethorphan 3.3 mg
guaifenesin 33.3 mg
Uses: Expectorant, antitussive

Vicks Pediatric Formula 44 m Multi-Symptom Cough & Cold Liquid:
pseudoephedrine 10 mg
chlorpheniramine 0.67 mg
dextromethorphan 5 mg
Uses: Adrenergic, antihistamine, antitussive

Vicodin:
acetaminophen 500 mg
hydrocodone 5 mg
Uses: Analgesic

Vicodin ES:
acetaminophen 750 mg
hydrocodone 7.5 mg
Uses: Analgesic

Vicodin HP:
hydrocodone 10 mg
acetaminophen 660 mg
Uses: Analgesic

VicodinTuss:
Per 5 ml:
hydrocodone 5 mg
guaifenesin 100 mg
Uses: Analgesic, expectorant

Vicoprofen:
hydrocodone 7.5 mg
ibuprofen 200 mg
Uses: Analgesic

Wigraine Suppositories:
ergotamine 2 mg
caffeine 100 mg
Uses: α-Adrenergic blocker

Yasmin 28:
ethinyl estadiol 30 mcg
dropirenone 3 mg
Uses: Oral contraceptive

Zestoretic 10/12.5:
lisinopril 10 mg
hydrochlorothiazide 12.5 mg
Uses: Antihypertensive

Zestoretic 20/12.5:
lisinopril 20 mg
hydrochlorothiazide 12.5 mg
Uses: Antihypertensive

Zestoretic 20/25:
lisinopril 20 mg
hydrochlorothiazide 25 mg
Uses: Antihypertensive

Ziac 2.5:
bisoprolol 2.5 mg
hydrochlorothiazide 6.25 mg
Uses: Antihypertensive

Ziac 5:
bisoprolol 5 mg
hydrochlorothiazide 6.25 mg
Uses: Antihypertensive

Ziac 10:
bisoprolol 10 mg
hydrochlorothiazide 6.25 mg
Uses: Antihypertensive

Ziks Cream:
methyl salicylate 12%
menthol 1%
capsaicin 0.025%
Uses: Analgesic, decongestant

Zydone:
hydrocodone 5 mg
acetaminophen 500 mg
Uses: Analgesic

Appendix j

High alert drugs

The Institute for Safe Medication Practices (ISMP) recently compiled a list of the medications with the greatest potential for patient harm if they are used in error. These high-alert medications include drugs in the 19 classes listed below, as well as the specific drugs listed below. To help nurses identify these drugs, in this book each specific drug monograph is highlighted with a light color screen. While care should be taken in giving any medication, nurses are advised to exercise extra precautions when administering these high-risk drugs.

Class/Category of Medications

adrenergic agonists, IV (e.g., epINEPHrine)
adrenergic antagonists, IV (e.g., propranolol)
anesthetic agents, general, inhaled and IV (e.g., propofol)
cardioplegic solutions
chemotherapeutic agents, parenteral and oral
dextrose, hypertonic, 20% or greater
dialysis solutions, peritoneal and hemodialysis
epidural or intrathecal medications
glycoprotein IIb/IIIa inhibitors (e.g., eptifibatide)
hypoglycemics, oral
inotropic medications, IV (e.g., digoxin, milrinone)
liposomal forms of drugs (e.g., liposomal amphotericin B)
moderate sedation agents, IV (e.g., midazolam)
moderate sedation agents, oral, for children (e.g., chloral hydrate)
narcotics/opiates, IV and oral (including liquid concentrates, immediate- and sustained-release)
neuromuscular blocking agents (e.g., succinylcholine)
radiocontrast agents, IV
thrombolytics/fibrinolytics, IV (e.g., tenecteplase)
total parenteral nutrition solutions

Individual Medications

abciximab
adenosine
aldesleukin
alteplase
amiodarone
anistreplase
antihemophilic factor
antithrombin III
ardeparin
argatroban
arsenic trioxide
asparaginase
atropine
basiliximab
bivalirudin
bleomycin
bretylium
busulfan
calfactant
carboplatin
carmustine
cisplatin

coagulation factor VIIa, recombinant
colchicine
cyclophosphamide
cytarabine
dacarbazine
daclizumab
dactinomycin
dalteparin
danaparoid
DAUNOrubicin
dezocine
digoxin
diltiazem
DOPamine
doxacurium
DOXOrubicin
droperidol
enoxaparin
epHEDrine
epINEPHrine
epirubicin
eptifibatide
etoposide
factor IX complex/factor IV
fentanyl
fentanyl/droperidol
fluorouracil
gallamine
gemtuzumab
heparin
hydromorphone
ibutilide
idarubicin
ifosfamide
inamrinone
insulin
irinotecan
ketamine
lepirudin
leuprolide
lidocaine
magnesium sulfate
melphalan
meperidine
methadone
methotrexate
milrinone
mitomycin
mitoxantrone
mivacurium
morphine
nalbuphine
nesiritide
nitroprusside
norepinephrine
oxycodone
oxymorphone
oxytocin
pancuronium
pegaspargase
pentazocine
pentobarbital IV
pentostatin
phenobarbital IV
pipecuronium
plicamycin
poractant alfa
potassium chloride inj concentrate
potassium phosphates inj
propofol
propoxyphene
remifentanil
rocuronium
secobarbital IV
sodium chloride inj, hypertonic
streptokinase
succinylcholine
sufentanil
tenecteplase
thiopental
tinzaparin
topotecan
trastuzumab
tubocurarine
urokinase
vecuronium
vinBLAStine
vinCRIStine
vinorelbine
warfarin

1. Cohen MR, Kilo CM: High-alert medications: safeguarding against errors. In Cohen MR, editor: *Medication errors,* Washington, DC, 1999, American Pharmaceutical Association.

2. High-alert medications and patient safety, *Sentinel Event Alert* 11, Nov 1999.

3. *ISMP's list of high-alert medications,* accessed 2/13/04 at http://www.ismp.org/msaarticles/highalert.htm.

Appendix k

Look-alike/sound-alike drug names

½ Halprin	Halfprin
Accolate	Accutane
Accupril	Accutane
Accupril	Aciphex
Accupril	Monopril
Accutane	Accolate
Accutane	Accupril
acetaZOLAMIDE	acetoHEXAMIDE
acetoHEXAMIDE	acetaZOLAMIDE
Achromycin	actinomycin
Achromycin	aureomycin
Aciphex	Accupril
actinomycin	Achromycin
Acular	ocular lubricants
Adderall	Inderal
adenosine	adenosine phosphate
adenosine phosphate	adenosine
Adriamycin	Aredia
Adriamycin	Idamycin
Aggrastat	Aggrenox
Aggrastat	argatroban
Aggrenox	Aggrastat
Akarpine	atropine
albuterol	atenolol
Aldara	Alora
aldesleukin	oprelvekin
Alkeran	Leukeran
Alkeran	Myleran
Allegra	Viagra
allopurinol	Apresoline
Alora	Aldara
alprazolam	lorazepam
Altace	alteplase
Altace	Amaryl
Altace	Amerge
Altace	Artane
Altenol	atenolol
alteplase	Altace
Alupent	Atrovent
amantadine	ranitidine
amantadine	rimantadine
Amaryl	Altace
Amaryl	Amerge
Ambien	Amen
Amen	Ambien
Amerge	Altace
Amerge	Amaryl
Amicar	Amikin
Amikin	Amicar
amiloride	amlodipine
amiodarone	amrinone (former nomenclature for inamrinone)
amitriptyline	nortriptyline
amlodipine	amiloride
amoxapine	amoxicillin
amoxapine	Amoxil
amoxicillin	amoxapine
amoxicillin	Amoxil
amoxicillin	Atarax
Amoxil	amoxapine
Amoxil	amoxicillin
amrinone (former nomenclature for inamrinone)	amiodarone
Anaprox	Avapro
Anaspaz	Antispas
Anfranil	enalapril
Ansaid	Asacol
antacid	Atacand
Antispas	Anaspaz
Anti-Xa	Arixtra
Anusol	Anusol-HC
Anusol-HC	Anusol
Apresoline	allopurinol
Aredia	Adriamycin
Aredia	Meridia
argatroban	Aggrastat
Arixtra	Anti-Xa
Artane	Altace
Asacol	Ansaid
Asacol	Os-Cal
asparaginase	pegaspargase
Atacand	antacid
Atarax	amoxicillin
Atarax	Ativan
Atarax	Marax
atenolol	albuterol

atenolol	Altenol
Atgam	ratgam (synonym for thymoglobulin)
Ativan	Atarax
atropine	Akarpine
Atrovent	Alupent
Atrovent	Natru-Vent
Attenuvax	Meruvax
aureomycin	Achromycin
Avandia	Coumadin
Avandia	Prandin
Avapro	Anaprox
Aventyl	Bentyl
Avinza	Invanz
azithromycin	erythromycin
Bactocil	Pathocil
Banthine	Brethine
Benadryl	Benylin
Bentyl	Aventyl
Bentyl	Proventil
Benylin	Benadryl
Benylin	Betalin
Benylin	Ventolin
Benzac W	Benzac W Wash
Benzac W Wash	Benzac W
bepridil	Prepidil
Betagan	Betagen
Betagan	Betoptic
Betagen	Betagan
Betalin	Benylin
Betapace	Betapace AF
Betapace AF	Betapace
Betoptic	Betagan
Betoptic	Betoptic S
Betoptic S	Betoptic
Bicillin	V-Cillin
Brethine	Banthine
Bretylol	Brevital
Brevibloc	Brevital
Brevital	Bretylol
Brevital	Brevibloc
Bumex	Buprenex
Bumex	Permax
bupivacaine	ropivacaine
Buprenex	Bumex
buPROPion	busPIRone
busPIRone	buPROPion
Cafergot	Carafate
Calan	Colace
Calciferol	calcitriol
calcitriol	Calciferol
Capitrol	captopril
captopril	Capitrol

captopril	carvedilol
Carafate	Cafergot
Carbatrol (carbamezapine in U.S.)	Carbrital (pentobarbitone sodium in Australia)
carboplatin	cisplatin
Carbrital (pentobarbitone sodium in Australia)	Carbatrol (carbamezapine in U.S.)
Cardene	Cardizem
Cardene	Cardura
Cardene	codeine
Cardene SR	Cardizem SR
Cardiem	Cardizem
Cardizem	Cardene
Cardizem	Cardiem
Cardizem CD	Cardizem SR
Cardizem SR	Cardene SR
Cardizem SR	Cardizem CD
Cardura	Cardene
Cardura	Coumadin
Cardura	Ridaura
carteolol	carvedilol
Cartia XT	Procardia XL
carvedilol	captopril
carvedilol	carteolol
Cataflam	Catapres
Catapres	Cataflam
Catapres	Catarase
Catarase	Catapres
Cedax	Cidex
cefaclor	cephalexin
cefazolin	cefprozil
Cefol	Cefzil
Cefotan	Ceftin
cefotaxime	ceftizoxime
cefotaxime	cefuroxime
cefprozil	cefazolin
cefprozil	cefuroxime
ceftazidime	ceftizoxime
Ceftin	Cefotan
Ceftin	Cefzil
Ceftin	Cipro
ceftizoxime	ceftazidime
ceftizoxime	cefotaxime
cefuroxime	cefotaxime
cefuroxime	cefprozil
cefuroxime	deferoxamine
Cefzil	Cefol
Cefzil	Ceftin
Cefzil	Kefzol
Celebrex	Celexa

Celebrex	Cerebra
Celebrex	Cerebyx
Celexa	Celebrex
Celexa	Cerebra
Celexa	Cerebyx
Celexa	Zyprexa
Centoxin	Cytoxan
cephalexin	cefaclor
cephalexin	ciprofloxacin
cephapirin	cephradine
cephradine	cephapirin
Cerebra	Celebrex
Cerebra	Celexa
Cerebyx	Celebrex
Cerebyx	Celexa
Chloromycetin	Chlor-Trimeton
chlorproMAZINE	chlorproPAMIDE
chlorproMAZINE	prochlorperazine
chlorproPAMIDE	chlorproMAZINE
Chlor-Trimeton	Chloromycetin
Chlor-Trimeton	Chlor-Trimeton (Nondrowsy)
Chlor-Trimeton (Nondrowsy)	Chlor-Trimeton
Cidex	Cedax
Cipro	Ceftin
ciprofloxacin	cephalexin
cisplatin	carboplatin
Citracal	Citrucel
Citrucel	Citracal
Claritin-D	Claritin-D 24-hour
Claritin-D 24-hour	Claritin-D
Clinoril	Clozaril
Clinoril	Oruvail
clomiPHENE	clomiPRAMINE
clomiPRAMINE	clomiPHENE
clomiPRAMINE	desipramine
clomiPRAMINE	Norpramin
clonazepam	clonidine
clonazepam	clorazepate
clonazepam	Klonopin
clonazepam	lorazepam
clonidine	clonazepam
clonidine	Klonopin
clorazepate	clonazepam
Clozaril	Clinoril
Clozaril	Colazal
codeine	Cardene
codeine	iodine
codeine	Lodine
Cognex	Corgard
Colace	Calan
Colazal	Clozaril
Combivir	Epivir
Compazine	Coumadin
Cordarone	Inocor
Corgard	Cognex
Cortane	Cortane-B
Cortane-B	Cortane
Cortef	Lortab
Coumadin	Avandia
Coumadin	Cardura
Coumadin	Compazine
Covera	Provera
Cozaar	Hyzaar
Cozaar	Zocor
cyclobenzaprine	cyproheptadine
cyclophosphamide	cycloSPORINE
cycloSERINE	cycloSPORINE
cycloSPORINE	cyclophosphamide
cycloSPORINE	cycloSERINE
cyproheptadine	cyclobenzaprine
cytarabine	Cytosar
cytarabine	Cytoxan
CytoGam	Gamimune N
Cytosar	cytarabine
Cytosar	Cytovene
Cytosar	Cytoxan
Cytosar-U	Neosar
Cytotec	Cytoxan
Cytovene	Cytosar
Cytoxan	Centoxin
Cytoxan	cytarabine
Cytoxan	Cytosar
Cytoxan	Cytotec
danazol	Dantrium
Dantrium	danazol
Darvon	Diovan
DAUNOrubicin	DOXOrubicin
Daypro	Diupres
DDAVP Nasal	DDAVP with Rhinal Tube
DDAVP with Rhinal Tube	DDAVP Nasal
Decaderm	Decadron
Decadron	Decaderm
Decadron	Percodan
deferoxamine	cefuroxime
Demerol	Desyrel
Demerol	Dilaudid
Demerol	Temaril
Denavir	indinavir
Depakote	Senokot
Depakote	Depakote ER
Depakote ER	Depakote
Depo-Estradiol	Depo-Testadiol
Depo-Medrol	Solu-Medrol
Depo-Testadiol	Depo-Estradiol

Deseril (methysergide maleate in Australia)	Desyrel (trazodone in U.S.)
Desferal	DexFerrum
desipramine	clomipramine
desipramine	imipramine
desipramine	nortriptyline
Desyrel	Demerol
Desyrel (Trazodone in U.S.)	Deseril (Methysergide Maleate in Australia)
DexFerrum	Desferal
DiaBeta	Zebeta
Dialose Plus (docusate potassium/ casanthranol)	Dialose Plus (docusate sodium/ phenolphthalein)
Dialose Plus (docusate sodium/ phenolphthalein)	Dialose Plus (docusate potassium/ casanthranol)
Diamox	Dobutrex
Diamox	Trimox
diazepam	Ditropan
diazepam	lorazepam
dicyclomine	diphenhydrAMINE
dicyclomine	dyclonine
Diflucan	Diprivan
Dilacor XR	Pilocar
Dilaudid	Demerol
Dilomine	Dyclone
Dilomine	dyclonine
dimenhyDRINATE	diphenhydrAMINE
Dioval	Diovan
Diovan	Darvon
Diovan	Dioval
Diovan	Zyban
Diphenatol	diphenidol
diphenhydrAMINE	dicyclomine
diphenhydrAMINE	dimenhyDRINATE
diphenidol	Diphenatol
Diprivan	Diflucan
Diprivan	Ditropan
Ditropan	diazepam
Ditropan	Diprivan
Diupres	Daypro
DOBUTamine	DOPamine
Dobutrex	Diamox
Dolobid	Slo-bid
DOPamine	DOBUTamine
doxepin	Doxidan
doxepin	doxycycline

Doxidan	doxepin
Doxil	Paxil
DOXOrubicin	DAUNOrubicin
DOXOrubicin	DOXOrubicin liposomal
DOXOrubicin	idarubicin
DOXOrubicin liposomal	DOXOrubicin
doxycycline	doxepin
Drisdol	Drysol
Drysol	Drisdol
Dyazide	Thiazide
Dyclone	Dilomine
dyclonine	dicyclomine
dyclonine	Dilomine
Dynabac	DynaCirc
Dynacin	DynaCirc
DynaCirc	Dynabac
DynaCirc	Dynacin
Echogen	Epogen
Edecrin	Eulexin
Efudex	Eurax
Efudex	Eurax
Elavil	Mellaril
Elavil	Oruvail
Elavil	Plavix
Eldepryl	enalapril
Eldopaque Forte	Eldoquin Forte
Eldoquin Forte	Eldopaque Forte
Elmiron	Imuran
enalapril	Anfranil
enalapril	Eldepryl
enalapril	ramipril
Enduron	Imuran
epHEDrine	epINEPHrine
epINEPHrine	epHEDrine
Epivir	Combivir
Epogen	Echogen
Equagesic	EquiGesic
EquiGesic	Equagesic
Erex	Urex
Erythrocin	Ethmozine
erythromycin	azithromycin
Eskalith	Estratest
esmolol	Osmitrol
Estraderm	Testoderm
Estratab	Estratest
Estratest	Eskalith
Estratest	Estratab
Estratest	Estratest HS
Estratest HS	Estratest
ethambutol	Ethmozine
Ethmozine	Erythrocin
Ethmozine	ethambutol

etidronate	etomidate
etidronate	etretinate
etomidate	etidronate
etretinate	etidronate
Eulexin	Edecrin
Eurax	Efudex
Eurax	Efudex
Eurax	Urex
Evista	E-Vista
E-Vista	Evista
Fam-Pren Forte	Parafon Forte
Femara	femhrt
femhrt	Femara
fentanyl	Sufenta
fentanyl citrate	sufentanil citrate
Fioricet	Fiorinal
Fiorinal	Fioricet
Fiorinal	Floricet
Flomax	Fosamax
Flomax	Volmax
Floricet	Fiorinal
flucytosine	fluorouracil
Fludara	FUDR
fludarabine	Flumadine
Flumadine	fludarabine
fluorouracil	flucytosine
flurazepam	temazepam
folic acid	folinic acid
folinic acid	folic acid
Foradil	Toradol
Fortovase (improved bioavailability saquinavir)	Invirase (low bioavailability saquinavir)
Fosamax	Flomax
FUDR	Fludara
furosemide	torsemide
Gamimune N	CytoGam
Gamulin Rh	MICRhoGAM
Garamycin	kanamycin
Gemzar	Zinecard
Gengraf	Prograf
gentamycin ophthalmic	gentian violet
gentian violet	gentamycin ophthalmic
glipiZIDE	glyBURIDE
Glucophage	Glutofac
Glucotrol	Glucotrol XL
Glucotrol	glyBURIDE
Glucotrol XL	Glucotrol
Glutofac	Glucophage
glyBURIDE	glipiZIDE
glyBURIDE	Glucotrol

Granulex	Regranex
guaifenesin	guanfacine
guanfacine	guaifenesin
Haldol	Stadol
Haldrone	Halodrin
Halfprin	½ Halfprin
Halodrin	Haldrone
haloperidol	Halotestin
Halotestin	haloperidol
Hemoccult	Seracult
heparin	Hespan
Herceptin	Perceptin
Hespan	heparin
Hexadrol	Hexalol
Hexalol	Hexadrol
Humalog, Insulin Human	Humulin, Insulin Human
Humulin, Insulin Human	Humalog, Insulin Human
Hycodan	Vicodin
hydrALAZINE	hydrOXYzine
hydrocodone	hydrocortisone
hydrocortisone	hydrocodone
hydromorphone	meperidine
hydromorphone	morphine
hydrOXYzine	hydrALAZINE
Hygroton	Regroton
Hypergel	MPM GelPad Hydrogel Saturated Dressing
Hytone	Vytone
Hyzaar	Cozaar
ibuprofen	Materna
Idamycin	Adriamycin
idarubicin	DOXOrubicin
IMDUR	Imuran
IMDUR	Inderal LA
IMDUR	K-Dur
Imferon	Imuran
Imferon	interferon
Imferon	Roferon-A
imipenem	Omnipen
imipramine	desipramine
Imovax	Imovax I.D.
Imovax I.D.	Imovax
Imuran	Elmiron
Imuran	Enduron
Imuran	IMDUR
Imuran	Imferon
Imuran	Tenormin
Inderal	Adderall
Inderal	Isordil
Inderal	Toradol

Inderal LA	IMDUR
indinavir	Denavir
inhibace (captopril in Israel)	inhibace (cilazapril in Switzerland and Japan)
inhibace (cilazapril in Switzerland and Japan)	inhibace (captopril in Israel)
Inocor	Cordarone
interferon	Imferon
Invanz	Avinza
Invirase (low bioavailability saquinavir)	Fortovase (improved bioavailability saquinavir)
iodine	codeine
iodine	Lodine
Isordil	Inderal
isotretinoin	tretinoin
kanamycin	Garamycin
Kaochlor	K-Lor
Kaopectate	Kayexelate
Kayexelate	Kaopectate
K-Dur	IMDUR
Kefzol	Cefzil
Klonopin	clonazepam
Klonopin	clonidine
K-Lor	Kaochlor
K-Lor	Klor-Con
Klor-Con	K-Lor
Kogenate	Kogenate-2
Kogenate-2	Kogenate
K-Phos Neutral	Neutra-Phos-K
Lacrilube	Surgilube
Lactacare (supplement)	Lacticare (lotion)
Lacticare (lotion)	Lactacare (supplement)
Lamicel	Lamisil
Lamictal	Lamisil
Lamictal	Lomotil
Lamictal	Ludiomil
Lamisil	Lamicel
Lamisil	Lamictal
Lamisil	Lomotil
lamivudine	lamotrigine
lamotrigine	lamivudine
Lanoxin	Lasix
Lanoxin	Levoxine
Lanoxin	Levoxyl
Lanoxin	Lomotil
Lanoxin	Lonox
Lanoxin	Xanax
Lantus, Insulin Human	Lente, Insulin Human
Lasix	Lanoxin
Lasix	Lomotil
Lasix	Luvox
L-Dopa	levodopa
L-Dopa	methyldopa
Lente, Insulin Human	Lantus, Insulin Human
leucovorin	Leukeran
leucovorin	Leukine
Leukeran	Alkeran
Leukeran	leucovorin
Leukeran	Leukine
Leukeran	Myleran
Leukine	leucovorin
Leukine	Leukeran
Levbid	Lithobid
Levbid	Lopid
Levbid	Lorabid
levobunolol	levocabastine
levocabastine	levobunolol
levodopa	L-Dopa
levodopa	methyldopa
Levoxine	Lanoxin
Levoxine	Levoxyl
Levoxine	Levsin
Levoxyl	Lanoxin
Levoxyl	Levoxine
Levoxyl	Luvox
Levsin	Levoxine
Librax	Librium
Librium	Librax
Lioresal	Lotensin
lisinopril	Risperdal
Lithobid	Levbid
Lithobid	Lithostat
Lithostat	Lithobid
Lodine	codeine
Lodine	iodine
Lomotil	Lamictal
Lomotil	Lamisil
Lomotil	Lanoxin
Lomotil	Lasix
Loniten	Lotensin
Lonox	Lanoxin
Lopid	Levbid
Lopid	Lorabid
Lopid	Slo-bid
Lopurin	Lupron
Lorabid	Levbid
Lorabid	Lopid
Lorabid	Lortab
Lorabid	Slo-bid

lorazepam	alprazolam
lorazepam	clonazepam
lorazepam	diazepam
Lortab	Cortef
Lortab	Lorabid
Lortab	Luride
losartan	valsartan
Lotensin	Lioresal
Lotensin	Loniten
Lotensin	lovastatin
Lotrimin	Lotrisone
Lotrimin	Otrivin
Lotrisone	Lotrimin
Lotronex	Lovenox
Lotronex	Protonix
lovastatin	Lotensin
Lovenox	Lotronex
Loxitane	Soriatane
Ludiomil	Lamictal
Lupron	Lopurin
Lupron	Nuprin
Luride	Lortab
Luvox	Lasix
Luvox	Levoxyl
Maalox	Marax
magnesium gluceptate	magnesium sulfate
magnesium sulfate	magnesium gluceptate
Marax	Atarax
Marax	Maalox
Materna	ibuprofen
Mazicon	Mivacron
Medigesic	Medi-Gesic
Medi-Gesic	Medigesic
Medrol ADT	Medrol Dosepak
Medrol Dosepak	Medrol ADT
medroxy-PROGESTERone	methyl-PREDNISolone
Megace	Reglan
Mellaril	Elavil
melphalan	Myleran
meperidine	hydromorphone
meperidine	meprobamate
meperidine	morphine
meprobamate	meperidine
Mepron (atovaquone in U.S.)	Mepron (meprobamate in Australia)
Meridia	Aredia
Meruvax	Attenuvax
Metadate CD	Metadate ER
Metadate ER	Metadate CD
methadone	methylphenidate

methotrexate	metolazone
methyldopa	L-Dopa
methyldopa	levodopa
methylphenidate	methadone
methyl-PREDNISolone	medroxy-PROGESTERone
methyl-PREDNISolone	predniSONE
methyl-PREDNISolone	methyl-TESTOSTERone
methyl-TESTOSTERone	methyl-PREDNISolone
metoclopramide	metolazone
metolazone	methotrexate
metolazone	metoclopramide
metoprolol	misoprostol
Miacalcin	Micatin
Micatin	Miacalcin
MICRhoGAM	Gamulin Rh
Micro-K	Micronase
Micronase	Micro-K
minoxidil	Monopril
MiraLax	Mirapex
Mirapex	MiraLax
misoprostol	metoprolol
mitomycin	mitoxantrone
mitoxantrone	mitomycin
Mivacron	Mazicon
Monoket	Monopril
Monopril	Accupril
Monopril	minoxidil
Monopril	Monoket
morphine	hydromorphone
morphine	meperidine
MPM GelPad Hydrogel Saturated Dressing	Hypergel
Murocel	Murocoll-2
Murocoll-2	Murocel
Mycelex	Myoflex
Mylanta Gas	Mylicon
Myleran	Alkeran
Myleran	Leukeran
Myleran	melphalan
Mylicon	Mylanta Gas
Myoflex	Mycelex
Naprelan	Naprosyn
Naprosyn	Naprelan
Narcan	Norcuron
Nasalcrom	Nasalide
Nasalide	Nasalcrom
Nasarel	Nizoral
Natru-Vent	Atrovent

Navane	Norvasc
Navelbine	Navoban
Navelbine	Navogan
Navoban	Navelbine
Navogan	Navelbine
Nebcin	Nubain
nelfinavir	nevirapine
Neocare	Neocate
Neocate	Neocare
Neoral	Neurontin
Neoral	Nizoral
Neosar	Cytosar-U
Neo-Synephrine	Neo-Synephrine 12 Hour
Neo-Synephrine 12 Hour	Neo-Synephrine
Nephrox	Niferex
Neumega	Neupogen
Neupogen	Neumega
Neurontin	Neoral
Neurontin	Noroxin
Neutra Phos K	K Phos Neutral
Neutra-Phos-K	K-Phos Neutral
nevirapine	nelfinavir
niacin	Niaspan
Niaspan	niacin
niCARdipine	NIFEdipine
niCARdipine	nimodipine
Nicobid	Nitro-Bid
Nicoderm	Nitroderm
NIFEdipine	niCARdipine
NIFEdipine	nimodipine
Niferex	Nephrox
Nimbex	Revex
nimodipine	niCARdipine
nimodipine	NIFEdipine
Nitro-Bid	Nicobid
Nitroderm	Nicoderm
Nizoral	Nasarel
Nizoral	Neoral
Norcuron	Narcan
Norflex	norfloxacin
Norflex	Noroxin
norfloxacin	Norflex
norfloxacin	Noroxin
Noroxin	Neurontin
Noroxin	Norflex
Noroxin	norfloxacin
Norpramin	clomipramine
Norpramin	nortriptyline
nortriptyline	amitriptyline
nortriptyline	desipramine
nortriptyline	Norpramin
Norvasc	Navane
Novolin 70/30	Novolin 70/30 PenFill Prefilled
Novolin 70/30 PenFill Prefilled	Novolin 70/30
Nubain	Nebcin
Nuprin	Lupron
Occlusal-HP	Ocuflox
Ocufen	Ocuflox
Ocufen	Ocupress
Ocuflox	Occlusal-HP
Ocuflox	Ocufen
Ocular Lubricants	Acular
Ocumycin	Ocu-Mycin
Ocu-Mycin	Ocumycin
Ocupress	Ocufen
Omnipen	imipenem
oprelvekin	aldesleukin
Oprelvekin	Proleukin
Organidin	Organidin NR
Organidin NR	Organidin
Orinase	Ornade
Ornade	Orinase
Ortho-Cept	Ortho-Cyclen
Ortho-Cyclen	Ortho-Cept
Oruvail	Clinoril
Oruvail	Elavil
Os-Cal	Asacol
Osmitrol	esmolol
Otrivin	Lotrimin
oxybutynin	OxyContin
oxycodone	OxyContin
OxyContin	oxybutynin
OxyContin	oxycodone
paclitaxel	paroxetine
paclitaxel	Paxil
Parafon Forte	Fam-Pren Forte
Paraplatin	Platinol
Parlodel	pindolol
Parlodel	Provera
paroxetine	paclitaxel
paroxetine	pyridoxine
Pathocil	Bactocil
Pavulon	Peptavlon
Paxil	Doxil
Paxil	paclitaxel
Paxil	Plavix
Paxil	Taxol
Pediapred	Pediazole
Pediaprofen	Pediazole
Pediaprofen	Prelone
Pediazole	Pediapred
Pediazole	Pediaprofen
pegaspargase	asparaginase
penicillamine	penicillin

penicillin	penicillamine
penicillin G potassium	penicillin G procaine
penicillin G procaine	penicillin G potassium
pentobarbital	phenobarbital
Peptavlon	Pavulon
Perative	Periactin
Perceptin	Herceptin
Percocet	Percodan
Percodan	Decadron
Percodan	Percocet
Percodan	Percorten
Percorten	Percodan
Periactin	Perative
Permax	Bumex
permethrin	pyrethrins, piperonyl butoxide
phenelzine	Phenylzin
Phenergan	Theragran
phenobarbital	pentobarbital
Phenylzin	phenelzine
Pilocar	Dilacor XR
pindolol	Parlodel
pindolol	Plendil
Pitocin	Pitressin
Pitressin	Pitocin
Platinol	Paraplatin
Plavix	Elavil
Plavix	Paxil
Plendil	pindolol
Plendil	Pletal
Plendil	Prilosec
Plendil	Prinivil
Pletal	Plendil
Pondimin	predniSONE
potassium phosphates	sodium phosphates
Prandin	Avandia
Pravachol	Prevacid
Pravachol	propranolol
PreCare	Precose
Precose	PreCare
prednisoLONE	predniSONE
predniSONE	methyl-PREDNISolone
predniSONE	Pondimin
predniSONE	prednisoLONE
predniSONE	Prilosec
predniSONE	primidone
Prelone	Pediaprofen
Premarin	Primaxin
Premarin	Provera
Premphase	Prempro
Prempro	Premphase
Prepidil	bepridil
Prevacid	Pravachol
Prevacid	Prinivil
Preven	Preveon
Preveon	Preven
Prilosec	Plendil
Prilosec	predniSONE
Prilosec	Prinivil
Prilosec	Prozac
Primaxin	Premarin
primidone	predniSONE
Prinivil	Plendil
Prinivil	Prevacid
Prinivil	Prilosec
Prinivil	Proventil
probenecid	Procanbid
Procanbid	probenecid
Procardia XL	Cartia XT
prochlorperazine	chlorproMAZINE
Proctocort	Proctocream HC
Proctocream HC	Proctocort
Profen	Profen II
Profen	Profen LA
Profen II	Profen
Profen II	Profen LA
Profen LA	Profen
Profen LA	Profen II
Prograf	Gengraf
Prokine	Proleukin
Proleukin	Oprelvekin
Proleukin	Prokine
Prolixin	Proloid
Proloid	Prolixin
promethazine	promethazine w/ codeine
promethazine w/codeine	promethazine
propranolol	Pravachol
propranolol	Propulsid
Propulsid	Propranolol
Proscar	ProSom
Proscar	Prozac
ProSom	Proscar
ProSom	Prozac
Protonix	Lotronex
Proventil	Bentyl
Proventil	Prinivil
Provera	Covera
Provera	Parlodel
Provera	Premarin
Provera	Provir
Provir	Provera

Prozac	Prilosec
Prozac	Proscar
Prozac	ProSom
Psorcon	Psorion
Psorion	Psorcon
pyrethrins, piperonyl butoxide	permethrin
pyridoxine	paroxetine
quinidine	quinine
quinine	quinidine
ramipril	enalapril
ranitidine	amantadine
ranitidine	rimantadine
ratgam (synonym for thymoglobulin)	Atgam
ReFresh (breath drops)	Refresh (lubricant eye drops)
Refresh (lubricant eye drops)	ReFresh (breath drops)
Reglan	Megace
Regranex	Granulex
Regroton	Hygroton
Relafen	Rezulin
Remegel	Renagel
Remeron	Zemuron
Renagel	Remegel
Renografin-60	Reno-M-60
Reno-M-60	Renografin-60
reserpine	Risperdal
reserpine	risperidone
Retrovir	ritonavir
Revex	Nimbex
Revex	ReVia
ReVia	Revex
Rezulin	Relafen
Ridaura	Cardura
rifabutin	rifampin
rifampin	rifabutin
rimantadine	amantadine
rimantadine	ranitidine
Risperdal	lisinopril
Risperdal	reserpine
Risperdal	risperidone
risperidone	reserpine
risperidone	Risperdal
Ritalin	ritodrine
Ritalin LA	Ritalin SR
Ritalin SR	Ritalin LA
ritodrine	Ritalin
ritonavir	Retrovir
Roferon-A	Imferon
ropivacaine	bupivacaine
Roxanol	Roxicet
Roxanol	Roxicodone
Roxicet	Roxanol
Roxicodone	Roxanol
Rynatan	Rynatuss
Rynatuss	Rynatan
Salbutamol	salmeterol
salmeterol	Salbutamol
Sarafem	Serophene
selegiline	Serentil
selegiline	sertraline
selegiline	Serzone
Senokot	Depakote
Seracult	Hemoccult
Serax	Xerac
Serentil	selegiline
Serentil	Seroquel
Serentil	sertraline
Serentil	Serzone
Serentil	Sinequan
Serophene	Sarafem
Seroquel	Serentil
Seroquel	Serzone
sertraline	selegiline
sertraline	Serentil
sertraline	Serzone
Serzone	selegiline
Serzone	Serentil
Serzone	Seroquel
Serzone	sertraline
Sinequan	Serentil
Sinequan	Singulair
Singulair	Sinequan
Slo-bid	Dolobid
Slo-bid	Lopid
Slo-bid	Lorabid
sodium phosphates	potassium phosphates
Solu-Medrol	Depo-Medrol
Soma	Soma Compound
Soma Compound	Soma
Soriatane	Loxitane
Stadol	Haldol
Sufenta	fentanyl
sufentanil citrate	fentanyl citrate
sulfADIAZINE	sulfiSOXAZOLE
sulfADIAZINE	sulfasalazine
sulfasalazine	sulfADIAZINE
sulfasalazine	sulfiSOXAZOLE
sulfiSOXAZOLE	sulfasalazine
sulfiSOXAZOLE	sulfADIAZINE
sumatriptan	zolmitriptan
Surgilube	Lacrilube
Symmetrel	Synthroid

Synagis	Synvisc
Synthroid	Symmetrel
Synvisc	Synagis
Tamiflu	Theraflu
Taxol	Paxil
Taxol	Taxotere
Taxotere	Taxol
Tegretol	Toradol
Temaril	Demerol
temazepam	flurazepam
Tenormin	Imuran
Tenormin	thiamine
Tenormin	Trovan
Testoderm	Estraderm
tetracycline	tetradecyl sulfate
tetradecyl sulfate	tetracycline
Theraflu	Tamiflu
Theragran	Phenergan
thiamine	Tenormin
Thiazide	Dyazide
Thyrar	Thyrolar
Thyrolar	Thyrar
tiagabine	tizanidine
Tiazac	Tigan
Tiazac	Ziac
Tigan	Tiazac
Timoptic	Viroptic
tizanidine	tiagabine
TNKase	t-PA (synonym for alteplase, recombinant)
TobraDex	Tobrex
Tobrex	TobraDex
TOLAZamide	TOLBUTamide
TOLBUTamide	TOLAZamide
Toradol	Foradil
Toradol	Inderal
Toradol	Tegretol
Toradol	Torecan
Toradol	tramadol
Torecan	Toradol
torsemide	furosemide
t-PA (synonym for alteplase, recombinant)	TNKase
tramadol	Toradol
tramadol	Voltaren
Trandate	Tridrate
tretinoin	isotretinoin
Triad (butalbital/ acetaminophen/ caffeine)	Triad (zinc oxide/ petroleum/ mineral oil)
Triad (zinc oxide/ petroleum/ mineral oil)	Triad (butalbital/ acetaminophen/ caffeine)
Triaminic	Triaminicin
Triaminicin	Triaminic
Tridrate	Trandate
trifluoperazine	trihexyphenidyl
trihexyphenidyl	trifluoperazine
Trimox	Diamox
Trimox	Tylox
Tri-Norinyl	Triphasil
Triphasil	Tri-Norinyl
Tronolane	Tronothane
Tronothane	Tronolane
Trovan	Tenormin
Tussi-Organidin	Tussi-Organidin DM
Tussi-Organidin DM	Tussi-Organidin
Tylox	Trimox
Tylox	Wymox
Tylox	Xanax
Ultane	Ultram
Ultram	Ultane
Ultram	Voltaren
Urex	Erex
Urex	Eurax
Uricit-K	Urised
Uridon	Vicodin
Urised	Uricit-K
Urised	Urispas
Urispas	Urised
valium	versed
valsartan	losartan
Vancenase	Vanceril
Vanceril	Vancenase
vancomycin	vecuronium
Vantin	Ventolin
V-Cillin	Bicillin
vecuronium	vancomycin
Ventolin	Benylin
Ventolin	Vantin
VePesid	Versed
verapamil	Verelan
Verelan	verapamil
Verelan	Virilon
Versed	valium
Versed	VePesid
Versed	Vistaril
Vexol	VoSol
Viagra	Allegra
Vicodin	Hycodan
Vicodin	Uridon
vinBLAStine	vinCRIStine

vinCRIStine	vinBLAStine
Vioxx	Zyvox
Viracept	Viramune
Viramune	Viracept
Virilon	Verelan
Viroptic	Timoptic
Viroptic	Timoptic
Vistaril	Versed
Vistaril	Zestril
Volmax	Flomax
Voltaren	tramadol
Voltaren	Ultram
VoSol	Vexol
Vytone	Hytone
Wymox	Tylox
Xanax	Lanoxin
Xanax	Tylox
Xanax	Zantac
xeloda	xenical
xenical	xeloda
Xerac	Serax
Yocon	Zocor
Yocon	Zyrtec
Zagam	Zyban
Zantac	Xanax
Zantac	Zofran
Zantac	Zyrtec
Zebeta	DiaBeta
Zemuron	Remeron
Zestril	Vistaril
Ziac	Tiazac
Zinacef	Zithromax
Zinecard	Gemzar
Zithromax	Zinacef
Zocor	Cozaar
Zocor	Yocon
Zocor	Zoloft
Zofran	Zantac
Zofran	Zosyn
zolmitriptan	sumatriptan
Zoloft	Zocor
Zonalon	Zone A Forte
Zone A Forte	Zonalon
Zosyn	Zofran
Zyban	Diovan
Zyban	Zagam
Zyprexa	Celexa
Zyprexa	Zyrtec
Zyrtec	Xanax
Zyrtec	Zantac
Zyrtec	Zyprexa
Zyvox	Vioxx

Appendix I

FDA pregnancy categories

A No risk demonstrated to the fetus in any trimester

B No adverse effects in animals, no human studies available

C Only given after risks to the fetus are considered; animal studies have shown adverse reactions, no human studies available

D Definite fetal risks, may be given in spite of risks if needed in life-threatening conditions

X Absolute fetal abnormalities; not to be used anytime during pregnancy

Note: **UK** = Unknown fetal risk (used in this text but not an official FDA pregnancy category).

Appendix m

Controlled substance chart

Drugs	United States	Canada
Heroin, LSD, peyote, marijuana, mescaline	Schedule I • High abuse potential • No currently accepted medical use	Schedule H
Opium (morphine), meperidine, amphetamines, cocaine, short-acting barbiturates (secobarbital)	Schedule II • High abuse potential; potentially severe psychologic or physical dependence • Currently accepted medical use but may be severely restricted • Telephone orders only in emergencies if written Rx follows promptly • No refills	Schedule G
Glutethimide, paregoric, phendimetrazine	Schedule III • Abuse potential less than the drugs/substances in Schedules I and II; potentially moderate or low physical dependence or high psychologic dependence • Currently accepted medical use • Telephone orders permitted • Prescriber may authorize limited refills	Schedule F

Drugs	United States	Canada
Chloral hydrate, chlordiazepoxide, diazepam, mazindol, meprobamate, phenobarbital (Canada—G)	Schedule IV • Low abuse potential relative to drugs/substances in Schedule III; potentially limited physical or psychologic dependence • Currently accepted medical use • Telephone orders permitted • Prescriber may authorize limited refills	Schedule F
Antidiarrheals with opium (Canada—G), antitussives	Schedule V • Lowest abuse potential; potentially very limited physical or psychologic dependence • Currently accepted medical use • Prescriber determines refills • Some products containing limited amounts of Schedule V substances (e.g., cough suppressants) available OTC to patients >18 yr	Schedule F

Appendix n

Abbreviations

AAS argininosuccinic acid synthetase
abd abdomen
ABG arterial blood gas
ac before meals
ACE angiotensin-converting enzyme
ADA American Diabetes Association
ADH antidiuretic hormone
ALT alanine aminotransferase
ANA antinuclear antibody
AP anteroposterior
APTT activated partial thromboplastin time
ASA acetylsalicylic acid, aspirin
ASHD arteriosclerotic heart disease
AST aspartate aminotransferase (SGOT)
AV atrioventricular
bid twice a day
BM bowel movement
BMR basal metabolic rate
B/P blood pressure
BPH benign prostatic hypertrophy
BPM beats per minute
BS blood sugar
BUN blood urea nitrogen
C Celsius (centigrade)
Ca cancer
CAD coronary artery disease
cap capsule
Cath catheterization or catheterize
CBC complete blood cell count
CC chief complaint
cc cubic centimeter
CHF congestive heart failure
cm centimeter
CNS central nervous system
CO_2 carbon dioxide
CONT continuous
COPD chronic obstructive pulmonary disease
CPAP continuous positive airway pressure
CPK creatine phosphokinase
CPR cardiopulmonary resuscitation
CPS carbamoyl phosphate synthetase
CrCl creatinine clearance
C&S culture and sensitivity
C sect cesarean section
CSF cerebrospinal fluid
CV cardiovascular
CVA cerebrovascular accident
CVP central venous pressure
D&C dilatation and curettage
DIC diffuse intravascular coagulation
DIR INF direct infusion
dr dram
D_5W 5% glucose in distilled water
ECG electrocardiogram (EKG)
EDTA ethylenediamine tetraacetic acid
EEG electroencephalogram
EENT ear, eye, nose, and throat
EPS extrapyramidal symptom
ESR erythrocyte sedimentation rate
EXT-REL extended release
EXTRA-STREN-SUSP extra strength suspension
FBS fasting blood sugar
FHT fetal heart tones
FSH follicle-stimulating hormone
g gram
GABA γ-aminobutyric acid
GI gastrointestinal

gr grain
GT glucose tolerance test
gtt drops
GU genitourinary
H_2 histamine$_2$
HCG human chorionic gonadotropin
Hct hematocrit
HDCV human diploid cell rabies vaccine
Hgb hemoglobin
H & H hematocrit and hemoglobin
5-HIAA 5-hydroxyindoleacetic acid
HIV human immunodeficiency virus (AIDS)
H_2O water
HOB head of bed
HR heart rate
hr hour
hs at bedtime
IgG immunolobulin G
IM intramuscular
INF infusion
INH inhalation
inj injection
I&O intake and output
INT intermittent
IPPB intermittent positive-pressure breathing
ITP idiopathic thrombocytopenic purpura
IUD intrauterine device
IV intravenous
IVP intravenous pyelogram
K potassium
kg kilogram
L liter
lb pound
LDH lactic dehydrogenase
LE lupus erythematosus
LFT liver function test
LH luteinizing hormone
LLQ left lower quadrant
LMP last menstrual period
LOC level of consciousness
LR lactated Ringer's solution
LT leukotriene
LUQ left upper quadrant
M meter
m minim
m^2 square meter
MAC monitored anesthesia care
MAOI monoamine oxidase inhibitor
mEq milliequivalent
mg milligram
MI myocardial infarction
min minute
ml milliliter
mm millimeter
mo month
Na sodium
neg negative
ng nanogram
NOS not otherwise specified
NPO nothing by mouth (Lat. *nulla per os*)
NS normal saline
O_2 oxygen
OBS organic brain syndrome
od right eye
OR operating room
os left eye
OTC over-the-counter
OU each eye
oz ounce
p̄ after
P56 plasma-lyte 56
$PaCO_2$ arterial carbon dioxide tension (pressure)
PaO_2 arterial oxygen tension (pressure)
PAT paroxysmal atrial tachycardia
PBI protein-bound iodine
pc after meals
PCWP pulmonary capillary wedge pressure
PEEP positive end-expiratory pressure
PERRLA pupils equal, round, react to light and accommodation
pH hydrogen ion concentration
PO by mouth
postop postoperative
PP postprandial
preop preoperative
prn as required
PT prothrombin time
PTT partial thromboplastin time

PVC premature ventricular contraction
pwd powder
qAM every morning
qd every day
qh every hour
q2h every 2 hours
q3h every 3 hours
q4h every 4 hours
q6h every 6 hours
q12h every 12 hours
qid four times daily
qod every other day
qPM every night
qs sufficient quantity
qt quart
R right
RAIU radioactive iodine uptake
RBC red blood cell count or red blood cell
RECT rectal
RLQ right lower quadrant
ROM range of motion
RUQ right upper quadrant
SC subcutaneous
SIMV synchronous intermittent mandatory ventilation
SL sublingual
SLE systemic lupus erythematosus
SOB shortness of breath
sol solution
ss one half
suppos suppository
SUS REL sustained release
syr syrup
T&A tonsillectomy and adenoidectomy
tab tablet
tbsp tablespoon
temp temperature
tid three times daily
tinc tincture
TPN total parenteral nutrition
top topical
TRANS transdermal
TSH thyroid-stimulating hormone
tsp teaspoon
TT thrombin time
UA urinalysis
UTI urinary tract infection
UV ultraviolet
vag vaginal
VMA vanillylmandelic acid
vol volume
VS vital sign
WBC white blood cell count
wk week
wt weight
yr year
> greater than
< less than
= equal
° degree
% percent
α alpha
β beta
γ gamma

- For a list of the Institute for Safe Medicine Practices (ISMP) error-prone abbreviations, symbols and dose designations, please see http://www.ismp.org/PDF/ErrorPhone.pdf.
- For frequently asked questions regarding the 2004 National Patient Safety Goals, please visit the Joint Commission on Accreditation of Healthcare Organizations (JCAHO) website at http://www.jcaho.org/accredited+organizations/patient+safety/04+npsg/04_faqs.htm

Appendix o

Weights and equivalents

METRIC SYSTEM

Weight

kilogram	=	kg	=	1000 grams
gram	=	g	=	1 gram
milligram	=	mg	=	0.001 gram
microgram	=	mcg	=	0.001 milligram

Volume

liter	=	L	=	1 L
milliliter	=	ml	=	0.001 L

AVOIRDUPOIS WEIGHT

1 ounce (oz) = 437.5 grains
1 pound (lb) = 16 ounces = 7000 grains

METRIC AND APOTHECARY EQUIVALENTS

Exact weight equivalents

Metric	*Apothecary*
1 mg	1/64.8 grain
64.8 mg	1 grain
324 mg	5 grains
1 g	15.432 grains
31.103 g	1 ounce = 480 grains

Exact volume equivalents

Metric	*Apothecary*		
1.00 ml	16.23 minims		
3.69 ml	1 fluidram	=	60 minims
29.57 ml	1 fluid ounce	=	480 minims
473.16 ml	1 pint	=	7680 minims
946.33 ml	1 quart	=	15,360 minims

Appendix p

Formulas for drug calculations

Surface area rule:

$$\text{Child dose} = \frac{\text{Surface area (m}^2)}{1.73\ \text{m}^2} \times \text{Adult dose}$$

Calculating strength of a solution:

Solution Strength: *Desired Solution:*

$$\frac{\text{x}}{100} = \frac{\text{Amount of drug desired}}{\text{Amount of finished solution}}$$

Calculating flow rate for IV:

$$\text{Rate of flow} = \frac{\text{Amount of fluid} \times \text{Administration set calibration}}{\text{Running time}}$$

$$\frac{x}{1} = \frac{\text{(ml) (gtt/min)}}{\text{min}}$$

Calculation of medication dosages:

Formula method:

$$\frac{\text{Amount ordered}}{\text{Amount on hand}} \times \text{Vehicle} = \text{Number of tablets, capsules, or amount of liquid}$$

Vehicle is the drug form or amount of liquid containing the dosage. Amounts used in calculation by formula must be in same system.

Ratio—proportion method:

1 tablet:tablet in mg on hand: : x tablet order in mg

Know or have: : Want to know or order

Multiply means and extremes, divide both sides by known amount to get x. Amounts used in equation must be in same system.

Dimensional analysis method:

$$\text{Order in mg} \times \frac{\text{1 tablet or capsule}}{\text{What 1 tablet or capsule is in mg}}$$

$$= \text{Tablets or capsules to be given}$$

If amounts are in different systems:

$$\text{Order in mg} \times \frac{\text{1 tablet or capsule}}{\text{What 1 tablet or capsule is in g}} \times \frac{1}{1000\ \text{mg}}$$

$$= \text{Tablets or capsules to be given}$$

Appendix q

Nomogram for calculation of body surface area

Place a straight edge from the patient's height in the left column to the patient's weight in the right column. The point of intersection on the body surface area column indicates the body surface area (BSA). (Reproduced in Behrman RE, Kliegman RM, Jenson HB: *Nelson textbook of pediatrics,* ed 17, Philadelphia, 2004, WB Saunders; Nomogram modified from data of E. Boyd by CD West.)

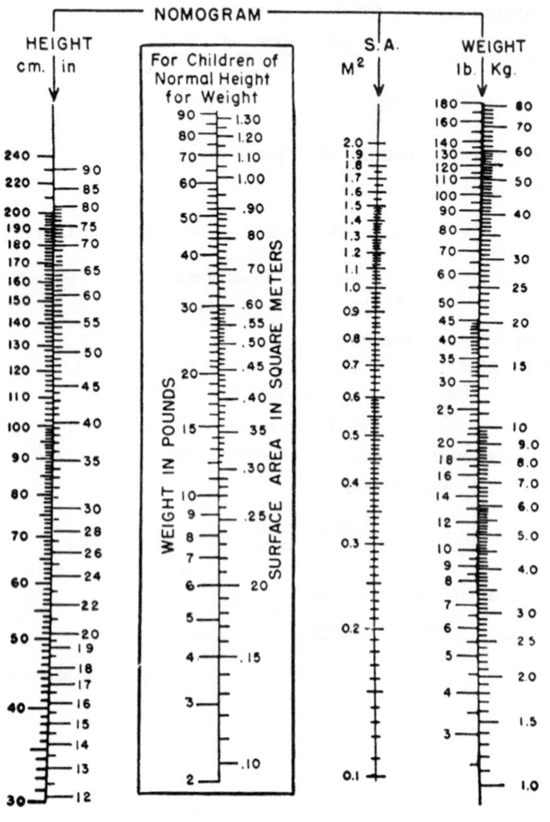

Index

Entries can be identified as follows: *Combination Products,* DISEASES/DISORDERS, *DRUG CATEGORIES,* generic names, Trade Names.

Entries can be identified as follows: *Combination Products,* DISEASES/DISORDERS, *DRUG CATEGORIES,* generic names, Trade Names.

Entries can be identified as follows: *Combination Products,* DISEASES/DISORDERS, *DRUG CATEGORIES,* generic names, Trade Names.

Entries can be identified as follows: *Combination Products,* DISEASES/DISORDERS, *DRUG CATEGORIES,* generic names, Trade Names.

Entries can be identified as follows: *Combination Products,* DISEASES/DISORDERS, *DRUG CATEGORIES,* generic names, Trade Names.

Entries can be identified as follows: *Combination Products,* DISEASES/DISORDERS, *DRUG CATEGORIES,* generic names, Trade Names.

Entries can be identified as follows: *Combination Products,* DISEASES/DISORDERS, *DRUG CATEGORIES,* generic names, Trade Names.

Entries can be identified as follows: *Combination Products,* DISEASES/DISORDERS, *DRUG CATEGORIES,* generic names, Trade Names.

Entries can be identified as follows: *Combination Products,* DISEASES/DISORDERS, *DRUG CATEGORIES,* generic names, Trade Names.

Entries can be identified as follows: *Combination Products,* DISEASES/DISORDERS, *DRUG CATEGORIES,* generic names, Trade Names.

Entries can be identified as follows: *Combination Products,* DISEASES/DISORDERS, *DRUG CATEGORIES,* generic names, Trade Names.

Entries can be identified as follows: *Combination Products,* DISEASES/DISORDERS, *DRUG CATEGORIES,* generic names, Trade Names.

Entries can be identified as follows: *Combination Products,* DISEASES/DISORDERS, *DRUG CATEGORIES,* generic names, Trade Names.

Entries can be identified as follows: *Combination Products,* DISEASES/DISORDERS, *DRUG CATEGORIES,* generic names, Trade Names.

Entries can be identified as follows: *Combination Products,* DISEASES/DISORDERS, *DRUG CATEGORIES,* generic names, Trade Names.

Entries can be identified as follows: *Combination Products,* DISEASES/DISORDERS, *DRUG CATEGORIES,* generic names, Trade Names.

Entries can be identified as follows: *Combination Products,* DISEASES/DISORDERS, *DRUG CATEGORIES,* generic names, Trade Names.

Entries can be identified as follows: *Combination Products,* DISEASES/DISORDERS, *DRUG CATEGORIES,* generic names, Trade Names.

Entries can be identified as follows: *Combination Products,* DISEASES/DISORDERS, *DRUG CATEGORIES,* generic names, Trade Names.

Entries can be identified as follows: *Combination Products,* DISEASES/DISORDERS, *DRUG CATEGORIES,* generic names, Trade Names.

Entries can be identified as follows: *Combination Products,* DISEASES/DISORDERS, *DRUG CATEGORIES,* generic names, Trade Names.

Mosby's DrugPro CD-ROM to accompany Mosby's 2005 Nursing Drug Reference

Use *Mosby's DrugPro to Accompany Mosby's 2005 Nursing Drug Reference* to find drug information fast! This four-in-one CD-ROM provides you with a drug interactions tool, patient teaching guides, herbal monographs, and calculators.

Mosby's DrugPro includes:

- **Drug Interactions Tool**
  Use this powerful drug interactions tool for instant access to drug-drug, drug-diet, and drug-lab test interactions.
- **Patient Teaching Guides**
  Select up-to-date English and Spanish patient teaching handouts for hundreds of the most commonly used drugs.
- **Herbal Monographs**
  Reliable, up-to-date, and detailed information on over 40 of the most commonly used herbs and natural supplements.
- **Calculators**
  Select from over 20 handy clinical calculators, including several IV and PO dosage calculators, and an IV dose rate calculator.

Contact Us
For further information, visit us at *www.mosby.com* or call us at (800) 545-2522.

Mini CD-ROM
This mini CD-ROM will work in your CD-ROM drive. Place it on the inner ring of the tray, as shown, and follow the on-screen installation instructions.

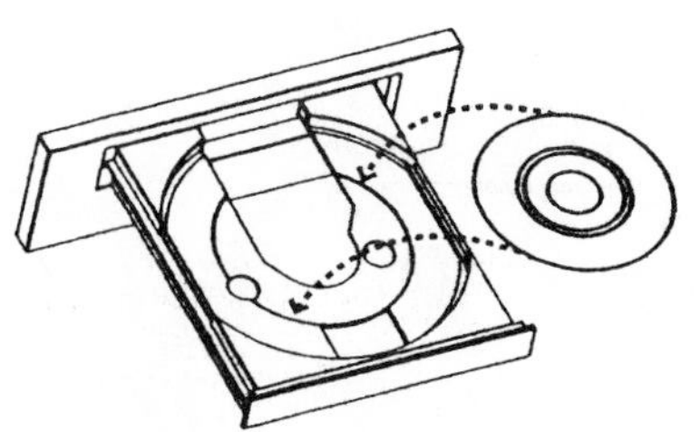

This mini-CD does not work in:
Floppy Drives
Slot Drives
Zip Drives
Stereos
Insert this mini-CD into your CD-ROM drive as shown at left.

Important
No credit or refund will be issued on this book if the CD envelope has been opened, torn, or otherwise tampered with.

Mosby's DrugPro CD-ROM to accompany *Mosby's 2005 Nursing Drug Reference*

MINIMUM SYSTEM REQUIREMENTS

Windows®
Windows® 98, 2000, NT, ME, or XP operating system
266 MHz Intel Pentium II processor or greater
64 MB or more of installed RAM
10 MB free hard disk space
2× or faster CD-ROM drive
800 × 600 monitor or larger
256 Colors

INSTALLATION INSTRUCTIONS

Windows®

1. Start Microsoft Windows® and insert the CD-ROM.
2. Click the *Start* button from the Taskbar and select the *Run* option.
3. Type d:\setup.exe (where "d:\" is your CD-ROM drive) and press *Enter.*
4. Follow the on-screen instructions for installation.

A program group folder named *Mosby's Drug Pro* will be created in the Windows Start menu and a shortcut will be placed on your desktop. Click on the icon labeled *Mosby's Drug Pro* on your desktop to run the program.

TECHNICAL SUPPORT

Technical support for this product is available between 7:30 AM and 7 PM CST, Monday through Friday. Before calling, make sure that your computer meets the minimum system requirements to run this software. Inside the United States, call (800) 692-9010. Outside the United States, call (314) 872-8370. You may also fax your questions to (314) 997-5080.

You may also contact Technical Support via e-mail at: technical.support@elsevier.com

For access to a list of *Frequently Asked Questions (FAQ),* as well as troubleshooting tips, please visit our website at **http://www.us.elsevierhealth.com/TechSupport**

Produced in the United States of America.

Part number: 9996004228

IV Drug/Solution Compatibility Chart

	D_5	D_{10}	D_5 $^1{}_2$S	D_5 S	NS	R	LR	OTHER
Acetazolamide	C	C	C	C	C	C	C	
Acyclovir	C							
$Alpha_1$-proteinase inhibitor								Sterile water for inj
Alprostadil	C	C			C			
Alteplase								Sterile water for inj
Amdinocillin	C	C	C	C	C	C	C	D_5 in R
Amikacin	C				C			
Aminocaproic acid			C	C	C	C		D in distilled water
Ammonium Cl					C			May add KCl to solution
Amphotericin B	C							
Ampicillin	C				C			
Amrinone lactate					C			0.45% saline
Antithrombin III	C				C			Sterile water for inj
Ascorbic acid	C				C	C	C	Sodium lactate
Atenolol	C				C			0.45% saline
Azlocillin	C		C		C			
Aztreonam	C	C			C	C	C	Normosol-R
Bretylium tosylate	C				C			
Cefamandole	C				C			
Cefazolin	C				C			
Cefotetan	C				C			
Cefoxitin	C	C			C	C	C	Aminosol
Ceftazidime	C		C	C	C	C	C	M/G Sodium lactate

This chart is not inclusive and is based on manufacturers recommendations.

Key

C = Compatible
D_5 = Dextrose 5%
D_{10} = Dextrose 10%
$D_5$$^1{}_2$S = Dextrose 5% in saline 0.45%
D_5S = Dextrose 5% in saline 0.9%
NS = Sodium chloride 0.9% (normal saline)
R = Ringer s solution
LR = Lactated Ringer s solution